Radiopathology of Organs and Tissues

Contributors

W. Alberti · K.K. Ang · W. Calvo · W. Gössner · H. Grosse-Wilde
T. Herrmann · F. Heuck · J.W. Hopewell · L. Keilholz · A. Keyeux
J. Kummermehr · H.-A. Ladner · A. Luz · M. Molls · W. Nothdurft
H.S. Reinhold · H. Reyners · R. Sauer · U.W. Schaefer · E. Scherer
T.E. Schultheiss · S. Schultz-Hector · L.C. Stephens · F.A. Stewart
C. Streffer · M. Stuschke · K.-R. Trott · D. van Beuningen
A.J. van der Kogel · M.V. Williams

Edited by

Eberhard Scherer, Christian Streffer,
and Klaus-Rüdiger Trott

Foreword by

Luther W. Brady, Martin W. Donner,
Hans-Peter Heilmann, and Friedrich Heuck

With 156 Figures

Springer-Verlag
Berlin Heidelberg New York
London Paris Tokyo
Hong Kong Barcelona Budapest

Professor (em.) Dr. EBERHARD SCHERER
Universitätsklinikum der Gesamthochschule
Radiologisches Zentrum, Strahlenklinik und Poliklinik
Hufelandstraße 55
W-4300 Essen 1, FRG

Professor Dr. CHRISTIAN STREFFER
Universitätsklinikum der Gesamthochschule
Institut für Medizinische Strahlenphysik und Strahlenbiologie
Hufelandstraße 55
W-4300 Essen 1, FRG

Professor Dr. KLAUS-RÜDIGER TROTT
Department of Radiation Biology
The Medical College of St. Bartholomew's Hospital
Charterhouse Square
London EC1M 6BQ, UK

MEDICAL RADIOLOGY · Diagnostic Imaging and Radiation Oncology

Continuation of
Handbuch der medizinischen Radiologie
Encyclopedia of Medical Radiology

ISBN 3-540-19094-5 Springer-Verlag Berlin Heidelberg New York
ISBN 0-387-19094-5 Springer-Verlag New York Berlin Heidelberg

Typesetting Best-set, Hong Kong
10/3130-543210 – Printed on acid-free paper

MEDICAL RADIOLOGY

Diagnostic Imaging and Radiation Oncology

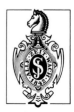

Foreword

The biologic effects of radiation on normal tissues and tumors represent a complex area for investigation. These effects are of far-reaching consequence to the diagnostic radiologist and the radiation oncologist having a significant impact not only in concepts relative to radiation protection but also in concepts relative to tumor biology and its response to radiation injury.

The volume edited by SCHERER, STREFFER, and TROTT represents an extension of basic radiation biology data into the effects of radiation in producing pathology in organs and tissues. The data presented by the multiple authors involved in this text cover essentially all tissues in the body with specific definition of radiopathology changes and their impact on clinical care of the patient. This volume represents an important and significant contribution toward a better understanding of these effects and the pathology produced by radiations.

L. W. BRADY   H.-P. HEILMANN   F. HEUCK   M. W. DONNER
Philadelphia   Hamburg   Stuttgart   Baltimore

Preface

This book represents an attempt to describe the clinical radiobiology of complications arising in different organs after radiotherapy of cancer patients. Since by their very nature malignant tumors infiltrate the organ in which they have arisen and the neighboring tissues, curative radiotherapy requires the planned irradiation of considerable amounts of healthy but potentially or microscopically involved normal tissues and organs with the full target dose. This may lead to early or late normal tissue radiation injury.

HOLTHUSEN (1936) was the first to discuss the problems of optimal dosage in cancer radiotherapy, balancing tumor control probability and complication risks. By comparing the dose-cure relationship of skin cancers with the dose-incidence relationship for late skin damage he concluded that the best dose in radiotherapy is one which causes a certain but acceptably low incidence of damage in cured patients. This implies that the various early and late side-effects and complications have to be considered a necessary price for the maximal chance of uncomplicated cure and that, unless their frequency becomes unacceptably high, the occurrence of complications does not per se indicate poor radiotherapeutic practice. On the contrary, the principle of cure-risk analysis would cause a very low or zero late complication rate after curative radiotherapy to be regarded as a certain indication of an overcautious approach precluding a chance of cure in many patients. Therefore, normal tissue radiation injury is an accepted, common feature of appropriate curative radiotherapy of cancer.

In many ways, this book is indebted to the fundamental, pioneering work written more than 20 years ago by a radiotherapist, P. RUBIN, together with a radiation biologist, G.W. CASARETT, which, under the title *Clinical Radiation Pathology*, summarized and defined in a beautiful way the state of knowledge of the day. We did not feel that any of us or anybody known to us would be able to write such a comprehensive analysis today. So we asked different experts to write about their field of expertise and, as editors, tried to make the individual contributions cohere into a systematic, comprehensible, and readable compendium of the radiopathology of organs and tissues.

Some side-effects or complications of radiotherapy develop during radiotherapy itself, and others arise soon after the completion of the treatment course. These are generally called early (or acute) responses and contrasted to late (or chronic) normal tissue injury, which develops later, i.e., after several months or years. The distinction is somewhat arbitrary and there are good reasons for subdividing the delayed complications further into subacute damage and late damage (RUBIN and CASARETT 1968). In addition to their time of appearance the early responses have various other features in common: they usually arise in rapidly proliferating tissues or tissue components (e.g., epithelia of organs), the proliferative damage causes a decrease in the number of specific cells and elicits an unspecific inflammatory response, and the acute response heals by proliferation of surviving stem cells. All this is suggestive of a specific pathogenetic mechanism which may be common to all early normal tissue responses.

Subacute and late normal tissue injury, however, is much more variable. It usually arises in tissues or tissue components which have a slow cell turnover and often involves diffuse or focal damage to the microvasculature and the stromal tissue of an affected organ. In contrast to the transient early responses it is often progressive and may get worse every year. At present, theories about the pathogenesis of subacute and late normal tissue radiation injury very widely.

It is by no means certain that the different effects of radiotherapy (i.e., the sterilization of tumor stem cells, which is the crucial effect with regard to tumor cure, the decreased cell production in rapidly proliferating normal tissues, which causes early radiation injury, and the ill-defined changes in stromal and parenchymal cells of different organs, which is responsible for the development of late normal tissue damage) are all consequences of the same primary radiation effect on the same cellular molecule or on the same molecular cell function. At various places within this book, such controversial questions in radiation biology have been addressed.

This book does not only attempt to summarize our present knowledge on the pathogenesis, the pathology, and the radiobiology of normal tissue radiation damage. The authors of the different chapters on the different organs and organ systems also place major emphasis on the clinical features of the various normal tissue responses, on observations in patients, and on data on dose-incidence and time-fractionation relationships derived from clinical information. Most authors in this book are practising radiotherapists but with a longstanding interest in clinical radiobiology; the radiobiologists who have made contributions have a long record of close cooperation with clinical radiotherapists. Therefore, in addition to providing the reader with an up-to-date description of knowledge on the clinical radiobiology of normal tissue responses in cancer radiotherapy, this book is also a product of fruitful interaction between radiobiologists and radiotherapists for the further development of effective treatment of cancer patients.

EBERHARD SCHERER   CHRISTIAN STREFFER   KLAUS-RÜDIGER TROTT

References

Holthusen H (1936) Erfahrungen über die Verträglichkeitsgrenze für Röntgenstrahlen und deren Nutzanwendung zur Verhütung von Schäden. Strahlentherapie 57: 254–269

Rubin P, Casarett GW (1968) Clinical Radiation Pathology, 2 volumes, Saunders, Philadelphia

Contents

1 Cellular Radiobiology

C. STREFFER and D. VAN BEUNINGEN

CONTENTS

1.1 Introduction

Just a few years after the discovery of x-rays and natural radioactivity several fundamental aspects of the biological effects of radiation were described, aspects which are still recognised today. Examples include the high radiosensitivity of lymphocytes, observed by HEINEKE (1904), and the inhibition of cell division. BERGONIE and TRIBONDEAU (1906) laid down the rule that the radiosensitivity of cells increases with increasing proliferation and decreases with increasing differentiation. Since then, problems pertaining to

Professor Dr. rer. nat. C. STREFFER, Universitätsklinikum der Gesamthochschule, Institut für Medizinische Strahlenphysik und Strahlenbiologie, Hufelandstraße 55, 4300 Essen 1, FRG

Professor Dr. D. VAN BEUNINGEN, Oberfeldarzt, Akademie des Sanitäts und Gesundheitswesen der Bundeswehr, Neuherbergstraße 11, 8000 München 45, FRG

cellular biology and, in particular, cell killing and the mechanisms responsible for it, have remained in the foreground of radiobiological research. Even so, these mechanisms, and above all their temporal sequence, are still not clear today.

While it has never been questioned that tumor destruction depends on the cell-killing effect of ionizing radiation, radiation-induced death in mammalians has not always been considered from this point of view. The studies by QUASTLER (1945) and others have clearly shown that the impairment of cell renewal in critical cell and organ systems after irradiation is the crucial factor in mammalian death. However, it must not be forgotten that numerous physiological factors, such as hormonal regulatory phenomena and age, can influence the radiosensitivity of tissues and organisms.

A variety of complex processes are involved prior to radiation-induced cell killing. The absorption of radiation energy by living material leads to ionization and excitation in the biomolecules concerned. These events are distributed over all regions of the irradiated cells and tissues. Intramolecular energy depositions, above all in macromolecules, finally result in relatively stable molecular changes. When, as described here, such effects are achieved through direct absorption of radiation energy by the biomolecule, they are described as "direct radiation effects" (DERTINGER and JUNG 1969; STREFFER 1969). Initially, however, radicals can also be produced (above all through energy absorption in the aqueous environment of the cell), which in turn react with the macromolecules in the cell. In this case, reference is made to "indirect radiation effects" (CHAPMAN and GILLESPIE 1981) (Fig. 1.1). Whereas previously "indirect radiation effects" were thought to be particularly important because of the high water content in mammalian cells, today they are considered to be less important in view of the fact that considerable amounts of water in the cell are bound to structures and macromolecules and are not freely available.

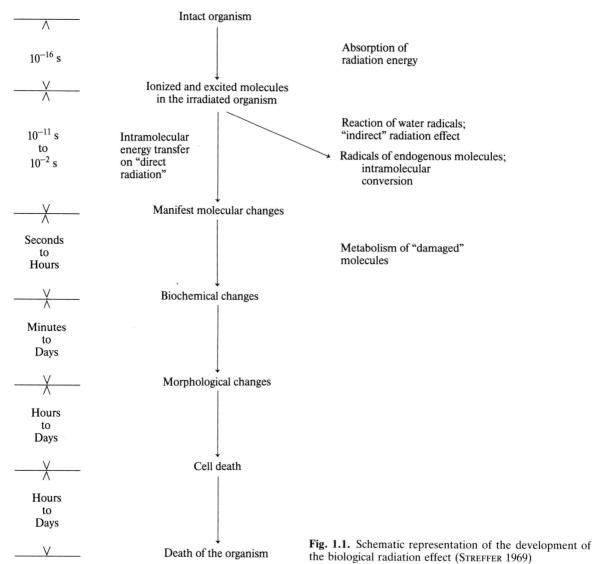

Fig. 1.1. Schematic representation of the development of the biological radiation effect (STREFFER 1969)

The molecular changes caused in this way are reflected in an altered metabolism. Thus, radiation-induced damage of the DNA has repercussions for the course of events in DNA synthesis. Whereas the physical processes of energy absorption, the physicochemical events of radical formation, and most chemical reactions involving radicals are completed in fractions of a second, biochemical changes generally take several hours or days to develop following irradiation (although in exceptional cases only minutes are required; Fig. 1.1). At the same time, morphological effects close to the cellular membrane structures can be observed. Finally, cell death occurs. If a consider-

able number of stem cells in a critical cell system are damaged in such a way that cell renewal is no longer possible, tissue failure or even death of the organism ensues. The causal relationships between these events of cell killing are not known in every detail, but the dose dependence of these effects has been studied for many cell systems and tissues. The present state of knowledge will be presented here, although the discussion will be restricted to the effects of radiation on mammalian cells.

1.2 Biochemical Effects and DNA Repair After Irradiation

As already mentioned above, radiation energy can be absorbed by all molecules in the cell, resulting in ionization, and these events are distributed over the entire irradiated material. Up to now, it has not been definitely shown which molecular changes are responsible for cell death. In spite of this, it can presently be assumed that radiation-induced DNA damage plays a decisive role. However, it has not been ascertained whether other molecular changes are involved in processes leading to cell death and, if so, which molecules or cell structures might be concerned. There is considerable discussion as to whether radiation-induced changes in the membranes and, in particular, the oxidation of unsaturated lipids, play a role.

The importance of DNA is indicated by the following consideration: The functional units of the cell genome, the genes, which contain DNA as a major component, are usually present as only a single copy or a few copies per haploid cell genome. A radiation-induced alteration of the DNA, and thus of one or more genes, will result in mutant or nonviable cells, so that relatively small doses of radiation can produce severe effects. By contrast, every enzyme protein per cell is usually present in multiple copies, so that many molecules must be destroyed in order to achieve a complete breakdown of the metabolic reaction concerned. However, since DNA forms the basis of the genetic material, enzyme proteins can be newly resynthesized even under these conditions if the protein-synthesizing system is undamaged.

The following types of damage in the DNA have been observed after irradiating isolated DNA or chromatin in vitro and also cells in vivo (STREFFER 1969; VON SONNTAG 1987):

1. Radiation absorption can lead to ionization in the polynucleotide chains, producing strand breaks. If only one of the polynucleotide chains is damaged in this manner, one refers to a single strand break. If, however, strand breaks occur in the complementary polynucleotide chains the DNA strands can dissociate following the disruption of hydrogen bonds. One then obtains a double strand break. The latter can result from independent events as well as from one particle passing through the DNA, in particular when using so-called densely ionizing radiation with high LET.
2. Radiochemical reactions can lead to modification or elimination of bases in the DNA. The genetic information of the DNA is thereby altered and structural changes in its conformation occur at the same time.
3. Cross-links between the two complementary DNA–poly-nucleotide strands can be formed at high radiation doses.

These forms of radiation-induced damage can impair two major processes that require DNA as a matrix: (a) replication (DNA synthesis) and (b) transcription (RNA synthesis).

A number of studies have shown that DNA synthesis is considerably more sensitive to radiation than RNA synthesis. Particularly in the case of radiosensitive cells, e.g., proliferating cells from lymphatic tissue, it has been observed that DNA synthesis can be impaired even at radiation doses of less than 1 Gy. This metabolic change is usually determined by measuring the incorporation of radioactively labeled precursors into the DNA. However, in general, the effect does not occur until several hours after irradiation with low doses (below 1 Gy). It is reversible and DNA synthesis may be completely restored after several hours. At higher doses, this radiation-induced change in DNA synthesis is observed earlier and lasts longer (ALTMAN et al. 1970; STREFFER 1969).

Investigations into the mechanism of DNA synthesis have shown that it commences at specific starting points. A number of such equivalent points, where DNA synthesis begins simultaneously, are to be found over the entire genome. This step is termed initiation, and involves specific processes. It is followed by the so-called elongation of the DNA strands, whereby the DNA polynucleotide chains are elongated. Investigations of these events after radiation insults have shown that initiation is much more radiosensitive than elongation (LITTLE 1970).

In addition, it has frequently been observed that protein synthesis, assessed by the general incorporation of amino acids into proteins, is comparable to RNA synthesis in terms of radiosensitivity and, as such, is much more radioresistant than DNA synthesis. Here, it is likely that the damage occurs above all at the level of formation of the corresponding messenger RNA (mRNA) and to a lesser extent involves inhibition of the translation process on the ribo-somes (HIDVEGI et al. 1978). This assumption is in agreement with the fact that the induction and synthesis of individual specific enzyme proteins can be inhibited by ionizing radiation to a greater extent than can protein synthesis in general. Studies on complex metabolic pathways, e.g., those of tryptophan and cholesterol biosynthesis, have thus shown that not all enzymatic steps of a metabolic pathway are damaged equally; rather those enzymatic steps are especially altered which are involved in the regulation of these metabolic pathways. These findings indicate that possibly not all structural genes possess the same radiosensitiv-ity (which is not only correlated to their size) but rather that particular specificities exist (STREFFER 1969; STREFFER and SCHAFFERUS 1971). There is good evidence that the induction of DNA damage is spatially nonrandom. This may be due to several factors: The compactness of DNA varies consider-ably. In actively transcribing regions the compact-ness is lower than in nontranscribing regions. Also microdosimetric distributions of ionizations may be responsible for the nonrandom distribution of DNA lesions. The ionizations produced by x- and γ-radiation are mainly induced by so-called δ-rays. At the ends of these δ-ray tracks, clusters of ionizations occur within a range of a few nanometers. Such clusters could be lethal events within the cell nucleus (GOODHEAD and BRENNER 1983; STEEL and PEACOCK 1989). Ion clusters would produce a number of damaged sites within a range of 10-15 DNA base pairs. Such sites have been termed local multiple damaged sites (LMDS) (WARD 1986).

Studies of the spatial distribution of ionizations lead to geometrical patterns which are analyzed with microdosimetry. According to these analyses the radiation dose is very heterogeneously distri-buted in microscopic scales of cells and tissues, especially with low doses and dose rates. With low LET radiation at radiation doses below 3 mGy, target volumes with a diameter of 8 μm (diameter of a cell nucleus) typically experience only one hit or even none. At lower doses the number of cell nuclei with hits decreases still further, but the energy deposited per hit remains constant. At low dose rates the period between two ionizing events increases to hours and days (BOOZ and FEINEN-DEGEN 1987).

It has further been shown that metabolic processes occurring in the cell nucleus are ex-tremely radiosensitive. Thus, a particularly large decrease in oxidative phosphorylation in nuclei has been observed after irradiation. Likewise, those enzymatic processes of nicotinamide-adenine dinucleotide (NAD) metabolism that are localized in the nucleus are disrupted even after radiation doses below 1 Gy in lymphatic tissue (Fig. 1.2) (STREFFER and BEISEL 1974). By con-trast, glycolysis in the cytoplasm and oxidative phosphorylation in the mitochondria have proven to be relatively resistant to ionizing radiation (ALTMAN et al. 1970; STREFFER 1969).

It has repeatedly been observed that lysosomal enzyme activities are increased in radiosensitive cells and tissues after irradiation. However, it has not been clarified whether this is directly related to the radiation effect or is merely a consequence of damaged cell structures.

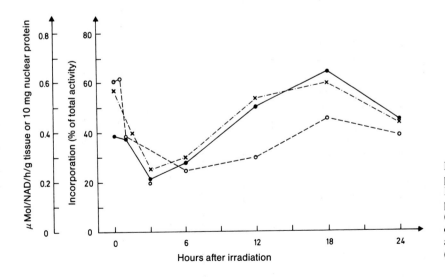

Fig. 1.2. DNA synthesis [incor-poration of ^{3}H-thymidine in the DNA (●)] and NAD pyrophos-phorylase [μmol NAD/h/g tissue (○) and μmol NAD/h/mg nu-cleoprotein (x)] in mouse spleen after x-irradiation with 0.5 Gy (STREFFER and BEISEL 1974)

It had already been reported in the 1940s that the amino acid cysteine can enhance radioresistance in mammals when administered prior to irradiation. It was then shown that a whole series of substances containing sulfhydryl groups could act as so-called radioprotective agents (BACQ 1965; MELCHING and STREFFER 1966; MÖNIG et al. 1989). On the other hand, radiochemical investigations have shown that sulfhydryl groups in enzyme proteins are extremely radiosensitive and that those enzymes containing such groups in their active centers are also very radiosensitive (SANNER and PIHL 1972). Based on such data it has been assumed that the intracellular sulfhydryl group content and, above all, the non-protein-bound fraction, decisively affects the radiosensitivity of cells (MICHAEL 1987; BIAGLOW et al. 1987). Such substances can act as radical scavengers and thus possibly reduce the amount of radicals on biomolecules (ELDJARN and PIHL 1960).

Several authors have been able to demonstrate a correlation between the radiosensitivity and the non-protein-bound sulfhydryl group content (REVESZ and MODIG 1965; BIAGLOW et al. 1987). It has further been observed that substances which react with sulfhydryl groups, e.g., N-methyl maleinimide or iodoacetamide, can greatly sensitize living cells towards ionizing radiation (SINCLAIR 1972; HAN et al. 1976). This sensitizing effect also appears to be correlated to the sulfhydryl group content. However, cell lines have been found where no such correlations seem to exist, so that this apparently is not a general phenomenon (SZUMIEL 1981). On the other hand, more recent studies have shown that cell lines in which glutathione synthesis is disturbed are relatively radiosensitive (GUICHARD et al. 1983). Further studies must clarify this matter.

In this respect it is of some interest that cAMP apparently exerts a regulatory effect on the sulfhydryl group content in cells (ISAACS and BINKLEY 1977). On the other hand cAMP can act as a radioprotective substance (LANGENDORFF and LANGENDORFF 1973; MITZNEGG et al. 1971). Enzymes important in the metabolism of cAMP are bound to the cytoplasmic membranes. It has already been mentioned that radiation-induced alterations to membranes are frequently considered to be an important event in radiation-induced cell death. In particular, the oxidation of lipids by oxygen radicals has been discussed. Oxygen is activated to yield superoxide radicals by radiochemical processes, and these superoxide radicals can react extremely well with unsaturated carbon bonds, for example. Such peroxides have been found to be increased in the membrane lipids. A further important finding in this direction has been obtained from investigations showing that vitamin E has a protective effect against radiation (FONCK and KONINGS 1978; KONINGS and DRIJVER 1979). Furthermore, it has been shown that superoxide dismutase (SOD), an enzyme capable of breaking down these superoxide radicals, can also increase the radioresistance of cells and tissues (LEUTHAUSER and OBERLEY 1978; PETKAU et al. 1976).

It was assumed for a long time that radiation-induced damage to the DNA was irreversible and could not be repaired. Studies initially carried out on micro-organisms have shown that living cells have very effective mechanisms at their disposal for repairing the above-mentioned molecular, radiation-induced changes in the DNA. It has been shown that such repair systems also exist in mammalian cells (HANAWALT et al. 1979; GENEROSO et al. 1980; FRIEDBERG and HANAWALT 1988).

Some of the single strand breaks in the polynucleotide chains can be repaired particularly rapidly by the enzyme polynucleotide ligase. However, DNA damage can only be repaired with the help of this relatively simple enzymatic step if a phosphodiester bond has been opened in the chain. If this is not the case, the damaged nucleotide must first be removed from the polynucleotide chain. In general, several nucleotides, including intact ones, are excised from the damaged chain by exonucleases. Because of the genetic information still available in the complementary polynucleotide strand, DNA repair is then possible. With the aid of this repair synthesis, the original base sequence is restored in the damaged polynucleotide strand. By means of a polynucleotide ligase the chain can finally be closed, so that even "complex" single strand breaks can be completely repaired in this way (Fig. 1.3). Kinetic studies have shown that there are apparently three different types of DNA single strand break, which are repaired at different rates (DIKOMEY and FRANZKE 1986).

In contrast to earlier assumptions, more recent studies have shown that double strand breaks can also be repaired to a certain extent (SMITH et al. 1987). For a long time it was thought that double strand breaks represent a lethal event, but in fact this is so in only a few cases.

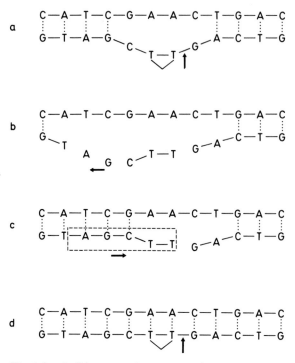

Fig. 1.3a–d. Diagrammatic representation of excision repair of DNA (Streffer 1969)

Radiochemically damaged DNA bases or other DNA structural defects, e.g., after elimination of a DNA base, can also be repaired with the help of similar repair systems. In this case, an additional enzymatic step is necessary. First, an incision of the damaged polynucleotide chain by an endonuclease must take place. The nucleotide with the damaged base can subsequently be removed. In general, during this process several nucleotides are excised from the polynucleotide chain by exonucleases. Again, DNA repair synthesis can be carried out (see above) to produce the original base sequence. The gap in the polynucleotide chain is finally closed by a polynucleotide ligase, so that the original DNA structure is completely renewed (Fig. 1.3).

It has been shown that these repair systems are needed not only to correct radiation-induced DNA damage but also to correct mistakes in the base sequence which occur during cell replication. Mistakes can occur during the DNA replication of about 3×10^9 base pairs in the genome of a mammalian cell and these need to be corrected so that identical cell renewal can take place. A "proof reading" occurs after DNA synthesis. These repair processes are regulated genetically.

The necessity of these events is particularly apparent in those persons with genetic defects who are able to carry out such DNA repair to only a limited degree. This applies especially to those suffering from xeroderma pigmentosum and ataxia telangiectasia (AT). In the former case, the incision by endonuclease is generally disturbed. Thus, in these cells, damage arising through the effects of ultraviolet light, for example, cannot be repaired. In persons with AT, repair following x-ray or γ-radiation is no longer possible or is severely restricted. Recent studies have demonstrated that AT cells are able to rejoin double strand breaks but that the fidelity of this repair is impaired. These processes have been studied in detail in cell lines isolated from persons afflicted with these syndromes (Hanawalt et al. 1979; Generoso et al. 1980; Debenham and Thacker 1987).

1.3 Cell Death After Irradiation

It has already been mentioned that according to the rule of Bergonié and Tribondeau, the proliferation rate of a cell population has a decisive influence on the radiosensitivity. On the other hand, very soon after this rule was set down (1906) it was shown that it is not of general validity; rather, there are exceptions to it.

1.3.1 Interphase Death

Peripherally circulating lymphocytes, which in general display only a low proliferation rate, have proved to be extremely radiosensitive (Heineke 1904). When these cells are irradiated with a dose of about 1–2 Gy or more, degenerative processes can be observed after several hours. A breakdown of macromolecules, in particular DNA, occurs. The effect of lysosomal enzymes is apparently of great significance (Streffer 1969; Altman et al. 1970; Hidvegi et al. 1978). Damage to the membrane systems and karyolysis were observed in electron microscopic studies (Braun 1965; Betz 1974). The cell volume is greatly decreased within a few hours (Ohyama et al. 1981) and the microvilli on the cell surface disappear (Yamada and Ohyama 1980). These cells are removed from the tissues by autolytic and phagocytic processes.

The question as to whether these events stem primarily from the cell nucleus or cytoplasm, however, is still unresolved. In electron microscopic studies on lymphocytes in the thymus following lethal radiation, BRAUN (1965) observed that the radiation damage was initiated by alterations to the nuclear membrane. By contrast, after sublethal radiation doses "dedifferentiation processes" were first seen in the cytoplasm. The whole cell can subsequently be taken up by macrophages (BRAUN 1967). Lasting biochemical changes are also observed. Hence, oxidative phosphorylation is considerably impaired, above all in the nucleus but also in the mitochondria (STREFFER 1969; HIDVEGI et al. 1978). OHYAMA and YAMADA have described in particular the radiation effect on glycolysis in association with cell death in lymphocytes. These authors observed that the allosteric regulation of phosphofructokinase was altered after irradiating thymocytes (OHYAMA and YAMADA 1973).

Cell death occurs before the cells can enter the next mitosis. Thus, this procedure is termed interphase death. Similar events are seen in mature oocytes over about the same dose range. Particularly in the case of lymphocytes, we are dealing with cells whose nucleocytoplasmic ratio is strongly shifted in favor of the nucleus. Relatively few mitochondria are found in the cytoplasm. Similar radiation effects can also be seen in other types of cells, although only after considerably higher doses.

1.3.2 Reproductive Cell Death

No interphase death is observed in proliferating mammalian cells after radiation doses of 1-2 Gy. In this case, cell damage usually only occurs after several cell divisions. At least one mitosis takes place after irradiation before the cell dies. This phenomenon is known as reproductive death. Such radiation effects can only, of course, be found in proliferating cells; however, nonproliferating cells are also able to express such radiation damage if they are stimulated to proliferate (ALPER 1979). For example, hepatocytes from liver tissue of adult animals, which generally do not proliferate, are relatively radioresistant with respect to cell killing. If, however, the proliferation of liver tissue after an exposure to radiation is stimulated by partial hepatectomy, there is an increase in cell death. Apparently, the radiation-induced damage can be expressed after a prolonged period under such conditions. Most radiobiological studies on the killing of proliferating cells have been undertaken on the basis of these phenomena.

In radiobiology, the technical term "reproductive cell death" therefore indicates that the cells involved have lost their reproductive integrity. Thus, the loss of unlimited division capability, e.g., in the case of stem cells of the hematopoietic system or of the crypts of Lieberkühn, is called cell death. The cells may still be metabolically active, capable of synthesizing proteins and RNA and fulfilling other functions, but they are no longer in a position to carry out their function as stem cells. By this definition, these cells are sterilized; they have not survived. Surviving cells have not lost the capability to proliferate and can form colonies; they are referred to as clonogenic.

Such events can be clearly observed in individual stem cells, e.g., during early mammalian embryogenesis. If, for example, one irradiates mouse embryos at the two-cell stage, with each cell still possessing the full potential to develop into a mammalian organism, then an initial delay in cell division is seen. However, after this delay mitosis starts and if mitosis has been completed then daughter cells can proliferate further despite exposure to 2 Gy x-rays. After the mitotic delay, a proliferation rate is observed which is similar to that of unirradiated embryos. Only after several cell divisions is there a loss of cells as a function of the radiation dose, so that the number of cells in the irradiated embryos is finally smaller than in the untreated ones (Fig. 1.4) (MOLLS et al. 1982; STREFFER and MOLLS 1987).

Such phenomena are also responsible for the observation that irradiation of tumors does not lead to immediate regression; instead further tumor growth is frequently observed over a substantial period of radiotherapy, although the tumor cells are damaged and a decrease in tumor volume later occurs (SUIT 1973; STREFFER 1980).

Cells damaged in the sense that reproductive cell death has occurred cannot generally be distinguished by morphological means or other criteria from those that have retained their capacity to proliferate and survive in accordance with the above-mentioned definition shortly after irradiation. Therefore, they must be evaluated by means of a functional test such as the colony-forming assay. In the case of micro-organisms, this has been a very long established method. Such

8

C. Streffer and D. van Beuningen

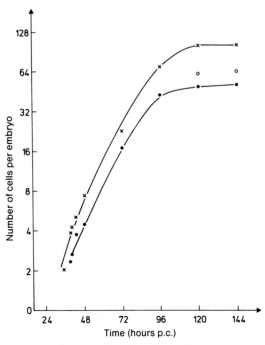

Fig. 1.4. Cell proliferation in preimplantation mouse embryos (in vitro culture) as a function of the time after conception (*p.c.*). x, controls; ●, after x-irradiation with 3.7 Gy; ○, after x-irradiation with 1.8 Gy (Molls et al. 1983)

procedures for mammalian cells were developed only in the 1950s, above all by Puck and Marcus (1955). Since then many mammalian cell lines have been studied in this way. Above all, dose–response curves have been set up with the help of colony formation.

1.3.3 Dose–Response Relationships

In order to obtain dose–response relationships for the clonogenic survival of mammalian cells using the colony formation test, cell populations in vitro are usually irradiated with various doses and the rate of colony formation of the irradiated cells determined. Since such dose–response curves for the survival of mammalian cells are the basis for the understanding of many radiobiological experiments, at this juncture an exception will be made in providing experimental details.

Established human melanoma cell lines, among others, are studied in our laboratories. The cells are usually grown in minimum essential medium with Earle's salts. First of all, 1% nonessential amino acids, 1 mM sodium pyruvate, and 15% fetal calf serum are added to the medium. The

medium is incubated with sodium bicarbonate and CO_2 at pH 7.4. Cells (5×10^5) are introduced into culture flasks with a growth surface of 25 cm^2. The cells grow on the bottom surface of the flask within 24 h and are then treated with various doses of irradiation. Directly after irradiation they are trypsinized; the trypsin is siphoned off after gentle centrifugation, and the cells are resuspended in a medium containing 20% fetal calf serum. They are then recentrifuged and, after decanting the medium, resuspended in fresh medium.

Usually a single cell suspension is then obtained. The cells in the suspension are counted and diluted accordingly. Control cultures contain 300 cells in 5 ml medium. These are placed into Petri dishes and incubated for 11 days at 37°C. The medium is then aspirated, the cultures washed once with ice-cold physiological saline, and the colonies fixed for 30 min with 80% alcohol. After allowing the cultures to dry, the colonies are stained with a 1% solution of crystal violet for 5 min. After removing the solution, the colonies can be counted under a stereoscopic microscope (Van Beuningen et al. 1981). Jung (1978) has presented an elegant method of counting. Numerous modifications of the colony formation test have been described.

Of the 300 cells from nontreated cultures seeded, about 100, i.e., 33%, are able to form colonies. This percentage represents the "plating efficiency."

If a culture is irradiated with a dose of 4 Gy in parallel, the following observations can be made after 11 days: Some cells have not divided at all, some have undergone one to three cell divisions and have formed microcolonies, and others have formed large colonies which cannot be distinguished from those of untreated cells. The latter are referred to as surviving cells since they have shown themselves to be clonogenic. In the case of irradiated cells, 3000 cells, rather than 300, are added to each Petri dish so that enough colonies can be counted. Here, 3000 cells per dish are given. Counting reveals that, again, 100 colonies have been formed.

Hence, the surviving fraction can be determined from the plating efficiency and the number of colonies. In the example given, the surviving fraction is 10%. This procedure is carried out in the same manner for other doses of radiation. The number of cells are adjusted in accordance with the dose so that a sufficient number of colonies are present after irradiation. Too few colonies would result in statistically inexact values and too many cannot be properly counted because of confluence.

It is customary to plot the logarithm of the surviving fraction on the ordinate against the radiation dose on the abscissa. In the case of a purely exponential decrease in cell survival with increasing dose, one would obtain a straight line. This dependence is expressed by the following equation:

$$N = N_0 \times e^{-aD} \qquad (1.1)$$

thus:

$$\ln \frac{N}{N_0} = -a \times D \qquad (1.2)$$

whereby $N_0 =$ is the number of clonogenic cells before irradiation, N is the number of clonogenic cells after irradiation with radiation dose D, and a is a constant.

Such dose responses are characterized by the parameter D_0. D_0 represents the dose needed to reduce the survival rate by the factor e, i.e., from 1 to $1/e = 0.37$ (37%). Such a simple dose–response relationship for cell survival is usually not obtained when mammalian cells are irradiated with loosely ionizing radiation x-rays, γ-rays, β-rays); rather, a complex function is obtained. In a semilogarithmic plot, a so-called shoulder curve is observed (Fig. 1.5).

In the case of an absolute exponential dose–response relationship, each dose interval results in the same biological effect, expressed in percent of the initial cell number. In the case of a shoulder curve, low radiation doses per dose interval are considerably less effective than higher doses. The significance of the shoulder will be discussed later. At higher doses the dose–response curve becomes exponential in many cases; a straight line is then obtained over this dose range. In order to describe such shoulder curves, the following parameters are usually given:

D_0: This is calculated from the slope of the linear part of the dose–response curve and, as in the case of a purely exponential function, gives the reduction in surviving cells still present by the factor $1/e = 0.37$. On average each cell receives a lethal hit which results in a survival rate of $1/e$.

n: If one extrapolates the linear part of the semilogarithmic dose–response curve to dose 0, the extrapolation number n is obtained from the point where the extrapolation meets the ordinate.

D_q: The dose D_q is a measure of the width of the shoulder in a dose–response curve. It is defined as that section of the abscissa where the extrapolated straight line meets the abscissa at the survival rate 1.0 (100%).

These parameters are related as follows:

$$D_q = D_0 \times \ln n \qquad (1.3)$$

In vitro studies involving many mammalian cell lines have shown that the D_0 values for dose–response relationships lie in a relatively close dose range (0.75–1.5 Gy), reflecting cell survival rates after treatment with loosely ionizing radiation, whereas the values for n or D_q vary considerably more (TROTT 1972; STREFFER 1980; MCNALLY 1982). If the survival rates of cells in tissues or cell aggregates are determined, the width of the shoulder is considerably greater than after irradiation in vitro (MCNALLY 1982). These phenomena are probably at least in part due to the fact that intercellular contacts increase radioresistance (DURAND and SUTHERLAND 1972; DERTINGER and HÜLSER 1981).

There are a number of formal presentations which describe the dose–response relationship based on considerations deriving from the target theory and others. These will not be treated in great detail here and the reader is referred to the literature (DERTINGER and JUNG 1969; ALPER 1979; KIEFER 1981).

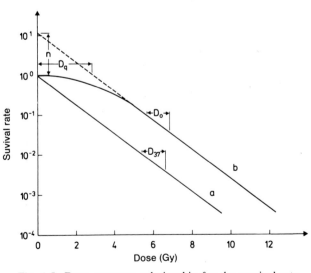

Fig. 1.5. Dose–response relationship for the survival rate of cells. *a*, exponential curve; *b*, shoulder curve

KELLERER and ROSSI (1972, 1978) have developed the so-called theory of dual radiation effect. This theory is formulated on the basis of fundamental microdosimetric concepts of energy deposition in order to explain the relationship between the relative biological effect and the radiation dose for high LET radiation, particularly neutrons. However, it is of a more general nature and has been applied not only to cell killing but also to other biological effects.

KELLERER and ROSSI assumed that the damage responsible for the biological effect results from the interaction of at least two sublesions. This assumption gives rise to the following relationship between dose and cell survival:

$$S = e^{-\alpha D - \beta D^2} \qquad (1.4)$$

This equation yields a dose–response relationship which contains a shoulder but does not end in a straight line. Numerous data from studies on cell survival rate after irradiation can be adequately described by this equation (BARENDSEN 1962; CHAPMAN et al. 1975). However, there are deviations, and a number of questions are thus left open. The two sublesions can arise from the penetration of one or two energy-rich particles. KELLERER and ROSSI assume that the distance over which interaction of sublesions can still occur is in the order of 1 μm.

These concepts have been placed somewhat in question by experiments using ultrasoft x-rays, which induce tracks in the order of several nanometers in biological material (McNALLY 1982). According to the theory of dual radiation effect, this radiation quality should not be more effective than ^{60}Co γ-radiation. However, ultrasoft x-rays, e.g., 1.5 keV aluminum K and 0.3 keV carbon K, are in fact more effective as regards both cell killing and the induction of chromosomal aberrations (GOODHEAD 1971, 1979; VIRSIK and HARDER 1981) (Fig. 1.6).

CHADWICK and LEENHOUTS (1973, 1981) have proposed a molecular biological basis for radiation-induced cell killing. These authors assume that the induction of DNA double strand breaks is the decisive damaging event leading to cell death. Double strand breaks can arise when a penetrating particle damages both DNA polynucleotide chains or when two single strand breaks, arising as a result of various penetrations in the complementary nucleotide chains, lie so close together that disruption of the adjacent hydrogen bonds occurs. Thus, loosely ionizing radiation, that

above all induces single strand breaks, is also in a position to induce double strand breaks. Thus, a correlation should exist between the number of single strand breaks and the rate of cell killing. DUGLE et al. (1976) have observed such an interrelationship in Chinese hamster cells. HESSLEWOOD (1978), however, found no difference in the number of single strand breaks either before or after DNA repair in two lymphoma cell lines with different radiosensitivity. Further examples arguing against the concepts of CHADWICK and LEENHOUTS have been reported (McNALLY 1982).

While CHADWICK and LEENHOUTS also arrive at

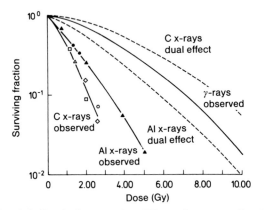

Fig. 1.6. Survival curves for Chinese hamster cells with x-rays, 1.5 keV Al (*solid symbols*), and 0.3 keV C (*open symbols*). The *broken curves* show the calculated curves for ultrasoft x-rays, corresponding to the dual radiation effect (GOODHEAD 1971)

the linear-quadratic formalism described by KELLERER and ROSSI (1972, 1978), the molecular biological assumptions as a basis for cell death are not convincing. However, it cannot be ruled out that such events may be relevant.

A similar form of presentation of dose–response relationships has been suggested by WIDEROE (1971, 1975). He distinguishes between an α-effect, which leads to direct cell killing without recovery, and a β-effect, where radiation damage is partially repaired. These ideas lead to the same formalism as was developed by KELLERER and ROSSI (1972, 1978).

1.4 Radiosensitivity and Cell Proliferation

1.4.1 Proliferating and Resting Cells

When mammalian cells are cultured, they will begin to proliferate after a certain delay. This delay is known as the lag phase. Thereafter, initially all cells are generally involved in proliferation. Assuming that the time interval from one mitosis to the next remains constant, so-called exponential growth is obtained under these conditions. The increase in cell numbers follows an exponential function.

If the logarithm of the cell number is plotted against time, one initially obtains a straight line, as shown in Fig. 1.4. With increasing incubation time, deviations from this exponential function are seen and the cell proliferation rate decreases. Finally, the curve generally enters the so-called plateau phase and the total number of cells in the culture does not change at this time. This plateau phase arises because the cells enter a resting phase to an increasing extent and are no longer active in cell proliferation. In addition, cell loss occurs in such cell cultures. A stationary equilibrium is reached in which cell renewal parallels cell loss.

Such equilibria also exist in tissues and cell systems of adults, whereby the equilibrium between proliferating and resting cells as well as the extent of cell loss is subject to tissue- and organ-specific regulation. Similar phenomena also occur in tumors, although in general an equilibrium is not reached, cell renewal tending to be greater than cell loss. In this connection, the proliferating cells are often referred to as the growth fraction (STREFFER 1980).

Exponential growth in vivo is only seen in exceptional cases, e.g., in the case of cell proliferation during very early prenatal development. As already mentioned, a situation is reached shortly after the start of in vitro cultures in which all cells participate in proliferation. By contrast, it is much more difficult to obtain a cell population consisting only of resting cells. In order to test the radiosensitivity of so-called plateau phase cells, the cells are irradiated in the plateau phase but must subsequently be induced to proliferate to permit an estimation of the survival rate via the colony formation test. As a consequence certain difficulties arise in trying to make experimental assessments of the radiosensitivity of resting cells, and

these difficulties lead to a number of contradictions when proliferating and resting cells are compared (ALPER 1979). It was at first assumed that the radiosensitivity of mammalian cells is the same during the various growth phases. However, MADOC-JONES (1964) was able to show that, as in the case of micro-organisms, the parameters D_0 and n from dose–response curves vary during the different growth periods. Thus, the highest values for the extrapolation number were obtained in the stationary (plateau) phase. By contrast, BERRY et al. (1970) observed that in the case of Chinese hamster and HeLa cells the extrapolation number n was identical for cells in the exponential growth and the plateau phase. This was also the case when the plateau phase cells were "postfed." In these experiments, fresh medium was given to the cell cultures in order to supply the cells with fresh nutrients. Both TAYLOR and BLEEHEN (1977) and MADOC-JONES (1964) observed a difference in radiosensitivity between the exponential growth and the plateau phase in EMT6 tumor cells cultured in vitro. In addition, however, these authors reported a difference between the early and late plateau phases.

1.4.2 Radiosensitivity in Various Phases of the Cell Cycle

Since the studies by HOWARD and PELC (1953) it has been known that proliferating cells pass through various separate phases during the time interval from one mitosis to the next. This can be shown very characteristically by means of DNA synthesis. Studies on this process have shown that it proceeds discontinuously during the above-mentioned time interval. DNA synthesis usually does not start for several hours after mitosis and then continues for about 6-8 h in mammalian cells. The total DNA in a cell is doubled during this time. Based on these phenomena, two phases of the so-called cell cycle can be determined relatively easily in experiments: (a) Mitosis, which can be observed under the microscope since the chromosomes become visible due to condensation. (b) The DNA synthesis phase, the so-called S phase; with the aid of radioactively labeled DNA precursors, incorporated into the DNA as selectively as possible, the DNA can be labeled when it is newly synthesized. With the aid of autoradiographic techniques it is possible to make those cells visible that have incorporated these radioactive precursors into the DNA.

Thus, a cycle arises, the so-called cell cycle, in which there is a gap between mitosis and the S phase and, likewise, another gap after the S phase up to the next mitosis. These two phases (gaps) are known as the G_1 and the G_2 phase, respectively. Today numerous processes are known to occur during these phases but they will not be dealt with here. Furthermore, so-called resting cells can be found in cell populations which cannot be distinguished from proliferating cells with the techniques described and these are frequently referred to as cells in the G_0 phase. In particular, this applies to differentiated, functional cells in tissues.

With the help of impulse cytophotometry it is nowadays possible to determine the distribution of cells within the cycle more easily and quickly. In this method, chromatin or DNA are coupled with dyes, usually fluorescent ones, as specifically as possible. The DNA content in each individual cell can then be determined by measuring the fluorescence excitation. As a result, the cells can be assigned to the various phases of the cycle; in the G_1 phase the cell genome is diploid (2n), in the S phase there is an increase in DNA content due to DNA replication so that the DNA content is doubled at the end of this phase, and the G_2 phase has a DNA content equivalent to a tetraploid genome. Finally, after mitosis the diploid cell genome is again obtained (Fig. 1.7) (Dittrich and Göhde 1969; see also Andreeff 1975).

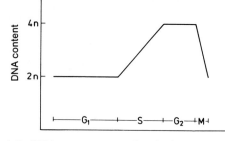

Fig. 1.7. DNA content per nucleus in the course of the cell cycle (2n $\hat{=}$ DNA content of diploid cells)

With an impulse cytophotometer, the fluorescence intensity of each single cell is determined with the aid of photomultipliers and the captured signals are sorted according to their size and arranged in groups (channels). One obtains a histogram showing the number of cells for each individual channel arranged according to the DNA content. The amount of cells in G_1, S, and G_2 phases can be determined from such histograms assuming that the peaks, representing the G_1 and G_2 phase cells, show a Gaussian distribution (Fig. 1.8). It is also possible to identify cells with an abnormal (aneuploid) DNA content as seen in tumors.

Thus, a very effective method has been developed to obtain these parameters relatively quickly from cell populations. With this method it

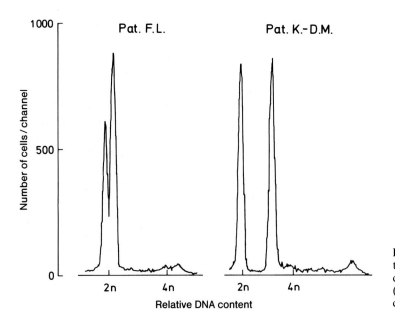

Fig. 1.8. DNA histograms measured with the impulse cytophotometer in two rectal carcinomas (patients F.L. and K.-D.M.) (2n $\hat{=}$ DNA content of diploid, normal cells)

also appears possible to distinguish the resting (G_0 phase) cells from proliferating cells, in particular the G_1 phase cells. In this case, not only the DNA content but also the RNA content per cell is measured and a so-called two parameter analysis is carried out (BAUER and DETHLEFSEN 1981).

Studies involving many cell populations in vivo and in vitro have shown, in general, that the S phase in the different cell populations has a relatively constant duration of about 6–8. In addition neither the G_2 phase nor mitosis appears to be subject to very large variations, mitosis lasting about 1–2 h in mammalian cells. By contrast, the G_1 phase shows very large variations. Very short G_1 phases (about 30–60 min) are observed in preimplantation mammalian embryos (STREFFER et al. 1980), whereas the G_1 phase can last several days in other cell populations (TUBIANA 1971). Up to now very little is known about the molecular biological regulatory processes, although there is some evidence that phosphorylation of proteins is important. The length of the total cell cycle for mammalian cells thus lies between 10 h and several days. However, during recent years it has been observed that phosphorylation of intracellular proteins increases at the onset of mitosis. The phosphorylation of histone III occurs during cell proliferation and the responsible protein kinase has been identified (LOHKA 1989). Several promoting factors for cell proliferation have been purified.

It has already been mentioned that the proportion of proliferating cells (growth fraction) can also vary considerably in individual tissues and cell systems. Organs and tissues that have a large growth fraction, such as skin, small intestine, and bone marrow, can thereby be differentiated from those with a low growth fraction, such as the liver or kidney, which, however, can be stimulated to proliferate again after injury. Furthermore there are organs with an extremely low growth fraction, e.g., the brain, where the cells cannot be stimulated to proliferate even after trauma. It has already been mentioned that there is an equilibrium between cell renewal and cell loss in proliferating organs. This balance can be disturbed by irradiation.

The cell populations whose behavior after irradiation has been reported up to now have always been very heterogeneous ones, distributed over all phases of the cell cycle at the time of irradiation. It has previously been pointed out that there is a mitotic delay after irradiation (TROTT

1972; STREFFER 1980). This mitotic delay is in part due to the fact that the cells are apparently arrested in the G_2 phase after irradiation, and this is termed G_2 block. The G_2 block can be considered to be a possible self-protective mechanism of the cell since recovery processes apparently take place preferentially or, indeed, only, when the cells have not gone through a mitosis after irradiation.

It has been shown in several studies that the radiosensitivity varies within the G_2 phase itself. Cells that are relatively close to mitosis react more strongly to radiation than those that have a much longer way to go before entering mitosis. This effect can be studied particularly impressively in mouse embryos at the two-cell stage, since these cells have a very long G_2 phase (about 12 h). MOLLS et al. (1982) found both the level of cell killing and the extent of chromosomal damage to be much lower after irradiation in the early G_2 phase than after the same dose in the late G_2 phase.

The radiation-induced extension of the cell cycle is dose dependent and apparently increases linearly with increasing dose. After radiation doses in the range 10–15 Gy the extension time is about the same as that of one cycle, although the lengths of cycle times have been very different in the cell lines studied (DENEKAMP 1975; STREFFER 1980).

Cell biological investigations, in which it is possible to obtain so-called synchronized cells, have enabled the radiosensitivity of mammalian cells to be studied specifically in the individual phases of the cell cycle. Cells that are in mitosis in "in vitro culture" become rounded, as a result of which their adhesion to the surface of the culture flask is considerably reduced, so that they can be loosened from the surface by shaking and obtained selectively, By collecting these cells it is possible to obtain a larger cell population in mitosis, which enters the G_1 phase synchronously. These cells pass through the cell cycle simultaneously and maintain their synchrony for some time (ELKIND and WHITMORE 1967).

Such synchronization can also be achieved by chemically inhibiting DNA synthesis in a cell culture. The cells traverse the other phases of the cycle and accumulate at the boundary between the G_1 and the S phase. Initially they cannot enter the S phase. Only when the block is removed is it possible for them to enter the S phase; they do so simultaneously and also complete the other phases in a synchronous manner (ELKIND and WHITMORE 1967).

The cells can now be irradiated in the various phases of the cycle and their survival rates or radiosensitivity can be determined with the aid of the colony formation test. Studies of this type have been carried out very extensively with HeLa and Chinese hamster cells (TERASIMA and TOLMACH 1963; SINCLAIR and MORTON 1966). The results are shown in Fig. 1.9. In these experiments synchronization was carried out during the mitotic phase. Further experiments have been reported by other authors.

Despite certain apparent differences from cell line to cell line, several common principles can be put forward with respect to radiosensitivity as measured by the survival rates (STREFFER 1980):

1. Cells irradiated during mitosis are the most sensitive.
2. In general, the cells are also radiosensitive during the early S phase and during the G_2 phase.
3. The radioresistance of cells increases during the course of the S phase.
4. If the G_1 phase is long, the cells are relatively resistant during the early G_1 phase. The radiosensitivity increases towards the end of the G_1 phase.

Dose–response relationships with very broad shoulders are seen particularly during the late S phase (Fig. 1.9). This is indicative of very pronounced recovery effects. By contrast, a purely

exponential dose–response relationship is frequently seen after irradiation during the mitotic phase. Apparently the recovery capacity of cells in this phase of the cell cycle is extremely limited.

These large differences in the radiosensitivity of mammalian cells in the various phases of the cell cycle mean that when a heterogeneous cell population is irradiated, those cells in the radiosensitive phases are killed initially, while the more resitant ones survive to a greater extent. Thus, a partial synchronization of cells is achieved after irradiation. In general, however, this effect is adjusted relatively quickly in the case of proliferating cells since synchronization disappears because of the varying lengths of the individual phases for single cells.

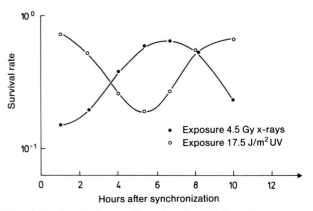

Fig. 1.10. Survival rate of synchronized Chinese hamster cells after exposure to x-rays or ultraviolet rays (HAN and ELKIND 1977)

Various authors have examined the aforementioned phenomena in response to ionizing radiation or ultraviolet light (DJORDJEVIC and TOLMACH 1967; HAN and ELKIND 1977). It could be shown that the radiosensitivity of cells during the course of the cell cycle did not vary in the same way with these forms of radiation (Fig. 1.10).

1.5 Recovery Phenomena After Irradiation

From the description of DNA repair synthesis it was shown that radiation damage to the DNA could be repaired by intracellular enzyme complexes. Likewise, dose-response relationships ex-

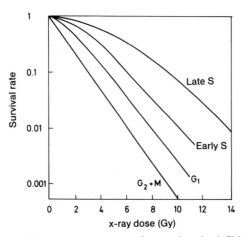

Fig. 1.9. Dose–response curves for synchronized Chinese hamster cells after x-irradiation (SINCLAIR 1968)

pressing a shoulder indicate that the relative radiation effect is smaller in the low than in the high dose range. This effect is also apparently due to recovery processes. Apart from these mechanisms, which are apparently based on intracellular processes, recovery in tissues can occur in such a way that unirradiated or undamaged cells can lead to a renewal of the cell system through cell replication. This process is generally called repopulation.

1.5.1 Recovery from Sublethal Radiation Damage

As long ago as the beginning of this century several authors observed that for the same dose the biological effect was considerably smaller after fractionated irradiation than after single-dose irradiation (KRÖNIG and FRIEDRICH 1918; REGAUD 1922; JÜNGLING and LANGENDORFF 1922). It was also observed that a reduction of the dose rate usually reduced the biological radiation effect (ALPER 1979). Especially ELKIND and co-workers have studied the recovery phenomena after a fractionated radiation dose at the cellular level (ELKIND and SUTTON 1960; ELKIND and WHITMORE 1967).

ELKIND and SUTTON (1960) observed a typical dose–response relationship with a shoulder after irradiation of Chinese hamster cells. After a single dose of 11.2 Gy, 0.1% of cells survived. In a second experiment, however, the cells were first irradiated with 5.05 Gy only, then incubated at 37°C for 18.1 h, and finally irradiated again with different doses of radiation. A typical shoulder curve was also seen in the second irradiation series. It was found that, for the same total radiation dose of 11.2 Gy, survival was about 0.5% when the dose was delivered in two fractions, as compared with the above-mentioned figure of 0.1% after single-dose irradiation (Fig. 1.11).

The shoulder of the second dose–response curve was identical to that after single-dose irradiation. This means that those cells that still survived after 5.05 Gy had regained their full recovery capacity during the time interval of 18.1 h and apparently behaved as unirradiated cells in relation to their survival rate. This effect is known as recovery from sublethal radiation damage or Elkind recovery. The width of the shoulder or D_q can be taken to be a relative measure of the intracellular recovery capacity from sublethal

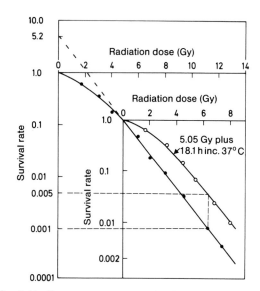

Fig. 1.11. Dose–response curve for Chinese hamster cells after single-dose irradiation (●) or fractionated irradiation (○) with a time interval of 18.1 h (ELKIND and SUTTON 1960)

radiation damage in this model. However, in the case of a larger number of fractions (10 × 1.5 or 2.0 Gy) it was observed that in Chinese hamster cells the full recovery no longer occurred after the last fractions (McNALLY and DeRONDE 1976). In the case of a purely exponential dose–response curve, it can be assumed that these cells are incapable of recovering from sublethal radiation damage.

It has already been mentioned that the values for D_q can be extremely different for various cell lines. This observation implies that recovery from sublethal radiation damage shows a very large range of variation in individual cell lines. If one considers different cell lines from the same tumor entity (e.g., melanoma cells), very different dose–response relationships can be observed even among these cell lines, particularly in the shoulder range (Fig. 1.12).

Fractionation experiments as carried out by ELKIND and SUTTON (1960) cannot be applied to all biological systems. This is only possible with cells in vitro and tissues or cell systems in vivo if a quantitative dose–response relationship can be established. For many tumors and normal tissues, recovery from sublethal radiation damage using the classical experiments of ELKIND et al. (1967) cannot be verified. However, in those tissues where this is not possible, a dose value corresponding to the D_q can be determined. This principle is demonstrated in Fig. 1.13.

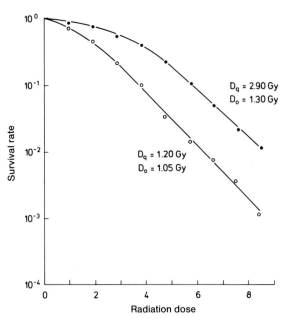

Fig. 1.12. Dose–response curves of two human melanoma cell lines after x-irradiation. ●, Bll; ○, MeWo. (unpublished data)

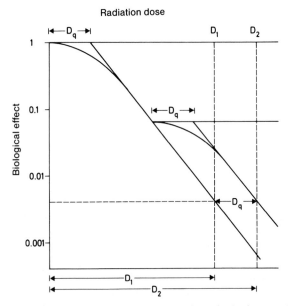

Fig. 1.13. Dose–response curves after single-dose and fractionated irradiation. Schematic representation of the difference $D_1 - D_2$

First of all the biological effect is measured after an experiment in which the total dose is fractionated in two equal radiation doses, separated by a sufficiently large time interval in order to allow for adequate recovery. The total dose of both fractions is designated as D_2. The dose that will lead to the same biological effect after single-dose irradiation is then determined and is designated as D_1. The difference D_2 minus D_1 is apparently equal to D_q as obtained from a dose–response relationship. Dutreix et al. (1973) carried out such recovery experiments on the skin of patients by irradiating skin fields with single doses or fractionated doses. (The data obtained after skin irradiation are described in more detail by Trott and Kummermehr, this volume, Chap. 2.) First, the authors applied single fractions and measured the biological effect which was acute desquamation. In parallel a second field was irradiated in which these single fractions were further divided into two dose fractions. The total dose D_2 was given over the same time period. The following relation is obtained for the same effects:

$$D_r = \frac{D_{2N} - D_{1N}}{N} \qquad (1.5)$$

Thus, the dose D_r additionally required when each dose fraction is again divided into two fractions can be calculated. The size of D_r is apparently that radiation dose which is compensated by recovery. Thus, recovery processes can be quantified. The value for the difference $D_2 - D_1$ has been determined for a number of normal tissues as well as tumors. Under oxic conditions, it lies between 3 and 6 Gy for loosely ionizing radiation. Very low values such as 1 Gy have been seen in the case of the hematopoietic system (Till and McCulloch 1963). The highest values were found for skin, small intestine, and lung (Withers 1967; Withers and Elkind 1969; Field and Hornsey 1974). On comparing the $D_2 - D_1$ values after irradiation in vivo with those after in vitro irradiation, the latter are seen to be significantly lower. Hornsey (1972) has estimated that the D_q values are below 2 Gy for the many cell lines investigated in vitro.

It is possible that intercellular contacts play a significant role in the recovery from sublethal radiation damage. If, for example, cells cultivated as multicellular spheroids are irradiated, the capacity to repair sublethal radiation damage is considerably greater than when the same cells are irradiated as a single cell suspension culture (DURAND and SUTHERLAND 1972). These data show how difficult it is to estimate the radiation effect in vivo from experiments carried out in vitro.

The intracellular recovery processes occur within a few hours. ELKIND et al. (1965) measured the survival rate of Chinese hamster cells after fractionated irradiation with varying time intervals between the dose fractions. When the cells were incubated at 24°C during the time interval, the survival rate increased rapidly with increasing interval between the dose fractions. This effect must be due to the intracellular recovery from sublethal radiation damage. As early as 2 h after the first dose fraction a "plateau" is achieved for the overall effect so that apparently the full recovery capacity has already been reached again at this time.

By contrast, if the cells are incubated at 37°C during the period between the two dose fractions, an increase in the survival rate is also initially observed because of the recovery effects. Subsequently, however, the survival rate again decreases. The authors interpret this effect to be due to a redistribution of cells within the cycle at the higher incubation temperature. On account of the previously described effects, particularly those cells that are in the radiosensitive phases of the cycle are killed by the first radiation exposure. On a subsequent incubation at 37°C the surviving cells from the more resistant cell cycle phases enter into the more radiosensitive ones so that an additional radiation dose will then be much more efficient in terms of cell killing.

The temporal course of these recovery processes can be different in various cell lines. Figure 1.14 shows the effect of fractionation of two x-ray doses of 3.76 Gy as a function of the time interval for two human melanoma cell lines. Whereas recovery is completed within a few minutes in one of the cell lines (Bevey), this can last for several hours in the second (MeWo).

HAHN et al. (1968) compared the effect of a single dose of 6 Gy with that of two dose fractions of 3 Gy each, administered at an interval of 3 h, on the survival rate of Chinese hamster cells in exponential growth and in the plateau phase. Whereas cells in the exponential growth phase showed the typical recovery from sublethal radiation damage, this capacity was decreased with increased duration in the plateau phase. By

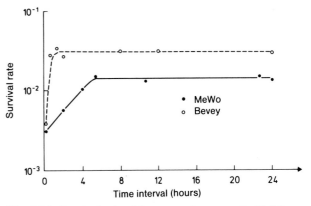

Fig. 1.14. Survival rate of human melanoma cells MeWo (●) and Bevey (○) after two 3.76 Gy irradiation doses, as a function of the time interval

contrast, HAHN and LITTLE (1972) also observed a distinct fractionation effect in plateau phase human liver cells. Apparently, considerable differences exist between individual types of cells. The contribution of repair to dose-rate effects was also observed with noncycling monolayer cultures of C_3H 10 $T_{1/2}$ cells irradiated with γ-rays at dose rates of 0.06 Gy/h to 55.8 Gy/h (BEDFORD 1987). A large reduction in effect per unit dose occurred when the dose rate was reduced to about 0.3 Gy/h, but no further reduction of cell killing was observed with lower dose rates. For lower dose rates (0.3 Gy/h and less) the dose–response curve is an exponential one and the slope is not significantly different from the "α-component" of survival curves after higher dose rates. These data also show that the D_q value is dependent on the dose rate. The D_q value apparently depends very much on the conditions of irradiation.

It is still not resolved which molecular processes are responsible for intracellular recovery from sublethal radiation damage. The very attractive view that repair of radiation-induced damage to DNA is of importance in relation to the recovery from sublethal radiation damage appears to be highly plausible. There are many indications for such a correlation, although the causality has not been proven up to now. Various inhibitors of DNA, RNA, and protein synthesis have been investigated with respect to their influence on the fractionation effect (ALPER 1979). Only actinomycin D, which in general inhibits the transcription of DNA but above all inhibits mRNA synthesis, decreases the recovery capacity of mammalian cells (ELKIND 1964). Investigations with inhibitors of energy metabolism have clearly shown that ATP is required for recovery (KIEFER 1971; JAIN and POHLIT 1973; REINHARDT and POHLIT 1976).

1.5.2 Recovery from Potentially Lethal Radiation Damage

A number of different factors, e.g., changes in the extracellular environment, can affect the survival rate of cells after irradiation. These phenomena were first reported by PHILLIPS and TOLMACH (1966). They found that when protein synthesis was inhibited with cycloheximide the survival rate of HeLa cells increased after irradiation. They suggested that this effect be considered as recovery from potentially lethal radiation damage. Apparently, some of the damage is repaired by the treatment after irradiation. Without such treatment this damage would have been lethal for the cells.

In contrast to recovery from sublethal radiation damage, this effect is studied by giving a single dose and measuring the modification of the survival rate induced by changes in the nutritional status of the cells after irradiation, without which these types of recovery process are not possible. All these subsequent treatments are associated with cessation of or a delay in cell cycle progression. Apparently the irradiated cell thus gains time to repair incurred damage to a greater extent.

As we have already mentioned, such repair phenomena are apparently no longer possible after cells have passed through mitosis. Thus, LITTLE (1970) showed that liver cells recovered from potentially lethal damage after irradiation when left in the same medium for 6–12 h, whereas recovery did not occur if the medium was changed after irradiation so that the cells were stimulated to proliferate again. Studies on the dose–response relationship revealed that, under these conditions, above all the D_0 was altered, not the extrapolation number n or the shoulder of the dose–response curve. Thus, the repair of sublethal radiation damage differs at least formally from that of potentially lethal damage.

Clearer experimental indications for such a distinction have arisen from studies on cell killing after irradiation and the effect of anisotonic culture media. RAAPHORST and DEWEY (1979) showed that hypertonic and hypotonic NaCl solutions can prevent recovery from potentially lethal radiation damage. Similar results were obtained

by UTSUMI and ELKIND (1979) from studies of cell death in Chinese hamster cells caused by x-rays. The survival rates after irradiation are strongly dependent on the osmolarity of the medium and temperature. It can be shown that the effects arise because of interference with the recovery from potentially lethal damage.

Both the rate and the extent of recovery decrease with fall in temperature. This is a clear indication that enzymatic processes are involved. Since hypo- and hypertonic solutions show this effect, it would appear that ion fluxes in the membranes are not a significant factor. By contrast, the recovery from sublethal radiation damage (dose fractionation experiments) is either not at all or only slightly affected by anisotonic solutions (UTSUMI and ELKIND 1979). Anisotonicity after irradiation apparently also leads to the expression of radiation damage which is normally repaired. The shoulder of the dose–response curve, however, is not affected. Thus, at least under the conditions in these studies, recovery from potentially lethal radiation damage appears to be independent of that from sublethal damage.

It is not yet clear which molecular processes are involved in recovery from potentially lethal damage. It has already been reported that the inhibitor of protein synthesis, cycloheximide, improves recovery, whereas inhibitors of DNA and RNA synthesis apparently have either no effect or an inhibitory effect on recovery (PHILLIPS and TOLMACH 1966; ELKIND et al. 1967; RAAPHORST and DEWEY 1979). More recent studies have indicated that cells from patients with ataxia telangiectasia as well as cells from those with xeroderma pigmentosum are unable to recover from potentially lethal damage after x- and UV irradiation, respectively (WEICHSELBAUM et al. 1978; SIMONS 1979). These results point to a correlation between the defective DNA repair processes and reduced cellular recovery from potentially lethal damage.

More recently CURTIS (1987) has developed the "lethal and potentially lethal" (LPL) lesion model. In this model it is assumed that two classes of radiation-induced molecular lesion occur: lethal and potentially lethal. The first type of lesion is not reparable. Such lesions lead directly to cell death and their extent is represented by the initial slope of the dose–response curve for cell killing. The second type of lesion can be repaired correctly by intracellular processes. However, these lesions can also interact with other molecular lesions to form a lethal lesion; CURTIS (1987) terms this "binary misrepair." Another possibility is "linear fixation." This process is assumed to occur by migration of the cell through a critical phase of the cell cycle, for instance mitosis. Linear fixation happens when repair has stopped and the remaining potentially lethal lesions become irreparable and, therefore, lethal.

The processes of "binary misrepair" enhance cell killing in the higher dose range. The dose dependence of these processes explains the shoulder of the dose–response curve for cell killing. If a longer time is available for repair, as in experiments with a low dose rate or experiments with dose fractionation, more potentially lethal lesions can be repaired. Thus, the interplay between the number of repaired lesions and binary misrepair of lesions can explain the modification of the shape of dose–response curves by changes in the time distribution of the radiation dose. The explanation by formation of sublethal damage and its accumulation appears unnecessary under these conditions. The linear–quadratic description of dose–response curves also can be understood by this model: The coefficients α and β depend on the cellular specific capacity of repair and on the available time for repair. The model can also explain why rapidly proliferating cells show a higher α/β ratio than slowly proliferating cells.

A similar model for cell killing by ionizing radiation has been proposed by WHEELER (1987). It is again assumed that the recovery from sublethal and partially lethal damage is correlated with the rate of repair and the metabolic state of the cells. WHEELER and his colleagues have measured the velocity of DNA repair and of recovery from partially lethal damage. They have calculated the half-times of these processes. It is suggested that at low radiation doses, when the number of repair complexes is higher than the number of DNA lesions, the rate of repair and of recovery increases with radiation dose and the half-time is constant. On the other hand at high radiation doses, when the number of repair complexes is lower than the number of DNA lesions (saturated conditions), the rate of repair and of recovery will be constant and the half-time for removal of the damage will increase with dose. These suggestions have been confirmed experimentally, but the experiments have had technical limitations; consequently more data are needed in order to prove the validity of these concepts.

On the basis of these and other considerations the above-mentioned linear–quadratic model is widely used for the interpretation of dose–response curves. The linear (α) component represents lethal events which cannot be repaired. These events determine the shape of the dose–response curve in the low dose range and after irradiation with low dose rates. The quadratic (β) component represents sublethal events which can be repaired in principle. In the high dose range with high dose rates interaction takes place between these events and the lesions become lethal. More and more damage therefore becomes irreparable, and the dose–response curve is determined by this component.

After high LET radiation the number of reparable lesions is reduced in relation to the irreparable damage. Therefore the α/β ratios are much higher after high LET radiation than after low LET radiation (HALL 1978; JUNG 1985). After exposures to high LET radiation fractionation or low dose rate exposures yield no or only little reduction of the biological effects in comparison to single-dose irradiation with high dose rates (STREFFER 1987).

1.5.3 Slow Repair

Apart from the recovery processes described up to now there is apparently another, very slow component. VAN DEN BRENK et al. (1974) and REINHOLD and BUISMAN (1975) have investigated the radiosensitivity of capillary endothelium. They stimulated the proliferation at various times after irradiation in this usually very slowly proliferating tissue. They observed recovery phenomena analogous to those of potentially lethal damage, but which were considerably slower. FIELD et al. (1976) have described two phases of recovery from sublethal damage in mouse lung by determining the difference $D_2 - D_1$. This increased with increasing interval between the two dose fractions. The course was biphasic and the second phase lasted about 100 times longer than the first. Apparently the slow recovery phase is not the result of cell proliferation (COULTAS et al. 1981).

1.5.4 Repopulation

Radiobiological studies have shown that cell proliferation initially decreases during protracted or continuous irradiation but can then return to normal and possibly even be enhanced. As mentioned previously, cell proliferation can play a role in tissue regeneration after a radiation insult. Oncologically orientated radiobiological studies have shown that the mean doubling times for lung metastases decrease from 53 to 12 days after irradiation (Malaise et al. 1972).

Tubiana (1973) calculated the number of clonogenic cells in a rhabdomyosarcoma during fractionated irradiation from the dose–response relationship obtained in vitro on the assumption that no cell proliferation occurred between the individual dose fractions. He then compared these values with those determined experimentally by Barendsen and Broerse (1970). It was shown that there was good agreement between the calculated and determined values during the first 2 weeks of radiation. During this time no proliferation had apparently taken place, which can be explained by division delay and cell death of proliferating cells. Subsequently, the experimentally determined value for surviving cells was clearly higher than the calculated value. This was apparently due to the fact that cell proliferation had again occurred and thus significantly more clonogenic cells were present in the tumor than was to be expected from the radiation dose. Such findings have also been observed with cells in culture when the interval between radiation fractions has been increased (Bedford 1987).

Similar findings have been obtained for proliferating normal tissues. In the skin, complete inhibition of mitotic activity was at first seen after fractionated irradiation, followed by a shortening of the cell cycle of surviving cells (Denekamp 1973). Withers and Elkind (1969) observed after irradiation a doubling time of 4–8 h in crypt cells in the small intestine of the mouse, after an initial division delay of 2.5 days. This rapid proliferation ceases when the number of crypt cells has reached normal values.

This compensatory cell proliferation is called repopulation. In this connection one must mention further processes, e.g., in hematopoiesis. The active bone marrow is widely distributed in the organism and hematopoietic stem cells are consequently located in all these regions. Following partial body irradiation, such stem cells can thus reach irradiated bone marrow regions from nonirradiated ones via the blood and again induce hematopoiesis through cell proliferation. Such processes will be described in more detail in the following sections.

The extent of repopulation varies greatly in tumors (Denekamp and Thomlinson 1971). In several normal tissues, such as skin and small intestine, repopulation is very high. These organs are very well able to compensate for a radiation insult from either protracted or continuous irradiation if the total dose is not too high. As in bone marrow, in skin this is due not only to the surviving cells in the irradiation zone but also to those in the unirradiated periphery. Why repopulation occurs has not been clarified up to now. Whether the surviving cells are able to recognize a reduction in the stem cell pool and thus induce enhanced proliferation or whether a reduction in differentiated cell compartments is the initiating factor is unresolved. In merely a few cell systems, such as the hematopoietic, has it been observed that stimulatory factors, e.g., glycoproteins, can enhance the proliferation of stem cells (Cairnie et al. 1976). On the other hand, the lung shows either only a slight or no tendency to repopulate (Coultas et al. 1981). The radiosensitivity of this organ is largely determined by intracellular recovery from radiation damage.

These examples show that the functional ability of an organ is restored or maintained through a compensatory proliferation (repopulation) on the one hand and by intracellular recovery processes on the other. The organs thus have two effective but fundamentally independent mechanisms at their disposal to compensate for radiation-induced damage. In order to estimate the risk of organic radiation damage, repopulation and intracellular recovery processes must be taken into consideration. The efficacy of these compensatory mechanisms is the reason why a severe loss of function only occurs after relatively high doses when fractionated irradiation is used (Table 1.1).

Experimentally, the amount of intracellular recovery can be distinguished from that of repopulation through differing intervals in fractionated irradiation and by changing the environmental conditions. With intervals shorter than 24 h, it is assumed that in the main, one observes intracellular recovery from radiation damage since this is completed within a few hours after irradiation. At intervals longer than 24 h, the dose required additionally to achieve the same effect as a single dose is considered to be that which "compensates" for the effect of repopulation. Under these conditions, the spared dose is a meas-

Table 1.1. Tolerance doses (TD) for various organs after conventional fractionated radiotherapy (Rubin and Casarett 1968)

Organ	Complications in 5 years	1%–5% TD$_{5/5}$ (Gy)	25%–50% TD$_{50/5}$ (Gy)	Volume/length
Skin	Ulcers, fibrosis	55	70	100 cm^3
Mouth mucous membrane	Ulcers, fibrosis	60	75	50 cm^3
Esophagus	Ulcers, constriction	60	75	75 cm^3
Stomach	Ulcers, perforation	45	50	100 cm^3
Small intestine	Ulcers, constriction	45	65	100 cm^3
Colon	Ulcers, constriction	45	65	100 cm^3
Rectum	Ulcers, constriction	55	80	100 cm^3
Pancreas	Xerostomia	50	70	50 cm^3
Liver	Liver failure, ascites	35	45	Whole
Kidney	Nephrosclerosis	23	28	Whole
Bladder	Ulcers, contraction	60	80	Whole
Ureter	Constriction, block	75	100	5–10 cm
Vagina	Ulcers, fistulas	90	<100	5 cm
Breast, adult	Atrophic necrosis	<50	<100	Whole
Lung	Pneumonitis, fibrosis	40	60	1 lung lobe
Capillaries	Telangiectasias, sclerosis	50–60	70–100	
Bone, adult	Necrosis, fracture	60	150	10 cm^3
Cartilage, adult	Necrosis	60	100	Whole
CNS (brain)	Necrosis	<50	<60	Whole
Spinal cord	Necrosis, paralysis	<50	<60	5 cm^3
Cornea	Keratitis	50	<60	Whole
Lens	Cataract	5	12	Whole
Bone marrow	Hypoplasia	20	40–50	localized
Lymph nodes	Atrophy	35–45	<70	–
Lymphatic organs	Sclerosis	50	<80	–

TD$_{5/5}$ is that dose leading to 5% damage after 5 years and the TD$_{50/5}$ is that dose leading to 50% damage after 5 years.

ure of repopulation. For skin the dose is between 0.3 and 0.9 Gy (Denekamp et al. 1969; Fowler et al. 1974; see also Trott and Kummermehr, this volume, Chap. 2).

The phenomenon of repopulation described up to now applies to rapidly proliferating tissue or to situations where cell proliferation can be stimulated within short periods. No such rapidly ensuing proliferation is known to occur in very slowly proliferating tissues such as liver or kidney. It is assumed that very slow repair takes place in these tissues in order to compensate for radiation damage (Denekamp 1973; Field and Hornsey 1977). This repair mechanism can be determined by extending the time interval between two doses from, for example, 5 to 55 days (Field et al. 1976).

1.5.5 Dose-Rate Effects

Given the findings described for recovery processes, it is understandable that the dose rate with which a dose of radiation is applied is of great importance for the extent of the biological effect. In general it can be stated that with decreasing dose rate the biological effect generally becomes smaller for the same dose. Fig. 1.15 shows the survival in mice that have received an identical radiation dose at different dose rates. Two completely different processes, discussed previously,

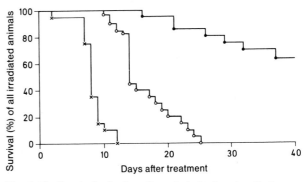

Fig. 1.15. Survival of mice after whole-body x-irradiation at various dose rates: x, 1 Gy/min; ○, 0.33 Gy/min; ●, 0.1 Gy/min. Dose: 7.61 Gy. (unpublished results)

are often responsible for the dose-rate effect: (a) intracellular recovery and (b) repopulation, which arises as a result of cell divisions during protracted irradiation.

It has been mentioned previously that the irradiated cells are able to repair sublethal damage after each single fraction of fractionated irradiation. If the dose–response relationship is determined, a dose–response curve with a shoulder for each dose fraction is then obtained. Ideally, a considerably flatter dose–response curve is obtained no longer containing a shoulder when the dose rate is reduced. Continuous irradiation at a lower dose rate can be thought of as a radiation exposure with an infinite number of small dose fractions. These situations have been described above.

LAJTHA and OLIVER (1961) have developed such model concepts. Their adopted survival curve for mammalian cells takes on a much flatter course and has no shoulder. These model concepts are in good agreement with the experimentally determined dose–response curves at low dose rates. Under these conditions, recovery from sublethal radiation damage occurs even during radiation exposure. If the dose rate is continually further reduced, then a point is reached at which all sublethal damage is repaired. A further lowering of the dose rate then results in no additional effect. The dose–response curve for cell killing is then determined by the linear term, while the β value becomes zero (BEDFORD 1987). In tissues with very rapidly dividing cells, proliferation may occur even during irradiation if the exposure time is long enough in comparison with that of the cell cycle. A further reduction in the biological radiation effect can occur because of this cellular progression during irradiation.

Various investigations have dealt with the effect of dose rate on cell killing or damage to organs (HALL 1972; BEDFORD and MITCHELL 1973; FU et al. 1975). At a low enough dose rate a situation can be reached where the radiation-induced cell killing or cell loss is in equilibrium with new cell formation during the period of irradiation. No radiation effect is then observed in the organ or cell system involved. The dose rate at which cell killing first exceeds new cell formation is referred to as the critical dose rate. The critical value in this sense is very organ specific.

Of all the different organs the testes are representative of one extreme: 0.02 Gy per day still

has no effect on spermiogenesis whereas a slight increase in the dose rate results in a considerable loss of cells (BROWN et al. 1964). The small intestine represents the other extreme: 4 Gy per day is the critical value (HALL 1978). This is associated with the high proliferative and recovery capacity of the crypts in the small intestine. Overall it can be stated that cells whose dose–response relationship shows a small shoulder and thus a low intracellular recovery capacity will also react sensitively to irradiation at a low dose rate. Among others, the stem cells of the hematopoietic system fall into this category.

A further aspect to be discussed is the dependence of this effect on the length of the cell cycle. As already mentioned, radiation exposure can lead to a prolongation of the cell cycle, on the one hand because of the G_2 block and on the other because an extended S phase can occur. The cells proliferate normally up to a critical dose rate. If the dose rate is increased then a point is reached at which division delay is greatly enhanced. The cell cycle becomes considerably longer. In turn, however, the dose per cell cycle also increases and cell division is finally totally inhibited so that the cell population is reduced. Thus, it has been discussed whether it may not be more meaningful to express the dose rate as dose per cell cycle duration rather than as dose per hour or minute.

HeLa cells have a cycle duration of 24 h. The critical dose at which cell divisions are inhibited is about 0.3 Gy/h (HALL 1972). Chinese hamster cells have a cycle duration of 11 h. In this case the critical dose is about 0.9 Gy/h. Intestinal crypt cells have a cycle lasting 10 h; their critical dose is about 0.8 Gy/h. In general, the critical dose per cell cycle duration is thus about 7–10 Gy. On the other hand it was observed that a similar dose (ca. 10 Gy) is necessary to achieve a division delay equivalent to the cell cycle time following irradiation with a high dose rate (DENEKAMP 1975). This conformity shows that the term "dose per cell cycle" apparently dose more justice to the biological facts with respect to the effects of radiation.

1.6 The Oxygen Effect

Molecular oxygen is an agent particularly well-known to modify the effects of radiation. When biological objects are irradiated with loosely ionizing radiation in the absence of oxygen, the effect is considerably smaller than for the same exposure in the presence of oxygen (HOLTHUSEN 1921). This phenomenon is generally described as the oxygen effect.

When the cell survival rates are determined from dose–response curves under anoxic or oxic conditions it is generally seen that the exponential part of the dose–response relationship is less steep under anoxia than with irradiation in the presence of oxygen, i.e., the D_0 is greater under anoxic conditions (ALPER 1979). The extrapolation number n of the dose–response relationship is altered to a lesser degree (ELKIND and WHITMORE 1967). However, LITTBRAND and REVESZ (1969) have also observed the complete disappearance of the shoulder in the dose–response curve under extremely low partial oxygen tensions.

This modification of the radiation effect by oxygen is apparently not due to its participation in metabolism. Instead, radiochemical processes are of importance. ALPER and HOWARD-FLANDERS (1956) have shown empirically that the radiosensitivity of living cells in dependence on the partial oxygen tension is expressed by the equation

$$\frac{S_p}{S_N} = \frac{m\,P + K}{P + K} = r \tag{1.6}$$

where S_N and S_p represent the radiosensitivity at partial oxygen tensions 0 or P; m and K are constants.

The relationship between S_p/S_N and the partial oxygen tension is shown in Fig. 1.16. At higher partial oxygen tensions the hyperbolic function converges towards a maximum saturation value for the oxygen effect, reaching a value m. This value is referred to as the oxygen enhancement

ratio (OER). Typical values for mammalian cells lie in the range 2.0–3.0, when these are exposed to loosely ionizing radiation. When the partial oxygen tension reaches the value K, the ratio S_p/S_N is equal to (m + 1)/2 (Fig. 1.16).

The above equation and its theoretical derivation as well as the question of its validity have been discussed by several authors, in particular by ALPER (1979).

In their review CULLEN and LANSLEY (1974) have checked the experimental results and the applicability of the equation. Most experimental data confirm the validity of the equation; this is particularly true for bacteria, but also for mammalian cells. K values of about 3.5 µM oxygen for mammalian cells, for chromosomal aberrations in Ehrlich ascites cells, and up to 12.5 µM for cell killing of HeLa cells have been reported (MOORE et al. 1972).

MILLAR et al. (1979) have investigated the radiosensitizing oxygen effect on the slope of the dose–response curve (D_0) for the survival rate of Chinese hamster cells as a function of the partial oxygen tension. At an O_2 concentration of 0.4–1.5 µM radiosensitization increases steadily and a plateau is reached in the range 1.5–7.0 µM (ca. 1%–5% O_2). Subsequently, with increasing O_2 concentrations, the oxygen effect again increases until a new plateau is obtained at high O_2 concentrations (28 µM = 20% and more). From such a biphasic course, it would follow that either two different target areas are involved in cell killing or that there are two mechanisms of cell killing, of which each single event has its own dependence on the partial oxygen tension.

With respect to the mechanism of radiation-induced cell killing it is interesting that the maximum number of DNA single strand breaks is

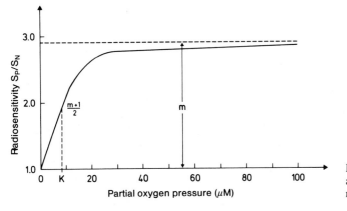

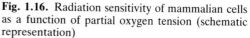

Fig. 1.16. Radiation sensitivity of mammalian cells as a function of partial oxygen tension (schematic representation)

reached at a lower partial oxygen tension than the maximum oxygen sensitization for cell killing (Adams et al. 1975).

The sensitization effect of oxygen only occurs when oxygen is present during or shortly after irradiation. Various techniques have been developed for investigating the tissue dependence of this effect (Alper 1979; Kiefer 1981). Michael et al. (1978) observed that radiation-induced radicals react very rapidly with oxygen and that the kinetics can be described by two exponential functions. After irradiating bacteria the half-lives were 0.4 and 4 ms. Similar studies have been undertaken for the kinetics of sensitization through oxygen in mammalian cells (Watts et al. 1978). Basically the same results have been obtained.

Using mammalian cells, Watts et al. (1978) found that the full OER was obtained when oxygen was present for 2 ms or more in the cell suspension prior to irradiation. When oxygen was added to the suspension after irradiation, the interval between irradiation and addition had to be less than 6–10 ms for oxygen sensitization to be observed. From this it can be concluded that the radicals reacting with oxygen must have a half-life of a few milliseconds.

These data support the theory that highly reactive free radicals induced by radiation are capable of reacting with oxygen and possibly form organic peroxides (Alper 1979). The role of unsaturated fatty acids has already been mentioned. Likewise, it has been reported that superoxide dismutase (SOD) can modify the radiosensitivity of cells. These findings indicate that superoxide radicals may be of great significance in such processes.

The oxygen effect plays a particular role in the radiotherapy of tumors (Suit 1973; Streffer 1980). The length of the diffusion pathway for oxygen in a tissue is about 150 μm from the oxygen supplying capillary. Cells lying beyond this range receive either only a poor supply of oxygen or no oxygen at all. Thus, so-called hypoxic cells will be found in tumors and must be assumed to be highly radioresistant (Thomlinson and Gray 1955). The possible consequences for tumor therapy will not be discussed here. The reader is referred to relevant reviews (Suit 1974; Streffer 1980).

From the discussion on the oxygen effect in dependence on the partial oxygen tension it emerges that the sensitizing effect reaches a saturation level. This occurs at a partial oxygen tension greater than 20–40 mmHg. The partial oxygen tension is usually not below this level in normal mammalian tissues. It can thus be assumed that maximum sensitization through oxygen is generally achieved in normal tissues.

1.7 Aspects of the Mechanism of Cell Killing

In the era of molecular biology it is pertinent to ask which molecular changes finally lead to cell death. Where are the molecules to be sought, the damage to which induces these processes? In this discussion, cell killing should be understood in terms of reproductive cell death. The irradiated cell itself and generally also daughter cells are usually able to complete mitoses but further cell divisions are no longer possible.

Surviving cells are those that retain their full reproductive capacity. In order to ensure this, the integrity of the genome must be maintained. Mutations giving rise to surviving cells are rare events. Under these preconditions, it is obvious that the genome and, in particular, the DNA with its possible radiation damage must be considered to play key roles. This is underlined by experimental data showing that irradiation of the cell nucleus is considerably more effective in cell killing than exposure of the cytoplasm to the same dose (Feinendegen 1979). Thus, tritium which is concentrated in the nucleus by the incorporation of ^{3}H-thymidine into DNA, is much more efficient than tritium in the form of tritiated water, which is distributed homogeneously over the entire cell (Streffer et al. 1977).

However, the question arises: Is the genome with its DNA the only sensitive region or are there other molecules whose radiation damage contributes to reproductive cell death? Cellular membrane systems and, in the case of mammalian cells, above all the nuclear membrane have frequently been mentioned in this connection (Alper 1979; Szumiel 1981). Studies on bacteria have shown that fatty acid composition and membrane fluidity have a marked effect on radiosensitivity (Yatvin 1976; Redpath and Patterson 1978). It has also been observed in mammalian cells that membranes are relatively sensitive to ionizing radiation when, for example, the peroxidation of lipids occurs, which can be reduced by vitamin E (Konings and Drijver 1979; Konings et al. 1979). A causal relationship between such radiation-induced changes and cell death has not been proven up to now.

ALPER (1979) assumed that nuclear membrane–DNA complexes and their radiation damage are of importance in eukaryotic cells. Experimental proof for such an assumption, as attractive as it may seem, is still awaited. WARTERS et al. (1977) compared the effects of ^{125}I selectively built into the DNA as ^{125}I-iododeoxyuridine or into membranes as ^{125}I-labeled concanavalin. The survival rate of cells was considerably more impaired by DNA-bound ^{125}I. All these results indicate that only radiation-induced damage to the DNA or chromatin is directly associated with cell death. However, it cannot be ruled out that damage to other molecules is involved. It has already been pointed out that sulfhydryl groups and, in particular, glutathione may be of importance (GUICHARD et al. 1983). Nevertheless, overall the experimental results have shown that a correlation between the sulfhydryl group content and radiosensitivity exists in only a few cases. (SZUMIEL 1981).

Even though there are many indications that the damage to the DNA is causally related to cell death, it has still not been ascertained which specific molecular changes are of significance. The idea that each DNA double strand break is representative of a lethal event (CHADWICK and Leenhouts 1981) has proved incorrect: various groups have shown that mammalian cells are capable of repairing double strand breaks (LANGE 1975; FRIEDBERG and HANAWALT 1988). Studies on mammalian cells in vitro have shown that a correlation apparently exists in a number of cell lines between the repair of radiation damage in the DNA and radiosensitivity with respect to cell killing.

Such a correlation is particularly evident in cell lines from patients with defective DNA repair, such as those with ataxia telangiectasia and Fanconi's anemia (HANAWALT et al. 1979). In other cells it has also been observed that repair of DNA strand breaks in radiosensitive cells is less efficient than in more resistant ones (KÖRNER et al. 1977). Such data, however, are not of a universal nature and there have been reports of cases where this correlation does not hold (CARR and FOX 1978). In all these studies only some aspects of DNA repair have been measured. DNA repair, however, is so multifaceted that measurement of all aspects is fraught with difficulties. More recent analyses of dose–response curves for cell survival have shown that radiosensitivities of tumor cells can vary considerably although the β-component of the mathematical model for cell killing is not very different (STEEL and PEACOCK 1989). Under such conditions the α-component becomes much more important, and this is especially so in the low dose range and with low dose rate irradiation.

Various authors have discussed the significance for radiosensitivity of the amount of DNA per cell but without reaching a satisfactory conclusion (STREFFER 1969; KIEFER 1981). By taking the chromosome volume into account, it has been shown that the volume of interphase chromosomes is inversely proportional to radiosensitivity in higher plants, amphibians, and insects but that no correlation exists for mammalian cells (UNDERBRINK and POND 1976). In mammalian cells there is apparently no relation between the degree of ploidy and radiosensitivity (SZUMIEL 1981). This observation is of considerable significance for tumor therapy since tetraploid tumor cell lines have not shown themselves to be more radiosensitive than diploid ones.

PHILBRICK and BURKI (cited in SZUMIEL 1981) investigated 34 cell lines with different numbers of chromosomes. These cells were obtained by cell fusion, among other techniques. The cells used were Chinese hamster and mouse lymphoma cells. With increased ratios of chromosome numbers to cell volume the radiosensitivity is enhanced. The more compact the chromatin, the higher are the rates of cell kill for the same radiation dose, yet even this interesting finding does not seem to be a general phenomenon. Thus, it has been observed that radiosensitivity is greater at the one-cell than the two-cell embryonic stage in the mouse, although the ratio of chromosome number to cell volume is smaller at the two-cell stage. (MOLLS et al. 1982).

Overall, however, it appears that the organization of the chromatin has a greater significance than used to be assumed. In this respect the finding of YAMADA et al. (1981) is of interest i.e., that following irradiation of thymocytes such DNA fragments appear as to suggest that their origin is primarily due to radiation-induced breakage of the DNA between the nucleosomes. This discussion leads to the problem of whether the manifest DNA damage is indeed merely stochastically distributed over the complete cell genome or whether specific sensitive sites in the DNA are favored. There is also good evidence that the repair of DNA lesions is nonrandomly distributed.

The repair of DNA damage in transcribing genes is much faster than in nontranscribing DNA regions (BOHR et al. 1987; FRIEDBERG and HANAWALT 1988).

The biophysical models developed to describe dose–response curves (e.g., KELLERER and ROSSI 1978) are of value for elaborating concepts on the effects of radiation. However, they have the disadvantage that biological phenomena such as recovery processes, of both an intra- and an intercellular nature, recede into the background in these discussions. In fact from the extensive data available it appears indisputable that these processes are of great importance for the extent of radiation effects. Apparently, the shoulder in dose–response relationships is an expression of the intracellular recovery capacity when the cell survival rate is plotted logarithmically against radiation dose. The vast majority of radiation events can be repaired after small radiation exposures. With increasing radiation doses the reparable proportion is decreased until the maximum recovery capacity is exhausted. In this case a "saturation" of repair systems is attained (ALPER 1979). The dose–response curve then shows a straight line under the above-described mode of plotting. The linear portion contains a slope corresponding to a dose–response relationship for complete inhibition of repair.

A good correlation can be observed between reproductive cell death and the appearance of chromosomal aberrations, in particular those of acentric and dicentric types (HOPWOOD and TOLMACH 1979). Acentric chromosomal aberrations can give rise to so-called micronuclei after mitosis (COUNTRYMAN and HEDDLE 1976). MIDANDER and REVESZ (1980) reported good agreement between the D_0 values for the survival rate and the number of cells without a micronucleus. Further studies, however, showed that this is only the case in the dose range up to about 5 Gy x-rays (VAN BEUNINGEN et al. 1981), and good agreement is only achieved for loosely ionizing rays. Cells with a micronucleus must be considered "dead" cells according to the definition of reproductive cell death. They are indeed able to carry out several cell divisions, but this is no longer possible in the succeeding generations. On the other hand, not all "dead" cells have acentric chromosomal aberrations or micronuclei, so that there must be other lethal events in the genome that lead to cell death (VAN BEUNINGEN et al. 1981).

This chromosomal damage, however, is not only expressed in the first mitosis after irradiation; instead further chromosomal aberrations can arise in the subsequent mitoses (HOPWOOD and TOLMACH 1979) and additional micronuclei can occur during the interphases (MOLLS et al. 1981). Apparently the radiation damage in the DNA of the genome is propagated further through DNA replication in the cell cycles after irradiation, so that additional chromosomal breaks can be observed. These phenomena have been studied very systematically with preimplantation mouse embryos. When these embryos are irradiated in the one-cell stage, it is possible clearly to identify the number of mitoses which have occurred after radiation exposure. It has been observed that new chromosome aberrations are formed during the second and third cell cycle after irradiation and are manifest at the second as well as the third mitosis after radiation (WEISSENBORN and STREFFER 1988).

As described previously, repair of genome radiation damage takes place within hours of irradiation. Apparently, this must occur above all prior to the first mitosis after irradiation in order to be successful. However, if mitosis has occurred, then the unrepaired damage becomes manifest. In this sense, one can consider the mitotic delay, along with the G_2 block, to act as a certain protective mechanism. Release of the G_2 block, e.g., by caffeine, enhances the radiation damage. The number of chromosomal aberrations is thus lower in those cells formed relatively late after irradiation, through cell division (MOLLS et al. 1981), and correspondingly such cells show a higher rate of survival (MOLLS et al. 1982).

In general an interplay of many phenomena leads to cell death after radiation exposure. The induction of DNA damage and its reparability seem to be most important. Reparable lesions can be converted into irreparable ones, which will modify the degree of cell killing.

References

Adams GE, Michael BD, Asquith JC, Shenoy MA, Watts ME, Williams DW (1975) Rapid-mixing studies on the time scale of radiation damage in cells. In: Nygaard OF, Adler HJ, Sinclair WK (eds) Radiation research, biomedical chemical and physical perspectives. Academic, New York. p 478

Alper T (1979) Cellular radiobiology. Cambridge University Press, Cambridge

Alper T, Howard-Flanders P (1956) The role of oxygen in modifying the radiosensitivity of *E. coli*. Nature 178: 978–979

Altman KJ, Gerber GB, Okada S (1970) Radiation biochemistry. Academic, New York

Andreeff M (1975) Impulscytophotometrie. Springer, Berlin Heidelberg New York

Bacq ZM (1965) Chemical protection against ionizing radiation. Thomas, Springfeld, Ill

Barendsen GW (1962) Dose-survival curves of human cells in tissue culture irradiated with α-, β-, 20 kV x-, and 200 kV x-radiation. Nature 193: 1153–1155

Barendsen GW, Broerse JJ (1970) Experimental radiotherapy of a rat rhabdomyosarcoma with 15 MeV neutrons and 300 kV x-rays. Eur J Cancer 6: 89–109

Bauer KD, Dethlefsen LA (1981) Control of cellular proliferation in HeLa-S3 suspension cultures. Characterization of cultures utilizing acridine orange staining procedures. J Cell Physiol 108: 99–112

Bedford JS (1987) The influence of proliferative status on responses to fractionated and low dose-rate irradiation. In: Fielden EM, Fowler FJ, Hendry JH, Scott D (eds) Radiation Research. Taylor & Francis, London, pp 461–467

Bedford JS, Mitchell JB (1973) Dose-rate effects in synchronous mammalian cells in culture. Radiat Res 54: 316–327

Bergonié J, Tribondeau L (1906) Une interpretation de quelques resultats de la radiothérapie et essai de fixation d'une technique rationelle. C R Acad Sci [D] (Paris) 143: 983–985

Berry RJ, Hall EJ, Cavanagh J (1970) Radiosensitivity and the oxygen effect for mammalian cells cultured in vitro in stationary phase. Br J Radiol 43: 81–90

Betz EH (1974) Morphologische Veränderungen des lymphatischen Systems nach Bestrahlung. In: Kärcher KH, Streffer C (eds) Die Strahlenwirkung auf das Lymphosystem. Springer, Berlin Heidelberg New York, p 29

Biaglow JE, Varnes ME, Clark EP, Epp ER (1987) Role of glutathione and other thiols in cellular response to radiation and drugs. In: Fielden EM, Fowler JF, Hendry JH, Scott D (eds) Radiation research. Taylor & Francis, London, pp 677–682

Bohr VA, Philips DH, Hanawalt PC (1987) Heterogeneous DNA damage and repair in the mammalian genome. Cancer Res 47: 6426–6436

Bond VP, Fliedner TM, Archambeau JO (1965) Mammalian radiation lethality: a disturbance in cellular kinetics. Academic, New York

Booz J, Feinendegen LE (1987) Application of microdosimetry. In: Fielden EM, Fowler FJ, Henry JH, Scott D (eds) Radiation research. Taylor & Francis, London, pp 331–337

Braun H (1965) Beiträge zur Histologie und Zytologie des bestrahlten Thymus. III. Mitteilung: Die Wirkung subletaler Dosen. Strahlentherapie 126: 236–246

Braun H (1967) Beiträge zur Histologie und Zytologie des bestrahlten Thymus. Strahlentherapie 133: 411–421

Brown SO, Krise GM, Pace HB, de Boer J (1964) Effect of continuous radiation on reproduction capacity and fertility of the albino rat and mouse. In: Carlson WD, Gasner FX (eds) Effects of ionizing radiation on the reproductive system. Pergamon, New York, p 1101

Cairnie AB, Lala PK, Osmond DG (1976) Stem cells of renewing cell populations. Academic, New York

Carr FJ, Fox BW (1978) Flow cytofluorimetric examination of changes in mammalian cell DNA denatured in situ following irradiation. Int J Radiat Biol 34: 549

Casarett GW (1964) Similarities and contrasts between radiation and time pathology. Adv Gerontol Res 1: 109–163

Chadwick KH, Leenhouts HP (1973) A molecular theory of cell survival. Phys Med Biol 18: 78–87

Chadwick KH, Leenhouts HP (1981) The molecular theory of radiation biology. Springer, Berlin Heidelberg New York

Chapman JD, Gillespie CJ (1981) Radiation-induced events and their time scale in mammalian cells. In: Lett JT, Adler H (eds) Advances in radiation biology, vol 9. Academic, New York, p 143

Chapman JD, Gillespie CJ, Reuvers AP, Dugle DL (1975) The inactivation of Chinese hamster cells by x-rays: the effects of chemical modifiers on single and double events. Radiat Res 64: 365–375

Coultas PG, Ahier RG, Field SB (1981) Effect of neutron and x-irradiation on cell proliferation in mouse lung. Radiat Res: 516–528

Countryman PJ, Heddle JA (1976) The production of micronuclei from chromosome aberrations in irradiated cultures of human lymphocytes. Mutat Res 41: 321–332

Cullen BM, Lansley I (1974) The effect of pre-irradiation growth conditions on the relative radiosensitivities of mammalian cells at low oxygen concentration. Int J Radiat Biol 26: 579–588

Curtis SB (1987) The cellular consequences of binary misrepair and linear fixation of initial biophysical damage. In: Fielden EM, Fowler FJ, Hendry JH, Scott D (eds) Radiation research. Taylor & Francis, London, pp 312–317

Debenham PG, Thacker J (1987) The luinian genetic disorder Ataxia-telangiectasia (A-T): New insights into the basis of radiosensitivity. In: Fielden EM, Fowler JF, Hendry JH, Scott D (eds) Radiation Research. Taylor & Francis, London, pp 437–442

Denekamp J (1973) Changes in the rate of repopulation during multifraction irradiation of mouse skin. Br J Radiol 46: 381–387

Denekamp J (1975) Changes in the rate of proliferation in normal tissues after irradiation. In: Nygaard OF, Adler HI, Sinclair WK (eds) Radiation research. Academic, New York, p 810

Denekamp J, Thomlinson RH (1971) The cell proliferation kinetics of four experimental tumours after acute x-irradiation. Cancer Res 31: 1279–1284

Denekamp J, Ball MM, Fowler JE (1969) Recovery and repopulation in mouse skin as a function of time after x-irradiation. Radiat Res 37: 361–370

Dertinger H, Hülser D (1981) Increased radioresistance of cells in cultured multicell spheroids. I. Dependence on cellular interaction. Radiat Environ Biophys 19: 101–107

Dertinger H, Jung H (1969) Molekulare Strahlenbiologie. Heidelberger Taschenbücher vol 57/58. Springer, Berlin Heidelberg New York

Dikomey E, Franzke J (1986) Three classes of DNA strand breaks induced by x-irradiation and internal β-rays. Int J Radiat Biol 50: 893–908

Dittrich W, Göhde W (1969) Impulsfluorometrie bei Einzelzellen in Suspension. Z Naturforsch [B] 24: 360–361

Djordjevic B, Tolmach LJ (1967) Responses of synchronous populations of HeLa cells to ultraviolet irradiation at selected stages of the generation cycle. Radiat Res 32: 327–346

Dugle DL, Gillespie CJ, Chapman JD (1976) DNA strand breaks, repair, and survival in x-irradiated mammalian cells. Proc Natl Acad Sci USA 73: 809–812

Durand RE, Sutherland RM (1972) Effects of intercellular contact on repair of radiation damage. Exp Cell Res 71: 75–80

Dutreix J, Wambersie A, Bounik C (1973) Cellular recovery in human skin reactions: application to dose fraction number overall time relationship in radiotherapy. Eur J Cancer 9: 159–167

Eldjarn L, Pihl A (1960) Mechanism of protective and sensitizing action. In: Errera M, Forssberg A (eds) Mechanisms in radiobiology, vol II. Academic, New York, p 231

Elkind MM, Sutton H (1960) Radiation response of mammalian cells grown in culture. I. Repair of x-ray damage in surviving Chinese hamster cells. Radiat Res 13: 556–593

Elkind MM, Whitmore GF (1967) The radiobiology of cultured mammalian cells. Gordon and Breach, New York

Elkind MM, Whitmore GF, Alescio T (1964) Actinomycin D: suppression of recovery in x-irradiated mammalian cells. Science 143: 1454–1457

Elkind MM, Sutton-Gilbert H, Moses WB, Alescio T, Swain RW (1965) Radiation response of mammalian cells grown in culture. V. Temperature dependence of the repair of x-ray damage in surviving cells (aerobic and hypoxic). Radiat Res 25: 359–376

Elkind MM, Sutton-Gilbert H, Moses WB, Kamper C (1967) Sublethal and lethal radiation damage. Nature 214: 1088–1092

Feinendegen LE (1979) Radiation problems in fusion energy production. In: Okada S, Imamura M, Terashima T, Yamaguchi Y (eds) Radiation research. Toppan, Tokyo, p 32

Field SB, Hornsey S (1974) Damage to mouse lung with neutron and X-rays. Eur J Cancer 10: 621–627

Field SB, Hornsey S (1977) Repair in normal tissues and the possible relevance to radiotherapy. Strahlentherapie 153: 371–379

Field SB, Hornsey S, Kutsutani Y (1976) Effects of fractionated irradiation on mouse lung and a phenomenon of slow repair. Br J Radiol 49: 700–707

Fonck K, Konings AWT (1978) The effect of vitamin E on cellular survival after X irradiation of lymphoma cells. Br J Radiol 51: 832–833

Fowler JF, Denekamp J, Delapeyre C, Harris SR, Skeldon PW (1974) Skin reactions in mice after multifraction x-irradiation. Int J Radiat Biol 25: 213–223

Friedberg EC, Hanawalt PC (1988) Mechanisms and consequences of DNA damage processing. Alan R. Liss, New York

Fu K, Phillips TL, Kane LJ, Smith V (1975) Tumor and normal tissue response to irradiation in vivo: variation with decreasing dose rates. Radiology 114: 709–716

Generoso WM, Shelby MD, de Serres FJ (1980) DNA repair and mutagenesis in eukaryotes. Plenum, New York

Goodhead DT (1971) Inactivation and mutation of cultured mammalian cells by aluminium characteristic ultra soft X-rays. III. Implications of the theory of dual radiation action. Int J Radiat Biol 32: 43–70

Goodhead DT (1979) Models of radiation inactivation and mutagenesis. In: Meyn RE, Withers HR (eds) Radiation biology in cancer research. Raven, New York, p 231

Goodhead DT, Brenner DJ (1983) Estimation of a single property of low LET radiations which correlates with biological effectiveness. Phys Med Biol 28: 485–492

Guichard M, Jensen G, Meister A, Malaise EP (1983) Depletion of glutathione synthesis by buthionine sulfoximine decreases the oxygen enhancement ratio of V79 cells. Radiat Res 94: 613

Hahn GM, Little JB (1972) Plateau phase cultures of mammalian cells. Curr Top Radiat Res 8: 39–83

Hahn GM, Stewart JR, Yang S-J, Parker V (1968) Chinese hamster cell monolayer cultures. I. Changes in cell dynamics and modifications of the cell cycle with the period of growth. Exp Cell Res 49: 285–292

Hall EJ (1972) Radiation dose-rate: a factor of importance in radiobiology and radiotherapy. Br J Radiol 45: 81–97

Hall EJ (1978) Radiobiology for the radiologist. Harper and Row, Hagerstown, Md

Han A, Elkind MM (1977) Additive action of ionizing and non-ionizing radiations throughout the Chinese hamster cell-cycle. Int J Radiat Biol 31: 275–282

Han A, Sinclair WK, Kimbler BE (1976) The effect of N-ethylmaleimide on the response to x-rays of synchronized HeLa cells. Radiat Res 65: 337–350

Hanawalt PC, Cooper PK, Ganesau AK, Smith CA (1979) DNA repair in bacteria and mammalian cells. Ann Rev Biochem 48: 783

Heineke H (1904) Über die Einwirkung der Röntgenstrahlen auf innere Organe. Muench Med Wochenschr 51: 785

Hesslewood JP (1978) DNA strand breaks in resistant and sensitive murine lymphoma cells detected by the hydroxylapatite chromatographic technique. Int J Radiat Biol 34: 461–469

Hidvegi EJ, Holland J, Streffer C, van Beuningen D (1978) Biochemical phenomena in ionizing irradiation of cells. In: Busch H (ed) Methods in cancer research, vol 25. Academic, New York, p 187

Holthusen H (1921) Beiträge zur Biologie der Strahlenwirkung. Untersuchungen an Askarideneiern. Pflugers Arch Ges Physiol 187: 1–24

Hopwood LE, Tolmach LJ (1979) Manifestation of damage from ionizing radiation in mammalian cells in the post-irradiation generations. In: Lett JT, Adler H (eds) Advances in radiation biology, vol 8. Academic, New York, p 317

Hornsey S (1972) The radiation response of human malignant melanoma cells in vitro and in vivo. Cancer Res 32: 650–651

Hornsey S (1973) The radiosensitivity of the intestine. In: Braun H, Henck F, Ladner H-A, Messerschmidt O, Musshoff K, Streffer C (eds) Strahlenempfindlichkeit von Organen und Organsystemen der Säugetiere und des Menschen. Thieme, Stuttgart, p 78

Howard A, Pelc SR (1953) Synthesis of DNA in normal and irradiated cells and its relation to chromosome breakage. Heredity 6: 261–273

Isaacs JT, Binkley F (1977) Cyclic-AMP-dependent control of the rat hepatic glutathione disulfdesulfhydryl ratio. Biochim Biophys Acta 498: 29–38

Jain VK, Pohlit W (1973) Influence of energy metabolism on the repair of x-ray damage in living cells. II. Split dose recovery, liquid holding reactivation and division delay reversal in stationary populations of yeast. Biophysik 9: 155–165

Jung H (1978) Eine einfache Anordnung zum Auszählen von Zellkolonien. Leitz-Mitt Wiss und Techn 4 (4): 102–103

Jung H (1985) Biologische Wirkungen dicht ionisierender Strahlen. In: Scherer E, Heuck F (eds) Strahlengefährdung und Strahlenschutz. Springer, Berlin Heidelberg New York (Handbuch der medizinischen Radiologie, vol XX, p 41)

Jüngling O, Langendorff H (1932) Über die Wirkung zeitlich verteilter Dosen auf den Kernteilungsablauf von *Vicia faba*. Strahlentherapie 44: 771–782

Kellerer AM, Rossi HH (1972) The theory of dual radiation action. Curr Top Radiat Res 8: 85–158

Kellerer AM, Rossi HH (1978) A generalized formulation of dual radiation action. Radiat Res 75: 471–488

Kiefer J (1971) The importance of cellular energy metabolism for sparing effect at dose fractionation with electrons and ultra-violet light. Int J Radiat Biol 20: 325–336

Kiefer J (1981) Biologische Strahlenwirkung. Springer, Berlin Heidelberg New York

Konings AWT, Drijver EB (1979) Radiation effects on membranes. I. Vitamin E deficiency and lipid peroxidation. Radiat Res 80: 494–501

Konings AWT, Damen J, Trieling WB (1979) Protection of liposomal lipids against radiation induced oxidative damage. Int J Radiat Biol 35: 343–350

Körner I, Walicka M, Malz W, Beer JZ (1977) DNA repair in two L5178 Y cell lines with different x-ray sensitivities. Stud Biophys 61: 141–149

Krönig S, Friedrich W (1918) Physikalische und biologische Grundlagen der Strahlentherapie. Sonderband Strahlentherapie. Urban & Schwarzenberg, München

Lajtha LG, Oliver R (1961) Some radiobiological considerations in radiotherapy. Br J Radiol 34: 252–257

Lange CS (1975) The repair of DNA double-strand breaks in mammalian cells and the organization of the DNA in their chromosomes. Basic Life Sci 5B: 677–683

Langendorff H, Langendorff M (1973) Weitere Untersuchungen über die Beziehungen der Strahlenempfindlichkeit eines höheren Organismus zum Adenylat-Cyclase-System seiner Zellen. Strahlentherapie 146: 436–443

Leuthauser SWC, Oberley LW (1978) Modification of radiation response of a solid tumor by superoxide dismutase. Radiat Res 74: 541–542

Littbrand B, Revesz L (1969) The effect of oxygen on cellular survival and recovery after irradiation. Br J Radiol 42: 914–924

Little JB (1970) Irradiation of primary human amnion cell culture: effects on DNA-synthesis and progression through the cell cycle. Radiat Res 44; 674–699

Little JB (1971) Repair of potentially lethal radiation damage in mammalian cells: enhancement by conditioned medium from stationary cultures. Int J Radiat Biol 20: 87–92

Lohka MJ (1989) Mitotic control by metaphase-promoting factor and cdc proteins. J Cell Science 92: 131–135

Madoc-Jones H (1964) Variations in radiosensitivity of a mammalian cell line with phase of growth cycle. Nature 203: 983–984

Malaise EP, Charbit A, Chavaudra N, Combes PF, Douchez J, Tubiana M (1972) Change in volume of irradiated human metastasis. Investigation of repair of sublethal damage and tumour repopulation. Br J Cancer 26: 43–52

McNally NJ (1982) Cell survival. In: Pizzarello DJ (ed) Radiation biology. CRC Press, Boca Raton, Fl, p 27

McNally NJ, de Ronde J (1976) The effect of repeated small doses of radiation on recovery from sublethal damage by Chinese hamster cells irradiation in the plateau phase of growth. Int J Radiat Biol 29: 221–234

Melching H-J, Streffer C (1966) Zur Beeinflussung der Strahlenempfindlichkeit von Säugetieren durch chemische Substanzen. In: Jucker E (ed) Fortschritte der Arznei-mittelforschung, vol 9. Birkhäuser, Basel, p 11

Michael BD (1987) Molecular and cellular aspects of the role of thiols in radiation response. In: Fielden EM, Fowler JF, Hendry JH, Scott D (eds) Radiation research. Taylor & Francis, London, pp 672–676

Michael BD, Harrop HA, Maughan RL, Patel KB (1978) A fast kinetics study of the modes of action of some different radiosensitizers in bacteria. Br J Cancer [Suppl 3] 37: 29–33

Midander J, Revesz L (1980) The micronucleus (MN) in irradiated cells as a measure of survival. Br J Cancer 41: 204

Millar BC, Fielden EM, Steele JJ (1979) A biphasic radiation survival response of mammalian cells to molecular oxygen. Int J Radiat Biol 36: 177–180

Mitznegg P, Heim F, Hach B, Säbel M (1971) The effect of ageing, caffeine treatment, and ionizing radiation on nucleic acid synthesis in the mouse liver. Life Sci Part II 10: 1281–1292

Mönig H, Messerschmidt O, Streffer C (1989) Chemical radioprotection in mammals and in man. In: Scherer E, Streffer C, Trott K-R (eds) Radiation exposure and occupational risks. Springer, Berlin Heidelberg New York, pp 97–132

Molls M, Streffer C, Zamboglou N (1981) Micronucleus formation in preimplanted mouse embryos cultured in vitro after irradiation with x-rays and neutrons. Int J Radiat Biol 39: 307–314

Molls M, Weißenborn U, Streffer C (1982) Bestrahlung von Mäuseembryonen des Pronukleus- und 2-Zell-Stadiums: die Abhängigkeit der Mikronukleusbildung und Zellvermehrung von DNA-Gehalt und Zellzyklusphase. Strahlentherapie 158: 504–512

Molls M, Streffer C, Fellner B, Weißenborn U (1984) Development of cytogenetic effects and recovery after irradiation of preimplantation mouse embryos. In: Streffer C, Patrick G (eds) Radiation Protection: "Effects of prenatal irradiation with special emphasis on late effects." EULEP Symposium, 29.7.1982, Bordeaux. Commission of the European Communities, pp 31–48

Moore JL, Pritchard JAV, Smith CW (1972) Oxygen equilibration in the determination of K for HeLa S$_3$ (OXF). Int J Radiat Biol 22: 149–158

Ohyama H, Yamada T (1973) X-ray modification of the allosteric functions of rat thymocyte phosphofructokinase. Biochim Biophys Acta 302: 261–266

Ohyama H, Yamada T, Watanabe I (1981) Cell volume reduction associated with interphase death in rat thymocytes. Radiat Res 85: 333–339

Petkau A, Chelack WS, Pleskach SD (1976) Protection of post-irradiated mice by superoxide dismutase. Int J Radiat Biol 29: 297–299

Phillips RA, Tolmach LJ (1966) Repair of potentially lethal damage in x-irradiated HeLa cells. Radiat Res 29: 413–432

Puck TT, Marcus PI (1955) A rapid method for viable cell titration and clone production with HeLa cells in tissue culture: the use of x-irradiated cells to supply conditioning factors. Proc Natl Acad Sci USA 41: 432–437

Quastler H (1945) Studies on roentgen death in mice. AJR 54: 449–456

Raaphorst GP, Dewey WC (1979) A study of the repair of potentially lethal and sublethal radiation damage in Chinese hamster cells exposed to extremely hypo- or hypertonic NaCl solutions. Radiat Res 77: 325–340

Redpath JL, Patterson LK (1978) The effect of membrane fatty acid composition on the radiosensitivity of E. coli. Radiat Res 75: 443–447

Regaud C (1922) Distribution chronologique rationelle d'un traitement de cancer épithélial par les radiation. C R Soc Biol (Paris) 86: 1085–1088

Reinhardt RD, Pohlit W (1976) Influence of intracellular adenosine-triphosphate concentration on survival of yeast cells following x-irradiation. In: Kiefer J (ed) Radiation and cellular control processes. Springer, Berlin Heidelberg New York, p 117

Reinhold HS, Buisman GH (1975) Repair of radiation damage to capillary endothelium. Br J Radiol 48: 727–731

Revesz L, Modig H (1965) Cysteamine-induced increase of cellular glutathione level: a new hypothesis of the radioprotective mechanism. Nature 207: 430–431

Rotblat J, Lindop P (1961) Long-term effects of a single whole-body exposure of mice to ionizing radiations. II. Causes of death. Proc R Soc Lond (Biol) 154: 350–368

Rubin P, Casarett GW (1968) Clinical radiation pathology. Saunders, Philadelphia

Sanner T, Pihl A (1972) Effect of X-rays on the regulatory functions of glutamate dehydrogenase from beef liver. Radiat Res 51: 155–166

Simons JWIM (1979) Development of a liquid-holding technique for the study of DNA-repair in human diploid fibroblasts. Mutat Res 59: 273–283

Sinclair WK (1972) Cell cycle dependence of the lethal radiation response in mammalian cells. Curr Top Radiat Res 7: 264–285

Sinclair WK, Morton RA (1966) X-ray sensitivity during the cell generation cycle of cultured Chinese hamster cells. Radiat Res 29: 450–474

Smith KC, Wang TC, Sharma RC (1987) Rec A dependent repair of DNA gaps and double-strand breaks after UV irradiation. In: Fielden EM, Fowler JF, Hendry JH, Scott D (eds) Radiation research. Taylor & Francis, London, pp 382–387

Steel GG, Peacock JH (1989) Why are some human tumours more radiosensitive than others? Radiother Oncol 15: 63–72

Streffer C (1969) Strahlen-Biochemie. Heidelberger Taschenbücher 59/60. Springer, Berlin Heidelberg New York

Streffer C (1980) Biologische Grundlagen der Strahlentherapie. In: Scherer E (ed) Strahlentherapie. Springer, Berlin Heidelberg New York, p 196

Streffer C (1987) Biologische Grundlagen der Strahlentherapie. In: Scherer E (ed) Strahlentherapie. Springer, Berlin Heidelberg New York, p 213

Streffer C, Beisel P (1974) Radiation effects on NAD- and DNA-metabolism in mouse spleen. FEBS Lett 44: 127–130

Streffer C, Molls M (1987) Cultures of preimplantation mouse embryos: a model for radiobiological studies. Adv Radiat Biol 13: 169–213

Streffer C, Schafferus S (1971) The induction of liver enzymes by cortisol after combined treatment of mice with x-irradiation and inhibitors of protein synthesis. Int J Radiat Biol 20: 301–313

Streffer C, van Beuningen D, Elias S (1977) Comparative effects of tritiated water and thymidine on the preimplanted mouse embryos in vitro. Curr Top Radiat Res 12: 182–193

Streffer C, van Beuningen D, Molls M, Zamboglou N, Schulz S (1980) Kinetics of cell proliferation in the preimplanted mouse embryo in vivo and in vitro. Cell Tissue Kinet 13: 135–143

Suit HD (1973) Radiation biology: a basis for radiotherapy. In: Fletcher GH (ed) Textbook of radiotherapy, 2nd edn. Lea and Febinger, Philadelphia, p 75

Szumiel I (1981) Intrinsic radiosensitivity of proliferating mammalian cells. In: Lett JT, Adler H (eds) Advances in radiation biology, vol 9. Academic, New York, p 281

Taylor IW, Bleehen NM (1977) Changes in sensitivity to radiation and ICRF 159 during the life of monolayer cultures of EMT 6 tumour line. Br J Cancer 35: 587–594

Terasima T, Tolmach LJ (1963) Variation in several responses of HeLa cells to X-irradiation during the division cycle. Biophys J 3: 11–33

Thomlinson RH, Gray LH (1955) The histological structure of some human lung cancers and possible implications for radiotherapy. Br J Cancer 9: 539–549

Till JE, McCulloch EA (1963) Early repair processes in marrow cells irradiated and proliferating in vivo. Radiat Res 18: 96–105

Trott K-R (1972) Strahlenwirkung auf die Vermehrung von Säugetierzellen. In: Diethelm L, Olson O, Strand F, Vieten H, Zuppinger A (eds) Handbuch der Medizinischen Radiologie. Springer, Berlin Heidelberg New York, p 43

Tubiana M (1971) The kinetics of tumour cell proliferation and radiotherapy. Br J Radiol 44: 225–247

Tubiana M (1973) Clinical data and radiobiological bases for radiotherapy. Curr Top Radiat Res 9: 109–118

Underbrink AG, Pond V (1976) Cytological factors and their predictive role in comparative radiosensitivity: a general summary. Curr Top Radiat Res 11: 251–306

United Nations Scientifc Committee on the Effects of Atomic Radiation (UNSCEAR) (1982) Ionizing radiation: sources and biological effects. United Nations, New York

Utsumi H, Elkind MM (1979) Potentially lethal damage versus sublethal damage: independent repair processes in actively growing Chinese hamster cells. Radiat Res 77: 346–360

van Beuningen D, Streffer C, Berthold G (1981) Mikronukleusbildung im Vergleich zur Überlebensrate von menschlichen Melanomzellen nach Röntgen-, Neutronenbestrahlung und Hyperthermie. Strahlentherapie 157: 600–606

van den Brenk HAS, Sharpington C, Orton C, Stone M (1974) Effects of X-radiation on growth and function of the repair blastema (granulation tissue). II. Measurements of angiogenesis in the Selye pouch in the rat. Int J Radiat Biol 25: 277–289

von Sonntag C (1987) The chemical basis of radiation biology. Taylor & Francis, London

Virsik RP, Harder D (1981) Statistical interpretation of the overdispersed distribution of radiation-induced dicentric chromosome aberrations at high LET. Radiat Res 85: 13–23

Ward J (1986) Mechanisms of DNA repair and their

potential modification for radiotherapy. Int J Radiat Oncol Biol Phys 12: 1027–1032

Warters RL, Hofer KG, Harris CR, Smith JM (1977) Radionuclide toxicity in cultured mammalian cells: elucidation of the primary site of radiation damage. Curr Top Radiat Res 12: 389–407

Watts ME, Maughan RL, Michael BD (1978) Fast kinetics of the oxygen effect in irradiated mammalian cells. Int J Radiat Biol 33: 195–209

Weichselbaum RR, Nove J, Little JB (1978) Deficient recovery from potentially lethal radiation damage in ataxia telangiectasia and xeroderma pigmentosum. Nature 271: 261–262

Weissenborn U, Streffer C (1988) Analysis of structural and numerical chromosomal anomalies at the first, second and third mitosis after irradiation of one-cell mouse embryos with X-rays or neutrons. Int J Radiat Biol 54: 381–394

Wheeler KT (1987) A concept relating DNA repair, metabolic states and cell survival after irradiation. In: Fielden EM, Fowler FJ, Hendry JH, Scott D (eds) Radiation research. Taylor & Francis, London, pp 325–330

Wideroe R (1971) Various examples from cellular kinetics showing how radiation quality can be analysed and calculated by the two-component theory of radiation. In: International Atomic Energy Agency (ed) Biophysical aspects of radiation quality. Vienna, p 311

Wideroe R (1975) Problems and trends in radiotherapeutic treatment of deep-seated tumors. Radiol Clin 44: 112–141

Withers HR (1967) The dose survival relationship for irradiation of epithelial cells of mouse skin. Br J Radiol 40: 187–194

Withers HR, Elkind MM (1969) Radiosensitivity and fractionation response of crypt cells of mouse jejunum. Radiat Res 38: 598–613

Yamada T, Ohyama H (1980) Changes in surface morphology of rat thymocytes accompanying interphase death. J Radiat Res 21: 190–196

Yamada T, Ohyama H, Kinjo Y, Watanabe M (1981) Evidence for the internucleosomal breakage of chromatin in rat thymocytes irradiated in vitro. Radiat Res 85: 544–553

Yatvin MB (1976) Evidence that survival of γ-irradiated *Escherichia coli* is influenced by membrane fluidity. Int J Radiat Biol 30: 571–575

2 Radiation Effects in Skin

K.-R. TROTT and J. KUMMERMEHR

CONTENTS

2.1 Introduction

The skin lies within the primary treatment field of radiotherapy more often than any other normal tissue. Its radiation response is immediately ob-

Professor Dr. K.-R. TROTT, Department of Radiation Biology, Medical College of St. Bartholomew's Hospital, University of London, Charterhouse Square, London ECIM 6BQ, UK

Dr. J. KUMMERMEHR, Institut für Strahlenbiologie, GSF-Forschungszentrum für Umwelt und Gesundheit, GmbH, 8042 Neuherberg, FRG

vious. Before megavoltage radiotherapy was introduced, skin tolerance limited the radiation dose that could be achieved in the tumor and, thus, overall treatment results in radiotherapy.

The clinical importance of radiation injury to skin has decreased since the introduction of megavoltage radiotherapy. Moreover, the pattern of skin injury has changed: severe acute radiodermatitis and dermal necrosis have become less frequent while chronic dermal and subcutaneous injury has become more frequent in relative and probably also in absolute terms. This is not due to different types of radiation effects from orthovoltage and from megavoltage radiations but to a different distribution of the radiation dose within the organ skin.

The progression of the acute skin reaction during and after radiotherapy with x-rays up to 250 kV has been well documented (e.g., STRAUSS 1925) and similar reactions may still be observed after high dose electron irradiation whereas with cobalt 60 γ-rays and megavoltage photons reactions are usually much milder. In the following discussion of clinical observations we shall, unless otherwise stated, refer to fractionated radiotherapy with cobalt 60 γ-rays with skin entrance doses up to 70 Gy and doses per fraction between 1.5 and 6 Gy.

2.2 Clinical Picture of Normal Skin Reactions During Radiotherapy

During radiotherapy, the skin reacts in a well-defined sequence with various waves of erythema which were described in detail by the early radiotherapists in the first half of this century, e.g., MIESCHER (1924).

No obvious radiation effects occur during the first 2 weeks of radiotherapy except for the occasional appearance of a faint erythema after the first few radiation doses and progressive dryness of the skin. After about 2 weeks epilation may start. The typical erythema, called the main erythema by the early radiotherapists, may gradually develop in the 3rd week: the skin turns red and becomes warm and edematous. The patient may report a sensation of burning and tenderness. The erythema is clearly limited to the radiation field. Depending on the treatment schedule, during the 4th and 5th weeks of radiotherapy radiodermatitis may progress from the phase of dry erythema (dry desquamation) to the exudative phase (moist desquamation). The dermis is denuded and responds with a marked inflammatory response and the oozing of serum. Patients may suffer from considerable discomfort during this period. About 1 week after the termination of radiotherapy, recovery and regeneration start from the margins or, occasionally, from regenerative foci in the center of the radiation field. Three weeks after the end of radiotherapy, recovery is usually complete.

With the presently used techniques of radiotherapy, large-scale exudative radiodermatitis is the exception. If epithelial denudation occurs it is usually limited to skin areas which are subject to additional stress, e.g., skin folds. The most common reaction today is exfoliative (dry) radiodermatitis and increased pigmentation which may be associated with a feeling of tenderness and itching for the last 2 weeks of radiotherapy. About 2 weeks later, these clinical signs and symptoms have usually cleared and the function of the sweat glands has recovered, too. The sebaceous skin glands, however, do not usually recover even after radiation doses which have not resulted in exudative radiodermatitis. Hair growth may be resumed again towards the end of the 2nd month after radiotherapy. Whereas in rodents regrowing hair is usually depigmented, in man it usually does not differ in color or structure from the preirradiation status. Occasionally the regrowing hair may be darker in fair- or white-haired patients (Ellinger 1957).

The radiosensitivity of the different skin annexes differs considerably. According to Borak (1936) the tolerance dose for a single radiation exposure is 1200 R for the sebaceous glands, 1600 R for the hair follicles, 2000 R for the epidermis, and 2500 R for the sweat glands.

The increased pigmentation usually apparent at the end of the course of radiotherapy will gradually disappear during the following months; in

colored people even focal depigmentation (vitiligo) may occur. The typical late stage of normal skin reaction after radiotherapy is mild skin atrophy with a somewhat glossy appearance. Due to the lack of the oily secretions from the sebaceous glands the skin is dry. After about 1 year, telangiectasia occasionally becomes visible, but it increases in frequency as time goes on (Turesson and Thames 1989). The incidence and severity of telangiectasia depends on the radiation dose, as described by Holthusen in 1936. The dose–response curve for the incidence of telangiectasia after radiotherapy was the first published dose–effect relationship for any chronic normal tissue injury (Fig. 2.1).

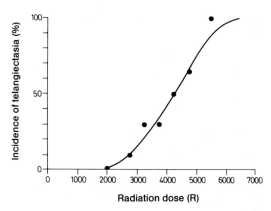

Fig. 2.1. The dependence of the incidence of telangiectasia on radiation dose (Holthusen 1936)

2.3 Skin Reaction After Radiation Doses Exceeding Skin Tolerance

After very high radiation doses the acute exudative skin reaction which may develop in the usual pattern will occasionally progress directly into acute dermal ulceration. More often, however, transient regeneration of the acute exudative reaction occurs, to be followed, after a variable latency time, by deep ulceration into the dermis and subcutis. Very often, skin necrosis is provoked by some minor trauma (mechanical, ultraviolet exposure, etc.) to the injured skin. During the first half of this century, the chronic radiation ulcer of skin was the major concern of radiotherapists. Its features have been described often and in great detail (Ellinger 1957). Although this type of skin necrosis does still occur today occasionally, especially after electron radiotherapy, the use of megavoltage photons has altered the clinical picture of the chronic skin reaction when skin tolerance has been exceeded. It is commonly called subcutaneous fibrosis. It appears as a hard plaque of scar tissue below the atrophic skin surface and is most commonly found at sites which have a thick layer of subcutaneous fat. Surprisingly few detailed descriptions have been published on the progression of this relatively frequent side-effect of curative radiotherapy. BIRKNER and HOFFMANN (1961) described the clinical features of the development of subcutaneous induration in 24 patients, of whom only three had displayed acute exudative radiodermatitis during the course of radiotherapy. Between 2 and 3 months later, a painful edematous swelling of the subcutaneous tissues was observed. Four months later, a very hard, wood-like plaque up to 3 cm thick was palpable under the intensely pigmented skin. The subcutaneous induration was sharply limited to the radiation field. During this acute phase, the induration was very tender and the patient avoided as far as possible any movement which might stress it. Gradually, pain became less severe but impairment of movement sometimes resulted from the mechanical restraint caused by the subcutaneous scar tissue.

Subcutaneous indurations had already been described after orthovoltage radiotherapy by MÜHLMANN and MEYER (1923) but they are more frequently seen today due to the different distribution of radiation dose in the skin. Sometimes, mauve coloration of the atrophic skin overlying the subcutaneous induration heralds imminent necrosis and ulceration (HOPEWELL et al. 1978). However, chronic skin ulcers are usually secondary to additional injuries like trauma, intensive ultraviolet light exposure, or poor hygiene. Chronic radiation ulcers do not heal well and require intensive and prolonged conservative dermatological treatment or even extensive plastic surgery. Moreover, the chronic atrophic and ulcerative changes in the irradiated skin require careful supervision as they have to be regarded as precancerous lesions (EHRING and HONDA 1967).

2.4 Histopathology of Acute and Chronic Radiation Injury in Skin

Acute radiodermatitis is primarily an inflammatory reaction of the skin (HEINEKE and BERTHES 1925). The early erythema which occurs within 1 day after high single doses is caused by dilatation of dermal capillaries and by interstitial edema. The erythema proper seems to be associated mostly with obstructive changes in arterioles (RUBIN and CASARETT 1968). Within a few days after the start of radiotherapy, endothelial swelling and proliferation can be observed. Arteriolar obstruction and capillary dilatation are associated with inflammatory infiltration of the dermis by neutrophils, and later by macrophages, eosinophilic granulocytes, and lymphocytes. Progressive cell degeneration in the epidermis leads to a decrease in epidermal thickness and flattening of the papillae, which is the typical feature of dry desquamation.

In the initial stages of exudative radiation dermatitis, intraepidermal blisters are formed which tend to coalesce and rupture. The inflammatory response in the dermis is more pronounced than with dry desquamation, and the denuded surface becomes covered with fibrin. The histological picture is similar to that of a second degree burn (FAJARDO and BERTHRONG 1981).

About a week or two after the sloughing of the epidermis, epithelial regeneration occurs from the margins and from surviving basal cells, most often in the hair follicles. After recovery from the acute radiation dermatitis, the histopathological picture of chronic atrophic skin develops gradually over many months. The epidermis is reduced in thickness to a few cell layers and the papillary protrusions are flattened out. Focal deposition of melanin is apparent in the superficial dermis (ZOLLINGER 1960). The hair follicles have disappeared with exception of the arrector muscles of hair, which are surrounded by collagen. The sebaceous glands are severely atrophic but the sweat glands appear normal. A conspicuous feature of the chronic atrophic skin changes is telangiectasia in the superficial dermis. Unless infection is complicating the picture there are no signs of inflammation (FAJARDO and BERTHRONG 1981). The pathological changes in the chronic phase show a rather focal pattern (ZOLLINGER 1960).

As time progresses, dermal and subcutaneous fibrosis becomes more prominent. The loose stromal net of the superficial dermis and the regular arrangement of fibers in the reticular dermis as well as the adipose tissue of the subcutis are gradually replaced by dense and irregular fibrous tissue. Fibrin exudation may still be found within the fibrous tissue. The number of elastic fibers is increased. The individual collagenous fibers appear enlarged and edematous. Whereas the clinical picture of subcutaneous fibrosis is very impressive, the microscopic picture is much less so. ZOLLINGER (1960) did not see any fundamental difference between these radiation-induced changes in the connective tissue of the dermis and subcutis and those changes occurring after healing of other defects. In the electron microscope, radiation fibrosis appears as thick bundles of collagen fibers, with the individual fibers looking normal but their number increased (FROMMHOLD and BUBLITZ 1967). Telangiectasia appears in the superficial dermis as grossly dilated and straightened capillaries. Endothelial proliferation in the arterioles can be observed even long after irradiation, leading to delayed arteriolar thrombosis (ZOLLINGER 1960).

2.5 Therapy for Radiation Injury in Skin

The normal radiation dermatitis which develops during radiotherapy does not require any specific treatment. The recommended measures are designed to relieve symptoms of inflammation and to prevent additional trauma and infection which may provoke acute or chronic ulceration. Patients are usually advised not to wash the marked radiation fields. Whereas alkaline soaps and vigorous brushing the skin may enhance the acute radiation reaction, neutral or acid detergents do not increase its severity. KÄRCHER (1958) described the dermatological principles of caring for the irradiated skin during radiotheraapy. A shower is preferable to a hot bath. During dry radiodermatitis, powders which are cooling as they increase the surface area and which may contain some anti-inflammatory drugs should be given; in contrast ointments should be avoided as they prevent heat exchange and thus may even increase the inflammatory reaction. During the phase of exudative radiation dermatitis, mild antiseptic

solutions like boric acid should be used. During the period of healing the skin requires treatment with only oily substances to alleviate the dryness caused by damage to the sebaceous glands.

Dermatological treatment of chronic ulcerations with local antibiotics and necrolytic measures may be successful. If conservative treatment fails, plastic surgery using myocutaneous flaps after wide excision of the necrotic and fibrotic area should be performed (LEMPERLE and KOSLOWSKI 1984; AL-SOUFI et al. 1986; TILKORN et al. 1986). The cosmetic sequelae of radiation-induced telangiectasia can be quite appalling and patients may insist on an attempt to treat them. GORDON et al. (1987) reported good results with injection sclerotherapy using tetradecyl sulfate sodium.

2.6 Heterogeneity of the Radiation Responses of Skin

The degree of radiation response of the skin during and after radiotherapy varies between different patients and between different sites in the same patient. It has long been realized that skin folds like the axilla and the groin are especially radiosensitive. KALZ (1941) classified the radiosensitivity of the different sites of the body with regard to the severity of acute skin reaction. The most radiosensitive regions are the anterior aspect of neck and the antecubital and popliteal spaces, followed in order of decreasing radiosensitivity by (a) the flexor surfaces of the extremities, (b) the chest and abdomen, (c) the nonpigmented face, (d) the back and the extensor surfaces of the extremities, (e) the pigmented face, (f) the nape of neck, (g) the scalp, and (h) the palms and soles.

The generally held opinion that fair-skinned people show a more pronounced acute skin reaction than pigmented people (ELLINGER 1957) was not confirmed in careful studies by CHU et al. (1960) and GLICKSMAN et al. (1960). However, they demonstrated a marked age dependence of the acute radiosensitivity of the skin. Children appeared to be less radiosensitive than adults; old people were more radioresistant again.

Various metabolic disorders have been claimed to cause an increased acute skin reaction, the best documented being thyrotoxicosis (STRAUSS 1925). Recently the emphasis has changed to identifying genetic factors as a major cause of increased skin radiosensitivity, yet except for homozygous ataxia telangiectasia no such genetic cause has been proven (ARLETT et al. 1989; PATERSON 1989). In vitro determination of the radiosensitivity of skin fibroblasts of these patients gave a decreased D_0 by a factor of 3. By decreasing the radiation dose to these patients to one-third, the acute radiation response was kept in the expected range. However, the contribution of homozygous and heterozygous genetic disorders to the observed heterogeneity of human skin reactions appears to be only marginal, as has been demonstrated by recent studies on a large number of patients whose fibroblasts, radiosensitivity was studied after an excessive acute skin reaction had been observed during radiotherapy (PATERSON 1989).

There are also great differences in the radiosensitivity of hair follicles at different sites of the body. According to ZOLLINGER (1960), radiosensitivity decreases from scalp, to axilla, to face, to pubic hair, with eyelashes and eyebrows being most radioresistant. To epilate eyelashes a 50% higher radiation dose is required than for scalp epilation (ELLINGER 1957).

Little is known about the heterogeneity of the radiosensitivity of different patients with regard to chronic radiation responses of the skin. However, the steepness of the published dose–response curves (e.g., POWELL-SMITH 1965) for subcutaneous fibrosis is a strong argument against the commonly held belief that there is greater heterogeneity between patients with regard to chronic as compared with acute radiation effects in the skin.

2.7 Pathogenesis of Radiation Effects in Skin

Of all organs in the body, the skin is best suited for the study of the complex interactions of radiation effects on tissue parenchyma and on tissue stroma which result, finally, in a clinical picture characterized by the typical interactive response of different tissue components. On the other hand, it is difficult to make extrapolations from experimental results on the pathogenesis and radiobiology of skin reactions in rodents, as the structure of the epidermis and its annexes (the parenchyma of skin), of the dermis and its vascular pattern, and of the subcutis is fundamentally different in mouse and man. This will affect the interactive response of the tissue as a whole more than the direct radiation effect on the critical tissue component.

2.7.1 Acute Radiation Effects

The first sign of an acute radiation effect in skin is the early erythema appearing on day 1 or 2, which is associated with increased capillary permeability (LAW 1981) and dilatation of the capillaries in the dermis at a time of complete structural and functional integrity of the epidermis. Thus the early erythema has to be regarded as being due to direct radiation effects on the dermal capillaries or as being mediated by radiation injury to other target cells which release vasoactive substances (JOLLES and HARRISON 1966).

The main erythema, however, appears to be a secondary inflammatory response of the dermis to epidermal radiation injury. This is proven by the appearance of a normal main erythema (affecting the entire depth of the dermis) after irradiation of human skin with alpha particles from thorium X, which do not penetrate beyond the epidermis and the superficial layers of the papillary dermis (ELLINGER 1957).

The epidermis is a typical example of a steady state self-renewing tissue with hierarchical organization of stem cells, transit cells, and functional end cells (MICHALOWSKI 1981). As discussed in detail by WHELDON et al. (1982), the response pattern of the epidermis which finally results in the acute radiation dermatitis is characterized by a dose-dependent decrease in the yield of proliferating stem cells and transit cells (cells in the basal and suprabasal compartment). As the life span of the postmitotic differentiating cells and differentiated cells is not altered by radiation, this leads to a progressive decrease in the number of epidermal cells and of epidermal thickness until, finally, denudation occurs (exudative radiation dermatitis) unless a new transit cell compartment has been reestablished from a sufficient number of surviving stem cells.

Cell proliferation and migration in skin are highly organized. Only 10% of the basal cells are stem cells, the other basal cells in mouse skin being proliferating transit cells. In the unperturbed state, these units of one stem cell and nine transit cells grow as independent proliferative units (epidermal proliferative units, EPUs) to form a distinctive hexagonal pattern on the skin surface which is related in a columnar pattern to the basal stem cells (POTTEN 1978, 1985). Cell division in the basal transit cells is usually polar, with one cell leaving the connection with the basal membrane and entering the spinocellular layer. Cells differentiate into prickle cells and further into keratinocytes to be shed from the surface after a total transit time of 21–45 days in human skin and of 11–21 days in mouse skin. The different values for the same species relate to different locations on the body surface.

Since cell turnover in the basal cell layer is slow, one does not observe any massive increase in cell pycnosis in the irradiated epidermis even after large single doses. Rather, in accordance with the slow turnover rate of the epidermis, cell injury like pycnosis and giant cell formation as well as cell depletion progresses slowly over weeks.

Two weeks after conventional fractionated radiotherapy most epidermal cells show various degrees of degeneration. It is at this stage of decreased epidermal thickness and increased epidermal cell degeneration that the dermal capillaries show distention and increased permeability leading to interstitial edema. The pathogenesis of this dermal inflammatory reaction to acute epidermal degeneration is poorly understood; however, it is likely that vasoactive substances like histamine, prostaglandins, and lysosomal enzymes are released from the disintegrating epidermal cells. This topic has been extensively reviewed by LAW (1981).

If the supply of new cells from the stem cell and transit cell compartments is depressed long enough, denudation of the dermis may occur, which will increase the dermal inflammatory reaction, especially if infection occurs. The delay and speed of regeneration of the thinned or absent epidermis depends primarily on the number of epidermal stem cells surviving the radiation treatment. In addition, secondary injury in the dermis, e.g., due to infection, may further delay regeneration of the epidermis. Various methods to determine the cellular radiosensitivity of epidermal stem cells have been developed. They are described in detail by POTTEN (1978, 1985). The average slope of the published exponential survival curves of murine epidermal stem cells has a D_0 of 1.35 Gy.

The delayed development of acute radiation dermatitis even after high single doses or accelerated treatment schedules is due to the slow cell turnover in the epidermis. Factors which speed up cell turnover in the epidermis, e.g., stripping the superficial layer of keratinocytes by adhesive tape or plucking the hair in mice, also lead to earlier development of the skin reaction (HEGAZY and FOWLER 1973 a,b). Irradiation itself does not stimulate cell proliferation in the epidermis. It is only at the time of onset of radiation dermatitis, when the epidermal layer has become thin and the inflammatory response in the dermis starts, that by some unknown homeostatic mechanism the basal cells of pig skin (MORRIS and HOPEWELL 1986; ARCHAMBEAU et al. 1988) (Fig. 2.2) and the stem

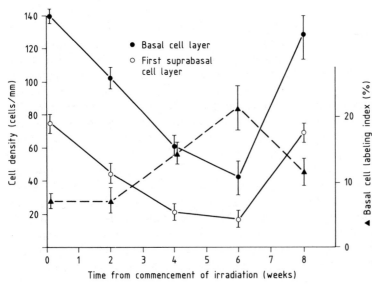

Fig. 2.2. Changes in cell density in the basal layer and the first suprabasal layer of pig skin during fractionated irradiation with 61.5 Gy in 30 fractions in 6 weeks and the proliferative response of the basal cells determined by the labeling index after intradermal injection of ³H-TdR (data from MORRIS and HOPEWELL 1986)

cells of mouse skin (DENEKAMP et al. 1976) are triggered into accelerated proliferation.

Acute radiation injury to the skin annexes such as hair (epilation), nails, and sebaceous glands shares the same pathogenetic mechanism (POTTEN 1978, 1985).

2.7.2 Chronic Radiation Effects

Acute radiation dermatitis heals by proliferation of surviving stem cells, leading to complete regeneration of the epidermis and also to the gradual fading of the inflammatory response of the dermis. Occasionally, the acute phase progresses directly into the chronic phase although this is usually due to additional secondary injury like infection or trauma. In most cases, chronic radiation injury develops only long after the acute radiation dermatitis is over. Yet severe chronic radiation injury to skin, such as skin necrosis and subcutaneous fibrosis, can also occur without any history of exudative radiation dermatitis (ISELIN 1912; STRAUSS 1925; LIEGNER and MICHAUD 1961; HOPEWELL 1980).

Whereas in acute radiation dermatitis the parenchyma of the skin, i.e., the epidermis, plays the leading role, it is the dermis and the subcutis which dominate the chronic phase of radiation injury to skin. The pathogenesis of the typical chronic reactions of the connective tissue in skin is controversial. Most certainly, direct radiation injury to the vessels, especially capillaries and arterioles, is of great importance. As early as 1899, GASSMANN described the typical radiation-induced alterations in the intimal layer of arteries near a radiation ulcer and regarded them as "the immediate cause of the ulcerations which would also explain the peculiar clinical features of radiation ulcers." The vascular changes in the dermis after irradiation are described by REINHOLD et al. in this volume (Chap. 8).

Besides the vascular radiation injury there is evidence that another independent mechanism may lead to dermal and subcutaneous fibrosis. The increase in fibrous tissue observed in the histological specimens is not necessarily an indication of an absolute increase in fibrous tissue. This is especially true for the "subcutaneous fibrosis," which above all is due to the atrophy of the adipose tissue, with the connective tissue between the fat cells remaining and being remodeled into hyaline tissue. HOPEWELL (1980) demonstrated

that in pig skin the clinical diagnosis of fibrosis is actually associated with a decrease in dermal and subcutaneous tissue thickness. Whether the dermal atrophy is due to impaired microcirculation in the dermis, to impaired proliferative potential of fibroblasts, or to a combination of both effects remains to be demonstrated.

ULLRICH and CASARETT (1977) assume a causal relationship between the early inflammatory reaction in the dermis (the erythema) and the later development of dermal fibrosis, as both can be reduced by a decrease in complement. LAW and THOMLINSON (1978) interpret their data on the deposition of fibrinogen in the tissue during the inflammatory response as supporting this hypothesis.

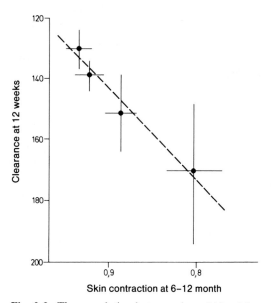

Fig. 2.3. The correlation between dermal blood flow at 12 weeks, determined by clearance of the radioactive tracer 99m Tc injected intradermally, and skin contraction at 6–12 months after irradiation, determined by the relative linear distance of tattooed markers (data from MOUSTAFA and HOPEWELL 1979)

In the pig, which of all experimental animals has a skin structure most similar to that of man, HOPEWELL et al. (1978) demonstrated that vascular injury preceded damage in the dermis and the subcutaneous adipose tissue. The decrease in blood perfusion in the dermis measured at 12 weeks after irradiation correlated well with the degree of dermal atrophy determined after 12 months (MOUSTAFA and HOPEWELL 1979) (Fig. 2.3). The transient decrease in vascular perfusion between weeks 10 and 16 was associated with a change in skin color into mauve and a decrease in skin temperature and, in histological specimens, with arteriolar thrombosis (Hopewell 1980).

2.8 Experimental Models of Radiation Injury in Skin

The pathogenesis of the various cutaneous reactions to radiation is very complex. Most cannot be fully explained by the direct radiation effects in the constituent cells. In order to perform quantitative analyses of the factors influencing the various radiation responses of skin, scoring systems which attribute numbers to different reactions are necessary, or specific response criteria (e.g., standard skin reaction) have to be defined. The effects of variations in the irradiation parameters are quantitated by comparing those radiation doses which produce the same effect, i.e., the same mean score of a graded response or the same incidence of a quantal response. These scores have been widely used in experimental animals as well as in patients. Up to about 1955, experimental studies were performed in patients treated for cancer but in skin areas not involved by cancer. Usually, many small fields in the same location (forearm, thigh) were treated with different doses and schedules and the development of the acute skin reactions was carefully recorded. These studies pioneered the field of normal tissue radiobiology and laid the ground for the science of experimental radiotherapy and clinical radiobiology.

2.8.1 Experimental Models of Acute Radiation Response

A milestone in the history of clinical radiobiology was the definition of the standard skin reaction after single dose irradiation (standard erythema dose, SED). Different investigators used different skin areas and field sizes. Seitz and Wintz (1920) defined the SED as "a pronounced early reaction which progresses into a marked main reaction peaking after 12 to 14 days and disappearing after 4 to 5 weeks." The smallest radiation dose which was just capable of producing this type of reaction homogeneously in a square field of about 1 inch side length in a defined localization of the body, most often the medial aspect of the thigh, was

taken as the biological unit of radiation dose in radiotherapy. Daily and total doses were quoted as fractions or multiples of the SED until reliable methods of physical and chemical dosimetry were introduced in the 1930s.

The precision of this biological dose meter is remarkably good. Kepp (1944) showed that, in the same patient, a dose difference of 10% can be clearly detected by the difference in the degree of the skin reaction. Holthusen (1925) estimated that, provided a well-standardized procedure is used, variability between different test persons is not more than 15%. However, if different investigators used different criteria, different field localizations, and different field sizes, variability in the SED was reported as being between 20% (Glasser 1925) and more than 40% (Heidenhain 1926).

The subjective method of visual scoring can be replaced by photometric (Nias 1963) or thermographic (White et al. 1975) measurements. The most extensive systematic study using photometric measurements of light reflection at wavelengths of 578 nm (for erythema) or 660 nm (for pigmentation) was performed by Turesson and Notter (1976, 1984, a,b,c, 1988) in breast cancer patients who received radiotherapy to both parasternal fields with different doses per fraction, different total doses, and different intervals between fractions. Fig. 2.4 demonstrates that using the symmetrical contralateral field as control, a dose difference of 5% leads to a significantly different skin response. A large body of important clinical data on the dose fractionation response of human skin has been collected in this way which, in precision and reliability, compares favorably with any data collected in animal experiments.

In animal experiments, the different acute reactions are recorded qualitatively and the various degrees of severity are then given numbers. The most commonly used scoring system was developed by Bewley et al. (1963) and Fowler et al. (1965) for pig skin. Various investigators adapted this system later to various sites in rodent skin, e.g., dorsum, foot, and ear (Table 2.1). The sensitivity of this semiquantitative scoring system is good enough to determine significant differences in effectiveness of doses differing by less than 10%.

Besides rodents like mice and rats, pigs are a favorite animal model for studying acute skin reactions since their histomorphology, and thus their radiation response pattern, is more similar to

Fig. 2.4. The time course of acute erythema in patients determined by photometric measurements of light reflection in two contralateral parasternal fields irradiated over 4 weeks with doses differing by 5% (data from TURESSON and NOTTER 1976)

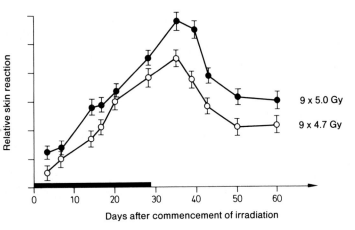

9 x 5.0 Gy

9 x 4.7 Gy

Relative skin reaction

Days after commencement of irradiation

Table 2.1. Mouse foot skin reactions

Score	Reaction
0.5	Slight hair loss and/or very slight reddening.
1.0	Severe reddening, often with distended blood vessels or slight swelling.
1.5	Scaly appearance with moist breakdown of *one* small area.
2.0	Breakdown of large area and/or toes stuck together.
2.5	Breakdown of about 50 per cent of the skin of the foot.
3.0	Breakdown of most of the skin.
3.5	Breakdown of entire skin of foot with severe moist exudation.

that of human skin than that of any other animal. Above all, acute dermal responses can be determined very precisely. As it is very difficult to diagnose or quantitate erythema in skin covered by a hairy coat, in mice the score is most reliable if exudative radiation dermatitis occurs in part of the field. In pigs, however, the intensity and the color of acute erythema can be used as the major response criterion.

In experimental studies on the acute skin reaction, animals are inspected at short intervals during the main response period, which, in most mouse strains, is the 2nd-5th week, and each field is given a score as shown in Table 2.1. From these data, a mean score for an experimental group over the period of the main reaction can be calculated and dose–response curves constructed (Fig. 2.5). However, since the scale attributes arbitrary numbers to effects, the differences between the numbers may not be proportional to different stem cell survival levels and often may relate to different pathogenetic mechanisms. Therefore, a quantal

analysis of these data is more appropriate. The proportion of animals which, during the period of the main reaction, exceed a certain threshold in their peak or mean reaction is related to the radiation dose (Fig. 2.6). The latter method is to be preferred as it makes fewer assumptions than scaling grades of severity and may even be used without attributing numbers to the different acute reactions, rather taking the clinical symptom

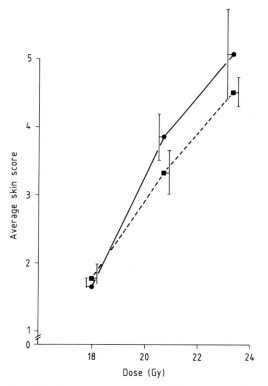

Fig. 2.5. Dose–response curve of the reaction of pig skin averaged over weeks 10–16 after single dose irradiation to a 16 cm² field (*squares*) or a 64 cm² field (*circles*) (data from HOPEWELL and YOUNG 1982)

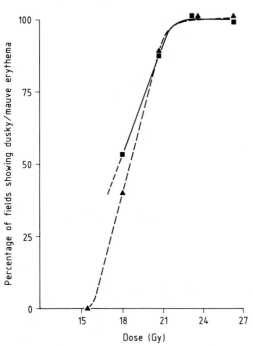

Fig. 2.6. Dose–response curve of the incidence of mauve erythema appearing between 10 and 16 weeks after single dose irradiation in pig skin of either 16 cm² or 64 cm² field area. Figures 2.5 and 2.6 show two different ways of analyzing the same data of Hopewell and Young (1982)

sebaceous glands on the cheeks of acne patients. After doses ranging from 300 to 1500 R, a rapid decrease in average gland size was recorded within as little as 1–2 weeks; however, the potential for regeneration was considerable. After a dose-dependent latency time (4 weeks after 400 R, 6 weeks after 800 R, and up to 1 year after 1500 R), complete recovery was observed.

2.8.2 Experimental Models of Chronic Radiation Response

While mouse skin is an adequate model for studying acute responses to radiation, it is less useful for the study of chronic responses. Hopewell (1980) discussed this problem extensively and related it to the different anatomical organization and vascular pattern of human and rodent skin. The most commonly used chronic endpoints for skin reactions in mice are scores quantitating foot deformity (Field 1969), skin contraction (Hayashi and Suit 1972; Masuda et al. 1980), and tail necrosis (Hendry et al. 1977). Some of these late sequelae of rodent skin irradiation may be late consequences of excessive, necrotizing, and nonhealing acute reactions which bear little relationship to the chronic skin reactions observed in patients after high dose radiotherapy. This possibility has been validated by a close correlation of acute and chronic skin reactions in individual animals of a large group of mice irradiated with single and fractionated doses (Denekamp 1977).

In patients, different types of chronic skin reaction may be scored in a semiquantitative way to study their dependence on dose and fractionation. Determining the thickness of subcutaneous fibrosis (Gauwerky and Langheim 1978) may involve some element of subjective assessment and, moreover, it quantitates the transgression of tolerance, which is uncommon with present treatment techniques. Counting the number of telangiectasias in the treatment field (Turesson and Notter 1976; Cohen and Ubaldi 1977) has become the most popular endpoint in studies in patients as it is well reproducible, can be objectively documented, and measures a biological effect which plays a direct role in the pathogenesis of the less well quantifiable chronic radiation effects like atrophy. Most important, this score is most sensitive at doses just below and just above tolerance. However, it has to be realized that the density of telangiectasias progresses over many

directly as the criterion (e.g., the proportion of animals which develop any exudative reaction). In addition, the duration of a response above a threshold may sometimes be a valuable additional response criterion.

The acute responses quantitated by these scores are generally assumed to be indicative of the level of survival of epidermal stem cells, equal scores indicating equal numbers of surviving stem cells (Thames and Hendry 1987). In rodents, in which stem cell survival can be determined directly (Withers 1967), this correlation seems justified.

Of the different skin annexes only hair has served as an experimental model in radiobiological research. At a defined time after irradiation (usually about 8 weeks) the number of hairs per unit of skin area is counted and related to dose (Vegesna et al. 1988). Griem et al. (1979) studied regenerating hair follicles, i.e., stem cell survival, rather than hair loss and determined a survival curve characterized by a D_0 of 1.35 Gy and a D_q of 5 Gy in anagen hair and 14 Gy in telogen hair. Strauss and Kligman (1960) performed a systematic study on the effect of x-rays on the size of

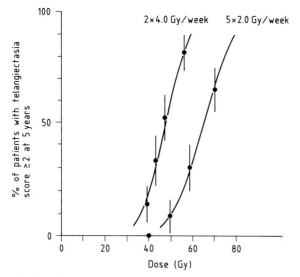

Fig. 2.7. Dose–response curves for telangiectasia score 2 or more at 5 years after either 5 × 2 Gy per week or 2 × 4 Gy per week (TURESSON and NOTTER 1986)

years. TURESSON and THAMES (1989) suggested taking the rate of progression, rather than the telangiectasia density at a given time, as a meaningful endpoint in such studies. Relating the proportion of radiation fields exceeding a certain level of telangiectasia density to radiation dose yields well-defined dose–response curves (Fig. 2.7).

During the era of orthovoltage radiotherapy, the occurrence of skin necrosis was of great clinical importance and a good model for investigating the dependence of this "late" skin reaction on dose fractionation. The "classical" studies of STRANDQVIST (1944) and ELLIS (1969) used this as their main criterion of skin tolerance for various fractionation schedules. Clinical and experimental studies have suggested that this criterion of chronic skin reaction is not suitable for describing the dose fractionation effects which occur after megavoltage radiotherapy and which arise mainly in the dermis and subcutis (BERRY et al. 1974b).

The most useful animal model for chronic radiation injury to the skin is the quantitation of dermal atrophy in pig skin by measuring field contraction (HOPEWELL et al. 1979). The size of the irradiated field is tattooed before irradiation. Even after radiation doses which do not lead to an acute exudative reaction, the field size decreases gradually and, after an observation period of a few months, well-defined dose–response curves are obtained either by determining mean field contraction (Fig. 2.8) or the proportion of fields exceeding a certain level of skin contraction (Fig. 2.9).

2.9 Dependence of Radiation Response on the Size of the Irradiated Skin Field

The severity of the skin reactions, acute erythema, exudative radiodermatitis, and late skin atrophy and necrosis, as well as the tolerated radiation doses, vary as the field size is altered. JOLLES and MITCHELL (1947) reported the experience with orthovoltage radiotherapy. The equations developed by VON ESSEN (1963, 1968) to relate tolerance dose to field size are mainly based on these data.

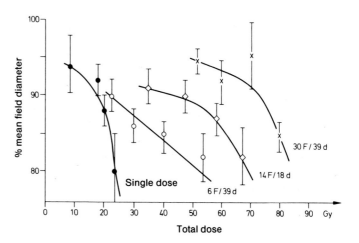

Fig. 2.8. Dose-response curves for skin contraction measured 6–12 months after irradiation of pig skin with various doses and fractionation schedules (data from HOPEWELL et al. 1979)

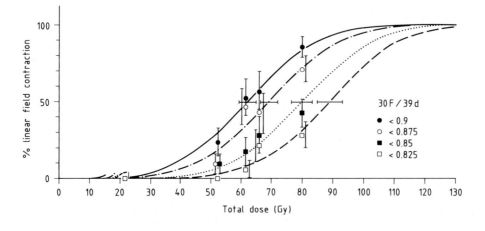

Fig. 2.9. Dose–response curves of the incidence of field contraction exceeding a certain level (between 10% and 17.5%) in pig skin fields irradiated with 30 fractions in 39 days. These curves show a quantal analysis of the same data as in Fig. 2.8 for the 30F/39 day group. (Hopewell et al., Annual Report CRC Normal Tissue Radiobiology Group 1985/86)

Table 2.2. Dependence of acute skin tolerance in man on field size (Joyet and Hohl 1955)

Skin area (cm)	Tolerance dose (Gy)
100	50 ± 4
16	58 ± 6
4	84 ± 7
1.7	200 ± 30
1	392 ± 100

The tolerated radiation dose depends on the field diameter according to

$$D = k / \sqrt[3]{d} \quad \text{(Von Essen 1963),} \tag{1}$$

with D as the tolerated dose, k a constant, and d the field diameter.

The tolerated radiation dose depends on the field area according to

$$D = k / A^{-0.16} \quad \text{(Von Essen 1968),} \tag{2}$$

A being the area of the field.

Joyet and Hohl (1955) performed the most systematic study on the dependence of acute skin tolerance on field size in patients, using exudative radiodermatitis which healed within 2–4 weeks as the response criterion on which basis isoeffective doses were determined. In seven patients who were given palliative radiotherapy for lung cancer, five different square fields on the back of the thorax with areas of 100, 16, 4, 1.7, and 1 cm² were given different total doses of 240 kV x-rays but with the same fractionation schedule of 18 fractions in 22–28 days. The tolerance doses increased as the field size decreased by the values in Table 2.2. These data do not conform to the clinically derived equations of Von Essen (1963, 1968). They demonstrate a much smaller increase in tolerance dose as the field size is decreased from 100 to 16 cm² than is predicted by the equations,

and a much steeper increase in tolerance at very small fields. In this study, the logarithm of the tolerance dose increases in proportion to the inverse of the field size.

Klostermann (1966) described the dependence of the incidence of late skin atrophy on the field size in a group of patients treated for hemangioma with three fractions of 500 R soft x-rays. No atrophy occurred in 27 fields smaller than 1 cm in diameter and only 1 of 22 fields of about 1.5 cm in diameter became atrophic, but five of eight fields of about 2.5 cm in diameter developed pronounced late atrophy and sclerosis.

Animal experiments on this problem were performed by the Oxford group in pig skin. Hopewell and Young (1982) compared isoeffective doses for acute skin reactions and late skin atrophy in fields of 16 and 64 cm². According to Von Essen's equation, tolerance doses should differ by 25%, yet no significant difference was observed (Figs. 2.5, 2.6); the data were consistent with only a 5% lower tolerance of the larger field. Further experiments using strontium 90 and thulium 170 plaques of different area (Coggle et al., 1984; Peel et al. 1984b; Hopewell et al. 1986) in pig and mouse skin supported the observations of Joyet and Hohl that a significant field size effect is

Table 2.3. ED$_{50}$ values (Gy) for acute tissue breakdown in the skin of pig and mouse after strontium or thulium irradiation (HOPEWELL et al. 1986)

Diameter (mm)	Strontium		Thulium	
	Pig	Mouse	Pig	Mouse
1	275	973	200	–
2	125	196	200	184
5	75	76	80	90
9	–	–	80	60
11	44	42	–	–
22.5	27.5	22	80	–

2.10 The Fractionation Response of Skin

observed only if the diameter of the field is below 2 cm (Table 2.3). These data are more consistent with the equation proposed by JOYET and HOHL than with that of VON ESSEN.

Although the incidence of objectively defined skin reactions depends on field size only if the field size is smaller than 16 cm^2, in clinical practice a field size effect can also be determined for larger fields using the clinical tolerance as the relevant criterion. Whereas exudative radiodermatitis of the entire field can be tolerated by the patient if the field size is very small (as in radiotherapy of skin cancer), it is definitely not well tolerated if the field is about 100 cm^2. The tolerated severity of the acute and chronic skin reactions clearly depends on the affected area. The equations of VON ESSEN are a rather successful attempt to relate the different tolerated effects to field size. They do not determine isoeffective doses in the radiobiological sense and, moreover, they grossly underestimate the increase in acute skin tolerance for very small fields.

The limiting role of skin tolerance in early cancer radiotherapy and the relative ease with which damage can be assessed explain why studies into dose–time relationships have long concentrated on this organ.

In the early days skin erythema was freely used as an experimental endpoint in humans. A systematic study was published in 1933 by REISNER, reporting among other data the effect of subdividing the radiation dose into 2–27 equal dose fractions, given daily to 2 × 2 cm fields on the frontal thigh. Using colorimetric measurement to follow the acute reaction, he established a curve that described the total isoeffective dose as a function of total treatment time. This curve, replotted in Fig. 2.10, demonstrates an increase in tolerance that is steep initially and levels off as the number of treatment days exceeds 15. REISNER's curve would readily have shown the impact of fraction number on tolerance, particularly when replotted as apparently recovered dose as a function of dose per fraction (insert in Fig. 2.10). At that time, however, treatment time was thought to be the major biological factor, continuously "diluting" the effect of previous dose fractions. In a subsequent study on human skin, MACCOMB and QUIMBY (1936) reported similar findings; some inconsistency in the data is explained by the threshold erythema used as the endpoint, but the results, expressed as fractionation factors (ratio of total over single dose), were largely the same. MACCOMB and QUIMBY explicitly

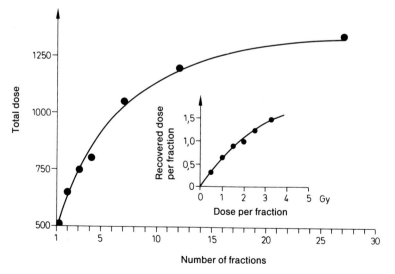

Fig. 2.10 Dependence of skin erythema dose on the number of equal daily dose fractions (data on human skin from REISNER 1933). *Insert*: Data replotted to show the recovered dose per fraction as a function of fraction size

concluded that treatment time (up to 5 days in their experiments) mattered more than fraction number and explained the less than cumulative effect by a gradual loss of tissue recuperation during daily fractionation.

The problems inherent in erythema were critically reviewed by later authors. For example, Nias (1963) repeated erythema measurements and concluded that fractionation factors of 1.2 and 1.6 could not reliably be separated by the early experiments. Some difficulties arising with erythema, e.g., variable sensitivity during the ascending limb of the reaction, were also recognized by Reisner; however, some of his data pertained to exudative radiodermatitis, and their time–dose relationship agreed well with the erythema results.

Strandqvist (1944), in his famous monograph, provided an interesting and quite modern discussion on the biological nature of these endpoints. He argued that exudative radiodermatitis reflects cell kill, an effect also critical for tumor cure; he also stressed that moist desquamation is a more relevant endpoint for assessing fractionation responses as it is indicative of the tolerance level to which skin is usually treated in radiotherapy of skin cancer. In his analysis of the time factor, however, he had to digress from the use of an isoeffective dose comparison for moist desquamation. Out of the total of 280 patients with lip or skin cancer (mostly basaliomas) reported in his publication, he selected 29 patients, treated within 14 days, who developed either a local recurrence or severe skin damage such as superficial necrosis or delayed healing. In a linear plot of total dose versus treatment time, parallel curves could be drawn above the complications and below the recurrences that encompassed a narrow band area of recommendable isoeffective doses for likely cure without complications (Fig. 2.11). Strandqvist concluded that these convex upward curves allowed fitting by several formalisms, but eventually chose to treat them as parabolae. The separation lines for skin tolerance and tumor cure thus became straight lines in a log-log plot, with slope 0.22, differing somewhat in tolerance dose but not in fractionation effect. His choice was partly based on the mathematical symmetry between his power function and Schwartzschild's law, which for photochemical reactions defines the fading effect with time. More specifically, the effect of time in protracted light treatment follows the formula.

$$const = I \times T^P; \tag{3}$$

Strandqvist equated I (intensity) with D/T for multifractionated irradiation, thus arriving at

$$D(\text{single dose}) = D(\text{total})/T(\text{total}) \times T^P \tag{4}$$

$$\text{or:} \quad D \ (total) = \ const \times T^{1-P} \tag{5}$$

Where p is 0.78, similar to Schwartzschild's exponent.

Thus in Strandqvist's opinion the parameter of importance was clearly time, as before. The historical importance of Strandqvist's choice was that the power function introduced linearity into the data analysis and possibly for this reason dominated the formal treatment of isoeffective data until very recently.

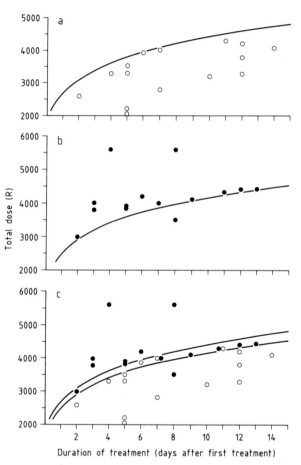

Duration of treatment (days after first treatment)

Fig. 2.11a-c. Response of skin cancer cases to radiotherapy, as originally published by Strandqvist (1944) to demonstrate the dependence of total dose on treatment time. The parabolic curve in **a** denotes the upper dose limit for recurrences (o), while the curve in **b** shows the lower dose limit for complications such as necrosis or delayed healing (x). When superimposed (**c**), the two curves define a narrow band in which tumor control without complication is most likely. (Strandqvist 1944)

It has to be realized that clinical radiotherapy at that time used a diversity of fractionation protocols that would nowadays be inconceivable. Clinical experience accrued indicating that the fractionation response of tumors and skin could not be entirely identical. COHEN (1949a, b) reanalyzed data of REISNER (1933), MACCOMB and QUIMBY (1936), ELLIS (1942), STRANDQVIST (1944), PATERSON (1948), and others and arrived at different slopes, i.e., 0.22 for tumor control and 0.33 for skin tolerance. As first pointed out by FLETCHER and BARKLEY (1974), this difference stems mainly from an inconsistent assignment of the treatment time for tumors and skin. COHEN followed STRANDQVIST in assigning to single dose treatment for tumors 0.35 days and to larger fraction numbers the time elapsed after the first fraction (e.g., 2 days for three daily fractions), while for skin he plotted total treatment time (e.g., 2 days for two daily fractions) and omitted the single dose data. Given the large proportion of data with few daily fractions, this divergent use of time made the curve steeper for skin tolerance than for cancer eradication, a difference not demonstrable with consistent handling of the data (FLETCHER and BARKLEY 1974). The biological explanation offered was a greater recovery *rate*. Quite generally the concept of time-dependent recovery persisted, and even in clinical data where the impact of fraction size or number was clearly realized, the deviation from STRANDQVIST's or COHEN's time factor was thought to arise from a slowing effect of large dose fractions on recuperation rate (TRAENKLE and MULAY 1960). All the same, COHEN's choice turned out to be important in the further search for differences in fractionation response and therapeutic gain.

In particular it was adopted by ELLIS (1968, 1969), who expanded the formalism by separating the influence of fraction number and treatment time into

$$D = \text{NSD} \times N^{0.24} \times T^{0.11} \qquad (6)$$

where D is the total isoeffective dose, N the number of (equal) fractions, T the total treatment time, and NSD the "nominal standard dose." The NSD cannot be taken as an equivalent single dose because in the formalism it is conceptually not possible to allot a real time T to a single fraction. The analysis was carried out on acutely and chronically necrotizing skin reactions, relying on mostly the same data as had been used by COHEN (1949a, b). Several arguments led ELLIS to differentiate between time and fractionation and to allocate the specific exponents. Firstly, intracellular recovery had been demonstrated in cells in vitro by ELKIND and SUTTON (1960), and although not translated in a quantitative way, suggested that fractionation was a tolerance factor on its own. Secondly, in pig skin experiments designed to differentiate between the importance of fraction number and time, FOWLER et al. (1963) had shown that time was less relevant. In their study five fractions given over 28 days required an isoeffective dose much closer to that of five fractions in 5 days than of 21 fractions in 28 days, and the exponents were compatible with those proposed in the NSD formula. In conclusion, ELLIS interpreted COHEN's exponents for skin *and* tumors as caused by a recovery exponent of 0.22, universally shared by all tissues, and a time exponent of 0.11, reflecting "homeostatic control," which was assumed to hold only for normal tissues. The biological nature of homeostatic control was not really identified in the papers of that time; it was sometimes equated with "slow repair" (as opposed to fast or ELKIND repair) or "tissue repair" (ELLIS 1971) or with repopulation, but such suggestions were not based on direct experimental evidence.

Several algebraic expansions of the NSD formula were subsequently published, such as the CRE or cumulative radiation effect formula of KIRK et al. (1971) and the TDF or time–dose factor system of ORTON and ELLIS (1973). A major advantage of these formulae is that they facilitate calculation of partial tolerance in the event of treatment interruptions, although again only in a formal way.

The NSD formula was never stretched to optimize a therapeutic margin between tumors and normal tissues although this is implicit in its framework. Its great attraction was that it seemingly allowed normalization of different fractionation protocols with regard to skin tolerance, and reduction of conventional schedules in a safe way. The boundaries within which this was possible were defined by ELLIS as a minimum fraction number of 4 and a minimum treatment time of 15 days.

However, soon after the institution of the NSD formula, its applicability even within the recommended limits was seriously questioned. A large body of evidence amassed from clinical studies in which for economic or practical reasons conventional fractionation was replaced by hypofractionation using two or even one weekly fraction instead of five.

The most extensive data were presented by TURESSON and NOTTER in a series of publications on postmastectomy patients who received mostly bilateral parasternal radiotherapy. Acute reactions were quantitated by reflectance spectrophotometry, recording erythema into the stage of dry desquamation, while late reactions were documented by a telangiectasia score (see p. 43). Protocols delivering either 5 × 2.16 Gy or 1 × 6.2 Gy per week over 22 days to the same CRE level of 15 resulted in comparable acute reactions, while the hypofractionated schedule produced excess telangiectasia, consistent with overdosing by about 7% (TURESSON and NOTTER 1976). Similarly, more extensive treatment schedules over 5 or 6 weeks contrasting conventional and twice weekly fractionation (CRE levels between 16 and 18) yielded considerably more telangiectasia in the twice weekly arms than predicted (TURESSON and NOTTER 1984b). The exponent to N derived from isoeffective doses delivered as 5 × 2 Gy or 2 × 4 Gy per week was as high as 0.35. Enhanced late effects (telangiectasia), but equal acute response, were also reported by SAUSE et al. (1981) for postmastectomy chest wall irradiation (7 MeV electrons) in 55 patients treated by 10 × 4 Gy in 5 weeks, as compared with conventional ^{60}Co treatment. BATES (1975) and BATES and PETERS (1975) similarly found that late effects of chest wall irradiation, including fibrosis, were increased when six fractions were given instead of 12. The dissociation of tolerance between early and late effects is a consistent finding in hypofractionation studies. Also for chest wall irradiation, more recently OVERGAARD et al. (1987) have stressed the particular risk of late damage when predictions are based on the NSD formula. Five times weekly and twice weekly irradiation to maximum NSD values of 1706 and 1756 rets, respectively, resulted in comparable early damage, but with the twice weekly regime there was a striking increase in the incidence of severe skin fibrosis from 5% to 67%. COHEN and UBALDI (1977) studied the severity and incidence of telangiectasia in 75 patients treated by one, two, or five fractions per week. A straightforward graphic plot gave a compound isoeffect slope of 0.40, while formal analysis by the complex cybernetic model of COHEN and SCOTT (1968)

rendered exponents to time and fraction number compatible with the NSD formula.

GAUWERKY and LANGHEIM (1978) reported data on 549 skin fields, irradiated with a great variety of doses per fraction (1–6 Gy, often given on alternate days) and range of treatment times (44% of all fields treated within less than 30 days or more than 50 days). Of the 549 fields, 144 developed severe induration within an observation period of 3–8 months. The most likely slope assessed from a regression analysis of log D vs log N was 0.42, but a rigid analysis is prevented as the individual dose–time parameters are not given.

The main conclusion from clinical investigations is that the NSD formula clearly tends to overestimate late but not early skin damage tolerance when the fraction number is reduced or the dose per fraction increased. This is also borne out by experiments on pig skin again designed mainly to test the predictive power of the NSD formula with regard to hypofractionation.

Data published by the Oxford group, contrasting 30 F/39 days to 6 F/18 days, demonstrated reasonably good agreement with the NSD prediction in dose groups that, as a continuation of early damage, developed necrosis within 3 months (BERRY et al. 1974a). However, true late damage presenting as skin contraction was clearly increased in the six-fraction regime and the estimated slope was 0.46 as opposed to a compound slope of 0.33 (BERRY et al. 1974b). Later experiments by this group, comparing 6 and 14 fractions in 18 days and 6, 14, and 30 fractions in 39 days, confirmed the greater than predicted fractionation response of late skin contraction, but in addition indicated that the exponent to N cannot be adequately described by a single figure. The trend showed a decline with increasing fraction number, but between 14 and 30 fractions both given in 39 days the exponent was still as high as 0.33 (HOPEWELL et al. 1979); conversely, the time exponent in the same analysis was negative, a fact tentatively explained by some degree of skin hypoxia. In minipig experiments WITHERS et al. (1978) studied early and late skin tolerance to protocols of either 32 or 13 fractions given in 6.5 weeks, i.e., given as five or two fractions per week. Tolerance for late skin contraction was grossly exceeded by the hypofractionated schedule when dose prediction was based on the NSD formula, and the actual exponent to fraction number was estimated to be 0.46 (Fig. 2.12). The acute responses behaved differently, with rather

Fig. 2.12. Relationship between isoeffective dose and fraction number for early (*solid lines*) and late (*dot-dashed lines*) skin response. Results include data on pig skin from WITHERS et al. (1978) (*W*) and HOPEWELL et al. (1979) (*H*), on mouse skin from FOWLER et al. (1974) (*F*), and clinical data from BRENNAN et al. (1976) (*B*) and DUTREIX et al. (1973) (*D*). (Redrawn with permission from HOPEWELL and VAN DEN AARDWEG 1988)

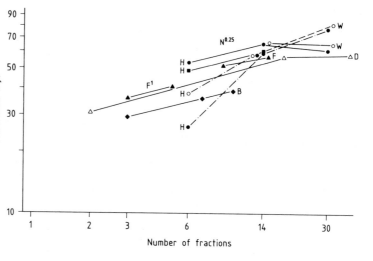

more pronounced effects in the conventional regime even at identical dose levels. Apart from again indicating a distinctly lower fractionation response of early damage, this finding points to changes caused by treatment times longer than 4 weeks, when rapid repopulation makes the epidermis more vulnerable to small repeated dose fractions than to twice weekly doses. A strikingly similar result, i.e., a decrease in acute tolerance, was seen in human parasternal fields when the treatment time was extended from 4 to 5 or 6 weeks, but not when an additional 3-week interval was allowed, presumably because the proliferative response subsided during that period (TURESSON and NOTTER 1984c).

A common pattern emerges from the clinical and experimental studies. The NSD formula predicts incorrectly for skin damage when unequivocal late effects are under consideration. The reason for this is that the target cells (tissue) underlying early and late effects differ in their capacity for sublethal damage repair and hence in their fractionation response. In principle the formal discrepancy could be improved by corrected exponents, but they would obviously have to be tissue specific and have to vary with dose per fraction used. Based on pig skin results TURESSON and NOTTER (1979c) have proposed such correction factors to the CRE values depending on fraction size, but the data base is too small to justify their values (HOPEWELL and GUNN 1981). A principal argument raised against the NSD formula concerns its very structure, i.e., the use of a power function for both fractionation and time dependence. The tolerance factor most directly associated

with time is repopulation. For late reacting tissues a proliferative response during treatment is questionable, while acutely reacting tissues will accelerate repopulation only after a lag period (see p. 55). In contrast to such a time course, the power function allots the same tolerance gain to an increase in treatment time from, for example, 2 to 4 days as to an increase from 20 to 40 days. The necessary adjustments in the formula would require the unreasonable task of further parametrization. As neither intracellular recovery nor time-dependent repopulation are adequately translated by a power function, the fitness of the empirical dose-time formulae must be questioned (PETERS and WITHERS 1981; FOWLER 1984; THAMES and HENDRY 1987).

2.10.1 Fractionation Response and Intracellular Repair

In contrast to the empirical formulae, modern approaches directly address defined biological processes associated with fractionation and treatment time, i.e., intracellular repair and repopulation. Consideration of these factors started soon after the experiments by PUCK and MARCUS (1956) that established survival curves of mammalian cells in vitro, and the demonstration of split-dose recovery by ELKIND and SUTTON (1960). Shortly thereafter FOWLER and STERN (1963) contrasted predictions based on split-dose recovery as demonstrable in vitro with experimental isoeffect curves. The main conclusion was that the multitarget cell survival curve with zero initial slope and

exponential tail was hard to reconcile with the
general shape of isoeffect curves derived for
tissues. In subsequent experimental and clinical
studies the opposite approach was chosen in that
isoeffective doses in vivo were used to reconstruct
the survival curve of the underlying target cells.

In an ingenious clinical experiment Dutreix et
al. (1973) used a dose-splitting protocol to quantitate intracellular recovery and its time course in
human skin. In 57 patients who underwent irradiation of cervical and inguinal lymph nodes with
palliative or curative intent, strictly symmetrical
fields were irradiated by *n* fractions in one field
and by *2n* fractions in the contralateral field (*n*
ranging from 1 to 8) over the same overall time;
intervals between the split fractions ranged from 2
to 24 h. When the incremental dose required by
fraction splitting (or recovered dose *D2–D1*) was
plotted as a function of dose per fraction, the
curve depicted in Fig. 2.13 resulted. It clearly
indicates that no additional recovery is obtained
once the dose per fraction is reduced to somewhere between 1 and 2 Gy. To obtain this
response the underlying cell survival curve must
have an exponential initial segment; within its
dose range subdividing the dose per fraction would
have no impact on the total dose required. As the
recovered dose with increasing dose fractions rises
in a sigmoid shape that seemingly saturates at the

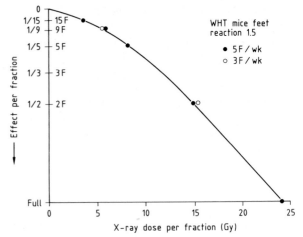

Fig. 2.14. A quasisurvival curve of the target cells responsible for early desquamation in mouse skin, reconstructed
from multifractionation data (redrawn with permission
from Fowler et al. 1974)

high dose end, consistent with an exponential tail,
the survival curve model proposed was a two-
component model combining an exponential and a
multitarget dose response. The time course of
repair assessed in the same study by giving 2 × 7.5
Gy within 2–24 h or 2 × 8.5 Gy within 6 h to 4
days indicated that "fast repair" was not complete
before 6 h; the longer intervals suggested a
possible maximum at 2 days that was lost at 4 days,
a fact that was best explained by redistribution. All results were based on acute responses
ranging from erythema to moist desquamation.

A similarly complex curve shape was derived
from experiments in the Gray laboratory using
early response of mouse foot skin (Fowler et al.
1974). Assuming that equal dose fractions produce
equal partial effect (when proliferation is excluded
by short overall times), the isoeffective doses were
converted into a so-called "quasi-survival curve,"
i.e., an unscaled dose–response curve that reflects
the relative response obtained with increasing
single dose (Fig. 2.14). The curve displayed an
initial and terminal exponential part separated by
a shoulder region, with a slope ratio of terminal
over initial slope of 2.5. The dose per fraction
at which fractionation saturated was lower than
2 Gy.

Following this deductive approach, Douglas
and Fowler (1976) presented a formal analysis of
fractionation data on desquamation in the mouse
foot that has led to a dose–relationship model now
widely accepted. The plot of reciprocal total dose

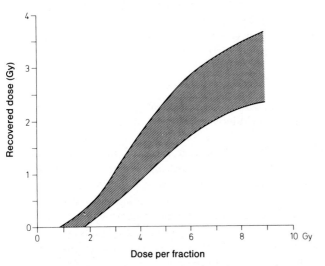

Fig. 2.13. Dependence of recovered dose on dose per
fraction, for early desquamation in human skin (Dutreix et
al. 1973). A dose-splitting technique was used (*n* vs *2n*
fractions) that allows direct comparison between small dose
fractions. Note the difference in shape from Fig. 2.10, where
all recovery increments are derived from comparing fractionated doses to the single dose

vs dose per fraction was shown to be well described by a linear curve down to the smallest dose per fraction of 1 Gy delivered with 64 fractions (Fig. 2.15). The linear relationship will be fulfilled when the survival curve follows a linear–quadratic dose relationship, where

$$sf = e(-\alpha d - \beta d^2) \tag{7}$$
$$\text{or } -\ln sf = (\alpha d + \beta d^2)n \tag{8}$$

where d is the fraction dose, n the number of fractions, and α and β are parameters of cellular sensitivity. The equation is easily transformed into the isoeffect relationship

$$1/D = \alpha/E + (\beta/E)\cdot d \tag{9}$$

where D is the total dose and E represents a defined biological effect assumed to be proportional to a fixed (though unknown) survival rate of the target cells. The linear–quadratic dose–response curve implies a component of irreparable damage linearly proportional to dose and a component that arises from the interaction of sublethal injury (quadratic term) and hence can be minimized by reducing the dose per fraction. Graphi-

cally such curves are continuously bending with a relative curvature defined by the single parameter α/β, which is sufficient to describe the fractionation response. This ratio, which has the dimension of a dose, is readily deduced from the isoeffect regression line by dividing the ordinate intercept at infinitely small doses (α/E) by the line slope (β/E). On statistical grounds more refined methods to calculate α/β and to test for fitness of the model have been proposed (TUCKER 1984), but its suitability for a large number of normal tissue endpoints has since been confirmed (THAMES and HENDRY 1987).

The remarkable finding from such analyses was that α/β values derived for early responses are systematically higher than those derived for late responses, indicating the greater relative importance of irreparable damage. For dry and moist desquamation in rodent skin, experimental α/β ratios were between 9 and 12 Gy (e.g., JOINER et al. 1983, 1984), in agreement with values of other acute tissue endpoints such as epilation, lip mucositis, and jejunal or colonic crypt survival (for a review see FOWLER 1984a; THAMES and HENDRY 1987). With regard to late damage in skin, experiments specifically designed to measure α/β ratios, i.e., including a large variety of fraction numbers or doses per fraction, have not been published; analysis of the available data has yielded values for late skin contraction of $0.3 < \alpha/\beta < 2.4$ Gy in the pig (WITHERS et al. 1978) and 4.6 Gy in the mouse (MASUDA et al. 1980). These values indicate a fractionation response similar to or slightly smaller than that of lung, kidney, or spinal cord (α/β ratios 1.6–4 Gy), and definitely greater than that of early skin damage.

The huge amount of material that has accrued from human postmastectomy radiotherapy studies reveals a similar difference. In a summarizing paper, based on a simultaneous analysis of 750 fields in 450 patients given one, two, or five fractions per week in the Gothenburg clinic trials since 1972, TURESSON and THAMES (1989) gave α/β values for early and late responses. For erythema and desquamation the best estimates were 7.5 and 11.2 Gy, respectively, for protocols that did not exceed treatment times of 4 weeks. Up to overall times as long as 6 weeks the α/β ratios unexpectedly rose to 18 and 34 Gy; this finding was tentatively explained either as reduced repair capacity or as a greater relative impact of redistribution in the daily fractionated arm, and so in either case was

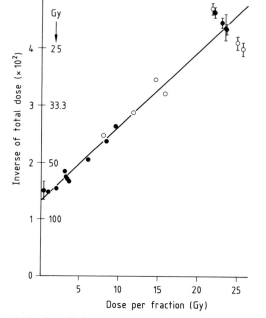

Fig. 2.15. So-called F_e plot of isoeffective doses for acute mouse skin response, evidencing a linear relationship between reciprocal total dose and dose per fraction (DOUGLAS and FOWLER 1976)

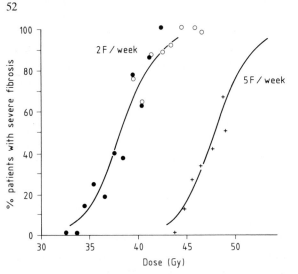

Fig. 2.16. Dose–response curves of subcutaneous fibrosis in postmastectomy patients treated by 2F/week or 5F/week protocols. Frequency of severe fibrosis is shown for supraclavicular (●) and axillary fields (o and +) as a function of dose at 4.1 mm depth. (Bentzen et al. 1987)

thought to arise as a consequence of accelerated proliferation. Evaluation of telangiectasia scores (distinct to severe levels) up to 5 years after therapy gave α/β ratios of between 2.8 and 4.3 Gy; surprisingly, a small but significant time factor became detectable when the model was expanded by a time-dependent term and this factor was held responsible for the higher α/β ratio quoted. From postmastectomy radiotherapy data, a large fractionation effect was derived by Bentzen et al. (1987) by contrasting regimes involving two fractions per week or five fractions per week (Fig. 2.16). The α/β ratios assessed for severe fibrosis ranged from 1.4 to 2.1 Gy, depending on the depth dose level considered; erythema and desquamation response conformed with an α/β of 12.3 Gy, albeit with large confidence limits due to their low incidence.

A question of practical importance is to what degree the linear–quadratic model can be used in routine clinical practice instead of the conventional time–dose formulae. Its application has been recommended for situations where planned treatment changes will not alter repopulation to a great extent and where the α/β ratio of the critical tissue is reasonably well known. In this case a new total dose or fraction number or dose per fraction can readily be calculated (Withers et al. 1984). Equating the effect of the new and the old treatment (see Eq. (8)) transforms to

$$D_1/D_2 = (d_2 + \alpha/\beta)/(d_1 + \alpha/\beta) \qquad (10)$$

where $D_{1,2}$ and $d_{1,2}$ are the total dose and dose per fraction of the new and the old protocol, respectively.

The finding that late-reacting normal tissues have greater split-dose recovery but less repopulation than tumors has stimulated unconventional protocols of accelerated hyperfractionation, where multiple small dose fractions are given per day. For the difference in repair capacity to be exploited it is crucial that the interfraction intervals are sufficiently long to allow for virtually complete repair. Severe skin fibrosis (among other more life-threatening sequelae) was reported after hyperfractionated irradiation of cervical nodes with 8×0.9 Gy per day over 5 successive days followed by a 2- or 4-week interval and another 5 treatment days (Nguyen et al. 1985); the protocol was slightly altered subsequently but an interfraction interval of only 2 h was maintained (Nguyen et al. 1988) and the rate of complications was still unacceptably high. Quantitative assessment of repair kinetics is difficult even from experimental data and it is as yet unclear whether the time course can be described by a single exponential component or whether it requires a more complex model (Thames and Hendry 1987; Hopewell and Van Den Aardweg 1988; Rojas et al. 1989). The apparent half-time of repair for acute skin desquamation in the mouse is about 1.3 h (Rojas et al. 1989). A half-time of ca. 1.5 h can be derived from data on pig skin erythema provided by Hopewell and Van Den Aardweg (1988), although the authors themselves favor a biexponential response with half-times of 15 min and 2.5 h, respectively. In their comprehensive analysis of postmastectomy radiotherapy data, Turesson and Thames (1989) also find evidence of a fast component ($T_{1/2}$ between 0.3 and -0.4 h) and a slow component ($T_{1/2}$ of 1.2 h for erythema/desquamation and 3.5 h for telangiectasia).

Despite the considerable uncertainty with regard to both half-times and model, current recommendations are to maintain interfraction intervals of at least 6 h, even between small dose fractions. It should be stressed that even for identical repair rates the amount of residual sublethal damage — and hence its interaction with a new dose fraction — will always be relatively greater in late-reacting tissue than in tumors, as is reflected in the relation of α to β. If the main rationale of hyperfractionation is a relative increase in late effect tolerance, inadequate fraction intervals that result in incomplete repair are counterproductive.

2.10.2 Effect of Low Dose Rate on Skin Tolerance

Percutaneous teletherapy by low dose rate (LDR) irradiation is a very old treatment modality. It was popularized by COUTARD in the 1920s as "protracted fractionated" irradiation and was the first modality to succeed in curing deepseated tumors (THAMES and HENDRY 1987). It was still practiced in the 1940s by ZUPPINGER (1941, 1949) with demonstrably good tolerance of skin for both acute and late effects. As was recognized quite early, the sparing effects of fractionation and LDR are not independent; for skin erythema WITTE (1942) demonstrated quite clearly that the fractionation effect declines and eventually disappears when the dose rate is lowered from 300 R/min down to 2 or 1 R/min, and vice versa. Similar experiences had been gathered in some clinical centers in the 1930s, i.e., it had been found that splitting the dose into small high dose rate (HDR) fractions rendered the same tolerance as COUTARD's technique (PAPE 1933; MACWHIRTER 1935; BORAK 1937; SCHINZ 1937). A compilation of the older literature has been given by HUG et al. (1966).

Conclusions regarding isoeffectiveness, i.e., the dependence of skin tolerance on dose rate and thus on treatment duration, were derived for continuous LDR irradiation, both from clinical studies (MITCHELL 1960; PATERSON 1963; ELLIS 1962) and from experiments on pig skin (ATKINS et al. 1972). Over a range of dose rates from 2.5 to 0.3 Gy/h the relationship between log tolerance dose and log exposure time is nearly linear, i.e., approximated by a power function, with exponents to exposure time of between 0.25 and 0.30. At either end of the range the curve must flatten out for theoretical reasons; the animal data indicate that this happens at levels around 10–40 Gy/h and 0.3 Gy/h, respectively (ATKINS et al. 1972; BAKER and LEITH 1977). All these data relate to early skin responses.

This exposure time exponent was incorporated in the CRE formula by KIRK et al. (1972, 1975) to define a normalized isoeffective skin dose CRE_c as

$$CRE_c = k \times D \times T^{-0.29}, \quad (11)$$

where D is the total dose and k is a constant normalizing factor of 0.80 introduced to ensure equivalence to the same CRE value delivered by HDR fractionated irradiation. TURESSON and NOTTER (1979a) have tested the validity of this constant in pig experiments using ^{137}Cs brachytherapy for both modalities. For the medium-term reaction (late erythema indicating prenecrotic damage level) the actual normalizing factor assessed was 0.57, which was markedly lower than that proposed by KIRK et al. In the same study a factor of 0.59 was derived for acute erythema. Using a factor of 0.80 would result in almost 40% overdosing when continuous LDR treatment is replaced, e.g., by hypofractionated HDR afterloading treatment.

A more analytical approach to equate continuous LDR and fractionated HDR irradiation was used by LIVERSAGE (1969). Building on the assumption that tissue-specific repair (proceeding at a constant rate) was expressed in the response to either modality, he derived a formula that allows calculation of the number of HDR fractions into which a given LDR dose has to be split to be isoeffective; for extrapolation to more practicable fraction numbers one then has to resort to empirical formulae. The longer treatment time that is inevitably required for complete recovery during multifractionated irradiation is accounted for by a dose correction of 0.25 Gy per day, to counteract repopulation. Although this correction and the assumed half-time of repair of 1.5 h both imply considerable uncertainty, the predictive value of the formula appeared to be quite good. In TURESSON and NOTTER's pig skin study (1979a), for example, the deviation from the experimental data was less than 10%. The formula was also tested in rat skin by KAL and SISSINGH (1974), who quantified the late contraction of preirradiated free skin grafts. The discrepancy was again within 10%, but the single dose HDR irradiation used necessitated large extrapolation.

The major biological factors that govern tissue response to LDR irradiation are repair of sublethal damage and changes in the distribution of cells in the various phases of the cell cycle. LDR irradiation can be more effective than acute irradiation in inducing a G2 block, with a concomitant increase in cellular radiosensitivity (MITCHELL et al. 1979). This effect pertains only to proliferating cells and hence should play a role only for acute effects. The impact may be relatively small, however, as even in rodent or pig skin the basal cells have intermitotic times of 4–6 days unless proliferation has been stimulated. There is no study that unequivocally demonstrates the effect of altered distribution.

In contrast to this, skin responses to LDR and HDR single dose or fractionated irradiation have been modeled quite consistently by mathematical approaches that consider only repair. As described in the preceding section, a constant repair rate independent of exposure conditions is most often assumed. One such attempt is Liversage's formula (see above). Along similar lines, Henkelman et al. (1980) analyzed acute responses of mouse foot to fractionated irradiation (dose rates 0.06–1.6 Gy/min) and calculated a half-time of repair of about 1.3 h that fitted all data well. The mathematical approach of Thames (1985) also allows repair parameters to be derived, including half-time from continuous or fractionated LDR irradiation.

2.10.3 Effect of Treatment Time on Skin Tolerance

The term "time factor" was originally introduced to denote any change in radiosensitivity (or effective radiation dose) that was observed when irradiation was spread out in time. After delineating the effect of fractionation itself, the impact of treatment time per se has to be reconsidered. Clinical data that lend themselves to a formal analysis of this parameter are scarce. In 1941 Zuppinger published a curve that for the late effects under consideration (telangiectasia) showed considerably greater recovery at longer treatment times than had previously been reported by Reisner (1933). However, this can also be explained by the smaller dose fractions that were associated with prolonged treatment. The considerable amount of work done to test the validity of the NSD formula concentrated on the importance of fraction number and therefore treatment time was often deliberately kept constant. As an exception, Durrant et al. (1977) compared the effect of a normalized dose of 1730 rets given in five fractions over 4, 10, or 28 days on acute responses in skin surrounding basaliomas. Protraction from 10 to 28 days resulted in a higher incidence of moist desquamation than predicted by a T exponent of 0.11. Similarly, for late contraction in pig skin the time exponent to equate 14 fractions in 18 or 39 days was definitely negative (Hopewell et al. 1979). Using medium-term

erythema the same group later reported some increase in tolerance with time between two fractions when the interval exceeded 28 days (van den Aardweg et al. 1988). In a recent analysis of the postmastectomy irradiation material from the Gothenburg clinic, Turesson and Thames (1989) computed a small sparing effect of treatment time for telangiectasia but no such effect for severe erythema, for overall treatment times between 3 and 6 weeks. This is difficult to interpret because unquestionable and long-standing clinical experience has proven that acute responses can readily be avoided by treatment protraction (Zuppinger 1941).

While the importance of treatment time for late skin effects is biologically unclear, acute responses (apart from early erythema) have long been recognized to be due to epithelial cell depletion caused by the inactivation of basal cells and the resulting lack of cell supply (see e.g. Strandqvist 1944). Rodent and pig skin studies have provided insight into the pattern of depletion and compensatory proliferation (for a review see Potten 1985). The typical reaction of renewal tissues to enhanced cell loss is an attempt to increase cell production. The signals that elicit such a reaction have not themselves been identified, but cell depletion in the functional compartment or the basal layer itself may act as the proper stimulus (pp. 38). As the life span of the differentiated layers is probably unaltered, and also because epidermal cell production is maintained for some time during fractionated and after single dose irradiation, critical levels of depletion are reached after a delay. This explains why both functional measurements and cell kinetic studies have demonstrated a biphasic time pattern of regeneration, with acceleration setting in after a time lag that is related to, but not identical with, the normal tissue turnover time.

In an extensive study into the dose–time relationship of acute skin response in rat foot, Moulder et al. (1975) and Moulder and Fischer (1976) clearly demonstrated these principles. In essence, schedules consisting of 3F/week, 5F/week, and 10F delivered in 9–63 days were compared. The dose–response curves of the ED_{50} doses required to produce partial denudation as a function of fraction number (and hence also of time) are shown in Fig. 2.17. Their initial convex shape is well explained by the increase in split-dose recovery as fraction number increases. The subsequent rise, occurring after 7F or 14 days in the 3F/week regime and 16F or 21 days in the 5F/week regime, indicates accelerated repopulation after well-defined lag periods. By comparing suitable data points the dose equivalent of repopulation can immediately be read off and, as demonstrated in Fig. 2.17, no less than 2.4 fractions of 4.25 Gy per week in the 3F/week protocol are compensated by regeneration. There is quite a lot of flexibility in this response, as discontinuous fractionation, i.e., 10 × 5.5 Gy in 3 days given at the beginning and end of a 4-week treatment period, seemed to elicit more repopulation than the same number of fractions spread out evenly (ANG et al. 1984).

In mouse skin DENEKAMP (1973) studied repopulation initiated by "clinical fractionation" with daily 3 Gy fractions given over 1, 2, or 3 weeks. Single top-up doses were delivered at intervals from zero to 14 days after the last 3 Gy fraction to measure repopulation. Accelerated repopulation first became detectable after nine fractions and it definitely further increased after 3 weeks, the daily dose equivalents or "repopulated doses" being 0.3–0.5 Gy. Using survival curves of epidermal stem cells in vivo (WITHERS 1967; EMERY et al. 1970), such dose increments can be converted to effective cell doublings. Following nine fractions the doubling rate was thus 0.52 extra doublings per day, increasing to 0.93 after 14

fractions or 3 weeks. This reflects a drastic shortening of the basal cell turnover time. While in normal mouse foot epidermis it is approximately 3–4 days, in the stimulated state it must have dropped to below 1 day after 3 weeks of fractionation, assuming that at least some natural attrition continues in irradiated epidermis. This estimate is backed by cell kinetic studies using continuous ^{3}H-TdR infusion, in which a shortening of basal cell turnover time from 111 h to 24 h was measured (DENEKAMP et al. 1976). In mouse skin stimulated by hair plucking, WITHERS (1967) measured an *effective* doubling time of 22 h and on the basis of the difference from the basal cell cycle time of 16 h concluded that 25% of the repopulating stem cells must have entered differentiation

Pig skin studies yielded similar results. In split-dose experiments VAN DEN AARDWEG et al. (1988) found no difference in total effective dose for time intervals between 1 and 14 days, while longer intervals (up to 63 days) necessitated dose increments equivalent to a daily repopulated dose of 0.74 Gy.

This increase in effective regeneration may be compared to changes in cell kinetics determined in the same pig strain. MORRIS and HOPEWELL (1988) found that after single doses of 15 and 20 Gy, a transitory depression in basal cell labeling index (LI) occurred, followed by an overshoot beyond the control LI of 7.5% after 2 weeks to reach a peak value of 20% after 4 weeks that subsequently declined but had not returned to control values at 8 weeks. During continuous fractionation over 6 weeks at daily doses between 1.74 and 2.67 Gy the LI also exceeded the control level after 2 weeks but subsequently rose more slowly to a peak value of around 20% by the end of treatment (MORRIS and HOPEWELL 1986) (Fig. 2.2). The average doubling times calculated for the basal cell population as a whole during the period of elevated LI were between one-half and two-thirds of control epithelium and would not fully explain the functional repopulation rate after or during treatment, but considerably shorter times were derived for microcolonies that became visible 3 weeks after single dose treatment or by the end of continuously fractionated treatment. This finding illustrates the general difficulty in correlating functional data and cell kinetic measurements in irradiated tissues where the great majority of the cells present are doomed. The doubling time separately derived for the microcolonies was 16–22 h, in accordance with

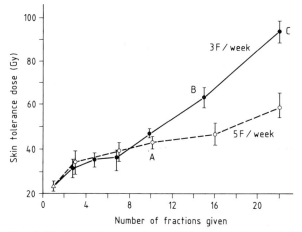

Fig. 2.17. Skin tolerance doses (ED$_{50}$ doses for partial desquamation in rat foot) for fractionation protocols delivering 3F/week (●) or 5F/week (o). Accelerated repopulation starts after 7F/14 days; its dose equivalent is best derived from comparing dose points A, B, and C, which all utilize a fraction size of 4.25 ± 0.05 Gy, to a total of 10F/11 or 15 days (A), 15F/32 days (B), and 22F/49 days (C). (Modified from MOULDER and FISCHER 1976)

a value of 20 h in basal cell colonies of Yorkshire pig epidermis (ARCHAMBEAU et al. 1979) and values of 25 h and 22 h obtained from colony growth measurements (AL-BARWARI and POTTEN 1976) or from functional measurements in irradiated plucked mouse skin (WITHERS 1967).

Particularly in pig skin attempts have been made to correlate radiation-induced repopulation or cell kinetics with morphological changes, in the search for a better understanding of how the homeostatic control is effected. Independent of the irradiation schedule, repopulation began to accelerate when extensive though by no means near-complete cell depletion in the basal layer had become manifest, i.e., when cellularity had dropped to values below 70% (Fig. 2.2) (MORRIS and HOPEWELL 1986, 1988) or below 50% (ARCHAMBEAU et al. 1988). In all these instances a near maximal repopulation rate was attained before tissue injury had developed into complete denudation.

2.10.4 Tolerance of Skin to Reirradiation

In many cases a second course of radiotherapy is the only treatment option when a tumor recurs after definitive local or regional irradiation. This may happen after disease-free intervals of between half a year and several years. Of major concern then is the dose level to which the normal tissues, and more specifically skin, can safely be treated.

There is no clear picture yet to what degree residual tolerance depends on the time interval or on the effective dose that was given in the first course. A modification of the NSD formula was proposed by ELLIS (1969) to calculate the effective dose (in rets) remaining after an interval G:

$$P' = P \left(T/(T + G) \right)^{0.11} \qquad (12)$$

The formula suggests that the biological damage (expressed as rets) decays with the same time exponent as used for a continuous course. This long-term recovery was somewhat arbitrarily supposed to terminate after 100 days, so that for longer intervals residual tolerance would become $P' = P \left(T/(T + 100) \right)^{0.11}$. In this case treatment duration of the first course will formally be the dominating factor, an assumption that has no biological or clinical basis.

Although the situation of retreatment must arise very often, clinical data on skin tolerance are scarce. HUNTER and STEWART (1977) studied 20 patients who underwent ^{60}Co treatment for squamous cell carcinoma of the upper aerodigestive tract some 5-15 years after irradiation for thyrotoxicosis. Although the majority presented with marked skin changes from the first course and the specified skin retreatment doses came close to tolerance levels, the early reactions were normal and no late sequelae occurred within a 4-year follow-up period. Similarly, SKOLYSZEWSKI et al. (1980) found acceptable tolerance in 20 patients retreated for recurrent head and neck tumor 6 months to 8 years after a full course of ^{60}Co therapy. Severe late sequelae (necrosis) were noted in four patients, all retreated with 50 Gy or more by conventional fractionation. LANGLOIS et al. (1985) have stressed the need to give 60 Gy or more for curative retreatment of head and neck carcinoma, and 16 out of their 35 patients received total doses greater than 120 Gy. Acute reactions were found to be normal; delayed necrosis was frequent (8/35 patients) but allegedly mostly due to tumor lysis. As mentioned by the authors, the short average survival in this patient group may have masked the true risk of late sequelae. However, favorable results in retreatment of nasopharyngeal carcinoma were reported by YAN et al. (1983), who, in 85 patients followed over more than 5 years, observed subcutaneous fibrosis in 16% as compared with 9% after a single course.

Two studies report complication rates associated with reirradiation of recurrent head and neck tumors with fast neutrons. ERRINGTON and CATTERALL (1986) studied 28 patients of whom 22 received a full neutron course of 15.6 Gy/12 F/26 days 1-24 months after first treatment. Necrosis occurred in 13 patients within 2 years after therapy, but considering the high frequency of cutaneous tumor infiltration (17/28 patients) and the large proportion of patients who had undergone additional surgical treatment and/or chemotherapy the authors claim that the complication rate was not greater than would have been expected from photon retreatment. The results reported by SKOLYSZEWSKI and KORZENIOWSKI (1988) regarding 20 similar cases of advanced head and neck cancers in relapse are less conclusive as only five patients received full retreatment, resulting in one case of limited skin necrosis.

Several experimental studies have been done to define residual tolerance and the biological parameters of interest. DENEKAMP (1975) studied the acute response of mouse foot skin to single and split test doses given 5–8 months after x-rays (10–30 Gy) or neutrons (9 Gy). The "remembered dose," quantified by the dose reduction necessary to give a fixed skin response, was as small as 10%; split-dose recovery was normal. In the same system BROWN and PROBERT (1975) found that the damage persisting 1–10 months after 10 × 3 Gy/11 days was almost nil, while after 10 × 5 Gy the required dose reduction was 21% after 1 month, subsiding to 9% after 10 months. Evaluation of late foot deformity in the same experiments (BROWN and PROBERT 1973, 1975) showed an alarmingly high level of persistence of latent damage, dependent on the priming dose and interval. While following 10 × 3 Gy residual damage was 21% after 1 month and then slightly decreased up to 8 months, following initial treatment with 10 × 5 Gy it was as high as 32% and even increased to somewhere between 36% and 50% over the same subsequent period. MASUDA et al. (1986) investigated early and late skin response in the mouse leg to a great variety of priming and challenging protocols, including single dose and multifractionated irradiation, with an interval between courses of 12 months. There was a tendency for acute reactions to set in earlier and to persist longer in preirradiated skin, but sensitivity as measured by peak reactions or mean scores (averaged over days 10–30) was lower than in agematched controls; a further unexpected finding was that in the challenging treatment the sparing effect of fractionation was extremely small (i.e., represented by a slope of 0.07). Leg contraction, taken as the late endpoint in this study, showed a complex response. When defining residual damage by the *net* response to secondary treatment, skin with persisting shrinkage from the initial treatment was seemingly more resistant even if the notable age-related decline in sensitivity was accounted for. However, this may simply reflect a reduced ability of preshrunk skin to respond, and may be misleading. When evaluating the total response as a function of test treatment it appears that skin pretreated to low damage (contraction prior to second course <10%) responded normally, while more effective pretreatment (contraction >10%) resulted in considerably enhanced contraction. In a recent reevaluation of these date, JINGU et al. (1989) gave explicit estimates of "remembered dose" that underline these conclusions. In agreement with the results of BROWN and PROBERT and MASUDA et al., more recently WONDERGEM and HAVEMAN (1987) found that in mouse foot residual

injury was greater for deformity than for acute skin response, as expressed by necessary dose reductions between 3% and 26% for desquamation and between 3% and 54% for severe deformity. Retreatment by heat (e.g., 90 min/44°C) revealed even more latent injury, while heat as a primary treatment was more readily "forgotten." Using radiation-induced necrosis of rat and mouse tail as the endpoint, HENDRY et al. (1977), and HENDRY (1978) assessed the necessary dose reduction to be about 10% in animals that 6 months earlier had not responded to fractionated x-ray or neutron doses around the 50% incidence dose level; a large variation of intervals from 6 weeks to 10 months was tested in the mouse experiments and found to have no influence. This system also allows measurement of basal cell survival by means of a macrocolony assay (HENDRY 1984), and in a later publication CHEN and HENDRY (1988) compared cellular radiosensitivity and overt tail necrosis; the dose reduction was similar in both endpoints and although an increase in cellular radiosensitivity cannot be excluded, the data are more likely explained by a reduction in clonogen number in preirradiated tail skin.

In summary, most studies suggest that damage responsible for early effects can be virtually eliminated in intervals of a few months. Biologically this is well explained by the great potential of the target cells, i.e., basal stem cells, to repopulate the epidermis. The issue is less clear for late damage, where results are more contradictory and the biology is still poorly understood. Some studies suggest that a first treatment course well within tolerance does not reduce tolerance to reirradiation, while others find quite large proportions of remembered though latent injury. Additional ambiguity is introduced by differences in study design that make it difficult to translate "remembered dose" into "remembered injury." For example, when test treatment is by single doses, a reduction specified as percent dose relates to the most effective (steepest) portion of the underlying dose–response curve. As a consequence the dose reduction factor *underestimates* residual injury. This is in contrast to the clinical situation, where dose reduction will usually be achieved through a *smaller number of equal dose fractions*, and thus be proportional to residual damage.

2.11 Skin Reaction to Densely Ionizing Radiations

During and after radiotherapy with fast neutrons, the skin reaction develops a similar clinical picture, following a similar time course, as during and after radiotherapy with x-rays or γ-rays provided the treatment time is similar. Qualitatively, densely ionizing radiations appear to be similar to sparsely ionizing radiations, yet quantitatively they differ and their relative biological effectiveness (RBE) is higher. The abundant data from animal experiments on acute skin reactions after fast neutron irradiation with single and fractionated doses have been summarized by Field (1976).

The data demonstrate a pronounced dependence of the RBE on the dose per fraction (Fig. 2.18). From these experiments in rodents and pigs (Bewley et al. 1963, 1967), formulas were developed for fast neutron radiotherapy in analogy to the NSD formula, maintaining the relative importance of the exponent of time but significantly reducing the exponent for the number of fractions (Field 1972, 1976). These formulas allowed matching of the acute skin reactions of patients treated with photons or fast neutrons; however, despite identical acute skin reactions, late skin injury such as atrophy and fibrosis was more severe in the neutron-treated patients. This was first seen in the series of patients treated in 1938 with fast neutrons in Berkeley (Sheline et al. 1971). Experiments in pigs (Withers et al. 1977,

1978b) using clinically relevant fractionation schedules yielded very similar results, which explained the disastrous outcome of the first neutron trial in 1938. Whereas for the acute skin reaction a 2 Gy dose fraction was equivalent to 0.75 Gy neutrons (giving an RBE of 2.7), this was less than the 0.65 Gy neutron dose for the chronic skin reaction, giving an RBE of more than 3.1. This means that if doses in fractionated radiotherapy with fast neutrons are scheduled to give the same acute skin reaction as with photons, an effective overdosage of about 20% will result for those tissues that lead to chronic skin damage. The higher RBE with regard to chronic as opposed to acute skin reactions is a direct consequence of the greater fractionation sensitivity (lower α/β value) of chronic radiation injury to low LET radiations as compared with acute radiation injury, whereas for neutrons this difference is very much reduced at clinically relevant doses per fraction.

Recently, the effects of pi-mesons on the skin of mice, pigs, and humans have been studied in preparation for the clinical application of pi-mesons in the treatment of various cancers. In mice, the acute moist desquamation after 1–20 fractions of x-rays and pi-mesons was compared (Raju et al. 1981; Chaplin et al. 1987). As with neutrons, the RBE increased as the dose per fraction was decreased; however, this effect was much less pronounced than with neutrons. Even at the lowest dose fraction studied, i.e., about 2 Gy pi-mesons, the RBE did not exceed 1.5. Since this is also the ratio of the α/β values in the linear

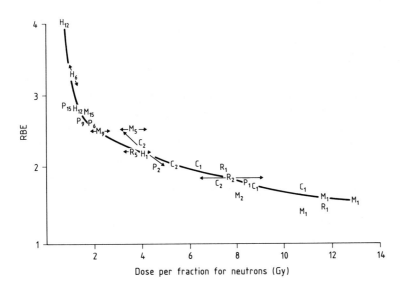

Fig. 2.18. The RBE for skin damage as a function of dose per fraction for neutrons produced by 16 MeV deuterons on beryllium, compiled by Field (1976). *H*, human; *P*, pig; *M*, mouse; *R* rat; *C* done counts in mouse skin

quadratic analysis, one would not expect any further increase with even lower dose fractions.

This value of a clinically applicable RBE of 1.5 for pi-mesons (in the peak region) was corroborated in studies with pigs (DOUGLAS et al. 1986) and also in two patients in whom the acute skin reactions after 13 fractions of pi-mesons or 100 kV x-rays given in 2 weeks to multiple skin nodules of breast cancer were compared (KLIGERMAN et al. 1977), an RBE of 1.44 being derived for pi-meson doses of less than 2 Gy. In the pig skin study (DOUGLAS et al. 1986) the same scoring system was used to quantitate the acute epidermal (4–8 weeks) and the "late dermal" (12–18 weeks) skin reaction, which is different to the criteria used in other pig skin experiments. A considerable spread of RBE values for individual animals both for the early and for the late reactions was obtained, with a mean of 1.5 at pi-meson dose fractions of 2.5–3.5 Gy. There was, in contrast to the data obtained for neutrons (WITHERS et al. 1978), no significant increase in RBE for late dermal damage as compared with that for early erythema and desquamation.

2.12 Radiation Response of Skin Grafts

There has been much controversy regarding the radiosensitivity of skin grafts. Pronounced differences occur in the reaction to radiation between normal and grafted skin sites. RUBIN and GRISE (1960) demonstrated greater radiosensitivity of skin grafts within the first 3 months after grafting; however, CRAM et al. (1958) did not see any increased response in split-skin grafts even as early as 4 days after grafting. Since no systematic clinical study on the radiation response of human skin grafts is available, the discussion concentrates on the results of two large experiments on the radiation response of full-thickness grafts and split-thickness grafts in pigs.

GRISE et al. (1960) drew the following conclusions from their study in two strains of pigs:

1. Fresh grafts tend to react to ionizing irradiation more vigorously and earlier than normal skin, and they recover more slowly.
2. Split-thickness grafts tend to react less vigorously than full-thickness grafts.

The variability of response of the graft is related to differences in the vascularization of grafted skin and normal skin. Therefore the greatest reaction in the graft is elicited by irradiation during the stage of vascularization, with excessive capillary sprouting and ingrowth of vessels. On the other hand, irradiation during the stage of cicatrization usually evokes no response in the graft, since vascularization is less than that in normal skin. If a reaction is elicited, the decreased vasculature may sufficiently compromise recovery that necrosis may ensue (RUBIN and CASARETT 1968).

In the study of YOUNG and HOPEWELL (1983) the clinically observed skin reaction in a split-skin graft was correlated to functional measurements of blood perfusion in the graft. Enhanced perfusion was measured for several months after revascularization of the graft had been completed, but irradiation in the 3rd week with single doses of 18–23 Gy resulted in a decreased acute skin reaction, less necrosis, and better blood perfusion as compared with normal skin.

In a separate experiment, the take rate of split-skin grafts grafted on a dermis which had been preirradiated 8 months previously with single doses between 18 and 23 Gy was investigated and a normal course of revascularization was observed. A second radiation dose to this graft 3 weeks later again did not lead to an enhanced acute skin reaction or necrosis during a follow-up period of 6 months.

Of special interest are studies by PATTERSON et al. (1972, 1975) on the viability of pedicled skin flaps in the flank of pigs which were mobilized and immediately afterwards sutured in again. If radiation doses which were just around the tolerance limit (e.g., an 18.8 Gy single dose or 38 Gy in six fractions in 18 days or 61 Gy in 30 fractions in 39 days) were given immediately before surgery, the surviving flap length was 10 cm of the original 16 cm. However, if the interval between irradiation and surgery was increased, the length of the surviving skin flap was reduced. Surgery 6 weeks after irradiation resulted in necrosis of more than two-thirds of the mobilized flap. No significant recovery was observed if the interval was further prolonged, although, before surgery, the skin showed normal blood perfusion 1–2 years after radiation.

Although the skin can maintain a normal blood perfusion the irradiated dermal vasculature has a permanently reduced capacity to respond to trauma. This is in agreement with clinical experience that late "radiation necrosis" of the skin is most often the consequence of secondary trauma to the chronically atrophic skin.

2.13 Influence of Chemotherapy on the Radiation Response of Skin

The acute skin reaction may be considerably increased by the simultaneous application of various cytostatic agents and irradiation. This has been demonstrated in experiments on mouse skin (Guigon et al. 1978; Redpath and Colman 1979; Von Der Maase 1986) and in numerous clinical reports which were summarized by Muggia et al. (1978) and by Phillips (1980). Increased acute skin reactions were observed especially if chemotherapy using actinomycin D, adriamycin, bleomycin, fluorouracil, and methotrexate was given during the course of radiotherapy. Most pronounced was the effect of actinomycin D, which may reduce acute skin tolerance in patients by as much as 50%. The increased tendency to develop an enhanced acute skin response may persist for many months after chemotherapy with actinomycin D, whereas the sensitizing effect of adriamycin disappears after an interval of about 1 week (Aristizabal et al. 1977). There is no convincing evidence that chronic skin reactions may be increased by the combination of chemotherapy and radiotherapy.

Actinomycin D (and to a lesser degree other cytostatic drugs) has been reported to elicit a peculiar effect when the drug is given some weeks or months after radiotherapy (i.e., when the acute response has completely cleared away) in that it may "recall" the acute radiation dermatitis, which remains limited to the irradiation field (D'Angio et al. 1959). The mechanism of this recall phenomenon is not known.

References

Al-Barwari SE, Potten CS (1976) Regeneration and dose-response characteristics of irradiated mouse dorsal epidermal cells. Int J Radiat Biol 30: 201–216
Al-Soufi A, Lemperle G, Exner K (1986) Plastic surgical procedures for the closure of radiation ulcers of the thoracic and pelvic regions. Br J Radiol [Suppl 19]: 134–137
Ang KK, Landuyt W, Riunders B, Van Der Schueren E (1984) Differences in repopulation kinetics in mouse skin during split course multiple fractions per day (MFD) or daily fractionated irradiations. Int J Radiat Oncol Biol Phys 10: 95–99
Arcangeli G, Friedman M, Paoluzi R (1974) A quantitative study of late radiation effect on human skin and subcutaneous tissues in human beings. Br J Radiol 47: 44–50
Archambeau JO, Bennett GW, Abata JJ, Brenneis HJ (1979) Response of swine skin to acute single exposures of x-rays: quantification of the epidermal cell changes. Radiat Res 79: 298–337
Archambeau JO, Hauser D, Shymko RM (1988) Swine basal cell proliferation during a course of daily irradiation, five days a week for six weeks (6000 rad). Int J Radiat Oncol Biol Phys 15: 1383–1388
Aristizabal SA, Miller RC, Schlichtemeier AL, Jones SE, Boone ML (1977) Adriamycin irradiation: cutaneous complications. Int J Radiat Oncol Biol Phys 2: 325–331
Arlett CF, Cole J, Green MHL (1989) Radiosensitive individuals in the population. In: Low Dose Radiation, Taylor and Francis, London
Atkins HL, Fairchild RG, Robertson JS (1972) Dose-rate effects on RBE of californium and radium reactions in pig skin. Radiology 103: 439–442
Baker DG, Leith JL (1977) Effect of dose rate on production of early and late radiation damage in mouse skin. Int J Radiat Oncol Biol Phys 2: 69–7
Bates TD (1975) A prospective clinical trial of post-operative radiotherapy delivered in three fractions per week versus two fractions per week in breast carcinoma. Clin Radiol 26: 297–304
Bates TD, Peters LJ (1975) Dangers of the clinical use of the NSD formula for small fraction numbers. Br J Radiol 48: 773
Bentzen SM, Christensen JJ, Overgaard J, Overgaard M (1987) Some methodological problems in estimating radiobiological parameters from clinical data. Acta Oncol 27: 105–116
Berry RJ, Wiernik G, Patterson TJS (1974a) Skin tolerance to fractionated x-irradiation in the pig — how good a predictor is the NSD formula? Br J Radiol 47: 185–190
Berry RJ, Wiernik G, Patterson TJS, Hopewell JW (1974b) Excess late cutaneous fibrosis after irradiation of pig skin, consequent upon the application of the NSD formula. Br J Radiol 47: 277–281
Bewley DK, Fowler J, Morgan RI, Silvester JL, Turner BA (1963) Experiments on the skin of pigs with fast neutrons and 8 MeV x-rays, including some effects of dose fractionation. Br J Radiol 36: 107–115
Bewley DK, Field SB, Morgan RL, Page BC, Parnell CJ (1967) The response of pig skin to fractionated treatments with fast neutrons and x-rays. Br J Radiol 40: 745–770
Birkner R, Hoffmann B (1961) Unterhautindurationen nach Telekobalttherapie. Strahlentherapie 116: 463–477
Borak J (1936) The radiation biology of the cutaneous glands. Radiology 27: 651–655
Borak J (1937) Spätergebnisse der fraktionierten Langbestrahlungsmethode. Strahlentherapie 58: 585–594
Brennan D, Young CMA, Hopewell JW, Wiernik G (1976) The effects of varied numbers of dose fractions on the tolerance of normal human skin. Clin Radiol 27: 27–32
Brown JM, Probert JC (1973) Long-term recovery of connective tissue after irradiation. Radiology 108: 205–207
Brown JM, Probert JC (1975) Early and late radiation changes following a second course of irradiation. Radiology 115: 711–716

Chaplin DJ, Douglas BG, Gruslkey W, Skarsgard LD, Lam G, Denekamp J (1987) The response of mouse epidermis to fractionated doses of π-mesons. Int J Radiat Oncol Biol Phys 13: 1199–1208

Chen F, Hendry JH (1988) Re-irradiation of mouse skin: similarity of dose reductions for healing and macrocolony endpoints. Radiother Oncol 11: 153–159

Choi CH, Suit HD (1975) Evaluation of rapid radiation treatment schedules utilizing two treatment sessions per day. Radiology 116: 703–707

Chu FCH, Conrad JT, Glicksman AS, Nickson JJ (1960) Quantitative and qualitative evaluation of skin erythema. I. Technic of measurement and description of the reaction. Radiology 75: 406–415

Chu FCH, Glicksman AS, Nickson JJ (1970) Late consequences of early skin reactions. Radiology 94: 669–672

Coggle, JE, Hansen, LS, Wells, I, Charles, MW (1984) Nonstochastic effects of different energy β emitters on the mouse skin. Radiat, Res 99: 336–345

Cohen L (1949a) Clinical radiation dosage. Br J Radiol 22: 160–163

Cohen L (1949b) Clinical radiation dosage. II. Interrelation of time, area and therapeutic ratio. Br J Radiol 22: 706–713

Cohen L, Scott MJ (1968) Fractionation procedures in radiation therapy: a computerised approach to evaluation. Br J Radiol 41: 529–533

Cohen L, Ubaldi SE (1977) Dose time relationships for post-irradiation cutaneous telangiectasia. Int J Radiat Oncol Biol Phys 2: 421–426

Cottier H (1966) Histopathologie der Wirkung ionisierender Strahlen auf höhere Organismen (Tier und Mensch). In: Zuppinger A (ed) Strahlenbiologie 2. Springer, Berlin Heidelberg New York (Handbuch der medizinischen Radiologie, Vol II/2, pp 35–272)

Coutard H (1932) Roentgentherapy of epitheliomas of the tonsillar region, hypopharynx and larynx from 1920 to 1929. AJR 103: 313–331, 343–348

Cram RW, Weder CH, Watson TA (1958) Tolerance of skin grafts to radiation; study of postmastectomy irradiated grafts. Ann Surg 149: 65–67

D'Angio GJ, Farber S, Maddock CL (1959) Potentiation of x-ray effects by actinomycin D. Radiology 73: 175–177

Denekamp J (1973) Changes in the rate of repopulation during multifractionation irradiation of mouse skin. Br J Radiol 46: 381–387

Denekamp J (1975) Residual radiation damage in mouse skin 5 to 8 months after irradiation. Radiology 115: 191–195

Denekamp J (1977) Early and late radiation reactions in mouse feet. Br J Cancer 36: 322–329

Denekamp J, Harris SR (1975) The response of mouse skin to multiple small doses of radiation. In: Alper T (ed) Cell survival after low doses of radiation. Wiley, London

Denekamp J, Stewart FA (1979) Evidence for repair capacity in mouse tumors relative to skin. Int J Radiat Oncol Biol Phys 5: 2003–2010

Denekamp J, Ball MM, Fowler JF (1969) Recovery and repopulation in mouse skin as a function of time after X-irradiation. Radiat Res 37: 361–370

Denekamp J, Stewart FA, Douglas BG (1976) Changes in the proliferation rate of mouse epidermis after irradiation: continuous labelling studies. Cell Tissue Kinet 9: 19–29

Devik F (1951) Histological and cytological changes produced by α-particles in the skin of mice. Acta Radiol 35: 149–155

Douglas BG (1982) Implications of the quadratic cell survival curve and human skin radiation 'tolerance doses' on fractionation and superfractionation dose selection. Int J Radiat Oncol Biol Phys 8: 1135–1142

Douglas BG, Fowler JF (1976) The effect of multiple small doses of x-rays on skin reactions in the mouse and a basic interpretation. Radiat Res 66: 401–426

Douglas BG, Grulkey WR, Chaplin DJ, Lam G, Skarsgard LD, Denekamp J (1986) Pions and pig skin: preclinical evaluation of RBE for early and late damage. Int J Radiat Oncol Biol Phys 12: 221–229

Durrant KR, Young MCA, Hopewell JW (1977) Effects of variation of overall treatment time on the radiation response of normal human skin. Radiobiological research and radiotherapy, vol I. IAEA, Vienna, pp 21–28

Dutreix J, Wambersie A, Bounik C (1973) Cellular recovery in human skin reactions: application to dose, fraction number, overall time relationship in radiotherapy. Eur J Cancer 9: 159–167

Ehring F, Honda M (1967) Das Basalzellkarzinom auf röntgenbelasteter Haut. Strahlentherapie 133: 198–207

Elkind MM, Sutton H (1960) Radiation response of mammalian cells grown in culture. I. Repair of x-ray damage in surviving Chinese hamster cells. Radiat Res 13: 556–593

Ellinger F (1957) Medical radiation biology. Thomas, Springfield

Ellis F (1942) Tolerance dosage in radiotherapy with 200 kV x-rays. Br J Radiol 15: 348–350

Ellis F (1968) Time, fractionation and dose rate in radiotherapy. Front Radiat Ther Oncol 3: 131–140

Ellis F (1969) Dose, time and fractionation: a clinical hypothesis. Clin Radiol 20: 1–7

Ellis F (1970) Time and dose relationships in radiation biology as applied to radiotherapy In: Bond (ed) National Cancer Institute-Atomic Energy Commission (NCI-AEC) Conference in Carmel, Upton, L.I. Brookhaven National Laboratory Report 50203 (C-57), pp 313–314

Ellis F (1971) Nominal standard dose and the ret. Br J Radiol 44: 101–108

Emery EW, Denekamp J, Ball MM, Field SB (1970) Survival of mouse skin epithelial cells following single and divided doses of x-rays. Radiat Res 41: 450–466

Errington RD, Catterall M (1986) Re-irradiation of advanced tumors of the head and neck with fast neutrons. Int J Radiat Oncol Biol Phys 12: 191–195

Fajardo LF, Berthrong M (1981) Radiation injury in surgical pathology. III. Salivary glands, pancreas and skin. Am J Surg Pathol 5: 279–296

Fertil B, Malaise EP (1981) Inherent cellular radiosensitivity as a basic concept for human tumor radiotherapy. Int J Radiat Oncol Biol Phys 7: 621–629

Field SB (1969) Early and late reactions in skin of rats following irradiation with x-rays or fast neutrons. Radiology 92: 381–384

Field SB (1972) The Ellis formula for x-rays and fast neutrons. Br J Radiol 45: 315–317

Field SB (1976) An historical survey of radiobiology and radiotherapy with fast neutrons. Curr Top Radiat Res 11: 1–86

Field SB, Law MP (1976) The relationship between early and late radiation damage in rodent skin. Int J Radiat Biol 30: 557–564

Field SB, Michalowski A (1979) Endpoints for damage to normal tissues. Int J Radiat Oncol Biol Phys 5: 1185–1196

Field SB, Morris C, Denekamp J, Fowler JF (1975) The response of mouse skin to fractionated x-rays. Eur J Cancer 11: 291–299

Field SB, Morgan RL, Morrison R (1976) The response of human skin to irradiation with x-rays or fast neutrons. Int J Radiat Oncol Biol Phys 1: 481–486

Fletcher GH, Barkley HT (1974) Present status of the time factor in clinical radiotherapy. I. The historical background of the recovery exponents. J Radiol Electrol 55: 443–450

Fowler JF (1971) Experimental animal results relating to time-dose relationships in radiotherapy and the "ret" concept. Br J Radiol 44: 81–90

Fowler JF (1984a) Review: total doses in fractionated radiotherapy — implications of new radiobiological data. Int J Radiat Biol 46: 103–120

Fowler JF (1984b) What next in fractionated radiotherapy? Br J Cancer 49 [Suppl IV]: 285–300

Fowler JF, Stern BE (1960) Dose-rate effects: some theoretical and practical considerations. Br J Radiol 33: 389–395

Fowler JF, Stern BE (1963) Dose-time relationships in radiotherapy and the validity of cell survival curve models. Br J Radiol 36: 163–173

Fowler JF, Morgan RL, Silvester JA, Bewley DK, Turner BA (1963) Experiments with fractionated x-ray treatment of the skin of pigs. I. Fractionation up to 28 days. Br J Radiol 36: 188–196

Fowler JF, Bewley DK, Morgan RL, Silvester JA (1965) Experiments with fractionated x-irradiation of the skin of pigs. II. Fractionation up to five days. Br J Radiol 38: 278–284

Fowler JF, Denekamp J, Delapayre C, Sheldon PW, Harris S (1974) Skin reactions in mice after multifraction x-irradiation. Int J Radiat Biol 25: 213–223

Frommhold W, Bublitz G (1967) Untersuchungen über Unterhautfibrosen nach Telekobaltterapie und ihre Behandlungsmöglichkeiten mit DMSO. Strahlentherapie 133: 529–538

Gassmann A (1899) Zur Histologie der Röntgenulcera. Fortschr Roentgenstr 2: 199–207

Gauwerky F, Langheim F (1978) Der Zeitfaktor bei der strahleninduzierten subkutanen Fibrose. Strahlentherapie 154: 608–616

Glasser O (1925) Erythemdosen in Röntgeneinheiten. Strahlentherapie 20: 141–144

Glicksman AS, Chu FCH, Bane HN, Nickson JJ (1960) Quantitative and qualitative evaluation of skin erythema. II. Clinical study in patients on a standardised irradiation schedule. Radiology 75: 411–415

Gordon AB, Harmer CL, O'Sullivan M (1987) Treatment of post-radiotherapy teleangiectasia by injection sclerotherapy. Clin Radiol 38: 25–26

Greco FA, Brereton HD, Kent H, Zimbler H, Merrill J, Johnson RE (1976) Adriamycin and enhanced radiation reaction in normal esophagus and skin. Ann Intern Med 85: 294–298

Griem ML, Malkinson FD (1967) Some studies on the effects of radiation and radiation modifiers on growing hair. Radiat Res 30: 431–443

Griem ML, Dimitrievich GS, Lee RM (1979) The effects of X-irradiation and adriamycin on proliferating and non-proliferating hair coat of the mouse. Int J Radiat Oncol 5: 1261–1264

Grise JW, Rubin P, Ryplansky A, Cramer L (1960) Factors influencing response and recovery of grafted skin to

ionizing irradiation; experimental observations. AJR 83: 1087–1096

Guigon M, Frindel E, Tubiana M (1978) Effects of the association of chemotherapy and radiotherapy on normal mouse skin. Int J Radiat Oncol Biol Phys 4: 233–238

Hayashi S, Suit HD (1972) Effect of fractionation radiation dose on skin contraction and skin reaction of Swiss mice. Radiology 103: 431–437

Hegazy MAH, Fowler JF (1973a) Cell population kinetics of plucked and unplucked mouse skin. I. Unirradiated skin. Cell Tissue Kinet 6: 17–23

Hegazy MA, Fowler JF (1973b) Cell population kinetics of plucked and unplucked mouse skin. II. Irradiated skin Cell Tissue Kinet 6: 587–602

Heidenhain L (1926) Das Problem der Röntgendosis. Strahlentherapie 21: 96–109

Heineke H, Perthes G (1925) Die biologische Wirkung der Röntgen- und Radiumstrahlen. In: Meyer H (ed) Lehrbuch der Strahlentherapie, vol 1. Urban & Schwarzenberg, Berlin, pp 725–882

Hendry JH The tolerance of mouse tails to necrosis after repeated irradiation with x-rays. Br J Radiol 51: 808–813

Hendry JH (1984) Correlation of the dose-response relationships for epidermal colony-forming units, skin reactions, and healing, in the x-irradiated mouse tail. Br. J Radiol 57: 909–918

Hendry JH (1987) Re-irradiation of tissues: dose-response relationships. Proc. 14th Int.Cancer Congr. Budapest 1986, vol 4, pp. 203–210, Karger, Basel/Akademiai Kiado, Budapest, 1987.

Hendry JH, Rosenberg I, Greene D, Stewart JG (1977) Reirradiation of rat tails to necrosis at six months after treatment with a "tolerance" dose of x-rays or neutrons. Br J Radiol 50: 567–572

Henkelman RM, Lam GKY, Kornelsen RO, Eaves CJ (1980) Explanation of dose-rate and split-dose effects on mouse foot reactions using the same time factor. Radiat Res 84: 276–289

Holthusen H (1925) Die qualitative und quantitative Messung der Röntgenstrahlen. In: Meyer H (ed) Lehrbuch der Strahlentherapie, vol 1. Urban & Schwarzenberg, Berlin, pp 287–360

Holthusen H (1936) Erfahrungen über die Verträglichkeitsgrenze für Röntgenstrahlen und deren Nutzanwendung zur Verhütung von Schäden. Strahlentherapie 57: 254–269

Hopewell JW (1980) The importance of vascular damage in the development of late radiation effects in normal tissues. In: Meyn RE, Withers HR (eds) Radiation biology in cancer research. Raven, New York, pp 449–459

Hopewell JW, Gunn Y (1981) Factors for correcting the CRE formula for late effects in normal tissues: how valid are they? Int J Radiat Oncol Biol Phys 7: 683–684

Hopewell JW, Van Den Aardweg GJMJ (1988) Current concepts of dose fractionation in radiotherapy. Normal tissue tolerance. Br J Radiol [Suppl 22]: 88–94

Hopewell JW, Young CMA (1982) The effect of field size on the reaction of pig skin to single doses of x-rays. Br J Radiol 55: 356–361

Hopewell JW, Foster JL, Gunn Y (1978) Role of vascular damage in the development of late radiation effects in the skin. In: Late biological effects of ionizing radiation. Proceedings of a Symposium, Vienna, March 1978. International Atomic Energy Agency publication STI/PUB/489, Vienna, pp 483–492

Hopewell JW, Foster JL, Young CMA, Wiernik G (1979) Late radiation damage to pig skin. Radiology 130: 783–788

Hopewell JW, Hamlet R, Peel D (1985) The response of pig skin to single doses of irradiation from strontium-90 sources of differing surface area. Br J Radiol 58: 778–780

Hopewell JW, Coggle JE, Wells J, Hamlet R, Williams JP, Charles MW (1986) The acute effects of different energy beta-emitters on pig and mouse skin. Br J Radiol [Suppl 19]: 47–50

Howes AE, Brown JM (1979) Early and late response of the mouse limb to multifractionated x-irradiation. Int J Radiat Oncol Biol Phys 5: 13–21

Hug O, Kellerer AM, Zuppinger A (1966) Der Zeitfaktor. In: Hug O, Zuppinger A (eds) Strahlenbiologie 1. Springer, Berlin Heidelberg New York (Handbuch der medizinischen Radiologie, vol II/1, pp 271–354)

Hunter RD, Stewart JG (1977) The tolerance to reirradiation of heavily irradiated human skin. Br J Radiol 50: 573–575

Iselin H (1912) Schädigung der Haut durch Röntgenlicht nach Tiefenbestrahlung (Aluminium). Kumulierende Wirkung. Münch Med Wochenschr 59: 2660–2663

Jingu K, Masuda K, Withers HR, Hunter N (1989) Radiosensitivity of pre-irradiated mouse skin to second courses of single and multifractionated irradiation — skin shrinkage. Radiother Oncol 14: 143–150

Joiner MC, Maughan RL, Fowler JF, Denekamp J (1983) The RBE for mouse skin irradiated with 3-MeV neutrons: single and fractionated doses. Radiat Res 95: 130–141

Joiner MC, Bremner JC, Denekamp J, Maughan RL (1984) The interaction between x-rays and 3 MeV neutrons in the skin of the mouse foot. Int J Radiat Biol 46: 625–638

Jolles B, Harrison RG (1966) Enzymatic processes and vascular changes in the skin irradiation reaction. Br J Radiol 39: 12–16

Jolles B, Mitchell RG (1947) Optimal skin tolerance dose levels. Br J Radiol 20: 405–409

Joyet G, Hohl K (1955) Die biologische Hautreaktion in der Tiefentherapie als Funktion der Feldgröße. Ein Gesetz der Strahlentherapie. Fortschr Roentgenstr 82: 387–400

Kal HB, Gaiser JF (1977) Tumour growth delay and normal tissue reactions induced by fractionated, low dose-rate irradiation. In: Radiobiological research and radiotherapy. IAEA, Vienna, vol 1, pp 11–19

Kal HB, Sissingh HA (1974) Effectiveness of continuous low dose-rate gamma-irradiation on rat skin. Br J Radiol 47: 673–678

Kalz F (1941) Theoretical considerations and clinical use of Grenz rays in dermatology. Arch Dermatol Syph 43: 447–472

Kärcher, KH (1958) Über die Nachbehandlung strahlenbelasteter Haut. Strahlentherapic 107: 453–461

Kepp RK (1944) Ergebnisse von Erythemversuchen mit fraktionierter Röntgenbestrahlung bei ungleicher Größe der Einzeldosen. Strahlentherapie 74: 331–339

Kim JH, Chu FCH, Hilaris B (1975) The influence of dose fractionation on acute and late reactions in patients with postoperative radiotherapy for carcinoma of the breast. Cancer 35: 1583–1586

Kirk J, Gray WM, Watson ER (1975) Cumulative radiation effect. Part IV. Normalization of fractionated and continuous therapy-area and volume correction factors. Clin Radiol 26: 77–88

Kirk J, Gray WM, Watson ER (1971) Cumulative radiation effect. Part I. Fractionated treatment regimes. Clin Radiol 22: 145–155

Kirk J, Gray WM, Watson ER (1975) Cumulative radiation effect. Part V. Time gaps in treatment regimes. Clin Radiol 26: 159–176

Kligerman MM, Smith A, Yuhas JM, Wilson S, Sternhagen CJ, Helland JA, Sala JM (1977) The relative biological effectiveness of pions in the acute response of human skin. Int J Radiat Oncol Biol Phys 3: 335–340

Klostermann GF (1966) Röntgenfolgen an der Haut nach Hämangiombestrahlung. Strahlentherapie: 130: 205–218

Langlois D, Eschwege F, Kramar A, Richard JM (1985) Reirradiation of head and neck cancers. Radiother Oncol 3: 27–33

Law MP (1981) Radiation-induced vascular injury and its relation to late effects in normal tissues. Adv Radiat Biol 9: 37–73

Law MP, Thomlinson RH (1978) Vascular permeability in the ear of rats after x-irradiation. Br J Radiol 51: 895–904

Lemperle G, Koslowski J (eds) (1984) Chirurgie der Strahlenfolgen. Urban & Schwarzenberg, Munich

Liegner LM, Michaud NJ (1961) Skin and subcutaneous reactions induced by supervoltage irradiation, AJR 85: 533–549

Liversage WE (1969) A general formula for equating protracted and acute regimes of radiation. Br J Radiol 42: 432–440

Liversage WE (1971) A critical look at the ret. Br J Radiol 44: 91–100

MacComb WS, Quimby EH (1936) The rate of recovery of human skin from the effects of hard or soft roentgen rays or gamma rays. Radiology 27: 196–207

Masuda K, Hunter N, Withers HR (1980) Late effect in mouse skin following single and multifractionated irradiation. Int J Radiat Oncol Biol Phys 6: 1539–1544

Masuda K, Matsuura K, Withers HR, Hunter N (1986) Response of previously irradiated mouse skin to a second course of irradiation: early skin reaction and skin shrinkage. Int J Radiat Oncol Biol Phys 12: 1645–1651

McWirther R (1935) 12th Annual Report, British Empire Cancer Campaign, pp 131–144

Michalowski, A (1981) Effects of radiation on normal tissues: hypothetical mechanisms and limitations of in situ assays of clonogenicity. Radiat Environ Biophys 19: 157–172

Miescher G (1924) Das Röntgenerythem. Strahlentherapie 16: 333–371

Mitchell JS (1960) Studies in radiotherapeutics. Blackwell, Cambridge, Oxford

Mitchell JB, Bedford JS, Bailey SM (1979) Dose-rate effects in mammalian cells in culture. III. Comparison of cell killing and cell proliferation during continuous irradiation for six different cell lines. Radiat Res 79: 537–551

Montague ED (1968) Experience with altered fractionation in radiation therapy of breast cancer. Radiology 90: 962–966

Morgan SA, Yarnold JR, Patterson D (1987) The severity of late skin damage related to fraction size in women treated by radiotherapy after mastectomy. Radiother Oncol 8: 315–319

Morris GM, Hopewell JW (1985) Pig epidermis: a cell kinetic study. Cell Tissue Kinet 18: 407–415

Morris GM, Hopewell JW (1986) Changes in the cell kinetics of pig epidermis after repeated daily doses of x-rays. Br J Radiol [Suppl 19]: 34–38

Morris GM, Hopewell JW (1987) Cell population kinetics in pig epidermis: further studies. Cell Tissue Kinet 20: 161–169

Morris GM, Hopewell JW (1988) Changes in the cell kinetics of pig epidermis after single doses of x-rays. Br J Radiol 61: 205–211

Moulder JE, Fischer JJ (1976) Radiation reaction of rat skin. Cancer 37: 2762–2767

Moulder JE, Fischer JJ, Casey A (1975) Dose-time relationships for skin reactions and structural damage in rat feet exposed to 250 kV x-rays. Radiology 115: 465–470

Moustafa HF, Hopewell JW (1979) Blood flow clearance changes in pig skin after single doses of x-rays. Br J Radiol 52: 138–144

Muggia FM, Cortes-Funes H, Wassermann TH (1978) Radiotherapy and chemotherapy in combined clinical trials: problems and promise. Int J Radiat Oncol Biol Phys 4: 161–171

Mühlmann E, Meyer O (1923) Beiträge zur Röntgenschädigung tiefgelegener Gewebe. Strahlentherapie 15: 48–64

Nguyen TD, Demange L, Froissart D, Panis X, Loirette M (1985) Rapid hyperfractionated radiotherapy. Clinical results in 178 advanced squamous cell carcinomas of the head and neck. Cancer 56: 16–19

Nguyen TD, Panis X, Froissart D, Legros M, Coninx P, Loirette M (1988) Analysis of late complications after rapid hyperfractionated radiotherapy in advanced head and neck cancers. Int J Radiat Oncol Biol Phys 14: 23–25

Nias AHW (1963) Some comparisons of fractionation effects in erythema measurements on human skin. Br J Radiol 36: 183–187

Notter G, Turesson I (1976) Prospective studies with the CRE formula of prolonged fractionation schedules. Radiology 121: 709–715

Orton CG, Ellis F (1973) A simplification in the use of the NSD concept in practical radiotherapy. Br J Radiol 46: 529–537

Overgaard M, Bentzen SM, Christensen JJ, Madsen EH (1987) The value of the NSD formula in equation of acute and late radiation complications in normal tissue following 2 and 5 fractions per week in breast cancer patients treated with postmastectomy irradiation. Radiother Oncol 9: 1–12

Pape R (1933) Zur Frage des Vergleichs der Hautreaktion unter verschiedenen Bestrahlungsbedingungen. Strahlentherapie 48: 73–96

Paterson R (1948) The treatment of malignant disease by radium and x-rays. Williams & Wilkins, Balimore

Paterson R (1963) The treatment of malignant disease by radiotherapy, 2nd edition. Edward Amold London

Paterson MC (1989) Human ill health, abnormal radiation induced cytotoxicity and aberrant DNA metabolism. In: Low Dose Radiation, Taylor and Francis, London, New York, Philadelphia

Patterson TJS, Berry RJ, Wiernik G (1972) The effect of x-radiation on the survival of skin flaps in the pig. Br J Plast Surg 25: 17–19

Patterson TJS, Berry RJ, Hopewell JW, Wiernik G (1975) The effect of x-radiation on the survival of experimental skin flaps. In: Grabb WC, Myers MB (eds) Skin flaps. Little, Brown & Co., Boston, pp 39–46

Peel DM, Hopewell JW, Simmonds RH, Dodd P, Meistrich ML (1984a) Split-dose recovery in epithelial and vascular-connective tissue of pig skin. Radiother Oncol 2: 151–157

Peel, DM, Hopewell, JW, Wells J, Charles, MW (1984b) Nonstochastic effects of different energy β emitters on pigskin. Radiat Res 99: 372–382

Peters LJ, Withers HR (1981) Factors for correcting the CRE formula for late effects in normal tissue: How valid are they? Int J Radiat Oncol Biol Phys 7: 684–685

Phillips TL (1980) Tissue toxicity of radiation-drug interaction. In: Sokol GH, Maickel RP (eds) Radiation-drug interactions in the treatment of cancer. Wiley, New York, pp 175–200

Potten CS (1978) The cellular and tissue response to single doses of ionizing radiation. Curr Top Radiat Res 13: 1–59

Potten CS (1985) Radiation and skin. Taylor & Francis, London

Powell-Smith C (1965) Factors influencing the incidence of radiation injury in cancer of the cervix. J Assoc Canad Radiol 16: 132–137

Probert JC, Brown JM (1974) A comparison of 3 and 5 times weekly fractionation on the response of normal and malignant tissues of the C3H mouse. Br J Radiol 47: 775–780

Puck TT, Marcus PI (1956) Action of x-rays on mammalian cells. J Exp Med 103: 273–283

Quimby EH (1937) Further studies on the rate of recovery of human skin from the effects of roentgen- or gamma-ray irradiation. Radiology 29: 305–312

Raju MR, Carpenter S, Tokita N, Dicello JF, Jackson D, Frolich E, von Essen C (1981) Effect of fractionated doses of pions on normal tissues: part I; mouse skin. Int J Radiat Oncol Biol Phys 6: 1663–1666

Redpath JL, Colman M (1979) The effect of adriamycin and actinomycin D on radiation-induced skin reactions in mouse feet. Int J Radiat Oncol Biol Phys 5: 483–486

Redpath JL, Peel DM, Dodd P, Simmonds RH, Hopewell JW (1985) Repopulation in irradiated pig skin: late versus early effects. Radiother Oncol 3: 173–176

Reisner A (1933) Hauterythem und Röntgenbestrahlung. Ergebnisse der Medizinischen Strahlenforschung 6: 1–60

Rojas A, Joiner MC, Johns H (1989) Recovery kinetics in mouse skin and CaNT tumours. Radiother Oncol 14: 329–336

Rubin P, Casarett GW (1968) Clinical radiation pathology. Saunders, Philadelphia

Rubin P, Grise JW (1960) The difference in response of grafted and normal skin to ionizing radiations. AJR 84: 645–655

Rubin P, Casarett G, Grise JW (1960) The vascular pathophysiology of an irradiated graft. AJR 83: 1097–1104

Sause WT, Stewart JR, Plenk HP, Levitt DD (1981) Late skin changes following twice-weekly electron beam radiation to post-mastectomy chest walls. Int Radiat Oncol Biol Phys 7: 1541–1544

Schinz HR (1937) Die fraktionierte und protrahiert-fraktionierte Bestrahlung. Zürcher Erfahrungen. Stralentherapic 58: 373–405

Seitz L, Wintz H (1920) Unsere Methode derr Röntgentiefentherapie und ihre Erfolge. Sonderband 5 der Strahlentherapie

Sheline GE, Phillips TL, Brennan SB (1971) Effects of fast neutrons on human skin. AJR 111: 31–41

Skolyszewski J, Korzeniowski S, Reinfuss M (1980) The reirradiation of recurrences of head and neck cancer. Br J Radiol 53: 462–465

Skolyszewski J, Korzeniowski S (1988) Re-irradiation of recurrent head and neck cancer with fast neutrons. Br J Radiol 61: 527–528

Smith KC, Hahn GM, Hopper RT, Earle JD (1980) Radiosensitivity in vitro of human fibroblasts derived from patients with a severe skin reaction to radiation therapy. Int J Radiat Oncol Biol Phys 6: 1573–1575

Stein G (1963) Röntgenfolgezustände im Bereich der Haut. Strahlentherapie 121: 247–258

Strandquist M (1944) Studien über die kumulative Wirkung der Röntgenstrahlen bei Fraktionierung. Acta Radiol [Suppl] 55: 1–300

Strauss O (1925) Schädigungen durch Röntgen-und Radiumstrahlen. In: Meyer H (ed) Lehrbuch der Strahlentherapie, vol I. Urban & Schwarzenberg, Berlin, pp 979–1060

Strauss, JS, Kligman, AM (1960) Effects of x-rays on sebaceous glands of the human face: radiation therapy of acne. J Invest Derm 32: 347–356

Thames, HD (1985) An 'incomplete-repair model' for survival after fractionated and continuous irradiation. Int J Radiat Biol 47: 319–339

Thames HD, Hendry JH (1987) Fractionation in radiotherapy. Taylor & Francis, London

Thames HD, Withers HR, Peters LJ, Fletcher GH (1982) Changes in early and late radiation responses with altered dose fractionation: implications for dose-survival relationships. Int J Radiat Oncol Biol Phys 8: 219–226

Tilkorn H, Drepper M, Ehring F (1986) Indications for the treatment by plastic surgery of the effects of radiation and radiolesions on the skin. Br J Radiol [Suppl 19]: 131–134

Traenkle HL, Mulay D (1960) Further observations on late radiation necrosis following therapy of skin cancer. Arch Dermatol 81: 908–913

Tucker SL (1984) Tests for the fit of the linear-quadratic model to radiation isoeffect data. Int J Radiat Oncol Biol Phys 10: 1933–1939

Turesson I, Notter G (1976) Control of dose administered once a week and three times a day according to schedules calculated by the CRE formula, using skin reaction as a biological parameter. Radiology 120: 399–404

Turesson I, Notter G (1979a) The response of pig skin to single and fractionated high dose-rate and continuous low dose-rate ^{137}Cs-irradiation — I: Experimental design and results. Int J Radiat Oncol Biol Phys 5: 835–844

Turesson I, Notter G (1979b) The response of pig skin to single and fractionated high dose-rate and continuous low dose-rate ^{137}Cs-irradiation — II: Theoretical considerations of the results. Int J Radiat Oncol Biol Phys 5: 955–963

Turesson I, Notter G (1979c) The response of pig skin to single and fractionated high dose-rate and continuous low dose-rate ^{137}Cs-irradiation — III: Re-evaluation of the CRE system and the TDF system according to the present findings. Int J Radiat Oncol Biol Phys 5: 1773–1779

Turesson I, Notter G (1984a) The influence of fraction size in radiotherapy on the late normal tissue reaction — I: Comparison of the effects of daily and once-a-week fractionation on human skin. Int J Radiat Oncol Biol Phys 10: 593–598

Turesson I, Notter, G (1984b) The influence of fraction size in radiotherapy on the late normal tissue reaction — II: Comparison of the effects of daily and twice-a-week fractionation on human skin. Int J Radiat Oncol Biol Phys 10: 599–606

Turesson I, Notter G (1984c) The influence of the overall treatment time in radiotherapy on the acute reaction: comparison of the effects of daily and twice-a-week fractionation on human skin. Int J Radiat Oncol Biol Phys 10: 607–618

Turesson I, Notter G (1988) Accelerated versus conventional fractionation. The degree of incomplete repair in human skin with a four-hour-fraction interval studied after postmastectomy irradiation. Acta Oncol 27: 169–179

Turesson I, Thames HD (1989) Repair capacity and kinetics of human skin during fractionated radiotherapy: erythema, desquamation, and telangiectasia after 3 and 5 years' follow-up. Radiother Oncol 15: 169–188

Ullrich RL, Casarett GW (1977) Interrelationship between the early inflammatory response and subsequent fibrosis after radiation exposure. Radiat Res 72: 107–121

Van Den Aardweg GJMJ, Hopewell JW, Simmonds RH (1988) Repair and recovery in the epithelial and vascular connective tissues of pig skin after irradiation. Radiother Oncol 11: 73–82

Van Rongen E, Kal HB (1984) Acute reactions in rat feet exposed to multiple fractions of x-rays per day. Radiother Oncol 2: 141–150

Von der Maase (1986) Experimental studies on interactions of radiation and chemotherapeutic drugs in normal tissues and a solid tumor. Radiother Oncol 7: 47–68

Vegesna V, Withers HR, Taylor JMG (1988) Epilation in mice after single and multifractionated irradiation. Radiother Oncol 12: 233–239

Von Essen CF (1963) A spatial model of time-dose-area relationship in radiation therapy. Radiology 81: 881–883

Von Essen CF (1968) Radiation tolerance of the skin. Acta Radiol Ther 8: 311–330

Von Essen CF (1972) Clinical radiation tolerance of the skin and upper aerodigestive tract. Front Radiat Ther Oncol 6: 148–159

Weichselbaum RR, Epstein J, Little JB (1976) In vitro radiosensitivity of human diploid fibroblasts derived from patients with unusual clinical responses to radiation. Radiology 121: 479–482

White RL, El-Mahdi AM, Ramirez HL (1975) Thermographic changes following preoperative radiotherapy in head and neck cancer. Radiology 117: 469–471

Wheldon TE, Michalowski AS, Kirk J (1982) The effect of irradiation on function in self-renewing normal tissues with differing proliferative organisation. Br J Radiol 55: 759–766

Wiernik G, Patterson TJS, Berry RJ (1974) The effect of fractionated dose-patterns of x-radiation on the survival of experimental skin flaps in the pig. Br J Radiol 47: 343–345

Wiernik G, Hopewell JW, Patterson TJS, Young CMA, Foster JL Response of pig skin to fractionated radiation doses. Radiobiological research and radiotherapy, vol I. IAEA, Vienna, 93–103

Withers HR (1967) Recovery and repopulation in vivo by mouse skin epithelial cells during fractionated irradiation. Radiat Res 32: 227–239

Withers HR, Flow BL, Huchton UI, Hussey DH, Jardine JH, Mason KA, Rauston GL, Smathers JB (1977) Effect of dose fractionation on early and late skin responses to γ-rays and neutrons. Int J Radiat Oncol Biol Phys 3: 227–233

Withers HR, Thames HD, Flow BL, Mason KA, Hussey DH (1978a) The relationship of acute to late skin injury in 2 and 5 fraction/week gamma-ray therapy. Int J Radiat Oncol Biol Phys 4: 595–601

Withers HW, Thames HD, Hussey DH, Flow BL, Mason KA (1978b) Relative biological effectiveness (RBE) of 50 MV (Be) neutrons for acute and late skin injury. Int J Radiat Oncol Biol Phys 4: 603–608

Withers HR, Thames HD, Peters LJ (1984) A new isoeffect curve for change in dose per fraction. Radiother Oncol 1: 187–191

Witte E (1941) Dosierung im biologischen Maß. Strahlentherapie 72: 177–194

Wondergem J, Haveman J (1987) The effect of previous treatment on the response of mouse feet to irradiation and hyperthermia. Radiother Oncol 10: 253–261

Yamaguchi T, Tabachnick J Cell kinetics of epidermal repopulation and persistent hyperplasia in locally β-irradiated guinea pig skin. Radiat Res 50: 158–180

Yan JH, Hu YH, Gu XZ (1983) Radiation therapy of recurrent nasopharyngeal carcinoma. Acta Radiol Oncol 22: 123–128

Young CMA. Hopewell JW (1983) The effects of preoperative x-irradiation on the survival and blood flow of pedicle skin flaps in the pig. Int J Radiat Oncol Biol Phys 9: 865–870

Zollinger HJ (1960) Radiohistologie und Radio-Histopathologie. In: Roulet F (ed) Strahlung und Wetter. Springer, Berlin Heidelberg New York (Handbuch der allgemeinen Pathologie, vol x/1), pp 127–287

Zuppinger A (1941) Spätveränderungen nach protrahiert-fraktionierter Röntgenbestrahlung im Bereich der oberen Luft und Speisewege. Strahlentherapie 70: 361–442

Zuppinger A (1949) Die Strahlenbehandlung der Larynx- und Pharynxtumoren. Strahlentherapie 78: 481–500

3 Bone

A. Luz, W. Gössner, and F. Heuck

CONTENTS

Professor Dr. A. Luz, GSF Forschungszentrum für Umwelt und Gesundheit, Institut für Pathologie, Ingolstädter Landstraße 1, 8042 Neuherberg, FRG

Professor Dr. W. Gössner, Institut für Allgemeine Pathologie und Pathologische Anatomie der Technischen Universität, Ismaninger Straße 22, 8000 München 80, FRG

Professor Dr. F. Heuck, Hermann-Kurz-Straße 5, 7000 Stuttgart 1, FRG

3.1 Introduction

The clinical–radiological assessment of radiation damage to bone is discussed in detail by Kolář and Vrabec (1976). This review also contains a comprehensive summary of the literature. Assessment of clinically relevant changes solely from the viewpoint of morphological pathology and radiology, however, can result in a considerable misrepresentation, since massive tissue damage does not necessarily result in severe functional defects. Clinical manifestation of damage necessarily depends on functional strain on the tissue. A knowledge of pathomorphological changes is necessary if patients are to be protected from severe damage. In this sense the description of the general pathological changes which are associated with radiation damage in bone is complementary to the chapter by Kolář and Vrabec (1976). An attempt will be made to emphasize the formal pathogenesis and the general principles it follows so as to convey an idea of the fate of the tissue after being challenged by radiation.

The pathological anatomy of radiation-damaged bone is described by Cottier (1966). The following publications provide useful reviews of the literature from a pathological–anatomical viewpoint: Desjardins (1930), Flaskamp (1930), Dahl (1936), Gates (1943), Heller (1948), Zollinger (1960), Rubin and Casarett (1968), Seelentag and Kistner (1969), Nilsson (1969), Thurner (1970), Jee (1971), Grimm (1971), Gössner (1972), Teft (1972), Parker (1972), Heuck and Gössner (1973), Vaughan (1973), and Parker and Berry (1976). Fajardo (1982) also gives a brief description of the pathology of the irradiated skeleton. The comprehensive description of pathological–anatomical changes by Heller (1948) remains one of the most important articles on the subject. Rubin and Casarett (1968) have tabulated the historically most important articles, providing a useful source of information for the interested reader.

3.2 Dose Burden

The local dose is of considerable importance in
radiation biology, so it is necessary first to consider
some of the special characteristics of the skeleton.

3.2.1 External Irradiation

X-irradiation below 1 MeV is increasingly more
absorbed in mineralized bone than in soft tissue
(SPIERS 1949; WACHSMANN 1949; WILSON 1950;
WOODARD 1957; literature review in PARKER 1972).
At 60 kV the dose rate in bone is six times that in
soft tissue (WACHSMANN 1949). The energy of
^{60}Co γ-irradiation is calculated using a conversion
factor of 0.93 rad/R (0.0093 Gy/R) (RANUDD
1966). At energy levels above 5 MeV there is again
increased absorption in bone (see PARKER 1972).
The dose rate to living cells in and around
mineralized bone also depends on the dimensions
of the cavities (for references see WILSON 1950;
WOODARD 1957). Measurements at the bone surface have shown a deviation from the theoretical
calculations (FOWLER 1957). LOBODZIEC and LUBAS
(1966) give a formal method for calculating the
radiation dose to tissue below the bone. HAZUKA
et al. (1988) have calculated correction factors for
dosimetry in the pelvic area when metal hip joint
prostheses are present. Areas of cartilage can be
expected to have the same energy absorption on
average as soft tissue areas, but with somewhat
higher absorption of longer-wave x-rays in the
zone of provisional calcification (DZIEWIATKOWSKI
and WOODARD 1959).

3.2.2 Internal Irradiation

VAUGHAN (1973) gives a review of the literature.
The primary distribution of incorporated osteotro-
pic radionuclides is determined by the chemistry of
the radionuclide (incorporation in mineral for
calcium-like behavior, i.e., bone volume seeker;
binding to the organic matrix for plutonium-type
behavior, i.e., bone surface seeker) and by age.
Thus in the growing organism the initial dose rate
in the metaphysis can be five times higher than
that in the area of the shaft (^{32}P, BLACKETT et al.
1959; ^{90}Sr, VAUGHAN and OWEN 1959). The
microdosimetry of bone-seeking radionuclides has
been described by PRIEST (1985). The influence of

age on this dosimetry has been described by
GERBER et al. (1987). Adults show a higher
retention of long-lived ^{239}Pu than do growing rats.
This results in a higher mean skeletal dose burden
for adults, especially in the vertebral column
(GAMER 1988). The radiation dose burden on cells
is determined by the range of the radiation (α, β)
and the geometry of the cavities. At all levels of
α-irradiation, the area which shows the highest
biological effect (LET 100–200 kev/μm) lies at the
bone surface within the 20-μm zone (SONTAG
1987). POLIG et al. (1988) calculated the following
relative values for the dose rate in the lumbar
vertebral region in the beagle dog following
incorporation of 355 kBq/kg ^{226}Ra: bone-lining
cells (3.1 μm), 1; osteoblasts (5.7 μm), 0.78;
progenitor cells (7.7 μm), 0.65; 0–10 μm, 0.33;
10–20 μm, 0.33; bone marrow, 0.20. The absolute
value of the dose rate for bone-lining cells was 271
Gy/day. The dose to growing cartilage is in general
lower than from external irradiation. The distribution of ^{239}Pu in the bone of the adult organism
appears to be determined by the vascularization
(SMITH et al. 1982) and the blood flow (HUMPHREYS
et al. 1982).

Changes in the distribution pattern of long-
lived radionuclides result in an unpredictable
situation. Interestingly, the mobility of radionuclides after deposition is relatively low so that , for
example, in cases of radium poisoning radium-free
areas of bone can also be found (HOECKER and
ROOFE 1951).

3.3 Growing Bone

3.3.1 Growth Plate

3.3.1.1 Normal Observations

The clinical and experimental aspects of the
growth plate have been reviewed recently by
UHTHOFF and WILEY (1988), and the morphology
and biochemistry of cartilage have been reviewed
by JOHNSON (1986). According to DODDS and
CAMERON (1934) (cited in GALL et al. 1940) the
growth plate can be divided into five zones: resting
cartilage, zone of proliferation, zone of hypertrophic cartilage, zone of provisional calcification,
and zone of cartilage removal and bone deposition. With improved fixation techniques it has
become clear that the hypertrophic chondrocytes
swell up but retain their nucleus and do not

actually degenerate right down to the border of the zone of cartilage removal and bone deposition. The actual increase in volume (factor 10) of hypertrophic chondrocytes is underestimated by normal fixation methods (COWELL et al. 1987; HUNZIKER et al. 1987). The highest level of type II collagen gene expression was detected in the chondrocytes of the lower proliferative and upper hypertrophic zones of cartilage. The levels of proα1 (I) collagen, TGF-β, and *c-fos* mRNAs are very high in perichondrium (SANDBERG et al. 1988).

KEMBER (1983) has summarized results describing the cell kinetics of the growth plate. Continuous intrauterine ^{3}H-thymidine labeling resulting in complete labeling of the cartilage cells has shown that postnatally the chondroid cells close to the epiphysis are the stem cells for the growth plate (KEMBER and LAMBERT 1981). Other ^{3}H-thymidine labeling experiments also indicate that all cells in the proliferation zone are involved in growth (KEMBER 1960). The DNA synthesis phase is approximately 7 h (WALKER and KEMBER 1972a,b), the generation phase approximately 1–3 days (KEMBER 1960, 1971; WALKER and KEMBER 1972a), and the time to pass through subsequent zones around 2–5 days (SISSONS 1956; KEMBER 1960; BLACKBURN and WELLS 1963). The increase in bone length can be calculated fairly well from the kinetic data on the position-dependent contribution to growth and the increase in cell size (WALKER and KEMBER 1972b). KEMBER and SISSONS (1976) calculated the generation time of human chondrocytes to be 20 days using morphometric investigations of the human growth plate and a comparison with experimental animals, but did not answer the question of whether there is a group of rapidly proliferating cells in the chondrocyte proliferation zone. Using fluorochrome labeling and morphometry, with good fixation (addition of ruthenium hexaminetrichloride) which allows retention of the correct cell volume, HUNZIKER et al. (1987) showed that on average eight chondrocytes are formed per day in each cartilage column in the growth zone of the proximal tibia in the rat. The kinetic data can best be explained by a regulation of growth in the growth plate by means of diffusion of regulating factors from the epiphyseal side, which is also the source of cell nutrition (KEMBER 1979). A chondrocyte growth factor has been described (AZIZKHAN and KLAGSBRUN 1980).

The growth cartilage in the mandibular condyle is part of the so-called secondary cartilage (for reviews see HALL 1981; JOHNSON 1986). The special characteristics, metabolism, and cell kinetics of the condyle have been described by SILBERMANN and FROMMER (1972a,b).

In vitro studies of the mouse mandibular condyle show the bipotential characteristics of the progenitor cell population of secondary cartilage, i.e., the ability to form cartilage or bone (SILBERMANN et al. 1983). Apparently the biomechanical effects of the musculature favor formation of cartilage (HALL 1981).

The histochemistry of normal cartilage and cartilage matrix development is described in GÖSSNER and SCHWABE (1971), MATSUZUWA and ANDERSON (1971), ENG and ESTERLY (1972), THYBERG (1972), THYBERG and FRIBERG (1972) and THYBERG et al. (1973).

3.3.1.2 Radiation Damage

The histological appearance of the growth plate in the early stages after irradiation has been described by BROOKS and HILLSTROM (1933), DAHL (1936), BISGARD and HUNT (1936), ENGEL (1938), GALL et al. (1940), HINKEL (1943a), BARR et al. (1943), REIDY et al. (1947), LEVY and RUGH (1952), GÜNSEL (1953), SISSONS (1956), DZIEWIATKOWSKI and WOODARD (1959), ZOLLINGER (1960), HELD (1960), HULTH and WESTERBORN (1960, 1962), MELANOTTE and FOLLIS (1961), BLACKBURN and WELLS (1963), BENSTED and COURTENAY (1965), KEMBER (1965), SAMS (1966b), KEMBER (1967), KEMBER and COGGINS (1967), GÖSSNER and SCHWABE (1968), RISSANEN et al. (1969b), KEMBER and SADEK (1970), KEMBER and WALKER (1971), and ANDERSON et al. (1979). These observations are based on experimental findings in rat, mouse, rabbit, dog, and hamster.

KEMBER (1983) has summarized the changes observed in the cell kinetics of the cartilage growth plate following external and internal irradiation.

The *mitotic activity* is reduced within the first hours of irradiation (BLACKBURN and WELLS 1963; KEMBER and SADEK 1970). The duration of inhibition is dose dependent: mitotic activity recovers during the 1st day after irradiation for doses up to 1000 R, with a return to normal values for doses up to 5 Gy and a return to about 50% normal activity for doses of 7.5 Gy (KEMBER and SADEK 1970).

The ^{3}H-thymidine labeling index in the growth

plate falls immediately after irradiation with 10 Gy (KEMBER 1983) and is zero after 24 h (ARGÜELLES et al. 1977). In vitro irradiation of chicken tibia with 10 Gy causes a 50% inhibition of ^{3}H-thymidine incorporation (DE RIDDER et al. 1988). In vitro irradiation of chick limb bud resulted in a reduction in formation of nodular islands of cartilage by approximately 20% 96 h after 0.96 Gy (GARRISON and UYEKI 1988).

Cell death is first observed in the proliferation zone (GÜNSEL 1953; ZOLLINGER 1960), 4 h after 20 Gy (DAHL 1936) and immediately after application of 80 000 R (given within 2 h 40 min) (LEVY and RUGH 1952). Cell death is already prominent in the proliferation zone after a dose of only 200 R (DAHL 1936). The frequency is dependent on the dose (SISSONS 1956; KEMBER and SADEK 1970). In vitro irradiation of chicken tibia with 200 Gy results in the death of all cartilage cells (DE RIDDER et al. 1988).

SISSONS (1956) investigated the quantitative *reduction in cell number* in the growth plate following irradiation. Table 3.1 shows these results expressed relative to control values. There can be a recovery in cell number up to 800 R, but at 1600 R there is a continual decrease in the number of cells in the growth zone, i.e., there is an irreversible numerical reduction in the proliferation pool.

The reduction of cartilage cells is accompanied by a *disturbance in the columnar organization* of the cartilage, the extent and time of occurrence of which are dose dependent. After 200 R, for example, the disturbance is focal and first appears after 15 days, whereas after 1540 R it is widespread from the 2nd day onwards (BISGARD and HUNT 1936).

After higher doses, recovery of proliferation in the growth plate takes place increasingly in the form of *cartilage cells clustered in club-shaped groups*, observed by HINKEL (1943a) as early as 1

Table 3.1. Number of cartilage cells per column in the growth plate (relative[a] to the control values) following local irradiation of the tibia in 30-day-old rats. (After SISSONS 1956)

Dose (R)	Time after irradiation			
	3 days	8 days	30 days	100 days
400	0.9	1.0	1.0	1.0
800	1.0	0.9	1.0	1.0
1200	0.8	0.7	0.7	Minimal
1600	0.6	0.4	<0.3	Minimal

[a] Calculated from data in SISSONS (1956).

week after 600 R. KEMBER (1967) counted these islands 25 days after irradiation with 1500–2300 R in order to assess the survival rate of the cartilage cells, and using the gradient of the semilogarithmic survival curve calculated a D_0 of 1.65 Gy, and a survival rate of 5% for cartilage cells after exposure to 800 R. Long-term (effectively permanent) sterilization of the growth plate probably takes place at a dose of around 1800 R (HOFFMANN 1923; DAHL 1936; KEMBER 1967).

It seems possible that ordered *restitution* of the growth plate can take place at radiation doses below 10 Gy. KEMBER and COGGINS (1967) observed such restitution 2–3 weeks after 9 Gy. Twelve weeks after continuous irradiation with 0.45 Gy/day (total 37.80 Gy) the cell population in the growth plate is only reduced to half the control values, whereas the ^{3}H-thymidine labeling index is considerably lowered (ANDERSON et al. 1979). Under similar conditions (0.5 Gy/day) a reduction is already observed in the size of the DNA-synthesizing cell columns within 35 days (KEMBER and WALKER 1971). Surprisingly, the productive capability, in the form of increase in length, was not affected following continuous irradiation with 0.45 Gy/day, at least not within the observation period (ANDERSON et al. 1979).

The radiation-induced disturbances in the cell population of the growth plate can be interpreted easily in terms of cell kinetics, and do not correlate with the relatively small, later-appearing effects in the blood vessels on the epiphyseal side which supply nutrients to the cartilage cells (KEMBER 1965; KEMBER and COGGINS 1967). It is not possible to describe precisely the changes in flow balance between new formation of cells and cell differentiation in the growth plate, because these are influenced by changes in the adjoining osteogenic tissue (described below).

Cell dystrophy is commonly observed in addition to the disturbances in cell formation, particularly in the zone of hypertrophic cartilage. Irregular swelling of cells results in a more varied cell appearance. Cell dystrophy has been observed as early as 24 h after 500 R (BROOKS and HILLSTROM 1933). The appearance of these abnormal cartilage cells is a useful measure of regression and can be used to show the effect of dose fractionation in reducing the extent of damage (BENSTED and COURTENAY 1965, see Table 3.2). Chondrocytes did not show any detectable morphological changes by either light or electron microscopy following in vitro irradiation of chicken tibia with

Table 3.2. The effect of dose fractionation on the frequency of dystrophic cellular changes in the cartilage plate. Experiments on 1- to 3-month-old rats. (After BENSTED and COURTENAY 1965)

Irradiation scheme	Frequency among investigated tibiae[a]
1 × 3000 R	80% (69/88)
3 × 1000 R (interval 2 weeks)	31% (8/26)
6 × 500 R (interval 2 weeks)	10% (6/58)

[a] Investigation of moribund and/or tumor-bearing animals.

doses up to 150 Gy (DE RIDDER et al. 1988). One expression of cell dystrophy is shown in changes in the location of glycogen-containing (PAS-positive) cells after irradiation, in particular the irregular loss of glycogen in cells in the hypertrophic zone (MELANOTTE and FOLLIS 1961; PUTZKE 1963). Particularly strongly swollen cartilage cells also show fatty degeneration (PUTZKE 1963).

Disturbances in matrix synthesis are shown by the reduced uptake of ^{35}S 21 days after 900 R (DZIEWIATKOWSKI and WOODARD 1959). Autoradiography shows that the loss of ^{35}S incorporation is due to loss of cartilage cells; the remaining swollen cells only incorporate ^{35}S in their peripheral areas and appear to give up ^{35}S-positive material at a slower rate (HULTH and WESTERBORN 1962). Surprisingly, continuous irradiation with 0.45 Gy/day for 12 weeks does not inhibit ^{35}S

incorporation or ^{35}S secretion in the remaining cells (ANDERSON et al. 1979). In vitro irradiation of chicken tibia with 150 Gy results in a 20% inhibition of ^{3}H-uridine incorporation and 40% inhibition of ^{3}H-proline incorporation in growth cartilage. After 200 Gy the metabolism of the cartilage is totally blocked (DE RIDDER et al. 1988).

Alkaline phosphatase, identified histochemically, is generally found in the zone of hypertrophic chondrocytes and disappears with increasing cellular dystrophy, although it can still be found in single swollen cells (MELANOTTE and FOLLIS 1961; PUTZKE 1963; SAMS 1966a). Even in the extreme case of complete stunting of growth following 3000 R, enzyme activity can still be observed in occasional cells 9 days after irradiation (Fig. 3.1; EURATOM-GSF 1967). Interestingly, after incorporation of the α-emitter ^{224}Ra at low doses (<25 μCi/kg) the enzyme activity only disappears within the range of the radiation (the source of which is located in the region of provisional calcification) (Fig. 3.2; GÖSSNER and SCHWABE 1968). When proliferative activity returns, alkaline phosphatase activity appears with increased strength in the

Fig. 3.1. Virtually complete loss of alkaline phosphatase-positive chondrocytes in the growth plate. Femur from a Wistar rat, 52 days after local x-irradiation with 3000 R at 6 weeks of age. Alkaline phosphatase (azo dye method), × 102

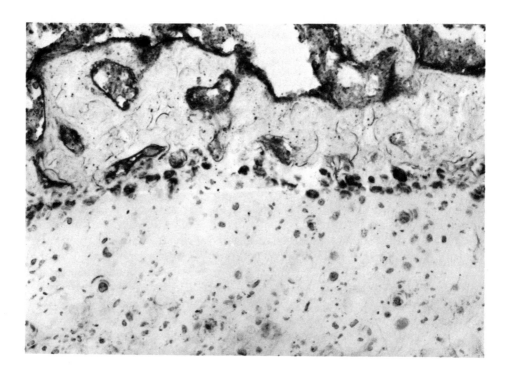

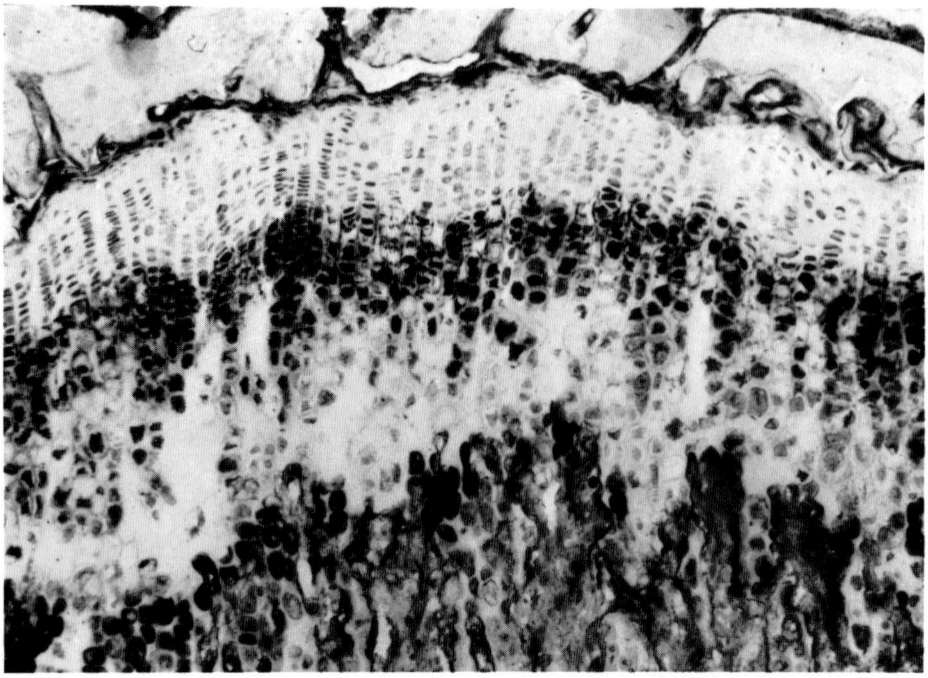

Fig. 3.2. Loss of alkaline phosphatase activity in those chondrocytes in the lower part of the growth plate which are within the range of the α-radiation. Femur from a Wistar rat, 9 days after i.p. injection of 16.3 μCi/kg ^{224}Ra (α-emitter, half-life 3.6 days) at 6 weeks of age. Alkaline phosphatase (azo dye method), × 80

regenerating cells, particularly in the cell islands (Fig. 3.3; PUTZKE 1963; SAMS 1966a; EURATOM-GSF 1967; GÖSSNER and SCHWABE 1968). Acid phosphatase activity is increased in cells in the radiation-damaged growth plate, presumably reflecting autophagia related to the dystrophic changes (GÖSSNER and SCHWABE 1968).

3.3.2 The Zone of Cartilage Erosion

The cartilage-derived growth factor which is produced by the chondrocytes not only stimulates the proliferation of the chondrocytes themselves; it also induces proliferation of endothelial cells and is chemotactic for endothelial cells (COWELL et al. 1987).

The capillaries in the zone of cartilage erosion have specialized characteristics. They do not have a basement membrane and the endothelial cells contain lysosomes. These cells are in direct contact with the cartilage cavity or capsule, or with

disrupting chondrocytes (ZINKERNAGEL et al. 1972). The study by HUNZIKER et al. (1987) cited in Sect. 3.3.1.1 showed that the hypertrophic chondrocytes do not degenerate. This had already been shown for hypertrophic chondrocytes in the mouse mandibular condyle (SILBERMANN and FROMMER 1972a,b). Despite this the chondrocytes disappear in the zone of cartilage removal and bone deposition (HUNZIKER et al. 1987). The cell kinetics of the transition from cartilage to bone during enchondral ossification is not fully understood. BALTADJIEV (1987) described the unclear situation as "mesenchymal complex in ossification." The histogenesis of ossification centers in cartilage corresponds formally to enchondral ossification. The ultrastructure of cells involved in this process was studied by COLE and WEZEMAN (1985). Their results indicate that in the area of cartilage removal and bone deposition transition may take place between chondrocytes and fibroblast-like cells. Polymorphic (pluripotent?) mesenchymal cells are found in a perivascular position (together with preosteoblasts and osteoblasts). Vacuolized macrophages and multinucleate chondroclasts remove the cartilage matrix.

Cell kinetic studies show that the proliferation rate of the endothelia is likely to be of the same order of magnitude as that of the other cells in the metaphysis (KEMBER 1971).

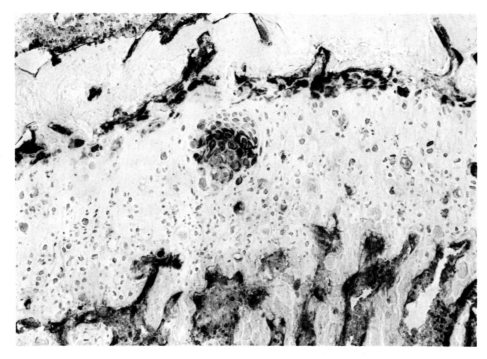

Fig. 3.3. Island-like cluster of regenerating cartilage cells in the growth plate. Rat tibia, 3 weeks after local x-irradiation with 2000 R at 6 weeks of age. Alkaline phosphatase (azo dye method), × 80

Damage to the capillaries in the zone of cartilage erosion has been studied using injection techniques (DAHL 1936; HINKEL 1943b; CARLSON et al. 1960; KEMBER and COGGINS 1967) as well as simple histological techniques (HINKEL 1943a; SISSONS 1956; HULTH and WESTERBORN 1960; MELANOTTE and FOLLIS 1961; MACPHERSON et al. 1962; LEVY and RUGH 1952). Initial dilation of the capillaries in the zone of cartilage erosion 2–3 days after irradiation with 2000 R was described as early as 1936 by DAHL.

Erythrocyte extravasation is seen at doses below 1000 R during the 1st week (HINKEL 1943a), and there is a raised permeability to thorium dioxide particles before the end of the 1st week after 1020 R (CARLSON et al. 1960). Erythrocyte extravasation is seen 3 days after ^{90}Sr incorporation, i.e., after a dose accumulation of 27 Gy (MACPHERSON et al. 1962). Whole body irradiation with 1500 R can lead to capillary dilation and erythrocyte extravasation after only 3 h (LEVY and RUGH 1952). MARQUART and GÖSSNER (1978) observed erythrocyte extravasation together with changes in the ultrastructure of the capillary endothelium as early as 2 h after incorporation of a relatively low activity (1.5 µCi/kg) of the short-lived α-emitter ^{224}Ra.

HINKEL (1943b) described a *reduction in the number of metaphyseal capillaries*, and a resultant serrated, discontinuous appearance of the line of capillary tufts (along the metaphyseal–cartilage junction), as early as 3 days after 950 R, although this type of change is not usually seen until 1 week after irradiation (DAHL 1936; KEMBER and COGGINS 1967). Complete or nearly complete loss of the capillaries in the zone of cartilage erosion is seen in the late phase after doses of 1000 R or more (MELANOTTE and FOLLIS 1961: 9 days after 1200 R and 1800 R; KEMBER and COGGINS 1967: 4 weeks after 18 Gy). This effect is observed within 9 days of ^{90}Sr incorporation when dose accumulation has reached 68 Gy (MACPHERSON et al. 1962).

At doses below 10 Gy it appears that after 1 month the arrangement of the capillaries has returned more or less to normal (HINKEL 1943a, b). Rebuilding of the line of cartilage erosion following division of the cartilage plate will be described later. The blood vessel system is considered to be a critical component with regard to the restoration of the complete biomechanism of enchondral ossification (HINKEL 1943a; JEE and ARNOLD 1961).

3.3.3 The Osteogenic Tissue

Reviews of the development and kinetics of these cells can be found in OWEN (1971), SIMMONS (1976), HEUCK (1976), OWEN (1978), VAUGHAN (1981), JOHNSON (1986), and MARKS and POPOFF (1988). MARKS and POPOFF (1988) also give a survey of growth and development factors in osteogenic tissue, the cytokines of osteogenic cells. In osteoblasts, production of TGF-β mRNA coincides with active type I collagen synthesis. The levels of proα1 (I) collagen, TGF-β, and c-*fos* mRNAs in periosteal fibroblasts are very high. Osteoclasts contain high levels of TGF-β and c-*fos* transcripts (SANDBERG et al. 1988). Interestingly, feedback between osteoblasts and proliferating cells can only take place via direct cell-to-cell contact (VAN DER PLAS and NIJWEIDE 1988). The relationship between chondrogenesis and osteogenesis, which is probably of importance for bone formation without direct skeletal contact, has been described in a review by TRIFFITT (1987). Molecular biological results describing the active morphogenetic protein which is involved have been published recently (WOZNEY et al. 1988). The chondrogenetic and osteogenetic potential of the progenitor cell population in the mandibular condyle has already been mentioned in Sect. 3.3.1.1. The time course of cell renewal is shown in Table 3.3 using the experimental data published by KEMBER (1960). According to current knowledge there seems to be a clear division between the developmental pathways of osteoclasts, on the one hand, and osteoblasts/osteocytes, on the other. For this reason the normal characteristics and radiation sensitivity of these cells will be described separately.

3.3.3.1 Osteoclasts

Developmental Pathway

The function of the osteoclast is to resorb vital bone, in contrast to dead bone which is resorbed by macrophages; thus the osteoclast cannot be simply classified in the phagocyte system (LOUTIT et al. 1982). Endocytotic uptake of peroxidase along the resorbing cell surface of the osteoclast (ruffled border) can be observed a short time after intravenous injection of the enzyme (LUCHT 1972). Even so, both SHIPLEY and MACKLIN (1916/17) and DAHL (1936) had already noticed that osteoclasts do not show storage of trypan blue a short time after injection. JEE and NOLAN (1963) finally found an increase in labeled osteoclasts at the end of the 2nd week after injection of a dextran sulfate–carbon suspension, in good agreement with the ³H-labeling experiments by KEMBER (1960) (see Table 3.3) but rejected by TONNA (1963) as an argument for the cytogenesis of osteoclasts. The first experiments which showed that it was likely that osteoclasts develop by fusion of monocytes, or at least cells from the myelomonocytic lineage, involved transplantation of bone marrow from mice with giant lysosomes into lethally irradiated animals without this genetic defect, and transplantation of healthy bone marrow into lethally irradiated animals with hereditary osteopetrosis (LOUTIT and TOWNSEND 1982a,b). Studies of cell surface markers, however, do not prove that osteoclasts are fused monocytes; both cells could also have a common precursor (JONES et al. 1981; LOUTIT and NISBET 1982; LOUTIT et al. 1982). HORTON (1988) recently reviewed the antigenic structure of osteoclasts as shown by experiments with monoclonal antibodies.

Table 3.3. Cell kinetics in the metaphysis. Number of labeled cells[a] in the proximal tibia metaphysis following single application of tritiated thymidine to rats weighing 100–120 g. (After KEMBER 1960)

Time following application of tritiated thymidine	Mesenchymal cells	Osteoblasts	Osteocytes	Osteoclasts
1 hour	**52**	9	0	0
1 day	**55**	29	0	1
2 days	41	**45**	0	2
3 days	32	22	0	2
5 days	34	33	6	5
7 days	23	8	17	5
14 days	3	9	21	4
21 days	7	2	**30**	**8**
28 days	0	1	14	4

[a] Calculated from a diagram.

When discussing osteoclast kinetics it is important to realize that in contrast to other systems these cells have a much less clearly defined lifetime; the half-life is of the order of 10 days but is dependent on the genetic background (LOUTIT and TOWNSEND 1982a,b). The youngest osteoclasts are found close to the cartilage plate (MILLER and MARKS 1982). During growth they move away from the cartilage plate together with the spongiosa (KIMMEL and JEE 1980b). In contrast to the osteoblasts, the osteoclasts are distributed fairly evenly over the primary and secondary spongiosa (KIMMEL and JEE 1980a). The number of osteoclasts is apparently determined at least partly by the resorption activity, since rats with hereditary osteopetrosis have more osteoclasts (MILLER and MARKS 1982).

The ultrastructure of osteoclasts is treated in JONES and BOYDE (1977) and HOLTROP and KING (1977).

Effect of Radiation

Changes in ultrastructure (chromatin condensation, dilation of cisternae of the endoplasmic reticulum, vacuolization of the Golgi complex, and, in particular, mitochondrial swelling) are observed as early as 2 h after incorporation of relatively low activities of ^{224}Ra (1.5 µCi/kg) (MARQUART and GÖSSNER 1978). The osteoclast population as such seems to be fairly radiation resistant; osteoclasts continue to resorb plutonium-containing bone even under these conditions of permanent irradiation (ARNOLD and JEE 1957).

No reduction is observed in the osteoclast population following external irradiation [e.g., DAHL 1936; LEVY and RUGH 1952; BLACKBURN and WELLS 1963; review by ZOLLINGER 1960; and with the exception of a report by HELLER (1948), a few hours after 1000 R whole body irradiation of chicken].

A reduction in the number of osteoclasts is seen at different times after incorporation of bone-seeking radionuclides (HELLER 1948; JEE and ARNOLD 1961). No reduction was observed in the number of osteoclasts in the metaphysis 12 weeks after incorporation of high activities of the short-lived α-emitter ^{227}Th (PÖMSL 1974). A transitional increase in the number of osteoclasts has been observed (GAMER 1988) 1 week after incorporation of 111 kBq/kg ^{239}Pu (accumulated mean skeletal dose, 0.338 Gy).

An increase in the number of giant cells in the zone of cartilage erosion and/or osteoclasts in the spongiosa has been reported to occur at very different times following external and internal irradiation (HINKEL 1943a; HELLER 1948; JEE and ARNOLD 1961; MACPHERSON et al. 1962). The same results were found following irradiation with 2000 R (SAMS 1966a) or incorporation of <25 µCi/kg, i.e., <7.5 Gy skeletal dose of ^{224}Ra (GÖSSNER and SCHWABE 1968), using detection of acid phosphatase as a marker. Repair mechanisms presumably play a role in this effect.

The close relationship between bone marrow and osteoclasts, including the time of appearance of radiation damage, has been shown by quantitative comparison of the two populations and by bone marrow transplantation (ANDERSON et al. 1979; GÜNGÖR et al. 1982). Thus it is readily understandable that local irradiation of bone does not necessarily lead to a reduction in the osteoclast population. Surprisingly, however, exposure to continuous whole body irradiation with 0.45 Gy/day leads to a 50% reduction in osteoclast density in the metaphysis after 10 weeks, even though the number of osteoblasts remains unchanged (ANDERSON et al. 1979). It has been shown in vitro that above a sort of threshold dose (D_q) of 1.85 Gy the bone marrow loses its ability to form osteoclasts (SCHEVEN et al. 1987).

3.3.3.2 Osteoblasts in the Metaphysis and Their Precursors

Normal Cell Kinetics

Osteoblast precursor cells cannot be distinguished from fibroblasts in the light microscope. The cell is characterized by its position close to osteoblasts and incorporation of ^{3}H-thymidine. The nuclear volume of the precursor cell is more than double that of osteoblasts (POLIG et al. 1984). In the literature the cells are described as "mesenchymal cells," "osteoprogenitor cells" (OPGCs), or "preosteoblasts" (see review literature cited in Sect. 3.3.3). The generation time of OPGCs in the metaphysis is given as approximately 1.5 days (KEMBER 1971; KIMMEL and JEE 1980b).

Surprisingly, even after repeated application of ^{3}H-thymidine only 50% of the OPGCs are labeled after 3 days, i.e., there must be a considerable reserve cell population among these cells (KEMBER 1960). A mitogenic regulating factor for osteogenic cells has been isolated from human bone (for literature see MAUGH II 1982). Looked at more precisely (for review see ASCENZI 1976), the cells described above as OPGCs should be called committed OPGCs, to differentiate them from the inducible OPGCs transmitted by bone marrow, which presumably play a role in metaplastic ossification. In contrast to bone marrow stem cells, it seems that the inducible OPGCs cannot be substituted by immigration from other regions (AMSEL and DELL 1972). The maximum number of labeled osteoblasts is found 2 days after single application of ^{3}H-thymidine (see Table 3.3, above). Occasional labeled osteoblasts are seen as soon as 1 h after injection, i.e., occasional osteoblasts are still dividing. Approximately one-quarter of osteoblasts are labeled 3 days after repeated ^{3}H-thymidine injection, i.e., the turnover time is about 12 days (KEMBER 1960). PRITCHARD (1972) has reviewed the physiology of osteoblasts. There are considerably more osteoblasts in the primary spongiosa than in the secondary spongiosa (KIMMEL and JEE 1980a).

Radiation Damage

Changes in ultrastructure (chromatin condensation, dilation of cisternae of the endoplasmic reticulum, vacuolization of the Golgi complex, and, in particular, swelling of mitochondria) have

been observed as early as 2 h after incorporation of ^{224}Ra (MARQUART and GÖSSNER 1978; Fig. 3.4).

Cell death is observed only a few hours after the start of irradiation in the OPGCs and osteoblast regions of the metaphysis (MACPHERSON et al. 1962; KEMBER and SADEK 1970), with a clear relationship to the radiation dose. Cell death precedes damage to the capillary system (MAC-PHERSON et al. 1962).

Mitotic activity is reduced – in a dose-dependent manner – during the 1st day after commencement of irradiation (MACPHERSON et al. 1962). The number of ^{3}H-thymidine labeled cells per unit area in the metaphysis is also reduced within the 1st day after irradiation. The values return to normal approximately 2 weeks after a dose of 17.5 Gy, but remain permanently low following abortive recovery after 35 Gy (KEMBER 1962). Interestingly, the number of DNA-synthesizing cells can be maintained at a reduced

Fig. 3.4. Early changes in osteoblast ultrastructure (detail of cytoplasm) following α-irradiation. The mitochondria (*m*) are swollen with a rarefied matrix and few cristae. The cisternae (*z*) of the rough endoplasmic reticulum are dilated. Tibia metaphysis from an NMRI mouse, 24 h after i.p. injection with 5 μCiμ/kg ^{224}Ra (α-emitter, half-life 3.6 days) at 4 weeks of age. (Sample and micrograph from Dr. K.-H. Marquart) × 20000

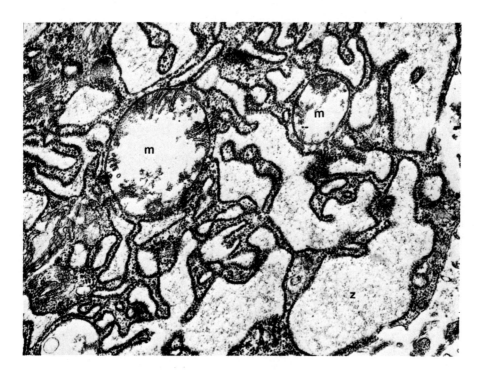

level for some time under conditions of continuous irradiation with 0.84 Gy/day (KEMBER 1962).

Following incorporation of ^{32}P there is a reduction in, and dose-dependent recovery of, DNA-synthesizing cells similar to that observed following external x-irradiation. The majority of labeled cells belong to the population of atypical spindle cells which is observed following loss of osteoblasts (see below) (KEMBER 1962). The loss of ^{3}H-thymidine labeled OPGCs has been shown to be dose dependent following incorporation of both the short-lived α-emitter ^{224}Ra (BECKER et al. 1972) and the long-lived α-emitter ^{226}Ra (KOF-RÁNEK et al. 1977). The number of spindle-shaped OPGCs per unit area remains unchanged after incorporation of 5 μCi/kg of the short-lived α-emitter ^{227}Th (half-life 18.7 days), which corresponds to an average initial maximum dose rate of 0.35 Gy/day, whereas the cell density falls to minimal values 4 weeks after 50 μCi/kg (3.5 Gy/day) (PÖMSL 1974).

Changes in the osteoblast population in the metaphysis have been studied under a variety of conditions (DAHL 1936; GALL et al. 1940; HINKEL 1943a; HELLER 1948; LEVY and RUGH 1952; ZOLLINGER 1960; HULTH and WESTERBORN 1960; JEE and ARNOLD 1961; MELANOTTE and FOLLIS 1961; MACPHERSON et al. 1962; BLACKBURN and WELLS 1963; BENSTED and COURTENAY 1965; PÖMSL 1974; ANDERSON et al. 1979; GAMER 1988; LÄNGLE 1988). In general there is a reduction in the number of osteoblasts within a week of irradiation or start of irradiation. The cell number is decimated within hours following a dose of 400–1000 R (HELLER 1948; HULTH and WESTERBORN 1960) or 80 000 R (LEVY and RUGH 1952).

Up to now the lowest dose which has been reported to cause a loss of osteoblasts is 400 R (HELLER 1948; MELANOTTE and FOLLIS 1961). The dose dependence of the phenomenon is best shown in experiments following internal irradiation. Thus incorporation of the long-lived β-emitter ^{90}Sr results in a reduction in the number of osteoblasts after 9 days with a dose rate of 0.08–0.09 Gy/h, and after 3 days with a dose rate of 0.35–0.36 Gy/h (MACPHERSON et al. 1962). The osteoblast population is maintained following internal α-irradiation with short-lived ^{227}Th (half-life 18.7 days) when applied so as to give a maximum initial dose rate of 0.35 Gy/day, but is greatly reduced within a week at a dose rate of 3.5 Gy/day (PÖMSL 1974). Surprisingly, the osteoblast population is maintained over a long period when subject

Table 3.4. Resistance of osteoblasts in the tibia metaphysis to chronic irradiation with 0.45 Gy/day ^{137}Cs γ-irradiation. Male C3H mice irradiated from 5 weeks of age. (After ANDERSON et al. 1979)

Time	No. of osteoblasts per field
0 (controls)	15
4 weeks	12
10 weeks	18
12 weeks	11
+4 weeks radiation-free recovery interval	14

to continuous irradiation with 0.45 Gy/day (see Table 3.4; ANDERSON et al. 1979).

MELANOTTE and FOLLIS (1961) have described a short-lived increase in the number of osteoblasts 1 h after irradiation (400–1800 R), whereas GALL et al. (1940) did not observe any changes in the osteoblast population even after 2400 R.

Spindle cells and/or newly formed fibers (peritrabecular fibrosis) appear in the region of trabeculae concomitant with the disappearance of active osteoblasts at doses above 1000 R/10 Gy (Fig. 3.5, DAHL 1936; HINKEL 1943a; LEVY and RUGH 1952; ZOLLINGER 1960; MACPHERSON et al. 1962; BENSTED and COURTENAY 1965). Following internal irradiation, fibrosis appears to be easier to induce with α-emitters (for literature see MACPHERSON et al. 1962). This phenomenon will be considered further in relationship to the disturbance of intramembranous ossification. Fractionation appears to reduce the effect of peritrabecular fibrosis (see Table 3.5; BENSTED and COURTENAY 1965). Peritrabecular fibrosis should be seen not only as a disturbance of the osteoblast system but also generally as a pathological effect of the intensely irradiated bone marrow region [see the early description by ENGEL (1938) following local

Table 3.5. The effect of dose fractionation on the frequency of radiation-induced peritrabecular fibrosis in the metaphysis. Experiments on 1- to 3-month-old rats. (After BENSTED and COURTENAY 1965)

Irradiation scheme	Frequency among investigated tibiae[a]
1 × 3000 R	45% (40/88)
3 × 1000 R (interval 2 weeks)	0% (0/26)
6 × 500 R (interval 2 weeks)	2% (1/58)

[a] Investigation of moribund and/or tumor-bearing animals.

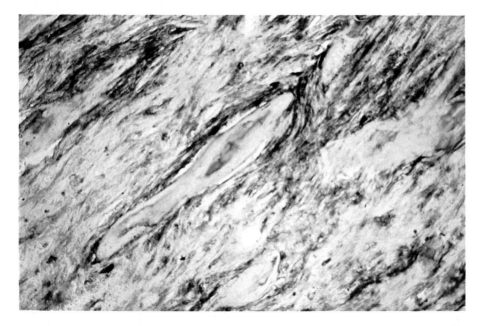

Fig. 3.5. Inter-and peritrabecular fibrosis showing clear alkaline phosphatase activity in the newly formed connective tissue. Femur from a Wistar rat, 10 days after i.p. injection of 75 μCi/kg ^{224}Ra (α-emitter, half-life 3.6 days) at 6 weeks of age. Alkaline phosphatase (azo dye method), × 100

radium irradiation, and descriptions by CALVO et al. (1978) and GÖSSNER et al. (1982) following whole body irradiation prior to bone marrow transplantation].

The reduction in the osteoblast population manifests as a disturbance in osteoid production, resulting in atrophy of the primary spongiosa (HINKEL 1943a; HULTH and WESTERBORN 1960). The complete separation of this spongiosa from the cartilage plate is described later (see Sect. 3.3.6.2).

Restitution of active osteoblasts is observed in the course of 3–4 weeks (HINKEL 1943a; JEE and ARNOLD 1961). The reduction in osteoblasts observed in chicken at doses below 1000 R appears to be much more short-lived (HELLER 1948).

3.3.3.3 Osteocytes in the Metaphysis

Young osteoblast-like osteocytes in the metaphysis show the same ultrastructural changes a short time after incorporation of low doses of ^{224}Ra as do osteoblasts (MARQUART 1977). Loss of a re-

cognizable fraction of this population generally appears to occur more than 3 days after irradiation with >10 Gy or incorporation of larger amounts of radionuclides (HELLER 1948; LEVY and RUGH 1952; MACPHERSON et al. 1962; BLACKBURN and WELLS 1963), in sufficient agreement with the production and maturation time of these cells (see Table 3.3, above). SAMS (1966b), however, did not observe any changes in metaphysis osteocytes following 2000 R irradiation of young rats.

3.3.4 Changes in Enzyme Activity

The enzyme histochemistry of bone tissue is reviewed in GÖSSNER and SCHWABE (1971).

The most important marker enzyme for bone production is alkaline phosphatase (BOURNE 1972). The enzyme is only directly inactivated in vitro at very high doses (NORRIS and COHN 1952). The activity of this enzyme in "in vivo" irradiation experiments was first studied in detail using biochemical methods and whole bone (WILKINS and REGEN 1934; REGEN and WILKINS 1936; WOODARD and SPIERS 1953; WOODARD and LAUGHLIN 1957; DZIEWIATKOWSKI and WOODARD 1959), although WOODARD and SPIERS (1953) did consider, comparing the enzyme histochemical preparations, that the zone of primary spongiosa was a region with particularly high activity. According to the authors cited above, the enzyme activity is reduced to a minimum in the 3rd week after a dose of 600 R. The effect shows a certain dependence on dose and radiation quality (WOODARD and SPIERS 1953), whereby the effects of 100–1000 kV x-irradiation must be considered identical on the basis of calculations of the dose actually absorbed in the enzyme-active region (WOODARD and LAUGHLIN 1957). There is a dose-dependent reduction (not strictly proportional) in alkaline phosphatase activity 24 h after the start of local irradiation (NORRIS and COHN 1952), which corresponds with the early loss of osteoblasts and chondrocytes seen by HELLER (1948). ENGSTRÖM et al. (1981) showed a reduction in activity in isolated tibia metaphysis as early as 1 day after a radiation dose of only 0.5 Gy.

The correlation between reduction in alkaline phosphatase in bone and serum 1 week after irradiation, and reduction in fixation of ^{45}Ca together with disappearance of the bone matrix, was already observed by COHN and GONG (1953b). These authors considered the results to be correlated with the loss of osteoblasts. WOODARD (1957) also observed a parallel reduction in alkaline phosphatase and ^{89}Sr uptake. Parallel biochemical and electron microscopic investigation of cell and matrix vesicle fractions in the skull of growing rats showed that the reduction in alkaline phosphatase activity and disturbance of mineralization are accompanied by breakdown of the vesicle membrane (SELA et al. 1982).

The high enzyme histochemical activity of alkaline phosphatase in active osteoblasts disappears parallel with the loss of these cells after both external and internal irradiation (PUTZKE 1963; GÖSSNER and SCHWABE 1968). SAMS (1966a), however, failed to observe such effects after 2000 R, and MELANOTTE and FOLLIS (1961) actually observed an increase in enzyme-active cells parallel to an increase in osteoblasts in the first days after 400–1800 R. Interestingly, the spindle cells which appear between the trabeculae in the metaphysis also react in the histochemical assay for alkaline phosphatase (BURSTONE 1952; PUTZKE 1963; GÖSSNER and SCHWABE 1968). These cells are rich in glycogen (BURSTONE 1952) – as are preosteoblasts (SCOTT and GLIMCHER 1971).

Acid phosphatase-positive cells are increased in the metaphysis in association with the appearance of repair processes (SAMS 1966a; GÖSSNER and SCHWABE 1968). At higher doses there seems to be a certain reduction in cells with histochemically

demonstrable acid phosphatase in the primary spongiosa (GÖSSNER and SCHWABE 1968). A small reduction in acid phosphatase has been shown in the matrix vesicles in growing skull bone 3 weeks after irradiation (SELA et al. 1982).

3.3.5 Disturbance of Mineralization in the Region of the Metaphysis

The mineralization of bone has been studied both with radiochemistry (e.g., WOODARD 1957; COHN and GONG 1953b; WILSON 1956a,b, 1957, 1958, 1959, 1960, 1961; COHN 1961; BLACKBURN and WELLS 1963; BABICKÝ and KOLÁŘ 1966) and using histochemical/autoradiographic methods (RISSANEN et al. 1969b; KUMMERMEHR 1971). KUMMERMEHR (1971) gives a review of the literature. No effects have been described following 100 or 250 R, but a reduction in mineralization is already observed in the 1st week (KUMMERMEHR 1971) after irradiation at doses above 500 R (BLACKBURN and WELLS 1963). In general the lowest levels of mineralization are observed 3–5 weeks after irradiation (see KUMMERMEHR 1971). There is a linear dose response relationship at doses above 1000 R (see Table 3.6; WILSON 1956b). Rapidly growing animals are the most sensitive (WILSON 1958). Fractionation reduces the effect (WILSON 1961), whereas the wavelength of x-irradiation has little influence (WILSON 1957). This is explained by the relative paucity of mineral close to mineralizing cells. Surprisingly, short-lived increases in ^{45}Ca uptake are observed in nonirradiated regions of the skeleton – presumably controlled by the nervous system (BABICKÝ and KOLÁŘ 1966). Whole body irradiation appears to inhibit mineralization more strongly than local irradiation (COHN 1961).

Table 3.6. Reduction in ^{32}P incorporation 4–8 weeks following irradiation of 6-week-old mice with 200 kV x-rays (HVL 1.0 mm Cu). (After WILSON 1956b)

Dose	^{32}P incorporation, tibia, % of control[a]
1000 R	85% ± 7%
1500 R	71% ± 6%
2000 R	57% ± 11%

[a] Values rounded up or down.

3.3.6 The Complex Disturbance of Enchondral Ossification

Apart from the interesting aspect of cell kinetics, the complex appearance of changes in enchondral ossification cannot be deduced quantitatively from the rules describing the changes in selected parts of the system. Thus in the following an attempt will be made to describe critical changes in their whole complexity. Normal enchondral ossification is characterized by a balance between cartilage growth/cartilage resorption/bone formation/bone remodeling. Radiation damage appears to affect the different phases in a different way, or at least at different times, leading on occasion to considerable disturbance of the equilibrium. This upset of equilibrium manifests itself in the phenomena of (a) expansion of the growth plate and increase in calcified remains of cartilage in the metaphysis, and (b) temporary separation of the growth plate and metaphysis and increase in metaphysis spongiosa with possible subsequent restoration of a functional connection between cartilage and metaphysis.

3.3.6.1 Disturbances in the Resorption of cartilase and Primary Spongiosa

The differentiation process in the cartilage cell columns in growth cartilage appears to continue independent of "growth pressure" – in the same way as other proliferative maturation systems (BOND et al. 1965). The entry of capillaries, which is upset by irradiation, appears to be an important step in the development of enchondral ossification (see discussion in MACPHERSON et al. 1962; SAMS 1966b). The effect is comparable to ischemia. *Thickening of the growth plate*, or at least of a large section of it, is often observed following external or internal irradiation (Fig. 3.6). SISSONS (1956) measured the dose response of this effect

Fig. 3.6. a Thickening of the growth plate and increase in nonresorbed remains of cartilage in the enriched metaphysis spongiosa. Tibia from an NMRI mouse, 7 days after i.p. injection of 75 µCi/kg [224]Ra (α-emitter, half-life 3.6 days) at 4 weeks of age. Toluidine blue, × 40. **b** Untreated control animal as comparison

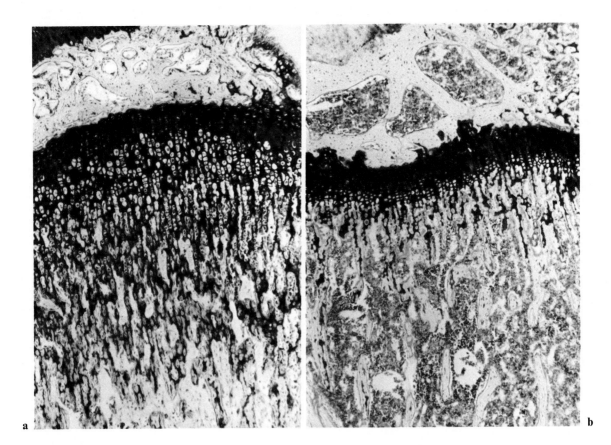

a   b

and, assuming a constant relationship between cartilage width and growth rate, calculated the increase in length of the phase of hypertrophy and degeneration of chondrocytes (see Table 3.7). He assumed, however, that widening of the plate was entirely due to increase in cell size, extension of the time for maturation, and increase in matrix, without taking into account processes in the zone of cartilage erosion. Widening of the growth plate has been described in numerous publications – following external irradiation by, for example, HOFFMANN (1923), BAUNACH (1935), BISGARD and HUNT (1936), ENGEL (1938), HINKEL (1943a), GÜNSEL (1953), SISSONS (1956), DZIEWIATKOWSKI and WOODARD (1959), BASERGA et al. (1961), BLACKBURN and WELLS (1963), BENSTED and COURTENAY (1965), SAMS (1966a,b), and KUMMER-MEHR (1971), and following internal irradiation by, among others, HELLER (1948), KOCH (1957), JEE and ARNOLD (1961), MACPHERSON et al. (1962), GÖSSNER and SCHWABE (1968), and PÖMSL (1974). α-Irradiation causes less damage to proliferating cartilage than to osteogenic tissue because of its short range. The available results do not allow the calculation of a simple relationship between dose and time for the appearance of a widened growth plate. In the majority of cases these changes are observed after the 2nd week following doses of around 1000 R and more. The changes observed after doses of 600 R or less have been described by HOFFMANN (1923), BISGARD and HUNT (1936), HINKEL (1943a), and BLACKBURN and WELLS (1963). HOFFMANN (1923) and HINKEL (1943a) found changes within the first weeks. HOFFMANN ascribed the early increase in growth

following 10%–20% SED (skin erythema dose) to widening of the growth plate.

The disturbance and delay in the zone of cartilage erosion can be followed by an increase in *calcified cartilage remains in the metaphysis* (see Fig. 3.6, above). Disturbances in the osteogenic tissue in the metaphysis (bone production and resorption) probably play an important role in this effect, i.e., the effect is also an expression of disturbances in the remodeling of the primary spongiosa such that the appearance of primary spongiosa is displaced to the level of the secondary spongiosa. Sometimes a widespread network of calcified cartilage can be seen (e.g., KOCH 1957); the calcified cartilage remains can protrude into the metaphysis in a tongue-like fashion so that the zone of cartilage erosion no longer lies along a boundary line (e.g., BROOKS and HILLSTROM 1933). Descriptions of the effect after external irradiation can be found in BROOKS and HILLSTROM (1933), BARR et al. (1943), HINKEL (1943a), SISSONS (1956), HULTH and WESTERBORN (1960), MELANOTTE and FOLLIS (1961), BLACKBURN and WELLS (1963), BENSTED and COURTENAY (1965), and ANDERSON et al. (1979), and after internal irradiation in HELLER (1948), KOCH (1957), VAUGHAN and OWEN (1959), BLACKETT et al. (1959), and BENSTED et al. (1961). Even though the dose-time relationship appears irregular, there are experiments which show that this is an effect found essentially at higher doses: for external irradiation above 1000 R (BARR et al. 1943; SISSONS 1956) and for large amounts of radionuclides (KOCH 1957; VAUGHAN and OWEN 1959; BLACKETT et al. 1959; BENSTED et al. 1961). Disturbances in the absorption mechanism also partly explain observations of increased ash weight of bone (HINKEL 1943a), increase in calcium content (DZIEWIATKOWSKI and WOODARD 1959), and disturbances in ^{32}P transport (GAUWERKY 1958).

Table 3.7. Relative widening of the cartilage plate, and relative lengthening of chondrocyte transit time, in the proximal epiphysis growth plate of the tibia following local irradiation. Rat, 30 days old at time of irradiation. (After SISSONS 1956)

Dose (R)	Lengthening of hypertrophic and degeneration period[a]	Relative change in plate width[b] after irradiation		
		8 days	30 days	100 days
400	×2	1.0	1.1	1.1
800	×4	1.1	0.9	1.2
1200	×4	1.0	1.1	1.3
1600	Cessation of growth	0.8	1.1	2.5

[a] Calculated by SISSONS (1956) from the change in relationship of plate width to growth rate on the 8th day after irradiation.
[b] Calculated from data in SISSONS (1956).

3.3.6.2 Loss of Connection Between the Cartilage Plate and the Metaphysis

The loss in equilibrium between cartilage formation, cartilage resorption, and bone formation can be partially restored during the recovery phase with stepwise resorption and formation (see, for example, descriptions in GÖSSNER and SCHWABE 1968; KUMMERMEHR 1971); equally there can be widespread disruption in continuity between the cartilage plate and the bone tissue. This phenomenon can result from two mechanisms. The first is a loss of interlinkage between the cartilage plate and the primary spongiosa in the early phase of radiation damage, presumably in part as an expression of *atrophy of the primary spongiosa.* (For published descriptions following external and internal irradiation see HELLER 1948; RUBIN et al. 1959; HULTH and WESTERBORN 1960; BENSTED et al. 1961; SAMS 1966b.) HELLER (1948) described this effect simply as "severance." Careful x-ray morphological and microradiographic studies by HULTH and WESTERBORN (1960) showed that the effect only appears at doses above 1000 R, and can then be observed in the first few days following irradiation in the form of a thin lucent zone in the x-ray. Microradiography shows atrophic watch-glass-shaped trabeculae profiles.

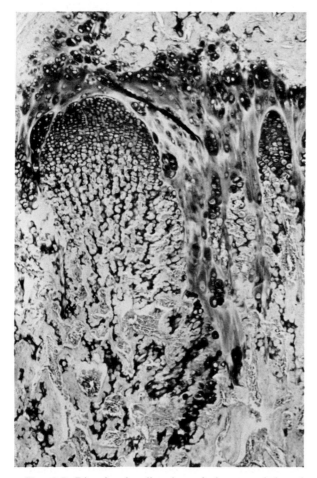

Fig. 3.7. Disordered splintering of the extended and damaged growth plate by proliferating connective tissue. Focal asbestos-like degeneration of the cartilage. Tibia from a Wistar rat, 26 days after i.p. injection of 25 µCi/kg [224]Ra (α-emitter, half-life 3.6 days) at 6 weeks of age. Azure eosin, × 20

The second mechanism leading to a disturbance in cartilage–bone continuity occurs in the restitution phase after disturbed enchondral ossification. The mechanisms which lead to *restoration of the zone of cartilage erosion* (see Figs. 3.7, 3.8) can result in horizontal division of the thickened growth plate. Descriptions of the effect following external and internal irradiation have been published in GALL et al. (1940), HINKEL (1943a), KOCH (1957), BASERGA et al. (1961), BENSTED and COURTENAY (1965), and SAMS (1966b). The limited results available indicate that the effect is first observed at doses clearly higher than 1000 R. Dose fractionation considerably reduces the frequency of the effect (BENSTED and COURTENAY 1965). The restoration of the zone of cartilage removal and bone deposition can also lead to simple displacement of devitalized metaphysis spongiosa, enriched with cartilage remains. Thus the appearance of nonresorbed spongiosa together with cartilage remains in the lower regions of the metaphysis and diaphysis may develop from different types of lesion. These displaced cartilage–bone boundary areas can arise as a result of calcification of the displaced lower half of a thickened growth plate; equally they can represent remains following complete displacement of a generation of primary spongiosa. Descriptions of such displaced cartilage–bone boundary regions following external or internal irradiation can be found in a number of publications, including DAHL (1936), RUBIN et al. (1959), BLACKETT et al. (1959), COTTIER (1961), BENSTED et al. (1961), JEE and ARNOLD (1961), BASERGA et al. (1961), and MACPHERSON et al. (1962). The temporary break in continuity between cartilage and primary spongiosa does not necessarily lead to development of new boundaries; it can just as well be followed by normal stepwise resorption of the spongiosa (HELLER 1948). Disturbances in the continuity between cartilage and bone at the level of provisional calcification appear in practice to play a very minor role. This effect was studied by RUBIN et al. (1959). Provisional calcification of cartilage was inhibited by uptake of the cartilage-seeking (chondrotropic) radionuclide ^{35}S and was also visible as a fine lucent zone in the x-ray.

3.3.6.3 Slipping of the Epiphysis

It is feasible that the loss of cartilage–bone continuity described in Sect. 3.3.6.2 could favor

Fig. 3.8. Duplication of the growth plate in the repair phase of radiation damage. Tibia from a Wistar rat, 53 days after i.p. injection of 75 μCi/kg ^{224}Ra (α-emitter, half-life 3.6 days) at 6 weeks of age. Alkaline phosphatase (azo dye method), × 50

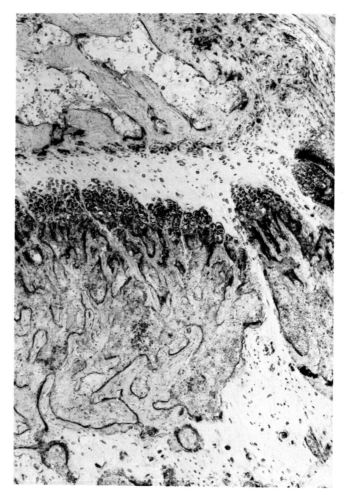

subsequent separation of the epiphysis and growth plate. RUBIN et al. (1957) were able to induce epiphyseal slippage by incorporation of ^{35}S in rats (i.e., by particularly high irradiation of cartilage and preferential disturbance of provisional calcification). SILVERMAN et al. (1981) summarized their clinical material on the subject and gave a detailed review of the literature. The risk of this effect occurring appears to be highest for children irradiated at an early age and with doses above 25 Gy (Table 3.8). The clinical phenomenon appears preferentially at an age of 8–10 years. The possible influence of chemotherapy (given in all

the cases in which epiphyseal slippage was observed) cannot be assessed from the available data.

3.3.6.4 Atypical Bone Formation in the Metaphysis

Even after active osteoblasts have disappeared from the metaphysis, formation of a hard substance can be observed in the areas of primary and secondary spongiosa, albeit with an unusual formal genesis and morphological appearance. On the one hand there can be direct transformation of nonresorbed cartilage into bone. The cartilage matrix becomes increasingly eosinophilic and it seems that erstwhile chondrocytes take on the form of active osteoblasts. A second possibility is the formation of a basophilic, coarsely fibrous material, generally poor in cells. In addition, when areas of devitalized metaphysis spongiosa are

Table 3.8. Slipping of the proximal femur epiphysis in irradiated children. Relationship to age and dose level. (After SILVERMAN et al. 1981)

	0–4 years	4–15 years
>25 Gy	47% = 7/15	5% = 1/21
≦25 Gy	0/25	0/22

present they can be surrounded by newly formed atypical or typical bone, instead of being resorbed, resulting in a reduction in the size of the bone marrow cavities. Descriptions of these processes are given in DAHL (1936), GALL et al. (1940), HINKEL (1943a), HELLER (1948), BURSTONE (1952), GÜNSEL (1953), RAY et al. (1956), KOCH (1957), VAUGHAN and OWEN (1959), ZOLLINGER (1960), BASERGA et al. (1961), KUMMERMEHR (1971), and PÖMSL (1974). Histochemistry shows that these atypical forms of bone are genuinely mineralized (BURSTONE 1952). The x-ray shows thickening of the metaphysis, sometimes described as "osteosclerosis." Both the coarsely fibrous cell-poor type of bone and the bone formed on a basis of devitalized spongiosa are likely to be particularly fragile — which can be significant when the atypical bone formation is displaced towards the diaphysis (see Sect. 3.3.6.2). Equally, the only remnants of this atypical bone can be a zone of thickened bone trabeculae.

3.3.6.5 The Pathology of "Growth Arrest Lines"

After growth has been resumed the processes described in Sects. 3.3.6.1, 3.3.6.2, and 3.3.6.4 can appear in the x-ray picture in the form of dense lines perpendicular to the longitudinal axis. Such "growth arrest lines" have long been recognized in roentgenology and are not specific for radiation damage (for a review of the literature see HINKEL 1943b; HEUCK 1976). HINKEL (1943a), BARR et al. (1943), and RUBIN et al. (1959) have all described the appearance of such lines in experimental situations following identification of the pathological–histological changes described above. The discrete lucent zone observed experimentally by HULTH and WESTERBORN (1960) appears not to be identifiable clinically. There are a number of clinical descriptions of groups of patients showing

Table 3.9. Lines of growth arrest in vertebrae of radiation-treated children in relation to age at time of irradiation and radiation dose. (After NEUHAUSER et al. 1952)

Radiation dose (R) at center of vertebra	<2 years	≧2 years	Sum
<1000	0/6	0/3	0/9
≦1000 <2000[a]	3/4	5/8	8/12

[a] Above 2000 R the phenomenon is overlaid by other major changes.

growth arrest lines following irradiation therapy (NEUHAUSER et al. 1952; VAETH et al. 1962; GUTJAHR et al. 1976; BLEHER and TSCHÄPPELER 1979). They all refer to children and juveniles treated with tumorigenic doses of radiation (see example in Table 3.9). Five of six of the patients with growth arrest lines described by BLEHER and TSCHÄPPELER (1979) had also received chemotherapy, which may be significant when considering the possible combination effects of radiation and chemotherapy.

3.3.7 Disturbed Enchondral Ossification Considered as a Whole

Among the review articles cited in the introduction, two give particularly good summaries of the histological changes which take place, GATES (1943) and RUBIN and CASARETT (1968). Experimental publications often deal with only isolated aspects. The complete process of enchondral ossification is considered in the following publications: after external irradiation by DAHL (1936), GALL et al. (1940), HINKEL (1943a), HELLER (1948), LEVY and RUGH (1952), HULTH and WESTERBORN (1960), MELANOTTE and FOLLIS (1961), and HORVÁTH et al. (1962), and after internal irradiation by HELLER (1948), KOCH (1957), RAY et al. (1956), and BENSTED et al. (1961).

Growing cartilage appears to be more sensitive than the processes involved in the generation of osteoblasts. Thus at dose levels below 1000 R the most prominent effect is that of reversible disturbance to cartilage formation, which is best recognized on the basis of changes in columnar arrangement and dystrophic swelling. At higher doses disorganization and loss of cells in the growth plate become more pronounced, followed by regeneration of the growth plate, occasionally in the form of islands. In addition at higher dose levels there is increasing inhibition of cartilage erosion and the osteoblast system, and thus of osteoid production. Spindle cells appear in the bone marrow cavities. These effects lead to an increase in a network of osteoid-poor calcified cartilage in the metaphysis, or even to persistence of an enlarged growth plate. The primary spongiosa can become separated from the cartilage. Finally the increased osteoid-poor primary spongiosa can be resorbed multifocally, or the thickened cartilage plate can be divided by a new line of cartilage erosion. This damage can persist over a long period. It is followed by development of interstitial fibrosis, formation of atypical, basophilic, coarsely fibrous bone, and/or direct cartilage ossification. If the metaphysis spongiosa has been devitalized this can be followed by extreme thickening of the trabecular network, possibly in the form of lamellar bone. In general at higher doses the atypical bone is displaced en masse, or in large chunks, towards the diaphysis. The inhibited resorption of spongiosa which is observed is compatible with the observation that the number of osteoclasts in the metaphysis spongiosa is reduced (GÖSSNER and SCHWABE 1968; ANDERSON et al. 1979).

3.3.8 Disturbance of Intramembranous Ossification

General reviews of normal intramembranous ossification are given in LEBLOND and WEINSTOCK (1971) and SISSONS (1971). The precise measurements made by SONTAG (1980) show that the form of the long bones is to a great extent determined by the different rates of cortical bone deposition. SONTAG (1986a,b) has also determined the age dependence of the deposition rate in rat femur. The generation time of endosteal and periosteal osteoprogenitor cells is longer than in the metaphysis (KEMBER 1971). ^{3}H-thymidine labeling shows that the periosteal stem cells are evenly distributed, i.e., growth is not restricted to the metaphysis region, rather the periosteum is evenly stretched in all segments (KEMBER and LAMBERT 1981).

Morphological studies of radiation damage to intramembranous ossification (both external and internal irradiation) have been described in BISGARD and HUNT (1936), HELLER (1948), LEVY and RUGH (1952), KOCH (1957), RUBIN et al. (1959), JEE and ARNOLD (1961), BLACKBURN and WELLS (1963), SAMS (1966a), and RISSANEN et al. (1969b). Basically the same effects are observed as in the metaphysis spongiosa. Active osteoblasts are reduced, spindle cells appear, and fibers are formed. This effect can be observed within a week. The damage which is critical in the long term, i.e., development of hyalinized fibrosis with reduced cell content, apparently develops later. As with deposition of atypical bone, there is a continuous transition to the osteoradionecrosis, which generally accompanies it. Disturbances in intramembranous ossification result in a thinning of the corticalis. The slimming of the central

portion of the long bones becomes more marked, i.e., the diameter of the diaphysis is reduced (RUBIN et al. 1959 after dose of 2400 R). On average the process of intramembranous ossification outside the metaphysis appears to be less radiation sensitive than that of enchondral ossification. This is shown in experiments by BLACKBURN and WELLS (1963) and SAMS (1966b) in which the two effects are compared. In contrast to these observations, LÄNGLE (1988) found that the increase in width of the femur diaphysis after incorporation of ^{239}Pu was more radiosensitive than the increase in length.

3.3.9 Disturbance to Growth

3.3.9.1 Dose Relationship

Radiation-induced growth disturbance is described in detail in KOLÁŘ and VRABEC (1976). The most important data came from x-ray morphology with its possibilities for measurement. In the following we will discuss some aspects of the biology of growth and the problem of determining threshold levels. When assessing the effect it is helpful to know that the nonirradiated epiphysis of an irradiated bone grows more than the corresponding epiphysis in the nonirradiated bone on the other side, resulting in a certain compensatory effect for damage to the growth zone (REIDY et al. 1947). This compensatory effect becomes greater with increasing radiation dose (GAUWERKY 1958). It is interesting to note the compensated total size in irradiated Hodgkin patients (see below). Growth on the nonirradiated opposite side of the body is not changed in comparison with that in completely nonirradiated control animals (COHN and GONG 1953a). When radiation-induced growth disturbance occurs, the normal linear relationship between the log of the body weight and bone length is lost and it is no longer possible to find a simple mathematical formula to describe bone growth (COHN and GONG 1953a).

Permanent strongly retarded growth first occurs above 1000 R. The relationship is clearly illustrated by SISSON's (1956) measurements (see Table 3.10). The minimum growth rate is already observed by 1 week after irradiation. The recovery rate is clearly dose dependent. Clinical experiments using x-irradiation on selected areas of the skeleton in order to induce early cessation of growth indicate that a dose of at least 3000 R

Table 3.10. Reduction in the daily growth of the tibia relative[a] to the control side at various times after irradiation. Rat, 30 days old at time of irradiation. (After Sissons 1956)

Dose (R)	Time after irradiation			
	3 days	8 days	30 days	100 days
400	0.6	0.4	1.0	0.7
800	0.6	0.4	0.5	0.5
1200	0.7	0.2	0.2	0.3
1600	0.3	0.2	0.3	0.3

[a] Calculated from data in Sissons (1956).

(fractionated) is needed in order to achieve the required effect (Judy 1941; Spangler 1941).

The results described by Aronson et al. (1976) are of fundamental importance when considering the problem of determining a threshold dose. They used roentgen stereophotogrammetric length measurements (error 43 µm) to show that 0.1 Gy irradiation of the tibia of 57-day-old rabbits has no effect on growth at least up to 75 days. Since small right–left differences are known to occur normally (Aronson et al. 1976), this dose is clearly at a subclinical level. This still leaves open the question of the lowest dose with a measurable effect on growth. Seventy days after local irradiation of rats with 80 R, Dahl (1936) measured a growth deficit of 0.2 mm in the femur diaphysis and 0.1 mm in the height of the epiphysis. He found no effect with 40 R in other animals and thus took 80 R (= 5%–7% of the dose which elicits an exudatory skin reaction) to be the lowest dose which induces growth damage. This threshold has since been directly or indirectly cited in the literature (Meier 1951; Günsel 1953; Fischer 1955; van Caneghem and Schirren 1956; Zollinger 1960; Seelentag and Kistner 1969; Kolář and Vrabec 1976). Wells (1969) measured the depression of growth in the mouse tibia after irradiation of one hind leg at 3 weeks of age with 250 kVp x-rays. The exposure–response curve is linear from 200 R down to 1000 R with a shoulder at 50–100 R. (The "length decrement," i.e. the fraction by which the ratio of the final lengths of the tibiae is less than unity, was 0.0099 per 100 R.) Gauwerky (1958) observed growth disturbance experimentally after 400–800 R. Careful measurements made by Hinkel (1942) on the femur of growing rats failed to reveal any effect below 500 R even in very young animals (less than 1 week old). Constine et al. (1987) observed tibia growth of 91%–95% of controls 80 days after irradiation of 4-week-old

rats with 6 Gy. Sonneveld and van Bekkum (1979) did not observe any clearly measurable growth deficit in the tibia of rhesus monkeys whole body irradiated with 4–5 Gy.

Rubin and Casarett (1972) considered that from a clinical viewpoint the TD 5/5 (tolerance dose, with 5% damage within 5 years after irradiation) for growing cartilage is 10 Gy.

The American College of Radiology (see Heaston et al. 1979) recommends a TD 5/5 of 8 Gy for children under 3 years of age. The careful retrospective study of patients irradiated as children for treatment of hemangiomas (Gauwerky 1960) showed growth deficits of more than 10% for one-quarter (2/8) of the cases at dose levels below 1000 R and for 64% (20/31) of cases with doses above 1000 R ($p = 0.054$). The dose calculations, however, contained some uncertainty. On the basis of both clinical and experimental experience, Gauwerky (1958) recommended that children's skeletons should not be exposed to doses above 600 R. Damage to single growth zones in the vertebral column is much less important for total body growth than is that in the long bones. Parker and Berry (1976) also observed that clinically relevant damage first occurs in the vertebral column at doses above 2000 R. The retrospective study of Hodgkin patients treated by irradiation (field dose 36–40 Gy) without chemotherapy, 2.5 or more years after start of treatment, showed normal size when standing for 3- to 12-year-olds, but differences of more than one standard deviation from average when sitting, for six of seven 3- to 8-year-olds and 10 of 16, 9- to 12-year-olds (Mauch et al. 1983).

The RBE (relative biological efficiency) for 14.4 Mev electrons was found to be 0.6 for growing rat tail (Hagemann 1970).

When considering possible combination treatment with hyperthermia, it is worth noting that disturbances resulting from radiation and heat are additive, not synergistic (Myers et al. 1980).

3.3.9.2 Time Factor and Radiation Quality

The reduction in the effect following dose fractionation was described in the classic paper by Dahl (1936). The depression of growth in the mouse tibia following total exposures of 2000 R or 1000 R given as two equal fractions (first irradiation at 21 days of age) is least when the fraction interval is 6–12 h. At longer intervals there is a partial recovery of efficiency which is more obvious after the smaller total exposure (WELLS 1969). GAUWERKY (1958) showed that there was an increase in the fractionation effect with dose, which he explained as resulting from the dose-dependent compensatory growth of the nonirradiated end of bone. "Hyperfractionation" (ten fractions/5 days instead of five fractions/5 days, total dose 20 or 25 Gy respectively) resulted in a 20% reduction in the growth deficit 200 days after irradiation of the tibia of 22-day-old rats (EIFEL 1988). The growth deficit is also lower after fractionation over 1 week, in place of a single irradiation, with whole body irradiation followed by bone marrow transplantation (SANDERS et al. 1986). With extreme fractionation (80 R/day whole body irradiation) no effect is observed even after a dose accumulation of 720 R (HELLER 1948). Similarly, 0.45 Gy/day over 12 weeks had no effect on growth rates in 5-week-old mice (ANDERSON et al. 1979). Further literature is cited in KOLÁŘ and VRABEC (1976).

SPIESS et al. (1986) investigated growth deficits in bone tuberculosis patients treated with ^{224}Ra at ages between 1 and 16 years (mean skeletal dose 7.72–14.27 Gy, decreasing with age at first injection). The measured values were compatible with the assumption that growth retardation is proportional to the product of the potential growth after irradiation and the dose. A growth-slowing factor of 2% potential growth after irradiation per 1 Gy was calculated for both sexes.

Significant shortening of the femur after incorporation of 111 kBq/kg ^{239}Pu in growing rats was not found until after 21 weeks (LÄNGLE 1988), i.e., after an accumulated dose of more than 3 Gy (GAMER 1988). The difference in length was 4%–5%.

3.3.9.3 Influence of Chemotherapy?

None of the collations of clinical data related to this problem has shown cytostatic therapy to have any additional effect (PROBERT and PARKER 1975; GUTJAHR et al. 1976; HEASTON et al. 1979). The growth curves of children given bone marrow transplants after preparative polychemotherapy and whole body irradiation with 9.4 Gy (acute leukemia cases) showed disturbances, whereas those from children pretreated with cyclophosphamide alone (aplastic anemia cases) did not (KOLB et al. 1982; Fig. 3.9).

3.3.9.4 Indirect, Hormone-Dependent (?) Growth Disturbance

A proportion of patients with growth disturbance following whole body irradiation and bone marrow transplantation have growth hormone deficits (SANDERS et al. 1986; LEIPER et al. 1987). Some of the patients reported in the aforementioned studies had also received radiation treatment to the head because of leukemia.

CLAYTON et al. (1988) found less marked growth disturbance in leukemia patients with irradiation to the head (18 Gy or 20 Gy) than in previous reports describing patients who also had growth hormone deficits. CLAYTON et al. considered that the reduced growth disturbance in their patients (0.84 standard deviations after 10 years) resulted from the lower doses of chemotherapy. They did not systematically investigate the effect of growth hormones. MÖELL and GARWICZ (1988), commenting on the publication by CLAYTON et al. (1988), noted the biphasic development of growth disturbance in their patient group: the growth deficit in girls irradiated with 24 Gy to the head resulted in a prepubertal growth loss of 0.5 standard deviations and a loss in early puberty of 1.0 standard deviations. The growth hormone first showed an abnormal reduction in puberty. The average age at menarche was 12.2 year, which is significantly lower than the expected 13.1 years (MÖELL et al. 1987).

3.3.9.5 Influence of Age

KOLÁŘ and VRABEC (1976) also considered this problem. GAUWERKY (1958) determined the age dependence of growth disturbance in rat tibia for animals up to 50 days old, and showed a considerable dose dependence for the influence of age. Since a prospective growth potential decreases with increasing age, both the absolute and the relative (with respect to the total length of the skeletal part) growth loss after irradiation treatment become less with increasing age. Similarly, growth inhibition is first observed after longer periods with increasing age – only large relative deficits can be detected. Thus the "minimum stunting dose" becomes higher with increasing age (HINKEL 1942). PHILLIPS and KIMELDORF (1966) give a formula for the influence of age on the radiation effect. The quantitative relationship given in Sect. 3.3.9.2 describing the growth deficit

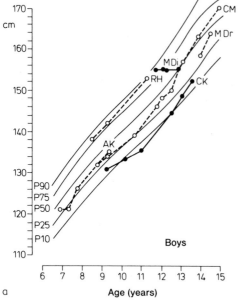
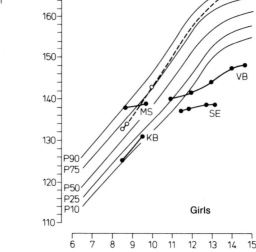

Fig. 3.9a,b. Growth curves of children with bone marrow transplantation after chemotherapy with or without whole body irradiation with 9.4 Gy. Normal percentile curves for comparison. **a** boys; **b** girls. *Continuous line with filled circles*: Patients with recurrence of acute leukemia treated with 2 × 200 mg/m² carmustine (BCNU), 5 × 200 mg/m² cytosine arabinoside, 2 × 60 mg/kg cyclophosphamide, and whole body irradiation with 9.4 Gy. *Broken line with open circles*: Patients with aplastic anemia. Conditioning treatment with cyclophosphamide alone. Divergence from the normal range is only seen after treatment with chemotherapy and whole body irradiation (leukemia patients). Patient M.Di. also had chronic graft-versus-host disease. (KOLB et al. 1982)

after ²²⁴Ra incorporation according to SPIESS et al. (1986) already takes the influence of age into account.

Smaller sizes when sitting were found only in Hodgkin patients irradiated up to age 12 years, and not in those irradiated at ages between 13 and 16 years. From a clinical viewpoint, growth disturbance in small children is certainly more relevant [see, for example, case in FRANTZ (1950) and the recommended dose levels in Sect. 3.3.9.1].

Survivors of the atomic bomb catastrophe irradiated in utero (see review by MOLE 1982) only show a slight reduction in skull size and no reduction in height (SHOHOJI and PASTERNAK 1973). Rats irradiated in utero with 0.4–0.8 Gy on the 17th day of gestation showed a growth deficit throughout life (calculated on the basis of weight). Postnatal growth was not affected by this treat-

ment; equally there was no compensatory increase in growth (JENSH and BRENT 1988).

3.3.10 Radiation-Induced Deformity

Since radiation-induced growth disturbance is a clearly delineated effect (RUBIN et al. 1959; BARNHARD and GEYER 1962), partial irradiation of parts of the skeleton would be expected to induce deformity (LANGENSKIÖLD 1988). A partially radiation-damaged growth plate can, from a clinical viewpoint, be classified as one of the roentgenological types of epiphyseal injury (with the corresponding traumatic consequences) (OGDEN 1988). According to the expected type of tumor irradiation in juveniles, this late effect is most likely to be associated with the vertebral column. More recent clinical data can be found in PROBERT and PARKER (1975), GUTJAHR et al. (1975, 1976), HÖRMANN et al. (1978), BLEHER and TSCHÄPPELER (1979), HEASTON et al. (1979), and SMITH et al. (1982). It is surprising that clinical defects requiring correction are observed only rarely. In the x-ray picture the appearance of the deformity is more striking. SMITH et al. (1982) observed vertebral column deformity in nephroblastoma patients after the lowest dose used (22 Gy). In the early observation period, megavolt irradiation seemed to induce the same changes as x-rays. The adolescent growth phase, however, was not included in the observation period. GUTJAHR et al. (1975), comparing two cases, suggested that chemotherapy might have an intensifying effect. In contrast SMITH et al. (1982) had the impression that chemotherapy did not increase damage; however, they did not have genuinely comparable data.

GAUWERKY (1958) described the presence of skull deformity in children irradiated for hemangioma.

The majority of Hodgkin patients irradiated at ages between 3 and 12 years showed shortening of the clavicula with corresponding changes in appearance (MAUCH et al. 1983).

Eight weeks after incorporation of 111 kBq/kg ^{238}Pu into young growing rats, LÄNGLE (1988) observed a significant increase in the angle of the femur neck.

3.3.11 Radiation-Induced Exostosis ("Osteochondroma")

VAUGHAN (1973), KOLÁŘ and VRABEC (1976), and SPIESS and MAYS (1979) have all reviewed the literature on observations of exostosis following irradiation of juveniles. Further reports can be found in POGRUND and YOSIPOVITCH (1976), GUTJAHR et al. (1975), HEASTON et al. (1979), and JAFFE et al. (1983). Among 200 long-term survivors of irradiation (dose burden to the bone, 15–55 Gy) for tumors in childhood (8 months to 11.5 years), JAFFE et al. (1983) found 6% with osteochondroma. Osteochondromas were already observed at doses below 10 Gy following external irradiation of the thymus in childhood (HEMPELMANN et al. 1975). Osteochondromas are fairly common after ^{224}Ra treatment of juveniles (see Table 3.11; SPIESS and MAYS 1979). Here it is particularly clear that the risk for induction is especially high for infants. Osteochondromas have

Table 3.11. Frequency of induction of exostoses by ^{224}Ra treatment (skeletal dose 3.43–49 Gy) depending on age at first injection. Total frequency 28/218. (After SPIESS and MAYS 1979)

Age at first injection	Males (%)	Females (%)
1– 5 years	53	12
6–10 years	17	11
11–15 years	18	9
16–20 years	0	0
Adults	0	0

also been described occasionally in animal experiments involving irradiation (KUZMA and ZANDER 1957; BASERGA et al. 1961; CASTENERA et al. 1971; DELGADO et al. 1985). DELGADO et al. (1985) showed that osteochondroma-like changes could be induced by doses of only 1.5 Gy if the irradiation field was limited to the perichondrial groove of Ranvier and the adjacent growth plate (rat distal radius). The osteochondromas ossified spontaneously and were integrated into the cortical bone of the diaphysis.

3.4 Induced Bone Formation

From a practical viewpoint the most important question is that of *fracture healing*. Regeneration in preirradiated bone has been investigated in quantifiable experimental systems. JACOBSSON et al. (1985) implanted a "bone growth chamber" in rabbit tibia immediately after irradiation. Four weeks later there was a dose-dependent deficit in bone regeneration compared with controls, the deficit being 20% after 5 and 8 Gy and 65%–75% after 11–25 Gy. Fracture repair in radiation-damaged bone is also one of the problems resulting from radiation-induced osteonecrosis (see Sect. 3.5.3). Clinical reports (BONFIGLIO 1953; KOK 1953) show that fracture healing can occur in radiation-damaged bone even after a radiation-induced spontaneous fracture.

The tissue affected by radiation after a fracture has a similar sensitivity to the region of the growth plate in the long bones (KOCH 1957; COOLEY and GOSS 1958, who also include a review of the literature; BONARIGO and RUBIN 1967; GREEN et al. 1969). Irradiation of the rat femur with 9 Gy 3 days after fracture resulted in a delay of 4 weeks in the restitution of biomechanical parameters (MARKBREITER et al. 1989). ARNOLD (1988) made a detailed study using the closing with bone of a drilled-out 1.2-mm hole (24 h before irradiation) in rat femur as a test model. ARNOLD (1988) used a test level of $ED_{50}/40\%$ – the radiation dose at which in 50% of animals the hole was less than 40% filled by bone after 6–7 weeks (at this time the hole was 76%–88% filled in nonirradiated controls). The $ED_{50}/40\%$ was 16.5 Gy for a single dose application 24 h prior to drilling. The $ED_{50}/40\%$ was not significantly different even when irradiation was performed up to 6 months prior to drilling. These studies also showed fractionation to have a strong influence. The $ED_{50}/40\%$ was 21.6 Gy following irradiation in two fractions (days 1 and 5) and 40.9 Gy after ten fractions (within 5 days) (in each case drilling was on day 7, i.e., 72 h after the last fraction). When the mandible is irradiated with 15–40 Gy immediately after induction of a bone defect there is a higher increase within 24 h in the histochemically identifiable enzyme activity (acid phosphatase, cytochrome oxidase, different dehydrogenases) in the area of the fracture than in nonirradiated controls (AITASALO 1986). Callus formation appears to be badly disturbed at doses above 2000 R. When rat jaw is irradiated with 1725 R 5 days after extraction of the molars, socket healing is somewhat delayed but not prevented (FRANDSEN 1962). UBIOS et al. (1986) measured morphometrically the delay in bony healing in the extraction cavity induced by 15 Gy irradiation immediately after molar extraction. The radiation-induced healing defect could be compensated 30 days after fracture by stimulating the osteoblast activity with ethane-1-hydroxy-1, 1-diphosphate.

The *ossification induced* by estrogen or implanted urothelium is markedly less sensitive, apparently because inducible osteoprogenitor cells can invade from outside (MORSE et al. 1974, and literature therein). This would explain why a bone defect produced by surgical operation in dog mandible 3 weeks after irradiation with 5000 R could be induced to heal by transplantation of autologous spongiosa (MARCIANI et al. 1977). In contrast, WEISS et al. (1982) have reported that fewer progenitor cells for late osteogenesis could be induced to proliferate in subcutaneous tissue following implantation of allogeneic bone matrix, apparently immediately after irradiation with 8.5 Gy. This might show that the local mesenchymal cells are, at least at first, the stem cells for this osteogenesis (WEISS et al. 1982).

Attempts have been made to suppress undesirable *heterotopic ossification* by irradiation with 2000 R immediately or 4–7 days after implantation of an artificial hip joint (LLOYD et al. 1979; REINING et al. 1988). SYLVESTER et al. (1988) did a follow-up study of patients with total hip replacement (and a high risk of heterotopic ossification) treated with 10 or 20 Gy. Clinically significant heterotopic ossification was only present in 3 of 27 patients (11%, historical control values 19%–28%). These patients were not irradiated until more than 4 days after the operation. No clinically significant heterotopic ossification was found when patients were irradiated less than 4 days after the operation. Treatment with 10 Gy had the same effect as treatment with 20 Gy. It is also interesting to note that although the morphogenetic activity of allogeneic bone can be reduced by sterilizing x-ray doses applied in vitro, this morphogenetic activity is not affected when irradiation is performed on decalcified bone (URIST and HERNANDEZ 1974). The latter can be explained on the basis of dosimetry, i.e., a lower dose is absorbed by the remaining nonmineralized tissue.

3.5 Mature Bone

3.5.1 Bone Remodeling

3.5.1.1 Normal Observations

General descriptions can be found in LACROIX (1971), VAUGHAN (1973), SIMMONS (1976), and JAWORSKI (1987). Bone remodeling is determined by mechanical and metabolic factors. CANALIS et al. (1988) and HUFFER (1988) both give a clear account of the control of remodeling by a multitude of local and differentiation factors and by the systemic effects of hormones. It is clear from these reviews that it is not possible to give a complete account of the mechanism of interaction between bone resorption and reconstruction. Normal remodeling affects not only the interplay between osteoblasts and osteoclasts but also bone formation by young osteocytes (YEAGER et al. 1975) and the resorption ability of osteocytes, which can be reactivated at any time (BÉLANGER 1971; SIMMONS 1976; HEUCK 1976). Even so, the osteocyte must be regarded as a terminally differentiated cell, since it apparently decays when released from its lacuna. Remains are found in the osteoclast cytoplasm (TONNA 1972; SOSKOLNE 1978). The local variation is striking (ANDERSON 1978; KIMMEL and JEE 1982). Even morphometric data are only reproducible when the sampling area is very precisely defined (HARDT and JEE 1982). Higher and lower formation rates correlate with areas of blood-forming marrow or fatty marrow in the corresponding skeletal regions (WRONSKI et al. 1981). SONTAG (1986a,b) measured the age dependence of the yearly remodeling rate in the rat diaphysis and found values of 424%/168% (males/females) in 100-day-old animals and 7.5%/10.1% in 900-day-old animals. There are reviews of the literature on age-associated osteoporosis in HEUCK (1976), MORGAN (1984), and SMITH (1987). RAISZ (1988) considers the role of local and systemic factors in detail. The osteoclastic activity is not significantly reduced with age (JOHNELL et al. 1977), which could be relevant for any radiation-induced effects. It appears to be the fractional area with deposition which is reduced with age, rather than the capacity of the active osteoblasts (MELSEN and MOSEKILDE 1978). The resultant change in spongiosa structure with age is different in the vertebral column and the neck of the femur, in correspondence with the different mechanical strain in these two parts (PESCH et al. 1977).

3.5.1.2 Effect of Radiation

From a clinical viewpoint the most important consideration is the pathogenesis of radiation-induced fractures of the neck of the femur. The development via radiation-induced osteoporosis is emphasized in reviews by ZOLLINGER (1960), GRIMM (1971), and KOLÁŘ and VRABEC (1976). Biopsies and autopsies have shown that atrophy of the trabeculae, i.e., osteoporosis, can be at the forefront of spontaneous fractures of the femur neck following irradiation: see STAMPFLI and KERR (1947), KOK (1953), BONFIGLIO (1953), STEPHENSON and COHEN (1956), and DE SÉZE et al. (1963). Analogous histological findings are also observed in the humerus (SENGUPTA and PRATHAP 1973).

HEUCK and LAURITZEN (1967) described the results of a long-term study of *mineral content* and *spongiosa structure* in the proximal femur following gynecological irradiation treatment. The average value of mineral content in the femur neck spongiosa (apatite values according to HEUCK and SCHMIDT 1960) was determined in 37 patients prior to irradiation and was again measured in 19 of these patients 1–3 years after radiation therapy. Only six patients showed the expected reduction in mineral content, while in a further six patients the values remained the same. Surprisingly three patients showed a slight and four a marked increase in mineral content in the femur neck spongiosa. The spongiosa structure in the head and neck of the femur in these patients was characterized by a regional spongiosclerosis (Figs. 3.10, 3.11). Clearly, the regenerative ability of the bone tissue was well maintained, so that neither osteoradionecrosis nor its precursor, structural changes in the spongiosa similar to osteoporosis,

could develop. Longer-term observations were made in two cases with pathological fracture of the neck of one femur as a result of osteoradionecrosis. In these cases the opposite femur had apatite values in the region of the femur neck spongiosa of 120 mg/ml and 170 mg/ml (Fig. 3.12). These values lie somewhat above the "critical apatite value" of 80–120 mg/ml. The critical apatite value is the average mineral concentration in an area of spongiosa at which static insufficiency with pathological fractures is often observed. A radiation dose of 2000 R appears not to influence the mineral content of the femur neck (DALÉN and EDSMYR 1974). No incorporation defects were observed at doses below 2000 R in a more recent study in which investigations were made using nuclear medicine techniques (^{99}Tc-methylene-diphosphonate) 4–6 months after bone doses of 450–6700 R (HATTNER et al. 1982). Interestingly, in an old man of 79 years the atrophy of the femur

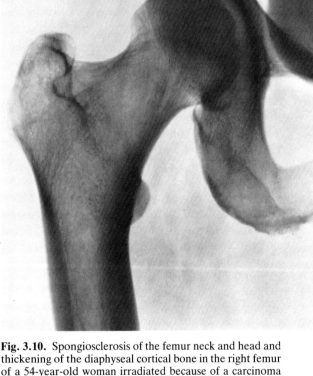

Fig. 3.10. Spongiosclerosis of the femur neck and head and thickening of the diaphyseal cortical bone in the right femur of a 54-year-old woman irradiated because of a carcinoma colli III. The average mineral content in the femur neck region (apatite value according to HEUCK and SCHMIDT 1960) was 380 mg/ml, i.e., clearly higher than the average for this age

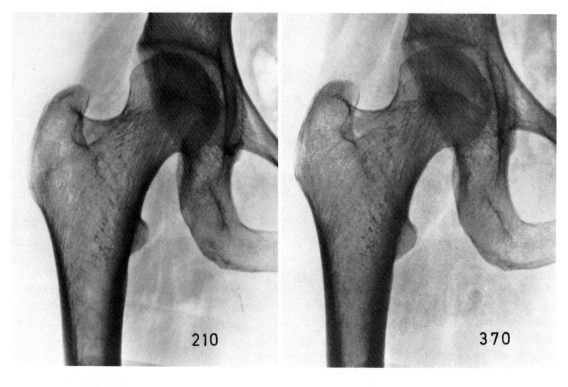

Fig. 3.11. Follow-up of the apatite value in the spongiosa of the femur neck in a 38-year-old woman showed an original value of 210 mg/ml before radiation treatment of a carcinoma colli II, rising to 370 mg/ml 18 months after treatment with accompanying mild spongiosclerosis

neck appeared to have reduced tolerance so that medial femur neck fractures appeared on both sides 15 months after a local dose of 1500 R. Kok (1953) also noted shorter latency times in patients over 70. Kok (1953) considered that age-associated and radiation-induced changes in the blood vessels played a key role. He showed that the highest local dose was in the area of the periosteal blood supply. Parker (1972) also supported this theory whereas Bonfiglio (1953) argued that blood vessels could not play an important role since he was not able to prevent fracture healing (see above). Bonfiglio also emphasized that the radiation dose lay below that necessary to induce osteonecrosis.

Radiation-induced osteoporosis also appears in other parts of the skeleton (Kolář and Vrabec 1976). Zollinger (1960) showed that the only damage observed after doses of 4000 R is a marked osteoporosis in the ribs, which can result in spontaneous fracture (his illustration shows an osteoporotic rib after 16 000 R). Zollinger (1960) also observed osteoporosis of the vertebral column. Clinical reports are given in Probert and Parker (1975), Gutjahr et al. (1975, 1976), Hörmann et al. (1978), and Bleher and Tschäppeler (1979). Wieland (1983) described a female patient with a metabolic, age-associated osteoporosis who developed compression in the region of the lower thoracic vertebrae following therapy with 70 Gy for carcinoma of the esophagus. The vertebral column mainly lay in the area of 80% – 70% isodosis so that this was presumably a combination effect.

Howland et al. (1975) observed bone atrophy in 47 of 49 patients (investigated on average 8 years after treatment) given radiation therapy (orthovoltage therapy) in the region of the shoulder girdle. Six patients had severe atrophy, and one of these developed fractures of the ribs and clavicula. Only mild forms of bone atrophy were observed in approximately 20% of cases following 25 MeV betatron photon irradiation and radiocobalt radiation.

Experimental studies of the morphology and functional morphology of disturbed skeletal remodeling following irradiation of nongrowing mature bone have been made by Levy and Rugh (1952), Birkner et al. (1956), Bures and Wuehrmann (1969a–c), Rissanen et al. (1969a), King

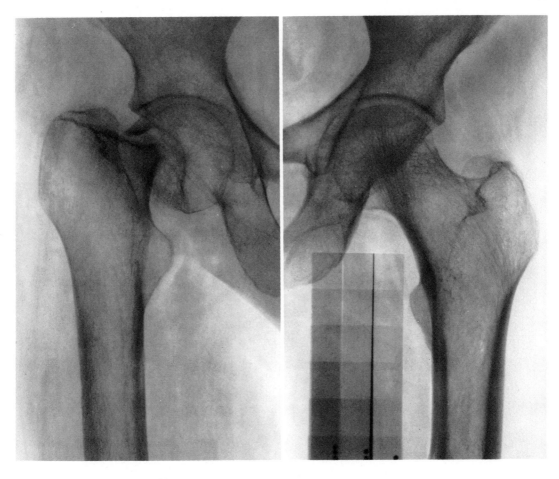

Fig. 3.12. Spontaneous fracture of the right femur neck, with pseudarthrotic healing. This severe osteoporosis accompanying osteoradionecrosis appeared after radiation treatment of a carcinoma colli II approximately 3 years previously. The apatite value of the spongiosa of the left femur neck was, at 170 mg/ml in a 57-year-old woman, clearly below the lower limit for the norm. The spongiosa structure of the right femur is clearly rarefied

et al. (1979, 1980), WRONSKI et al. (1980), and MAEDA et al. (1988).

The most striking morphological feature is the appearance of loss of osteoblasts and peritrabecular fibrosis (LEVY and RUGH 1952; BIRKNER et al. 1956). Enzyme histochemical investigation of deposition and resorption shows that remodeling is less sensitive than bone growth (SAMS 1966a). The loss of bone substance at doses above 2000 R is shown in measurements of dry weight 8 months after irradiation (CUTRIGHT and BRADY 1971), whereby vascularization was reduced many months earlier. The increased uptake of ^{32}P on the 7th day after irradiation of adult rats with 3000 R is difficult to interpret (MARINELLI and KENNEY 1941). The latter results, however, showed a marked variability and were called preliminary by the authors. In this context it is interesting to note that KUMMERMEHR (1971) observed increased incorporation of ^{45}Ca in the spongiosa of epiphysis and patella 1 week after irradiation of growing rats with 2000 R. COHN and GONG's observations (1953a) are similarly interesting: irradiation of tibia in young rats with 2000 R did not induce any change in the relative ash weight up to 160 days (end of observation period), i.e., there was no loss of mineral. KUMMERMEHR (1971) observed a reduction in diffuse ^{45}Ca incorporation in the diaphysis region at longer times after irradiation with 2000 R. KING et al. (1979) made a very precise study of bone deposition and resorption and blood circulation in cortical and trabecular bone of adult rabbit following application of the "minimum tolerance dose" (17.56 Gy). A phase of hyperemia is followed after 1 month by a reduction in remodel-

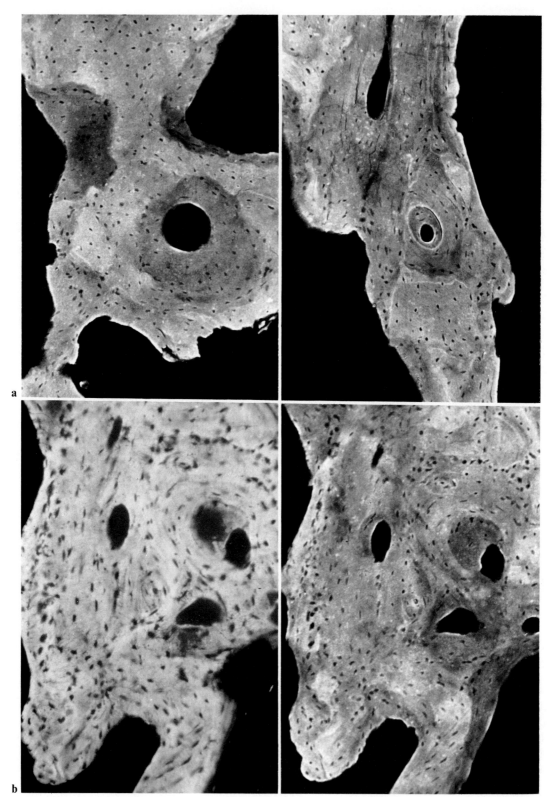

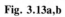
Fig. 3.13a,b

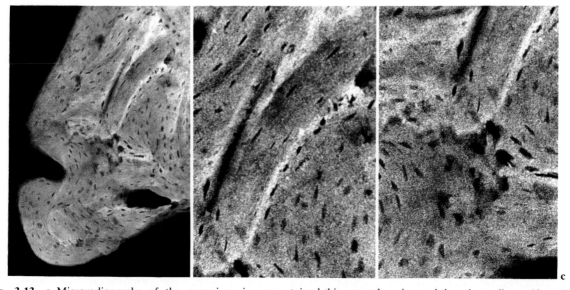

Fig. 3.13. a Microradiographs of the spongiosa in an osteoradionecrotic region. The adjacent processes of resorption and formation (Howship's lacunae, poorly mineralized bone) are clear. Highly mineralized cement lines and wide areas of sclerosis (50 μm thin-ground). **b** An undecalcified 50 μm thin-ground section from the border of the region of necrosis showing discrete areas of bone resorption, newly formed areas of poorly mineralized bone and osteoid (recognizable at the *lower right* in the fuchsin-stained thin-ground section and the microradiograph), and an inhomogeneous low mineral concentration in the tela ossea in the microradiograph. The osteocyte lacunae are variable in size and irregularly dispersed in the bone. **c** The newly formed bone in the peripheral spongiosclerosis shows irregular mineralization with "buried osteoid seams," highly mineralized band-like regions, and variable osteocyte lacunae with focal perilacunar demineralization spreading into the surrounding area

ing and later (after 3 months) by an increased remodeling rate. KING et al. (1980) also followed the effect using nuclear medicine techniques. A similar increase in remodeling after 3 months, followed by a reduction after 12 months, was seen following 46.5 Gy fractionated over 3 weeks (1756 ret). BURES and WUEHRMANN (1969a,b) investigated the relationship between periosteal and endosteal deposition up to 60 days after irradiation of rat mandible or tibia with 4500 R. Periosteal deposition was reduced whereas endosteal deposition was increased. Incorporation of ^{32}P equivalent to a dose of 4.33 Gy (within the same observation period of 60 days) did not affect endosteal bone formation but did result in a reduction in periosteal bone formation (BURES and WUEHRMANN 1969c).

MAEDA et al. (1988) observed a reduced periosteal deposition rate in a morphometric study of rat femur 6–8 weeks after irradiation with 35 Gy. After 14–18 weeks there was no significant difference between bone formation (osteoid seam/mm^2) and resorption spaces in irradiated and nonirradiated femur from the same animal. Surprisingly both values were significantly higher than in nonirradiated controls. The porosity of the corti-calis was significantly increased in irradiated femur.

GAMER (1988) showed that 4 weeks after incorporation of 37 kBq/kg ^{239}Pu (accumulated skeletal dose, 0.672 Gy) into young adult rats, the bone volume density in the fourth lumbar vertebra was less than 60% of that in controls.

Clinically both reactive sclerosis and deposition effects in areas of necrosis have been observed, in addition to bone atrophy, following disturbance of bone remodeling in radiation-damaged bone (HEUCK and GÖSSNER 1973). Microradiograms of nondecalcified thin-ground sections of bone from the same area of spongious bone enable deposition and resorption processes to be seen adjacent to one another at the microscopic level. The well-preserved activity of the bone cells is shown by periosteocytic demineralization followed by osteolysis directly adjacent to areas of active bone formation, with highly mineralized cement lines and interstitial lamellae which result from the biological potency of the tela ossea (Fig. 3.13).

Incorporation of long-lived α-emitting bone-seeking radionuclides results in a different type of disturbance of bone remodeling in which resorption processes appear to be more strongly

affected, resulting in increased formation of thickened trabeculae (ARNOLD and JEE 1959; JEE and
ARNOLD 1961; WRONSKI et al. 1980; POLIG et al.
1988). After incorporation of radium, mature
bone shows structural changes similar to osteoporosis, with widening of the haversian systems to
form lacunae, and histologically there is fibrosis of
marrow areas with osteosclerotic foci resulting
from bone apposition. Apposition of bone is
observed in the subperiosteal bone region. High
radium concentrations are found wherever the
bone structure appears particularly irregular
(ROWLAND et al. 1958, 1959a; ROWLAND and
MARSHALL 1959; ENGSTRÖM 1964). Microradiograms of the bone area show a varied picture (Fig.
3.14), with mineralization defects in the region of
the tela ossea adjacent to highly mineralized zones
(HEUCK and GÖSSNER 1973). The cement lines are
rarely highly mineralized. The inner layer of the
haversian systems show bone apposition, with
higher mineralization of the tela ossea. There are
certain parallels with the results observed after
radiation treatment of bone, which show an
increase in average mineral content (apatite value)
and sclerosis of the spongiosa. WEGENER (1970)
appears to be describing a similar process in his
case of "osteodystrophy" in a Joachimstal miner,
with narrowing of marrow areas and a mosaic
structure similar to that found in Paget's disease.
Fibro-osseous foci have been observed in the
mouse skeleton after incorporation of ^{224}Ra (LUZ
et al. 1979) and low activities of ^{239}Pu (HUMPHREYS
and LOUTIT 1980). These probably reflect a type of
radiation-induced dysplasia. The phenomenon of

bizarre bone resorption in ^{226}Ra-burdened bone
above a whole body dose of 1 µCi also seems to be
related to osteonecrosis, since haversian systems
closed by calcification are described in this case
too (ROWLAND et al. 1959b).

3.5.2 Osteoradionecrosis

A comprehensive survey of the literature on this
topic can be found in KOLÁŘ and VRABEC (1976),
together with a large collection of their own
clinical observations. Development of osteoradionecrosis is not as such necessarily critical from
a clinical point of view. The clinical significance
results from unusual mechanical loading of the
bone with subsequent fracture, and from open
contact with the environment resulting in
osteomyelitis (PARKER and BERRY 1976). Thus the
localization of osteoradionecrosis is of decisive
importance for the fate of the patient; this aspect is
considered in detail in KOLÁŘ and VRABEC (1976).

The genesis of osteoradionecrosis is sometimes
considered to be purely vascular (AXHAUSEN 1954;
RUBIN and CASARETT 1968). However, widespread
clinical and experimental experience indicates that

Fig. 3.14. Different areas of microradiographs from a 50
µm thin-ground section from the proximal diaphysis following radium deposition in the tela ossea. Irregular different-
sized osteons are present, which are inhomogeneously
mineralized and cell poor. In the interstitial lamellae there
are very dense, more mineralized regions in the form of
broad areas, strips, and patches

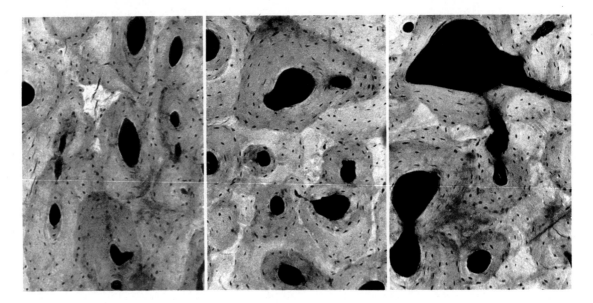

Bone

97

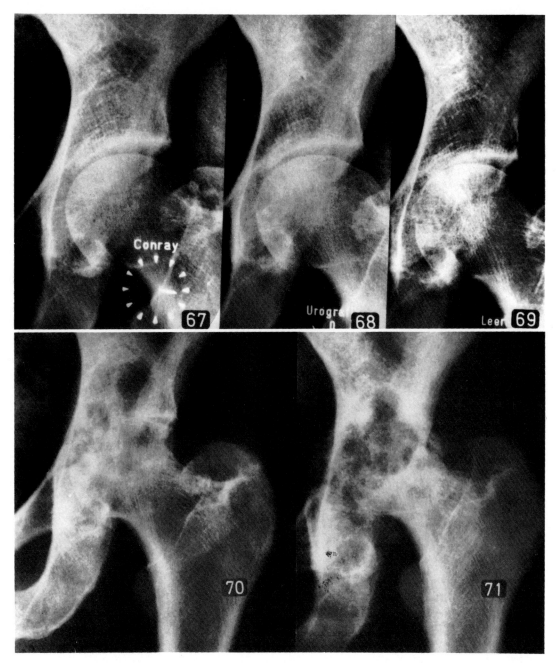

both direct destruction of osteocytes and indirect damage via radiation-induced vasculopathy are possible (NILSSON 1969; THURNER 1970; GRIMM 1971; JEE 1971; VAUGHAN 1973; ROHRER et al. 1979). GRIMM (1971) differentiates in his review between an early necrosis, which appears to be a primary radiation effect, and a late form of necrosis, which appears to result from secondary vascular damage.

Fig. 3.15. Development and follow-up of osteoradionecrosis in the region of the left proximal femur (femur head and neck) and the left acetabulum over a period of 4 years in a 60-year-old woman following intense radiation (cobalt therapy) for a carcinoma colli II. Reactive spongiosclerosis can be seen along the border areas of the necrotic decaying bone, particularly in the neck of the femur and spongiosa of the os ileum

Osteoradionecrosis is not identifiable radiologically prior to the appearance of clinical symptoms (GRIMM 1971). In general, increased uptake in the scintigram, resulting from osteonecrosis (shown using the experimental caisson disease), is first seen after 3 weeks. This finding also appears earlier than any roentgen morphological change (GREGG and WALDER 1980). The clinical result is explained by the start of reparative bone formation (Fig. 3.15). Retrospective analysis of x-ray pictures indicates the presence of positive findings prior to the appearance of clinical symptoms (TIMOTHY et al. 1978). The study by DAMBRAIN et al. (1988) makes a useful contribution to understanding these changes. They compared microradiographs with the histological findings in irradiated cat mandible. Zones which were still devitalized appeared normal in the microradiograms. The bone in the microradiographically identifiable remodeling areas was vital. DAMBRAIN and DHEM (1984) found similar results in mandible samples from patients following radiation therapy.

In histological assessments it is important to recognize that a certain loss of osteocytes is physiologically normal (SHERMAN and SELAKOVICH 1957). Experiments in which osteocytes were counted after irradiation of bone show very variable results. MAEDA et al. (1988) observed a reduced number of osteocytes 2 weeks after irradiation of rat femur with 35 Gy (whereby the nonirradiated femur also showed a reduced number of osteocytes in comparison with femur from a nonirradiated animal). JACOBSSON et al. (1987) did not observe any reduction in osteocytes in rabbit tibia even 22 weeks after irradiation, using enzyme histochemical identification. The study of cat mandible by DAMBRAIN et al. (1988) shows clearly the important role of local factors: osteocyte loss after irradiation was particularly marked in the basal and dorsal mandibular regions.

Histological findings of osteoradionecrosis in humans without radiation-induced changes in the blood vessels have been reported by EWING (1926), PHEMISTER (1926), BONFIGLIO (1953), and SENGUPTA and PRATHAP (1973). Primary, i.e., not vascular-dependent, osteoradionecrosis has also been observed experimentally: see BIRKNER et al. (1956), UEBERSCHÄR (1959) (in the first weeks after 5000 R beginning in the center of the compact bone), and ROSENTHALL and MARVIN (1957) (2 weeks after fractionated irradiation with 9000 R, 140 kV). Similar results after internal irradiation have been reported by HELLER (1948) (5 months

after incorporation of 0.06 µCi/g radium), JEE and ARNOLD (1961) (2 months after plutonium incorporation, restricted to the irradiation area of the alpha particles), and MACPHERSON et al. (1962) (5% empty osteocyte lacunae after 9 days ^{90}Sr, corresponding to 15–25 Gy, and 11% empty lacunae after 90 days, corresponding to 240 Gy).

When considering the possibility of primary osteonecrosis it is interesting to note that TANNOCK and HAYASHI (1972) failed to observe appreciable damage to or regeneration processes in capillary endothelium in bone up to 22 days after irradiation, in experiments using 20 or 40 Gy. RAY (1976) gives a general description of the normal blood supply in bone. The microvasculature is described in RHINELANDER (1972). Experimental results which indicate a relationship between disturbances in blood supply and osteocyte destruction, or changes in blood vessels at dose levels which induce osteonecrosis, have been variously described: see BIRKNER et al. (1956); UEBERSCHÄR (1959) (disruption of blood supply to the compact bone 20 days after 5000 R; fibrosis of the periosteum and vessel-poor marrow fibrosis; these authors consider that the key role of vascular damage lies not in the development of osteoradionecrosis but in its influence on the fate of this lesion); KOLLATH (1964) (loss of osteocytes 7 weeks after 5000 R at a time when the periosteum is already hyalinized and the arteriolar lumina are narrowed); KOLLATH (1965) (complete osteonecrosis and thrombotic vascular occlusions 10 days after 10 000 R); SAMS (1963, 1965a,b) (6 weeks after 2000 R empty osteocyte lacunae in the central two-thirds of the compact bone associated with cell-poor marrow and disturbed blood supply); HORN et al. (1974) (only functional and clinical tests; clear disturbance of circulation in the irradiated extremities 10 weeks after 6000–7000 R; spontaneous amputation not until after 35 weeks); MAEDA et al. (1988) (loss of osteocytes 2 weeks after 35 Gy, together with hyaline thrombi in the blood vessels). Plugging of the haversian canals with mineralized material is observed as a long-term effect after internal irradiation (JEE and ARNOLD 1961; ARNOLD and JEE 1959).

The TD 5/5 (tolerance dose with 5% damage within 5 years of irradiation) for radiation-induced osteonecrosis is generally taken to be 60 Gy, which is very close to the values given for the tolerance dose for damage to the capillary bed (RUBIN and CASARETT 1972). The value of 60 Gy is in good agreement with the threshold values observed following irradiation of the os temporale (Wang and Doppke 1976) but differs from values given in earlier reports (Greve 1952: 3800–4300 R; Woodard and Spiers 1953: 5000 R). Von Rottkay (1985) has discussed the possibility that irradiation schemes with more than one fraction per day raise the risk of osteonecrosis. He described two cases in which radionecrosis was observed in the region of the vertebrae after 52–62 Gy following irradiation twice a day with 1.8 Gy.

The possibility of lowered bone tolerance following combination radiotherapy and chemotherapy is particularly feared in cases of malignant lymphoma (sometimes treated in addition with steroids!) (Timothy et al. 1978; Prosnitz et al. 1981; Engel et al. 1981). According to the experience of Rossleigh et al. (1986), 1.6% of patients with Hodgkin's disease and 0.12% of patients with non-Hodgkin's lymphoma develop osteoradio-

necrosis. Patients treated by steroid-containing multiple drug therapy are at the highest risk.

Bricout et al. (1985) also attributed the appearance of (rarely observed) humerus head necrosis following irradiation with 50 Gy to the additional effects of accompanying chemotherapy.

3.5.3 The Fate of Osteoradionecrosis

Experience of osteoradionecrosis in lymphoma patients indicates that these lesions do not enlarge (Rossleigh et al. 1986). The main complication associated with osteoradionecrosis is the appearance of *spontaneous fractures* following appropriate strain on the bone (Fig. 3.16). This effect has been observed experimentally (e.g., Ueberschär 1959; Baserga et al. 1961; Jee and Arnold 1961). The area at highest risk seems to be the boundary region between the necrosis and nonirradiated healthy bone in which repair mechanisms develop (Ueberschär 1959). The stimulation of osteogenic tissue following the appearance of spontaneous fracture is striking (Ueberschär 1959). The reader is referred to the reviews by Grimm (1971) and Kolář and Vrabec (1976) for clinical reports of

Fig. 3.16. Osteoradionecrosis in the right clavicula which has led to a pathological fracture with formation of pseudarthrosis. Result of radiation treatment in a 53-year-old woman treated approximately 4 years earlier for a supraclavicular metastasizing tumor

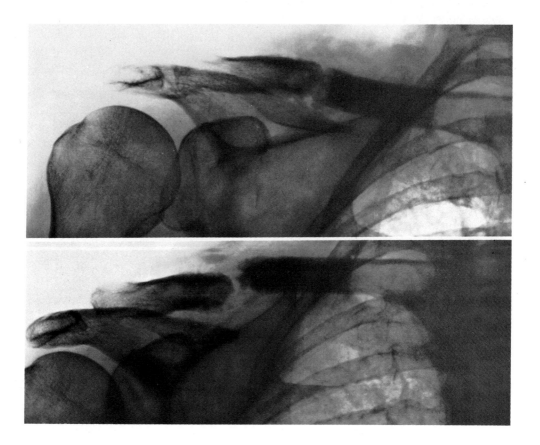

the condition. The accompanying condition of obliterative endarteritis is often mentioned when discussing the appearance of femur neck fractures (Gates 1943). The often surprisingly good healing – also mentioned in the discussion on osteoporosis – indicates that the blood vessels do not play an important role in the development of the fracture, in contrast to the situation of fracture of the femur neck in old people. It is still open to discussion whether fractures which heal really well were in fact complete necroses. Birkner (1953) reported, for example, that healing followed in two cases after 3000 R and 3000–3200 R but not in a third case after 5500 R.

Spontaneous fracture after osteoradionecrosis is not restricted to the femur neck, which is exposed to extreme mechanical strain; it can also occur in other bones (Rosenstock et al. 1978). The latter report concerns young patients with Ewing's sarcoma. The authors ascribe the increased risk of fracture after 40 Gy to the additional burden of chemotherapy. Osteoradionecrosis with bone destruction in the non-load-bearing shoulder girdle can appear after very long latency times, as in the case described by Barak et al. (1984) (22 years after 120 Gy). The latter authors also cited other reports giving latency times of up to 29 years.

The most common fate of osteoradionecrosis –

as with other forms of osteonecrosis – is probably stepwise substitution beginning with *apposition of new bone* along the devitalized skeletal region (Figs. 3.17, 3.18; Zollinger 1960). After irradiation this begins with the appearance of the atypical basophilic cell-poor coarsely woven type of bone, that is if the osteoblast system has not yet recovered. During the course of this slow reactive build-up of hard substance, the osteonecrosis becomes visible in the x-ray picture. Heuck and Lauritzen (1967) performed parallel histological and microradiographic investigations of spongious bone in the region of fragmentation and debris in the neck of the femur in cases of osteoradionecrosis. In addition to bone resorption, they observed formation of new bone along the old trabecules. The mineral concentration in the newly formed bone varied and was sometimes incomplete. The wide osteoid seam could only be seen histologically. Perilacunar halos of bone with lesser density,

Fig. 3.17. Osteoradionecrosis; appearance 8 months after i.p. injection of 50 µCi/kg ^{227}Th (α-emitter, half-life 18.7 days), equivalent to an average skeletal dose of 100 Gy. Part of a thoracic vertebra from an NMRI mouse. Empty osteocyte lacunae in extended regions of bone. The devitalized bone is partially covered by a thin band of atypical basophilic bone substance along the marrow surface. The bone marrow is aplastic. HE, × 125

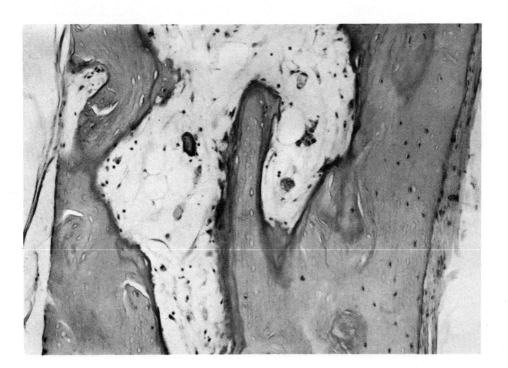

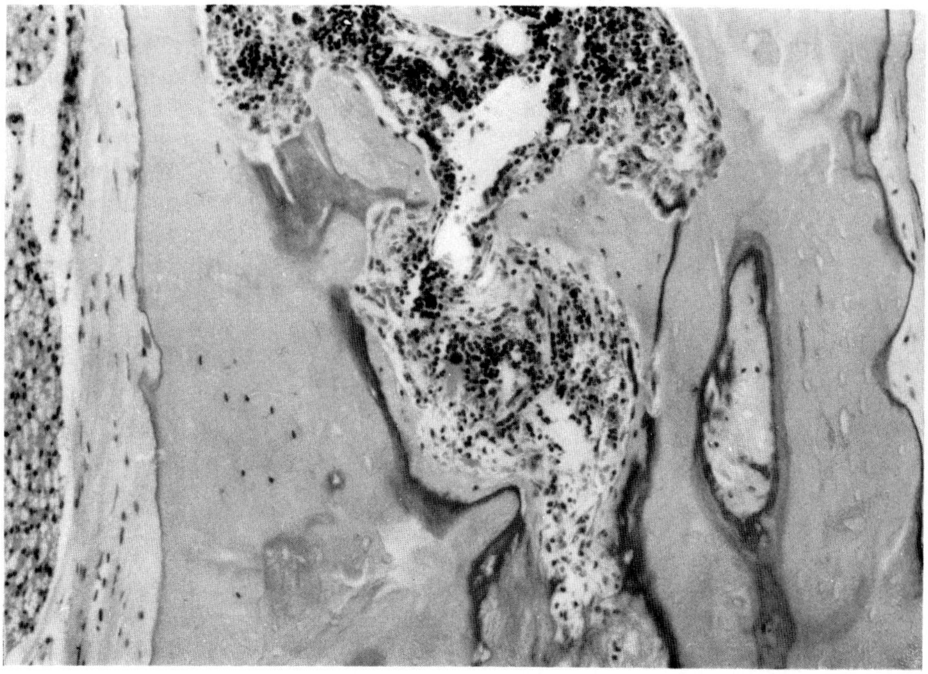

Fig. 3.18. Osteoradionecrosis; appearance 12 months after i.p. injection of 100 μCi/kg ^{227}Th (α-emitter, half-life 18.7 days), equivalent to an average skeletal dose of 200 Gy. Part of a thoracic vertebra from an NMRI mouse. There is irregular bone formation on the marrow surface, and below it, directly adjacent to the devitalized bone, is a thin band of atypical basophilic bone substance. HE, × 125

resulting from the reduced mineral concentration in the tela ossea, were rather conspicuous and can be seen as an expression of increased metabolism in the bone cells. The same skeletal region shows areas of clear bone formation adjacent to those with bone resorption and signs of bone necrosis. The reactive sclerosis of the bone which is observed is easily understandable on the basis of this varied picture (see Figs. 3.15, 3.16, above).

Reactive new bone formation associated with osteoradionecrosis was first described in detail in human material by EWING (1926), who named it "radiation osteitis." BLOOM and BLOOM (1949) give a classic description of the experimental appearance of the effect following radium incorporation in adult mice. Atypical bone formation – presumably as a result of chronic radiation effects – is the most striking feature in these experiments (ZOLLINGER 1960). In our experiments we have even seen this type of atypical bone 1 year after incorporation of large amounts of a short-lived α-emitter (^{227}Th, half-life 18.7 days) (see Fig. 3.18, above). UEBERSCHÄR (1959) even observed callus-type bone formation in the marrow region adjacent to necrosis after external irradiation with 5000 R. JEE and ARNOLD (1961) observed new formation of bone after plutonium incorporation in the dog. In addition they observed a focal resorption of bone which almost certainly generally accompanies bone repair processes (ZOLLINGER 1960). ALBREKTSSON et al. (1980) followed the stepwise substitution of devitalized bone in rabbits after irradiation with 15 Gy. The original bone was to a great extent replaced 10 weeks after irradiation. BIRKNER et al. (1956) and UEBERSCHÄR (1959) described resorption processes occurring approximately 1 month after irradiation with 5000 R. These processes first come to a halt as result of subsequent fibrosis and disturbance of blood circulation and then restart, after a considerable interval, in the form of a "progressive lacunar osteolysis." GRIMM (1971) observed large numbers of osteoclasts on the surface of devitalized bone in rabbit jaw 16 days after a surface dose of 5000 R, followed after 4 months by irregular apposition of osteoid and new formation of lamellar bone. DAMBRAIN et al. (1988) showed the regional differences in substitution after radionecrosis in the lower jaw of the cat 12 months after irradiation with 80 Gy. The alveolar region shows osteolysis and deposition of vital bone, whereas the peripheral area mainly retains devitalized bone. Similar results are seen in mandible samples from patients following radiation therapy and are explained by the authors as resulting from vascular factors (DAMBRAIN and DHEM 1984). In the case of chronic internal irradiation, peritrabecular fibrosis can form a barrier to further remodeling of devitalized trabeculae (JEE and ARNOLD 1961).

If a *soft tissue necrosis* develops above the osteoradionecrosis it can lead to infection, osteomyelitis, and sequestration of the bone. PHEMISTER (1926) reported two such cases which developed in the long bones during experiments with dogs. It appears that entry of pyogenic organisms by way of skin defects in the auditory canal is a prerequisite for clinical manifestation of the rare cases of osteoradionecrosis of the os temporale. In one report the effect was secondary to a brain abscess (WURSTER et al. 1982).

For practical reasons the main region likely to be affected by osteomyelitis and sequestration of complete parts of the skeleton as a consequence of osteoradionecrosis is that of the jaw bones, and in particular the area of the mandible (GRIMM 1971; PARKER 1972). Surgical operations and defects in the mucous membrane favor such a development. GRIMM (1971) did not observe any age dependence, even though the blood supply in the mandible changes with age to a more centrifugal or centripetal direction (BRADLEY 1972).

Early primary osteoradionecrosis of the jaw bone can be shown experimentally after irradiation with 5000 R or 45 Gy (GRIMM 1971; ROHRER et al. 1979), and even with 20 Gy (LIND and NATHANSON 1977). Radiation-induced vascular occlusion, which occurs later, does not seem to play any decisive role. The remodeling processes which follow radiation-induced necrosis are still not identifiable in rabbit skull 8 weeks after irradiation (LIND and NATHANSON 1977). Osteoradionecrosis of the jaw has been studied histologically in detail by CHAMBERS et al. (1958), NG et al. (1959), GOWGIEL (1960), and COFFIN (1983). CHAMBERS et al. (1958) observed simultaneous mucous membrane ulceration and osteomyelitis. The inflammation spread from the periodontium. Osteonecrosis was never seen without osteomyelitis (up to 8000 R). The effect seemed to develop less often when tooth extraction was performed 16 days prior to irradiation. FRANDSEN (1962) observed osteomyelitis in approximately half of the cases following extraction of rat molars 8 days after irradiation with 1725 R. GOWGIEL (1960) showed that in rhesus monkey jaw tooth extraction 2 months or more after irradiation only led to complications at doses above 8500 R. In these investigations, too, clinically relevant changes were never seen when the gingiva was intact. The tooth only becomes an important point of entry for infection at higher doses; no complications were seen below 60 Gy (BEDWINEK et al. 1976; REGEZI et al. 1976; MORRISH et al. 1981). MURRAY et al. (1980) emphasized the fact that in their experience the tooth itself does not pose a threat unless it is extensively carious. Accordingly, BEDWINEK et al. (1976) observed the lowest complication rates when only teeth which were considered unsalvageable were extracted before radiation therapy, particularly as when all teeth are extracted before therapy there is often insufficient time left for the wound to heal before starting irradiation. MARX's (1983) investigations indicated that pathogenic micro-organisms of the sort observed in osteomyelitis are not important for the development of osteoradionecrosis of the jaw. According to COFFIN (1983) the most important prophylactic measure against manifestation of osteoradionecrosis is avoidance of surgical procedures on bone both before and after irradiation therapy, except when the irradiated bone is removed en bloc.

The effect of alcohol in triggering clinical complications following osteoradionecrosis is not negligible (REGEZI et al. 1976).

GOWGIEL (1960) emphasized the direct primary effect of radiation on osteocytes. The changes in blood vessels (observed at doses above 8500 R) only play a role in the subsequent worsening of the condition. More than half of the clinical complications associated with osteoradionecrosis of the jaws were observed in the 1st year after irradiation (BEDWINEK et al. 1976; REGEZI et al. 1976).

3.6 Cartilage of the Joints and Larynx

The reader is referred to KOLÁŘ and VRABEC (1976) for a review of the degenerative changes which can occur in the joints. When histological biopsy results are available the condition is referred to as chondritis dissecans (KOLÁŘ and VRABEC 1959). BARR et al. (1943) studied the rat knee joint up to 36 weeks after irradiation with 665–1800 R, as a part of their study of radiation-induced growth disturbance. They did not observe any degenerative changes. Similarly, BUDRAS et al. (1986) observed no morphological changes following irradiation with five fractions of 1.5 Gy within 5 weeks. In the clinical literature spondylosis-like lesions have been observed following radiation therapy of children (PROBERT and PARKER 1975; BLEHER and TSCHÄPPELER 1979). PARKER (1972) did not observe any clinically relevant cartilage necrosis with 65–70 Gy applied with standard fractionation. BAHOUS and MÜLLER (1976) considered the problem of radiation-induced damage to the joints following radionuclide treatment of chronic arthritis, taking into account published reports, their own experience, and the results of animal experiments. Yttrium 90 penetrates cartilage by up to 8.5 mm. Despite this, cartilage damage appeared only to a very limited extent in animal experiments. But the authors consider that premature development of degenerative osteoarthritis might occur. The presence of bone atrophy associated with chronic arthritis could cause the damage to become critical: in one case a severe inflammatory lesion in the knee joint, with destruction of the tibia surface, was observed following ^{90}Y treatment. In the mouse intra-articular injection of ^{90}Y resulted in a slight loss of chondrocytes after 33 days, but only when given at high doses (approximately 20 times the therapeutic dose). However, the treatment did cause complete loss of subchondral osteocytes (DE VRIES et al. 1984).

As in the case of osteonecrosis of the jaw, mucous membrane defects appear to be the trigger for critical damage to the larynx cartilage (GOODRICH and LENZ 1948; ZOLLINGER 1960). MACIEJEWSKI et al. (1983) observed late complications in 25% of patients with irradiated larynx carcinoma. The effects only appeared in patients treated with a total dose of 56 Gy or more. The risk of damage was independent of the length of the treatment period.

Irradiation of the larynx in juveniles can, as a result of the subsequent cessation of growth, lead to the appearance of stenoses in adulthood. This type of complication has been described following irradiation therapy for juvenile larynx papillomatosis (SALINGER 1942; RABBETT 1965).

Acknowledgments. The authors wish to thank Dr. A. Beatrice Murray for the English translation and Ms. W. Pedit for preparing the manuscript and compiling the list of references.

References

Aitasalo K (1986) Effect of irradiation on early enzymatic changes in healing mandibular periosteum and bone. A histochemical study on rats. Acta Radiol Oncol 25: 207–212

Albrektsson T, Jacobsson M, Turesson I (1980) Irradiation injury of bone tissue. A vital microscopic method. Acta Radiol Oncol 19: 235–239

Amsel S, Dell ES (1972) Bone formation by hemopoietic tissue: separation of preosteoblast from hemopoietic stem cell function in the rat. Blood 39: 267–273

Anderson C (1978) Bone-remodeling rates of the beagle: a comparison between sites on the same rib. Am J Vet Res 39: 1763–1765

Anderson ND, Colyer RA, Riley LH Jr (1979) Skeletal changes during prolonged external irradiation: alterations in marrow, growth plate and osteoclast populations. Johns Hopkins Med J 145: 73–83

Argüelles F, Gomar F, Garcia A, Esquerdo J (1977) Irradiation lesions of the growth plate in rabbits. J Bone Joint Surg [Br] 59: 85–88

Arnold JS, Jee WSS (1957) Bone growth and osteoclastic activity as indicated by radioautographic distribution of plutonium. Am J Anat 101: 367–394

Arnold JS, Jee WSS (1959) Autoradiography in the localization and radiation dosage of Ra^{226} and Pu^{239} in the bones of dogs. Lab Invest 8: 194–203

Arnold M (1988) Der Einfluß von Strahlendosis und Dosisfraktionierung auf die knöcherne Heilung eines definierten Bohrlochdefektes im Rattenfemur. Dissertation, Tierärztliche Fakultät der Ludwig-Maximilians-Universität München

Aronson AS, Gustafsson M, Selvik G (1976) Bone growth in the rabbit after irradiation. Acta Radiol [Diagn] (Stockh) 17: 838–844

Ascenzi A (1976) Physiological relationship and pathological interferences between bone tissue and marrow. In: Bourne GH (ed) The biochemistry and physiology of bone, vol IV, 2nd edn. Academic, New York, pp 403–444

Axhausen G (1954) Die Ernährungsunterbrechungen am Knochen. Erg Allg Pathol 37: 207–257

Azizkhan JC, Klagsbrun M (1980) Chondrocytes contain a growth factor that is localized in the nucleus and is associated with chromatin. Proc Natl Acad Sci USA 77: 2762–2766

Babicky A, Kolář J (1966) Generalized skeletal response to local radiation injury. Radiat Res 27: 108–118

Bahous I, Müller W (1976) Die lokale Behandlung chronischer Arthritiden mit Radionukliden. Schweiz Med Wochenschr 106: 1065–1073

Baltadjiev G (1987) Stereological characteristics of the mesenchymal complex in the degenerative-osteogenic zone of the growth cartilage of the tibia of premature neonates. Anat Anz 163: 243–248

Barak F, Werner A, Walach N, Horn Y (1984) Extensive late bone necrosis after postoperative orthovoltage irradiation of breast carcinoma. Report of a case. Acta Radiol Oncol 23: 485–488

Barnhard HJ, Geyer RW (1962) Effects of x-radiation on growing bone. Radiology 78: 207–214

Barr JS, Lingley JR, Gall EA (1943) The effect of roentgen irradiation on epiphyseal growth. I. Experimental studies upon the albino rat. 49: 104–115

Baserga R, Lisco H, Cater DC (1961) The delayed effects of external gamma irradiation on the bones of rats. Am J Pathol 39: 455–472

Baunach A (1935) Über den Einfluß von Dosis und Rhythmus auf den Grad der Wachstumsschädigung des Knochenwachstums bei Röntgenstrahlungen. Strahlentherapie 54: 52–67

Becker G, Lepp C, Pömsl H, Luz A (1972) Störung des Knochen-wachstums nach Incorporation von Ra-224 (Thorium X) bei der Maus. Verh Dtsch Ges Pathol 56: 448–452

Bedwinek JM, Shukovsky LJ, Fletcher GH, Daley TE (1976) Osteonecrosis in patients treated with definitive radiotherapy for squamous cell carcinomas of the oral cavity and naso- and oropharynx. Radiology 119: 665–667

Bélanger LF (1971) Osteocytic resorption. In: Bourne GH (ed) The biochemistry and physiology of bone, 2nd edn, vol III. Academic, New York, pp 239–270

Bensted JPM, Courtenay VD (1965) Histological changes in the rat bone after varying doses of x-rays with particular reference to bone tumour production. Br J Radiol 38: 261–270

Bensted JPM, Blackett NM, Lamerton LF (1961) Histological and dosimetric considerations of bone tumour production with radioactive phosphorus. Br J Radiol 34: 160–175

Birkner R (1953) 3 Fälle von Spontanfrakturen am Becken und Schenkelhals als Strahlenschädigungsfolge. Ideale Spontanheilung in 2 Fällen. Strahlentherapie 92: 297–307

Birkner R, Frey J, Ueberschär K-H (1956) Frühveränderungen am Knochen erwachsener Meerschweinchen nach Röntgenbestrahlung. Strahlentherapie 100: 574–590

Bisgard JD, Hunt HB (1936) Influence of roentgen rays and radium on epiphyseal growth of long bones. Radiology 26: 56–64

Blackburn J, Wells AB (1963) Radiation damage to growing bone: the effect of x-ray doses of 100 to 1,000r on mouse tibia and knee-joint. Br J Radiol 36: 505–513

Blackett NM, Kember NF, Lamerton LF (1959) The measurement of radiation dosage distribution by autoradiographic means with reference to the effects of bone-seeking isotopes. Lab Invest 8: 171–178

Bleher EA, Tschäppeler H (1979) Spätveränderungen an der Wirbelsäule nach Strahlentherapie und kombinierter Behandlung bei Morbus Hodgkin im Kindes- und Adoleszentenalter. Strahlentherapie 155: 817–828

Bloom MA, Bloom W (1949) Late effects of radium and plutonium on bone. Arch Pathol 47: 494–511

Bonarigo BC, Rubin P (1967) Nonunion of pathologic fracture after radiation therapy. Radiology 88: 889–898

Bond VP, Fliedner TM, Archambeau JO (1965) Mammalian radiation lethality. Academic, New York

Bonfiglio M (1953) The pathology of fracture of the femoral neck following irradiation. Am Roentgenol 70: 449–459

Bourne GH (1972) Phosphatase and calcification. In: Bourne GH (ed) Biochemistry and physiology of bone, vol I, 2nd edn. Academic, New York, pp 79–120

Bradley JC (1972) Age changes in the vascular supply of the mandible. Br Dent J 132: 142–144

Bricout PB, Simanovsky M, Feldman MI, Mattii R (1985) Necrosis of the humeral head following postoperative supervoltage irradiation and chemotherapy in carcinoma of the breast. Br J Radiol 58: 562–563

Brooks B, Hillstrom HT (1933) Effect of roentgen rays on bone growth and bone regeneration. An experimental study. Am J Surg 20: 599–614

Budras K-D, Hartung K, Münzer BM (1986) Licht- und elektronenmikroskopische Untersuchungen über den Einfluß von Röntgenbestrahlung auf das Stratum synoviale des entzündeten Kniegelenks. Berl Münch Tierärztl Wochenschr 99: 148–152

Bures MF, Wuehrmann AH (1969a) Bone-remodeling dynamics following local x-irradiation: I. J Dent Res 48: 376–384

Bures MF, Wuehrmann AH (1969b) Bone remodeling dynamics following local x-irradiation: II. J Dent Res 48: 904–908

Bures MF, Wuehrmann AH (1969c) Bone remodeling dynamics after intraperitoneal administration of radioactive sodium phosphate (^{32}P). J Dent Res 48: 909–912

Burstone MS (1952) A histochemical study of irradiated bone. Am J Pathol 28: 1133–1141

Calvo W, Fliedner TM, Steinbach I, Alcober V, Nothdurft W, Fache I (1978) Development of fibrosis in dogs as a late consequence of whole-body x-irradiation. In: Late biological effects of ionizing radiation, vol II. International Atomic Energy Agency, Vienna, pp 127–136

Canalis E, McCarthy T, Centrella M (1988) Growth factors and the regulation of bone remodeling. J Clin Invest 81: 277–281

Carlson HC, Williams MMD, Childs DS, Dockerty MB, Janes JM (1960) Microangiography of bone in the study of radiation changes. Radiology 74: 113–114

Castenera TJ, Jones DC, Kimeldorf DJ (1971) The effect of age at exposure to a sublethal dose of fast neutrons on tumorigenesis in the male rat. Cancer Res 31: 1543–1549

Chambers F, Ng E, Ogden H, Coggs G, Crane J (1958) Mandibular osteomyelitis in dogs following irradiation. Oral Surg 11: 843–859

Clayton PE, Shalet SM, Morris-Jones PH, Price DA (1988) Growth in children treated for acute lymphoblastic leukaemia. Lancet I: 460–462

Coffin F (1983) The incidence and management of osteoradionecrosis of the jaws following head and neck radiotherapy. Br J Radiol 56: 851–857

Cohn SH (1961) Effect of aging and x-irradiation on the kinetics of skeletal metabolism in the rat. Radiat Res 15: 355–365

Cohn SH, Gong JK (1953a) Effect of 2000 roentgen local x-irradiation on the growth of rat bone. Growth 17: 7–20

Cohn SH, Gong JK (1953b) Effect of 2000 roentgens local x-irradiation on metabolism and alkaline phosphatase activity of rat bone. Am J Physiol 173: 115–119

Cole AA, Wezeman FH (1985) Perivascular cells in cartilage canals of the developing mouse epiphysis. Am J Anat 174: 119–129

Constine LS, Rubin P, Gregory P (1987) The differential protection by WR2721 of skin versus growing cartilage following irradiation in weanling rats. Radiat Res 110: 61–71

Cooley LM, Goss RJ (1958) The effects of transplantation and x-irradiation on the repair of fractured bones. Am J Anat 102: 167–181

Cottier H (1961) Strahlenbedingte Lebensverkürzung. Springer, Berlin Göttingen Heidelberg

Cottier H (1966) Histopathologie der Wirkung ionisierender Strahlen auf höhere Organismen (Tier und Mensch). In: Zuppinger A (ed) Strahlenbiologie 2. Springer, Berlin Heidelberg New York (Handbuch der medizinischen Radiologie, vol II/2, pp 35–272)

Cowell HR, Hunziker EB, Rosenberg L (1987) The role of

hypertrophic chondrocytes in endochondral ossification and in the development of secondary centers of ossification. J Bone Joint Surg [Am] 69: 159–161

Cutright DE, Brady JM (1971) Long-term effects of radiation on the vascularity of rat bone – quantitative measurements with a new technique. Radiat Res 48: 402–408

Dahl B (1936) De l'effet des rayons x sur les os longs en développement et sur la formation de cal. Étude radiobiologique et anatomique chez le rat. Skrifter utgitt av det Norske Videnskaps-Akademi i Oslo I. Matematisk-Naturvidenskapelig Klasse 1: 1–149

Dalén N, Edsmyr F (1974) Bone mineral content of the femoral neck after irradiation. Acta Radiol [Ther] (Stockh) 13: 97–101

Dambrain R, Dhem A (1984) Bone vitality in induced radionecrosis of the mandible estimated by osteocytic population counting. Strahlentherapie 160: 39–44

Dambrain R, Dhem A, Gueulette J, Wambersie A (1988) Bone vitality in the cat's irradiated jaw. Histological study. Strahlenther Onkol 164: 351–356

Delgado E, Rodriguez JI, Serrada A, Tellez M, Paniagua R (1985) Radiation-induced osteochondroma-like lesion in young rat radius. Clin Orthop 201: 251–258

De Ridder L, Thierens H, Cornelissen M, Segaert O (1988) Effects of ionizing radiation on the metabolism and longitudinal growth of cartilaginous embryonic chick tibiae in vitro. Int J Radiat Biol 53: 965–975

De Séze S, Ryckewaert A, Lequesne M, Freneaux B (1963) La hanche radiothérapique formes classiques et formes méconnues. Rev Rhum Mal Osteoartic 30: 695–705

Desjardins AU (1930) Osteogenic tumor; growth injury of bone and muscular atrophy following therapeutic irradiation. Radiology 14: 296–307

De Vries B, van den Berg WB, van der Putte LBA (1984) The effects of colloidal yttrium-90 silicate on the knee-joint of the mouse. Agents Actions 15: 101–103

Dodds GS, Cameron HC (1934) Studies on experimental rickets in rats. I. Structural modifications of the epiphyseal cartilages in the tibia and other bones. Am J Anat 55: 135–165 (cited after Gall et al. 1940)

Dziewiatkowski DD, Woodard HQ (1959) Effect of irradiation with x-rays on the uptake of S^{35} sulfate by the epiphyseal cartilage of mice. Lab Invest 8: 205–212

Eifel PJ (1988) Decreased bone growth arrest in weanling rats with multiple radiation fractions per day. Int J Radiat Oncol Biol Phys 15: 141–145

Eng W, Esterly JR (1972) Histochemical localization of enzymes in cartilage in neonatal and adult rats. Arch Pathol 94: 291–297

Engel D (1983) An experimental study of the action of radium on developing bones. Br J Radiol 11: 779–803

Engel IA, Straus DJ, Lacher M, Lane J, Smith J (1981) Osteonecrosis in patients with malignant lymphoma. A review of twenty-five cases. Cancer 48: 1245–1250

Engström A (1964) Der Einfluß strahlender Energie auf das Knochengewebe. Ergeb Allg Pathol Anat 45: 1–22

Engström H, Turesson I, Waldenström J (1981) The effect of 50 kV x-ray irradiation on the alkaline phosphatase activity of growing rat bone. Int J Radiat Biol 40: 659–663

Euratom-GSF (1967) Pathogenese genetischer und somatischer Strahlenschäden. Jahresbericht 1965, p 26 EUR 3270. d

Ewing J (1926) Radiation osteitis. Acta Radiol (Stockh) 6: 399–412

Fajardo LF (1982) Pathology of radiation injury. Masson, New York

Fischer E (1955) Zur Häufigkeit der Skelettwachstumshemmung bei Strahlenbehandlung der Hämangiome. Strahlentherapie 97: 599–607

Flaskamp W (1930) Über Röntgenschäden und Schäden durch radioaktive Substanzen. Strahlentherapie (Sonderb) 12: 1–354

Fowler JF (1957) Absorbed dose near bone: a conductivity method of measurement. Br J Radiol 30: 361–366

Frandsen AM (1962) Effects of roentgen irradiation of the jaws on socket healing in young rats. Acta Odontol Scand 20: 307–353

Frantz CH (1950) Extreme retardation of epiphyseal growth from roentgen irradiation. Radiology 55: 720–724

Gall EA, Lingley JR, Hilcken JA (1940) Comparative experimental studies of 200 kilovolt and 1000 kilovolt roentgen rays. I. The biological effects on the epiphysis of the albino rat. Am J Pathol 16: 605–618

Gamer AO (1988) Histomorphologische und -morphometrische Untersuchungen von frühen Knochenschäden nach Inkorporation optimal kanzerogener Dosen von 239-Plutonium an männlichen Ratten verschiedenen Alters. Kernforschungszentrum Karlsruhe, KfK 4380

Garrison JC, Uyeki EM (1988) The effects of gamma radiation on chondrogenic development in vitro. Radiat Res 116: 356–363

Gates O (1943) Effects of radiation on tissues. XII. Effects on bone, cartilage and teeth. AMA Arch Pathol 35: 323–340

Gauwerky F (1958) Strahlenbedingte Wachstumsstörungen am Gesichtsschädel und deren Verhütung auf Grund biologischer Untersuchungen und klinischer Erfahrungen. Fortschr Kiefer Gesichtschir 4: 33–43

Gauwerky F (1960) Über die Strahlenschädigung des wachsenden Knochens. Strahlentherapie 113: 325–350

Gerber GB, Métivier H, Smith H (eds) (1987) Age-related factors in radionuclide metabolism and dosimetry. Martinus Nijhoff, Dordrecht

Goodrich WA, Lenz M (1948) Laryngeal chondronecrosis following roentgen therapy. Am J Roentgenol 60: 22–28

Gössner W (1972) Grundlagen und allgemeine pathologische Anatomie der Strahlenschäden. Verh Dtsch Ges Pathol 56: 168–187

Gössner W, Schwabe M (1968) Histochemische Untersuchungen am Knochen nach Inkorporation von Ra-224 (Thorium X). Verh Dtsch Ges Pathol 52: 334–338

Gössner W, Schwabe M (1971) Enzymhistochemie des Knochengewebes. Z Orthop 109: 212–230

Gössner W, Calvo W, Zurcher C (1982) Pathological findings in lethally irradiated and reconstituted dogs. In: Fliedner TM, Gössner W, Patrick G (eds) Late effects after therapeutic whole-body irradiation. Commission of the European Communities. Luxembourg, pp 89–98 EUR 8070 EN

Gowgiel JM (1960) Experimental radio-osteonecrosis of the jaws. J Dent Res 39: 176–197

Green N, French S, Rodriquez G, Hays M, Fingerhut A (1969) Radiation-induced delayed union of fractures. Radiology 93: 635–641

Gregg PJ, Walder DN (1980) Scintigraphy versus radiography in the early diagnosis of experimental bone necrosis. J Bone Joint Surg [Br] 62: 214–221

Greve W (1952) Spontanfrakturen nach Röntgentiefenbestrahlung. Strahlentherapie 86: 617–621

Grimm G (1971) Klinische und experimentelle Untersuchungen über die radiogene Knochenschädigung am Kieferapparat. Nova Acta Leopoldina (Abhandlungen der Deutschen Akademie der Naturforscher Leopoldina), NF 36: 196

Güngör T, Hedlund T, Hulth A, Johnell O (1982) The effect of irradiation on osteoclasts with or without transplantation of hematopoietic cells. Acta Orthop Scand 53: 333–337

Günsel E (1953) Die Strahlenschäden am wachsenden Knochen. Strahlentherapie 91: 595–601

Gutjahr P, Greinacher I, Kutzner J (1975) Ergebnisse der kombinierten Wilmstumor-Behandlung unter besonderer Berücksichtigung der therapiebedingten Skelettveränderungen. Strahlentherapie 149: 119–130

Gutjahr P, Greinacher I, Kutzner J (1976) Spätfolgen der Tumortherapie. Form- und Strukturveränderungen der Wirbelsäule im Röntgenbild. Dtsch Med Wochenschr 101: 988–992

Hagemann G (1970) Die Wirkung ionisierender Strahlen auf proliferierendes Knorpelgewebe, Dissertation. Fakultät für Mathematik und Naturwissenschaft, Technische Univ Hannover

Hall BK (1981) Intracellular and extracellular control of the differentiation of cartilage and bone. Histochem J 13: 599–614

Hardt AB, Jee WSS (1982) Trabecular bone structural variation in biopsy sites of the beagle ilium. Calcif Tissue Int 34: 391–395

Hattner RS, Hartmeyer J, Wara WM (1982) Characterization of radiation-induced photopenic abnormalities on bone scans. Radiology 145: 161–163

Hazuka MB, Ibbott GS, Kinzie JJ (1988) HIP protheses during pelvic irradiation: effects and corrections. Int J Radiat Oncol Biol Phys 14: 1311–1317

Heaston DK, Libshitz HI, Chan RC (1979) Skeletal effects of megavoltage irradiation in survivors of Wilm's tumor. Am J Roentgenol 133: 389–395

Held F (1960) Die Bedeutung der Strahlenqualität für die schädigende Wirkung ionisierender Strahlung auf die Tibia-Epiphysenfuge der Albinoratte. Radiobiol Radiother (Berl) 1: 151–158

Heller M (1948) Bone. In: Bloom W (ed) Histopathology of irradiation from external and internal sources. McGraw-Hill, New York, pp 70–161

Hempelmann LH, Hall WJ, Phillips M, Cooper RA, Ames WR (1975) Neoplasms in persons treated with x-rays in infancy: fourth survey in 20 years. J Natl Cancer Inst 55: 519–530

Heuck F (1967) Allgemeine Radiologie und Morphologie der Knochenkrankheiten. In: Diethelm L (ed) Röntgendiagnostik der Skeletterkrankungen. Springer, Berlin Heidelberg New York (Handbuch der medizinischen Radiologie, vol V/1, pp 3–303

Heuck F, Gössner W (1973) Strahlenempfindlichkeit der Knochen. In: Braun H von, Heuck F, Ladner HA, Messerschmidt O, Musshoff K, Streffer C (eds) Strahlenempfindlichkeit von Organen und Organsystemen der Säugetiere und des Menschen. Thieme, Stuttgart (Strahlenschutz in Forschung und Praxis, vol XIII, pp 153–171

Heuck F, Lauritzen C (1967) Veränderungen von Mineralgehalt und Struktur des Femur nach gynäkologischer Strahlentherapie. Deutscher Röntgenkongress 1967, part B. Strahlentherapie [Sonderb] 66: 87–92

Heuck F, Schmidt E (1960) Die quantitative Bestimmung des Mineralgehaltes der Knochen aus dem Röntgenbild. Fortschr Roentgenstr 93: 523–554

Hinkel CL (1942) The effect of roentgen rays upon the growing long bones of albino rats. I. Quantitative studies of the growth limitation following irradiation. Am J Roentgenol 47: 439–457

Hinkel CL (1943a) The effect of roentgen rays upon the growing long bones of albino rats. II. Histopathological changes involving endochondral growth centers. Am J Roentgenol 49: 321–348

Hinkel CL (1943b) The effect of irradiation upon the composition and vascularity of growing rat bones. Am J Roentgenol 50: 516–526

Hoecker FE, Roofe PG (1951) Studies of radium in human bone. Radiology 56: 89–98

Hoffmann V (1923) Über Erregung und Lähmung tierscher Zellen durch Röntgenstrahlen. II. Experimentelle Untersuchungen an wachsenden Knochen von Kaninchen und Katzen. Strahlentherapie 14: 516–526

Holtrop ME, King GJ (1977) The ultrastructure of the osteoclast and its functional implications. Clin Orthop 123: 177–196

Hörmann D, Kamprad F, Hofmann V, Willnow U (1978) Wachstumsstörungen des kindlichen Skeletts im Röntgenbild nach kombinierter Therapie von Wilms-Tumoren und Neuroblastomen. Kinderärztl Prax 9: 475–488

Horn NL, Thompson M, Howes AE, Brown JM, Kallman RF, Probert JC (1974) Acute and chronic effects of x-irradiation on blood flow in the mouse limb. Radiology 113: 713–722

Horton MA (1988) Osteoclast-specific antigens. ISI atlas of science: immunology, pp 35–43

Horváth J, Horváth F, Juhász E, Urbányi L (1962) Über die Strahlenschädigungen wachsender Knochen. Strahlentherapie 118: 462–478

Howland WJ, Loeffler RK, Starchman DE, Johnson RG (1975) Postirradiation atrophic changes of bone and related complications. Radiology 117: 677–685

Huffer WE (1988) Morphology and biochemistry of bone remodeling: possible control by vitamin D, parathyroid hormone, and other substances. Lab Invest 59: 418–442

Hulth A, Westerborn O (1960) Early changes of the growth zone in rabbit following roentgen irradiation. Acta Orthop Scand 30: 155–168

Hulth A, Westerborn O (1962) Early changes of the growth zone in the rabbit following roentgen irradiation: autoradiographic investigation after the administration of radiosulphate. Br J Exp Pathol 43: 137–141

Humphreys ER, Loutit JF (1980) Lesions in CBA mice from nanocurie amounts of ^{239}Pu. Int J Radiat Biol 37: 307–314

Humphreys ER, Green D, Howells GR, Thorne MC (1982) Relationship between blood flow, bone structure, and ^{239}Pu deposition in the mouse skeleton. Calcif Tissue Int 34: 416–421

Hunziker EB, Schenk RK, Cruz-Orive L-M (1987) Quantitation of chondrocyte performance in growth-plate cartilage during longitudinal bone growth. J Bone Joint Surg [Am] 69: 162–173

Jacobsson M, Jönsson A, Albrektsson T, Turesson I (1985) Dose response for bone regeneration after single doses of ^{60}Co irradiation. Int J Radiat Oncol Biol Phys 11: 1963–1969

Jacobsson M, Kälebo P, Tjellström A, Turesson I (1987) Bone cell viability after irradiation. An enzyme histochemical study. Acta Oncol 26: 463–465

Jaffe N, Ried HL, Cohen M, McNeese MD, Sullivan MP (1983) Radiation induced osteochondroma in long-term survivors of childhood cancer. Int J Radiat Oncol Biol Phys 9: 665–670

Jaworski ZFG (1987) Does the mechanical usage (MU) inhibit bone "remodeling"? Calcif Tissue Int 41: 239–248

Jee WSS (1971) Bone-seeking radionuclides and bones. In: Berdijs CC(ed) Pathology of irradiation. Williams & Wilkins, Baltimore, pp 186–212

Jee WSS, Arnold JS (1961) The toxicity of plutonium deposited in skeletal tissues of beagles. Lab Invest 10: 797–825

Jee WSS, Nolan PD (1963) Origin of osteoclasts from fusion of phagocytes. Nature 200: 225–226

Jensh RP, Brent RL (1988) The effect of low level prenatal x-irradiation on postnatal growth in the Wistar rat. Growth Dev Aging 52: 53–62

Johnell O, Wiklund PE, Hulth A (1977) Osteoclast counting in crista biopsies. Acta Orthop Scand 48: 566–571

Johnson DR (1986) The genetics of the skeleton. Animal models of skeletal development. Clarendon, Oxford

Jones SJ, Boyde A (1977) Some morphological observations on osteoclasts. Cell Tissue Res 185: 387–397

Jones SJ, Hogg NM, Shapiro IM, Slusarenko M, Boyde A (1981) Cells with Fc receptors in the cell layer next to osteoblasts and osteoclasts on bone. Metab Bone Dis Rel Res 2: 357–362

Judy WS (1941) An attempt to correct asymmetry in leg length by roentgen irradiation. A preliminary report. Am J Roentgenol 46: 237–240

Kember NF (1960) Cell division in endochondral ossification. J Bone Joint Surg [Br] 42: 824–839

Kember NF (1962) Kinetics of population of bone-forming cells in the normal and irradiated rat. In: Dougherty F et al. (eds) Some aspects of internal irradiation. Pergamon, Oxford, pp 309–316

Kember NF (1965) An in vivo cell survival system based on the recovery of rat growth cartilage from radiation injury. Nature 207: 501–503

Kember NF (1967) Cell survival and radiation damage in growth cartilage. Br J Radiol 40: 496–505

Kember NF (1971) Cell population kinetics of bone growth: the first ten years of autoradiographic studies with tritiated thymidine. Clin Orthop 76: 213–230

Kember NF (1979) Proliferation controls in a linear growth system: theoretical studies of cell division in the cartilage growth plate. J Theor Biol 78: 365–374

Kember NF (1983) Cytotoxic effects on cartilage growth plates. In: Potten CS, Hendry JH (eds) Cytotoxic insult to tissue. Churchill Livingstone, Edinburgh, pp 353–367

Kember NF, Coggins J (1967) Changes in the vascular supply to rat growth cartilage during radiation injury and repair. Int J Radiat Biol 12: 143–151

Kember NF, Lambert BE (1981) Slowly cycling cells in growing bone. Cell Tissue Kinet 14: 327–330

Kember NF, Sadek M (1970) Mitotic suppression in gut and growth cartilage by x-irradiation in vivo. Int J Radiat Biol 17: 19–23

Kember NF, Sissons HA (1976) Quantitative histology of human growth plate. J Bone Joint Surg [Br] 58: 426–435

Kember NF, Walker KVR (1971) Control of bone growth in rats. Nature 229: 428–429

Kimmel DB, Jee WSS (1980a) A quantitative histologic analysis of the growing long bone metaphysis. Calcif Tissue Int 32: 113–122

Kimmel DB, Jee WSS (1980b) Bone cell kinetics during

longitudinal bone growth in the rat. Calcif Tissue Int 32: 123–133

Kimmel DB, Jee WSS (1982) A quantitative histologic study of bone turnover in young adult beagles. Anat Rec 203: 31–45

King MA, Casarett GW, Weber DA (1979) A study of irradiated bone: I. Histopathologic and physiologic changes. J Nucl Med 20: 1142–1149

King MA, Weber DA, Casarett GW, Burgener FA, Corriveau O (1980) A study of irradiated bone. Part II: Changes in Tc-99m pyrophosphate bone imaging. J Nucl Med 21: 22–30

Koch W (1957) Die spezifische Strahlenreaktion des Knochens. In: Graul EH (ed) Fortschritte der Angewandten Radioisotopie und Grenzgebiete, vol II. Hüthig, Heidelberg, pp 102–193

Kofránek V, Pařizek O, Svoboda V, Bubeniková D, Machek J (1977) ^{3}H-TDR labelling of osteoprogenitor cells after ^{226}Ra incorporation in mice. Acta Radiol Ther Phys Biol 16: 232–240

Kok G (1953) Spontaneous fractures of the femoral neck after the intensive irradiation of carcinoma of the uterus. Acta Radiol (Stockh) 40: 511–527

Kolár J, Vrabec R (1959) Gelenkknorpelschäden nach Röntgenbestrahlung. Forschr Roentgenstr 90: 717–721

Kolář J, Vrabec R (1976) Strahlenbedingte Knochenschäden. In: Diethelm L (ed) Röntgendiagnostik der Skeletterkrankungen. Springer, Berlin Heidelberg New York (Handbuch der medizinischen Radiologie, vol V/1, pp 389–512)

Kolb HJ, Bender-Götze C, Janka G et al. (1982) Late radiation effects in patients treated with chemotherapy, total body irradiation and allogeneic bone marrow transplantation for relapsed, acute leukemia. In: Fliedner TM, Gössner W, Patrick G (eds) Late effects after therapeutic whole-body irradiation. Commission of the European Communities, Luxembourg, pp 27–33, EUR 8070 EN

Kollath J (1964) Radiogene Schäden der Knochen, des Knochenmarks und der Gefäße nach Telekobaltbestrahlung. I. Mitteilung: Experimente an Meerschweinchen, Bestrahlungen mit 5000 R Co^{60}. Strahlentherapie 123: 614–622

Kollath J (1965) Radiogene Schäden der Knochen und der umgebenden Weichteile nach Telekobaltbestrahlung. II. Mitteilung: Experimente an Meerschweinchen, Bestrahlungen mit 10000 R Co^{60}. Strahlentherapie 126: 432–448

Kummermehr J (1971) Mikroradiographische Untersuchungen über den Einbau und die Retention von Calcium-45 im Kniegelenk der Ratte nach lokaler Röntgenbestrahlung. Dissertation, Med Fakultät Ludwig-Maximilian-Universität München

Kuzma JF, Zander G (1957) Cancerogenic effects of Ca-45 and Sr-89 in Sprague Dawley rats. AMA Arch Pathol 63: 198–206

Lacroix P (1971) The internal remodeling of bones. In: Bourne GH (ed) The biochemistry and physiology of bone, vol III, 2nd edn. Academic, New York, pp 119–144

Langenskiöld A (1988) Growth plate regeneration. In: Uhthoff HK, Wiley JJ (eds) Behavior of the growth plate. Raven, New York, pp 47–54

Längle UW (1988) Frühe Knochenveränderungen nach Inkorporation kleiner Mengen von Alphastrahlern bei männlichen Ratten. Kernforschungszentrum Karlsruhe, KfK 4473

Leblond CP, Weinstock M (1971) Radioautographic studies of bone formation. In: Bourne GH (ed) The biochemistry and physiology of bone, vol III, 2nd edn. Academic, New York, pp 181–200

Leiper AD, Stanhope R, Lau T, Grant DB, Blacklock H, Chessells JM, Plowman PN (1987) The effect of total body irradiation and bone marrow transplantation during childhood and adolescence on growth and endocrine function. Br J Haematol 67: 419–426

Levy BM, Rugh R (1952) The effect of total body roentgen irradiation on the long bones of hamsters. Am J Roentgenol 67: 974–979

Lind MG, Nathanson A (1977) ^{99}Tc^{m}-DP accumulation in rabbit skull bones after ^{60}Co gamma irradiation. Acta Radiol [Ther] (Stockh) 16: 489–496

Lloyd KW, Keys H, Hubbard L, Thomas F, Evarts C (1979) Use of irradiation after total hip replacement to prevent heterotopic bone formation (abstract). Int J Radiat Oncol Biol Phys [Suppl 2] 5: 208

Lobodziec W, Lubas B (1966) Influence of transverse dimensions of bone on roentgen dose distribution for different qualities of primary radiation. Acta Radiol Ther Phys Biol 4: 471–480

Loutit JF, Nisbet NW, (1982) The origin of osteoclasts. Immunobiology 161: 193–203

Loutit JF, Townsend KMS (1982a) Longevity of osteoclasts in radiation chimaeras of beige and osteopetrotic microphthalmic mice. Br J Exp Pathol 63: 214–220

Loutit JF, Townsend KMS (1982b) Longevity of osteoclasts in radiation chimaeras of osteopetrotic beige and normal mice. Br J Exp Pathol 63: 221–223

Loutit JF, Marshall MJ, Nisbet NW, Vaughan JM (1982) Versatile stem cells in bone marrow. Lancet II: 1090–1093

Lucht U (1972) Absorption of peroxidase by osteoclasts as studied by electron microscope histochemistry. Histochemie 29: 274–286

Luz A, Schäffer E, Erfle V et al. (1979) Vor- und Frühstadien des strahleninduzierten Osteosarkoms der Maus. Verh Dtsch Ges Pathol 63: 433–437

Maciejewski B, Preuss-Bayer G, Trott K-R (1983) The influence of the number of fractions and of overall treatment time on local control and late complication rate in squamous cell carcinoma of the larynx. Int J Radiat Oncol Biol Phys 9: 321–328

Macpherson S, Owen M, Vaughan J (1962) The relation of radiation dose to radiation damage in the tibia of weanling rabbits injected with strontium 90. Br J Radiol 35: 221–234

Maeda M, Bryant MH, Yamagata M, Li G, Earle JD, Chao EYS (1988) Effects of irradiation on cortical bone and their time-related changes. J Bone Joint Surg [Am] 70: 392–399

Marciani RD, Gonty AA, Giansanti JS, Avila J (1977) Autogenous cancellous-marrow bone grafts in irradiated dog mandibles. Oral Surg 43: 365–372

Marinelli LD, Kenney JM (1941) Absorption of radiophosphorus in irradiated and non-irradiated mice. Am J Roentgenol 37: 691–697

Markbreiter LA, Pelker RR, Friedlaender GE, Peschel R, Panjabi MM (1989) The effect of radiation on the fracture repair process. A biomechanical evaluation of a closed fracture in a rat model. J Orthop Res 7: 178–183

Marks SC Jr, Popoff SN (1988) Bone cell biology: the regulation of development, structure, and function in the skeleton. Am J Anat 183: 1–44

Marquart K-H (1977) Early ultrastructural changes in osteocytes from the proximal tibial metaphysis of mice after the incorporation of ^{224}Ra. Radiat Res 69: 40–53

Marquart K-H, Gössner W (1978) Histopathology of early effects of ^{224}Ra on bone tissue. In: Müller WA, Ebert HG (eds) Biological effects of ^{224}Ra. Nijhoff, The Hague, pp 149–157

Marx RE (1983) Osteoradionecrosis: a new concept of its pathophysiology. J Oral Maxillofac Surg 41: 283–288

Matsuzuwa T, Anderson HC (1971) Phosphatases of epiphyseal cartilage studied by electron microscopic cytochemical methods. J Histochem Cytochem 19: 801–808

Mauch PM, Weinstein H, Botnick L, Belli J, Cassady JR (1983) An evaluation of long-term survival and treatment complications in children with Hodgkin's disease. Cancer 51: 925–932

Maugh II TH (1982) Human skeletal growth factor isolated. Science 217: 819

Meier A (1951) Einwirkung der Radiumstrahlen auf den wachsenden menschlichen Knochen. Strahlentherapie 84: 587–600

Melanotte PL, Follis RH (1961) Early effects of x-irradiation on cartilage and bone. Am J Pathol 29: 1–15

Melsen F, Mosekilde L (1978) Tetracycline double-labeling of iliac trabecular bone in 41 normal adults. Calcif Tissue Res 26: 99–102

Miller SC, Marks SC Jr (1982) Osteoclast kinetics in osteopetrotic (ia) rats cured by spleen cell transfers from normal littermates. Calcif Tissue Int 34: 422–427

Möell C, Garwicz S (1988) Growth in children treated for acute lymphoblastic leukaemia. Lancet I: 1335

Möell C, Garwicz S, Westgren U, Wiebe T (1987) Disturbed pubertal growth in girls treated for acute lymphoblastic leukemia. Pediatr Hematol Oncol 4: 1–5

Mole RH (1982) Consequences of pre-natal radiation exposure for post-natal development. A review. Int J Radiat Biol 42: 1–12

Morgan DB (1984) Osteoporosis. Surv Synth Pathol Res 3: 442–456

Morrish RB, Chan E, Silverman S, Meyer J, Fu KK, Greenspan D (1981) Osteonecrosis in patients irradiated for head and neck carcinoma. Cancer 47: 1980–1983

Morse BS, Giuliani D, Giuliani ER (1974) Effects of radiation on bone formation: a functional assessment. Radiat Res 60: 307–313

Murray CG, Daly TE, Zimmerman SO (1980) The relationship between dental disease and radiation necrosis of the mandible. Oral Surg 49: 99–104

Myers R, Robinson JE, Field SB (1980) The relationship between heating time and temperature for inhibition of growth in baby rat cartilage by combined hyperthermia and x-rays. Int J Radiat Biol 38: 373–382

Neuhauser EBD, Wittenborg MH, Berman CZ, Cohen J (1952) Irradiation effects of roentgen therapy on the growing spine. Radiology 59: 637–650

Ng E, Chambers FW, Ogden HS, Coggs GC, Crane JT (1959) Osteomyelitis of the mandible following irradiation. Radiology 72: 68–74

Nilsson A (1969) Der Effekt der ionisierenden Strahlung auf das Skelett. In: Dobberstein J, Pallaske G, Stünzi H (eds) Handbuch der Spez Path Anat der Haustiere, vol I, 3rd edn. Parey, Berlin, pp 456–487

Norris WP, Cohn SH (1952) The effect of injected radium on the alkaline phosphatase activity of bone and tissues. J Biol Chem 196: 255–264

Ogden JA (1988) Skeletal growth mechanism injury patterns. In: Uhthoff HK, Wiley JJ (eds) Behavior of the growth plate. Raven, New York, pp 85–96

Owen M (1971) Cellular dynamics of bone. In: Bourne GH (ed) The biochemistry and physiology of bone, vol III, 2nd edn. Academic, New York, pp 271–298

Owen M (1978) Histogenesis of bone cells. Calcif Tissue Res 25: 205–207

Parker RG (1972) Tolerance of mature bone and cartilage in clinical radiation therapy. Front Radiat Ther Oncol 6: 312–331

Parker RG, Berry HC (1976) Late effects of therapeutic irradiation on the skeleton and bone marrow. Cancer 37: 1162–1171

Pesch H-J, Henschke F, Seibold H (1977) Einfluß von Mechanik und Alter auf den Spongiosaumbau in Lendenwirbelkörpern und im Schenkelhals. Virchows Arch [A] 377: 27–42

Phemister DB (1926) Radium necrosis of bone. Am J Roentgenol 16: 340–348

Phillips RD, Kimeldorf DJ (1966) Age and dose dependence of bone growth retardation induced by x-irradiation. Radiat Res 27: 384–396

Pogrund H, Yosipovitch Z (1976) Osteochondroma following irradiation. Isr J Med Sci 12: 154–157

Polig E, Kimmel DB, Jee WSS (1984) Morphometry of bone cell nuclei and their location relative to bone surfaces. Phys Med Biol 29: 939–952

Polig E, Jee WSS, Dell RB, Johnson F (1988) Microdistribution and local dosimetry of ^{226}Ra in trabecular bone of the beagle. Radiat Res 116: 263–282

Pömsl H (1974) Frühschäden and Tibia und Wirbel der Maus nach Inkorporation von Thorium-227 und Radium-224. Dissertation, Fakultät für Medizin der Technischen Universität München

Priest ND (ed) (1985) Metals in bone. MTP, Lancaster

Pritchard JJ (1972) The osteoblast. In: Bourne GH (ed) The biochemistry and physiology of bone, vol I, 2nd edn. Academic, New York, pp 21–43

Probert JC, Parker BR (1975) The effects of radiation therapy on bone growth. Radiology 114: 155–162

Prosnitz LR, Lawson JP, Friedlander GE, Farber LR, Pezzimenti JF (1981) Avascular necrosis of bone in Hodgkin's disease patients treated with combined modality therapy. Cancer 47: 2793–2797

Putzke HP (1963) Histochemische Untersuchungen der Tibiaepiphyse der Ratte nach Röntgen- und Kobaltbestrahlung. Acta Histochem 15: 241–250

Rabbett WF (1965) Juvenile laryngeal papillomatosis. The relation of irradiation to malignant degeneration in this disease. Ann Otol Rhinol Laryngol 74: 1149–1163

Raisz LG (1988) Local and systemic factors in the pathogenesis of osteoporosis. N Engl J Med 318: 818–828

Ranudd NE (1966) Dose distribution studies in external irradiation of carcinoma colli uteri. Acta Radiol Ther Phys Biol 4: 353–362

Ray RD (1976) Circulation and bone, In: Bourne GH (ed) The biochemistry and physiology of bone, vol IV, 2nd edn. Academic, New York, pp 385–402

Ray RD, Thompson DM, Wolf NK, LaViolette D (1956) Bone metabolism. II. Toxicity and metabolism of radioactive strontium in rats. J Bone Joint Surg [Am] 38: 160–174

Regen EM, Wilkins WE (1936) Influence of roentgen irradiation on rate of healing of fractures and phosphatase activity of callus of adult bone. J Bone Joint Surg [Am] 18: 69–79

Regezi JA, Courtney RM, Kerr DA (1976) Dental managements of patients irradiated for oral cancer. Cancer 38: 994–1000

Reidy JA, Lingley JR, Gall EA, Barr JS (1947) Effect of roentgen irradiation on epiphyseal growth. J Bone Joint Surg [Am] 29: 853–873

Reining J, Heß F, Pfab R (1988) Strahlenbehandlung nach Hüfttotalendoprothese gegen periartikuläre Verknöcherungen. Dtsch Ärztebl 85: C–1031

Rhinelander FW (1972) Circulation of bone. In: Bourne GH (ed) Biochemistry and physiology of bone, vol II, 2nd edn. Academic, New York, pp 2–77

Rissanen P, Rokkanen P, Paatsama S (1969a) The effect of Co^{60} irradiation on bone in dogs, part I. Mature bone. Strahlentherapie 137: 162–169

Rissanen P, Rokkanen P, Paatsama S (1969b) The effect of Co^{60} irradiation on bone in dogs, part II. Growing bone. Strahlentherapie 137: 344–354

Rohrer MD, Kim Y, Fayos JV (1979) The effect of cobalt-60 irradiation on monkey mandibles. Oral Surg 48: 424–440

Rosenstock JG, Jones PM, Pearson D, Palmer MK (1978) Ewing's sarcoma, adjuvant chemotherapy and pathologic fracture. Eur J Cancer 14: 799–803

Rosenthall L, Marvin JF (1957) The effect of roentgen-ray quality on bone growth and cortical bone damage. Am J Roentgenol 77: 893–898

Rossleigh MA, Smith J, Straus DJ, Engel IA (1986) Osteonecrosis in patients with malignant lymphoma. A review of 31 cases. Cancer 58: 1112–1116

Rowland RE, Marshall JH (1959) Radium in human bone, the dose in microscopic volumes in bone. Radiat Res 11: 299–313

Rowland RE, Jowsey J, Marshall JH (1958) Structural changes in human bone containing ^{226}Ra. Proc 2nd UN Int Conf on the Peaceful Uses of Atomic Energy, Geneva. 22: 242–246

Rowland RE, Jowsey J, Marshall JH (1959a) Microscopic metabolism of calcium in bone. III. Microradiographic measurements of mineral density. Radiat Res 10: 234–242

Rowland RE, Marshall JH, Jowsey J (1959b) Radium in human bone, the microradiographic appearance. Radiat Res 10: 323–334

Rubin P, Casarett GW (1968) Clinical radiation pathology, vol II. Saunders, Philadelphia

Rubin P, Casarett G (1972) A direction for clinical radiation pathology. Front Radiat Ther Oncol 6: 1–16

Rubin P, Brace KC, Gump H, Swarm R, Andrews JR (1957) The radiotoxic effects of S^{35} in growing cartilage. Radiology 69: 711–719

Rubin P, Andrews JR, Swarm R, Gump H (1959) Radiation induced dysplasias of bone. Am J Roentgenol 82: 206–216

Salinger S (1942) Arrested development of the larynx following irradiation for recurring papillomas. Ann Otol Rhinol Laryngol 51: 273–277

Sams A (1963) Effect of x-irradiation on the circulatory system of the hind limb of the mouse. Int J Radiat Biol 7: 113–129

Sams A (1965a) Histological changes in the larger blood vessels of the hind limb of the mouse after x-irradiation. Int J Radiat Biol 9: 165–174

Sams A (1965b) The long term effects of 2000 r of x-rays on the bone marrow of the mouse tibia. Br J Radiol 38: 914–919

Sams A (1966a) The effect of 2000 r of x-rays on the acid

and alkaline phosphatase of mouse tibiae. Int J Radiat Biol 10: 123–140

Sams A (1966b) The effect of 2000 r of x-rays on the internal structure of the mouse tibia. Int J Radiat Biol 11: 51–68

Sandberg M, Vuorio T, Hirvonen H, Alitalo K, Vuorio E (1988) Enhanced expression of TGF-β and c-*fos* mRNAs in the growth plates of developing human long bones. Development 102: 461–470

Sanders JE, Pritchard S, Mahoney P et al. (1986) Growth and development following marrow transplantation for leukemia. Blood 68: 1129–1135

Scheven BAA, Wassenaar A-M, Kawilarang-de Haas EWM, Nijweide PJ (1987) Comparison of direct and indirect radiation effects on osteoclast formation from progenitor cells derived from different hemopoietic sources. Radiat Res 111: 107–118

Scott BL, Glimcher MJ (1971) Distribution of glycogen in osteoblasts of the fetal rat. J Ultrastruct Res 36: 565–586

Seelentag W, Kistner G (1969) Erzeugung von Krankheiten des Skeletts durch Strahlung. In: Eichler O (ed) Stütz- und Hartgewebe. Springer, Berlin Heidelberg New York (Handbuch der experimentellen Pharmakologie, vol XVI/8, pp 96–169)

Sela J, Deutsch D, Bodner L, Bab I, Waschler Z, Muhlrad A (1982) Effect of x-ray irradiation on primary mineralization in rat alveolar bone. Virchows Arch [A] 398: 11–18

Sengupta S, Prathap K (1973) Radiation necrosis of the humerus. A report of three cases. Acta Radiol [Ther] (Stockh) 12: 313–320

Sherman MS, Selakovich WG (1957) Bone changes in chronic circulatory insufficiency. A histopathology study. J Bone Joint Surg [Am] 39: 892–901

Shipley PG, Macklin CC (1916/17) Some features of osteogenesis in light of vital staining. Am J Physiol 42: 117–123

Shohoji T, Pasternak B (1973) Adolescent growth patterns in survivors exposed prenatally to the A-bombs in Hiroshima and Nagasaki. Health Phys 25: 17–27

Silbermann M, Frommer J (1972a) Vitality of chondrocytes in the mandibular condyle as revealed by collagen formation. An autoradiographic study with ³H-proline. Am J Anat 135: 359–370

Silbermann M, Frommer J (1972b) Further evidence for the vitality of chondrocytes in the mandibular condyle as revealed by ³⁵S-sulfate autoradiography. Anat Rec 174: 503–512

Silbermann M, Lewinson D, Gonen H, Lizarbe MA, von der Mark K (1983) In vitro transformation of chondroprogenitor cells into osteoblasts and the formation of new membrane bone. Anat Rec 206: 373–383

Silverman CL, Thomas PRM, McAlister WH, Walker S, Whiteside LA (1981) Slipped femoral capital epiphyses in irradiated children: dose, volume and age relationships. Int J Radiat Oncol Biol Phys 7: 1357–1363

Simmons DJ (1976) Comparative physiology of bone. In: Bourne GH (ed) The biochemistry and physiology of bone, vol IV, 2nd edn. Academic, New York, pp 445–516

Sissons HA (1956) Experimental study of the effect of local irradiation of bone growth. In: Mitchell JS (ed) Proc 4th Intern Conf on Radiobiol 1955, Cambridge. Oliver & Boyd, Edinburgh pp 436–448

Sissons HA (1971) The growth of bone. In: Bourne GH (ed) The biochemistry and physiology of bone, vol III, 2nd edn. Academic, New York, pp 145–180

Smith JM, Miller SC, Jee WSS (1982) The microdistribution and local dosimetry of plutonium: effects of bone marrow microvasculature (abstract). Radiat Res 91: 297

Smith R (1987) Osteoporosis: cause and management. Br Med J 294: 329–332

Smith R, Davidson JK, Flatman GE (1982) Skeletal effects of orthovoltage and megavoltage therapy following treatment of nephroblastoma. Clin Radiol 33: 601–613

Sonneveld P, van Bekkum DW (1979) The effect of whole-body irradiation on skeletal growth in rhesus monkeys. Radiology 130: 789–791

Sontag W (1980) An automatic microspectrophotometric scanning method for the measurement of bone formation rates in vivo. Calcif Tissue Int 32: 63–68

Sontag W (1986a) Quantitative measurements of periosteal and cortical-endosteal bone formation and resorption in the midshaft of female rat femur. Bone 7: 55–62

Sontag W (1986b) Quantitative measurements of periosteal and cortical-endosteal bone formation and resorption in the midshaft of male rat femur. Bone 7: 63–70

Sontag W (1987) Dosimetry of alpha-emitting radionuclides in bone – a practical approach. Health Phys 53: 495–501

Soskolne WA (1978) Phagocytosis of osteocytes by osteoclasts in femora of two week-old rabbits. Cell Tissue Res 195: 557–564

Spangler D (1941) The effect of x-ray therapy for closure of the epiphyses: preliminary report. Radiology 37: 310–314

Spiers FW (1949) The influence of energy absorption and electron range on dosage in irradiated bone. Br J Radiol 22: 521–533

Spiess H, Mays CW (1979) Exostoses induced by ²²⁴Ra (ThX) in children. Eur J Pediatr 132: 271–276

Spiess H, Mays CW, Spiess-Paulus E (1986) Growth retardation in children injected with ²²⁴Ra. In: Gössner W, Gerber GB, Hagen U, Luz A (eds) The radiobiology of radium and thorotrast. Urban & Schwarzenberg, Munich

Stampfli WP, Kerr HD (1947) Fractures of femoral neck following pelvic irradiation. Am J Roentgenol 57: 71–83

Stephenson WH, Cohen B (1956) Post-irradiation fractures of the neck of the femur. J Bone Joint Surg [Br] 38: 830–845

Sylvester JE, Greenberg P, Selch MT, Thomas BJ, Amstutz H (1988) The use of postoperative irradiation for the prevention of heterotopic bone formation after total HIP replacement. Int J Radiat Oncol Biol Phys 14: 471–476

Tannock IF, Hayashi S (1972) The proliferation of capillary endothelial cells. Cancer Res 32: 77–82

Teft M (1972) Radiation effect on growing bone and cartilage. Front Radiat Ther Oncol 6: 289–311

Thurner J (1970) Iatrogene Pathologie. Urban & Schwarzenberg, Munich

Thyberg J (1972) Ultrastructural localization of arylsulfatase activity in the epiphyseal plate. J Ultrastruct Res 38: 332–342

Thyberg J, Friberg U (1972) Electron microscopic enzyme histochemical studies on the cellular genesis of matrix vesicles in the epiphyseal plate. J Ultrastruct Res 41: 43–59

Thyberg J, Lohmander S, Friberg U (1973) Electron microscopic demonstration of proteoglycans in guinea pig epiphyseal cartilage. J Ultrastruct Res 45: 407–427

Timothy AR, Tucker AK, Park WM, Cannell LB (1978)

Osteonecrosis in Hodgkin's disease. Br J Radiol 51: 328–332

Tonna EA (1963) Origin of osteoclasts from fusion of phagocytes. Nature 200: 226–227

Tonna EA (1972) An electron microscopic study of osteocyte release during osteoclasis in mice of different ages. Clin Orthop 87: 311–317

Triffitt JT (1987) Initiation and enhancement of bone formation. A review. Acta Orthop Scand 58: 673–684

Ubios AM, Guglielmotti MB, Cabrini RL (1986) Effect of diphosphonate on the prevention of x-irradiation-induced inhibition of bone formation in rats. J Oral Pathol 15: 500–505

Ueberschär K-H (1959) Tierexperimentelle Untersuchungen über Verlauf und Reparation der radiogenen Knochenschädigung. Strahlentherapie 110: 529–540

Uhthoff HK, Wiley JJ (eds) (1988) Behavior of the growth plate. Raven, New York

Urist MR, Hernandez A (1974) Excitation transfer in bone. Deleterious effects of cobalt 60 radiation-sterilization of bank bone. Arch Surg 109: 486–493

Vaeth JM, Levitt SH, Jones MD, Holfreter C (1962) Effects of radiation therapy in survivors of Wilms' tumor. Radiology 79: 560–568

van Caneghem P, Schirren CG (1956) Tierexperimentelle Untersuchungen zur Frage der Röntgenstrahlenempfindlichkeit von Knochenwachstumszonen. Strahlentherapie 100: 433–444

van der Plas A, Nijweide PJ (1988) Cell-cell interactions in the osteogenic compartment of bone. Bone 9: 107–111

Vaughan JM (1973) The effects of irradiation on the skeleton. Clarendon, Oxford

Vaughan J (1981) Osteogenesis and haematopoiesis. Lancet II: 133–136

Vaughan J, Owen M (1959) The use of autoradiography in the measurement of radiation dose-rate in rabbit bones following the administration of Sr^{90}. Lab Invest 8: 181–191

von Rottkay P (1985) Bericht über zwei Fälle von strahleninduzierten Knochennekrosen an Brustwirbelkörpern bei Bronchialkarzinomen nach akzelerierter Bestrahlung. Strahlentherapie 161: 704–705

Wachsmann F (1949) Ausblick auf die Anwendung'smöglichkeiten der Elektronenschleuder in der Medizin und bisherige Versuchsergebnisse mit ultraharten Strahlungen. Acta Radiol (Stockh) 32: 146–158

Walker KVR, Kember NF (1972a) Cell kinetics of growth cartilage in the rat tibia. I. Measurements in young male rats. Cell Tissue Kinet 5: 401–408

Walker KVR, Kember NF (1972b) Cell kinetics of growth cartilage in the rat tibia. II. Measurements during ageing. Cell Tissue Kinet 5: 409–419

Wang CC, Doppke K (1976) Osteoradionecrosis of the temporal bone – consideration of nominal standard dose. Int J Radiat Oncol Biol Phys 1: 881–883

Wegener K (1970) Osteodystrophy after inhalation of radon-222. Virchows Arch [A] 350: 179–182

Weiss JF, Catravas GN, Reddi AH (1982) Influence of radiation on matrix-induced endochondral bone differentiation (abstract). Radiat Res 91: 353

Wells AB (1969) The effect of acute and fractionated doses of x-rays on the growth of the mouse tibia. Br J Radiol 42: 364–371

Wieland C (1983) Wirbelveränderungen nach Bestrahlung eines Ösophaguskarzinoms. Strahlentherapie 159: 211–213

Wilkins WE, Regen EM (1934) The influence of roentgen rays on the growth and phosphatase activity of bone. Radiology 22: 674–677

Wilson CW (1950) Dosage of high voltage radiation within bone and its possible significance for radiation therapy. Br J Radiol 23: 92–100

Wilson CW (1956a) The uptake of ^{32}P by the kneejoint and tibia of six-week-old mice and the effect of x-rays upon it. Variation of uptake with time after a dose of 2000 r of 200 kV x-rays. Br J Radiol 29: 86–573

Wilson CW (1956b) The effect of x-rays on the uptake of ^{32}P by the knee-joint and tibia of six-week-old mice: relation of depression of uptake to x-ray dose. Br J Radiol 29: 571–573

Wilson CW (1957) The effects of x-rays on the uptake of ^{32}P by the knee joint and tibia of six-week-old mice. A comparison of the effects produced by equal doses of 200 kV and 2 MeV x-rays. Br J Radiol 30: 92–94

Wilson CW (1958) The effect of x-rays upon the uptake of ^{32}P by the knee joint of the mouse. Relation between the depression of ^{32}P uptake and the age of animal. Br J Radiol 31: 384–386

Wilson CW (1959) Effect of x-rays on uptake of ^{32}P by the mouse knee joint when the x-ray dose is given in two carefully spaced fractions. Br J Radiol 32: 547–551

Wilson CW (1960) Effect of x-rays on the uptake of phosphorus 32 by the mouse knee joint. Dependence upon the spacing interval of the effect produced by two spaced equal dose fractions. Br J Radiol 33: 636–639

Wilson CW (1961) Effect of spaced x-ray dose fractions on ^{32}P uptake by the mouse knee joint. Dependence upon size of fractions and their spacing intervals. Br J Radiol 34: 454–457

Woodard HQ (1957) Some effects of x-rays on bone. Clin Orthop 9: 118–130

Woodard HQ, Laughlin JS (1957) The effect of x-rays of different qualities on the alkaline phosphatase activity of living mouse bone. II. Effects of 22.5 Mevp x-rays. Radiat Res 7: 236–252

Woodard HQ, Spiers FW (1953) The effect of x-rays of different qualities on the alkaline phosphatase of living mouse bone. Br J Radiol 26: 38–46

Wozney JM, Rosen V, Celeste AJ et al. (1988) Novel regulators of bone formation: molecular clones and activities. Science 242: 1528–1534

Wronski TJ, Smith JM, Jee WSS (1980) The microdistribution and retention of injected ^{239}Pu on trabecular bone surfaces of the beagle: implications for the induction of osteosarcoma. Radiat Res 83: 74–89

Wronski TJ, Smith JM, Jee WSS (1981) Variations in mineral apposition rate of trabecular bone within the beagle skeleton. Calcif Tissue Int 33: 583–586

Wurster CF, Krespi YP, Curtis AW (1982) Osteoradionecrosis of the temporal bone. Otolaryngol Head Neck Surg 90: 126–129

Yeager VL, Chiemchanya S, Chaiseri P (1975) Changes in size of lacunae during the life of osteocytes in osteons of compact bone. J Gerontol 30: 9–14

Zinkernagel R, Riede UN, Schenk RK (1972) Ultrastrukturelle Untersuchungen der juxtaepiphysären Kapillaren nach Perfusionsfixation. Experientia 28: 1205–1206

Zollinger HU (1960) Radio-Histologie und Radio-Histopathologie In: Roulet F (ed) Strahlung und Wetter. Springer, Berlin Göttingen Heidelberg (Handbuch der allgemeinen Pathologie, vol 10/1, pp 127–287)

4 Bone Marrow

W. NOTHDURFT

Professor Dr. W. NOTHDURFT, Universität Ulm, Institut für Arbeits- und Sozialmedizin, Albert-Einstein-Allee 11, 7900 Ulm, FRG

4.1 Introduction

The hematological consequences of exposures of the human body to ionizing radiation under different conditions can be understood only on the basis of the biology of this complex organ system. Therefore, this article will begin with a short description of the anatomical structure and functional organization of the bone marrow and its various tissue components. Until the recent past radiation hematology mainly focused on the cellular events (see reviews by HENDRY and LORD 1983; FLIEDNER and NOTHDURFT 1986). In fact, the dividing immature hemopoietic cells are the true targets of radiation, and the mature end cells produced by them are the essential functional elements which contribute to a homeostatic state.

On the other hand, cellular (and also extracellular) elements not belonging to the hemopoietic tissue are involved in the regulation of blood cell formation. Furthermore, the importance of humoral regulators for hemopoietic cell function has been well established for some 30–40 years, since the description of erythropoietin (BONSDORFF and JALAVISTO 1948) and thrombopoietin (see review by McDONALD 1988). However, decisive progress in understanding the role of soluble factors in the regulation of hemopoietic cell production under normal or pathological conditions has been made during the last few years. Various hemopoietic growth factors and synergizing factors (grouped under the term "cytokines") have been characterized and are now available in large quantities for experimental and clinical studies.

Thus, this survey will give a detailed and comprehensive description and analysis of the cellular events in the bone marrow after irradiation. The regulatory processes involved can be described only in a rather concise fashion. Whenever possible, emphasis will be laid on the radiation effects on the human bone marrow. However, in certain areas the only data available derive from experimental animals.

4.2 Anatomical Organization and Distribution

After birth the hemopoietic tissue in man is exclusively located in the bone cavities (WINTROBE 1974). Under normal circumstances no extramedullary hemopoiesis is present in any of the organs that are active in certain periods during fetal life, e.g., liver, spleen, and thymus (KELEMEN et al. 1979; MORGENSTERN 1988). However, these organs may develop hemopoietic activity under pathophysiological conditions such as myelofibrosis (VAN DYKE and ANGER 1965) or after extended-field radiotherapy or total body irradiation followed by bone marrow transplantation (see Sects. 4.11.3.3 and 4.13.3).

In the bone marrow, the hemopoietic tissue forms a parenchyma of free cells included within the meshes of the so-called stroma, which consists of different types of fixed but quite flexible cells and various types of fibers and filaments (VON HEYDEN 1978; VON KEYSERLINGK 1978; LICHTMAN 1981; TAVASSOLI and FRIEDENSTEIN 1983; FLIEDNER et al. 1985). In the adult the active (or red) marrow is distributed over a large number of bones of the axial skeleton, the proximal ends (heads) of the humeri and of the femora, and some bones of the skull (VON KEYSERLINGK 1978). Quantitative data on active bone marrow distribution were established by ELLIS (1961), ATKINSON (1962), and HASHIMOTO and YAMAKA (1964). In general there is little difference between the data from the first two sources (Table 4.1). Certain deviations observed in the fractional distribution as reported by HASHIMOTO and YAMAKA (1964) may reflect some racial characteristics and in part

be due to methodological differences. Further data, including age-dependent changes in the bone marrow distribution, are given by SHLEIEN (1973) and in ICRP Report No. 23 (1974), in which it is stated (p. 90) that the data provided by ELLIS constitute "the generally accepted distribution pattern for red marrow" (e.g., KEREIAKES et al. 1972; THIERRY et al. 1985). However, there is obviously much variation, and in the female the hemopoietic marrow may occupy up to half or two-thirds of the shaft of the femur.

4.3 Functional Structure

The two main tissues constituting the bone marrow organ are quite different with respect to their cytokinetic status. The hemopoietic tissue is a cell-renewal system. In contrast, most of the different cell types forming the stroma, in which the hemopoietic cells are embedded, have quite a low mitotic activity, if any under normal circumstances.

4.3.1 Hemopoiesis

The formation of functional blood cells takes place along an extremely hierarchically organized system by multiple divisions and differentiation of progenitor cells and maturation of precursor cells and their progeny. According to this organization hemopoiesis has to be grouped with the "continually replacing tissues" (POTTEN 1986) or "type H" ("H" for hierarchical) populations (MICHALOWSKI 1981), together with the surface epithelia of the skin and the gastrointestinal tract, the testicular epithelia, and some glandular epithelia

Table 4.1. Active bone marrow distribution (in %) in adults

Bone (site)	ELLIS (1961)[a]	ATKINSON (1962)[a]	HASHIMOTO and YAMAKA (1964)
Head	13	15	7
Upper limb girdle	8[b]	9	7
Sternum	2	2	3
Ribs	8	7	14
Vertebrae, cervical	4	} 30	3
thoracic	14		13
lumbar	11		11
Sacrum	14		9
		} 37	
Lower limb girdle	26[c]		33
Extremities	–	–	–

[a] 40 years of age.
[b,c] Including the heads of the humeri and femora, respectively.

(for further details see THAMES and HENDRY 1987).

A general scheme of hemopoiesis is presented in Fig. 4.1. The blood cell formation along the different cell lineages originates in a common population of pluripotent stem cells and generally follows the same principle. As can be seen from Fig. 4.1, the basic structure shows a certain compartmentalization. Differentiation of pluripotent stem cells leads to cytologically unidentifiable progenitor cells of the different lineages capable of several divisions. The progenitor cells feed into maturing, cytologically identifiable precursors which, after a limited number of divisions, give rise to nondividing maturing cells. For more details see HENDRY and LORD (1983), CRONKITE (1985), and POTTEN (1986).

Figure 4.2 presents the hierarchy of the progenitor cells and the main cellular pathways leading to functional blood cells along with the cytokines (growth factors and synergizing factors) controlling the cell development. These factors are produced by several types of cell, including those of the stroma (cf. Sect. 4.5).

It is important to notice that pluripotent stem cells and the progenitor cells of the different lineages not only are present in the bone marrow but also in the peripheral blood at any time, though at comparatively low concentrations, i.e. in the range from 10 to 200 per ml (reviews by NOTHDURFT and FLIEDNER 1979, FLIEDNER and NOTHDURFT 1986, McCARTHY and GOLDMAN 1983).

4.3.1.1 Pluripotent Stem Cells

The pluripotent stem cell is capable of self-replication as well as producing all the different cell lineages referred to above, including eosinophilic granulocytes, lymphopoietic cells, osteo-

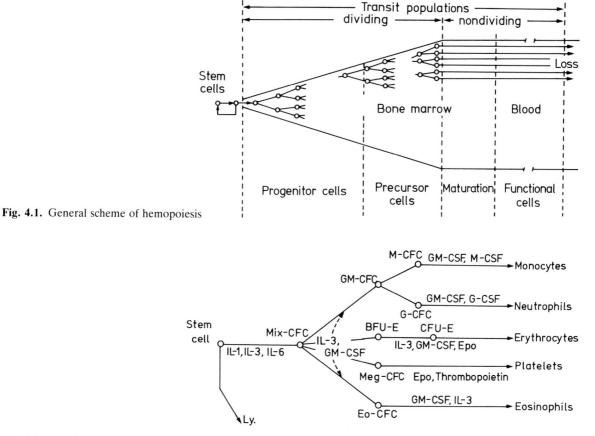

Fig. 4.1. General scheme of hemopoiesis

Fig. 4.2. The hierarchy of hemopoietic progenitor cells and the cytokines controlling the cell development along the different lineages. *Ly*, lymphopoiesis; *GM-CFC, G-CFC*, and *M-CFC*, granulocyte/macrophage, granulocyte, and macrophage progenitor cells; *Mix-CFC*, multipotent progenitor cells; *BFU-E* and *CFU-E*, erythroid progenitor cells; *Meg-CFC*, megakaryocyte progenitor cells; *Eo-CFC*, eosinophil progenitor cells; *IL-1, IL-3*, and *IL-6*, interleukin-1, -3, and -6; *GM-CSF, G-CSF*, and *M-CSF*, granulocyte/macrophage, granulocyte, and macrophage colony-stimulating factors; *Epo*, erythropoietin (QUESENBERRY 1986; CLARK and KAMEN 1987; SIEFF 1987; LORD and TESTA 1988; HERRMANN and MERTELSMANN 1989)

clasts, tissue mast cells, and epidermal Langerhans cells (LORD and TESTA 1988).

The stem cell population can be defined as "the population of cells in a given tissue which are ultimately responsible for all cell replacement in that tissue throughout life" (POTTEN 1986). Serial bone marrow transplantations performed in mice revealed that a stem cell population is able to maintain its repopulating capacity over at least five murine generations (HENDRY and LORD 1983; Ross et al. 1982). Clinical practice has shown that in human patients long-term hemopoietic reconstitution is achieved with bone marrow transplants corresponding to 1% of the total bone marrow stem cell population (see Sect. 4.11).

The stem cells can be assayed and functionally characterized only in the mouse and, to a more limited extent, in the rat.

Pluripotent Stem Cells in the Mouse

In the mouse those cells in the hemopoietic tissues (the bone marrow, the spleen, the fetal liver) and in the peripheral blood which, after intravenous injection into lethally irradiated mice, seed to the spleen and form macroscopic hemopoietic colonies, i.e., the "colony-forming units in the spleen" (CFU-S; TILL and MCCULLOCH 1961), have been considered as representative of pluripotent stem cells. However, data have accumulated indicating that CFU-S subpopulations with different self-renewal capacities may be assayed by this technique depending on the day of colony counting (see reviews by CRONKITE 1985; QUESENBERRY 1986), although this has been questioned recently (BLACKETT 1987). Obviously, stem cells more primitive than CFU-S exist as well (review by OGAWA et al. 1983). For more details with respect to proposed models of stem cell renewal and commitment and the control of proliferation by stimulators and inhibitors, various papers and reviews may be consulted (e.g., SCHOFIELD 1978, 1979; LAJTHA 1979; TILL and MCCULLOCH 1980; MCCULLOCH 1985; PHARR and OGAWA 1985; LORD 1986; POTTEN 1986; LORD and TESTA 1988).

The total number of pluripotent stem cells with CFU-S properties present in the bone marrow of normal mice has been estimated to vary from 362 600 to 1 780 711 depending on the strain. In the spleen there are between 18 000 and 42 000 CFU-S (COGGLE and GORDON 1975). The concentration of stem cells in the bone marrow is in the range of 0.25%–0.4% (POTTEN 1986; LORD and TESTA 1988). The fraction of potential CFU-S that actually settle in the spleen of the recipient after injection of a bone marrow cell suspension (i.e., seeding efficiency or "f" factor) varies from 1/20th to 1/5th (HENDRY and LORD 1983; CRONKITE 1985).

Under steady state conditions there is little proliferation within the CFU-S population, as is indicated by the usually low S-phase fraction of between 1/50th and 1/10th (BECKER et al. 1965; LAJTHA et al. 1969; GIDALI et al. 1974; review by POTTEN 1986). However, though there is good evidence for the existence of CFU-S subpopulations in different proliferative states, i.e., cycling or prolonged G_0/G_1 (CILLO et al. 1985), and for a primitive pre-CFU-S in a G_0 state (HODGSON and BRADLEY 1979), the exact cytokinetic nature of the stem cells is not completely understood (for reviews see CRONKITE 1985; LORD 1986; POTTEN 1986). Obviously CFU-S not in DNA synthesis have a preference for seeding in the spleen, whereas S-phase cells have a higher affinity for the bone marrow (see review by CRONKITE 1985).

Besides the bone marrow and spleen, CFU-S are also present in the peripheral blood of the normal mouse, though at rather small concentrations, in the range of 6–24 CFU-S per ml (without correcting for the "f" factor) (COGGLE and GORDON 1975; review by NOTHDURFT and FLIEDNER 1979).

Pluripotent Progenitor Cells in Man

A culture system that allows the assessment of multipotent progenitor cells in hemopoietic tissues of man in analogy to the murine situation (MCLEOD et al. 1976; JOHNSON and METCALF 1977) was developed by FAUSER and MESSNER (1978). These cells are able to produce mixed colonies consisting of at least four different lineages, i.e., neutrophilic granulocytes, erythrocytes, macrophages, and megakaryocytes, and were therefore named GEMM-CFC (FAUSER and MESSNER 1979a). The cloning efficiencies obtained under appropriate culture conditions are 10–15 GEMM-CFC per 10^5 bone marrow cells plated (MESSNER and FAUSER 1980; ASH et al. 1981), and the S-phase fraction is in the range of 10%–35% (FAUSER and MESSNER 1979b; LEPINE and MESSNER 1983). GEMM-CFC can also be found in the blood of normal persons at concentrations of about 5 per 10^5 cells plated (ASH et al. 1981; LEPINE and MESSNER 1983).

As could be shown more recently, the functional repertoire of GEMM-CFC is not restricted to multilineage hemopoiesis; rather it may extend to lymphopoiesis under appropriate growth conditions (MESSNER 1986).

In the mouse, GEMM-CFC and CFU-S seem to be partly overlapping populations (see review by OGAWA et al. 1983).

4.3.1.2 Granulocytopoiesis/Monocytopoiesis

The granulocyte/macrophage progenitor cell (GM-CFC) population is the common source of both cell lineages. The GM-CFC and their descendents, the granulocyte progenitor cell (G-CFC) and the macrophage progenitor cell (M-CFC), are well characterized (METCALF 1977; METCALF and BURGESS 1982). The number of GM-CFC found under normal circumstances in conventional cultures per 10^5 bone marrow cells ranges from 50 to 100 in man and from 100 to 200 in the mouse (METCALF 1977) and the dog (NOTHDURFT et al. 1984, 1986). The heterogeneous GM-CFC population is composed of subpopulations in a different kinetic state (DRESCH et al. 1979; CILLO et al. 1985; CROSSEN et al. 1986.) The overall S-phase fraction is rather similar for different species, e.g., 31%–45% in man (RICKARD et al. 1974; TEBBI et al 1976; LOHRMANN 1978), 30%–50% in the mouse (ISCOVE et al. 1970; METCALF 1977), and 25%–40% in the dog (NOTHDURFT et al. 1984, 1986). Under conditions of bone marrow regeneration the S-phase fraction may increase to up to 80% in the mouse (METCALF 1977) and 60% in the dog (NOTHDURFT et al. 1986).

The more mature progenitors, G-CFC, at least give rise to the myeloblasts, the earliest cytologically recognizable precursor cells, and after a further four or five divisions and maturation the neutrophilic granulocytes will arise (for details see ROBINSON and MANGALIK 1975; DANCEY et al. 1976; WALKER and WILLEMZE 1980; CRONKITE 1985).

The main growth factors directly involved in granulocyte/macrophage formation are IL-3, GM-CSF, G-CSF, and M-CSF. In vitro they have been shown to be essential for survival of the progenitor cells and their proliferation, but also to affect the functions of the mature end cells (for reviews see METCALF 1986a,b; QUESENBERRY 1986; BROXMEYER 1986; CLARK and KAMEN 1987; NICOLA 1987; SIEFF 1987; LORD and TESTA 1988; HERRMANN and MERTELSMANN 1989).

4.3.1.3 Erythropoiesis

There are two different stages of progenitor cells in the hierarchy that can be clearly distinguished. The erythroid burst-forming unit, BFU-E (AXELRAD et al. 1974), sometimes subdivided into two compartments, represents a more primitive class of progenitor cells than the erythroid colony-forming unit (CFU-E) (STEPHENSON et al. 1971). The growth of BFU-E in vitro has been found to require high concentrations of erythropoietin together with the synergistic action of burst-promoting activity (ISCOVE 1978a), supplied by either IL-3 or high concentrations of GM-CSF (for reviews see LORD 1986; METCALF 1986b; QUESENBERRY 1986; CLARK and KAMEN 1987).

The concentration of BFU-E in the bone marrow ranges from 25 to 100 per 10^5 nucleated cells in aspirates from human marrow (NISHIHIRA and KIGASAWA 1981; TAKEICHI et al. 1987), from 11 to 55 per 10^5 cells in the mouse (KREJA and SEIDEL 1982), and from 30 to 120 per 10^5 cells in the dog, depending on the culture conditions (SCHWARTZ et al. 1986; KREJA et al. 1988). The S-phase fraction of BFU-E has been reported to range from 30% to 35% in the mouse (HARA and OGAWA 1977; ISCOVE 1977), and from 25% to 35% in man (LIPTON and NATHAN 1980).

The CFU-E are present at much higher concentrations in all the species (ISCOVE 1978b; SCHWARTZ et al. 1986; LIPTON and NATHAN 1981), and they are rapidly cycling, as indicated by their S-phase fraction of between 71% and 75% (HARA and OGAWA 1977; ISCOVE 1977).

In the precursor compartment four further mitoses are completed before erythrocyte formation (for more details see FLIEDNER et al. 1978; HENDRY and LORD 1983; CRONKITE 1985).

4.3.1.4 Megakaryocytopoiesis/thrombocytopoiesis

Megakaryopoiesis originates from the compartment of committed progenitor cells, Meg-CFC. Their concentration in normal human bone marrow as assessed in vitro under appropriate culture conditions is approximately 5–10 per 10^5 cells (GEWIRTZ and HOFFMAN 1985; DE ALARCON 1989). The number of doublings at the level of Meg-CFC is low (PAULUS et al. 1980) in comparison to GM–CFC and BFU-E. Intermediate between the proliferative Meg-CFC and the early megakaryocytes is a pool of nonproliferating cells that, however, are capable of undergoing endoreduplication, over five generations at the maximum. Thus, platelet-producing megakaryocytes arise with ploidy values between 8N and 64N (EBBE 1980; NAKEFF 1982; BURSTEIN and HARKER 1983; MAZUR 1987).

IL-3 and GM-CSF are growth factors that control the development of Meg-CFC (HERRMANN and MERTELSMANN 1989; LORD and TESTA 1988). A humoral component operationally defined as thrombopoietin that is present in the plasma of thrombocytopenic animals and patients has been shown to act on the megakaryocyte precursors, to significantly shift the megakaryocyte ploidy upward and to affect platelet production (GEWIRTZ and HOFFMAN 1985; MAZUR 1987; McDONALD 1988). This regulator seems to be produced in the kidney, but also in other organs, perhaps the liver (GEWIRTZ and HOFFMAN 1985).

4.3.2 Organization and Function of the Stroma

The bone marrow stroma (in the strict sense) is composed of several types of fixed cells and the extracellular matrix containing glycosaminoglycans, fibronectin, and collagen. Together with other cellular elements operationally termed accessory cells (for review see TOROK-STORB 1988), it represents what more than 20 years ago was defined as the "hemopoietic-inductive microenvironment" (HIM) (CURRY et al. 1967).

Evidence for, or proof of, the essential role that the stroma and the accessory cells play as the HIM comes from several sources: the specific association of cells of the different hemopoietic cell lineages with certain stromal and accessory cells in situ (see reviews by WEISS and CHEN 1975; LICHTMAN 1981; TAVASSOLI and FRIEDENSTEIN 1983); genetic diseases in experimental animals associated with either defects in stromal functions or hemopoietic dysfunctions (see reviews by RUSSEL 1979; TRENTIN 1978); heterotopic transplantations of fragments of hemopoietic organs of different origin, e.g., red marrow, spleen, or yellow marrow (see review by TAVASSOLI 1975; PATT et al. 1982); and in vitro studies on long-term bone marrow cultures demonstrating the requirement of hemopoietic cell development for certain stromal elements (see reviews by ALLEN and DEXTER 1984; TOROK-STORB 1988).

There are three major nonhemopoietic components of the bone marrow structure: (a) vasculature and microvasculature (sinuses) consisting of endothelial cells and adventitial reticular cells, apposing the abluminal surface of the vascular sinus; (b) the network of reticular cell cytoplasmic processes and fibers in the intersinal space, integrating fat cells and fibroblastoid cells, both often in a parasinal location, upon which the hemopoietic cells are arranged ("hemopoietic cords"); and (c) neural structures, e.g., nerve fibers and Schwann cells (see review by WEISS and CHEN 1975; LICHTMAN 1981; TAVASSOLI and FRIEDENSTEIN 1983).

The kinetics of the cells organizing the stroma have mainly been studied in rodents. The populations of differentiated reticular cells, endothelial cells, and the fat cells in the rat show no or only an extremely slow turnover (CAFFREY et al. 1966; HAAS et al. 1971). Similarly, the ^{3}H-thymidine (^{3}H-TdR) labeling indices of about 2%–2.4% for murine bone marrow endothelial cells and those in the Haversian canals of the bone, and the low incidence of mitotic figures, also indicate that only a small proportion of these elements is in cycle under normal circumstances (TANNOCK and HAYASHI 1972; LANGDON and BERMAN 1975). This is in general agreement with the findings in other tissues (see review by HOPEWELL 1983). Obviously the reticular and endothelial cells can be recruited from the normal $G_0(G_1)$ state into S under certain conditions such as by successive injections of urethane (LANGDON and BERMAN 1975) or after fracture of the bone (TANNOCK and HAYASHI 1972).

Access to quantitative studies of stromal function was achieved by the establishment of an assay for clonogenic cells (FRIEDENSTEIN et al. 1970; review by FRIEDENSTEIN 1976). These cells give rise to large adherent fibroblast (or fibroblastoid) colonies. The fibroblastoid colony forming units (CFU-F) are heterogeneous with respect to their proliferative potential and commitment to varying differentiation pathways, including osteogenesis (FRIEDENSTEIN 1976; PATT et al. 1982; TAVASSOLI and FRIEDENSTEIN 1983).

In the bone marrow of the adult the CFU-F is quiescent, as shown for guinea pigs (FRIEDENSTEIN 1976), mice (BEN-ISHAY et al. 1986), and man (CASTRO-MALASPINA et al. 1980; DA et al. 1986).

CFU-F type cells are present in the circulation under normal circumstances in several mammals, including man (see FRIEDENSTEIN 1976). However, recent studies indicate that the role attributed to these cells as pioneers for hemopoietic regeneration after perturbations such as treatment of mice with phenylhydrazine (PIERSMA et al. 1985) or partial body irradiation (WERTS et al. 1980) has been overestimated (see MALONEY et al. 1985).

4.4 Spatial Organization of the Hemopoietic Tissue

Using different experimental (and theoretical) approaches several authors have been able to show that in the bone marrow of the femur of the mouse the CFU-S, GM-CFC, BFU-E, CFU-E, and even CFU-F exhibit distinct distributions across the radial axis of the marrow cavity (LORD et al. 1975; LORIMORE and WRIGHT 1987; for details see HENDRY and LORD 1983; LORD and TESTA 1988). The significance of these murine data for the human situation (trabecular bones) is discussed in more detail by LORD (1988) and LORD and TESTA (1988).

A model with distinctly different stromal functions in a radially organized fashion has been presented by LAMBERTSEN and WEISS (1984). However, the experimental data were not obtained under steady state conditions but from irradiated bone marrow space.

The implications for radiation dose distribution of different locations of hemopoietic cells in the axial area or the marginal zone, e.g., in close proximity to the bone surface, are considered by HENDRY and LORD (1983), LORD (1988), and LORD and TESTA (1988).

4.5 Origin of Cytokines

The cytokines are substances produced by cells present in all organs (Table 4.2). Some of these cells belong to the stroma (e.g., endothelial cells and fibroblasts), whereas others belong to the group of accessory cells of lymphohemopoietic origin (e.g., T cells, macrophages, and monocytes) (see reviews by LORD and TESTA 1988; SEGAL and BAGBY 1988; TOROK-STORB 1988; ZIPORI 1988; HERRMANN and MERTELSMANN 1989). There is a complex network of cytokine interactions between the different cell types producing the various factors, among them the CSFs and the synergizing factors that both at least act on the hemopoietic cells and their progeny as the targets (reviews by SIEFF 1987; CRONKITE 1988; LORD and TESTA 1988; HERRMANN and MERTELSMANN 1989).

4.6 Effects of Irradiation on Hemopoietic Cells

Knowledge concerning the response of mammalian pluripotent hemopoietic stem cells to ionizing radiation is almost exclusively restricted to the murine species. It is only in this species (and under certain circumstances in the rat) that the clonal growth of pluripotent stem cells can be studied in vivo based on the spleen colony technique, i.e., the assay measures CFU-S.

4.6.1 Pluripotent Stem Cells in Mice

It has to be kept in mind that the spleen colony technique measures those stem cells that seed to and proliferate in the spleen. Among the various modifications of the spleen colony technique that allow radiation dose-response curves for the CFU-S to be established, the exogenous techniques requiring stem cell transplantations are the most common (see HENDRY 1985a). The cell populations to be assayed can be irradiated in vivo in the

Table 4.2. Growth factors (or colony-stimulating factors, CSFs) and synergizing factors[a]

Factor-producing cell	Growth factors				Synergizing factors	
	GM-CSF	G-CSF	M-CSF	IL-3	IL-1	IL-6
Endothelial cell	+	+	+			
Fibroblast	+	+	+			+
Monocyte/macrophage		+	+		+	
T cell	+			+		

[a] Data from different sources (see text).

donor mice with different doses before sampling and transfusion into the preirradiated recipient mice, but they also can be exposed in vitro before or in vivo after injection into the preirradiated recipients. On the other hand the endogenous assay measures the CFU-S survival in the irradiated mouse itself, i.e., it is a direct in situ assay requiring no further perturbations of the hemopoietic tissue (TILL and McCULLOCH 1963). However, this method can be used over a limited range of doses only and poses some other problems, as considered in more detail by HENDRY and LORD (1983).

Several recent compilations review the response of CFU-S to low LET radiation under different exposure conditions, i.e., in vitro or in vivo, acute or protracted irradiations (SONG et al. 1981; GLASGOW et al. 1983; HENDRY and LORD 1983; FLIEDNER and NOTHDURFT 1986).

4.6.1.1 Response to Acute Doses

A typical set of survival data obtained for CFU-S after irradiation in vivo and the shouldered curve originally fitted to the data are shown in Fig. 4.3. The radiation dose–response relationship was defined by the D_0 value and the extrapolation number n, i.e., parameters of the multitarget model, $S = 1 - [1 - \exp(-D/D_0)]^n$, though the data

are also compatible with the existence of a negative initial slope. Furthermore, it has been shown that CFU-S survival data such as are presented in Fig. 4.3. also can be fitted by other models, for example a continuously bending curve type $S = \exp -(\alpha D + \beta D^2)$ (HENDRY 1979; KELLERER et al. 1980).

A compilation of values of D_0 and n as reported for murine CFU-S after irradiation in vivo or in vitro with γ-rays, x-rays, or fast electrons at various dose rates ranging from 0.3 Gy/min to 6 Gy/min (240 Gy/min for fast electrons) is given in Table 4.3.

From such compilations the following conclusions can be drawn (see the extensive review by HENDRY and LORD 1983 for more detailed information):

1. The survival curves obtained for high dose rates exhibit a small shoulder, as reflected by an extrapolation number of about 1.8 (extreme range 0.92–10).
2. CFU-S that are irradiated in vivo show a similar response irrespective of whether they are irradiated in the donor or in the recipient after transplantation.
3. According to some studies there is no detectable effect on CFU-S of in vitro or in vivo irradiation with low doses of γ-rays or x-rays up to 0.2 Gy, i.e., a "threshold" dose (HANKS 1972; HENDRY and LORD 1983; CRONKITE et al. 1987). In contrast, more recently it has been stated by HENDRY (1988) "that with doses down to 0.05 Gy there was no evidence for significant deviation from an exponential decline in survival with dose given using a wide range of dose rates."
4. Differences obtained between CFU-S survival curves after irradiation of the cells in vitro or in vivo are not uniform and their causes are unclear.
5. There is a clear difference in the sensitivity of murine femoral CFU-S to x-rays and γ-rays (at comparable dose rates). The mean D_0 values reported by HENDRY and LORD (1983) for 200–300 kV x-rays and 0.6–1.3 MeV γ-rays are 0.77 ± 0.03 Gy and 1.00 ± 0.03 Gy, respectively. The mean RBE value of 0.77 ($D_{0,R}/D_{0,\gamma}$) of the γ-rays is small compared with those for other biological systems. The RBE of 15 MeV electrons may also approach a value of approximately 0.8. The reasons for this low RBE value are not clear.

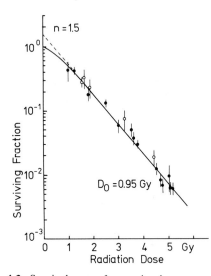

Fig. 4.3. Survival curve for murine bone marrow CFU-S after irradiation in vivo with ^{60}Co γ-rays. $\bigcirc$, irradiated in the femora of the donor mice before transplantation; $\bullet$, irradiated after transfusion into the recipient mice. (After McCULLOCH and TILL 1962)

Table 4.3. Survival curve parameters D_o and n of murine femoral CFU-S after irradiation with acute doses of γ-rays, x-rays, and fast electrons

Radiation source	Irradiation		Parameter		RBE $D_0(x)/D_0(\gamma)$	Reference
	Dose rate (Gy/min)	Exposure of cells	D_0 (Gy)	n		
γ-rays	3.30	In vitro	1.15 ± 0.08	~ 2		TILL and McCULLOCH (1961)
^{60}Co, ^{137}Cs	0.55, ~ 3.0	In vitro	1.05 ± 0.13	2.5		McCULLOCH and TILL (1962)
	0.55	In vivo (d)[a]	0.95 ± 0.09	1.5		McCULLOCH and TILL (1962)
	0.55	In vivo (r)[b]	0.95 ± 0.09	1.5		McCULLOCH and TILL (1962)
	0.293 (R/100)	In vivo (d)[a]	0.90 ± 0.10 (R/100)	1.93		KREBS and JONES (1972)
	6.00	In vitro	0.94 ± 0.05	2.2 ± 0.5		TESTA et al. (1973)
	0.5×10^{-3}	In vivo (d)[a]	0.92 ± 0.04	0.8 ± 0.1		TESTA et al. (1973)
	1.39 (R/100)	In vitro	1.00 (R/100)	~ 1.6		GIDALI et al. (1974)
	2.74	In vivo (d)[a]	0.80	1.0		FU et al. (1975)
	0.36	In vivo (d)[a]	1.13	1.0		FU et al. (1975)
		In vitro	1.22	1.06		BOERSMA (1983)
	0.9	In vivo (d)[a]	1.01	1.17		BOERSMA (1983)
	5.20	In vitro	1.00 (from 0 to 2 Gy)	1 up to 10		HENDRY (1979)
		In vivo (d)[a]	down to 0.66 (for doses > 2 Gy)			
x-rays						
250 kV	1.05 (R/100)	In vivo (r)[b]	0.72 ± 0.03 (R/100)	2.4		PURO and CLARK (1972)
280 kV	0.50	In vitro	0.87	~ 2.3		SCHNEIDER and WHITMORE (1963)
300 kV	1.50	In vitro	0.671 ± 0.073	2.24 ± 1.23		HENDRY (1972)
^{137}Cs γ	6.00	In vitro	0.925 ± 0.069	1.90 ± 0.83	0.73	HENDRY (1972)
300 kV	0.60, 1.50	In vivo (d)[a]	0.722 ± 0.017	2.47 ± 0.28		BROERSE et al. (1971)
^{137}Cs, ^{60}Co γ	0.09, 0.52 6.00	In vivo (d)[a]	0.907 ± 0.024	2.47 ± 0.28	0.80 ± 0.02	BROERSE et al. (1971)
Electrons						
15 MeV	240	In vivo (d)[a]				
		6 weeks	0.939 ± 0.046	2.47 ± 0.64		PROUKAKIS and LINDOP (1967)
		30 weeks	1.262 ± 0.060	1.42 ± 0.33		PROUKAKIS et al. (1969)
		100 weeks	1.187 ± 0.036	0.92 ± 0.11		PROUKAKIS et al. (1969)

[a] Irradiation of the cells in the donor (d).
[b] Irradiation of the cells in the recipient (r), i.e., after transplantation.

The survival curve parameters D_0 and n are useful for comparative purposes. However, as mentioned before, there are several observations indicating that the femoral CFU-S survival data after in vivo and in vitro irradiation may be represented best by a curve with an initial slope for doses in the range from 0 to 2 Gy and showing a tendency toward increased sensitivity at high doses.

Such a curve fitted by HENDRY (1979) to his own data is represented by the parameters $_1D_0 = 1$ Gy for the initial slope, and a D_0 of 0.66 Gy for the terminal slope. The application of the α, β model of cell inactivation resulted in $\alpha = 0.9$ Gy^{-1} and $\beta = 0.04$ Gy^{-2} (HENDRY 1985a). As pointed out, (a) this value of β is similar to that for clonogens of other tissues, and (b) both values are compatible with the increasing split-dose effect on CFU-S with

increasing dose (HENDRY 1979) and with the clear dose-rate effect obtained at higher doses using the LD$_{50/30}$ as a criterion (see Sect. 4.9.2.1). The initial slope of the femoral CFU-S survival curve with $_1D_0 = 1$ Gy, or $\alpha = 1$ Gy^{-1}, is extremely steep when compared with clonogenic cells of other tissues such as jejunal mucosa ($_1D_0 = 2.8$ Gy), gastric mucosa ($_1D_0 = 5.5$ Gy), or spermatogonia ($_1D_0 = 4.9$ Gy) (HENDRY 1985a).

4.6.1.2 Proliferative State and Cell Cycle

Various experimental approaches have been used to study to what extent the radiation response of murine bone marrow CFU-S varies with the cell cycle phase and whether the radiation response of the whole population is influenced by its proliferative state. The results are not uniform, probably due to the fact that some of the methods applied may have had an impact on the assay itself.

The results reported by Boggs and Boggs (1973) suggest that in a CFU-S population under steady state conditions the S-phase cells are less "sensitive" than the cells in the other phases of their cycle. On the other hand, Gerber and Maes (1981) could detect no differences in the radiation response between a CFU-S population in total and cell suspensions from which the S-phase cells had been eliminated before irradiation. Significant fluctuations in the radiation response were reported for CFU-S in the early phase of stimulated proliferation, probably due to partial synchronization (McCulloch and Till 1964; Chaffey and Hellman 1971). For rapidly (asynchronously) proliferating CFU-S an increase in D_0 was observed (compared with steady state CFU-S) by a factor of 1.1 for x-rays (in vivo and in vitro), associated with decreases in the extrapolation numbers from $n = 2.5$ to $n = 1.34$ (Hendry 1972).

It has been stated by Thames and Hendry (1987) that generally the radiosensitivity of cells from renewal systems such as the bone marrow, hair follicles, and intestinal mucosa does not depend markedly on the proliferative state (resting or growing) of the cells at the time of irradiation.

4.6.1.3 Potentially Lethal Damage Repair

While clonogenic cells from several tissues (e.g., of the rat) show a considerable capacity for potentially lethal damage repair (PLDR) in transplantation assays when the assay is delayed for several hours ("in situ" repair according to Gould and Clifton 1979; review by Hendry 1985a; Thames and Hendry 1987), murine CFU-S behave differently. CFU-S survival decreases further when the bone marrow transplantation is performed later than 2 h after doses above 1 Gy (Thomas and Gould 1982), and the survival curves obtained for CFU-S transplanted 16 or 24 h after the exposure are nearly exponential (Thames and Hendry 1987). This decrease in survival has been explained by PLDR inhibition caused by postirradiation in situ holding (Thomas and Gould 1982). Other possible explanations for the observed reduction in CFU-S are induced differentiation and/or a normal differentiation rate

during a period of mitotic delay (for review see Hendry 1985a; Thames and Hendry 1987).

4.6.1.4 Effects of Dose Rate

In the last two decades several studies have been performed in which the effects of different dose rates in the range 0.01–2 Gy/min (i.e., the range of clinical interest) have been evaluated. Based on compilations such as that in Table 4.4, it has generally been concluded that there is little dependence of CFU-S survival on dose rate (Hendry and Lord 1983; Steel and Horwich 1988). Glasgow et al. (1983), referring to data collected from ten different studies, came to a similar conclusion for femoral marrow CFU-S irradiated in situ at dose rates in the range 0.05–1 Gy/min, with doses less than 5 Gy. However, as was pointed out by these authors, there is a clear dose-rate effect in the study by Puro and Clark (1972), which showed a progressive increase in D_0 (associated with a decrease in n) with decreasing dose rates. Since this study was the only one in which the CFU-S were irradiated in the recipient mice and not in the donors, the different techniques obviously have a significant influence on the results. For further details see Glasgow et al. (1983).

Puro and Clark (1972) were able to establish similar dose-rate effects for the endogenous CFU-S in the exposure range from 450 to 850 R, i.e., for large doses. On the other hand, at exposures below 200 R the survival levels remained the same and there was no demonstrable exposure-rate effect.

4.6.2 Progenitor Cells

The radiation response characteristics of the different types of progenitor cell have been studied quite intensively in the mouse and in man, and to a lesser extent in the dog. For previous reviews see Hendry and Lord (1983) and Fliedner and Nothdurft (1986).

In most cases the irradiations were performed in vitro and the cells were cultured thereafter in semisolid medium. It has to be stressed that survival and the proliferation of these clonogens in vitro is essentially dependent on the presence of specific growth factors (see Sect. 4.3.1.2). The proliferative capacity of irradiated cells seems to be particularly dependent on the concentration of

Table 4.4. Radiation dose-rate effect on the survival of normal murine bone marrow CFU-S

Radiation source	Irradiation		Parameter		Remarks	Reference
	Dose rate (Gy/min)	Exposure of cells	D_0 (Gy)	n		
γ-rays [137]Cs	6.00	d[a]	0.857 ± 0.045	3.12 ± 0.73	No effect of dose rate	BROERSE et al. (1971)
γ-rays [60]Co	0.52	d	0.982 ± 0.094	1.74 ± 0.60		BROERSE et al. (1971)
γ-rays [60]Co	0.096	d	0.968 ± 0.063	1.81 ± 0.48		BROERSE et al. (1971)
γ-rays [60]Co	0.292 (R/100)	d[a]	0.901 (R/100)	1.93	No differences in	KREBS and JONES (1972)
γ-rays [60]Co	0.032 (R/100)	d	0.929 (R/100)	1.83	survival parameters	KREBS and JONES (1972)
x-rays 250 kV	1.05 (R/100)	r[c]	0.72 ± 0.03 (R/100)	2.4	"Higher exposure	PURO and CLARK (1972)
x-rays 250 kV	0.116 (R/100)	r	0.79 ± 0.04 (R/100)	1.8	rates were clearly	PURO and CLARK (1972)
x-rays 250 kV	0.054 (R/100)	r	0.85 ± 0.11 (R/100)	1.7	more efficient . . . for	PURO and CLARK (1972)
x-rays 250 kV	0.029 (R/100)	r	0.99 ± 0.05 (R/100)	1.7	dosages above 200 R"	PURO and CLARK (1972)
γ-rays [137]Cs	2.74	d[a]	0.80	1	Little change in D_0;	FU et al. (1975)
γ-rays [137]Cs	0.36	d	1.13	1	puzzling results	FU et al. (1975)
γ-rays [137]Cs	0.045	d	0.87	1		FU et al. (1975)
γ-rays [137]Cs	0.0092	d	0.76/0.95	1/∼ 0.15		FU et al. (1975)
γ-rays [137]Cs	0.0054	d				
γ-rays [60]Co	0.45	d[a]	1.163 ± 0.069	1.17 ± 0.29		BELLETTI et al. (1979)
γ-rays [60]Co	0.101	d	1.165 ± 0.147	1.20 ± 0.47		BELLETTI et al. (1979)
γ-rays [60]Co	0.050	d	1.097 ± 0.091	1.17 ± 0.31	No differences	BELLETTI et al. (1979)
γ-rays [60]Co	0.0165	d	1.241 ± 0.128	0.72 ± 0.22	between	BELLETTI et al. (1979)
γ-rays [60]Co	0.0083	d	1.330 ± 0.210	0.52 ± 0.21	D_0 values	BELLETTI et al. (1979)
γ-rays [60]Co	1.03	d[b]	0.617 ± 0.034	0.65 ± 0.15	No differences	GLASGOW et al. (1983)
γ-rays [60]Co	0.45	d[b]	0.649 ± 0.018	0.87 ± 0.08	between	GLASGOW et al. (1983)
γ-rays [137]Cs	0.08	d	0.690 ± 0.020	0.72 ± 0.08	the parameters	GLASGOW et al. (1983)
x-rays 250 kV	0.80	d[a]	0.80	1	Little effect of dose	TARBELL et al. (1987)
x-rays 250 kV	0.05	d	0.85	2	rate	TARBELL et al. (1987)

[a] Cells irradiated in the donor < 2–3 h before transplantation.
[b] Cells irradiated in the donor 24 h before transplantation.
[c] Cells irradiated in the recipient 2–3 h after transplantation.

the stimulators in the cultures (BROXMEYER et al. 1976; SUGAVARA et al. 1980). Usually an undefined cocktail of growth factors obtained as conditioned medium from cell cultures or as "conditioned" serum from pretreated animals has been added to the cultures as a source of colony-stimulating activity (CSA). As a consequence, due to the heterogeneity of these stimulators on the one hand and the heterogeneity of the various progenitor cell populations on the other hand (see Sect. 4.3.1.2), the cell populations assayed by different authors (under otherwise comparable conditions) may not have been identical, which would explain the large differences observed in the dose–response curves reported for the same species. Some of the progenitor cells can also be assayed "in vivo" as diffusion chamber implants. (For

more detailed consideration of the biological relevance of the different assays, see the review by HENDRY 1985a.) Most of the survival curves obtained for unselected progenitor cell populations are nearly exponential but this does not exclude the possibility that some subpopulations may have survival curves with a shoulder (ELKIND 1988).

4.6.2.1 Progenitor Cells in the Mouse

Most survival curves obtained for different types of progenitor cell from unfractionated bone marrow under the influence of the crude stimulators from natural sources (Table 4.5) are exponential or nearly exponential.

Table 4.5. Survival characteristics of hemopoietic progenitor cells in murine bone marrow after irradiation with acute doses

Cell type	Radiation source	Irradiation		Parameter		Reference
		Dose rate (Gy/min)	Exposure of cells	D_0 (Gy)	n	
Mix-CFC	x-rays 200 kV	0.60	In vivo[b]	1.44 ± 0.30	1.03	Imai and Nakao (1987)
BFU-E	γ-rays ^{137}Cs	1.15	In vitro	0.73 ± 0.12	1.6	Wagemaker et al. (1979)
	x-rays 200 kV	0.60	In vivo[b]	0.69 ± 0.90	0.85	Imai and Nakao (1987)
CFU-E	—	—	In vitro	Steady state: 0.70	Slightly > 1	Monette et al. (1978)
	—	—	In vitro	Regenerating: 1.15	?	Monette et al. (1978)
	γ-rays ^{137}Cs	1.12	In vivo[c]	0.66	~ 1.3	Nakeff et al. (1979)
	x-rays 200 kV	0.60	In vivo[b]	0.53 ± 0.03	0.76	Imai and Nakao (1987)
Meg-CFC	γ-rays ^{137}Cs	1.12	In vivo[c]	1.28	1.0	Nakeff et al. (1979)
GM-CFC$_{DC}$[a]	γ-rays ^{60}Co	—	DC in mice	1.39 ± 0.05	1.02 ± 0.04	Gordon (1975)
GM-CFC	x-rays 235 kV	1.10	In vivo[d]	0.85	1.3	Robinson et al. (1967)
	γ-rays ^{137}Cs	1.16	In vitro	1.60	1.0	Senn and McCulloch (1970)
	γ-rays ^{137}Cs	6.00	In vitro	1.60 ± 0.15	1.0 ± 0.2	Testa et al. (1973)
	γ-rays ^{60}Co	—	In vivo[e]	1.37 ± 0.03	1.18 ± 0.54	Gordon (1975)
	γ-rays ^{60}Co	1.5 (R/100)	In vitro	1.90 (R/100)	$0.94 - 0.89$	Wu et al. (1978)
	γ-rays ^{60}Co		In vivo	1.74–2.37 (R/100)	$0.92 - 0.59$	Wu et al. (1978)
	γ-rays ^{137}Cs	1.12	In vivo[c]	1.28	1.0	Nakeff et al. (1979)
	γ-rays ^{60}Co	1.50	In vivo	0.74	4	Peacock et al. (1986)
	γ-rays ^{60}Co	0.03	In vivo	~ 1.25	~ 1	Peacock et al. (1986)
	γ-rays ^{137}Cs	0.005	In vivo	~ 1.6	~ 1	Peacock et al. (1986)
	x-rays 200 kV	0.60	In vivo[b]	1.57 ± 0.11	1.09	Imai and Nakao (1987)

[a] GM-CFC assessed in diffusion chambers.
[b] Cells harvested within 2 h after TBI.
[c] Cells harvested and cultured 24 h after irradiation.
[d] Cells harvested and cultured 48 h after irradiation.
[e] Cells harvested and cultured 3–4 h after irradiation.

1. GM-CFC (assessed in total) are less sensitive (D_0 values of 1.28–1.90 Gy) than the BFU-E and CFU-E and perhaps the Meg-CFC, for which no data exist after in vitro irradiation.
2. A dose-rate effect was reported for GM-CFC (in contrast to CFU-S!) under conditions of in vivo irradiation (Peacock et al. 1986). However, in these studies irradiation of the donor-mice at a dose rate of 1.5 Gy/min resulted in a survival curve with one of the steepest slopes ($D_0 = 0.74$ Gy) reported, but with a relatively high value of $n = 4$.
3. Mix-CFC, which are considered to be heterogeneous multipotential progenitor cells with subpopulations closely related to GM-CFC or Meg-CFC (Imai and Nakao 1987), show survival characteristics similar to GM-CFC.

Recently Baird et al. (1988) reported that for in vitro irradiated bone marrow cells cultured in the presence of different purified growth factors a variety of survival curves were obtained, their shapes depending on the factor or the combination of different factors applied (see Table 4.6). However, only when the irradiated cells were grown under the influence of IL-3 was the extrapolation number clearly >1. The authors concluded that the progenitor cells become increasingly more radiosensitive as they progress along the hierarchy.

4.6.2.2 Progenitor Cells in the Dog

In this species radiation survival data are limited to the granulocyte/macrophage and the erythroid lineage (Table 4.7). They allow the following conclusions:

1. Most of the experimental data reported can be fitted by a simple exponential function, i.e., n ~0.8–1.1.

Table 4.6. Survival characteristics of different subpopulations of progenitor cells in the GM lineage(s) (data from BAIRD et al. 1988)

Cell type	Radiation source	Irradiation		Growth factor	Parameter	
		Dose rate (Gy/min)	Exposure of cells		D_0 (Gy)	n
Bone marrow	γ-rays ^{137}Cs		In vitro	G-CSF	0.4	1
				M-CSF	1.0	1
				GM-CSF	1.3	1
				IL-3	1.2	1.9
				IL-1 + IL-3	1.2	1
				IL-1 + M-CSF	1.2	1
				IL-1 + IL-3 + M-CSF	Biphasic[a]	

[a] D_0 value of 1.7 Gy for the resistant population (60%).

Table 4.7. Survival characteristics of hemopoietic progenitor cells in canine bone marrow after irradiation with acute doses

Cell type	Radiation source	Irradiation		Parameter		Reference
		Dose rate (Gy/min)	Exposure of cells	D_0 (Gy)	n	
BFU-E	x-rays 250 kV	1.70	In vitro	0.26 ± 0.09		SCHWARTZ et al. (1986)
	x-rays 280 kV	0.72	In vitro	0.15 ± 0.02	1.05 ± 0.28	KREJA et al. (1989)
CFU-E	x-rays 250 kV	1.70	In vitro	0.61 ± 0.05		SCHWARTZ et al. (1986)
GM-CFC	γ-rays ^{60}Co	0.024 (R/100)	In vivo[a]	~ 0.70 (R/100)	~ 0.8	WILSON et al. (1978)
	γ-rays ^{60}Co		In vitro	0.59 − 0.67 (R/100)	1.09 − 0.98	WU et al. (1978)
	γ-rays ^{60}Co	0.05 (R/100)	In vitro	0.35 (R/100)	~ 1.3	KOLB et al. (1981)
	γ-rays ^{60}Co	0.25 (R/100)	In vitro	0.68 ± 0.03 (R/100)	1.1 ± 0.1	SEED et al. (1982)
	x-rays 250 kV	0.56	In vitro	0.61 ± 0.01 or 0.55 ± 0.02	1 / 1.2 ± 0.1	NOTHDURFT et al. (1983)

[a] Cells harvested and cultured 24 h after TBI.

2. BFU-E clearly are more radiosensitive than CFU-E and GM-CFC. However, there is an unexplained difference between the D_0 values for BFU-E by a factor of 1.7. Improvements in culture technique may well reduce the D_0 under certain circumstances (see review by HENDRY 1985a).

3. Except for one value the GM-CFC data show less variations in slope ($D_0 = 0.55$ Gy to approx. 0.7 Gy) than those reported for the mouse and the human. Under certain experimental conditions an increase in the extrapolation number has been found, associated with a decrease in D_0 (NOTHDURFT et al. 1983).

4. The effect of 1 Gy given in vitro does not depend on the exposure rate in the range 0.005–0.55 Gy/min (KOLB et al. 1981).

5. When compared with the human and the mouse the progenitor cells of the dog clearly are the most radiosensitive except, perhaps, for the CFU-E.

4.6.2.3 Progenitor Cells in Man

No data are available for CFU-E and Meg-CFC.

From the data presented in Table 4.8 the following features can be deduced for unfractionated progenitor cell populations:

1. The survival curves obtained in the dose range 3–10 Gy, i.e., comprising 1.5–3 logs of cell inactivation, are exponential in most cases, i.e., $n = 0.9–1.1$.

2. The D_0 values for GM-CFC show considerable variations, from 0.83 to 1.60 Gy, and extrapolation numbers range from 3.5 to 0.75. There is a tendency for the lower D_0 values to be associated with higher n values. Whether the low D_0

values reported in some of the studies are due to the fact that the cells were irradiated after plating, i.e., preincubation in the agar environment at 37°C for several hours (Bromer et al. 1982; Kimler at al. 1984, 1985), is an open question. The CSA in the cultures has a definite influence on GM-CFC survival in cultures of unfractionated bone marrow cells (Broxmeyer et al. 1976; Sugavara et al. 1980). In the experiments by Broxmeyer et al. the survival curve obtained after elimination of the S-phase cells by pretreatment with hydroxyurea showed an unchanged $D_0 = 1.65$ Gy but a significant shoulder ($n = 1.5$) when compared with the exponential curve for the total population. Biphasic (exponential) curves (Bøyum et al. 1978; Kimler et al. 1984, 1985) and, to an even greater extent, heterogeneous survival data mostly fitted by simple exponential curves (Fitzgerald et al. 1986) indicate that subpopulations with different radiosensitivities are assessed by the assay in question. The few data available for GM-CFC after in vivo irradiation (Bromer et al. 1982) are in accordance with the in vitro data but do not allow deductions about the dose–response relationship.

For GM-CFC irradiated in the steady state in vitro there seems to be little dependence of survival on dose rate between 0.05 and 2 Gy/min (Fitzgerald et al. 1986).

3. The pluripotent progenitor cell population GEMM-CFC seems to be the most radiosensitive among the different progenitor cells (Neumann et al. 1981). However, more data are needed before definite conclusions can be drawn.
4. GM-CFC$_{DC}$, considered representative of a relatively immature population of the compartment, seem to be comparable in sensitivity to GEMM-CFC. Again, for further proof more data are needed from studies using separated GM-CFC subpopulations in combination with specific growth conditions.
5. BFU-E obviously are not much different from GM-CFC with respect to their radiation response characteristics.
6. Human BFU-E are obviously slightly more resistant than murine BFU-E, whereas GM-CFC and GEMM-CFC are somewhat more sensitive than their murine equivalents.

4.7 Progenitor Cells of the Stroma

Survival data are available for CFU-F from the bone marrow of the mouse, the dog, and the human, obtained after in vitro or in vivo irradiation using γ-rays or x-rays (Table 4.9). Most of the in vitro irradiations were performed on bone marrow cell suspensions before plating, at temperatures of + 4°C or in the range of 20°C. In cases where CFU-F survival was assessed after total body irradiation, collection of the bone marrow took place either 1–2 h (Werts et al. 1980; Imai and Nakao 1987) or 24 h (Wilson et al. 1978) after the exposure. Culture methods and the criteria for defining clonogenicity, i.e., survival, were rather different. Keeping these variables in mind, variations in the survival curve parameters reported are to be expected. However, it can be seen from the data in Table 4.9 that for CFU-F, in contrast to (unseparated) hemopoietic progenitor cells, there is a tendency for n to exceed 1, independent of the species. Consequently, in some cases a shoulder can be observed with values of $D_q \sim$ 0.8–1 Gy, indicating the capacity of sublethal damage accumulation or PLDR. There is also a dose-rate effect for human bone marrow CFU-F (Fitzgerald et al. 1986). Perhaps there may be more capacity for repair to CFU-F in situ than the different assays allow to appear. (For more details about the biological relevance of the different clonogenic assays, see Hendry 1985a.) Based on the data available it may be concluded that x-rays and γ-rays have similar efficiency.

The D_0 values obtained for murine CFU-F mostly are in the range 2.1–2.6 Gy. However, rather different survival curves were obtained depending on whether fresh culture medium ($D_0 = 1.6$ Gy, $n = 2.7$) or medium stored for 15 days ($D_0 = 3.9$ Gy, $n = 1.2$) was used, suggesting selection of a radioresistant subpopulation in the latter case (Xu et al. 1983, see Table 4.9). The CFU-F in the dog seem to be more resistant ($D_0 > 2.4$ Gy) than those in the mouse. However, the high D_0 values reported by Klein et al. (1984, 1985) in part may be due to the fact that small clusters were included in the colony counts, and that a simple exponential function was fitted to the inhomogeneous sets of data (see Greenberg et al. 1984).

CFU-F from human bone marrow obviously are more radiosensitive ($D_0 \sim$1–2.68 Gy at dose rates >0.05 Gy/min) than CFU-F from murine or

Table 4.8. Survival characteristics of hemopoietic progenitor cells in human bone marrow after irradiation with acute doses

Cell type	Radiation source	Irradiation		Parameter		Reference
		Dose rate (Gy/min)	Exposure of cells	D_0 (Gy)	n	
GEMM-CFC	γ-rays ^{60}Co	–	In vitro	0.91 ± 0.07	~1	NEUMANN et al. (1981)
BFU-E	γ-rays ^{137}Cs	1.16	In vitro	1.13 ± 0.08	1.5 ± 0.15	TEPPERMAN et al. (1974)
	x-rays 280 kV	0.62	In vitro	1.27 ± 0.11	1	GRILLI et al. (1982)
GM-CFC$_{DC}$[a]	γ-rays ^{60}Co	–	DC in mice	0.852 ± 0.45	0.96 ± 0.10	GORDON (1975)
GM-CFC	γ-rays ^{137}Cs	1.16	In vitro	1.37	~1	SENN and McCULLOCH (1970)
	x-rays 240 kV	0.48 (R/100)	In vitro	1.27 (R/100)	1.1	RICKARD et al. (1974)
	γ-rays ^{137}Cs	1.12	In vitro	1.60 ($\rightarrow$0.40)	1.0	BROXMEYER et al. (1976)
	x-rays 250 kV	0.25	In vitro	~1.17 ($\pm$0.05)	~1	BØYUM et al. (1978)
	–	–	In vitro	0.83 ± 0.11[b]	3.5 ± 0.7	ZWAAN et al. (1980)
	–	–	In vitro	1.91 ± 0.29[c]	1.5 ± 0.01	ZWAAN et al. (1980)
	γ-rays ^{60}Co	–	In vitro	1.14 ± 0.08	–	NEUMANN et al. (1981)
	x-rays 6 MV	2.00	In vitro	0.84	1.18	BROMER et al. (1982)
	same?		In vivo	~0.84?	~1.18?	BROMER et al. (1982)
	x-rays 280 kV	0.62	In vitro	1.36 ± 0.09	1	GRILLI et al. (1982)
	x-rays 6 MV	2.00	In vitro	0.86	1.2	KINSELLA et al. (1984)
	γ-rays ^{60}Co	0.72 or 3.0	In vitro	0.88 to 0.79	0.82 to 1	KIMLER et al. (1984)
	x-rays 6 MV	0.72 or 3.0	In vitro	0.85 to 0.75	0.75 to 1	KIMLER et al. (1985)
	γ-rays ^{137}Cs	1.00	In vitro	1.15	1.0	LAVER et al. (1986)
	x-rays 250 kV	2.0	In vitro	1.02 ± 0.05[d]	1.59 ± 0.21	FITZGERALD et al. (1986)
	x-rays 250 kV	0.05	In vitro	1.07 ± 0.03[d]	1.50 ± 0.04	FITZGERALD et al. (1986)
	x-rays 250 kV	2.0	In vitro	1.13 ± 0.03[e]	1.43 ± 0.03	FITZGERALD et al. (1986)
	x-rays 250 kV	0.05	In vitro	1.16 ± 0.04[e]	1.34 ± 0.05	FITZGERALD et al. (1986)

[a] GM-CFC assessed in diffusion chambers.
[b] Colonies.
[c] Clusters (aggregates with <20 cells).
[d] colonies counted at day 7, i.e., GM-CFC-day 7.
[e] colonies counted at day 14, i.e., GM-CFC-day 14.

Table 4.9. Survival characteristics of CFU-F from the bone marrow of the human, the dog, and the mouse

Species	Radiation source	Irradiation		Remarks	Parameter		Reference
		Dose rate (Gy/min)	Exposure of cells		D_0 (Gy)	n	
Mouse	γ-rays ^{60}Co	0.3 (R/100)	In vitro		2.16 ± 0.36 (R/100)	1.13	FRIEDENSTEIN et al. (1976)
	x-rays 250 kV	0.80	In vitro		2.30	1.20	WERTS et al. (1980)
	x-rays 250 kV	0.80	In vivo		2.15	1.60	WERTS et al. (1980)
	x-rays 300 kV	1.54	In vitro	Fresh medium	1.6 ± 0.1	2.7 ± 0.2	XU et al. (1983)
	x-rays 300 kV	1.54	In vitro	Stored medium	3.9 ± 0.8	1.2 ± 0.4	XU et al. (1983)
	x-rays 200 kV	0.60	In vivo[a]		2.57 ± 0.62	1.06	IMAI and NAKAO (1987)
Dog	γ-rays ^{60}Co	0.024 (R/100)	In vivo[b]		~4? (R/100)		WILSON et al. (1978)
	x-rays	1.8	In vitro		4.24 ± 0.30[c]	1	KLEIN et al. (1984)
	x-rays	1.8	In vitro		3 to 5.5 (6.7)	1	KLEIN et al. (1985)
	x-rays 280 kV	0.72	In vitro	Iliac crest	2.41 ± 0.38	1.38 ± 0.62	KREJA et al. (1989)
	x-rays 280 kV	0.72	In vitro	Humerus	2.61 ± 0.40	1.04 ± 0.42	KREJA et al. (1989)
Human	γ-rays ^{137}Cs	1.00	In vitro	Iliac crest	1.30	1.3	LAVER et al. (1986)
	γ-rays ^{137}Cs	1.00	In vitro	Iliac crest, passaged	1.10	1.4	LAVER et al. (1986)
	x-rays 250 kV	2.00	In vitro		0.99	1.03	FITZGERALD et al. (1986)
	x-rays 250 kV	0.05	In vitro		1.45	2.00	FITZGERALD et al. (1986)
	–	–	In vitro	Normal persons	2.68[c]	~0.98	GREENBERG et al. (1984)
	–	–	In vitro	Patients with ANLL	4.61[c]	~1.06	GREENBERG et al. (1984)

[a] Cells harvested and cultured within 1–2 h after TBI.
[b] Cells harvested and cultured 24 h after TBI.
[c] Counting of aggregates consisting of ≥5 cells after 4–14 days.

canine bone marrow; on the other hand their D_0 is rather similar to the values reported for CFU-F from human skin and lung (see review by Hendry and Lord 1983).

The D_0 value of 2.68 Gy as reported by Greenberg et al. (1984) for CFU-F from normal human bone marrow appears unusually high. However, their survival data indicate considerable heterogeneity in radiation response, probably because the colony counts included small clusters. Consequently, a shoulder curve could be fitted to the data in the dose range up to 7 Gy as well, resulting in a D_0 of about 2 Gy, and an n of 1.5. It is interesting to note that CFU-F obtained from the bone marrow of patients with acute nonlymphocytic leukemia (ANLL) were found to be significantly more radioresistant, i.e., $D_0 = 4.61$ Gy.

4.8 General Aspects of Bone Marrow Radiation Pathophysiology

Understanding of the acute response of the bone marrow organ to irradiations under different conditions of exposure and the development of subacute and possible late effects has to be based on:

- The cytokinetics of hemopoiesis on the one hand and the stroma on the other, and the essential differences between them
- The intrinsic "radiosensitivity" of the cellular components with respect to their specific functions
- The actual anatomical distribution of the active marrow
- The functional status of the exposed marrow sites at the time of irradiation
- Possible influences of accessory cell systems and organs or tissues involved in the control of blood cell production

It is well documented that the kinetics of a tissue are an essential determinant of its response to irradiation (Patt and Quastler 1963; Bond et al. 1965; Rubin and Casarett 1968; Michalowski 1981; Wheldon et al. 1982; Michalowski et al. 1984; Rubin 1984).

4.8.1 Hemopoiesis

Radiation leads to mitotic delay and a loss of the reproductive capacity at all levels in the hierarchy of proliferating cells, including the stem cell compartment, in which the proliferation rate is rather low under normal circumstances. Acute radiation doses of 0.5 Gy and less have been shown to cause injury to the hemopoietic tissue in a given bone marrow site (Unscear 1982; review by Fliedner and Nothdurft 1986). On the other hand, the mature end cells of the various lineages are quite resistant to radiation, maintaining their cytological integrity and specific functional properties, as shown in the case of neutrophilic granulocytes, erythrocytes, and platelets after irradiation with single doses of 50 Gy (Holley et al. 1974; Button et al. 1981). For monocytes, survival in vitro and the rate of microbial (*Listeria monocytogenes*) killing were somewhat decreased after radiation doses of 25 or 50 Gy, whereas certain enzymatic activities remained unchanged (Buescher and Gallin 1984). On the other hand, Kwan and Norman (1978) found a significant decrease in survival of human blood monocytes after irradiation in vitro even at doses down to 0.5 Gy.

The kinetic pattern of the postirradiation events in the hemopoietic tissue leading to changes in the blood cell concentration of the different lineages in the mammalian organism in general and the human in particular has been described and analyzed in detail in a number of articles and monographs (Patt and Quastler 1963; Bond et al. 1965; Langham 1967; Fliedner 1969; Wald 1971; Cronkite and Fliedner 1972; Prasad 1974; Fliedner and Nothdurft 1986; Fliedner et al. 1988).

The time-related pattern of development of injury in the form of clinically critical blood cell concentrations depends on the time required by the cells of the different lineages for their transit through the compartments of the proliferating and the nondividing maturing cells in the bone marrow and the life span of the mature functional elements in the peripheral blood or solid tissues. Due to the short life span of the neutrophilic granulocytes [half-disappearance time 7 h or approximately 17 h, depending on the method applied (Steinbach et al. 1979)] and of the platelets (about 9.5 days), granulocytopenia and thrombocytopenia will occur within some 5–8 days to about 3–4 weeks, depending on the degree of damage to the proliferating compartments and the stem cell population (for references see preceding paragraph), characterizing the bone marrow as an early-responding organ.

Besides the cellular kinetics as a determinant of the radiation response of the hemopoietic tissue, its pathophysiology has to be considered, with reference to its anatomical structure and distribution. Each site of the hemopoietic tissue can primarily be understood as a partially autonomous subunit of the whole organ in which proliferation and differentiation are controlled by short-range regulatory mechanisms (PHARR and OGAWA 1985; LORD 1986; LORD and TESTA 1988). But in addition, all parts of the hemopoietic tissue are interconnected with each other via the bloodstream, which serves as a vehicle for humoral regulators with long-range action such as erythropoietin (CRONKITE 1985) and other growth factors and for the traffic of progenitor cells and stem cells (see review by NOTHDURFT and FLIEDNER 1979) and different types of accessory cell (TOROK-STORB 1988). Consequently, due to the persistent interchange of signals and the cellular traffic between all the bone marrow sites, the hemopoietic tissue in the whole skeleton is able to respond as a single entity to any damage, whether local or involving the whole body.

Due to its kinetic organization and the cytoarchitecture of the bone marrow organ, the hemopoietic tissue is able to respond to enhanced demand in several ways:

- By enhanced proliferation of stem cells and progenitor cells due to recruitment of quiescent cells and/or shortening of the cell cycle of slowly proliferating cells (see reviews by POTTEN 1986; LORD 1986; METCALF 1986a)
- By completing more divisions in certain compartments than under normal conditions (see reviews by HENDRY and LORD 1983; CRONKITE 1985, 1988)
- By compensatory hyperplasia, i.e., by increasing the hemopoietic cell number per unit volume at the expense of the lipid content of fat cells within those sites normally containing active marrow (ICRP No. 23, 1974; WINTROBE 1974; FORDHAM and ALI 1981; see review by TAVASSOLI 1984)
- By extension of active marrow into the marrow space of the long bones at the expense of inactive fatty marrow (VAN DYKE and ANGER 1965; WINTROBE 1974; FORDHAM and ALI 1981;

see review by TAVASSOLI 1984)
- By the development of extramedullary hemopoiesis, particularly in the spleen but also in the liver and lymph nodes, which under certain extreme conditions may supplement bone marrow hemopoiesis (ICRP No. 23, 1974; VAN DYKE and ANGER 1965; WINTROBE 1974)

However, whatever the mechanism might be, the hemopoietic response is dependent on the functional status of the stroma and the accessory cell systems and the organs involved in the regulatory processes.

In this context a question of major importance is the identity of the target cell for bone marrow failure and the cell(s) from which the repopulation of the radiation-damaged bone marrow will originate.

4.8.1.1 The Target Cell Problem

In the murine system, the CFU-S assessed by colony counting between day 7 and day 10 has long been considered to represent the target cell for radiation toxicity. Indeed, there are several correlations between CFU-S and lethality (determined as the $LD_{50/30}$) for various conditions of exposure to total body irradiation, e.g., with respect to split-dose effects of low LET radiation (as will be shown in Sect. 4.9.3) and RBE of neutrons of different mean energies (see reviews by NOTHDURFT 1985; FLIEDNER and NOTHDURFT 1986). More recently, THAMES and HENDRY (1987) came to the conclusion that "the simplest and most useful interpretation is that haematopoietic stem cells (i.e. CFU-S [the author]) or another closely related cell population with very similar radiosensitivity, form the true target cell population for the bone marrow syndrome in the mouse." However, the GM-CFC is likely to play an important role in animal survival, too, though it is the stem cells that are the target cells for long-term recovery.

On the other hand, several other observations suggest that at least part of the CFU-S population is not identical with cells exhibiting marrow-repopulating capability or life-rescuing ability (BRADLEY et al. 1985; PLOEMACHER and BRONS 1988a,b). Furthermore, the 30–day survival of lethally irradiated mice is not related to the cellular repopulation of the bone marrow by injected bone marrow cells, supporting the importance of the spleen for survival in rodents

(Ploemacher and Brons 1988a,b; see also Noth-durft 1985). These facts may explain some of the discrepancies between murine lethality and the D_0 value of bone marrow CFU-S or endogenous colonies in the bone marrow as observed in the analyses by Thames and Hendry (1987).

Besides CFU-S or related cells that are mobile, certain other cells have been discussed as potential stem cells. Mesenchymal cells residing in the Haversian system in the bone cortex have been suggested as primordial cells from which local regeneration of the bone marrow may originate in the case of complete CFU-S depletion (Maloney and Patt 1969; Rubin and Scarantino 1978). Such cells are supposed also to reside in the bone cortex of man and possibly to initiate extension of the bone marrow into the long bones by their ingrowth into protected bone cavities and perhaps into irradiated sites also (Rubin 1984). However, with respect to the location there is no need to postulate a special mesenchymal colony-forming cell (CFUm) since CFU-S also can be found in the endosteal region and perhaps associated with the Haversian spaces in the bone (see reviews by Patt and Maloney 1975; Schofield 1979).

On the other hand, there is no question that seeding of circulating stem cells can be involved in hemopoietic regeneration after partial body irradiation and even after total body irradiation, depending on the damage received by the various irradiated sites (see review by Nothdurft and Fliedner 1979; Fliedner and Nothdurft 1986).

4.8.2 Stroma and Accessory Cells

On the basis of the slow turnover of the different cell populations, the stroma is expected to show only moderate acute structural alterations due to mitotic cell death. In principle, as a type F organized tissue (Michalowski 1981) or conditional renewing tissue (according to Potten 1986), the stroma has to be considered as a late-responding tissue as far as the possible cellular depletion and associated functional defects are concerned. However, due to the complex cytoarchitecture of the marrow organ as a whole, any damage to the hemopoietic tissue will influence the stromal integrity, too.

With respect to the accessory cells, radiation quite well may cause some early functional damage in some of these cell populations at fairly small doses since some of them are rather radiosensitive,

e.g., certain T-cell subsets and B lymphocytes (Stewart et al. 1988) and progenitors of monocytes/macrophages (see Sect. 4.6.2). However, the consequences of these effects for hemopoietic function and regeneration are not well defined.

In the following the general aspects of the radiation pathophysiology of the stroma are considered. More details will be given in the separate sections dealing with the different radiation exposures.

Experimental studies in rodents have shown that after acute radiation doses in the range of several grays the stroma experiences considerable early damage, but also that it has a high capacity for reconstruction and reorganization.

In the bone marrow of mice which had received a radiation dose of 8.5 Gy the severe progressive hypoplasia within the first 3 days was found to be accompanied by alterations in the stroma, most evident as microvascular damage of different degrees depending on the bone marrow site (Lambertsen and Weiss 1983, 1984). Stromal regeneration progressed within 3–6 days after exposure. The transient occurrence of lipid-containing elements (reticular cells), besides others, seemed to be a stabilizing element in the phase of hypoplasia and regeneration. Based on studies of the acute ultrastructural alterations and the associated hemodynamic disturbances of the microcirculation in the bone marrow of the rat after irradiation with a dose of 8.25 Gy, Niu et al. (1988) classified the sinuses in the marrow as ultrasensitive when compared with other organs (lymphatics, spleen, intestinal wall, liver), this ultrasensitivity being due to certain structural characteristics. In rabbits local irradiation of the femoral bone marrow with a dose of 10 Gy first caused an increased blood flow from day 4 to day 21 after exposure, followed by a depression to day 120 at least (Maloney and Patt 1972).

Some studies on the kinetics of the long-lived elements in the stroma in the first weeks after irradiation revealed uniform results. In the bone marrow of rats and mice no increase could be observed in the proliferation rate of reticulum and endothelial cells in the first 2–3 weeks after doses in the range from 3 to 40 Gy (Caffrey et al. 1966; Haas et al. 1971; Tannock and Hayashi 1972).

On the other hand, moderate to high doses of radiation may cause both a long-lasting reduction in the number of clonogenic progenitors of the stroma, i.e. CFU-F, and late mitotically-connected cell loss among the different types of stromal elements, once they eventually go into division. However, at low dose rates and during fractionated irradiations with small doses per fraction the stromal elements exhibit more sparing than the hemopoietic elements (HENDRY 1985b; GALLINI et al. 1988).

4.9 Total Body Irradiation

4.9.1 Short Single Exposures

4.9.1.1 Lethality

Total body irradiation (TBI) results in systemic damage to the bone marrow organ. The disturbance of hemopoiesis determines the symptomatology of acute radiation sickness and its associated lethality following the lower doses that represent critical and possibly lethal exposures. For short exposures the dose range for the bone marrow syndrome is about 1–12 Gy for mammalian species in general (BOND 1969; BOND et al. 1965; MORRIS and JONES 1988). Radiation doses beyond this range will cause the gastrointestinal syndrome, which occurs earlier than the bone marrow syndrome. However, there is considerable overlap in the symptoms and mechanisms of death for both syndromes (BOND et al. 1965; AFRRI 1979; UN-

SCEAR 1982). For the human the threshold dose for the gastrointestinal syndrome is given as 5 Gy (RUBIN and CASARETT 1968).

The sequelae of damage to the hemopoietic tissue are granulocytopenia associated with susceptibility to infection, thrombocytopenia with susceptibility to diffuse hemorrhage, and possibly anemia due to suppression of erythrocyte production and/or hemorrhage (BOND et al. 1965; FLIEDNER 1969).

Species Differences in Radiation Tolerance

The hemopoietic tolerance of mammalian species shows considerable variation, as is reflected by their median lethal dose ($LD_{50/30}$) values, which range from approximately 1.6 Gy (cattle and sheep) to about 10 Gy and even higher (certain strains of mice) for short exposures to low LET radiation (see review by MORRIS and JONES 1988). Such differences become evident from the data of Table 4.10, representing some of the species most often used in experimental studies.

Generally, the $LD_{50/30}$ values are below 3.5 Gy for large species and above 5.4 Gy for smaller ones (BOND et al. 1965; BOND 1969; UNSCEAR 1982); however, there are some exceptions to this, for example the monkey (SCOTT et al. 1988). Recently, the applicability of LD_{50} as a species-dependent

Table 4.10. $LD_{50/30}$ for various species following whole-body irradiation with acute doses of x-rays or γ-rays

Species	Type of radiation	Dose rate (Gy/min)	$LD_{50/30}$ ± 1 SEM	Mean survival time (days)	References
Mouse	x-rays 200 kV		6.40	~10	BOND et al. (1965)
Mouse, CBA T6	x-rays 300 kV	1.25	7.00		VRIESENDORP and van BEKKUM (1984)
Mouse, SAS 10 weeks old	x-rays 15 MV	4.00 (R/100)	8.26 ± 0.20 (R/100)		CROSFILL et al. (1959)
Mouse, CBA × C75Bl	x-rays 250 kV	~0.06	7.35 ± 0.05		BROERSE (1969)
Mouse, CBA × C75Bl	γ-rays ^{137}Cs	~0.06	9.38 ± 0.11		BROERSE (1969)
Rat, Brown Norway × Lewis	x-rays 300 kV	1.42	6.75[a]		VRIESENDORP and van BEKKUM (1984)
Rat	x-rays 250 kV		7.14	~12	BOND et al. (1965)
Rat, different strains	x-rays 200–250 kV	0.03–0.30 (R/100)	4.26–8.07[b]		MORRIS and JONES (1988)
Monkey, *Macaca mulatta*	x-rays 300 kV	0.06	5.25[c]		VRIESENDORP AND van BEKKUM (1984)
Monkey, *Macaca mulatta*	x-rays 250 kV		5.32 ± 0.13[d]		LANGHAM (1967)
Monkey, *Macaca mulatta*	x-rays 250 kV		6.00	~14	BOND et al. (1965)
Dog	x-rays 250 kV				LANGHAM (1967)
Dog, mongrel and beagle	x-rays 50–250 kV	~0.06–0.48 (R/100)	2.31 ± 0.03		MacVITTIE et al. (1984)
Dog, mongrel and beagle	x-rays 1–2 MV	~0.10–0.60 (R/100)	2.06–2.60[b]		MacVITTIE et al. (1984)
Dog, mongrel and beagle	γ-rays ^{60}Co	~0.06–0.30 (R/100)	~2.56–2.68[b]		MacVITTIE et al. (1984)
Dog, beagle	x-rays 300 kV	0.16	3.70[c]		VRIESENDORP and van BEKKUM (1984)

[a] Calculated value for 300-kV x-rays, derived from determinations of $LD_{50/30}$ with ^{137}Cs γ-rays using an RBE of 0.85 for the latter.
[b] Range of values obtained by different groups for the range of dose rates indicated.
[c] Animals had received supportive treatment.
[d] Composite data from two sources; data obtained with 2-MV x-rays were normalized to 250-kV x-rays using an RBE of 0.8.

constant has been questioned, at least for some of the larger animals, due to the marked lack of homogeneity among LD_{50} values within species (BAVERSTOCK et al. 1985). It has been shown for different strains of mice or rats that within the same species the LD_{50} can vary considerably as a consequence of genetic factors (see reviews by CARSTEN 1984; MORRIS and JONES 1988). The differences in radiosensitivity have given rise to speculation about the underlying mechanisms and to different approaches to resolve this problem.

Some authors have considered species-specific differences in the kinetics of hemopoiesis as one possible cause for the different $LD_{50/30}$ values (BOND and ROBINSON 1967; PATT 1969). The model proposed by VRIESENDORP and VAN BEKKUM (1984) is based on a comparative evaluation of the stem cell numbers required for survival after irradiation with a dose equal to the $LD_{50/30}$ or to rescue 50% of the animals with autologous bone marrow transplants after supralethal TBI. The authors conclude (p. 51) "that the differences in susceptibility between species for hematological toxicity of TBI are best explained by assuming high concentrations of hemopoietic stem cells per kg body weight in radioresistant species and low concentrations of hemopoietic stem cells in radiosensitive species." However, this model is based on survival curves of pluripotent stem cells with the same values of $D_0 = 0.6$ Gy and $n = 1$ for the different species such as the mouse, the rat, the rhesus monkey, and the dog. A more recent study based on the analysis of the slopes of the dose–response curves for marrow failure in different species suggests that differences in cell sensitivity between species also may be an important factor in determining animal lethality (THAMES and HENDRY 1987).

Based on CFU-S data, calculations can be performed with respect to the radiation tolerance of the stem cell population in the mouse. An $LD_{50/30}$ at the level of 6–8 Gy will reduce the CFU-S to a survival fraction of approximately 5×10^{-3} to 1×10^{-4}. Accordingly, the absolute numbers of CFU-S surviving in the bone marrow and spleen of mice that have received radiation doses in the range of 6–8 Gy will be of the order of 40–2000 or 180–9000, depending on whether the normal CFU-S number in a mouse of the given strain is 4×10^5 or 18×10^5 (COGGLE and GORDON 1975). PROUKAKIS et al. (1969) have calculated that in 6- and 30-week-old mice, 420 CFU-S will survive an $LD_{80/30}$ (7.2 and 9 Gy, respectively).

Radiation Quality and RBE

RBE values of 0.72–0.89 have been reported for ^{137}Cs and ^{60}Co γ-rays and 15 MV x-rays relative to orthovoltage x-rays for the bone marrow syndrome in mice using the $LD_{50/30}$ values (CROSFILL et al. 1959; BROERSE 1969; LANGENDORFF et al. 1970). Thus, there is good agreement with the values obtained from the respective CFU-S survival curves (see Sect. 4.6.1.1).

$LD_{50/60}$ of Man

For obvious reasons there are no data on the tolerance of the hemopoietic system to TBI in previously healthy persons receiving no medical treatment that are comparable to the $LD_{50/30}$ values of other mammalian species. However, estimates of human $LD_{50/60}$ have been made by different groups and institutions concerned with civil defence in nuclear conflict and the consequences of radiation accidents. Some such estimates from the last 35 years are presented in Table 4.11. As is evident from this table, the data analyzed in the different studies were obtained from only a few, and often identical, sources.

According to the most recent estimates, the $LD_{50/60}$ of normal man after TBI could be of the order of 4.5 Gy; and the gradient of mortality with dose will probably lie in the dose range from 3 to 6 Gy to the bone marrow, assuming survival will not be influenced by medical treatment. Interestingly, calculations by VRIESENDORP and VAN BEKKUM (1984) based on their model (mentioned above) also resulted in a value of 4.5 Gy as the $LD_{50/60}$ of man.

The blood cell changes in the human will reach critical levels later than in other mammalian species, i.e., between 3 and 6 weeks after TBI with doses in the range 3–6 Gy (FLIEDNER 1969).

4.9.1.2 Regeneration of the Stem Cells and Progenitor Cells

The early changes in the pluripotent stem cell and the progenitor cell populations and their regeneration after TBI with acute single doses have been studied quite intensively in mice using radiation doses up to 8 Gy. Less information is available for large mammals, including man, and the information we do have is restricted to progenitor cell data due to the lack of a true stem cell assay.

Table 4.11. Estimates of dose–lethality relations for the bone marrow syndrome in man for uniform exposure to acute doses of low-LET radiation

Source	Parameter and dose (Gy)	Remarks	References
Radiation therapy patients, atomic bomb casualties	$L_{50/60}$, ~ 3.0		WARREN and BOWERS (1950)
Marshallese observations, large animal studies	$LD_{50/60}$, ~ 3.6	Midline dose, no treatment	CRONKITE and BOND (1960)
Radiation therapy patients, accident cases	$LD_{50/60}$ (± 1 SEM), 2.86 ± 0.25	For total treatment times up to 1 day	LANGHAM (1967)
Radiation therapy patients, accident cases	$LD_{50/60}$, 3.0 (range: 2.6–3.25)	Midline dose	NCRP Report No. 39 (1974)
Marshallese observations, radiation therapy patients	$LD_{50/60}$, 3.4 LD_{10}, ~2.5; LD_{90} ~4.2	Minimal medical treatment	Wash-1400 (1975)
In part data from LANGHAM (1967)	$LD_{50/60}$, 3.5; threshold dose, 2 LD_{90}, ~5	No medical treatment	IAEA Safety Series No. 47 (1978)
Data from various sources	Threshold lethality dose, 1–3 $LD_{50/60}$, 3–5; LD_{100}, 4–6	Brief exposure; protraction over 1 days supposed to increase the LD_{50} by ~ 1Gy	SMITH (1983)
Radiation therapy patients, accident cases	Threshold lethality dose, ≥3 Minimal 100% lethality, ~ 6	Adult healthy man, no medical treatment	Medical Research Council's Committee on Effects of Ionizing Radiation (1984)
Radiation therapy patients, accident cases	$LD_{50/60}$, 4.5	Bone marrow dose, minimal specific treatment	MOLE (1984)
Human data, extrapolation from animal data	Gradient of mortality with dose between 3 and 6	Bone marrow dose	BAVERSTOCK et al. (1985)

Regeneration Events in the Mouse

Pluripotent Stem Cells. Several reviews provide detailed information on pluripotent stem cells (HENDRY and LORD 1983; NOTHDURFT 1985; FLIEDNER and NOTHDURFT 1986), so the following discussion can be restricted to the essentials.

Within the first 2–4 h after exposure the absolute numbers of CFU-S are reduced according to the dose–response curves, as described in Section 4.6.1.1. There is a further reduction to approximately 50% of the initial value (see Sect. 4.6.1.3). Repopulation will commence within the following 24 h, with a mean doubling time of approximately 28 h within the first 8–12 days after doses greater than 3 Gy. Typical curves are presented in Fig. 4.4. The cell cycle time in this period might be as short as 7 h (see review by SCHOFIELD 1979). HENDRY and LORD (1983) found no difference in the regeneration kinetics between CFU-S that had survived irradiation and unirradiated CFU-S grafted in primary recipients.

Repopulation slows down quite markedly as the cell numbers approach normal levels; this occurs between day 10 and day 24 after the exposure, depending on the radiation dose (see Fig. 4.4). The proliferation rate may be rather low at the end of this early phase (NEČAS and ZNOJIL 1988). In any case, it has to be considered that besides CFU-S repopulation there is an interfering need for differentiation (BOGGS and BOGGS 1975; see

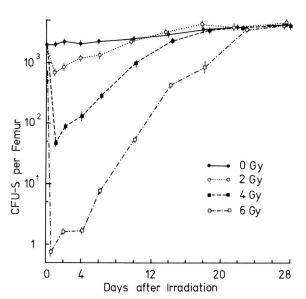

Fig. 4.4. Regeneration of the CFU-S population in the femur of the mouse (SAS/4) after TBI with ^{60}Co γ-rays given as acute incremental doses (after COGGLE 1980)

review by CRONKITE 1985). It has been postulated that self-renewal of stem cells is performed at the expense of differentiation as long as the stem cell compartment has not reached 10% of its original size (CHERVENICK and BOGGS 1971).

Analysis of 13 regeneration curves of bone marrow CFU-S after doses in the range from 3 to 8 Gy indicates that some 18 days to several months after TBI the CFU-S numbers may have attained between 50% and 100% (mean value 83% ± 7%) of their normal values, but that there is no evidence of an overshoot (Hendry and Lord 1983). Interestingly, after a small dose of 0.5 Gy causing an initial reduction in CFU-S to 60% of control, repopulation in the femur and the lumbar vertebrae was considerably delayed, the normal levels not being reached until days 55–65 (Scho-field and Dexter 1982).

Recently, the persistence of slightly subnormal CFU-S numbers in the femur for 1 year was reported for mice which had received a dose of 1.5 Gy (300 kV x-rays, or ^{60}Co γ-rays) given at dose rates in the range from 0.06 to 4 Gy/min. However, after 1.5 Gy given at 0.0005 Gy/min the CFU-S numbers were found to be normal 1 year after the exposure (Gallini et al. 1988). Furthermore, the CFU-S number per colony indicated a decrease in the self-renewal capacity for more than 100 days after the exposure. In mice showing somewhat reduced CFU-S numbers in their femora 6 or 36 months after TBI with a dose of 5 or 4.5 Gy the cycling rate was found to be significantly increased (Croizat et al. 1979; Te-jero et al. 1988). In other experiments a decreased proliferative ability of spleen-seeding cells from donors irradiated with 5 Gy, in parallel with a reduced CFU-S concentration, was present 12 weeks after exposure and persisted for longer periods (von Wangenheim et al. 1986).

In young mice which at the age of 6 or 9 days were exposed to 150 or 500 R, regeneration of the bone marrow CFU-S was severely delayed when compared with regeneration in adult animals (Gerber and Maes 1980).

Repopulation curves of the bone marrow CFU-S have to be interpreted with some reservations, since in the mouse, besides the bone marrow, the spleen is involved in hemopoiesis, and regeneration of CFU-S in the spleen is faster than that of CFU-S in the bone marrow at each dose level (Till 1963; Guzman and Lajtha 1970; Lahiri 1976; Gerber and Maes 1980). Thus, there is the possibility that the bone marrow–spleen interdependence in the donors as well as in the lethally irradiated recipients might influence the regeneration of bone marrow CFU-S.

The anatomical–topographical aspect of stem cell regeneration was studied by Micklem et al. (1975). These authors showed that after radiation doses up to 3.5 Gy, causing 95% stem cell depletion, hemopoietic regeneration is mainly of "local" origin, i.e., it starts from resident stem cells. On the other hand, stem cell migration over longer distances is significantly involved in the regeneration process after larger doses, e.g., 6 Gy, at which the survival fractions are in the range of 10^{-3}.

Hemopoietic Progenitor Cells. Simultaneous assessments of three or more types of progenitor cell and CFU-S were performed in the studies by Nakeff et al. (1979) and Imai and Nakao (1987).

In the experiments by Imai and Nakao (1987) hemopoietic regeneration was studied after acute doses of 1.5 and 3.0 Gy. After either radiation dose the number of cells per femur was found to be maximally depressed from day 1 to day 2 in the order: CFU-E > BFU-E> CFU-S-day 10 > Mix-CFC > GM-CFC. The regeneration as expressed by the length of time required to reach normal or nearly normal values progressed in the following order: CFU-E < GM-CFC < BFU-E < Mix-CFC < CFU-S-day 10. However, as is shown in Fig. 4.5 for the higher dose of 3.0 Gy, BFU-E, Mix-CFC, and CFU-S-day 10 in part did not reach normal levels even after day 28.

In the experiments by Nakeff et al. (1979) mice were irradiated with 5.0 Gy. At day 1 or day 2 (the time of maximum depression) the relative progenitor cell number was (in the order of degree of depression): CFU-E: 0.05%; CFU-S: 0.4%; Meg-CFC: 2%; and GM-CFC: 8%. The regeneration was fastest for CFU-E, which reached normal levels at about day 7. GM-CFC were normal at day 14, whereas by this time the Meg-CFC and the CFU-S had recovered to only 60% and 50% of the normal values, respectively.

The results reported by others for GM-CFC and CFU-S after doses in the range 0.5–4.5 Gy are either concordant with the above results (Chen and Schooley 1970) or in part show considerable deviations with respect to the relative initial depression of CFU-S and GM-CFC and the relation between their recovery curves (Schofield and Dexter 1982; Hendry and Lord 1983).

Progenitor Cells of the Stroma. Some curves representing the regeneration of CFU-F in the bone marrow of guinea pigs and mice after irradiation with varying doses are presented in the review by Hendry and Lord (1983). The repopulation of CFU-F is dose dependent, as has been confirmed by Imai and Nakao (1987). Recent studies have shown that after single doses in the range of 4.5 Gy given at dose rates of 0.06 Gy/min or 0.7 Gy/min the CFU-F may show a transient recovery to near normal values several weeks after the exposure but that thereafter their numbers decrease again (GALLINI et al. 1988).

Hemopoietic Progenitor Cells in Large Mammals

Information about progenitor cell changes and regeneration in large animals is available from canine studies. Since in such studies the bone marrow is collected by aspiration, it is only the concentration of the progenitor cells per unit number of bone marrow cells that is determined, not the absolute progenitor cell number in a defined volume of the bone marrow cavity. However, during regeneration, both the progenitor cell number per unit volume as well as the number of cells they produce will change with time after irradiation.

In dogs which received homogeneous TBI with incremental doses of 0.78, 1.57, and 2.4 Gy, the recuperation of the GM-CFC concentration in the bone marrow was dose dependent up to day 21 after the exposure (NOTHDURFT and FLIEDNER 1982; NOTHDURFT et al. 1984; BALTSCHUKAT and NOTHDURFT 1990). As is evident from the curves in Fig. 4.6, the GM-CFC concentration reached or approached the normal levels at day 28 but showed some fluctuations thereafter. The concentration of GM-CFC in the blood (GM-CFC/ml) exhibited a strong depression in the first 15 days

even after a dose of 0.4 Gy (NOTHDURFT and FLIEDNER 1982) and failed to recover to the normal levels within more than 100 days after the higher doses (NOTHDURFT et al. 1984; BALTSCHUKAT and NOTHDURFT 1990). Recently, regeneration curves were also established for BFU-E in dogs that had received TBI with doses of 1.6 or 2.4 Gy. In accordance with the canine progenitor cell survival curves (Sect. 4.6.2.2) and the murine data, the BFU-E concentration was far more strongly depressed than the GM-CFC concentration; however, beyond day 14 the regeneration of BFU-E was faster. On the other hand, the BFU-E recovery was delayed in dogs which had received the higher dose of 2.4 Gy (BALTSCHUKAT et al. 1989b).

The regeneration curves reported by MacVittie et al. (1984) for GM-CFC in the bone marrow and blood in dogs which had received ^{60}Co γ-irradiation with a dose of 1.5 Gy (0.1 Gy/min) are quite similar to those mentioned before for 1.57 Gy x-ray irradiated dogs, except for certain differences observed in the early phase of bone marrow regeneration. Such differences might be due to differences in the preparation of the bone marrow cell suspensions.

4.9.2 Low Dose Rates

The dose rates to be considered in this section are within the range of practical interest in radiotherapy, i.e., from approximately 2 Gy/min to about 0.01 Gy/min. For even lower dose rates the reader is referred to other reviews and compilations, e.g., BATEMAN et al. (1962), HENDRY and LORD (1983), and SCOTT et al. (1988).

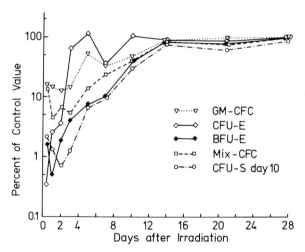

Fig. 4.5. Regeneration of the different types of hemopoietic progenitor cells and pluripotent stem cells CFU-S-day 10 in the femur of the mouse [(DBA/2 × C57B1) F₁] following TBI with 200 kV x-rays given as an acute dose of 3 Gy (after IMAI and NAKAO 1987)

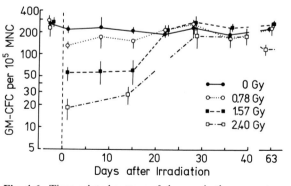

Fig. 4.6. Time-related pattern of changes in the concentration of GM-CFC in the bone marrow of the beagle after TBI with 300 kV x-rays given as three incremental doses. The concentration of GM-CFC is expressed per 10^5 mononuclear bone marrow cells (*MNC*). (NOTHDURFT et al. 1984; BALTSCHUKAT and NOTHDURFT 1990)

The influence of dose rate on the radiation tolerance of the hemopoietic system has been studied from two angles: (a) the lethality from bone marrow failure at the level of the median lethal dose, $LD_{50/30}$, and (b) parameters of stem cell survival. $LD_{50/30}$ data on the dose-rate effect are available for several mammalian species.

4.9.2.1 Murine Experiments

A large amount of information is available regarding the variation of $LD_{50/30}$ with dose rate, and there are a considerable number of experiments in which stem cell survival has been determined. However, there are very few experiments in which both parameters have been studied (Krebs and Jones 1972; Puro and Clark 1972). $LD_{50/30}$ data from different sources have been repeatedly reviewed. In the compilation by Hall and Bedford (1964) of nine sets of $LD_{50/30}$ data for mice (and rats) in the dose-rate range from 1 Gy/min to 0.01 or 0.02 Gy/min, an increasing dose-rate effect below 0.1 Gy/min was evident in most cases.

On the basis of more recent reviews (Page 1968; Peters et al. 1979; Dutreix et al. 1979) it can be concluded that reduction in dose rate to between 0.1 and 0.05 Gy/min may add between 10% and 15% to the $LD_{50/30}$ compared with a high dose-rate exposure at about 1 Gy/min (see Fig. 4.7A). The $LD_{50/30}$ will further increase by 15%–25% (of the value at approximately 0.1 Gy/min) if the dose rate is further reduced to 0.02 Gy/min, i.e., there will be a total increase in $LD_{50/30}$ by a factor of 1.3–1.4 if the dose rate is lowered from 1 Gy/min to 0.02 Gy/min. However, there may also be exceptions to this, with an increase in LD_{50} only below 0.01 Gy/min (e.g., Scott al. 1988).

The effect of dose rate on survival of normal murine bone marrow CFU-S has been considered in detail in Sect. 4.6.1.4. Based on the values obtained for D_0 and/or the extrapolation number of the survival curves, most authors have come to the conclusion that there appears to be little if any effect of dose rate on murine CFU-S within the dose-rate range of interest (see also Steel et al. 1986; Steel and Horwich 1988). Using other measures, such as the respective survival fractions for a given dose of 5 Gy, leads to the same conclusions (Fig. 4.7B). It is evident that there is no uniform correlation between the assay of bone marrow CFU-S and the changes in the $LD_{50/30}$. The heterogeneous picture does not change signi-

ficantly for higher dose levels, for which a dose-rate effect might be expected to be more pronounced on the basis of the single-dose survival curve (Thames and Hendry 1987).

Obviously, correlations between $LD_{50/30}$ data and stem cell survival, as obtained in the study by Puro and Clark (1972), are exceptions among the available data. Consequently, the role of the exogenous CFU-S as the target cell has to be questioned or, alternatively, the properties of the CFU-S may have changed due to the modifications in the CFU-S assay. Indeed, the endogenous CFU-S has been assumed to be a candidate target cell for survival (Puro and Clark 1972). Another possibility is that only a small subpopulation of the bone marrow CFU-S is responsible for animal survival, and that this subpopulation cannot be detected in the standard assays. Biexponential survival curves, as sometimes reported (Fu et al. 1975; Belletti et al. 1979), point in this direction.

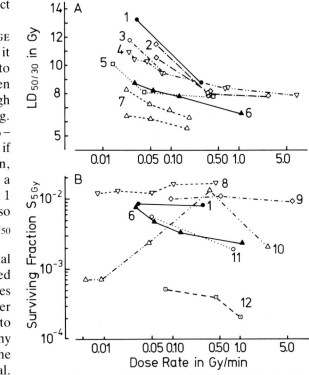

Fig. 4.7. Dose-rate dependence of **A** $LD_{50/30}$ values for the mouse, and **B** the surviving fraction of femoral CFU-S after a dose of 5 Gy (S_{5Gy}). ●—● 1 (Krebs and Jones 1972); ◇---◇ 2 (Feola et al. 1974); ○---○ 3 (Broerse 1969); ▽----▽ 4 (Neal 1960); □----□ 5 (Thomson and Tourtellotte 1953); ▲—▲ 6 (Puro and Clark 1972); △---△ 7 (Kallman 1962); ▽---▽ 8 (Belletti et al. 1979); ◇---◇ 9 (Broerse et al. 1971); △----△ 10 (Fu et al. 1975); ○----○ 11 (Tarbell et al. 1987); ■---■ 12 (Glasgow et al. 1983)

GM-CFC have also been discussed as possible target cells (see Sect. 4.8.1.1).

As compared with the murine $LD_{50/30}$ data, other acutely responding tissues such as the intestine, the epidermis, and the testis generally are characterized by a more pronounced increase in the isoeffective doses (ED_{50}) or the D_0 values of the survival curves for their clonogens with decreasing dose rate over the dose-rate range of interest, i.e., from 1 to 0.01 Gy/min (DUTREIX et al. 1979; see review by STEEL et al. 1986). The same holds true when comparison is with the lung as a late responding tissue (STEEL et al. 1986; THAMES and HENDRY 1987).

4.9.2.2 Large Mammals

Low dose-rate data for large mammals such as dogs, swine, goats, and sheep derived from different sources were first reviewed by PAGE (1968) and have been reanalyzed by SCOTT et al. (1988). The curves fitted to the LD_{50} data in relation to dose rate over the range from 0.5 to 0.0001 Gy/min seem to form a family with diverging LD_{50} values at dose rates below 0.005 Gy/min. At higher dose rates, however, the LD_{50} values seem to be independent of species (SCOTT et al. 1988) (see also Sect. 4.9.1.1 and BAVERSTOCK et al. 1985). Overall, there is little increase in the LD_{50} values for the bone marrow syndrome of large mammals with decreasing dose rate within the dose-rate range of clinical interest. Perhaps with the exception of the swine the time factor is between 1.1 and 1.3.

4.9.3 Recovery from Radiation Injury – Split-Dose Effects

The recovery of the hemopoietic cells from sublethal damage after acute doses of radiation has been studied (a) on the level of the stem cells and progenitor cells, and (b) in animal lethality studies; in both cases the split-dose technique has been used.

4.9.3.1 Stem Cells and Progenitor Cells

The response of hemopoietic cells to split acute doses has been studied by several authors for CFU-S using both the endogenous and the exoge-

nous technique, in the latter case with the irradiations performed either in the donor or the recipient. (For a discussion of the radiobiological implications of the two exogenous assay methods, see HENDRY and HOWARD 1971).

Some of the curves are presented in Fig. 4.8, illustrating both conformity and divergence between the various reports. In general a clear sparing effect of splitting the dose can be observed, with the occasional exception where the single-dose survival curve already exhibits no shoulder (e.g., PEACOCK et al. 1986).

For CFU-S that were irradiated in the steady state the first peak generally occurred at 4–5 h, and sometimes earlier, after the first fraction. The curves that were obtained for bone marrow CFU-S by the exogenous technique and with split-dose irradiations given to the recipients resulted in a survival ratio (= recovery factor) between 1.5 and 2.8 after two equal fractions of 1.8 or 2 Gy each (TILL and McCULLOCH 1963, 1964; PHILLIPS 1968), the CFU-S from 3-month-old mice showing the higher values when compared with 25- to 27-month-old mice (CHEN 1974).

Exposures to equal doses of 1.5 or 2 Gy per fraction given to the donor resulted in survival ratios of 1.5–1.7 at 4–5 h (HENDRY 1973; FU et al. 1975). However, when corrections are made for the loss of CFU-S from the femoral marrow ("dip," see Sect. 4.6.1.3) within the interval

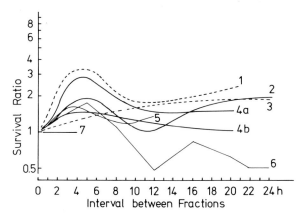

Fig. 4.8. Recovery factor for murine bone marrow CFU-S following split-dose irradiation as a function of the time interval between the two fractions. ---- 1, 4 + 3 (3.5) Gy, endogenous assay; — 2, 2 + 2 Gy, 1 h after transplantation (TILL and McCULLOCH 1964); --- 3, 500 + 250 R, endogenous assay (CHAFFEY and HELLMAN 1969); — 4, 200 + 200 R, 1 h after transplantation; (a) age 3 months, (b) age 2 years (CHEN 1974); — 5, 180 + 180 R, 2 h after transplantation (PHILLIPS 1968); — 6, 2 + 2 Gy, irradiation in the donor (HENDRY 1973); — 7, 1.5 + 1.5 Gy, irradiation in the donor (PEACOCK et al. 1986)

between the two exposures the survival ratio amounts to approximately 3 (HENDRY 1973).

At lower doses per fraction a lower survival ratio was obtained than after the larger doses in the range of 2 Gy, e.g., approximately 1.4 and 1.5 after 50 + 50 R or 75 + 75 R (HANKS 1972). Furthermore, as shown by others, the split-dose effect in terms of additional dose ($D_2 - D_1$) required is negligible when doses of less than about 1 Gy are split, and there is an increasing survival ratio with increasing total doses up to at least 6 Gy (HENDRY 1979; HENDRY and LORD 1983). These features are characteristic of continuously bending survival curves as reported for the majority of stem cell types in other tissues, but are not in accordance with a survival curve characterized by a small shoulder and a terminal exponential slope, i.e., usually characterized by n and D_0 (HENDRY 1979; HENDRY and LORD 1983).

The endogenous technique, which requires higher doses than the former technique, resulted in survival ratios of 2, 2.8, and 3.4, respectively, after split doses of 250 + 500 R (CHAFFEY and HELLMAN 1969), 3.6 + 3.6 Gy (PHILLIPS 1968), and 4 + 3–3.5 Gy (TILL and McCULLOCH 1964) (Fig. 4.8). Split-dose versus time–response curves obtained after 250 + 500 R, or the inverse sequence, 500 + 250 R, showed remarkable differences, especially beyond 12 h (CHAFFEY and HELLMAN 1969).

The D_0 values of the survival curves obtained at the time of the first peak, i.e., 3–5 h after the first fraction, have been reported to remain unchanged (TILL and McCULLOCH 1963; CHEN 1974) or to show some increase (FRINDEL et al. 1966; PHILLIPS and HANKS 1968; HENDRY and HOWARD 1971; CHEN 1974).

The split-dose response of rapidly proliferating CFU-S (determined in regenerating femoral marrow 6 days after TBI with 4.5 Gy) is less pronounced than for normal CFU-S, which is in accordance with the smaller shoulder to the single-dose survival curve of the former (HENDRY 1973). On the other hand, no split-dose effect was obtained for a CFU-S population supposed to be in a non-cycling state due to pretreatment of the donor mice with vinblastine (HANKS 1972).

Data for split-dose effects on GM-CFC are available from a few sources. The changes obtained in experiments with murine GM-CFC resulted in a survival ratio of about 3.6 between 1 and 2 h, followed by a considerable decrease thereafter (BRIGANTI and MAURO 1979). An in-

crease in the survival ratio to approximately 4 was reported by PEACOCK et al. (1986) after split doses of 3 + 3 Gy given to the donors at an interval of 4 h. In both studies the single-dose survival curves were of the shoulder-curve type.

No split-dose effects could be observed when human bone marrow GM-CFC were irradiated in vitro after plating (in agar cultures) and preincubation at 37°C for 4–24 h, using a dose of 0.5 Gy as the first fraction and 0.5–2.5 Gy as the second fraction (KIMLER et al. 1984). This was to be expected, given the lack of a shoulder on the single-dose survival curve. However, when GM-CFC that had been irradiated with 2 Gy received a second fraction 3 h later with increasing doses the slope of this latter curve showed a significant decrease ($D_0 = 1.39$ Gy) when compared with the single-dose curve ($D_0 = 0.66$ Gy). One may speculate that such an "anomalous" effect is due to the split-dose response of a relatively radioresistant GM-CFC subpopulation. A similar observation was reported for HL-60 human leukemia cells (LEHNERT et al. 1986; see also ELKIND 1988).

4.9.3.2 Animal Lethality Studies

There are several reviews of animal lethality studies (CASARETT 1969; BAUMANN and MUTH 1977; KINDT and SATTLER 1977; AINSWORTH et al. 1984) to which reference must be made for details, such as variations with species, strain, sex, and size of the first dose.

In the mouse the changes in the $LD_{50/30}$ within the first 48 h (or longer) after an acute dose, the "conditioning dose," have been tested repeatedly. Using a dose in the range 1.5–5 Gy at the first exposure the main features of the results obtained with orthovoltage x-rays or γ-rays are rather uniform (KALLMAN and SILINI 1964; HORNSEY 1967; MOLE 1975). As is reflected by the curves in Fig. 4.9, there is a discontinuous increase in the $LD_{50/30}$ (of the second exposure) within 48 h after the various conditioning doses.

Comparison with the split-dose response curves of the bone marrow CFU-S reveals a clear temporal coincidence between the first maximum and the decrease thereafter and the following changes in the curves for the CFU-S and the $LD_{50/30}$ values. As can be seen from Fig. 4.9, the value of the "effective D_q" [corresponding to ($D_2 - D_1$), MOLE 1975] at the first maximum, i.e., 4–6 h after the first exposure, may reach approximately 0.5

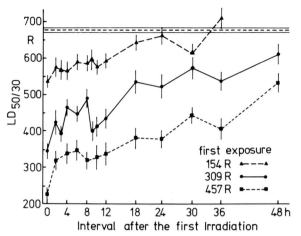

Fig. 4.9. Changes in second dose $LD_{50/30}$ for mice over time after preirradiation at three different exposure levels. The *horizontal bar* represents the $LD_{50/30} \doteq 676$ R $\pm$ 1 SEM for normal mice. (After KALLMAN and SILINI 1964)

Gy for a conditioning dose of about 1.5 Gy, and 1.2 Gy for the highest conditioning dose of about 4.5 Gy. Furthermore, the hemopoietic damage experienced at the smaller conditioning doses not only may have disappeared 24 h later; rather even some "overrecovery" is possible (see reviews by PAGE 1968; CASARETT 1969; KINDT and SATTLER 1977), mainly due to proliferation and possibly associated effects of redistribution.

The pattern of changes over time in the $LD_{50/30}$ of large animals following irradiation has been studied for conditioning doses mainly between one-half and two-thirds of the LD_{50} for single-dose exposures (see reviews by PAGE 1968; CASARETT 1969; KINDT and SATTLER 1977; AINSWORTH et al. 1984). However, in all of these studies the minimum time interval between the two exposures has been at least 2–3 days. Consequently virtually no information is available about the kinetics of recovery from sublethal damage occurring within a few hours after the first fraction.

Generally, the regeneration processes observed in large animals, e.g., the dog, sheep, goat, swine, burro, and monkey (*Macaca mulatta*), within the first 10 days or at least 20 days after exposure, show extremely variable kinetics see review by AINSWORTH et al. (1984).

Three weeks after irradiation the LD_{50} has been found to be quite normal in sheep, goat, and dog, i.e., the same as in previously unirradiated animals, indicating 100% regeneration from the first dose. On the other hand, only moderate or slow regeneration has been found in the monkey or the burro within the first 14 days or after longer

intervals. Phases of transient "overrecovery" (LD_{50} values higher than for normal animals) have been observed in dog, sheep, and swine at about day 20 after the first exposure. However, the goat and the monkey show a return to a radiosensitive state after a phase of transient increase in the LD_{50}.

4.9.4 Fractionation

The influence of fractionation on hemopoietic tolerance has been studied in considerable detail in mice for different fractionation regimes involving variations in dose per fraction, dose rate, length of interfraction interval, and overall treatment time. $LD_{50/30}$ data and CFU-S survival have been used as isoeffect endpoints.

4.9.4.1 $LD_{50/30}$ and CFU-S Data

Figure 4.10 depicts the results from some of the experiments in which the cumulative $LD_{50/30}$ for treatments with daily fractions or five fractions per week with exposures to 25–400 R per fraction (120 kV or 250 kV x-rays, 25–45 R/min) was determined (KAPLAN and BROWN 1952; MOLE 1957; KREBS and BRAUER 1964). There is a clear increase in the LD_{50} with increasing number of fractions and overall treatment time. In the log-log plot the relationship can be approximated by straight lines according to standard Strandqvist functions (KAPLAN and BROWN 1952; MOLE 1975).

In other experiments (MOLE 1975) in which mice received several fractions either of 1.5 Gy at 3-day intervals or 3 Gy at 6-day intervals the radiation tolerance (measured as total cumulative LD_{50}) first showed a relatively steep increase for each regime, followed by a more flattened segment. With the 3 Gy per fraction regime this increase could be observed within 6 days after the first fraction, whereas for the 1.5 Gy per fraction regime a total dose of 4.5 Gy and a 9-day interval were required to attain the same effect. Rapid proliferation was initiated after the first exposures, and the larger dose per fraction was more efficient than the smaller one. Further experiments clearly showed that the response to fractionated irradiation is governed by recovery from sublethal damage, proliferation (i.e., cell multiplication), and the associated age distribution of the target cells.

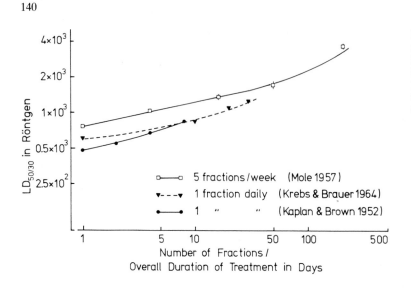

Fig. 4.10. Increase in LD$_{50/30}$ for mice as a function of fractionation. *Abscissa*: log number of fractions for daily fractions (data of KAPLAN and BROWN 1952; KREBS and BRAUER 1964) or total treatment time in days for five fractions/week (data of MOLE 1957)

The response of the femoral CFU-S to fractionation has been studied for different regimes. The most important features are summarized by HENDRY and LORD (1983) and HENDRY and POTTEN (1988).

At dose fractions below 2 Gy little effect of fractionation is observed for several days. Later the repopulating ability of the rapidly proliferating cells will come into play. Isoeffect curves for 1% or 10% survival of bone marrow CFU-S during irradiation with daily fractions (× 5/week) indicate that little additional dose is required for isoeffective CFU-S reduction until more than four fractions have been given. In this respect the curves for bone marrow CFU-S are different from most such curves for other tissues. On the other hand, the slope exponent of 0.65 characterizing the steep increase for more than four fractions, due to the rapid repopulating ability of the CFU-S, is very large when compared with the slope exponents of 0.35 for the epidermis and up to 0.58 for the jejunum.

4.9.4.2 α/β Ratio Values for LD$_{50/30}$

Even though they were not designed for such purposes, some of the multifraction experiments considered above permit α/β ratio values to be derived. Estimates of the value of α/β for LD$_{50/30}$ as a parameter defining the overall hemopoietic functional tolerance were performed by FOWLER (1983) on the basis of results obtained from several sources and applying some essential corrections (subtraction of effect of time, etc.). The estimates

of α/β values lie between 7 and 35 Gy. Such values are within the range of those for acute functional effects in other murine organs, and higher than the values for late-responding tissues as cited in the same paper (1–2.5 Gy to 4.4–6.3 Gy).

Interestingly, the α/β values of approximately 9 Gy (THAMES et al. 1982) or 8.9 (7.5–10.9) Gy (THAMES and HENDRY 1987) obtained from multifraction isoeffect data for endogenous spleen colony forming cells are lower than most obtained for the LD$_{50/30}$ as the overall functional parameter. The value obtained for survival of bone marrow CFU-S when irradiated in the steady state with single doses, i.e., α/β = 23 Gy, and the operational value of α/β = 16 Gy for the target cell for animal lethality, derived from dose-incidence data at low dose rates (HENDRY and MOORE 1985), are in the middle of the 7- to 35-Gy range deduced by FOWLER (1983) from the fractionation LD$_{50/30}$ data. At present it is an open question whether α/β ratios are different for stem cells irradiated in the steady state and stem cells irradiated when they are rapidly cycling (HENDRY and POTTEN 1988).

4.10 Low-Dose Fractionated Total Body Irradiation for Therapy

Due to the high responsiveness of some malignancies, and with the intention of keeping the hematological toxicity as low as possible, fractionated TBI with small doses per fraction has been applied as systemic therapy. The malignancies in question include chronic lymphocytic leukemia

(CLL), neuroblastoma, multiple myeloma, and non-Hodgkin's lymphoma (NHL) (DEACON et al. 1984; FERTIL and MALAISE 1985; MARUYAMA and FEOLA 1987). The following discussion will focus on the results in patients treated for CLL and NHL because they are representative of this mode of systemic treatment and the hematological sequelae.

4.10.1 Chronic Lymphocytic Leukemia

A detailed review of the hematological findings obtained in 66 patients with previously untreated CLL who were treated between 1964 and 1972 was given by JOHNSON and RÜHL (1976) and was later updated by JOHNSON (1979). The method consisted in administering 0.05–0.10 Gy per day at three to five exposures per week. The total dose given for initial induction treatment was individually adjusted to the response of the disease and the hematological toxicity. The initial course of treatment was delivered in courses of 0.5 Gy in a large number of patients, interrupted for 4–8 weeks to avoid undue bone marrow depression. The total induction doses ranged from 1 to 4 Gy (median 2 Gy). It is important to note that approximately 50% of the patients were anemic at diagnosis, as is common in CLL. Mild to moderate thrombocytopenia caused by hypersplenism was relatively common too. Consequently, anemia and thrombocytopenia constituted major problems in 5% and 15% of the patients, respectively, whereas neutropenia was not a limiting factor for treatment. On the other hand, many patients experienced improvement of progressive anemia and/or thrombocytopenia as a consequence of therapy. Overall, the toxicity of TBI in CLL was found to be acceptable if considered in context with those pathophysiological processes inherent in CLL.

The excellent results reported by JOHNSON (1979) for treatment of active CLL with TBI could not be confirmed in other studies performed by the Eastern Cooperative Oncology Group (RUBIN et al. 1981). Of 11 patients treated according to a prescribed protocol consisting of three treatment courses with a total dose of 1.5 Gy each given over 5 weeks, with three fractions of 0.10 Gy per week, seven completed one course and only three were able to receive a second course. In another group of 15 patients treated with courses of 0.5 Gy given in five fractions of 0.05 Gy per week, 14 were able to complete the first course, and only four began a third course. Thrombocytopenia or granulocy-topenia associated with partial response was the most common reason for discontinuing TBI.

4.10.2 Non-Hodgkin's Lymphoma

CONSTINE and RUBIN (1988) have reviewed the various treatment plans employed in NHL, which have consisted of two, three or five fractions per week of 0.15 or 0.10 Gy each with a total dose of 1.0 Gy to be given within somewhat more than 3 weeks, or 1.5 Gy in 3–5 weeks. Where daily fractions of 0.15 Gy have been applied five times a week, the total dose has been limited to 0.75 Gy per course. In most cases a second course has been planned to commence 2 weeks, 4–6 weeks, or even 8–12 weeks after the termination of the first one. However, in a high percentage of patients treatment has not been performed in accordance with the original plans, i.e., the total doses achieved per course have been lower than intended because of hematological complications.

Though in some treatment groups the granulo-cytes have shown considerable depression (quite often only the total leukocyte count is mentioned), the primary problems have arisen from thrombocytopenia (platelet counts below $10^5/\mu l$ blood, $5 \times 10^4/\mu l$, or even $1.5 \times 10^4/\mu l$.) requiring interruption or termination of treatment and associated with the need for blood transfusions and even hospitalization (THAR and MILLION 1978). The nadirs in the blood granulocyte and platelet counts generally have been observed some 2–3 weeks after termination of one course (Fig. 4.11). Therefore, it is impossible to make any predictions of the response during the treatment itself.

Persistent thrombocytopenia has been observed after TBI on certain occasions in previously untreated patients (CARABELL et al. 1979). CHAFFEY et al. (1975) reported that the decrease in the blood thrombocyte concentration following a second course of TBI was more severe than that observed after the first course. Patients showing a reduced bone marrow reserve (i.e., anemia, gra-nulocytopenia, and thrombocytopenia) before treatment were found to be more sensitive than patients with normal blood cell counts (LABETZKI et al. 1980). Also, patients with involvement of the bone marrow and/or a palpably enlarged spleen were at a higher risk for bone marrow suppression than patients without these conditions (CHAFFEY et al. 1975; THAR and MILLION 1978; VAN DIJK-MILATZ 1979).

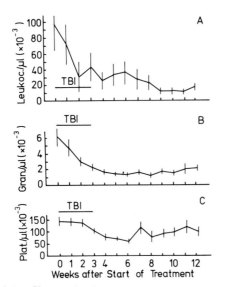

Fig. 4.11. Changes in the concentration of **A** the leuko-cytes, **B** the granulocytes, and **C** the thrombocytes in the blood of patients with lymphoma after fractionated TBI with an average total dose of 1.1 Gy (after LABETZKI et al. 1982)

The acute toxicity of radiotherapy was found to be less severe than that of chemotherapy in some studies (JOHNSON et al. 1978). In patients treated with chemotherapy leukopenia was more common and more severe than thrombocytopenia, in contrast to the findings in patients treated with fractionated TBI (YOUNG et al. 1977; JOHNSON et al. 1978). Combination chemotherapy (CVP, B-CVP, BA-CVP)[1] or single agent treatment with cyclophosphamide following relapse in previously whole body irradiated patients who often had received additional boost irradiation to local fields, generally was well tolerated (JOHNSON et al. 1978; VAN DIJK-MILATZ 1979; ÖHL et al. 1979; CARABELL et al. 1979). Similar observations were reported for patients who had received local radiotherapy prior to chemotherapy at least 6 weeks before they received TBI.

GM-CFC determinations that perhaps could help to detect an unusual radiation response at the progenitor cell level have been performed on certain occasions in patients with lymphoma. In the studies by BULL et al. (1975) the concentration of GM-CFC in bone marrow aspirates from patients with mixed histiocytic-lymphocytic or lymphocytic lymphoma with a nodular disease

---
[1] CVP = cyclophosphamide, vincristine, prednisone; B-CVP = bleomycin-CVP; BA-CVP = bleomycin-adriamycin-CVP.

pattern was not significantly different from the normal median. In contrast, patients with diffuse lymphoma showed GM-CFC concentrations clearly below the normal range. However, GM-CFC concentrations in the marrow did not differ according to the presence or absence of tumor invasion of the marrow. Clearly subnormal GM-CFC values before treatment, ranging from 1 to 25 per 10^5 bone marrow cells (normal values: 50–100/10^5), were reported by LABETZKI et al. (1982) in patients exhibiting marrow infiltration. After treatment with a mean total dose of 1.1 Gy there was no uniform pattern of changes within the following 6–10 weeks and the GM-CFC indices remained generally low. The subnormal bone marrow GM-CFC compartment was reflected by the low blood granulocyte values at the same time. However, the results obtained from the GM-CFC assay in bone marrow aspirates from such patients are difficult to interpret because both the GM-CFC and, perhaps to an even greater extent, the atypical lymphocytes in the bone marrow are affected by the irradiation.

4.10.3 Animal Studies

Some studies have been performed in experimental animals using treatment regimes similar to those applied therapeutically. In mice which had received fractions of 0.2 or 0.5 Gy twice a week for 5 weeks, i.e., total doses of 2 or 5 Gy, no clear changes were observed in the platelet counts in either of the irradiated groups; the hematocrit values also remained quite normal (MELAMED et al. 1980). The leukocytes remained within the normal range in animals that were treated with 0.2 Gy per fraction, whereas they dropped to 40% of normal in animals that received three fractions with 0.5 Gy per fraction, but thereafter showed stabilization. On the other hand, the GM-CFC were found initially to be depressed in both groups of mice in a dose-dependent fashion; however, they showed an increase even during treatment in those mice which were irradiated with a dose of 0.2 Gy per fraction.

Multifractionation studies performed by others (HENDRY 1985b) indicate that with daily fractions of 0.1 Gy a slight but long-lasting reduction in the femoral CFU-S is obtained after total doses in the range of 1.5 Gy. With 0.3 Gy per fraction the level of the CFU-S remained at 50% of normal between 2 and 6 months after irradiation with a total dose of 4.5 Gy. Such results are in accordance with the CFU-S data reported by MELAMED et al. (1980).

In rabbits which were treated with fractions of 0.1 Gy three or five times per week, with cumulative doses of 15 or 10 Gy given over 50 or 20 weeks respectively, only a slight decrease in the total blood leukocyte count occurred after initiation of the treatment (RUBIN et al. 1984). With daily fractions of 0.25 Gy a significant depression of the blood leukocyte count took place toward a cumulative dose of 10 Gy and continued to the 25-Gy level. However, in all cases a recovery or even a rebound occurred within 3–4 weeks following the treatment. No changes could be observed in the hematocrit in any of the treatment groups. The erythrocyte counts showed an increase during irradiation and the GM-CFC assay indicated a hyperactive state of the progenitor cell compartment.

COWALL et al. (1981) studied the hematological effects of fractionated TBI with two fractions of 0.15 Gy per week given over 5 weeks in normal beagles and dogs with diffuse lymphomas. The changes observed in the blood cell counts of the normal beagles (no data are presented for the lymphoma dogs) were minimal for the total leukocytes, whereas the thrombocytes showed a reduction to about 60% of the normal value about

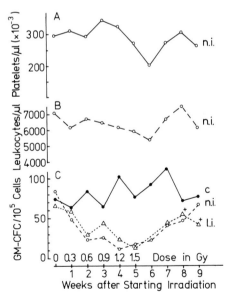

Fig. 4.12. Changes in the concentration of **A** the thrombocytes and **B** the leukocytes in the blood, and **C** the GM-CFC in the bone marrow of dogs after fractionated TBI with a total dose of 1.5 Gy. *n.i.*, normal dogs, irradiated; *l.i.*, dogs with lymphoma, irradiated; *c*, control, not irradiated; +, data from 1 dog. (Data of COWALL et al. 1981)

10 days after termination of the treatment (Fig. 4.12). The bone marrow cellularity remained within normal limits. On the other hand, the GM-CFC concentration in the bone marrow showed a continuous and nearly parallel reduction in both groups of dogs, a gradual recovery occurring within the first weeks following the treatment. Furthermore, the bone marrow GM-CFC compartment in irradiated normal beagles clearly showed a reduced proliferation response to endotoxin 2 weeks after TBI when compared with nonirradiated animals. On the other hand, the increase in serum CSA as measured 2 h after the injection of endotoxin was substantially the same in the previously irradiated dogs and the unirradiated controls.

Given that such animal studies unequivocally show that TBI with small fractional radiation doses involves less hematological toxicity than single large doses, the severe bone marrow depression occurring in patients with lymphomas and CLL certainly seems puzzling, as emphasized by others (RUBIN et al. 1981, 1984; CONSTINE and RUBIN 1988). In fact hematological toxicity may not entail a direct radiation effect on the stem cells and/or progenitor cells. In patients with CLL, inhibitors released by either the destroyed lymphocytes or the irradiated, diseased marrow have been considered as possible causes of the toxicity (RUBIN et al. 1981). More recently it has been suggested that in patients with CLL and NHL imbalances occur in stimulating and inhibitory factors related to both granulocytopoiesis and megakaryocyto-/thrombocytopoiesis (RUBIN et al. 1984), and that defects arise in the production of colony-stimulating factors in parallel with the onset of leukopenia (CONSTINE and RUBIN 1988).

The observation that in CLL patients it is the platelet system that is more affected by this treatment than granulocytopoiesis needs special attention. In this respect the results obtained from the experiments performed with rodents are obviously different. Such differences in the blood cell changes between small mammals and human patients during the course of extended fractionated irradiation in part may be due to the differences in the generation time of hemopoietic cells and the associated proliferation, which will play a role if exactly the same fractionation regimes are applied in each case. However, considerable variations in the radiation tolerance between individual patients indicate that other factors also may be important, such as disease-related reductions in stem cell and progenitor cell population size and perturbations in the micro-ecology in the bone marrow specifically affecting megakaryocytopoiesis and platelet production and/or in accessory cell systems in other tissues producing essential stimulators.

4.11 High-Dose Total Body Irradiation and Bone Marrow Transplantation

Bone marrow suppression is the most important dose-limiting acute toxic effect for most antineo-plastic agents, including systemic radiotherapy. However, substantial dose escalation can be achieved if treatments are followed by rescue with normal bone marrow cells. High dose TBI in combination with bone marrow transplantation (BMT) was originally applied in the management of hematological diseases such as acute leukemias (see reviews by GALE and CHAMPLIN 1986; THOMAS 1986), but has found increasing use during the last decade in the systemic treatment of a variety of other lymphohematological disorders or malignan-cies and solid tumors such as multiple myeloma, neuroblastoma, and oat cell carcinoma of the lung (see reviews by CHAMPLIN and GALE 1984; BLUME 1986; GALE and CHAMPLIN 1986; BARRETT 1987). The total radiation doses given are usually in the range 7.5–15 Gy, but may even be as high as 17.5 Gy (see reviews by BARRETT 1982; CHAMPLIN and GALE 1984). Usually they are administered in combination with single cytotoxic agents or mul-tidrug treatment (see review by BARRETT 1987).

The hemopoietic cells to be grafted are obtained from one of the following three possible sources depending on the nature of the disease and other important circumstances:

1. Syngeneic bone marrow from a genetically identical twin
2. Autologous bone marrow cryopreserved before transplantation
3. Allogeneic bone marrow from sibling donors or otherwise related individuals who are HLA-identical or partially HLA-matched

Under syngeneic or autologous conditions, successful transplantation is obtained with approx-imately $1 \times 10^7 - 5 \times 10^7$ bone marrow cells/kg body weight, whereas for transplantation of allogeneic cells $1 \times 10^8 - 3 \times 10^8$ bone marrow cells/kg are required (CHAMPLIN and GALE 1984;

VRIESENDORP and VAN BEKKUM 1984; MESSNER and YAMASAKI 1988). A cell number of 2×10^8/kg has been estimated to be about 1%–1.5% of the normal marrow content (BARRETT 1984; FAILLE et al. 1981), or somewhat more (MESSNER and YAMASAKI 1988).

In the last 5 years increasing evidence has been presented that in certain diseases blood derived stem cells can be used as an alternative source of stem cells for hemopoietic reconstitution under autologous conditions (e.g. KÖRBLING et al. 1986; KESSINGER et al. 1988).

When given as the only treatment modality or in combination with antineoplastic drugs, TBI can fulfil the following functions (BARRETT 1982):

1. Elimination of the malignant stem cells from the body; this will be the more successful the greater the reduction in malignant cells achieved by preceding chemotherapy
2. Immune suppression, which will allow the grafted bone marrow cells to take
3. Bone marrow ablation, providing the space that is needed by the transplanted cells to become established

In patients with aplastic anemia the only essen-tial function of TBI is to suppress the resistance to marrow engraftment.

Besides complications that are common for all types of BMT (i.e., whether syngeneic, auto-logous, or allogeneic), such as the acute toxicity of the conditioning chemoradiotherapy, long-lasting immunodeficiency and associated infections, in-terstitial pneumonitis, and delayed hemopoietic recovery, in the case of transplantations of allogeneic bone marrow cells there is also the problem of the complex reciprocal balance be-tween the mechanisms responsible for graft rejec-tion and those involved in the graft versus host disease (GVHD) with which the pretransplant TBI may interfere. Additionally, it is well documented that there is an antileukemia ("graft-versus-leukemia") effect under conditions of allogeneic BMT, and there is evidence that certain T cells in the donor marrow may be involved (see reviews by GALE and CHAMPLIN 1986; GALE and REISNER 1986).

Estimates of the response of hemopoietic cells to different TBI protocols, i.e., involving different dose rates or fractions, have mainly been based on either murine pluripotent stem cell (CFU-S) data or LD_{50} studies. It is generally concluded that for hemopoietic cells no significant dose sparing will be achieved if, instead of a single exposure at a high dose rate, i.e., > 0.3 Gy/min, TBI is given in several fractions or at low dose rates, i.e., below 0.1 Gy/min (PETERS et al. 1979; PETERS 1980; TRAVIS et al. 1985; STEEL et al. 1986). On the other hand, SONG et al. (1981) concluded after a reexamination of a variety of survival data for normal hemopoietic cells that these cells have a substantial repair capacity which is usually underestimated.

4.11.1 The Role of Total Body Irradiation (TBI) in T Cell-Depleted Bone Marrow Transplantation (BMT)

Allogeneic BMT is followed by moderate to severe GVHD in 45% of recipients of HLA-identical grafts and in 75% of recipients of HLA-mismatched transplants (see reviews by GALE 1987; BARRETT 1987). GVHD can be significantly reduced in both incidence and severity if the bone marrow is depleted of T lymphocytes before transplantation (O'REILLY et al. 1985; SULLIVAN 1986). On the other hand, T cell depletion is associated with an increased risk of graft failure and more frequent leukemia relapse (see review by BUTTURINI and GALE 1988). The "graft-versus-leukemia" effect present under conditions when unseparated allogeneic cells are transplanted obviously is mediated by T cells (GALE and REISNER 1986). Recently VOSS et al. (1988) reported that in patients receiving T cell-depleted marrow the relapse rate was lower if, for conditioning, fractionated TBI with a total dose of 12 Gy was given instead of a single dose of 10 Gy. However, hyperfractionated TBI with total doses of 13.2 or 14.4 Gy in combination with cyclophosphamide, which resulted in a comparatively low relapse rate in good-risk patients with acute myeloblastic or acute lymphocytic leukemia who had received unseparated bone marrow (BROCHSTEIN et al. 1987), was associated with more frequent relapse in some groups of patients transplanted with T cell-depleted marrow (KERNAN et al. 1987). On the other hand, in patients with malignant hemopathies who were transplanted with T cell-depleted marrow cells from HLA-identical donors and were treated beforehand with hyperfractionated TBI with a total dose of 14.4 Gy given in combination with cyclophosphamide, the rate of graft rejection reached 10% (O'REILLY et

al. 1985; KERNAN et al. 1987; LATINI et al. 1988). However, the results reported by MARTIN et al. (1985) suggest that this rate could perhaps be reduced by increasing the dose of cyclophosphamide and/or the irradiation dose. At present it is not clear whether additional doses of TBI or total lymphoid irradiation (TLI) could be effective in decreasing graft rejection (BUTTURINI and GALE 1988), particularly in patients grafted with marrow from HLA-nonidentical donors (O'REILLY et al. 1985).

Viable and potentially functional T lymphocytes that may mediate graft rejection could be obtained from the blood of patients after they had received pretransplant conditioning with TBI given as a single dose (10 Gy) or in fractions (total dose 13.5 Gy) in combination with chemotherapy, and in some cases additional TLI (BUTTURINI et al. 1986). Obviously such T cells are rather resistant to what is termed an escalating conditioning regime.

4.11.2 Partial Chimerism and Autochthonous Regeneration

Evidence is accumulating that the different types of escalating conditioning regimens alone are insufficient to be ablative for pluripotent lymphohemopoietic stem cells. Surviving normal hemopoietic stem cells may lead to partial (i.e., mixed) chimerism or even complete autochthonous repopulation of the bone marrow.

PETZ et al. (1987), using several genetic markers, observed mixed hemopoietic chimerism in 29 of 172 patients who were treated for hematological malignancies with cyclophosphamide, cytosine arabinoside (ara-C), and TBI with a single dose of 10 or 7.5 Gy and thereafter were transplanted with unseparated bone marrow cells form HLA-identical donors. Some of the patients had severe GVHD, and 24 of the patients with mixed chimerism were in complete remission for up to 116 months after BMT. Obviously, hemopoietic chimerism is not rare after BMT for hematological malignancies and, as was concluded by the authors, its presence is compatible with long-term disease-free survival.

On the other hand, in dogs which had received TBI with a single dose of 11.7 Gy and thereafter were transplanted with allogeneic blood-derived cell suspensions, no surviving cell clone of reci-

146

pient type could be found in a long-term follow-up (CARBONELL et al. 1984). However, dogs which had received transplants from which the immune cells had been eliminated showed a long-lasting coexistence of lymphohemopoietic cells of both donor and host origin. Interestingly, none of the animals of this latter group showed any sign of GVHD, in contrast to the dogs in the former group, which all suffered from GVHD.

More detailed analyses showed that among patients transplanted with HLA-identical bone marrow from which the T cells had been eliminated, a high percentage bore mixed hemopoietic chimerism independent of whether TBI was given in a single dose or in fractions with a higher total dose (MASCRET et al. 1986; JANSSEN et al. 1986; BERTHEAS et al. 1988). Mixed chimerism obviously is more frequent in the blood lymphocytes than in marrow cells (HEINZE et al. 1987; BERTHEAS et al. 1988).

Based on an analysis of clinical data, DE WITTE et al. (1987) came to the conclusion that under conditions of histocompatible transplantations "mixed chimaerism occurs more frequently than previously believed, but may not necessarily be associated with a higher relapse rate." Generally, omission of TBI or fractionated TBI is associated with more recurrent host hemopoiesis; the absence of GVHD and T cell depletion of the donor marrow accounts for an increased incidence of mixed chimerism.

Under certain circumstances complete autochthonous hemopoietic reconstitution may occur after graft rejection (PATTERSON et al. 1986). This was confirmed in two patients who were transplanted for leukemia with T cell-depleted marrow from HLA-haploidentical donors after conditioning with cyclophosphamide and fractionated TBI with a total dose of 12.0 or 13.2 Gy (SONDEL et al. 1986).

These recent observations are not unexpected in the light of some reports from the early 1960s. In 1961, THOMAS et al. reported complete autochthonous bone marrow recovery in a 5-month-old infant who had received protracted TBI with a dose of 8.09 Gy (dose rate, 0.0054 Gy/min) and then undergone multiple allogeneic transplants of fetal liver cells and intensive supportive treatment. At the same time it was shown that in a dog, endogenous repopulation of the bone marrow occurred several weeks following TBI with a dose of 10 Gy and subsequent intensive transfusion support (HAGER et al. 1961).

4.11.3 Bone Marrow Regeneration

The repopulation of the bone marrow and the reestablishment of the normal functional properties after BMT following high dose chemoradiotherapy will depend on a variety of variables and their possible interactions.

Generally the integrity of the hemopoietic supportive stroma and the accessory cell systems of the recipient and their tolerance to the treatment are of major importance for engraftment of the transplanted cells, unless these elements are transplantable and able to grow in the recipient's marrow spaces similar to the hemopoietic stem cells. The same holds true for the stroma of the lymphatics, to which essential accessory cells belong, e.g., T cells. At least under allogeneic conditions GHVD may interfere with hemopietic regeneration.

4.11.3.1 Stromal Components

Based on their findings in long-term cultures that were prepared from bone marrow samples obtained from patients between 14 and 490 days after BMT, KEATING et al. (1982) concluded that the in vitro microenvironment in long-term cultures generated from marrow transplant recipients was donor derived. Comparable results, i.e., maintenance of donor-type CFU-F for at least 4 weeks in the marrow of lethally irradiated and bone marrow transplanted mice, were reported by PIERSMA et al. (1982). However, it is not the fact but the biological relevance of the presence of donor-type stromal elements in the host stroma (probably in small numbers) that has been questioned (MALONEY et al. 1985). Results obtained from murine transplantation models performed in combination with long-term bone marrow cultures have repeatedly shown that the progenitors of stromal fibroblastoid cells are not transplantable by intravenous injection (CHERTKOV et al. 1985; LENNON and MICKLEM 1986).

Recently, it was shown for bone marrow samples obtained from patients between 55 days and 3 years after transplantation that marrow-derived stromal cells proliferating in long-term cultures were of host genotype, whereas adherent macrophages in these cultures were of donor origin (SIMMONS et al. 1987). Such findings have been confirmed by others (RASKIND et al. 1988).

The changes in the bone marrow CFU-F in patients treated for leukemia with cyclophosphamide and fractionated TBI (with total doses of 12 or 14 Gy) and thereafter receiving HLA-identical sibling marrow transplants were studied by DA et al. (1986). At day 21 the number of CFU-F per ml bone marrow (aspirate) was found to be reduced to about 30% of the pretreatment value, but it had recovered to the normal range by day 42 after transplantation. Obviously, the regeneration kinetics of the CFU-F were not influenced by the presence of GVHD or immunosuppressive treatment (i.e., by methotrexate or cyclosporine). On the other hand, no apparent CFU-F reconstitution was reported in another study (REYNOLDS and MCCANN 1986). The possible implications of stromal dysfunctions for graft failure are considered in detail by PRZEPIORKA et al. (1988).

4.11.3.2 Hemopoietic Regeneration

The features of hemopoietic regeneration following BMT and the spectrum of abnormalities and complications observed, including experimental analyses of factors influencing engraftment, have been reviewed by BURAKOFF et al. (1983), BARRETT (1987), EMERSON and GALE (1987), MESSNER and YAMASAKI (1988), and PRZEPIORKA et al. (1988).

Peripheral blood granulocyte values generally increase after 2–3 weeks and normalize within 1 or 2 months. On the other hand, platelet recovery shows wide variations among individuals and is extremely delayed in many patients (BURAKOFF et al. 1983; ARNOLD et al. 1986; EMERSON and GALE 1987). Whether patients were conditioned with TBI or with a combination of busulfan and cyclophosphamide did not affect time from transplantation to engraftment (REYNOLDS and MCCANN 1986). Similarly, no differences in the recovery kinetics of the blood cell counts were found according to whether patients received transplants of unseparated bone marrow for either leukemia or aplastic anemia (ARNOLD et al. 1986).

Despite the normalization of the peripheral blood cell counts, the bone marrow cellularity, which showed a rapid increase during the first 56 days, was found to be subnormal in a high percentage of patients for more than 1 year, although it sometimes eventually attained the normal range after 3–5 years (ARNOLD et al. 1986; RUBIN et al. 1988). In contrast, others have reported that in most of their patients the bone marrow cellularity recovered to normal within 40 days and was stable thereafter (ATKINSON et al. 1982; LI et al. 1985). Indeed, the repopulation of the bone marrow in recipients is dependent on the cell number transfused if unseparated bone marrow is transplanted (BIANCO et al. 1986; MESSNER and YAMASAKI 1988); however, the reasons for the aforementioned differences remain unclear.

Delayed recovery of hemopoietic progenitor cells in the bone marrow and long-lasting persistence of subnormal concentrations have been reported by several groups as follows: for GM-CFC and CFU-E (REYNOLDS and MCCANN 1986), for GM-CFC, including a loss in their proliferative capacity in vitro (BARRETT and ADAMS 1981), for GM-CFC, BFU-E, and CFU-E (ARNOLD et al. 1986), for GM-CFC but not BFU-E (LI et al. 1985), and for GEMM-CFC, Meg-CFC, GM-CFC, and BFU-E (MESSNER and YAMASAKI 1988). Reports such as that by ATKINSON et al. (1982), showing the progenitor cell values to be somewhat reduced only in a minority of patients in the long term, are obviously rare.

No significant differences were observed in the kinetics of the blood cell recovery after fractionated TBI and HLA-identical BMT between patients who received unseparated and patients who received T cell-depleted bone marrow (O'REILLY et al. 1985). In another study the recovery of the bone marrow cellularity was found to be delayed in patients who had been transplanted with bone marrow from which the T cells had been eliminated by the antibody Campath-1 (ARNOLD et al. 1987) and in patients who had received transplants of unseparated bone marrow but were treated with methotrexate for GVHD prophylaxis (ARNOLD et al. 1986). Obviously, the granulocyte recovery in patients of the former group was depressed due to late complications.

The reasons for the reduced progenitor cell numbers in the bone marrow are not yet completely understood. A defect at the stem cell level has been suggested (ARNOLD et al. 1986), possibly due to impaired host factors (ARNOLD et al. 1982; BARRETT and ADAMS 1981). This would be in accordance with observations that in patients with acute leukemia the incidence of the pluripotent progenitor cells GEMM-CFC in bone marrow cell cultures is extremely low and increases after complete remission are achieved; however, the GEMM-CFC incidence remained subnormal in most of the bone marrow transplant recipients in whom engraftment was successful (MESSNER

1984). From recent studies it is evident that patients undergoing BMT show a reduced concentration of the various progenitor cells in the bone marrow even before treatment (MESSNER and YAMASAKI 1988). The reduced numbers of hemopoietic progenitors and their enhanced cycling over a long period of time after BMT (MESSNER and YAMASAKI 1988) need special attention if additional treatment is required.

The important role of accessory cells, either as part of the transplant, i.e., derived from the donor, or residing in the recipient, in regulating hemopoietic regeneration has become evident from clinical observations and experimental studies. Particularly T cell-mediated inhibition but also enhancement of colony-forming ability of progenitor cells in vitro could be established (for details see reviews by EMERSON and GALE 1987; TOROK-STORB 1988). Whether the same effects are operative in situ remains an open question. EMERSON et al. (1987) were able to show that adherent cells obtained from patients after BMT often produced near-normal functional burst-promoting activity (BPA) and granulocyte–macrophage colony-stimulating acticity (GM-CSA), but the Fc receptor-positive cells and T cells produced little if any BPA or GM-CSA in comparison with cells of the donor. The reason for such accessory cell dysfunctions is not clear.

4.11.3.3 Atypical Sites of Hemopoietic Activity

Extramedullary hemopoiesis and extension of hemopoietic tissue into the marrow space of the long bones are common features after BMT (ARNOLD et al. 1985). However, both are obviously not specifically associated with TBI since these abnormalities can also be observed in patients conditioned with cyclophosphamide only. Extramedullary hemopoiesis was found to be most pronounced in the spleen within the first 2 weeks after transplantation and was also present in the lymph nodes and the liver, i.e., at precisely the same time as the bone marrow stroma showed considerable damage. It thus may be speculated that the expansion of the hemopoietic tissue by extramedullary hemopoiesis is a compensatory event. However, the late extramedullary hemopoiesis in the spleen and the lymph nodes and also the persistence of hemopoietic activity in the femur shaft for at least 8–12 months, i.e., at times

when there seems to be sufficient hemopoiesis in regular medullary sites, remains unexplained. Reactivation of fetal-type stroma and stem cell functions was considered a possible reason by ARNOLD et al. (1985); however, damage to the stroma caused by the disease and/or the treatment might also have some influence.

4.11.3.4 Colony-Stimulating Activity

Recently, GEISSLER et al. (1988) studied the CSA in serum samples from patients undergoing BMT with respect to granulopoietic, erythropoietic, and megakaryopoietic stimulators. The results show that in patients who had received autologous transplants the levels of CSA in the serum generally remained low during the whole post-transplantation period. In contrast, sera obtained from patients who had undergone allogeneic BMT revealed a clear transient increase between day 8 and day 15 after treatment, inversely correlated with the blood granulocyte count. These findings demonstrate an adequate feedback mechanism during this period. Some other findings suggest that G-CSF (and not GM-CSF) might be particularly beneficial in stimulating granulocyto-/monocytopoiesis within the first few days after BMT.

The reason for the observed differences between patients receiving allogeneic transplants and those receiving autologous bone marrow are not clear. The defects may be due to the disease, and can be reversed by transplants from a normal donor. Interestingly, the same pattern of CSA changes as is observed in human allogeneic transplant recipients has been reported previously for dogs after TBI with a single dose of 11.7 Gy and transfusions of autologous blood-derived stem cells (NOTHDURFT et al. 1978).

4.12 Half Body Irradiation

4.12.1 Application for Systemic Therapy

In the early 1970s a wide field irradiation technique was introduced as an innovative approach to the palliative management of patients with advanced cancer. To meet the requirements for such treatment, namely to encompass as much disease as possible and to use a single dose as large as possible, but also to avoid compromising the hemopoietic tolerance, irradiation was limited to one half of the body. Half body irradiation (HBI) was given to the upper half of the body (UHBI) or to the lower half (LHBI) (FITZPATRICK and RIDER 1976a,b; SALAZAR et al. 1978).

Initially, bone marrow tolerance was expected to be the major limiting factor with this technique. The fraction of the bone marrow within the field during UHBI has been calculated to be approximately 57%–64% for an individual with normal bone marrow distribution (for references see NOTHDURFT et al. 1986, 1989; HERRMANN et al. 1988).

The first experience reported for patients with advanced cancer (FITZPATRICK and RIDER 1976a) was that UHBI with single doses of up to 8 or even 10 Gy (^{60}Co γ-rays, dose rate 0.5 Gy/min, or 25 MV x-rays, dose rate 2 Gy/min) was well tolerated by the bone marrow and that blood cell counts returned to pretreatment levels within 3–5 weeks. Similar observations were made in patients receiving the same doses for LHBI. Moreover, most of the patients in these initial trials could receive treatment of the other half of the body after an interval of 4–6 weeks. However, problems were encountered with sequential HBI when the second half of the body was irradiated before the blood cell counts had recovered to their normal range, e.g., at day 28 after the first exposure. Consequently blood cell counts were introduced as a guideline for therapy planning, and the second treatment was not given until the blood cell concentrations had reached their normal range (FITZPATRICK and RIDER 1976b). These studies clearly showed that sequential HBI allowed treatment of the whole body with single doses exceeding by far those that can be tolerated hematologically if given as TBI in single or multiple fractions.

SALAZAR et al. (1978), employing HBI to treat patients with occult or overt metastases from different types of cancer (lung, breast, multiple myeloma, lymphoma, etc.), reported transitory hematological toxicity in 91% of the patients after UHBI with a single dose of 8 Gy. But they also found that when the blood cell counts had returned to normal 6–8 weeks after the first exposure the other half of the body could be irradiated with the same dose without significant consequences. More recently, a report from the Radiation Therapy Oncology Group has summarized the hematological consequences of single dose HBI

applied for palliation in patients with multiple bone metastases (SALAZAR et al. 1986). After either LHBI or UHBI with doses of 8–10 Gy and 6–8 Gy, respectively, severe hematological toxicity and complications were observed only in those patients (10% and 32%, respectively) who had received prior chemotherapy courses and generally had very low baseline peripheral blood cell counts before irradiation. HERRMANN et al. (1988) reported a somewhat faster recovery of the blood granulocyte values after LHBI than after UHBI. These differences in the blood cell changes are in accordance with the different bone marrow volumes involved, i.e., approximately 40% for LHBI and 60% for UHBI.

In sequential HBI the second treatment is given when the granulocyte and the platelet counts have recovered from the first treatment or still are subnormal but at an acceptable level. This was generally found to require some 6–8 weeks (SALAZAR et al. 1978; QUASIM 1981; URTASUN et al. 1983; HÜTTNER et al. 1988), and 3–4 weeks at the least (STANDKE 1988) (see Fig. 4.13). However, LHBI as the second treatment caused a relatively more severe decrease in the blood granulocyte values than UHBI, and the recovery of the granulocytes and the platelets was sometimes delayed for as long as several months after the second exposure (QUASIM 1981; HERRMANN et al. 1988; STANDKE 1988; HÜTTNER et al. 1988). This indicates that the bone marrow in the upper half of the body had not completely recovered from the damage received from UHBI. However, no ob-

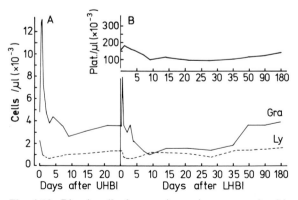

Fig. 4.13. Blood cell changes in patients treated with sequential HBI. **A** UHBI was given in two fractions of 4 Gy each separated by 6h; **B** LHBI was given as a single dose of 8 Gy. *Gra*, granulocytes; ---- *Ly*, lymphocytes; Platelets, after LHBI only. (After STANDKE 1988)

vious persistent damage could be detected in the bone marrow 6–8 weeks after the exposure (Salazar et al. 1978).

Because of the initial success achieved in palliation, HBI has been explored as consolidation therapy in combination with multiagent chemotherapy in patients with small cell carcinoma of the lung (Mason et al. 1982; Urtasun et al. 1983; Powell et al. 1985), breast cancer, gastrointestinal tumors, Ewing's sarcoma (Lombardi et al. 1982; Berry et al. 1986), and multiple myeloma (Jaffe et al. 1979; Thomas et al. 1984; Rostom 1988).

In patients who were treated for small cell carcinoma of the lung with HBI and multiagent chemotherapy, an increased incidence of bone marrow toxicity was observed. However, the intensive induction chemotherapy had already caused severe though transient leukopenia and thrombocytopenia at the time of UHBI; thus only a few patients were able to receive maintenance chemotherapy without delay (Mason et al. 1982). An increased incidence of bone marrow toxicity was also reported by Urtasun et al. (1983), who treated their patients with fractionated sequential HBI with a total dose of 10 Gy, given in four equal fractions. Powell et al. (1985) treated 41 patients with multiagent chemotherapy followed by sequential HBI with single doses of 6 Gy. Myelosuppression usually was the limiting toxicity, with thrombocytopenia (platelet values $<75 \times 10^3/\mu l$) leading to a delay in therapy in 27% of the patients.

In Ewing's sarcoma sequential HBI has been employed in patients with metastatic disease suffering a relapse after initial radiotherapy and chemotherapy (Lombardi et al. 1982), or as consolidation treatment following adjuvant chemotherapy for nonmetastatic disease (Berry et al. 1986). Lombardi et al. (1982) reported that myelosuppression is rarely severe. In patients initially treated with LHBI using a relatively low dose of 6 Gy there was no evidence of significant marrow depression. However, when UHBI was employed as the first treatment, some patients showed variable degrees of leuko- and/or thrombocytopenia. More severe decreases in the blood cell counts were observed in two patients who initially showed involvement of their marrow. Similarly, in the study performed by Berry et al. (1986) the treatment was not accompanied by dose-limiting bone marrow toxicity. However, after the second HBI the recovery of the blood cell concentration to normal levels was extremely delayed in some of the patients.

Interestingly, more severe bone marrow toxicity and hematological complications than usual resulted from HBI in patients with multiple myeloma refractory to standard chemotherapy (Rubin et al. 1985). Of interest are the observations by Jaffe et al. (1979) that UHBI resulted in greater hematological toxicity than LHBI, whether it was administered first or second. Thomas et al. (1984) treated seven patients with sequential HBI with a dose of 8 Gy for each exposure separated by an interval of 5–6 weeks. After LHBI, employed first, the hematological complications were mild. In contrast UHBI (as the second treatment) caused a strong depression in marrow function. Bone marrow recovery was achieved in five patients, but one died after 5 months from marrow aplasia. In the study reported by Rostom (1988) a decrease in hemoglobin was noted in half of the cases after the second treatment, and 40% of the patients required transfusions to correct anemia. All patients developed thrombocytopenia and nearly all developed leukopenia as well. These patients had been treated with UHBI and LHBI with single doses of 8.5 Gy separated by an interval of 4–6 weeks. Similar results had been reported by Tobias et al. (1985). Thus, the problems observed are the same as those reported for patients with lymphoma treated with fractionated TBI (see Sect. 4.10.2).

The return of the blood cell counts (granulocytes and thrombocytes) to the normal range after either UHBI or LHBI is taken to indicate that the previously irradiated bone marrow sites have recovered to such an extent that the second treatment given to the other half of the body will also be tolerated. However, it has to be considered that increased cell proliferation in the protected bone marrow (possibly associated with transient hyperplasia) is to some extent responsible for the recovery of the blood cell counts during the first weeks after irradiation (see Sect. 4.12.2).

4.12.2 Studies in Experimental Animals

The results from experimental studies using rabbits, mice, and dogs will provide some insight into how the bone marrow is able to compensate for the damage caused to large fractions of the whole organ, especially when sequential HBI is used.

In rabbits receiving radiation of the lower part of the body with single doses of 5 or 10 Gy, the GM-CFC concentration in the exposed femur was strongly depressed in a dose-dependent fashion immediately after irradiation (SCARANTINO et al. 1984). Recovery during the first 7 days was quite rapid after both radiation doses, and after 10 Gy there was even an overshoot in the GM-CFC (expressed as the ratio of GM-CFC numbers in irradiated and unirradiated femur) in the first weeks after irradiation. However, these latter results are difficult to interpret in light of the findings from the murine and canine studies.

In mice UHBI with a dose of 10 Gy caused a continuous decrease in the cellularity (i.e., degeneration) in the irradiated bone marrow up to day 4 (BRAUNSCHWEIG and STANDKE 1987). This was followed by a strong increase, leading to a peak value at day 8 after treatment. However, beyond day 10 the bone marrow cellularity remained stable at a subnormal level. In the protected bone marrow UHBI caused a strong compensatory increase in bone marrow cellularity with a predominance of granulocytopoiesis. After LHBI given as the second treatment, there was a decrease in cellularity in the previously unirradiated half of the body within the following 10 days. The recovery thereafter was quite fast. On the other hand, in contrast to what has been observed after UHBI given as the first exposure, there was no significant compensatory increase in bone marrow cellularity in sites of the upper body that remained protected during LHBI. This may be due to a significant contribution of the spleen to the compensatory response after LHBI performed as the second treatment. Furthermore, it is evident from these studies that in the mouse the hemopoietic regeneration is quite fast.

In canine studies UHBI and LHBI involved approximately 70% and 30%, respectively, of the total active marrow (NOTHDURFT et al. 1986, 1989; BALTSCHUKAT et al. 1989a). The general pattern of events in the GM-CFC compartment after UHBI or LHBI with single doses of 11.7 Gy each was similar; the same holds true for sequential HBI where LHBI was given as the second treatment 56 days after UHBI. The GM-CFC alterations in the bone marrow after UHBI are shown in Fig. 4.14. The dose of 11.7 Gy caused a reduction of the GM-CFC in the irradiated sites to unmeasurably low numbers, as expected. A first phase of repopulation occurred from day 7 to day 21, followed by a stabilization of the GM-CFC at clearly subnormal levels beyond day 120. At least 1 year after the exposure the GM-CFC values had returned to the normal range or were slightly subnormal. In the protected bone marrow the GM-CFC showed an immediate decrease, probably due to enhanced differentiation, and a transient compensatory increase thereafter due to enhanced proliferation. After LHBI involving only 30% of the total bone marrow mass the recovery of the GM-CFC in the irradiated sites was also extremely delayed, though in the initial phase of repopulation they attained slightly higher levels than after UHBI (BALTSCHUKAT et al. 1989a). However, due to the small volume irradiated the changes in the blood granulocyte values and thrombocyte counts were only marginal.

The experimental results obtained from sequential HBI of dogs (NOTHDURFT et al. 1989) can be summarized as follows: At day 56 after UHBI the GM-CFC in the irradiated bone marrow had recovered to between 30% and 40% of the pretreatment values. Despite this incomplete repopulation the GM-CFC compartment responded to LHBI in a fashion similar to the GM-CFC in the protected marrow after UHBI, i.e., with a transient increase in proliferation for at least 21 days, thus effectively compensating for the ablation of the bone marrow in the lower part of the body.

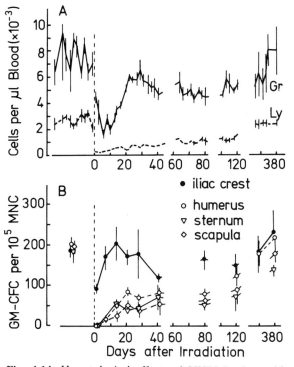

Fig. 4.14. Hematological effects of UHBI in dogs with a single dose of 11.7 Gy. **A** Changes in the concentration of the blood granulocytes (*Gr*) and lymphocytes (*Ly*). **B** Changes in the GM-CFC concentration in the bone marrow from the protected iliac crest (●), and from the irradiated humeri (○), sternum (▽), and scapulae (◇). (NOTHDURFT et al. 1986)

However, the LHBI caused a more severe depression in the blood granulocyte and thrombocyte counts than in dogs which had received LHBI as the only treatment. These findings are in accordance with the clinical observations mentioned previously, clearly indicating that at 8 weeks after UHBI when the second irradiation was performed the marrow had not completely recovered. Damage to the stroma has been considered as the most likely reason for these alterations (NOTHDURFT et al. 1989).

The initial repopulation at least within the first week of the highly irradiated bone marrow sites after either half body or sequential half body irradiation most probably is due to early seeding of circulating stem cells from the protected marrow sites (NOTHDURFT et al. 1986; 1989).

The kinetics of the bone marrow repopulation after HBI as observed in dogs suggest that in man, too, at least 3 or even 4 weeks are needed for the irradiated bone marrow (if not compromised by prior treatment) to attain a degree of regeneration that will allow an effective compensatory response when the other half of the body is irradiated. The clinical observations are in accordance with this assumption. On the other hand, the results from the canine studies suggest that after UHBI the bone marrow may recover faster in animals which have received additional LHBI than in those treated with UHBI alone.

4.13 Large-Field Irradiations in the Treatment of Malignant Lymphoma

Extended-field irradiation or sequential segmental irradiation as employed in the treatment of Hodgkin's disease (HD) or non-Hodgkin's lymphoma (NHL) involves irradiation of large fractions of the total active bone marrow with large total doses. The role of radiotherapy in the treatment of these diseases has been considered and evaluated in several articles and monographs, e.g., KAPLAN (1980), WASSERMAN and TUBIANA (1988), and HOPPE (1988).

The fraction of the bone marrow located in the fields may well equal or even exceed that irradiated under HBI. The bone marrow fractions receiving direct irradiation from the primary beam have been calculated to be 20%–30% for the mantle field, 30%–40% for an inverted-Y field, and approximately 50% for subtotal nodal irradia-

tion (including the mantle field, the para-aortic, and the spleen fields) (DROZ et al. 1978; PARMENTIER et al. 1988). Total nodal irradiation (TNI) involves 60%–75% of the total bone marrow mass (RUBIN et al. 1973; PARMENTIER et al. 1988) provided there is a normal anatomical distribution. The total doses given to a certain field or segment amount to 35–47 Gy and are delivered in five daily fractions of 1.5–2.0 Gy per week (COIA and HANKS 1988; HOPPE 1988; PARMENTIER et al. 1988; PROSNITZ 1988). It is important to note that in bone marrow outside the primary beam, scattered radiation may give 0.02–0.04 Gy per 2-Gy fraction with 6-MeV photons, or 0.10–0.20 Gy per 2-Gy fraction with ^{60}Co γ-rays; this has to be taken into account when considering bone marrow toxicity (RUBIN et al. 1973; PARMENTIER et al. 1988).

4.13.1 Changes in the Blood Cell Counts

The general features of the changes in the blood cell counts have been described in considerable detail by KAPLAN (1980) and can be summarized as follows. A cumulative dose of 40 Gy given to the mantle field over 4 weeks will generally cause a decrease in the platelet counts and the granulocyte values to approximately 50% of the pretreatment levels by the end of the treatment course. Immediate continuation of the treatment with the irradiation now given to the para-aortic and spleen fields very likely will cause only a moderate further reduction in the blood cell counts. However, further extension of the treatment to the pelvic field usually causes an additional drop in the white blood cell and/or the platelet count, to approximately 50% of the level attained at the completion of the mantle field treatment. Experience has shown that if a rest period of 2–4 weeks is permitted between the completion of the initial field and the resumption of irradiation to the other major field(s), leukopenia and/or thrombocytopenia may not develop or, if they do develop, may be moderate.

After sequential segmental irradiation, recovery of the platelet and white blood cell counts to normal levels may occur within 1 or 2 months (RUBIN et al. 1973), but this may also take 4 months or even longer (KAPLAN 1980). Recently, COIA and HANKS (1988) have reported that in 883 patients treated with infradiaphragmatic irradiation a total of 135 complications of any severity occurred, including 29 of a hematological nature that necessitated alterations in the planned course of therapy. The hematological toxicity described for TNI or less extensive irradiations was less in some studies (SLANINA et al. 1977) than in others (TIMOTHY et al. 1979).

Severe anemia obviously is less frequent than other hematological complications (SLANINA et al. 1977; KAPLAN 1980), but it may occur 1–2 months after TNI and persist for several months (PARMENTIER et al. 1983). WEIDEN et al. (1973) reported three patients who had been treated with sequential segmental irradiation alone or in combination with multiagent chemotherapy and who, between 1 month and 3 years later, had developed pancytopenia terminating in leukemia.

In individuals receiving chemotherapy before or during sequential segmental irradiation severe depression of the blood cell counts may occur, and recovery may be extremely delayed, by 6–7 months (RUBIN et al. 1973).

Blood granulocyte and platelet counts consistently higher than normal have been observed in patients subjected to splenectomy. Interestingly, in such patients the blood cell counts are less likely to decrease during treatment to such critical levels that modifications of the prescribed treatment are required (KAPLAN 1980). On the other hand, splenectomy has no obvious influence on the pattern of bone marrow regeneration (see review by PARMENTIER et al. 1988).

4.13.2 Bone Marrow

Analyses of the compensatory response of the bone marrow in nonirradiated areas and the in-field regeneration after extended-field irradiations or TNI are based on radioisotope whole body scanning, on ferrokinetic studies, including surface counting, on histological bone marrow evaluations, and in a few cases on progenitor cell determinations. The results of such investigations indicate that the response of the bone marrow is influenced by many factors.

The problems associated with the use of the various radioisotopes usually applied in bone marrow studies, such as ^{59}Fe (or ^{52}Fe), ^{99m}Tc-sulfur colloid, and ^{111}In, are discussed by PARMENTIER et al. (1988). A considerable body of data obtained from bone marrow analyses has been considered and reviewed by RUBIN et al. (1973), KAPLAN (1980), and PARMENTIER et al. (1988).

Whereas bone marrow scanning using Fe or ^{111}In and bone marrow examinations through biopsy usually revealed normal bone marrow activity (RUBIN et al. 1973; DEGOWIN et al. 1974; KNOSPE et al. 1976; HILL et al. 1980), the GM-CFC concentration obviously is subnormal in most of the patients (BULL et al. 1975; DROZ et al. 1978).

Suppression of the uptake of the radioisotopes in the irradiated fields and little or no activity at the completion of irradiation with total doses ranging from 30–50 Gy has been reported for extended-field irradiation, sequential segmental irradiation, and TNI, regardless of whether ^{99m}Tc-sulfur colloid (RUBIN et al. 1973), ^{59}Fe (DEGOWIN et al. 1974), or ^{111}In (SACKS et al. 1978) was applied. Furthermore, the GM-CFC were found to be reduced to undetectable numbers (DROZ et al. 1978).

4.13.2.1 Compensatory Responses

Based on the results obtained from bone marrow scanning, RUBIN et al. (1973) concluded that in the early postirradiation period the nonirradiated iliac crests and the heads of the humeri and the femora are the major sites of hemopoietic function. A compensatory increase in erythropoietic activity in the nonirradiated areas which are normally hemopoietic (iliac crest, sacrum) was also established by PARMENTIER et al. (1983) at least 2 months after irradiation, and interestingly the hyperactivity in these sites persisted for up to 13 years after treatment. STEERE et al. (1979) also observed that in patients who showed a decreased marrow uptake of ^{52}Fe in the irradiated region there was a compensatory increased uptake in the areas of nonirradiated normally active marrow. Such hyperactivity was found within a few months after completion of the treatment and persisted for 6 years or more in those patients who showed delayed in-field recovery of hemopoietic activity. DEGOWIN et al. (1974) suggested that hyperplasia of hemopoietic tissue in the axial skeleton (including the ribs) may compensate for the ablation of vertebral and pelvic marrow. Though no data are available just for these irradiation conditions, it is legitimate to assume that the compensatory mechanisms in the nonirradiated areas are similar to those already described for HBI, i.e., enhanced cycling of hemopoietic progenitors, possibly associated with local hyperplasia, and that these mechanisms will become operative during the course of treatment.

Extension of hemopoietic tissue to previously inactive areas (containing fat marrow), such as the long bones of the extremities, is an additional way of compensating for the damage to large fractions of the bone marrow in the axial skeleton. Knospe et al. (1976) found extension of active marrow, as measured by ^{52}Fe marrow scanning, 3–12 months after irradiation, followed by regression. In contrast, Rubin et al. (1973) reported marrow extension to some degree in 50% of patients, appearing after the 1st year following treatment. Hill et al. (1980) observed marked peripheral extension of the marrow in 57% of the patients with marrow activity in the irradiated volume at 9 months or more following irradiation. Interestingly, the incidence of marrow extension was lower among those patients who showed no bone marrow activity in the irradiated volume. Parmentier et al. (1983) reported extension of the hemopoietic tissue into distal bones up to 8 years or more after mantle field irradiation. In four of six patients who had been treated with irradiation to the mantle and the inverted-Y field, ^{59}Fe scintigraphy revealed bone marrow extension from 26 months to 10.5 years after irradiation. An expanded bone marrow space associated with decreased cellularity was observed in a patient developing pancytopenia (Weiden et al. 1973). However, in contrast to the above findings, Steere et al. (1979) could detect no extension of active bone marrow up to 8 years after treatment under comparable conditions.

4.13.2.2 In-field Regeneration and Tolerance Doses

A progressive increase in the percentage of bone marrow volumes that did not incorporate ^{99m}Tc-sulfur colloid was observed by Hill et al. (1980) within the first 6 months after treatment of the field in question with doses in the range of 40 Gy. Thereafter in the period up to 1 year following irradiation the proportion of completely inactive marrow volume decreased from 100% to approximately 50% and remained at that level up to 3 years. After 12 years of treatment the fraction of completely inactive bone marrow volumes had been further reduced to 30%. A somewhat faster recovery (though also measured with ^{99m}Tc-sulfur colloid) was reported by Rubin et al. (1973) for bone marrow sites that in the course of

extended-field or sequential segmental irradiation had received doses from 40 to 50 Gy.

Using ^{52}Fe scanning, Knospe et al. (1976) found suppression of erythropoiesis in most irradiation fields treated with doses of 40–44 Gy, with the maximum occurring in patients scanned less than 6 months after treatment. Some recovery of erythropoietic activity was observed from 6 to 12 months after irradiation. During the following 12 months and more, progressive improvement of hemopoietic function took place. In contrast, DeGowin et al. (1974) reported a delayed recovery of erythropoietic activity for 1–3 years in fields that had received total doses of 35–40 Gy. Similarly, Steere et al. (1979) observed that 1 year appears to be the minimum time before the uptake of Fe in the marrow in fields that have received radiation doses of 30–40 Gy begins to recover. Furthermore, these authors found that in some patients the iron uptake in the marrow returned to nearly normal levels within 1–3 years, but that in other patients the erythropoietic activity recovered slowly within 6 years after completion of treatment. Limited recovery of erythropoietic function within 10–13 years after treatment was reported by Parmentier et al. (1983) for bone marrow areas that had been irradiated with total doses in the range of 40 Gy.

Sacks et al. (1978), using ^{111}In for scanning, observed that after TNI with total doses from 30 to 50 Gy most regenerative activity takes place within the first year, and that over the following 5 years and beyond there is a slight trend toward increased regeneration; this is in general agreement with the data of Hill et al. (1980) and Parmentier et al. (1983).

The results from these studies indicate delay of hemopoietic recovery for several years in sites located in fields treated with total doses from 30 to 50 Gy. However, there are obviously some quantitative differences between the results reported from different studies. In part these discrepancies may be due to the fact that the tests using the different radioisotopes do not reflect the microscopic appearance of the regenerating bone marrow. Histological studies of bone marrow aspirates obtained from sites that had been irradiated 3 years before with doses from 35 to 46 Gy revealed various degrees of hypocellularity and a patchy appearance of partially regenerated marrow, but no normal appearances (DeGowin et al. 1974; Knospe et al. 1976). Slanina et al. (1977) reported quantitative data derived from cytological examinations of aspirates from the irradiated sternum of 73 patients treated with doses between 26 and 46 Gy. Normal marrow was found in 4% of these patients, and hypoplastic marrow in 16%; in the remaining 80% there was evidence of aplastic marrow. The extent of bone marrow damage was similar in patients controlled within the first 5 years after treatment and those controlled at later intervals. Furthermore, cytologically normal bone marrow was observed only after doses below 40 Gy.

Owing to differences in the range of doses employed, the techniques applied for measuring bone marrow activity, and the criteria used for defining bone marrow recovery, it is difficult to compare the results from the different studies. However, there is general agreement over the conclusions drawn with respect to bone marrow tolerance.

RUBIN et al. (1973) stated that it is reasonable to conclude that bone marrow recovery is achieved consistently at levels of 40 Gy and is time dependent as well as dose dependent. According to KNOSPE et al. (1976), it appears that the dose required to consistently cause permanent aplasia is well over 44 Gy. STEERE et al. (1979) pointed to the large variations in bone marrow recovery and concluded that there is no sharp threshold in the dose range from 30 to 40 Gy at which the bone marrow can no longer recover. Summarizing the essential results of their studies, HILL et al. (1980) similarly concluded that no threshold dose for ablation or regeneration can be demonstrated in the dose range from 35 Gy to as much as 50 Gy. However, in the studies by SACKS et al. (1978) there appeared to be a sharp decrease in the extent of bone marrow regeneration at doses larger than 40 Gy in patients who had received TNI, in contrast to the findings in those who had received limited-field irradiation only.

4.13.3 Extramedullary Hemopoiesis

In three patients, PARMENTIER et al. (1983) found extramedullary erythropoiesis in the liver or spleen or both 4 months to 13 years after treatment to the mantle field. Among 24 patients who received irradiation to the mantle and inverted-Y fields, 19 showed extramedullary erythropoiesis between 1 month and 10 years after irradiation. However, STEERE et al. (1979), who also applied quantitative scanning (^{52}Fe), did not find any evidence of extramedullary erythropoiesis.

4.13.4 Factors Influencing Hemopoietic Regeneration

KNOSPE et al. (1976) observed that after TNI bone marrow regeneration in the pelvic bones was more delayed than in bone marrow sites located in the mantle field. However, whether these differences were due to anatomical differences in the sensitivity remained open, since usually the pelvic field was the last to be irradiated. Based on a more thorough analysis of various factors that might influence bone marrow regeneration, SACKS et al. (1978), using ^{111}In scanning, reported the following findings:

1. In patients who had undergone limited-field irradiation, the extent of regeneration observed at various dose levels was less than that in the irradiated bone marrow of patients who had received TNI (Fig. 4.15). Such observations were confirmed for recovery of erythropoietic function (PARMENTIER et al. 1983) as well as for granulocytopoiesis as assessed by GM-CFC determinations (MORARDET et al. 1978).
2. Bone marrow function in patients under the age of 20 years invariably recovered to normal or nearly normal levels irrespective of the radiation dose, unlike in older patients (Fig. 4.15). Some observations by STEERE et al.

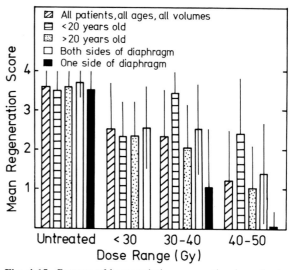

Fig. 4.15. Pattern of hemopoietic regeneration in patients treated for Hodgkin's disease as a function of the dose ranges employed. The influence of the volume treated and age at the time of treatment is shown separately.
(From SACKS et al. 1978, with modifications; with permission of J.B. Lippincott Company, Philadelphia, and the authors)

(1979) also suggest a somewhat faster hemopoietic recovery in individuals under the age of 26 years than in older ones.

3. Analysis of the temporal pattern of bone marrow recovery indicated that most regenerative activity took place within the first 12 months following treatment and that in the period thereafter there was only a slight trend toward further regeneration. These observations are in accordance with the reports by HILL et al. (1980) and PARMENTIER et al. (1973), but are at variance with the data reported by RUBIN et al. (1973), KNOSPE et al. (1976), and STEERE et al. (1979).

Recovery of the bone marrow function in irradiated areas is not stimulated by adjuvant chemotherapy or chemotherapy given for treatment of relapse several years after radiotherapy (STEERE et al. 1979; PARMENTIER et al. 1983). On the other hand, it has been shown that hemopoietic tolerance to chemotherapy improves with time after extensive radiotherapy (CURRAN and JOHNSON 1970; HASKELL and PARKER 1980).

Taken together, all the observations in patients during and after extended-field and sequential segmental irradiation clearly indicate that the bone marrow has to be considered as one organ despite its wide anatomical distribution. Destruction of the hemopoietic tissue in irradiated areas is compensated primarily by prolonged increases in activity in nonirradiated areas that are normally active (such as the iliac crests, the heads of the humeri and the femora, and the ribs) (RUBIN et al. 1973; DEGOWIN et al. 1974; KNOSPE et al. 1976; STEERE et al. 1979; PARMENTIER et al. 1983). Any damage to these sites by scattered radiation will reduce their compensatory capacity. Extension of the hemopoietic tissue into marrow spaces normally inactive in the adult and, perhaps, extramedullary hemopoiesis appear to play a role at later times in maintaining sufficient hemopoietic activity, possibly for a limited period only (RUBIN et al. 1973; KNOSPE et al. 1976; HILL et al. 1980; PARMENTIER et al. 1983).

The aforementioned facts offer an explanation for the apparent paradox of hemopoietic regeneration after irradiation with large doses. That is, if limited fields are irradiated and small bone marrow fractions are involved, there is less hemopoietic regeneration than after TNI, where a major fraction of the bone marrow is destroyed (see above). In this latter case the fraction of nonirradi-

ated marrow is too small to maintain hemopoietic equilibrium, even if there is maximal compensatory hyperactivity.

4.14 Radiation Sensitivity of Bone Marrow Cells in Patients with Genetic Disorders

Certain human genetic disorders are associated with a high incidence of malignancy. Furthermore, some of these syndromes are characterized by an excessive sensitivity of the individuals to ionizing radiation [e.g., the autosomal recessive disease ataxia telangiectasia (AT)], giving rise to severe complications if radiotherapy is employed at conventional doses (ABADIR and HAKAMI 1983; PRITCHARD et al. 1982).

Recently, HART et al. (1987) estimated the radiation dose for the treatment of a medulloblastoma in a patient with AT on the basis of the radiation response characteristics of GM-CFC obtained from his bone marrow. When irradiated in vitro the GM-CFC showed a considerably higher radiosensitivity ($D_0 = 0.32$ Gy) than GM-CFC from normal donors ($D_0 = 0.98$ Gy). Based on these findings, the fraction size and total radiation dose employed were reduced by a factor of nearly 3. The skin reaction in this patient was similar to that in normal patients receiving the standard treatment schedule. The patient was doing well at least for more than 6 months after radiation therapy, showing that determinations of the radiosensitivity of hemopoietic progenitor cells can be essential for individual treatment planning.

4.15 Modulation of Hemopoietic Recovery by Treatment with Cytokines

One of the most important advances in the field of hematological research has been the biochemical and biological characterization of hemopoietic growth factors and their molecular cloning. Several of the various factors produced by modern gene techniques, i.e., recombinant or derived from their natural sources, have now been tested in experimental animals and administered to patients to accelerate bone marrow recovery after irradiation and high dose TBI followed by BMT.

Recombinant human granulocyte-macrophage colony-stimulating factor, rhGM-CSF (reviewed recently by CLARK 1988), when given continuously over several days, has been shown to shorten the period of neutropenia and thrombocytopenia and to accelerate bone marrow recovery in monkeys after TBI and autologous BMT (NIENHUIS et al. 1987; MONROY et al. 1987). Furthermore, treatment of monkeys with this factor after inhomogeneous TBI led to a faster autochthonous recovery of the bone marrow GM-CFC when compared with animals receiving no such treatment (MONROY et al. 1988).

Treatment of patients involved in the Brazil radiation accident of September 1987 with rhGM-CSF similarly caused prompt increases in the blood granulocyte values and the bone marrow cellularity (BUTTURINI et al. 1988); and daily infusions for 2 weeks of GM-CFC also led to increased granulocyte counts and increased bone marrow cellularity associated with GM-CFC activity in patients with secondary bone marrow failure resulting from chemotherapy or radiotherapy (VADHAN-RAJ et al. 1988). Continuous administration over 14–21 days of rhGM-CSF to patients treated for ALL, Hodgkin's disease, or non-Hodgkin's lymphoma with chemotherapy alone or with chemotherapy in combination with TBI (8.5 or 12 Gy, fractionated) and autologous bone marrow transplants caused an earlier and faster neutrophil recovery when compared with untreated controls (BLAZAR et al. 1988; LINK et al. 1988).

Another factor of this class, rhG-CSF, was also found to be effective in monkeys in reducing the phase of neutropenia after TBI and autologous BMT when administered over 4 weeks (WELTE et al. 1988).

Interleukin-1 (IL-1) (see reviews by DINARELLO 1988, PANTEL and NAKEFF 1989) has been shown to increase survival in lethally irradiated mice if given as a single injection within a certain time interval before irradiation (NETA et al. 1986). Furthermore, when IL-1 was injected in combination with GM-CSF there was a clear synergistic effect on survival, though the GM-CSF was completely ineffective if given alone at the same dose (see review by HENNEY 1988). Recently, SCHWARTZ et al. (1988) showed that injection of IL-1 promotes an earlier recovery of mature cells in the blood, and of CFU-S, GM-CFC, BFU-E, and CFU-E in the bone marrow. IL-1 was also found to accelerate the hemopoietic recovery in mice when it was

given for several days after irradiation (MORRISSEY et al. 1987).

These results in experimental and clinical studies indicate that under the given conditions without treatment of the growth factors the hemopoietic cell populations are obviously not operating at the maximum of their regenerative capacity.

Acknowledgment. This work was supported in part by the Bundesminister für Umwelt, Naturschutz und Reaktorsicherheit (St. Sch 1.029) and the Commission of the European Communities [Contract BI-6-0061-1 (B)].

References

Abadir R, Hakami N (1983) Ataxia telangiectasia with cancer. An indication for reduced radiotherapy and chemotherapy doses. Br J Radiol 56: 343–345

Ainsworth EJ, Leong GF, Alpen EL (1984) Early radiation mortality and recovery in large animals and primates. In: Broerse JJ, MacVittie TJ (eds) Response of different species to total body irradiation. Martinus Nijhoff, Boston, pp 87–111

Allen TD, Dexter TM (1984) The essential cells of the hemopoietic microenvironment. Exp Hematol 12: 517–521

Armed Forces Radiobiology Research Institute (AFRRI) (1979) Medical effects of nuclear weapons. Bethesda

Arnold R, Heit W, Heimpel H, Frickhofen N, Schmeiser T, Kubanek B (1982) The reconstitution of haemopoietic precursors after bone marrow transplantation. Exp Hematol 10 [Suppl 10]: 79–82

Arnold R, Calvo, Heymer B, Schmeiser T, Heimpel H, Kubanek B (1985) Extramedullary haemopoiesis after bone marrow transplantation. Scand J Haematol 34: 9–12

Arnold R, Schmeiser T, Heit W, Frickhofen N, Pabst G, Heimpel H, Kubanek B (1986) Hemopoietic reconstitution after bone marrow transplantation. Exp Hematol 14: 271–277

Arnold R, Wiesneth M, Raghavachar A et al. (1987) Haemopoietic reconstitution after BMT: comparison of the influence of two different methods of GVHD prophylaxis. Bone Marrow Transplantation 2 [suppl 1]: p 183

Ash RC, Detrick RA, Zanjani ED (1981) Studies of human pluripotential hemopoietic stem cells (CFU-GEMM) in vitro. Blood 58: 309–316

Atkinson HR (1962) Bone marrow distribution as a factor in estimating radiation to the blood-forming organs: a survey of present knowledge. J Coll Radiol Aust 6: 149–154

Atkinson K, Norrie S, Chan P, Biggs J (1982) Bone marrow cellularity and blood and marrow myeloid and erythroid stem cell colony growth during the first three months after allogeneic marrow transplantation for severe aplastic anaemia or acute leukaemia. Exp Hematol 10 [Suppl 11]: p 34 (abstract)

Axelrad AA, McLeod DL, Shreeve MM, Heath DS (1974) Properties of cells that produce erythrocytic colonies in vitro. In: Robinson WA (ed) Hemopoiesis in culture. Grune & Stratton, New York, pp 226–234

Baird MC, Hendry JH, Testa NG (1988) The radiosensitivity of different sub-populations of colony forming cells in the haemopoietic hierarchy. Int J Radiat Biol 53: 1004 (abstract)

Baltschukat K, Nothdurft W (1990) Hematological effects of unilateral and bilateral exposures of dogs to 300 KVp x-rays. Radiat Res 123: 7–16

Baltschukat K, Fliedner TM, Nothdurft W (1989a) Hematological effects in dogs after irradiation of the lower part of the body with a single myeloablative dose. Radiother Oncol 14: 239–246

Baltschukat K, Kreja L, Nothdurft W, Weinsheimer W (1989b) Acute and long-term alterations of erythroid burst forming units (BFU-E) in dogs after total body irradiation. 22nd Annual Meeting of the European Society Radiation Biology, Brussels, 11–16 Sept 1989. Book of Abstracts, abstract p 127

Barrett A (1982) Total body irradiation before bone marrow transplantation: a review. Clin Radiol 33: 131–135

Barrett A (1984) Total body irradiation and LD 50 in man. In: Broerse JJ, MacVittie TJ (ed) Response of different species to total body irradiation. Martinus Nijhoff, Boston, pp 205–208

Barrett AJ (1987) Bone marrow transplantation. Cancer Treat Rev 14: 203–213

Barrett AJ, Adams J (1981) A proliferative defect of human bone marrow after transplantation. Br J Haematol 49: 159–164

Bateman JL, Bond VP, Robertson JS (1962) Dose-rate dependence of early radiation effects in small mammals. Radiology 79: 1008–1114

Baumann B, Muth H (1977) Zur Frage der Erholungsfähigkeit von Säugetieren nach akuter subletaler Ganzkörperbestrahlung mit energiereichen Strahlen unter Berücksichtigung des jugendlichen Organismus. In: Messerschmidt O, Möhrle G, Zimmer R et al. (eds) Vorsorgemedizin und Strahlenschutz (Risiko/Nutzen-Analyse). Erholungsvorgänge nach Strahleneinwirkung. Medizinische Aspekte der Strahlenschutzgesetzgebung in verschiedenen europäischen Ländern. Strahlenschutz Forsch Prax XVIII: 35–45

Baverstock KF, Papworth DG, Townsend KMS (1985) Man's sensitivity to bone marrow failure following whole body exposure to low LET ionizing radiation: inferences to be drawn from animal experiments. Int J Radiat Biol 47: 397–411

Becker AJ, McCulloch EA, Siminovitch L, Till JE (1965) The effects of differing demands for blood cell production on DNA synthesis by hemopoietic colony-forming cells of mice. Blood 26: 296–308

Belletti S, Gallini RE, Magno L (1979) The effects of dose rate on hematopoietic stem cells: preliminary results. Int J Radiat Oncol Biol Phys 5: 403–405

Ben-Ishay Z, Prindull G, Sharon S, Borenstein A (1986) Pre-CFU-f: young-type stromal stem cells in murine bone marrow following administration of DNA inhibitors. Int J Cell Cloning 4: 126–134

Berry MP, Jenkin RDT, Harwood AR, Cummings BJ, Quirt IC, Sonley MJ, Rider WD (1986) Ewing's sarcoma: a trial of adjuvant chemotherapy and sequential half-body irradiation. Int J Radiat Oncol Biol Phys 12: 19–24

Bertheas MF, Maraninchi D, Lafage M et al. (1988) Partial chimerism after T-cell-depleted allogeneic bone marrow transplantation in leukemic HLA-matched patients: a cytogenetic documentation. Blood 72: 89–93

Bianco P, Arcese W, Papa G et al. (1986) Histopathological patterns of marrow failure in allogeneic bone marrow transplantation for CML. Bone Marrow Transplantation 1 [Suppl 1]: 242–243

Blackett NM (1987) Haemopoietic spleen colony growth: a versatile, parsimonious, predictive model. Cell Tissue Kinet 20: 393–402

Blazar BR, Widmer MB, Kersey JH et al. (1988) Recombinant granulocyte/macrophage colony stimulating factor in human and murine bone marrow transplantation. Behring Inst Mitt 83: 170–180

Blume KG (1986) A review of bone marrow transplantation. Int J Cell Cloning 4 [Suppl 1]: 3–10

Boersma WJA (1983) Radiation sensitivity and cycling status of mouse bone marrow prothymocytes and day 8 colony forming units spleen (CFUs). Exp Hematol 11: 922–930

Boggs SS, Boggs DR (1973) Cell cycling characteristics of exogenous spleen colony-forming units. J Lab Clin Med 82: 740–753

Boggs SS, Boggs DR (1975) Earlier onset of hematopoietic differentiation after expansion of the endogenous stem cell pool. Radiat Res 63: 165–173

Bond VP (1969) Radiation mortality in different mammalian species. In: Bond VP, Sugahara T (eds) Comparative cellular and species radiosensitivity. Igaku Shoin, Tokyo, pp 5–19

Bond VP, Robinson CV (1967) A mortality determinant in nonuniform exposures of the mammal. Radiat Res [Suppl] 7: 265–275

Bond VP, Fliedner TM, Archambeau JO (1965) Mammalian radiation lethality. A disturbance in cellular kinetics. Academic, New York

Bonsdorff E, Jalavisto E (1948) A humoral mechanism in anoxic erythrocytosis. Acta Physiol Scand 16: 150–170

Bøyum A, Carsten AL, Chikkappa G, Cook L, Bullis J, Honikel L, Cronkite EP (1978) The r.b.e. of different-energy neutrons as determined by human bone-marrow cell-culture techniques. Int J Radiat Biol 34: 201–212

Bradley TR, Hodgson GS, Kriegler AB, McNiece IK (1985) Generation of CFU-S$_{13}$ in vitro. In: Cronkite EP, Dainiak N, McCaffrey RP, Palek J, Quesenberry PJ (eds) Hematopoietic stem cell physiology. Alan R. Liss, New York, pp 39–56

Braunschweig R, Standke E (1987) Knochenmarkveränderungen nach Halbkörperbestrahlung. Radiobiol Radiother (Berl) 28: 465–472 (summary in English)

Briganti G, Mauro F (1979) Differences in radiation sensitivity in subpopulations of mammalian multicellular systems. Int J Radiat Oncol Biol Phys 5: 1095–1101

Brochstein JA, Kernan NA, Groshen S et al. (1987) Allogeneic bone marrow transplantation after hyperfractionated total-body irradiation and cyclophosphamide in children with acute leukemia. Engl J Med 317: 1618–1624

Broerse JJ (1969) Dose-mortality studies for mice irradiated with x-rays, gamma-rays and 15 MeV neutrons. Int J Radiat Biol 15: 115–124

Broerse JJ, Engels AC, Lelieveld P et al. (1971) The survival of colony-forming units in mouse bone-marrow after in vivo irradiation with D-T neutrons, x- and γ-radiation. Int J Radiat Biol 19: 101–110

Bromer RH, Mitchell JB, Soares N (1982) Response of human hematopoietic precursor cells (CFUc) to hyperthermia and radiation. Cancer Res 42: 1261–1265

Broxmeyer HE (1986) Biomolecule-cell interactions and the regulation of myelopoiesis. Int J Cell Cloning 4: 378–405

Broxmeyer HE, Galbraith PR, Baker FL (1976) Relationship of colony-stimulating activity to apparent kill of human colony-forming cells by irradiation and hydroxyurea. Blood 47: 403–411

Buescher ES, Gallin JI (1984) Radiation effects on cultured human monocytes and on monocyte–derived macrophages Blood 63: 1402–1407

Bull JM, De Vita VT, Carbone PP (1975) In vitro granulocyte production in patients with Hodgkin's disease and lymphocytic, histiocytic and mixed lymphomas. Blood 45: 833–842

Burakoff SJ, Lipton JM, Nathan DG (1983) Recapitulation of the immune response and haematopoietic system in bone marrow transplantation. Clin Haematol 12: 695–720

Burstein SA, Harker LA (1983) Control of platelet production. Clin Haematol 12: 3–22

Button LN, DeWolf WC, Newburger PE, Jacobsen MS, Kevy SV (1981) The effects of irradiation on blood components. Transfusion 21: 419–426

Butturini A, Gale RP (1988) T cell depletion in bone marrow transplantation for leukemia: current results and future directions. Bone Marrow Transplantation 3: 185–192

Butturini A, Seeger RC, Gale RP (1986) Recipient immune-competent T lymphocytes can survive intensive conditioning for bone marrow transplantation. Blood 68: 954–956

Butturini A, Gale RP, Lopes DM et al. (1988) Use of recombinant granulocyte-macrophage colony stimulating factor in the Brazil radiation accident Lancet II: 471–475

Caffrey RW, Everett NB, Rieke WO (1966) Radioautographic studies of reticular and blast cells in the hemopoietic tissues of the rat. Anat Rec 155: 41–58

Carabell SC, Chaffey JT, Rosenthal DS, Moloney WC, Hellman S (1979) Results of total body irradiation in the treatment of advanced non-Hodgkin's lymphomas. Cancer 43: 994–1000

Carbonell F, Calvo W, Fliedner TM et al. (1984) Cytogenetic studies in dogs after total body irradiation and allogeneic transfusion with cryopreserved blood mononuclear cells: observations in long-term chimeras. Int J Cell Cloning 2: 81–88

Carsten AL (1984) Acute lethality – the hemopoietic syndrome in different species. In: Broerse JJ, MacVittie TJ (eds) Response of different species to total body irradiation. Martinus Nijhoff, Boston, pp 59–86

Casarett GW (1969) Pattern of recovery from large single-dose exposure to radiation. In: Bond VP, Sugahara T (eds) Comparative cellular and species radiosensitivity. Igaku Shoin, Tokyo, pp 42–52

Castro-Malaspina H, Gay RE, Resnick G et al. (1980) Characterization of human bone marrow fibroblast colony forming cells (CFU-F) and their progeny. Blood 56: 289–301

Chaffey JT, Hellman S (1969) Radiation fractionation as applied to murine colony-forming cells in differing proliferative states. Radiology 93: 1167–1172

Chaffey JT, Hellman S (1971) Differing responses to radiation of murine bone marrow stem cells in relation to the cell cycle. Cancer Res 31: 1613–1615

Chaffey JT, Rosenthal DS, Pinkus G, Hellman S (1975) Advanced lymphosarcoma treated by total body irradiation. Br J Cancer 31 [Suppl II]: 441–449

Champlin RE, Gale RP (1984) Role of bone marrow transplantation in the treatment of hematologic malignancies and solid tumors: critical review of syngeneic, autologous, and allogeneic transplants. Cancer Treat Rep 68: 145–161

Chen MG (1974) Impaired Elkind recovery in hematopoietic colony-forming cells of aged mice. Proc Soc Exp Biol Med 145: 1181–1186

Chen MG, Schooley JC (1970) Recovery of proliferative capacity of agar colony-forming cells and spleen colony-forming cells following ionizing radiation or vinblastine. J Cell Physiol 75: 89–96

Chertkov JL, Drize NJ, Gurevitch OA, Samoylova RS (1985) Origin of hemopoietic stromal progenitor cells in chimeras. Exp Hematol 13: 1217–1222

Chervenick PA, Boggs DR (1971) Patterns of proliferation and differentiation of hematopoietic stem cells after compartment depletion. Blood 37: 568–580

Cillo C, Sekaly RP, Magli MC, Odartchenko N (1985) Early hemopoietic progenitor cells: direct measurement of cell cycle status. In: Bond VP, Chandra P, Rai KR (eds) Hematopoietic cellular proliferation. Ann NY Acad Sci 459: 150–161

Clark SC (1988) Biological activities of human granulocyte-macrophage colony-stimulating factor. Int J Cell Cloning 6: 365–367

Clark SC, Kamen R (1987) The human hematopoietic colony-stimulating factors. Science 236: 1229–1237

Coggle JE (1980) Absence of late radiation effects on bone marrow stem cells. Int J Radiat Biol 38: 589–595

Coggle JE, Gordon MY (1975) Quantitative measurements on the haemopoietic systems of three strains of mice. Exp Hematol 3: 181–186

Coia LR, Hanks GE (1988) Complications from large field intermediate dose infradiaphragmatic radiation: an analysis of the Patterns of Care Outcome Studies for Hodgkin's disease and seminoma. Int J Radiat Oncol Biol Phys 15: 29–35

Constine LS, Rubin P (1988) Total body irradiation: normal tissue effects. In: Bleehen NM (ed) Radiobiology in radiotherapy. Springer, London Berlin Heidelberg New York, pp 95–121

Cowall DE, MacVittie TJ, Parker GA, Weinberg SR (1981) Effects of low-dose total-body irradiation on canine bone marrow function and canine lymphoma. Exp Hematol 9: 581–587

Croizat H, Frindel E, Tubiana M (1979) Long term radiation effects on the bone marrow stem cells of C_3H mice. Int J Radiat Biol 36: 91–99

Cronkite EP (1985) Regulation and structure of hemopoiesis: its application in toxicology. In: Irons RD (ed) Toxicology of the blood and bone marrow. Raven, New York, pp 17–38

Cronkite EP (1988) Analytical review of structure and regulation of hemopoiesis. Blood Cells 14: 313–328

Cronkite EP, Bond VP (1960) Diagnosis of radiation injury and analysis of the human lethal dose of radiation. US Armed Forces Med J 11: 249–260

Cronkite EP, Fliedner TM (1972) The radiation syndromes. In: Hug O, Zuppinger A (eds) Strahlenbiologie 3. Springer, Berlin Heidelberg New York (Handbuch der medizinischen Radiologie, vol II/3, pp 299–339)

Cronkite EP, Bond VP, Carsten AL, Inoue T, Miller ME, Bullis JE (1987) Effects of low level radiation upon the hematopoietic stem cell: implications for leukemogenesis. Radiat Environ Biophys 26: 103–114

Crosfill ML, Lindop PJ, Rotblat J (1959) Variation of sensitivity to ionizing radiation with age. Nature 183: 1729–1730

Crossen PE, Durie BGM, Trent JM (1986) Generation time (GT) of human bone marrow cells cultured in the CFC-gm assay. Cell Tissue Kinet 19: 533–538

Curran RE, Johnson RE (1970) Tolerance to chemotherapy after prior irradiation for Hodgkin's disease. Ann Intern Med 72: 505–509

Curry JL, Trentin JJ, Wolf N (1967) Hemopoietic spleen colony studies. II. Erythropoiesis. J Exp Med 125: 703–720

Da W-M, Ma DDF, Biggs JC (1986) Studies of hemopoietic stromal fibroblastic colonies in patients undergoing bone marrow transplantation. Exp Hematol 14: 266–270

Dancey JT, Deubelbeiss KA, Harker LA, Finch CA (1976) Neutrophil kinetics in man. J Clin Invest 58: 705–715

Deacon J, Peckham MJ, Steel GG (1984) The radioresponsiveness of human tumors and the initial slope of the cell survival curve. Radiother Oncol 2: 317–323

De Alarcon PA (1989) Megakaryocyte colony-stimulating factor (Mk-CSF): its physiologic significance. Blood Cells 15: 173–185

DeGowin Rl, Chaudhuri TK, Christie JH, Callis MN, Mueller AL (1974) Marrow scanning in evaluation of hemopoiesis after radiotherapy. Arch Intern Med 134: 297–303

de Witte T, Schattenberg A, Salden M, Wessels J, Haanen C (1987) Mixed chimerism and the relation with leukaemic relapse after allogeneic bone marrow transplantation. Bone Marrow Transplantation 2 [Suppl 1]: 11–12

Dinarello CA (1988) Biology of interleukin 1. The FASEB Journal 2: 108–115

Dresch C, Faille A, Poirier O, Balitrand N, Najean Y (1979) Hydroxyurea suicide study of the kinetic heterogeneity of colony forming cells in human bone marrow. Exp Hematol 7: 337–344

Droz JP, Parmentier C, Morardet N, Maraninchi D, Gardet P, Tubiana M (1978) Effects of radiotherapy on the bone marrow granulocytic progenitor cells (CFUc) of patients with malignant lymphomas. I. Short-term effects. Int J Radiat Oncol Biol Phys 4: 845–851

Dutreix J, Wambersie A, Loirette M, Broisserie G (1979) Time factors in total body irradiation. Pathol Biol (Paris) 27: 365–369

Ebbe S (1980) Megakaryocytopoiesis in vivo. In: Evatt BL, Levine RF, Williams NT (eds) Megakaryocyte biology and precursors: in vitro cloning and cellular properties. Elsevier North-Holland, New York, pp 1–13

Elkind MM (1988) The initial part of the survival curve: does it predict the outcome of fractionated radiotherapy? Radiat Res 114: 425–436

Ellis RE (1961) The distribution of active bone marrow in the adult. Phys Med Biol 5: 255–258

Emerson SG, Gale RP (1987) The regulation of hematopoiesis following bone marrow transplantation. Int J Cell Cloning 5: 432–449

Emerson SG, Sieff CA, Gross RG, Rozans MK, Miller RA, Rappeport JM, Nathan DG (1987) Decreased hematopoietic accessory cell function following bone marrow transplantation. Exp Hematol 15: 1013–1021

Faille A, Maraninchi D, Gluckman E, Devergie A, Balitrand N, Ketels F, Dresch C (1981) Granulocyte progenitor compartments after allogeneic bone marrow grafts. Scand J Haematol 26: 202–214

Fauser AA, Messner HA (1978) Granuloerythropoietic colonies in human bone marrow, peripheral blood, and cord blood. Blood 52: 1243–1248

Fauser AA, Messner HA (1979a) Identification of megakaryocytes, macrophages, and eosinophils in colonies of human bone marrow containing neutrophilic granulocytes and erythroblasts. Blood 53: 1023–1027

Fauser AA, Messner HA (1979b) Proliferative state of human pluripotent hemopoietic progenitors (CFU-GEMM) in normal individuals and under regenerative conditions after bone marrow transplantation. Blood 54: 1197–1200

Feola JM, Song CW, Khan FM, Levitt SH (1974) Lethal response of C57BL mice to 10 MeV X-rays and to ^{60}Co gamma-rays. Int J Radiat Biol 26: 161–165

Fertil B, Malaise EP (1985) Intrinsic radiosensitivity of human cell lines is correlated with radioresponsiveness of human tumors: analysis of 101 puplished survival curves. Int J Radiat Oncol Biol Phys 11: 1699–1707

FitzGerald TJ, McKenna M, Rothstein L, Daugherty C, Kase K, Greenberger JS (1986) Radiosensitivity of human bone marrow granulocyte-macrophage progenitor cells and stromal colony-forming cells: effect of dose rate. Radiat Res 107: 205–215

Fitzpatrick PJ, Rider WD (1976a) Half-body radiotherapy of advanced cancer. J Can Assoc Radiol 27: 75–79

Fitzpatrick PJ, Rider WD (1976b) Half body radiotherapy. Int J Radiat Oncol Biol Phys 1: 197–207

Fliedner TM (1969) A cytokinetic comparison of hematological consequences of radiation exposure in different mammalian species. In: Bond VP, Sugahara T (eds) Comparative cellular and species radiosensitivity. Igaku Shoin, Tokyo, pp 89–101

Fliedner TM, Nothdurft W (1986) Cytological indicators: haematopoietic effects. In: Kaul A, Dehos A, Bögl W et al. (eds) Biological indicators for radiation dose assessment. Biologische Indikatoren zum Nachweis von Strahlenexpositionen. bga-Schriften 2/86. MMV Medizin, Munich, pp 123–152 (discussion, pp 153–156)

Fliedner TM, Hoelzer D, Steinbach KH (1978) Physiologische und pathologische Regulation der Erythropoese. Verh Dtsch Ges Inn Med 84: 15–27

Fliedner TM, Calvo W, Klinnert V, Nothdurft W, Prümmer O, Raghavachar A (1985) Bone marrow structure and its possible significance for hematopoietic cell renewal. In: Bond VP, Chandra P, Rai KR (eds) Hematopoietic cellular proliferation. Ann NY Acad Sci 459: 73–84

Fliedner TM, Nothdurft W, Steinbach KH (1988) Blood cell changes after radiation exposure as an indicator for hemopoietic stem cell function. Bone Marrow Transplantation 3: 77–84

Fordham EW, Ali A (1981) Radionuclide imaging of bone marrow. Semin Hematol 18: 222–239

Fowler JF (1983) Dose response curves for organ function or cell survival. Br J Radiol 56: 497–500

Friedenstein AJ (1976) Precursor cells of mechanocytes. Int Rev Cytol 47: 327–359

Friedenstein AJ, Chailakhjan RK, Lalykina KS (1970) The development of fibroblast colonies in monolayer cultures of guinea-pig bone marrow and spleen cells. Cell Tissue Kinet 3: 393–403

Friedenstein AJ, Gorskaja UF, Kulagina NN (1976) Fibroblast precursors in normal and irradiated mouse hematopoietic organs. Exp Hematol 4: 267–274

Frindel E, Charruyer F, Tubiana M, Kaplan HS, Alpen EL (1966) Radiation effects on DNA synthesis and cell division in the bone marrow of the mouse. Int J Radiat Biol 11: 435–443

Fu KK, Phillips TL, Kane LJ, Smith V (1975) Tumor and normal tissue response to irradiation in vivo: variation with decreasing dose rates. Radiology 114: 709–716

Gale RP (1987) T cells, bone marrow transplantation, and immunotherapy: use of monoclonal antibodies. In: Fahey JL (moderator) Immune interventions in disease (UCLA conference). Ann Intern Med 106: 263–267

Gale RP, Champlin RE (1986) Bone marrow transplantation in acute leukaemia. Clin Haematol 15: 851–872

Gale RP, Reisner Y (1986) Graft rejection and graft-versus-host disease: mirror images. Lancet I: 1468–1470

Gallini R, Hendry JH, Molineux G, Testa NG (1988) The effect of low dose rate on recovery of hemopoietic and stromal progenitor cells in γ-irradiated mouse bone marrow. Radiat Res 115: 481–487

Geissler D, Niederwieser D, Aulitzky WE, Tilg H, Grünewald K, Huber C, Konwalinka G (1988) Serum colony stimulating factors in patients undergoing bone marrow transplantation: enhancing effect of human GM-CSF. Behring Inst Mitt 83: 289–300

Gerber GB, Maes J (1980) Stem cell kinetics in spleen and bone marrow after single and fractionated irradiation of infant mice. Radiat Environ Biophys 18: 249–256

Gerber GB, Maes J (1981) The in vitro radiosensitivity of hemopoietic stem cells from control and preirradiated infant mice. Radiat Environ Biophys 19: 173–179

Gewirtz AM, Hoffman R (1985) Megakaryocytopoiesis. In: Golde DW, Takaku F (eds) Hematopoietic stem cells. Marcel Dekker, New York, pp 81–121

Gidali J, Feher I, Antal S (1974) Some properties of circulating hemopoietic stem cells. Blood 43: 573–580

Glasgow GP, Beetham KL, Mill WB (1983) Dose rate effects on the survival of normal hematopoietic stem cells of BALB/c mice. Int J Radiat Oncol Biol Phys 9: 557–563

Gordon MY (1975) A comparison of the radiosensitivity and o.e.r. of human and mouse progenitor cells cultured in agar diffusion chambers. Int J Radiat Biol 28: 285–290

Gould MN, Clifton KH (1979) Evidence for a unique in situ component of the repair of radiation damage. Radiat Res 77: 149–155

Greenberg BR, Wilson FD, Woo L, Klein AK, Rosenblatt LS (1984) Increased in vitro radioresistance of bone marrow fibroblastic progenitors (CFU-F) from patients with acute non-lymphocytic leukemia. Leuk Res 8: 267–273

Grilli G, Nothdurft W, Fliedner TM (1982) Radiation sensitivity of human erythroid and granulopoietic progenitor cells in the blood and in the bone marrow. Int J Radiat Biol 41: 685–687

Guzman E, Lajtha LG (1970) Some comparisons of the kinetic properties of femoral and splenic haemopoietic stem cells. Cell Tissue Kinet 3: 91–98

Haas RJ, Bohne F, Fliedner TM (1971) Cytokinetic analysis of slowly proliferating bone marrow cells during recovery from radiation injury. Cell Tissue Kinet 4: 31–45

Hager EB, Mannick JA, Thomas ED, Ferrebee JW (1961) Dogs that survive "lethal" exposures to radiation. Radiat Res 14: 192–205

Hall EJ, Bedford JS (1964) Dose rate: its effect on the survival of HeLa cells irradiated with gamma rays. Radiat Res 22: 305–315

Hanks GE (1972) Recruitment and altered recovery in noncycling bone marrow stem cells. Radiology 103: 691–693

Hara H, Ogawa M (1977) Erythropoietic precursors in mice under erythropoietic stimulation and suppression. Exp Hematol 5: 141–148

Hart RM, Kimler BF, Evans RG, Park CH (1987) Radiotherapeutic management of medulloblastoma in a pediatric patient with ataxia telangiectasia. Int J Radiat Oncol Biol Phys 13: 1237–1240

Hashimoto M, Yamaka K (1964) Distribution of red bone marrow and its weight. Annual Report of Scientific Research Grants, 1963, Ministry of Education

Haskell CM, Parker R (1980) Hodgkin's disease. In: Haskell CM (ed) Cancer treatment. WB Saunders, Philadelphia, pp 866–905

Heinze B, Arnold R, Kratt E, Heit W, Heimpel H, Fliedner TM (1987) Cytogenetic studies in leukaemic patients after transplantation of T cell-depleted bone marrow cells. Bone Marrow Transplantation 2 [Suppl 1]: p 152

Hendry JH (1972) The response of haemopoietic colony-forming units and lymphoma cells irradiated in soft tissue (spleen) or a bone cavity (femur) with single doses of x-rays, γ-rays or D-T neutrons. Br J Radiol 45: 923–932

Hendry JH (1973) Differential split-dose radiation response of resting and regenerating haemopoietic stem cells. Int J Radiat Biol 24: 469–473

Hendry JH (1979) The dose-dependence of the split-dose response of marrow colony-forming units (CFU-S): similarity to other tissues. Int J Radiat Biol 36: 631–637

Hendry JH (1985a) Review: survival curves for normal-tissue clonogens: a comparison of assessments using in vitro, transplantation or in situ techniques. Int J Radiat Biol 47: 3–16

Hendry JH (1985b) The cellular basis of long-term marrow injury after irradiation. Radiother Oncol 3: 331–338

Hendry JH (1988) Survival of cells in mammalian tissues after low doses of irradiation: a short review. Int J Radiat Biol 53: 89–94

Hendry JH, Howard A (1971) The response of haemopoietic colony-forming units to single and split doses of γ-rays or D-T neutrons. Int J Radiat Biol 19: 51–64

Hendry JH, Lord BI (1983) The analysis of the early and late response to cytotoxic insults in the haemopoietic cell hierarchy. In: Potten CS, Hendry JH (eds) Cytotoxic insult to tissue. Effects on cell lineages. Churchill Livingstone, Edinburgh, pp 1–66

Hendry JH, Moore JV (1985) Deriving absolute values of α and β for dose fractionation, using dose-incidence data. Br J Radiol 58: 885–890

Hendry JH, Potten CS (1988) α/β ratios and the cycling status of tissue target cells (letter to the editor). Radiother Oncol 12: 79–83

Henney CS (1988) Hematopoietic activities of interleukin 1. Behring Inst Mitt 83: 165–169

Herrmann F, Mertelsmann R (1989) Polypeptides controlling hematopoietic cell development and activation. I. In vitro results. Blut 58: 117–128

Herrmann T, Knorr A, Lesche A, Koch R (1988) Hämatologische Befunde nach einzeitiger hochdosierter Halbkörperbestrahlung in Abhängigkeit von Dosis, Körperhälfte und Sequenz. Radiobiol Radiother (Berl) 29: 336–338

Hill DR, Benak SB, Phillips TL, Price DC (1980) Bone marrow regeneration following fractionated radiation therapy. Int J Radiat Oncol Biol Phys 6: 1149–1155

Hodgson GS, Bradley TR (1979) Properties of haematopoietic stem cells surviving 5-fluorouracil treatment: evidence for a pre-CFU-S-cell? Nature 281:381–382

Holley TR, Van Epps DE, Harvey RL, Anderson RE, William RC Jr (1974) Effect of high doses of radiation on human neutrophil chemotaxis, phagocytosis and morphology. Am J Pathol 75: 61–68

Hopewell JW (1983) Radiation effects on vascular tissue. In: Potten CS, Hendry JH (eds) Cytotoxic insult to tissue. Effects on cell lineages. Churchill Livingstone, Edinburgh, pp 228–257

Hoppe RT (1988) The contemporary management of Hodgkin's disease. Radiology 169: 297–304

Hornsey S (1967) The recovery process in organized tissue. In: Silini G (ed) Radiation research. North-Holland, Amsterdam, pp 587–603

Hüttner J, Grunau H, Merkle K, Radunz W, Buth K (1988) Hämatologische Reaktionen nach hochdosierter sequentieller Halbkörperbestrahlung bei Patienten mit kleinzelligem Bronchialkarzinom. Radiobiol Radiother (Berl) 29: 343–348

IAEA Safety Series No.47 (1978) Manual on early medical treatment of possible radiation injury with an appendix on sodium burns. International Atomic Energy Agency, Vienna

Imai Y, Nakao I (1987) In vivo radiosensitivity and recovery pattern of the hematopoietic precursor cells and stem cells in mouse bone marrow. Exp Hematol 15: 890–895

International Commission on Radiological Protection No.23 (1974) IV. Report of the task group on reference man. Pergamon, Oxford, pp 85–98

Iscove NN (1977) The role of erythropoietin in regulation of population size and cell cycling of early and late erythroid precursors in mouse bone marrow. Cell Tissue Kinet 10: 323–334

Iscove NN (1978a) Erythropoietin-independent stimulation of early erythropoiesis in adult marrow cultures by conditioned media from lectin-stimulated mouse spleen cells. In: Golde DW, Cline MJ, Metcalf D, Fox CF (eds) Hematopoietic cell differentiation. Academic, New York, pp 37–52

Iscove NN (1978b) Regulation of proliferation and maturation at early and late stages of erythroid differentiation. In: Saunders GF (ed) Cell differentiation and neoplasia. Raven, New York, pp 195–209

Iscove NN, Till JE, McCulloch EA (1970) The proliferative states of mouse granulopoietic progenitor cells. Proc Soc Exp Biol Med 134: 33–36

Jaffe JP, Bosch A, Raich PC (1979) Sequential hemi-body radiotherapy in advanced multiple meyeloma. Cancer 43: 124–128

Janssen J, Drenthe – Schonk A, van Dijk B, Bloo J, Kunst V, de Witte T (1986) Erythrocyte repopulation after allogeneic bone marrow transplantation using lymphocyte depleted marrow from histocompatible siblings. Bone Marrow Transplantation 1 [Suppl 1]: 239–240

Johnson RE (1979) Treatment of chronic lymphocytic leukemia by total body irradiation alone or combined with chemotherapy. Int J Radiat Oncol Biol Phys 5: 159–164

Johnson GR, Metcalf D (1977) Pure and mixed erythroid colony formation in vitro stimulated by spleen conditioned medium with no detectable erythropoietin. Proc Natl Acad Sci USA 74: 3879–3882

Johnson RE, Rühl U (1976) Treatment of chronic lymphocytic leukemia with emphasis on total body irradiation. Int J Radiat Oncol Biol Phys 1: 387–397

Johnson RE, Canellos GP, Young RC, Chabner BA, DeVita VT (1978) Chemotherapy (cyclophosphamide, vincristine, and prednisone) versus radiotherapy (total body irradiation) for stage III-IV poorly differentiated lymphocytic lymphoma. Cancer Treat Rep 62:321–325

Jones TD (1977) CHORD operators for cell-survival models and insult assessment to active bone marrow. Radiat Res 71: 269–283

Kallman RF (1962) The effect of dose rate on mode of acute radiation death of C57BL and BALB/C mice. Radiat Res 16: 796–810

Kallman RF, Silini G (1964) Recuperation from lethal injury by whole-body irradiation. I. Kinetic aspects and the relationship with conditioning dose in C57BL mice. Radiat Res 22: 622–642

Kaplan HS (1980) Hodgkin's disease, 2nd edn. Harvard University Press, Cambridge MA

Kaplan HS, Brown MB (1952) Mortality of mice after total-body irradiation as influenced by alterations in total dose, fractionation, and periodicity of treatment. J Natl Cancer Inst 12: 765–775

Keating A, Singer JW, Killen PD et al. (1982) Donor origin of the in vitro haematopoietic microenvironment after marrow transplantation in man. Nature 298: 280–283

Kelemen E, Calvo W, Fliedner TM (1979) Atlas of human hemopoietic development. Springer, Heidelberg Berlin New York

Kellerer AM, Chmelevsky D, Hall EJ (1980) Nonparametric representation of dose-effect relations. Radiat Res 84: 173–188

Kereiakes JG, Riet W Van de, Born C, Ewing C, Silberstein E, Saenger EL (1972) Active bone-marrow dose related to hematological changes in whole-body and partial-body ^{60}Co gamma radiation exposures. Radiology 103: 651–656

Kernan NA, Collins NH, Cunningham I et al. (1987) Prevention of GVHD in HLA-identical marrow grafts by removal of T cells with soybean agglutinin and SRBCs. Bone Marrow Transplantation 2 [Suppl 2]:13–17

Kessinger A, Armitage JO, Landmark JD, Smith DM, Weisenburger DD (1988) Autologous peripheral hematopoietic stem cell transplantation restores hematopoietic function following marrow ablative therapy. Blood 71: 723–727

Kimler BF, Park CH, Yakar D, Mies RM (1984) Lack of recovery from radiation-induced sublethal damage in human haematopoietic cells. Br J Cancer 49 [Suppl VI]: 221–225

Kimler BF, Park CH, Yakar D, Mies RM (1985) Radiation response of human normal and leukemic hemopoietic cells assayed by in vitro colony formation. Int J Radiat Oncol Biol Phys 11: 809–816

Kindt A, Sattler E-L (1977) Literaturübersicht zur Frage der Erholung nach Ganzkörperbestrahlung. Zivilschutzforschung, vol 6. Osang, Bad Honnef

Kinsella TJ, Mitchel JB, McPherson S, Miser J, Triche T, Glatstein E (1984) In vitro radiation studies on Ewing's sarcoma cell lines and human bone marrow: application to the clinical use of total body irradiation. Int J Radiat Oncol Biol Phys 10: 1005–1011

Klein AK, Rosenblatt LS, Stitzel KA, Greenberg B, Woo L (1984) In vitro radiation response studies on bone marrow fibroblasts (CFU-F) obtained from normal and chronically irradiated dogs. Leuk Res 8: 473–481

Klein AK, Dyck JA, Shimizu JA, Stitzel KA, Wilson FD, Cain GR (1985) Effect of continuous, whole-body gamma irradiation upon canine lymphohematopoietic (CFU-GM, CFU-L) progenitors and a possible hematopoietic regulatory population. Radiat Res 101: 332–350

Knospe WH, Rayudu VMS, Cardello M, Friedman AM, Fordham EW (1976) Bone marrow scanning with ^{52}iron (^{52}Fe). Regeneration and extension of marrow after ablative doses of radiotherapy. Cancer 37: 1432–1442

Körbling M, Dörken B, Ho AD, Pezzutto A, Hunstein W, Fliedner TM (1986) Autologous transplantation of blood-derived hemopoietic stem cells after myeloablative therapy in a patient with Burkitt's lymphoma. Blood 67: 529–532

Kolb HJ, Bodenberger U, Geyer S et al. (1981) Total body irradiation regimens before bone marrow transplantation in dogs. In: Touraine JL, Gluckman E, Griscelli C (eds) Bone marrow transplantation in Europe, vol 3. Excerpta Medica, Amsterdam, pp 38–41

Krebs JS, Brauer RW (1964) Comparative accumulation of injury from X-, gamma and neutron irradiation – the position of theory and experiment. In: International Atomic Energy Agency (ed) Biological effects of neutron and proton irradiations, vol II. IAEA, Vienna, pp 347–364

Krebs JS, Jones DCL (1972) The LD$_{50}$ and the survival of bone marrow colony-forming cells in mice: effect of rate of exposure to ionizing radiation. Radiat Res 51: 374–380

Kreja L, Seidel H-J (1982) Differences in BFU-E growth in different mouse strains after stimulation with a mixed lymphocyte culture supernatant (MLC-BPA). Stem Cells 2: 177–188

Kreja L, Baltschukat K, Nothdurft W (1988) Growth of erythroid burst forming units (BFU-E) in cultures of canine bone marrow and blood cells. Effect of serum from irradiated dogs. Exp Hematol 16: 647–651

Kreja L, Baltschukat K, Nothdurft W (1989) In vitro studies of the sensitivity of canine bone marrow erythroid burst forming units (BFU-E) and fibroblast colony forming units (CFU-F) to x-irradiation. Int J Radiat Biol 55: 435–444

Kwan DK, Norman A (1978) Radiosensitivity of large human monocytes. Radiat Res 75: 556–562

Labetzki L, Frommhold H, Illiger J, Grauthoff H (1980) Zur hämatologischen Toxizität der Ganzkörperbestrahlung. Strahlentherapie 156: 30–34

Labetzki L, Schmidt RE, Hartlapp JH, Illiger HJ, Frommhold H, Boldt I (1982) Ganzkörperbestrahlung bei malignen Lymphomen niedriger Malignität. Strahlentherapie 158: 195–201

Lahiri SK (1976) Kinetics of haemopoetic recovery in endotoxin-treated mice. Cell Tissue Kinet 9: 31–39

Lajtha LG (1979) Stem cell concepts. Differentiation 14: 23–34

Lajtha LG, Pozzi LV, Schofield R, Fox M (1969) Kinetic properties of haemopoietic stem cells. Cell Tissue Kinet 2: 39–49

Lambertsen RH, Weiss L (1983) Studies on the organization and regeneration of bone marrow: origin, growth, and differentiation of endocloned hematopoietic colonies. Am J Anat 166: 369–392

Lambertsen RH, Weiss L (1984) A model of intramedullary hematopoietic microenvironments based on stereologic study of the distribution of endocloned marrow colonies. Blood 63: 287–297

Langdon HL, Berman I (1975) An autoradiographic and morphological study of mouse bone marrow littoral cells during and after treatment with urethane. Cell Tissue Kinet 8: 285–292

Langendorff H, Langendorff M, Metzner R, Mönig H, Steinbach K-H, Tumbrägel G (1970) Radiobiological investigations with fast neutrons. I. Comparative investigations on the mortality of male mice after an irradiation with 15 MeV-neutrons and ^{60}Co-γ-rays. Atomkernenergie 16: 255–260

Langham WH (ed) (1967) Radiobiological factors in manned space flight. National Academy of Sciences, National Research Council, Washington DC

Latini P, Checcaglini F, Maranzano E et al. (1988) Hyperfractionated total body irradiation for T-depleted HLA identical bone marrow transplants. Radiother Oncol 11: 113–118

Laver J, Ebell W, Castro-Malaspina H (1986) Radiobiological properties of the human hematopoietic microenvironment: contrasting sensitivities of proliferative capacity and hematopoietic function to in vitro irradiation. Blood 67: 1090–1097

Lehnert S, Rybka WB, Suissa S, Giambattisto D (1986) Radiation response of haematopoietic cell lines of human origin. Int J Radiat Biol 49: 423–431

Lennon JE, Micklem HS (1986) Stromal cells in long-term murine bone marrow culture: FACS studies and origin of stromal cells in radiation chimeras. Exp Hematol 14: 287–292

Lepine J, Messner HA (1983) Pluripotent hemopoietic progenitors (CFU-GEMM) in chronic myelogenous leukemia. Int J Cell Cloning 1: 230–239

Li S, Champlin R, Fitchen JH, Gale RP (1985) Abnormalities of myeloid progenitor cells after "successful" bone marrow transplantation. J Clin Invest 75: 234–241

Lichtman MA (1981) The ultrastructure of the hemopoietic environment of the marrow: a review. Exp Hematol 9: 391–410

Link H, Freund M, Kirchner H et al. (1988) Recombinant human granulocyte-macrophage colony stimulating factor (rhGM-CSF) after bone marrow transplantation. Behring Inst Mitt 83: 313–319

Lipton JM, Nathan DG (1980) Cell-cell interactions in in vitro erythropoiesis. Blood Cells 6: 645–663

Lohrmann H-P (1978) Thymidine-suicide of human granulocytic progenitor cells (CFU-C). Biomedicine 28: 319–323

Lombardi F, Lattuada A, Gasparini M, Gianni C, Marchesini R (1982) Sequential half-body irradiation as systemic treatment of progressive Ewing sarcoma. Int J Radiat Oncol Biol Phys 8: 1679–1682

Lord BI, Testa NG, Hendry JH (1975) The relative spatial distributions of CFU-S and CFU-C in the normal mouse femur. Blood 46: 65–72

Lord BI (1986) Controls on the cell cycle. Int J Radiat Biol 49: 279–296

Lord BI (1988) The distribution of potential leukaemogenic cells in bone marrow. Int J Radiat Biol 53: 523–524 (extended abstr)

Lord BI, Testa NG (1988) The hemopoietic system. Structure and regulation. In: Testa NG, Gale RP (eds) Hematopoiesis. Long-term effects of chemotherapy and radiation. Marcel Dekker, New York (Hematology, vol 8, pp 1–26)

Lorimore SA, Wright EG (1987) Stem cell maintenance and commitment to differentiation in long-term cultures of murine marrow obtained from different spatial locations in the femur. Cell Tissue Kinet 20: 427–434

MacVittie TJ, Monroy RL, Patchen ML, Darden JH (1984) Acute lethality and radiosensitivity of the canine hemopoietic system to cobalt-60 gamma and mixed neutron-gamma irradiation. In: Broerse JJ, MacVittie TJ (eds) Response of different species to total body irradiation. Martinus Nijhoff, Boston, pp 113–129

Maloney MA, Patt HM (1969) Origin of repopulating cells after localized bone marrow depletion. Science 165: 71–73

Maloney MA, Patt HM (1972) Persistent marrow hypocellularity after local x-irradiation of the rabbit femur with 1000 rad. Radiat Res 50: 284–292

Maloney MA, Lamela RA, Patt HM(1985) The question of bone marrow stromal fibroblast traffic. In: Bond VP, Chandra P, Rai KR (eds) Hematopoietic cellular proliferation. Ann NY Acad Sci 459: 190–197

Martin PJ, Hansen JA, Buckner CD et al. (1985) Effects of in vitro depletion of T cells in HLA-identical allogeneic marrow grafts. Blood 66: 664–672

Maruyama Y, Feola JM (1987) Relative radiosensitivities of the thymus, spleen, and lymphohemopoietic systems. In: Lett JT, Altman KI (eds) Relative radiation sensitivities of human organ systems. Academic, New York (Advances in radiation biology, vol 12, pp 1–82)

Mascret B, Bertheas MF, Lafage M, Blaise D, Maraninchi D, Fraisse J, Carcassone Y (1986) Cytogenetic evidence of partial chimaerism after T-cell depleted allogeneic transplantation in leukaemic matched patients. Bone Marrow Transplantation 1 [Suppl 1]: 235–236

Mason BA, Richter MP, Catalano RB, Creech RB (1982) Upper hemibody and local chest irradiation as consolidation following response to high-dose induction chemotherapy for small cell bronchogenic carcinoma – a pilot study. Cancer Treat Rep 66: 1609–1612

Mazur EM (1987) Megakaryocytopoiesis and platelet production: a review. Exp Hematol 15: 340–350

McCarthy DM, Goldman JM (1983) Transfusion of circulating stem cells. CRC Critical Review in Clinical Laboratory Sciences 20: 1–24

McCulloch EA (1985) Normal stem cells and the clonal hemopathies. Prog Clin Biol Res 184: 21–38

McCulloch EA, Till JE (1962) The sensitivity of cells from mouse bone marrow to gamma radiation in vitro and in vivo. Radiat Res 16: 822–832

McCulloch EA, Till JE (1964) Proliferation of hemopoietic colony-forming cells transplanted into irradiated mice. Radiat Res 22: 383–397

McDonald TP (1988) Thrombopoietin: its biology, purification, and characterization. Exp Hematol 16: 201–205

McLeod DL, Shreeve MM, Axelrad AA (1976) Induction of megakaryocytic colonies with platelet formation in vitro. Nature 261: 492–494

Medical Research Council's Committee on Effects of Ionizing Radiation (1984) Lethality from acute and protracted radiation exposure in man. Int J Radiat Biol 46: 209–217

Melamed JS, Chen MG, Brown JW, Katagiri CA (1980) Acute hematological tolerance to multiple fraction whole body, low dose irradiation in an experimental murine system. Radiology 134: 503–506

Messner HA (1984) Human stem cells in culture. Clin Haematol 13: 393–404

Messner HA (1986) The role of CFU-GEMM in human hemopoiesis. Blut 53: 269–277

Messner HA, Fauser AA (1980) Culture studies of human pluripotent hemopoietic progenitors. Blut 41: 327–33

Messner HA, Yamasaki K (1988) Conditions affecting the growth of hemopoietic progenitors after bone marrow transplantation. In: Testa NG, Gale RP (eds) Hematopoiesis. Long-term effects of chemotherapy and radiation. Marcel Dekker, New York (Hematology, vol 8, pp 377–388)

Metcalf D (1977) Hemopoietic colonies: in vitro cloning of normal and leukemic cells. Recent results in cancer research, vol 61, Springer, Berlin Heidelberg New York

Metcalf D (1986a) Molecular control of granulocyte and macrophage production. In: Baserga R, Foa P, Metcalf D, Polli EE (eds) Biological regulation of cell proliferation. Raven, New York, pp 67–73

Metcalf D (1986b) The molecular biology and functions of the granulocyte macrophage colony-stimulating factors. Blood 67: 257–267

Metcalf D, Burgess AW (1982) Clonal analysis of progenitor cell commitment to granulocyte or macrophage production. J Cell Physiol 111: 275–283

Michalowski A (1981) Effects of radiation on normal tissues: hypothetical mechanisms and limitations of in situ assays of clonogenicity. Radiat Environ Biophys 19: 157–172

Michalowski A, Wheldon TE, Kirk J (1984) Can cell survival parameters be deduced from non-clonogenic assays of radiation damage to normal tissues? Br J Cancer 49 [Suppl VI]: 257–261

Micklem HS, Ogden DA, Evans EP, Ford CE, Gray JG (1975) Compartments and cell flows within the mouse haemopoietic system. II. Estimated rates of interchange. Cell Tissue Kinet 8: 233–248

Mole RH (1957) Quantitative observations on recovery from whole-body irradiation in mice. II. Recovery during and after daily irradiation. Br J Radiol 30: 40–46

Mole RH (1975) Deductions about survival-curve parameters from iso-effect radiation regimes: observations on lethality after whole-body irradiation of mice. In: Alper T (ed) Cell survival after low doses of radiation: theoretical and clinical implications. The Institute of Physics. Wiley, Bristol, pp 299–307

Mole RH (1984) The LD_{50} for uniform low LET irradiation of man. Br J Radiol 57: 355–369

Monette FC, Kent RB, Weiner EJ, Livanis EC, Lydon PJ (1978) Cell cycle properties and proliferation kinetics of late erythroid progenitor cells. Exp Hematol 6 [Suppl 3]: 12 (abstr)

Monroy RL, Skelly RR, MacVittie TJ, Davies TA, Sauber JJ, Clark SC, Donahue RE (1987) The effect of recombinant GM-CSF on the recovery of monkeys transplanted with autologous bone marrow. Blood 70: 1696–1699

Monroy RL, Skelly RR, Taylor P, Dubois A, Donahue RE, MacVittie TJ (1988) Recovery from severe hematopoietic suppression using recombinant human granulocyte-macrophage colony-stimulating factor. Exp Hematol 16: 344–348

Morardet N, Parmentier C, Hayat M, Charbord P (1978) Effects of radiotherapy on the bone marrow granulocytic progenitor cells (CFUc) of patients with malignant lymphomas. II. Long-term effects. Int J Radiat Oncol Biol Phys 4: 853–857

Morgenstern GR (1988) Bone marrow-structure and function. Int J Radiat Biol 53: 522–523

Morris MD, Jones TD (1988) A comparison of dose-response models for death from hematological depression in different species. Int J Radiat Biol 53: 439–456

Morrissey PJ, Charrier K, Bressler L, Alpert A (1987) The influence of IL-1 treatment on the reconstitution of the hemopoietic and immune systems following sublethal radiation. J Immunol 140: 4204–4210

Nakeff A (1982) Megakaryocytopoiesis: progenitor pool. In: Trubowitz S, Davis S (eds) The human bone marrow:

anatomy, physiology, and pathophysiology, vol I. CRC Press, Boca Raton, pp 209–243

Nakeff A, McLellan WL, Bryan J, Valeriote FA (1979) Response of megakaryocyte, erythroid, and granulocyte-macrophage progenitor cells in mouse bone marrow to gamma-irradiation and cyclophosphamide. In: Baum SJ, Ledney GD (eds) Experimental hematology today 1979. Springer, New York Heidelberg Berlin, pp 99–104

NCRP Report No. 39 (1974) Basic radiation protection criteria, 2nd reprinting. National Council on Radiation Protection and Measurements, Washington DC 20014

Neal FE (1960) Variation of acute mortality with dose-rate in mice exposed to single large doses of whole-body x-irradiation. Int J Radiat Biol 2: 295–300

Nečas E, Znojil V (1988) Bone marrow response to single small doses of irradiation: implications for stem cell functional organization. Exp Hematol 16: 871–875

Neta R, Douches S, Oppenheim JJ (1986) Interleukin 1 is a radioprotector. J Immunol 136: 2483–2485

Neumann HA, Löhr GW, Fauser AA (1981) Radiation sensitivity of pluripotent hemopoietic progenitors (CFU_{GEMM}) derived from human bone marrow. Exp Hematol 9: 742–744

Nicola NA (1987) Granulocyte colony-stimulating factor and differentiation-induction in myeloid leukemic cells. Int J Cell Cloning 5: 1–15

Nienhuis AW, Donahue RE, Karlsson S et al. (1987) Recombinant human granulocyte-macrophage colony-stimulating factor (GM-CSF) shortens the period of neutropenia after autologous bone marrow transplantation in a primate model. J Clin Invest 80: 573–577

Nishihira H, Kigasawa H (1981) Growth of human erythroid and erythroid-granulocytic colonies in culture without addition of exogenous erythropoietin. Br J Haematol 49: 563–566

Niu T, Fengying L, Yuying L (1988) Radiosensitivity of microvessels and its relation to damage of parenchymal cells. In: Zhang Q-X, Wu D-C (eds) Radiation biological effects. Modifiers and treatment. Proceedings of the International Conference on Biological Effects of Large Dose Ionizing and Non-Ionizing Radiation. Hangzhou, 29 March–1 April 1988. Society of Radiation Medicine and Protection, Chinese Medical Association, Beijing, pp 296–303

Nothdurft W (1985) Knochenmark. In: Diethelm L, Heuck F, Olson O, Strnad F, Vieten H, Zuppinger A (eds) Strahlengefährdung und Strahlenschutz. Springer, Berlin Heidelberg New York (Handbuch der medizinischen Radiologie, vol xx, pp 235–264)

Nothdurft W, Fliedner TM (1979) Stem cell migration after irradiation. In: Okada S, Imamura I, Terasima T, Yamaguchi H (eds) Radiation research. Toppan, Tokyo, pp 657–663

Nothdurft W, Fliedner TM (1982) The response of the granulocytic progenitor cells (CFU-C) of blood and bone marrow in dogs exposed to low doses of x-irradiation. Radiat Res 89: 38–52

Nothdurft W, Fliedner TM, Weindler M, Wurzberger R (1978) Correlations of blood levels of CSA with degenerative and regenerative changes of the granulopoietic cell renewal system in 1200 R whole-body x-irradiated dogs given autologous stem-cell transfusion. XVII Congress of the International Society of Hematology, Paris, 27–28 July 1978. Book of abstracts II: 878

Nothdurft W, Steinbach KH, Fliedner TM (1983) In vitro studies on the sensitivity of canine granulopoietic prog-enitor cells (GM-CFC) to ionizing radiation: differences between steady state GM-CFC from blood and bone marrow. Int J Radiat Biol 43: 133–140

Nothdurft W, Steinbach KH, Fliedner TM (1984) Dose- and time-related quantitative and qualitative alterations in the granulocyte/macrophage progenitor cell (GM-CFC) compartment of dogs after total-body irradiation. Radiat Res 98: 332–344

Nothdurft W, Calvo W, Klinnert V, Steinbach KH, Werner C, Fliedner TM (1986) Acute and long-term alterations in the granulocyte/macrophage progenitor cell (GM-CFC) compartment of dogs after partial-body irradiation: irradiation of the upper body with a single myeloablative dose. Int J Radiat Oncol Biol Phys 112: 949–957

Nothdurft W, Baltschukat K, Fliedner TM (1989) Hematological effects in dogs after sequential irradiation of the upper and lower part of the body with single myeloablative doses. Radiother Oncol 14: 247–259

Ogawa M, Porter PN, Nakahata T (1983) Renewal and commitment to differentiation of hemopoietic stem cells. Blood 38: 823–829

Öhl S, Bamberg M, Holfeld H, Höffken K, Schmidt CG, Scherer E (1979) Behandlung von Non-Hodgkin-Lymphomen niedriger Malignität mit Ganzkörperbestrahlung und kombinierter Chemotherapie. Blut 38: 181–183

O'Reilly RJ, Collins NH, Kernan N et al. (1985) Transplantation of marrow-depleted T cells by soybean lectin agglutination and E-rosette depletion: major histo-compatibility complex-related graft resistance in leukemic transplant recipients. Transplant Proc 17: 455–459

Page NP (1968) The effect of dose-protraction on radiation lethality of large animals. In: Proceedings of a Symposium on Dose Rate in Mammalian Radiation Biology, CONF-680410, 1968, pp 12.1–12.23

Pantel K, Nakeff A (1989) Lymphoid cell regulation of hematopoiesis. Int J Cell Cloning 7: 2–12

Parmentier C, Morardet N, Tubiana M (1983) Late effects on human bone marrow after extended field radiotherapy. Int J Radiat Oncol Biol Phys 9: 1303–1311

Parmentier C, Morardet N, Tubiana M (1988) Long-term bone marrow damage after treatment of lymphomas. In: Testa NG, Gale RP (eds) Hematopoiesis. Long-term effects of chemotherapy and radiation. Marcel Dekker, New York, (Hematology, vol 8, pp 301–324)

Patt HM (1969) Species differences in leukocyte regeneration after irradiation. In: Bond VP, Sugahara T (eds) Comparative cellular and species radiosensitivity. Igaku Shoin, Tokyo, pp 112–122

Patt HM, Maloney MA (1975) Bone marrow regeneration after local injury: a review. Exp Hematol 3: 135–148

Patt HM, Quastler H (1963) Radiation effects on cell renewal and related systems. Physiol Rev 43: 357–396

Patt HM, Maloney MA, Flannery ML (1982) Hematopoietic microenvironment transfer by stromal fibroblasts derived from bone marrow varying in cellularity. Exp Hematol 10: 738–742

Patterson J, Prentice HG, Brenner MK et al. (1986) Graft rejection following HLA matched T-lymphocyte depleted bone marrow transplantation. Br J Haematol 63: 221–230

Paulus JM, Deschamps JF, Prenant M, Casals EJ (1980) Kinetics of platelets, megakaryocytes, and their precursors: what to measure? Blood Cells 6: 215–255

Peacock JH, Steel GG, Stephens TC (1986) Radiation dose-rate dependent differences in cell kill and repopulation in murine bone-marrow CFU-S and CFU-C. Br J Cancer 53 [Suppl VII]: 171–173

Peters L (1980) Discussion: the radiobiological bases of TBI. Int J Radiat Oncol Biol Phys 6: 785–787

Peters LJ, Withers HR, Cundiff JH, Dicke KA (1979) Radiobiological considerations in the use of total-body irradiation for bone-marrow transplantation. Radiology 131: 243–247

Petz LD, Yam P, Wallace RB et al. (1987) Mixed hematopoietic chimerism following bone marrow transplantation for hematologic malignancies. Blood 70: 1331–1337

Pharr PP, Ogawa M (1985) Pluripotent stem cells. In: Golde DW, Takaku F (eds) Hematopoietic stem cells. Marcel Dekker, New York, pp 3–18

Phillips TL (1968) Qualitative alteration in radiation injury under hypoxic conditions. Radiology 91: 529–536

Phillips TL, Hanks GE (1968) Apparent absence of recovery in endogenous colony-forming cells after irradiation under hypoxic conditions. Radiat Res 33: 517–532

Piersma AH, Ploemacher RE, Brockbank KGM (1982) Transplantation of stromal progenitor cells (CFU-F) in mice. Exp Hematol 10 [Suppl 11]: 82

Piersma AH, Ploemacher RE, Brockbank KGM, Nikkels PGJ, Ottenheim CPE (1985) Migration of fibroblastoid stromal cells in murine blood. Cell Tissue Kinet 18: 589–595

Ploemacher RE, Brons NHC (1988a) Isolation of hemopoietic stem cell subsets from murine bone marrow: I. Radioprotective ability of purified cell suspensions differing in the proportion of day-7 and day-12 CFU-S. Exp Hematol 16: 21–26

Ploemacher RE, Brons NHC (1988b) Isolation of hemopoietic stem cell subsets from murine bone marrow: II. Evidence for an early precursor of day-12 CFU-S and cells associated with radioprotective ability. Exp Hematol 16: 27–32

Potten CS (1986) Cell cycles in cell hierarchies. Int J Radiat Biol 49: 257–278

Powell BL, Jackson DV, Scarantino CW et al. (1985) Sequential hemibody and local irradiation with combination chemotherapy for small cell lung carcinoma: a preliminary analysis. Int J Radiat Oncol Biol Phys 11: 457–462

Prasad KN (1974) Human radiation biology. Harper and Row, Hagerstown

Pritchard J, Sandland MR, Breatnach FB, Pincott JR, Cox R, Husband P (1982) The effects of radiation therapy for Hodgkin's disease in a child with ataxia telangiectasia. A clinical, biological and pathological study. Cancer 50: 877–886

Prosnitz LR (1988) Radiation complications for Hodgkin's disease and seminoma: assessing the risk:benefit ratio. Int J Radiat Oncol Biol Phys 15: 239–241

Proukakis C, Lindop PJ (1967) Age dependence of radiation sensitivity of haemopoietic cells in the mouse. Nature 215: 655–656

Proukakis C, Coggle JE, Lindop PJ (1969) Effect of age at exposure on the bone-marrow stem-cell population in relation to 30-day mortality in mice. In: Sikov MR, Mahlum DD (eds) Radiation biology of the fetal and juvenile mammal. US Atomic Energy Commission, Oak Ridge, pp 603–612

Przepiorka D, Torok-Storb B, Simmons PJ (1988) The origin of bone marrow stroma after transplantation. Implica-

tions for graft failure. In: Testa NG, Gale RP (eds) Hematopoiesis. Long-term effects of chemotherapy and radiation. Marcel Dekker, New York, pp 357–376

Puro EA, Clark GM (1972) The effect of exposure rate on animal lethality and spleen colony cell survival. Radiat Res 52: 115–129

Quasim MM (1981) Half body irradiation (HBI) in metastatic carcinomas. Clin Radiol 32: 215–219

Quesenberry PJ (1986) Synergistic hematopoietic growth factors. Int J Cell Cloning 4: 3–15

Raskind WH, Singer JW, Morgan CA, Fialkow PJ (1988) Host origin of marrow stromal cells obtained from marrow transplant recipients and transformed in vitro by simian virus-40. Exp Hematol 16: 827–830

Reynolds M, McCann SR (1986) Effect of conditioning regimen on bone marrow progenitors following allogeneic bone marrow transplantation. Bone Marrow Transplantation 1 [Suppl 1]: 249

Rickard KA, Brown R, Kronenberg H (1974) Radiation and the human agar colony forming cell. Pathology 6: 169–181

Robinson WA, Mangalik A (1975) The kinetics and regulation of granulopoiesis. Semin Hematol 12: 7–25

Robinson WA, Bradley TR, Metcalf D (1967) Effect of whole body irradiation on colony production by bone marrow cells in vitro. Proc Soc Exp Biol Med 125: 388–391

Ross EAM, Anderson N, Micklem HS (1982) Serial depletion and regeneration of the murine hematopoietic system. Implications for hematopoietic organization and the study of cellular aging. J Exp Med 155: 432–444

Rostom AY (1988) A review of the place of radiotherapy in myeloma with emphasis on whole body irradiation. Hematol Oncol 6: 193–198

Rubin A, Thompson IW, Mackinnon S, Goldman JM, Lampert IA (1988) Reduced cellularity of bone marrow following transplantation for chronic myeloid leukaemia. J Pathol 154: p 53 A (abstr)

Rubin P (1984) The Franz Buschke Lecture: late effects of chemotherapy and radiation therapy: a new hypothesis. Int J Radiat Oncol Biol Phys 10: 5–34

Rubin P, Casarett GW (1968) Clinical radiation pathology, vols I and II. WB Saunders, Philadelphia

Rubin P, Scarantino CW (1978) The bone marrow organ: the critical structure in radiation-drug interaction. Int J Radiat Oncol Biol Phys 4: 3–23

Rubin P, Landman S, Mayer E, Keller B, Ciccio S (1973) Bone marrow regeneration and extension after extended field irradiation in Hodgkin's disease. Cancer 32: 699–711

Rubin P, Bennett JM, Begg C, Bozdech MJ, Silber R (1981) The comparison of total body irradiation vs chlorambucil and prednisone for remission induction of active chronic lymphocytic leukemia: an ECOG study. Part I: total body irradiation — response and toxicity. Int J Radiat Oncol Biol Phys 7: 1623–1632

Rubin P, Constine LS III, Scarantino CW (1984) The paradoxes in patterns and mechanism of bone marrow regeneration after irradiation. 2. Total body irradiation. Radiother Oncol 2: 227–233

Rubin P, Salazar OM, Zagars G, Constine LS, Keys H, Poulter CA, van Ess JD (1985) Systemic hemibody irradiation for overt and occult metastases. Cancer 55: 2210–2221

Russel ES (1979) Hereditary anemias of the mouse: a review for geneticists. Adv Gen 20: 357

Sacks EL, Goris ML, Glatstein E, Gilbert E, Kaplan HS (1978) Bone marrow regeneration following large field radiation. Influence of volume, age, dose, and time. Cancer 42: 1057–1065

Salazar OM, Rubin P, Keller B, Scarantino C (1978) Systemic (half-body) radiation therapy: response and toxicity. Int J Radiat Oncol Biol Phys 4: 937–950

Salazar OM, Rubin P, Hendrickson FR et al. (1986) Single-dose half-body irradiation for palliation of multiple bone metastases from solid tumors. Final Radiation Therapy Oncology Group Report. Cancer 58: 29–36

Scarantino CW, Rubin P, Constine LS III (1984) The paradoxes in patterns and mechanism of bone marrow regeneration after irradiation. 1. Different volumes and doses. Radiother Oncol 2: 215–225

Schneider DO, Whitmore GF (1963) Comparative effects of neutrons and x-rays on mammalian cells. Radiat Res 18: 286–306

Schofield R (1978) The relationship between the spleen colony-forming cell and the haemopoietic stem cell. A hypothesis. Blood Cells 4: 7–25

Schofield R (1979) The pluripotent stem cell. Clin Hematol 8: 221–237

Schofield R, Dexter TM (1982) CFU-S repopulation after low-dose whole-body radiation. Radiat Res 89: 607–617

Schwartz GN, Vigneulle RM, MacVittie TJ (1986) Survival of erythroid burst-forming units and erythroid colony-forming units in canine bone marrow cells exposed in vitro to 1 MeV neutron radiation or x-rays. Radiat Res 108: 336–347

Schwartz GN, Neta R, Vigneulle RM, Patchen ML, MacVittie TJ (1988) Recovery of hematopoietic colony-forming cells in irradiated mice pretreated with' interleukin 1 (IL–1). Exp Hematol 16: 752–757

Scott BR, Hahn FF, McClellan RO, Seiler FA (1988) Risk estimators for radiation-induced bone marrow lethality in humans. Risk Analysis 8: 393–402

Seed TM, Kaspar LV, Tolle DV, Fritz TE (1982) Hemopathologic predisposition and survival time under continuous gamma irradiation: responses mediated by altered radiosensitivity of hemopoietic progenitors. Exp Hematol 10 [Suppl 12]: 232–248

Segal GM, Bagby GC Jr (1988) Vascular endothelial cells and hematopoietic regulation. Int J Cell Cloning 6: 306–312

Senn JS, McCulloch EA (1970) Radiation sensitivity of human bone marrow cells measured by a cell culture method. Blood 35: 56–60

Shleien B (1973) A review of determinations of dose to the active bone marrow from diagnostic x-ray examinations. DHEW Publication (FDA) 74–8007. U.S. Department of Health, Education, and Welfare, Public Health Service, Food and Drug Administration, Bureau of Radiological Health, Rockville, Maryland 20852

Sieff CA (1987) Hematopoietic growth factors. J Clin Invest 79: 1549–1557

Simmons PJ, Przepiorka D, Thomas ED, Torok-Storb B (1987) Host origin of marrow stromal cells following allogeneic bone marrow transplantation. Nature 328: 429–432

Slanina J, Musshoff K, Rahner T, Stiasny R (1977) Long-term side effects in irradiated patients with Hodgkin's disease. Int J Radiat Oncol Biol Phys 2: 1–19

Smith H (1983) Problems in defining dose-mortality relationships for early effects in man following brief exposure to a few Gray of low LET radiation. In: Broerse JJ, Barendsen GW, Kal HB, van der Kogel AJ (eds) Radiation research. Somatic and genetic effects. Martinus Nijhoff, Boston, abstract C 1–31

Sondel PM, Hank JA, Trigg ME et al. (1986) Transplantation of HLA-haploidentical T-cell-depleted marrow for leukemia: autologous marrow recovery with specific immune sensitization for donor antigens. Exp Hematol 14: 278–286

Song CW, Kim TH, Khan FM, Kersey JH, Levitt SH (1981) Radiobiological basis of total body irradiation with different dose rate and fractionation: repair capacity of hemopoietic cells. Int J Radiat Oncol Biol Phys 7: 1695–1701

Standke E (1988) Klinische Verträglichkeit und hämatologische Langzeiterholung nach sequentieller oberer und unterer Halbkörperbestrahlung. Radiobiol Radiother (Berl) 29: 338–340

Steel GG, Horwich A (1988) Radiation resistance and the dose-rate effect: experimental. In: Bleehen NM (ed) Radiobiology in radiotherapy. Springer, London Berlin Heidelberg New York, pp 73–79

Steel GG, Down JD, Peacock JH, Stephens TC (1986) Dose-rate effects and the repair of radiation damage. Radiother Oncol 5: 321–331

Steere HA, Lillicrap SC, Clink HM, Peckham MJ (1979) The recovery of iron uptake in erythropoietic bone marrow following large field radiotherapy. Br J Radiol 52: 61–66

Steinbach KH, Schick P, Trepel F et al. (1979) Estimation of kinetic parameters of neutrophilic, eosinophilic, and basophilic granulocytes in human blood. Blut 39: 27–38

Stephenson JR, Axelrad AA, McLeod DL, Shreeve MM (1971) Induction of colonies of hemoglobin-synthesizing cells by erythropoietin in vitro. Proc Natl Acad Sci USA 68: 1542–1546

Stewart CC, Stevenson AP, Habbersett RC (1988) The effect of low-dose irradiation on unstimulated and PHA-stimulated human lymphocyte subsets. Int J Radiat Biol 53: 77–87

Sugavara S, Tsuneoka K, Shikita M (1980) Colony-stimulating factor and the proliferation of x-irradiated myeloid stem cells. Biochem Biophys Res Commun 96: 1488–1493

Sullivan KM (1986) Acute and chronic graft-versus-host disease in man. Int J Cell Cloning 4 [Suppl 1]: 42–93

Takeichi N, Umemura T, Katsuno M, Nishimura J, Motomura S, Ibayashi H (1987) Regulatory roles of burst-promoting activity (BPA) from bone marrow cells during human regenerating hemopoiesis. Exp Hematol 15: 790–796

Tannock IF, Hayashi S (1972) The proliferation of capillary endothelial cells. Cancer Res 322: 77–82

Tarbell NJ, Amato DA, Down JD, Mauch P, Hellman S (1987) Fractionation and dose rate effects in mice: a model for bone marrow transplantation in man. Int J Radiat Oncol Biol Phys 13: 1065–1069

Tavassoli M (1975) Studies on hemopoietic microenvironments. (Report of a Workshop held in La Jolla, California, 8–9 August 1974) Exp Hematol 3: 213–226

Tavassoli M (1984) Marrow adipose cells and hemopoiesis: an interpretative review. Exp Hematol 12: 139–146

Tavassoli M, Friedenstein A (1983) Hemopoietic stromal microenvironment. Am J Hematol 15: 195–203

Tebbi K, Rubin S, Cowan DH, McCulloch EA (1976) A comparison of granulopoiesis in culture from blood and bone marrow cells of nonleukemic individuals and patients with acute leukemia. Blood 48: 235–243

Tejero C, Hendry JH, Testa NG (1988) Persistent dose-dependent increases in cycling of haemopoietic precursor cells after irradiation. Cell Tissue Kinet 21: 201–204

Tepperman AD, Curtis JE, McCulloch EA (1974) Erythro-poietic colonies in cultures of human marrow. Blood 44: 659–669

Testa NG, Hendry JH, Lajtha LG (1973) The response of mouse haemopoietic colony formers to acute or continuous gamma irradiation. Biomedicine 19:183–186

Thames HD, Hendry JH (1987) Fractionation in radiotherapy. Taylor and Francis, London New York Philadelphia

Thames HD, Withers HR, Peters LJ, Fletcher GH (1982) Changes in early and late radiation responses with altered dose fractionation: implications for dose-survival relationships. Int J Radiat Oncol Biol Phys 8: 219–226

Thar TL, Million RR (1978) Total body irradiation in non-Hodgkin's lymphoma. Cancer 42: 926–931

Thierry D, Jullien D, Rigaud O, Hardy M, Vilcoq JR, Magdelenat H (1985) Human blood granulocyte macrophage progenitors (GM-CFU) during extended field radiation therapy. Acta Radiol Oncol 24: 521–526

Thomas ED (1986) Long-term results of marrow transplantation for leukemia. Bone Marrow Transplantation 1 [Suppl 1]: 175–176

Thomas ED, Herman EC, Cannon JH, Sahler OD, Ferrebee JW, Kay HEM, Constanoulakis M (1961) Autogenous recovery of marrow function. Recovery after general exposure to 1082 roentgens of Co^{60} radiation at 36 roentgens per hour. Arch Intern Med 107: 395–400

Thomas F, Gould MN (1982) Evidence for the repair of potentially lethal damage in irradiated bone marrow. Radiat Environ Biophys 20: 89–94

Thomas PJ, Daban A, Bontoux D (1984) Double hemi-body irradiation in chemotherapy-resistant multiple myeloma. Cancer Treat Rep 68: 1173–1175

Thomson JF, Tourtellotte WW (1953) The effect of dose rate on the LD$_{50}$ of mice exposed to gamma radiation from cobalt 60 sources. Am J Roentgenol 69: 826–829

Till JE (1963) Quantitative aspects of radiation lethality at the cellular level. AJR 90: 917–927

Till JE, McCulloch EA (1961) A direct measurement of the radiation sensitivity of normal mouse bone marrow cells. Radiat Res 14: 213–222

Till JE, McCulloch EA (1963) Early repair processes in marrow cells irradiated and proliferating in vivo. Radiat Res 18: 96–105

Till JE, McCulloch EA (1964) Repair processes in irradiated mouse hematopoietic tissue. Ann NY Acad Sci 114: 115–125

Till JE, McCulloch EA (1980) Hemopoietic stem cell differentiation. Biochim Biophys Acta 605: 431–549

Timothy AR, Sutcliffe SB, Wrigley FM, Jones AE (1979) Hodgkin's disease: combination chemotherapy for relapse following radical radiotherapy. Int J Radiat Oncol Biol Phys 5: 165–169

Tobias JS, Richards JDM, Blackman GM, Joannides T, Trask CWL, Nathan JI (1985) Hemibody irradiation in multiple myeloma. Radiother Oncol 3: 11–16

Torok-Storb B (1988) Cellular interactions. Blood 72: 373–385

Travis EL, Peters LJ, McNeill J, Thames HD, Karolis C (1985) Effect of dose-rate on total body irradiation: lethality and pathological findings. Radiother Oncol 4: 341–352

Trentin JJ (1978) Hemopoietic microenvironments. Transplantation Proc 10: 77–82

UNSCEAR (1982) Ionizing radiation: sources and biological effects. 1982 Report to the General Assembly

Annex J: non-stochastic effects of irradiation. United Nations, New York

Urtasun RC, Belch A, Bodnar D (1983) Hemibody radiation, an active therapeutic modality for the management of patients with small cell lung cancer. Int J Radiat Oncol Biol Phys 9: 1575–1578

Vadhan-Raj S, Buescher S, LeMaistre A et al. (1988) Stimulation of hematopoiesis in patients with bone marrow failure and in patients with malignancy by recombinant human granulocyte-macrophage colony-stimulating factor. Blood 72: 134–141

van Dijk-Milatz A (1979) Total-body irradiation in advanced lymphosarcoma. Br J Radiol 52: 568–570

Van Dyke D, Anger HO (1965) Patterns of marrow hypertrophy and atrophy in man. J Nucl Med 6: 106–120

von Heyden HW (1978) Die ortsständigen Knochenmark-zellen. In: Queißer W (ed) Das Knochenmark — Morphologie Funktion Diagnostik. Thieme, Stuttgart, pp 99–107

von Keyserlingk DG (1978) Anatomie des Knochenmarks. In: Queißer W (ed) Das Knochenmark — Morphologie Funktion Diagnostik. Thieme, Stuttgart, pp 78–95

von Wangenheim K-H, Peterson H-P, Feinendegen LE (1986) Residual radiation effect in the murine hemato-poietic stem cell compartmant. Radiat Environ Biophys 25: 93–106

Voss A-L, Heit W, Müller F, Schlimok G, Wannenmacher M, Wiesneth M (1988) Erste Ergebnisse der fraktionier-ten gegenüber der Einzeit-Ganzkörperbestrahlung als Konditionierungsmaßnahme bei der allogenen Knochen-marktransplantation. Radiobiol Radiother (Berl) 29: 295–296

Vriesendorp HM, van Bekkum DW (1984) Susceptibility to total body irradiation. In: Broerse JJ, MacVittie TJ (eds) Response of different species to total body irradiation. Martinus Nijhoff, Boston, pp 43–57

Wagemaker G, Peters MF, Bol SJL (1979) Induction of erythropoietin responsiveness in vitro by a distinct population of bone marrow cells. Cell Tissue Kinet 12: 521–537

Wald N (1971) Haematological parameters after acute radiation injury. In: International Atomic Energy Agency (ed) Manual on radiation hematology, technical reports series No. 123. IAEA, Vienna, pp 253–264

Walker R, I Willemze R (1980) Neutrophil kinetics and the regulation of granulopoiesis. Rev Infect Dis 2: 282–292

Warren S, Bowers JZ (1950) The acute radiation syndrome in man. Ann Intern Med 32: 207–216

Wash-1400 (1975) Reactor safety study. Appendix F. US Nuclear Regulatory Commission

Wasserman TH, Tubiana M (1988) Lymphoma: radiation therapy in lymphoma treatment. Int J Radiat Oncol Biol Phys 14 [Suppl 1]: 187–201

Weiden PL, Lerner KG, Gerdes A, Heywood JD, Fefer A, Thomas ED (1973) Pancytopenia and leukemia in Hodgkin's disease: report of three cases. Blood 42: 571–577

Weiss L, Chen LT (1975) The organization of hematopoietic cords and vascular sinuses in bone marrow. Blood Cells 1: 617–638

Welte K, Bonilla MA, Gillio AP, Gabrilove JL, O'Reilly RJ, Souza LM (1988) Recombinant human granulocyte-colony stimulating factor: in vivo effects on myelopoiesis in primates. Behring Inst Mitt 102–106

Werts ED, Gibson DP, Knapp SA, DeGowin RL (1980) Stromal cell migration precedes hemopoietic repopulation of the bone marrow after irradiation. Radiat Res 81: 20–30

Wheldon TE, Michalowski AS, Kirk J (1982) The effect of irradiation on function in self-renewing normal tissues with differing proliferative organisation. Br J Radiol 55: 759–766

Wilson FD, Stitzel KA, Klein AK et al (1978) Quantitative response of bone marrow colony-forming units (CFU-C and PFU-C) in weanling beagles exposed to acute whole body γ irradiation. Radiat Res 74: 289–297

Wintrobe MM (1974) Clinical hematology, 7th edn. Lea and Febiger, Philadelphia

Wu C-T, Xue H-H, Chu J-P (1978) Comparison of radio-sensitivity of the murine and canine haemopoietic stem cells. Acta Physiol Sin 30: 121–128 (abstr in English)

Xu CX, Hendry JH, Testa NG, Allen TD (1983) Stromal colonies from mouse marrow: characterization of cell types, optimization of plating efficiency and its effect on radiosensitivity. J Cell Sci 61: 453–466

Young RC, Johnson RE, Canellos GP, Chabner BA, Brereton HD, Berard CW, DeVita VT (1977) Advanced lymphocytic lymphoma: randomized comparisons of chemotherapy and radiotherapy, alone or in combination. Cancer Treat Rep 61: 1153–1159

Zipori D (1988) Hemopoietic microenvironments. In: Testa NG, Gale RP (eds) Hematopoiesis. Long-term effects of chemotherapy and radiation. Marcel Dekker, New York, pp 27–62

Zwaan FE, Goselink H, Veenhof W (1980) CFU-c in human peripheral blood; a rapid method for purification and various in vitro properties. Exp Hematol 8 [Suppl 7]: 99 (abstr)

5 Lymphatic System

H. Grosse-Wilde and U.W. Schaefer

5.1 Definition of the Lymphatic System

Central roles of the immune system are to encounter, recognize, and destroy foreign soluble substances and particular microbes. Furthermore, the immune system has to discriminate between structures which belong to the body (self) and those which do not (nonself), and to regulate throughout life the dynamic process of immune responses. A third feature is the capacity of the immune system to learn and build up a memory with the consequence that a second encounter with a foreign structure results in an accelerated specific immune

reaction (Nossal 1987). More recently a further field of responsibility was found for the immune system in its regulatory role in hematopoiesis and other differentiation processes (Sachs 1987).

5.1.1 Anatomy

Although the lymphatic system has a less organoid structure, one can define organs with a predominant immune function. The bone marrow and the thymus are labeled as primary lymphatic organs, where immune cells proliferate in an antigen-independent fashion. Secondary lymphatic organs are the lymph nodes, spleen, tonsils, Peyer's patches of the intestine, and lymphatic tissue associated with the bronchi of the lung. The secondary lymphatic organs are the typical sites where the antigen-dependent proliferation of immune cells takes place.

The major cellular components of the lymphatic organs are lymphocytes, monocytes or macrophages, and accessory cells. Except for the latter, one specific character of the immune cells is their mobility throughout the body. The ubiquitous presence of immune cells seems to be sensible, given the above-mentioned general function of the immune system. Between the primary and secondary lymphoid organs there exists a constant recirculation of immune cells. For this traffic two main routes are used, the blood vessels and the lymphatic vessels with afferent and efferent channels. The central efferent lymph vessel is the thoracic duct draining into the venous system at the angulus sterni.

5.1.2 Morphology

Lymphocytes are small mononucleated cells with a dense nucleus and a thin cytoplasmic border. Under the light microscope no further differentiation is possible. Electron microscopically, how-

H. Grosse-Wilde, Professor Dr., Institut für Immungenetik, U.W. Schaefer, Professor Dr., Klinik und Poliklinik für Knochenmarktransplantation, Universitätsklinikum Essen, Hufelandstraße 55, 4300 Essen 1, FRG

ever, two subpopulations are discernible. Thymus-derived lymphocytes (i.e., T cells) have a smooth cell membrane, whereas bone marrow-derived lymphocytes (i.e., B cells) appear as numerous villi-studded cells, the villi enlarging the cell surface enormously.

Monocytes, the second mononuclear cell lineage, are larger than lymphocytes; their nucleus is typically U-shaped. These distinctive features allow differentiation even under a light microscope. In addition, in contrast to lymphocytes, monocytes have the capacity for surface adherence, active locomotion, and phagocytosis.

5.1.3 Function

The immune system exerts its complex functions in the healthy individual in a discreet, nearly invisible fashion. Only in the disease state do clinical signals of immune reactions become apparent, e.g., fever, rubor, and tumefaction of secondary lymphatic organs. The mediators of these reactions can be classified according to the criteria: soluble or cellular bound, and antigen specific or non-antigen specific. This categorization is indeed a simplistic representation of the complex interaction of the different immune mediators.

At the beginning of a specific immune reaction stand the encounter with and correct recognition of the foreign substance or particle. In the naive state of the immune system, i.e., when the host has never seen the intruding antigen before, the scenario starts with an unspecific deposition of the antigen on the membrane of a so-called antigen-presenting cell (APC), which is mostly a monocyte/macrophage. This unspecific antigen contact induces the APC to phagocytose and enzymatically digest the foreign structure or part of the structure into peptide fragments. This energy-dependent step is called antigen processing. Some of the peptides (obviously the immunodominant ones) are complexed intracellularly with glycoproteins and then together displayed on the surface of the APC (von Boehmer and Kisielow 1990).

Today we know that these glycoproteins are the gene products of the major histocompatibility complex (MHC), which in man are named HLA (human leukocyte antigens). According to their molecular structure they are subdivided into HLA class I antigens and HLA class II antigens. Peptides derived from exogenous foreign struc-

tures (e.g., soluble antigens and intruding microbes) are predominantly complexed with HLA class II molecules, whereas peptides from endogenous antigens (e.g., virus encoded structures) form a complex with HLA class I molecules (Sprent et al. 1990).

A peptide-presenting monocyte has to find a particular T cell displaying the corresponding peptide-specific receptor on its membrane. This T cell receptor (TCR) resembles the molecular structure of an antibody, with variable regions for the specific binding of the peptide–HLA complex and constant regions for the insertion in the cell membrane and further signal transduction.

For an intimate physical interaction between an APC and a T cell there exists a series of distinct surface molecules which behave in a ligand–receptor fashion. Besides the TCR recognizing the peptide–HLA complex there are at least three further pairs of interacting surface structures: The CD4 molecule of a T helper cell or the CD8 molecule of a T suppressor/cytotoxic cell binds to the constant part of the HLA class II or class I molecule, respectively, on the APC; the CD2 antigen (formerly the E-rosette receptor) of the T cell is the receptor for the CD58 antigen on the APC; and CD54 and the pair of CD11a and CD18 mutually present on the APC and the T cell interact to stabilize the close contact between the peptide-recognizing T cell and the peptide-presenting monocyte. This is then the signal for the APC to secrete a cytokine termed interleukin-1 (IL-1) and for the T cell to pass through further activation steps resulting in the expression of distinct receptors and the secretion of cytokines like IL-2 through IL-4 and IL-6, as well as interferon-γ (Henney 1989).

The secretion of IL-2 together with the expression of a high affinity IL-2 receptor (CD25) enables the T cell to enter an autocrine proliferation loop which results in a clonal expansion of this particular cell. The recruitment of specific immune cells by growth hormone-driven clonal proliferation is a distinctive feature of the immune response. Clonal proliferation is not restricted to the amplification of a T helper cell clone after the initial recognition of a foreign structure. The same holds true for the recruitment of cytotoxic or suppressor T cells and B lymphocytes, which may differentiate into antibody-secreting plasma cells (Cooper 1987; Royer and Reinherz 1987). The antigen- or, more precisely, peptide-dependent specific proliferation takes place preferentially in the above-described secondary lymphatic organs. Besides this T cell-dependent immune response a subpopulation of B cells can be induced to antibody production without the help of T cells by substances like soluble polysaccharides. These substances are designated as T cell-independent antigens.

Immunocompetent lymphocytes are derived from pluripotent stem cells which reside in the bone marrow but can also be found at low frequency in the peripheral blood. The differentiation and amplification are under the regulation of a series of growth hormones or cytokines which are labeled lymphokines or interleukins, if they are secreted predominantly from lymphocytes (DINARELLO and MIER 1987).

Under the influence of IL-1 and IL-3 some of the pluripotent stem cells become committed to the lymphatic lineage, from which a certain number enter the thymus to differentiate into thymocytes and later into immunocompetent T cells with their subtypes T helper cells, T suppressor cells, and cytotoxic T cells. Other lymphatic stem cells remain in the bone marrow to become B lymphocytes, which later also populate the secondary lymphatic organs like spleen and lymph nodes. T lymphocytes are the effector cells mediating the so-called specific cellular immune response whereas B lymphocytes are the progenitors for plasma cells mediating, via antibody formation and secretion, the so-called specific humoral immune response. Both activated B and activated T cells can revert to resting lymphocytes with a specific memory for the recognized antigen-derived peptide structure. Upon rechallenge these memory cells can mount a specific immune response more rapidly. Whereas plasma cells exist for only a few days, memory cells can last a lifetime.

Most structural genes of the above-described cytokines or interleukins and their chromosomal location are now identified and even cloned and transfected in eukaryotic hosts to produce so-called genetically recombinant cytokines in abundant quantities and high purity. These modern molecular technologies enabled immunohematological research to study the biological functions of cytokines more deeply. One common feature of all cytokines is their pleiotropic effect, i.e., they act not only on lymphatic cells but also on cells, e.g., of the hematopoietic lineages.

5.1.4 Markers of Differentiation

B lymphocytes carry membrane-bound immunoglobulins or antibodies forming the antigen-specific B cell receptor. Thymocytes and mature T cells, on the other hand, express a receptor for sheep red blood cells (SRBCs). These two characteristics were for a long time the only markers to identify and enumerate B and T cells.

Since the advent of the technology to produce monoclonal antibodies of a more or less desired specificity this picture has changed dramatically. Within approximately 10 years typing of subpopulations of immune cells with marker-specific monoclonal antibodies has become a routine method. At present nearly 80 distinct membrane markers are officially recognized and labeled according to a WHO nomenclature as cluster of differentiation (CD) antigens. Typical CD antigens on all mature T cells are CD2 (SRBC receptor) and CD3, whereas CD4 and CD8 mark the T helper and T suppressor/cytotoxic subpopulations respectively (KNAPP et al. 1989).

Very similar differentiation antigens with comparable expression on immune cells of experimental animals like mouse, rat, dog, swine, and primates have been described. This points to the fact that the immune systems of nonhuman mammals function in general very similarly and, furthermore, that these membrane structures are indispensable for an effective immune reaction. These similarities add further support to the concept that immunological research data from experimental animal studies can be applied to the human situation.

5.1.5 Assessment of Immunocompetence

According to the above classification into four areas of immune reactions or immune mediators, the in vitro or in vivo tests for immunocompetence can be presented as follows:

5.1.5.1 Specific Humoral Immune Defense

Plasma cell derived antibodies are the principle mediators of an antigen specific humoral immune response. If present in sufficient quantity and specificity they can eliminate foreign intruders within minutes or hours. Antibodies are com-

174

H. Grosse-Wilde and U.W. Schaefer

plexed globular glycoproteins and have a Y-shaped form. Each antibody possesses at least two antigen binding sites (Fab part) and one Fc-part. The latter dictates the physico-chemical properties and the membership to distinct classes of immunoglobulins (Ig), which is another denomination of antibodies according to their overall molecular structure. In man we know IgA, IgD, IgE, IgG, and IgM. In the peripheral blood IgG is the predominant immunoglobulin followed by IgM and IgA. In healthy individuals IgD and IgE have an extremely low concentration.

A specific humoral immune response will normally not alter the overall concentration of Ig. If, however, antigen specific antibodies are determined, in the primary immune response the occurence of IgM type followed by IgG type antibodies can be observed. In a second immune response against the same antigen the production of IgM antibodies is small, but IgG antibodies occure more rapidly and in higher concentration. If the whole plasma cell or B-cell compartment of specific lineages of B-lymphocytes is affected, the blood levels of whole Ig or their classes and subclasses are found reduced and increased respectively.

For the precise quantification and specification of immunoglobulins or antibodies there nowadays exists a battery of various in vitro tests. The reader is referred to specific textbooks for further details (Bier et al. 1986; Paul 1986).

5.1.5.2 Unspecific Humoral Immune Defense

Since a specific immune response and especially the primary one takes days to become effective, the body needs defense mechanisms which act more rapidly. The complement system with the components of the alternative pathway of activation is a typical and most important mediator of humoral immune reaction without antigen specificity. Solely the encounter of lipopolysaccharides on the membrane of, for example, bacteria is sufficient to trigger the complement components of the alternative pathway, which results finally in conglutination and opsonization of the microbes, enabling granulocytes or macrophages to phagocytose and destroy the intruders.

Another example of unspecific but effective humoral immune defense is the action of interferons blocking the virus replication. Furthermore, interferons, especially interferon-α and interferon-γ, have the capacity to increase the expression of HLA molecules on immune and accessory cells, to induce the expression of HLA on other somatic cells, and to activate monocytes. Thus interferon can augment indirectly the specific and unspecific cellular defense mechanisms. Similar effects are described for other cytokines like tumor necrosis factor (TNF).

5.1.5.3 Specific Cellular Immune Defense

As already described for antigen recognition, the monocytes and the T lymphocytes are the key cells. In addition B cells can function as APCs by capturing the antigen via their membrane-bound antibodies, engulfing this antigen–antibody complex, performing intracellular processing like the monocyte, and presenting the peptide with HLA class II molecules to the respective T cell.

In the recognition phase antigen-specific T helper cells are operative, recruiting either B cells or further T cells for the effector phase of the immune response. B cells are directed to proliferate clonally and differentiate into determined immune cells producing and secreting as plasma cells one type of antigen-specific antibody per cell. Especially for elimination of virus-infected cells, T helper cells instruct precursors of cytotoxic T cells to amplify and then destroy their targets by cell-mediated cytotoxicity. Antibody-dependent cell-mediated cytotoxicity represents a combination of humoral and cellular specific immune response where the antibody determines the specificity of binding and the complement-independent target destruction is executed by a cytotoxic effector cell.

Immunocompetent cells circulating in the peripheral blood can be enumerated according to their surface markers and in vitro can be stimulated by mitogens and antigens to enter blast transformation and mitosis. In healthy individuals, two-thirds of peripheral blood mononuclear cells (PBMCs) are T cells carrying the pan-T markers CD2 and CD3. The T cell fraction can be subdivided into CD4-positive (approx. 40%) and CD8-positive cells (approx. 20%). This relation is commonly expressed as the CD4:CD8 ratio, which is therefore 2:1. B cells carrying membrane Ig represent approximately 10% of PBMCs.

In vitro transformation of PBMCs under cell culture conditions by mitogens leads to polyclonal activation of immunocompetent T cells and, in some cases, also B cells. In most cases monocytes are indispensable for this proliferation. If PBMCs are confronted in vitro with soluble antigens like tetanus toxoid or tuberculin, memory T cells will, with the aid of APCs, recognize these antigens and start to proliferate in a clonal fashion which can be measured quantitatively. Cell-mediated cytotoxicity can be assessed by incubating cytotoxic T cells with the respective target cells labeled with an appropriate tracer. If the target cells are lysed the released tracer can be measured accordingly.

Cell-mediated immunity can also be estimated in vivo by skin tests. Very similar to the in vitro lymphocyte transformation test, T cells with antigen-specific memory accumulate and proliferate at the site where the antigen is deposited. This antigen-specific proliferation is visible and semi-quantitatively measurable as skin induration.

5.1.5.4 Unspecific Cellular Immune Defense

Like the humoral defense mechanisms, cellular immune surveillance has unspecific mediators. The so-called natural killer cells or large granular lymphocytes belong to a still undefined lineage, but mount very effective reactions towards, for example, tumor cells without prior sensitization (TIMONEN et al. 1981; HERBERMAN and ORTALDO 1981).

5.2 Effects of Irradiation on the Lymphatic System

The effects of irradiation on immune responses have been extensively investigated during the past 50 years. Most of these experiments have concentrated on the effects of ionizing radiation given at a high dose rate on the production of specific antibodies after injection of antigens into animals. More recent investigations have attempted to determine dose–response curves of a given cell population or a physiological function, using various doses of absorbed radiation.

After high doses of ionizing radiation the number of lymphocytes decreases in the peripheral blood. Several authors have reported differences in the radiosensitivity of the different subpopulations of lymphocytes, causing alterations in the relative proportions of these subpopulations. Lymphocytes removed from mice

subjected to whole-body x-irradiation show dose-time dependent functional and morphological changes.

5.2.1 Cytomorphological and Histological Changes

Of all mammalian tissues, lymphocytes (but not all subsets) and sperm cells are most sensitive to irradiation and have the lowest D_0 of 0.25–0.35 Gy (ANDERSON and WARNER 1976; et al. 1986; NAPARSTEK and SLAVIN 1988; HALL 1988; BETZ 1974; DEHOS et al. 1986; BERDJIS 1971). Moreover, while most cells exposed to irradiation do not die until they attempt to undergo mitosis, most lymphocytes are killed without entering the mitotic cycle. The immediate death of lymphocytes after small doses of irradiation is thus nonmitotic or "interphase."

In rats this radiosensitivity of lymphocytes to irradiation results in a rapid decrease in the number of circulating lymphocytes after 1 Gy whole body exposure, so that after 4 h only 25% remain (SCHREK 1961). Within 1 h after exposure to an LD_{50} dose of x-rays, necrosis of various lymphoid tissues is evident and within a few days the lymphoid tissues are almost devoid of lymphocytes (JORDAN 1967). There is a remarkable variability in radiosensitivity of various lymphoid organs and various areas of the same organ. The microenvironmental cell mass is less radiosensitive than the lymphoid cells (ANDERSON et al. 1974, 1977; DURKIN and THORBECKE 1972; TROWELL 1965). Therefore the weight loss of the spleen after irradiation is less pronounced than that of the thymus, in which the microenvironmental cell mass is much smaller. As shown histologically and by immunofluorescence, non-thymic-dependent areas are extremely radiosensitive, resulting in greater and faster depletion of B cells from B-dependent areas than from T-dependent areas (DURKIN and THORBECKE 1972). Thymus lymphocytes already show alterations in their morphology after exposure to 0.05 Gy (ANDERSON and WARNER 1976), while the stroma cells are not altered even after 50 Gy (TROWELL 1961). Following low dose irradiation (1.5–2 Gy) the thymus regains its initial weight within 12 days. After higher doses there is an initial recovery, presumably due to regeneration of radioresistant subsets of intrathymic precursors, and later an influx of lymphocytes from regenerating bone marrow (KATAOKA and SATO 1975; TOKADA et al. 1969).

Computer-assisted morphometric analysis of the arrangement and texture of the chromatin of lymphocytes from irradiated mice reveals that the optical density values in the chromatin shift toward lower values, indicating lighter staining chromatin, as radiation dose increases (Olson et al. 1982; Olson and Bartels 1984).

5.2.2 Chromosomal Aberrations and Micronucleus Formation

The analysis of radiation-induced chromosome aberrations in human peripheral lymphocytes is a very sensitive method for biological determination of body doses. Total body doses in excess of about 0.25 Gy can be detected in this way. Abnormal chromosomes have been found as early as 2 min and as late as 40 years after exposure (Hall 1988; Wald and Conner 1988; Lloyd et al. 1982; Lloyd 1984; Bauchinger 1972, 1984; Guedeney et al. 1988; Hakoda et al. 1988; Kakati et al. 1986; Scheid et al. 1988).

The basis for a cytogenetic dose estimation is dose–effect curves for radiation-induced chromosome aberrations obtained by in vitro γ-irradiation and fitted by a linear-quadratic relationship (Sato et al. 1974; Bauchinger 1984).

Another method to determine chromosomal damage in lymphocytes is the micronucleus test (Hogstedt 1984; Countryman and Heddle 1976). Micronuclei are found in interphase cells which have passed through at least one mitosis after irradiation. It is assumed that they derive from acentric chromosomal fragments which are incorporated into daughter nuclei during mitosis. A correlation between radiation-induced formation of micronuclei and cell death has been described. Increased frequencies of micronuclei in lymphocytes were found in various human populations, including occupationally exposed individuals, patients who had undergone diagnostic radiological procedures or radiotherapy, and atomic bomb survivors (Almassy et al. 1987; Fenech and Morley 1985; Huber et al. 1989; Prosser et al. 1988). However, in vitro experiments with x-rays revealed that this biological dosimetry method is not sensitive enough at low dose levels (<0.3 Gy) because of an high background frequency of micronuclei (Bauchinger 1984; Huber et al. 1989).

5.2.3 Mechanisms of Functional Changes After Irradiation

Measurement of the influence of γ-irradiation on immunocompetence is based on the different sensitivity of the above-described subpopulations of lymphocytes and accessory cells. Although it has now been known for more than 20 years that among somatic cells lymphocytes are the most sensitive to lethal effects of irradiation (Anderson and Warner 1976), the precise mechanisms responsible for this sensitivity are still not well defined.

Radiobiological research has utilized in vivo and in vitro experiments to monitor the discrete changes in immune cell functions after experimental irradiation of animals or radiotherapy of patients suffering from various diseases (Bazin and Platteau 1984; Anderson and Williams 1977; Birkeland 1978).

There is general agreement that resting lymphocytes are most sensitive to irradiation. These cells die in the absence of further mitoses, so-called interphase radiation death. Although the mechanism is still unclear, the most dramatic intracellular change after irradiation with $1-5$ Gy is the degradation of DNA. This DNA fragmentation is thought to be mediated by activation of topoisomerases and endogenous endonucleases cleaving DNA into oligonucleosome-length fragments of approximately 200 base pairs (Johnston and McNerney 1985; Sellins and Cohen 1987). As in the case of immature thymocytes, the activation of endonucleases can be induced by an increase in cytosolic Ca^{2+} levels due to cell membrane alteration or damage caused by irradiation. In this mechanism of programmed cell death or apoptosis in naive or resting immune cells it is interesting to note that protein kinase C (PKC) blocks the Ca^{2+}-dependent activation of endonucleases and that interleukin-1 (IL-1) is a typical PKC inhibitor (McConkey et al. 1990). In the mouse model it was shown that IL-1 acts as a radioprotector (Neta et al. 1986). Since this cytokine is produced mainly in monocytes or macrophages after incubation with microbial agents such as lipopolysaccharides, muramyl dipeptide, and BCG, all known to have immunomodulatory and radioprotective properties (Langendorff et al. 1971; Smith et al. 1957), it is tempting to speculate that the mechanism of radioprotection is the secretion of IL-1 (Behling 1983; Manori et al. 1986; Morrissey et al. 1987). Via activation of PKC the radiation-induced apoptosis is inhibited by blocking endogenous endonuclease activity.

This apoptosis is restricted to resting immune cells. Primed, i.e., ligand-activated B cells or T cells are relatively resistant to low dose irradiation (LOWENTHAL and HARRIS 1985; CIRKOVIC 1970; JAMES et al. 1983; STEFANI 1966; STEFANI and SCHREK 1963). A comparative analysis, however, shows that B cells are more sensitive than T cells (ANDERSON and WARNER 1976). With regard to radiosensitivity, B cells can be subdivided into thymus-dependent and thymus-independent subpopulations (LEE and WOODLAND 1985). Among the thymus-independent B cells the surface amount of IgM in comparison to IgG seems to play a role in radiosensitivity, since IgM > IgG B cells are more sensitive than IgM < IgG ones (RIGGS et al. 1988). Clinical analysis in humans has shown that, in general, thymus-dependent B cells are more prone to radiation damage than thymus-independent ones (KOTZIN and STROBER 1984; TANAY and STROBER 1984). Plasma cells are relatively radioresistant but physiologically possess a short life span.

As regards T cells, there is general agreement that they are more resistant to irradiation than B cells (SPRENT et al. 1974; ANDERSON and WARNER 1976; DURUM and GENGOZIAN 1978; PROSSER 1976). Especially activated (e.g., by lectins or specific antigens) T cells or T cell clones show no significant DNA fragmentation or loss of viability even at doses of 30 Gy (ASHWELL et al. 1986; SANDERSON and MORLEY 1986). Results regarding the radiosensitivity of CD4-positive T helper cells and CD8-positive T suppressor cells are controversial (FARNSWORTH et al. 1988; NAPARSTEK and SLAVIN 1988; AGAROSSI et al. 1978; ANDERSON et al. 1986; GERBER et al. 1985). Based on numerous reports of quantitative measurements of circulating T cell subsets showing that after total lymphoid irradiation or whole-body irradiation in man and animals the CD4-positive subset becomes diminished, it seems reasonable to conclude that T helper cells are more radiosensitive than T suppressor cells (FUKS et al. 1976; STROBER et al. 1979; HASEGAWA et al. 1988; AMAGAI et al. 1987). The T helper subset can be further subdivided into IL-2 and IL-4 secreting cells (TH1 and TH2 respectively). There is evidence that the IL-4 releasing CD4 subset is more radioresistant (COSULICH et al. 1986; BASS et al. 1989).

In vitro, the typical changes of T or B cells after radiation are reduced or abrogated with regard to antigen presentation capacity and response to mitogens like phytohemagglutinin (PHA) or concanavalin A (ConA), and also specific antigens like purified protein derivative (PPD) (tuberculin) (NAPARSTEK and SLAVIN 1988; ANDERSON and LEFKOVITS 1980a). However, the differential effects of radiation on T cell subsets, mostly judged upon their quantitative changes in the peripheral blood, could well be an epiphenomenon. Irradiation may also alter the homing and recirculation behavior of lymphocytes by influencing their microenviroment and accessory cells. Thus, the generally reported observation that after local or whole-body irradiation of patients or experimental animals the CD4 subset decreases and the CD8 subset becomes the predominant T cell fraction does not represent definite proof that CD8-positive cells are more radioresistant than CD4-positive cells.

Accessory cells for the immune response, such as monocytes, macrophages, and dendritic cells, are relatively radioresistant even at high doses of more than 20 Gy. Furthermore, their typical cytokine IL-1 secreted after stimulation by substances like lipopolysaccharides (LPS) has recently been shown to act as a potent radioprotective agent that can rescue mice subjected to lethal doses of irradiation (MANORI et al. 1986; NETA et al. 1986). In addition, γ-irradiation of more than 10 Gy can augment the expression of MHC class I molecules on macrophages and render them susceptible for triggering signals, like LPS interaction, to acquire a tumoricidal status (LAMBERT and PAULNOCK 1987).

Another type of immune cells mediating unspecific response is the spontaneous natural killer (NK) cells or large granular lymphocytes (LGLs). The precise role of NK cells/LGLs in vivo is uncertain, but NK cell activity is believed to play a significant role in surveillance against tumors, the response to viral infections, and graft versus host disease after allogeneic marrow transplantation (TALMADGE et al. 1980). In man, there obviously exists a polymorphic x-linked codominant trait for radiation sensitivity of NK cell function (SCHACTER et al. 1985). Irradiation of NK cells with 30 Gy discriminates the population into approximately 90% sensitive and 10% resistant individuals (PIERCE et al., 1986). In the murine system, the data indicate that NK cell activity is under the influence of H-2 linked factors (SADO et al. 1985). Doses below 10 Gy resulted in an augmentation of NK cell activity.

Functional changes in the immune response after radiation are immediate and remarkable, but not uniform. Given that unprimed T cells undergo a programmed cell death even at low radiation doses, it is understandable that in vitro stimulation experiments with various lectins, such as PHA, ConA, and pokeweed mitogen (PWM), to induce polyclonal T cell proliferation, revealed a marked reduction in reagibility (Baral and Blomgren 1976; Anderson and Lefkovits 1980a; Birke-land 1978; Kotzin et al. 1984; Sieber et al. 1985; Zarcone et al. 1989). Similar irradiation-associated immune derangements were observed using specific antigen preparations like PPD for in vitro stimulation of committed T cells or dinitro-chlorobenzene for skin tests assessing T cell-dependent delayed-type hypersensitivity (Fuks et al. 1976; Naparstek and Slavin 1988). The humoral immune response based on the plasma level of immunoglobulins is not seriously affected, since the antibody-secreting plasma cells are relatively radioresistant.

This general statement, however, must be modified since in vivo irradiation encounters for the most part not a uniform and static but rather a complex and dynamic status of immune reactions. From animal experiments we know that the timing of antigenic stimulation and irradiation dictates the outcome: If the antigenic challenge precedes the irradiation, the specific antibody production may not be seriously affected and may even be enhanced, whereas postirradiation antigen application will decrease antibody formation (Dixon et al. 1952; Dixon and McConahey 1963; Graham et al. 1956; Tagliaferro and Tagliaferro 1970; Takada et al. 1971; Tanay and Strober 1984; Zan-Bar et al. 1978). Different radiation doses may have opposing effects on antibody secretion (Anderson and Lefkovits 1979; Anderson et al. 1980). A number of studies reported enhancement of the humoral immune response when antigen administration was restricted to a particular part of the body (Eltringham 1984); however, many of these results were not substantiated by other investigators. Given the above-mentioned differential radiosensitivity of immune cells participating in the process and recent descriptions of distinct subpopulations of CD4 helper cells with a relatively radioresistant (TH2) fraction secreting predominantly IL-4, this in some ways paradoxical humoral immune response can be explained by a preponderance of these helper cells inducing via IL-4 augmented B cell proliferation

and differentiation into plasma cells, including the selection of immunoglobulin isotypes. In addition, low dose irradiation inducing apoptosis of uncommitted immune cells, sparing the primed ones, will simply result in more available space in the lymphatic tissue for the proliferating B cell clones (Bier et al. 1986).

In general, and this also holds true for other immunosuppressive regimens, the irradiation effect is more profound in the primary cellular and humoral immune response (the secondary response is only slightly affected by irradiation). This apparent rule can be explained by the above-described differential radiosensitivity of unprimed and primed immune cells and has substantial implications for therapeutic irradiation protocols.

5.3 High Dose Total Body Irradiation

Data on the acute systemic effects of whole body exposure to ionizing radiation can be drawn from animal experiments, from nuclear plant accidents, from atomic bomb casualties, and from therapeutic exposures of patients with malignant disorders (Barrett 1988; Constine and Rubin 1988). It is generally accepted that in humans the whole body $LD_{50/60}$ is around 4.5 Gy for acute exposure (Vriesendorp and van Bekkum 1984; Constine and Rubin 1988).

5.3.1 Atomic Bomb Casualties

An increased frequency of malignant diseases has been observed in atomic bomb survivors (Kato and Schull 1982; Schull 1984; Beebe et al. 1978; Finch 1984). Reports on the immune functions in atomic bomb survivors are rare (Akiyama et al. 1983; Bloom et al. 1983; Yamada et al. 1985). Akiyama et al. (1983) and Bloom et al. (1983) investigated some immune parameters in such individuals. Akiyama et al. studied the percentage of T cells and PHA responses in 1047 survivors 30–33 years after exposure. Of these, 900 were apparently healthy without evidence of malignant tumors or chromosomal abnormalities. These individuals were presumably exposed to doses between 0 and over 2 Gy. Decreased responsiveness to PHA was demonstrated years later and was more severe in apparently healthy persons with a chromosomal abnormality. The study of Bloom et al. comprised a population exposed to doses of less than 0.5 Gy. In this group of 189 survivors, natural cell-mediated cytotoxicity was significantly higher than in normal controls. Likewise, interferon production and responsiveness to PHA also tended to be higher. The increase in cell-mediated immunity following low dose irradiation may be explained by abrogation of the normal negative feedback, mediated by suppressor cells, as demonstrated in experimental animal models.

The earliest laboratory finding after single-dose total body exposure is lymphopenia, absolute lymphocyte levels reaching below 1000/ml within the first 48 h after potentially lethal exposure (ANDERSON et al. 1986). The lymphocytes appear to have two types of radiation response. About 80% die a prompt intermitotic death while some lymphocytes survive. Their response depends on the class of lymphocytes involved, the extent of cell proliferations required, cell traffic, and the balance between inhibiting (suppressor) and stimulatory (helper) systems involved.

5.3.2 Bone Marrow Transplantation

Bone marrow transplant recipients are another group of patients exposed to high doses of total body irradiation. The purpose of bone marrow transplantation is to provide the recipient with a new, permanently functioning hematopoietic system. Total body irradiation is used to enable the homing of the graft by creating space in the bone marrow and by suppressing the allogeneic resistance (CHAMPLIN and GALE 1984; GRATWOHL et al. 1987; SCHAEFER and BEELEN 1989; VAN BEKKUM and DE VRIES 1967; VAN BEKKUM and LÖWENBERG 1985; THOMAS et al. 1975, 1982).

5.3.2.1 Host-Versus-Graft Reaction

An unprepared healthy marrow recipient will oppose engraftment of allogeneic bone marrow cells by a host-versus-graft (HvG) reaction. The need for suppression of the HvG reaction in addition to the need for space is illustrated by the experience with allogeneic bone marrow transplants in patients with hypoplastic marrow due to severe aplastic anemia. However, lasting engraftment after intravenous injection of allogeneic bone marrow cells can only be obtained if the donor is histocompatible.

5.3.2.2 Graft-Versus-Host Reaction

After the take of an allogeneic bone marrow graft another immunological reaction can occur, caused by the T lymphocytes transferred with the graft itself or by T lymphocytes which develop from grafted precursor cells. This graft-versus-host (GvH) reaction is directed against the tissue antigens of the recipient, leading to pathological changes in many organs, the skin, the intestinal tract, and the liver being most frequently and severely affected. The outcome of allogeneic bone marrow transplantation is the end result of competing HvG and GvH reactions (GALE and REISNER 1986). This two-way reactivity is a feature unique to the transplantation of hematopoietic cells. After a successful allogeneic marrow transplant all cells of the hematopoietic system will be of donor type.

Bone marrow transplant patients as well as other severely immunocompromised patients are at risk for transfusion-associated GvH disease. In humans, whole blood, packed red cells, pooled platelet concentrates, platelets prepared by apheresis, and granulocytes have enough viable lymphocytes to lead to transfusion-associated GvH disease (ANDERSON and WEINSTEIN 1990). Fresh plasma with as few as 10^4 lymphocytes per kilogram of the recipient's body weight can cause the disease (RUBINSTEIN et al. 1973). A useful measure to prevent transfusion-associated GvH disease is to irradiate all blood products before transfusion. The results of most recent studies suggest that irradiation with 15–20 Gy can reduce mitogen-responsive lymphocytes by 10^{-5} to 10^{-6} as compared to non-irradiated control samples (DROBYSKI et al. 1989). BUTTON et al. (1981) examined the function of blood components after radiation doses of 5–200 Gy and demonstrated that doses as high as 50 Gy decreased mitogen-induced stimulation by 98.5% but did not compromise the function of other cells. However, the observation that a small percentage of lymphocytes survive irradiation of 10–20 Gy, coupled with a single reported case of apparently transfusion-related GvH disease in a bone marrow transplant recipient who received only blood components irradiated with 20 Gy (DROBYSKI et al. 1989), suggests that existing guidelines for the irradiation of blood products may require reassessment (LEITMAN and HOLLAND 1985).

5.3.2.3 Immune Reconstitution
in Transplant Patients

The recovery of both hematological and immuno-logical functions following bone marrow trans-plantation has been found to take much longer in patients receiving allogeneic (HLA-identical sibl-ing) marrow than in those treated with syngeneic or autologous marrow (Witherspoon et al. 1982, 1984; Tsoi et al. 1984; van Bekkum and Löwen-berg 1985). All immunological parameters show pronounced impairment for the first few months to a year following transplantation. Although both the number of circulating lymphocytes and the ab-solute number of T and B cells reach near-normal levels about 3 months after transplantation, severely abnormal in vivo and in vitro functions of lymphoid subsets are the rule. Serum immuno-globulin levels reach normal values within 3 months after bone marrow transplantation, yet the humor-al response, both in vivo and in vitro, demons-trates marked impairment. In the presence of GvH disease it takes longer for most immune reactions to normalize (Tsoi et al. 1984; van Bekkum et al. 1985; Mori et al. 1983). Because of the severe impairment of all cellular and humoral responses shortly after transplantation the patients are extremely susceptible to life-threatening infections.

Histology of the lymphatic tissues of transplant patients has been obtained from autopsies of patients who died from a variety of complications. The current conditioning regimens of high dose total body irradiation and intravenous infusion of high dose cyclophosphamide induce a complete or near-complete depletion of lymphocytes from the lymphatic tissues. In a series of patients described by Woodruff and co-workers (1976), clear signs of lymphatic reconstitution were found after day 30, consisting primarily in a repopulation of the B lymphocyte areas. The T lymphocyte areas in the spleen and the lymph nodes remained poorly populated as late as 215 days after transplantation, although in most patients the T lymphocytes in the peripheral blood reached normal values after 2–3 months. Beschorner et al. (1978, 1981) investigated several lymphatic organs in marrow recipients. Severe atrophy in the thymus, peripheral lymph nodes, spleen, Peyer's plaques, and mesenteric lymph nodes was found in marrow recipients dying within 1–4 months after trans-plantation. After 2–3 months, signs of reconstitu-tion were seen in the different lymphatic organs.

The pathology of the radiation chimera has been studied systematically in the mouse, the rat, the rabbit, the rhesus monkey, and the dog. The reader is referred to the recent review of Zurcher and van Bekkum (1985). This and the data in human patients treated with total body irradiation and bone marrow transplantation have resulted in a fairly complete understanding of the characteris-tic pathology of GvH disease, which has to be clearly differentiated from pathologies due to irradiation or infections. The syndrome which is now known as GvH disease was originally termed secondary disease because it developed in mice grafted with allogeneic hematopoietic cells after the primary disease (i.e. the bone marrow syn-drome following high dose total body irradiation) had resolved.

5.3.2.4 Immune Reconstitution in Animal Models

In most animal species bone marrow aplasia following lethal irradiation develops in about 2–3 days.

In the lymphatic tissues of the lymph nodes, spleen, intestinal tract, and thymus atrophy de-velops. After 24 h depletion of lymphoid cells is pronounced and the lymphatic follicles have dis-appeared. However, even after a supralethal dose small numbers of mature lymphoid cells may be found dispersed in the reticular stroma, and a further decrease in cellularity occurs during the following days. In a proportion of the animals large reticular cells and histiocytes with swollen nuclei and prominent nucleoli, sometimes display-ing abnormal mitoses, are found in the follicular remnants. Frequently the surrounding tissue and the medullary cords are heavily infiltrated with plasma cells. The lymphatic sinusoids are dilated and filled at first with histiocytic cells, and after the 1st week with erythrocytes, which are sometimes engulfed by macrophages. Sometimes small groups of lymphoblasts are found at the end of the 1st week, probably representing abortive regen-eration.

The time and the extent of the regeneration of the lymphatic tissues are dependent on both the number of lymphoid cells contained in the grafted cell suspension and the host–donor combination. Compared with the repopulation of lymphatic tissue in mice, that in monkeys occurs relatively early if the time of bone marrow recovery is taken into account. This finding can be explained by the much higher proportion of lymphoid cells in monkey's bone marrow as compared to bone marrow of the mouse. In a number of allogeneic or semiallogeneic parent to F1 combinations in mice, complete regeneration of the lymphatic tissues occurs in about a month. In other strict allogeneic combinations in mice or in allogeneic combinations in rats, rabbits, monkeys, and man, the initial regeneration is followed by secondary changes due to GvH reaction (ZURCHER and VAN BEKKUM 1985).

5.3.2.5 Graft Rejection

In animals in which the graft is rejected, a peculiar granulomatous reaction has been observed in the lymphatic tissues. Massive proliferation of reticuloendothelial cells of an epithelioid type occurs in the red pulp of the spleen, the lymph nodes, and the bone marrow (CONGDON et al. 1957). In addition, multinucleated cells of the foreign-body type are seen. It is not known whether the epithelioid cell reaction is primarily connected with the antibody response against the graft, or whether it represents a non-specific histiocytic response to cellular disintegration.

In human patients with aplastic anemia in whom sustained engraftment was not obtained, no histological features were observed which could be considered characteristic for rejection (Naijm et al. 1978).

The phenomenon of marrow rejection following supralethal radiochemotherapy was explained in the past mainly by non-T cell mechanisms known to be resistant to high dose irradiation.

In murine models two major lymphocyte subpopulations have been implicated in bone marrow rejection. NK cells have been extensively studied in this context. In particular, CUDKOWICZ and co-workers (CUDKOWICZ and BENNET 1971; KIESSLING et al. 1977; LOTZOVÁ and CUDKOWICZ 1974) have shown that these radioresistant cells are involved in the hybrid-resistance phenomenon. On the other hand, radioresistant T cells were suggested to be involved in allogeneic inhibition of colony forming units in the spleen (VON MELCHNER and BARLETT 1983; SCHWARTZ et al. 1987). REISNER et al. (1986) investigated whether clonable T lymphocytes can be detected in primates after supralethal radiochemotherapy and allogeneic bone marrow transplantation. Only minute numbers of mononuclear cells were obtained

from the blood and spleen of these lethally treated monkeys. However, in every such experiment, a significant number of T cells was found by the E-rosette assay with sheep erythrocytes. Interestingly, the majority of T cells at day 0, the day of marrow infusion, were found in the blood, whereas on day 5 they were concentrated in the spleen. These cells surviving the heavy irradiation and chemotherapy were still capable of clonal expansion in response to the appropriate mitogenic stimulus.

In addition to the radioresistant alloreactive T cells surviving in supralethally irradiated marrow recipients ($\geqslant 15$ Gy), lymphoid subpopulations in the marrow graft itself also may play a role in the engraftment of allogeneic marrow cells. If T cell-depleted bone marrow is grafted a significantly higher rejection rate is observed as compared to unmanipulated bone marrow (O'REILLY et al. 1985; BUTTURINI and GALE 1988).

The complex biological mechanisms after total body irradiation and allogeneic bone marrow transplantation have been extensively discussed by VAN BEKKUM in his books *Radiation Chimaeras* (VAN BEKKUM and DE VRIES 1967) and *Bone Marrow Transplantation* (VAN BEKKUM and LÖWENBERG 1985).

5.4 Total Lymphoid Irradiation

The rationale for using total lymphoid irradiation (TLI) as an immunosuppressive treatment originated from studies of patients with Hodgkin's disease, in which TLI is an accepted form of therapy (KAPLAN 1980). This radiotherapy regimen was noted to induce profound immunological abnormalities, and yet was well tolerated and had few long-term side-effects (FUKS et al. 1976).

A vast amount of experimental data in animals and humans suggest that TLI may be used alone or in combination with other immunosuppressive modalities for the treatment of drug-resistant autoimmune disorders and in organ transplantation.

5.4.1 Total Lymphoid Irradiation in Autoimmune Disease

The situation where immune cells of a given individual attack structures of that individual's own somatic cells is labeled as an autoimmune or, better, an autoaggressive status. The recognition steps and effector mechanisms in an autoaggressive response are the same as in the physiological response to foreign antigens, i.e., specific activation of T cells and B cells as well as amplification and differentiation into T effector cells and antibody-secreting plasma cells. The only difference is that the specific targets are now self-structures (Sinha et al. 1990; von Boehmer and Kisielow 1990). Although it is believed and for some steps proven that a certain level of autoaggression is present in every individual, the incidence of clinically manifest autoimmune diseases is increasing. Typical diseases are systemic lupus erythematosus (SLE), multiple sclerosis, and rheumatoid arthritis.

Due to the unique immunosuppressive effect of TLI and the clinical experience that some autoimmune diseased patients are, to varying degrees, resistant to classical antiinflammatory or immunosuppressive drugs, it was suggested that TLI may be a rational alternative therapy. Clinical experiences with TLI have been reported especially for intractable rheumatoid arthritis, SLE, and multiple sclerosis.

5.4.1.1 Animal Models

In mice strains like NZB/NZW and MRL/1 prone to develop autoaggressive diseases, extensive and very promising studies using TLI have been reported (Dixon et al. 1980). The autoimmune features closely resemble those in human SLE, with antinuclear antibodies and fatal immune complex nephritis. Besides the well-known efficacy of immunosuppressive drugs in preventing the outbreak of the lupus-like disease in NZBxW, TLI was shown to reverse even the well-expressed murine SLE, resulting in a survival rate similar to that of control animals (Kotzin and Strober 1979; Slavin 1979). The autoimmune disease could not be reinduced by transferring large numbers of murine cells from mice suffering from active disease. This indicates that TLI resulted in an active defense mechanism towards the autoimmune process in the treated animals (Kotzin and Strober 1984). Another autoimmune disease spontaneously develops in MRL/1 mice, with massive nonmalignant T cell proliferation resulting in lymph node hyperplasia, splenomegaly, and severe glomerulonephritis, which leads to death in nearly 50% of the animals at approximately 6 months of age. If TLI is administered at approx-

imately 3 months of age, the typical time of disease onset, 100% of the animals are still alive at 9 months. Autoantibodies against native and single-stranded DNA, however, are not significantly influenced by TLI (Theofilopoulos et al. 1980).

A further, but artificially induced autoimmune model is adjuvant arthritis in rats, resembling clinical signs of rheumatoid arthritis in man. In rats this disease develops after injection of *Mycobacterium butyricum* in mineral oil. The best clinical improvements were seen in those rats receiving TLI plus local paw irradiation. Arthritis scores and x-ray findings markedly improved in the animals with no signs of relapse (Schurman et al. 1981).

These experimental data clearly indicate that fractionated TLI has a long-lasting beneficial effect on murine SLE and related disorders as well as arthritis, although the precise mechanisms are still unclear. Nevertheless, these preclinical results were one of the main arguments for introducing TLI in the treatment of similar diseases in man (Slater et al. 1976; Slavin et al. 1977a,b).

5.4.1.2 Clinical Results

Total lymphoid irradiation was administered to patients suffering from rheumatoid arthritis (Kotzin et al. 1981, 1983, 1984; Trentham et al. 1981; Field et al. 1983; Tanay et al. 1984, 1987; Soden et al. 1989; Nuesslein et al. 1985; Herbst et al. 1986; Harris 1990), SLE (Kotzin et al. 1984; Terr et al. 1987; BenChetrit et al. 1986), or multiple sclerosis (Cook et al. 1987; Troiano et al. 1988; Kolar and Hornback 1986). Several feasibility studies demonstrated significant improvement in clinical disease activity in some patients resistant to conventional therapy.

Total lymphoid irradiation produced a significant reduction in the absolute number of T cells (Harris et al. 1985). This reduction was associated with a marked decrease in CD4-positive T cells and their in vitro function and only a slight decrease in CD8-positive T cells (Field et al. 1984; King et al. 1981). TLI also resulted in marked alterations of in vitro lymphocyte functions. The proliferative responses of peripheral lymphocytes to the mitogens PHA, ConA, and PWM were profoundly decreased after TLI. A marked decrease in the response to allogeneic cells in mixed lymphocyte culture has also been demonstrated (Weigensberg et al. 1984).

In studies on the effect on T cell-dependent and- independent humoral immune responses in patients with rheumatoid arthritis, TLI appeared to selectively decrease T helper cell-dependent antibody response (i.e., response to diphtheria or tetanus toxoid) while leaving intact or even augmenting T helper cell-independent antibody responses (i.e., response to pneumococcal polysaccharide) (TANAY and STROBER 1984).

In a randomized controlled trial comparing high dose TLI (10 × 2 Gy) and low dose TLI (10 × 0.2 Gy), significant improvements in the clinical symptoms in patients with rheumatoid arthritis occurred only after the high dose TLI. As expected, marked changes in in vitro lymphocyte functions were noted in the high dose group (KOTZIN and STROBER 1984).

Despite improvement in disease activity, TLI did not induce changes in serum rheumatoid factor titer, antinuclear antibodies, and IgE levels (TERR et al. 1987). The long-term efficacy of TLI is controversial. Several reports demonstrate clinical improvement, especially with high dose fractionated TLI, but the sometimes severe and even fatal side-effects cannot be ignored (NUESSLEIN et al. 1985; ORDER 1981).

In drug-resistant SLE with severe nephrotic syndrome, fractionated TLI was chosen as an ultimate treatment. There was improvement of kidney function (decrease in protein loss, increase in serum albumin) and reduction of cortisol dosage in most of the patients. However, TLI-related side-effects such as varicella zoster were reported. Among patients with chronic progressive multiple sclerosis, those who received TLI showed at least a clinically better course than sham-treated controls.

As in the studies in rheumatoid arthritis, in SLE and multiple sclerosis a number of alterations of cellular immune functions were noted after TLI: a decrease in the total number of T cells, a decrease in T helper cells, a decrease in the mitogen response, a decrease in the reactivity against allogeneic cells in the mixed lymphocyte culture, and a decrease in in vitro PWM-stimulated immunoglobulin production.

In summary, TLI is not generally accepted as an alternative immunosuppressive regimen for the treatment of autoimmune diseases; rather its use is confined to severe, drug-resistant disease.

5.4.2 Total Lymphoid Irradiation in Organ Transplantation

As long as 40 years ago it was shown that irradiation will prolong the survival of allogeneic skin grafts (DEMPSTER et al. 1950) and in the late 1950s it was regarded as the most hopeful approach to immunosuppression in organ transplantation (CALNE 1982).

In animal models TLI was shown to achieve tolerance towards specific antigens, a central goal of immunologists and clinicians in transplantation medicine (ZAN-BAR et al. 1978, 1979; SLAVIN et al. 1976, 1978, 1980; RYNASIEWICZ et al. 1981).

5.4.2.1 Experimental Models

In mice TLI was found to prolong skin allograft survival approximately fivefold even in strong H-2 incompatible donor–recipient combinations (SLAVIN et al. 1976, 1977a,b). This fractionated TLI-induced immunosuppression was related to the cumulative radiation dose, since skin graft survival was markedly reduced when 14 Gy was given to the recipients instead of 20 Gy.

For preclinical allogeneic organ transplantation larger experimental animals like dogs, pigs, and monkeys were studied. In heart allografts between mongrel dogs, STROBER et al. (1984) found a synergy of TLI and administration of rabbit anti-dog thymocyte globulin (ATG) in a 10-day posttransplant course, leading to an allograft-specific tolerance for more than 1 year in 40% of the animals in spite of the fact that no further immunosuppressive drug was given. A similar effect of TLI plus ATG or immunosuppressive drugs on heart graft survival was observed in rhesus primates (BIEBER et al. 1979; PENNOCK et al. 1981). The allospecific tolerance was documented by a prompt rejection of a third party graft.

For kidney and liver transplantation in baboons, long-lasting and specific acceptance of the allograft was produced by TLI in approximately half of the animals (MYBURGH et al. 1984a,b). However, it was not possible to predict at the time of grafting or in the initial posttransplant period whether an individual baboon would be rendered tolerant or not (WAER et al. 1984).

Since permanent tolerance of skin or heart allografts is induced in rodents after TLI only if donor marrow cells are transfused at the time of transplantation, the same regimen was studied in the dog (KORETZ et al. 1981; STROBER et al. 1984). If concomitant marrow transfusion was omitted, rejection occurred at an higher frequency although much later than in controls.

5.4.2.2 Clinical Results

Based on the experimental finding that TLI can induce immunological tolerance if used together with ATG, the TLI regimen was introduced in clinical renal transplantation (MYBURGH et al. 1987; NAJARIAN et al. 1981; WAER et al. 1984; LEVIN et al. 1985; SAMPSON et al. 1985: WOODRUFF et al. 1963). Despite the fact that TLI had an azathioprine- and cortisol-sparing effect, the overall results were not so impressive that this regimen was generally accepted. The long-lasting immunosuppressive effect in patients given TLI resulted in an increased incidence of viral infections (cytomegalovirus, varicella zoster virus, etc.) (WAER et al. 1984). Also local irradiation of the allograft had no significant beneficial effect in reducing the rejection episodes (PILEPICH et al. 1983; HUME and WOLF 1967). The same situation was true for other large organs like liver and heart.

With regard to the unprimed cellular immune response capacity mediated by NK cells, this important cell function is maintained or even enhanced in patients subjected exclusively to TLI, explaining the low incidence of malignancy in this group of patients (GRAY et al. 1989). Because TLI-treated patients are more prone to viral infections, which also augment NK cell activity (WAER et al. 1984), it is difficult to decide whether such augmentation is secondary to the viral infections or not.

Despite the equivocal depressive effect on the general immune response, the disappointing clinical results in allogeneic organ transplantation may be explained by the fact that in most cases the patients were already immunized by blood transfusions and/or prior rejected allografts (NAJARIAN et al. 1981; SUTHERLAND et al. 1983). Although TLI allowed a drastic reduction of steroids, no clinical sign or immunological test was able to predict whether the TLI radiation dose given would be sufficient for an individual patient, and it is obviously difficult to find the optimal clinical TLI schedule (WAER et al. 1984).

As stated above, irradiation exerts its major effect on the primary immune response, and abrogation of the memory response needs radiation doses above the tolerated level in humans. In the light of new and relatively specific immunosuppressive drugs like cyclosporin A (KAHAN 1989) and more recently FK-506 (STARZL et al. 1989), which in general have tolerable side-effects, one has to state that TLI or local irradiation (HUME and WOLF 1967) is now to be regarded as a historical episode in the manipulation of the immune system of solid organ recipients.

In clinical bone marrow transplantation TLI is used to reduce the morbidity associated with total body irradiation or to increase the immunosuppressive effect of the chemotherapeutic conditioning regimen. Combination of 7.5 Gy single-dose TLI and intravenous cyclophosphamide can prevent graft rejection in multiply transfused patients suffering from severe aplastic anemia (RAMSAY and KERSEY 1984). Sensitized patients pretreated by cyclophosphamide alone reject the transplant in up to 60% of cases, whereas consistent takes of the allografts can be achieved using TLI (RAMSAY and KERSEY 1984).

The use of fractionated TLI in clinical bone marrow transplantation was introduced in 1979 by SLAVIN et al. (1983a,b, 1985, 1986; SLAVIN and SEIDEL 1982). There is some indication that fractionated TLI can reduce the enhanced risk of graft rejection when T lymphocyte-depleted allogeneic marrow is grafted.

5.5 Regional Irradiation

Local and extended field irradiation has become a treatment of choice for a variety of localized tumors. It appears that even localized radiation has a marked delayed effect on the immune system. Analysis of radiation-induced changes of immune parameters is difficult because the malignant disease itself, the age of the patient, other comorbid conditions, and cytotoxic chemotherapy can produce changes in cellular and functional immune mechanisms.

A voluminous literature exists describing effects of locoregional irradiation on the immune response of patients with malignant tumors. The interested reader is referred to DU BOIS et al. (1981), ELTRINGHAM et al. (1984), and NAPARSTEK and SLAVIN (1988). Radiation-induced changes have usually been assessed in patients with clinically localized cancers of the breast, prostate, testis, lung, or uterine cervix. Persistent and prolonged decrease in the number of lymphocytes, particularly circulating T lymphocytes, is a most constant finding years after termination of the therapy. Many have reported a functional decrease in PHA response. A decrease in or absence of cell-mediated skin reactivity to T cell-mediated antigens was documented by some investigators as late as 12 years following radiation therapy (HOPPE et al. 1977).

The significance of these changes and the ultimate impact on outcome are not entirely clear (ALEXANDER 1976). Emotive controversies have erupted in the literature about the possibility of enhanced growth of distant metastases. However, none of these studies showed any correlation between the severity of the immunological derangements and the probability of relapse or cure.

References

Agarossi G, Pizzi L, Mancini C, Doria G (1978) Radiosensitivity of the helper cell function. J Immunol 121: 2118–2121

Akiyama M, Yamakido M, Kobuke K, Dock DS, Hamilton HB, Awa AA, Kato H (1983) Peripheral lymphocyte response to PHA and T cell population among atomic bomb survivors. Radiat Res 93: 572–580

Alexander P (1976) The bogey of the immuno-suppressive action of local radiotherapy. Int J Rad Oncol Biol Phys 1: 369–371

Almassy Z, Krepinsky AB, Bianco A, Koteles GJ (1987) The present state and perspectives of micronucleus assay in radiation protection. A review. In: Applied radiation and isotopes. Int J Radiat Applic Instrument P. A, 38 (4): 241–249

Amagai T, Kina T, Hirokawa K, Nishikawa S, Imanishi J, Katsura Y (1987) Dysfunction of irradiated thymus for the development of helper T cells. J Immunol 139: 358–364

Anderson KC, Weinstein HJ (1990) Transfusion-associated graft-versus-host disease. N Engl J Med 323: 315–321

Anderson RE, Lefkovits I (1979) In vitro evaluation of radiation-induced augmentation of the immune response. Am J Pathol 97: 456–472

Anderson RE, Lefkovits I (1980) Effects of irradiation on the in vitro immune response. Exp Cell Biol 48: 255–278

Anderson RE, Warner NL (1975) Radiosensitivity of T and B lymphocytes. III. Effects of radiation on immunoglobulin production by B cells. J Immunol 115: 161–169

Anderson RE, Warner NL (1976) Ionizing radiation and the immune response. Adv Immunol 24: 215–335

Anderson RE, Williams WL (1977) Radiosensitivity of T and B lymphocytes vs effects of whole body irradiation on numbers of recirculating T cells and sensitization to primary skin grafts in mice. Am J Pathol 89: 367–378

Anderson RE, Sprent J, Miller JPAF (1974) Radiosensitivity of T and B lymphocytes. I. Effect of irradiation on cell migration. Eur J Immunol 4: 199–203

Anderson RE, Olson GB, Autry JR, Howarth JL, Troup GM, Bartels PH (1977) Radiosensitivity of T and B lymphocytes. IV. Effect of whole body irradiation upon various lymphoid tissues and numbers of recirculating lymphocytes. J Immunol 118: 1191–1200

Anderson RE, Lefkovits I, Troup GM (1980) Radiation induced augmentation of the immune response. Contemp Top Immunobiol 11: 245–274

Anderson RE, Standefer JC, Tokuda S (1986) The structural and functional assessment of cytotoxic injury of the immune system with particular reference to the effects of ionizing radiation and cyclophosphamide. Br J Cancer 53 [Suppl VII]: 140–160

Ashwell JD, Schwartz RH, Mitchell JB, Russo A (1986) Effect of gamma radiation on resting B lymphocytes. I. Oxygen-dependent damage to the plasma membrane results in increased permeability and cell enlargement. J Immunol 136: 3649–3656

Baral E, Blomgren H (1976) Response of human lymphocytes to mitogenic stimuli after irradiation in vitro. Acta Radiol Ther Phys Biol 15: 149–161

Barrett A (1988) Total body irradiation: clinical aspects. In: Bleehen NM (ed) Radiobiology in radiotherapy. Springer, London Berlin Heidelberg New York, pp 123–127

Bass H, Mosmann T, Strober S (1989) Evidence for mouse Th1- and Th2-like helper T cells in vivo. Selective reduction of Th1-like cells after total lymphoid irradiation. J Exp Med 170: 1495–1511

Bauchinger M (1972) Strahleninduzierte Chromosomenaberrationen. In: Hug O, Zuppinger A (eds) Handbuch der medizinischen Radiologie, vol II. Springer, Berlin Heidelberg New York, pp 127–180

Bauchinger M (1984) Cytogenetic effects in human lymphocytes as a dosimetry system. In: Eisert WG, Mendelsohn ML (eds) Biological dosimetry. Springer, Berlin Heidelberg New York

Bazin H, Platteau B (1984) Immunohistological observations on the spleen B lymphocyte populations from whole body irradiated rats. Int J Radiat Biol 45: 321–329

Beebe GW, Kato H, Land CE (1978) Mortality experience of atomic bomb survivors 1950–1974. Radiat Res 75: 138–201

Behling UH (1983) The radioprotective effect of bacterial endotoxin. In: Nowotny A (ed) Beneficial effects of endotoxin. Plenum, New York, pp 127–135

BenChetrit E, Gross DJ, Braverman A, Weshler Z, Fuks Z, Slavin S, Eliakim M (1986) Total lymphoid irradiation therapy in refractory systemic lupus erythematosus. Ann Intern Med 105: 58–60

Berdjis CC (1971) Pathology of irradiation. Williams & Wilkins, Baltimore

Beschorner WE, Hutchins GM, Elfenbein GJ, Santos GW (1978) The thymus in patients with allogeneic bone marrow transplants. Am J Pathol 92: 173–181

Beschorner WE, Yardley JH, Tutschka PJ, Santos GW (1981) Deficiency of intestinal immunity with graft-versus-host disease im humans. J Infect Dis 144: 38–46

Betz EH (1974) Morphologische Veränderungen des lymphatischen Systems nach Bestrahlung. In: Kärcher KH, Streffer C (eds) Die Strahlenwirkung auf das Lymphsystem. Unter besonderer Berücksichtigung der kleinen Dosen. Springer, Berlin Heidelberg New York, pp 29–36

Bieber CP, Jamieson S, Raney A et al. (1979) Cardiac allograft survival in rhesus primates treated with combined total lymphoid irradiation and rabbit antithymocyte globulin. Transplantation 28: 347–350

Bier OG, Dias da Silva WD, Götze D, Mota J (eds) (1986) Fundamentals of immunology. Springer, New York Berlin Heidelberg, pp 401–440

Birkeland SA (1978) In vitro radiosensitivity of human T and B lymphocytes evaluated using lymphocyte transformation tests and rosette formation tests. Int Arch Allergy Appl Immunol 57: 425–434

Bloom ET, Korn EL, Tagasugi M, Toji DS, Onari K, Makinodan T (1983) Immune function in ageing atomic bomb survivors residing in the USA. Radiat Res 96: 399–410

Button LN, DeWolf WC, Newburger PE, Jacobson MS, Kevy SV (1981) The effects of irradiation on blood components. Transfusion 21: 419–426

Butturini A, Gale RP (1988) T cell depletion in bone marrow transplantation for leukemia: current results and future directions. Bone Marrow Transplant 3: 185–192

Calne R (1982) The initial study of the immunosuppressive effects of 6-mercaptopurine and a few words on cyclosporin A. World J Surg 6: 637–640

Champlin RE, Gale RP (1984) Role of bone marrow transplantation in the treatment of hematologic malignancies and solid tumors: critical review of syngeneic, allogeneic, autologous, marrow stem cells. Int J Radiat Biol 38: 589–595

Cirkovic D (1970) Protection by phytohemagglutinin of human blood lymphocytes irradiated in vitro. Strahlentherapie 140: 318–324

Congdon CC, Makinodan T, Gengozian N (1957) Effect of injection of rat bone marrow on reticular tissues of mice exposed to x-radiation in the midlethal dose range. J Natl Cancer Inst 18: 603–613

Constine LS, Rubin P (1988) Total body irradiation: normal tissue effects. In: Bleehen NM (ed) Radiobiology in radiotherapy. Springer, London Berlin Heidelberg New York, pp 95–121

Cook SD, Devereux C, Troiano R et al. (1987) Total lymphoid irradiation in multiple sclerosis: blood lymphocytes and clinical course. Ann Neurol 22: 634–638

Cooper M, (1987) B lymphocytes-normal development and function. N Engl J Med 317: 1452–1456

Cosulich ME, Risso H, Canomia GW, Bargellesi A (1986) Functional characterization of a regulatory human T-cell subpopulation increasing during autologous MLR. J Immunol 57: 265–273

Countryman P, Heddle J (1976) The production of micronuclei from chromosome aberrations in irradiated cultures of human lymphocytes. Mutat Res 41: 321–331

Cudkowicz G, Bennet M (1971) Peculiar immunobiology of bone marrow allografts. I. Graft rejection by irradiated responder mice. J Exp Med 134: 83–102

Dehos G, Hinz G, Schwarz E-R (1986) Changes in number and function of the lymphocyte populations as a biological indicator for ionizing radiation. In: Kaul A, Dehos A, Bögl W, Hing G, Kossel F, Schwarz E-R, Stamm A, Stephan G (eds) Biological indicators for radiation dose assessment. Biologische Indikatoren zum Nachweis von Strahlenexpositionen. MMV Medizin, München, pp 298–301

Dempster WH, Lennox B, Doag FW (1950) Prolongation of survival of skin homotransplantation in the rabbit by irradiation of the host. Br J Exp Pathol 31: 670–679

Dinarello CA, Mier JW (1987) Lymphokines. N Engl J Med 317: 940–945

Dixon FJ, McConahey PJ (1963) Enhancement of antibody formation by whole body x-radiation. J Exp Med 117: 833–847

Dixon FJ, Talmage DW, Maurer PH (1952) Radiosensitive and radioresistant phases in the antibody response. J Immunol 68: 693–700

Dixon FJ, Theofilopoulos AN, Izui S, McCapakey PJ (1980) Murine SLE – aetiology and pathogenesis. In: Fongereau M, Dausset J (eds) Progress in immunology IV Academic, London pp 959–995

Drobyski W, Thibodeau S, Truitt RL et al. (1989) Third-party-mediated graft rejection and graft-versus-host disease after T-cell depleted bone marrow transplantation, as demonstrated by hypervariable DNA probes and HLA-DR polymorphism. Blood 74: 2285–2294

Dubois JB, Serrou B, Rosenfeld C (eds) (1981) Immunopharmacologic effects of radiation therapy. Monograph series of the European organization for research on treatment of cancer, vol 8. Raven, New York

Durkin HG, Thorbecke GJ (1972) Preferential destruction of germinal centers by prednisolone and x-irradiation. Lab Invest 26: 53–62

Durum SK, Gengozian N (1978) The comparative radiosensitivity of T and B lymphocytes. Int J Radiat Biol 34: 1–15

Ekstrand KE, Dixon RL (1982) Lymphocyte chromosome aberrations in partial-body fractionated radiation therapy. Phys Med Biol 27: 407–411

Eltringham JR (1984) Effects of regional irradiation on immune responses. Clin Immunol Allergy 4: 359–376

Farnsworth A, Wotherspoon JS, Dorsch SE (1988) Postirradiation recovery of lymphoid cells in the rat. Transplantation 46: 418–425

Fenech M, Morley AA (1985) Measurement of micronuclei in lymphocytes. Mutat Res 147: 29–36

Field EH, Strober S, Hoppe RT et al. (1983) Sustained improvement of intractable rheumatoid arthritis after total lymphoid irradiation. Arthritis Rheum 26: 937–946

Field EH, Engleman EG, Terrell CP, Strober S (1984) Reduced in vitro immune responses of purified human Leu-3 (helper/inducer phenotype) cells after total lymphoid irradiation. J Immunol 84: 1031–1035

Finch SC (1984) Leukemia and lymphoma in atomic bomb survivors. In: Boice JD Jr, Fraumeni JF Jr (eds) Radiation carcinogenesis: epidemiology and biological significance. Raven, New York, pp 21–36

Fuks Z, Strober S, Bobrove AM et al. (1976) Long-term effects of radiation on T and B lymphocytes in peripheral blood of patients with Hodgkin's disease. J Clin Invest 58: 803–814

Gale RP, Reisner Y (1986) Graft rejection and graft-versus-host disease: mirror images. Lancet I: 1468–1470

Gerber M, Ball D, Michel F, Crastes de Paulet A (1985) Mechanism of enhancing effect of irradiation on production of IL-2. Immunol Lett 9: 279–283

Graham JB, Graham RM, Nori, Wright KA (1956) Enhanced production of antibodies by local irradiation. I. Measurement of circulating antibodies. J Immunol 76: 103–109

Gratwohl A, Hermans J, Lyklema A, Zwaan FE (1987) Bone marrow transplantation for leukaemia in Europe. Report from the Leukaemia Working Party 1987. Bone Marrow Transplantation 2 [Suppl 1]: 15–18

Gray CM, Smit JA, Myburgh JA (1989) Function and numbers of natural killer (NK) cells in patients conditioned with total lymphoid irradiation (TLI). Transplant Proc 21: 1800–1801

Gross UM, Herms J (1965) Das Verhalten des aktivierten Mäuselymphkotens nach Röntgenbestrahlung. Beitr Pathol Anat 131: 200–219

Guedeney G, Grundwald D, Malarbet JL, Doloy MT (1988) Time dependence of chromosomal aberrations induced in human and monkey lymphocytes by acute and fractionated exposure to ^{60}Co. Radiat Res 116: 254–262

Hakoda M, Akiyama M, Kyoizumi S, Awa AA, Yamakido M, Otake M (1988) Increased somatic cell mutant frequency in atomic bomb survivors. Mutat Res 201: 39–48

Hall EJ (1988) Radiobiology for the radiologist. JB Lippincott, Philadelphia

Harris ED (1990) Rheumathoid arthritis. Pathophysiology and implications for therapy. N Engl J Med 322: 1277–1289

Harris G, Cramp WA, Edwards JC et al. (1985) Radiosensitivity of peripheral blood lymphocytes in autoimmune disease. Int J Radiat Biol 47: 689–699

Hasegawa Y, Nakashima I, Ando K et al. (1988) Dynamics of cytotoxic T lymphocyte precursors in vivo assessed by change in the radiation sensitivity. Evidence for development of radiation-sensitive memory cells without clonal expansion. Scand J Immunol 28: 43–53

Henney CS (1989) The interleukins as lymphocyte growth factors. Transpl Proc 21: 22–25

Herberman RB, Ortaldo JR (1981) Natural killer cells: their role in defenses against disease. Science 214: 24–29

Herbst M, Fritz H, Sauer R (1986) Total lymphoid irradiation of intractable rheumatoid arthritis. Br J Radiol 59: 1203–1207

Hogstedt B (1984) Micronuclei in lymphocytes with preserved cytoplasm. A method for assessment of cytogenetic damage in man. Mutat Res 130: 63–72

Hoppe RT, Fuks ZY, Strober S, Kaplan HS (1977) The long-term effects of radiation on T and B lymphocytes in the peripheral blood after regional irradiation. Cancer 40: 2071–2078

Huber R, Braselmann H, Bauchinger M (1989) Screening for interindividual differences in radiosensitivity by means of the micronucleus assay in human lymphocytes. Radiat Environ Biophys 28: 113–120

Hume DM, Wolf JS (1967) Modification of renal homograft rejection by irradiation. Transplantation 5: 1174–1191

James SE, Arlett CF, Green MHL (1983) Radiosensitivity of human T-lymphocytes proliferating in long term culture. Int J Radiat Biol 44: 417–422

Johnston A, McNerney R (1985) Changes in topoisomerase I activity after irradiation of lymphoid cells. Biosci Rep 5: 907–912

Jordan SW (1967) Ultrastructural studies of spleen after whole body irradiation of mice. Exp Mol Pathol 6: 156–171

Kahan BD (1989) Cyclosporine. N Engl J Med 321: 1725–1738

Kakati S, Kowalczyk JR, Gibas Z, Sandberg AA (1986) Use of radiation induced chromosomal damage in human lymphocytes as a biological dosimeter is questionable. Cancer Genet Cytogenet 22: 137–141

Kaplan HS (1980) Hodgkin's disease, 2nd edn. Harvard University Press, Cambridge

Kataoka Y, Sato T (1975) The radiosensitivity of T and B lymphocytes in mice. Immunology 29: 121–130

Kato H, Schull WJ (1982) Studies of the mortality of A-bomb survivors. Report 7. Mortality 1950–1978. Part I. Cancer mortality. Radiat Res 90: 395–432

Kiessling R, Hochman PS, Haller D, Shearer GM, Wigzell H, Cudkowicz G (1977) Evidence for a similar or common mechanism for natural killer cell activity and resistance to hemopoetic grafts. Eur J Immunol 7: 655–663

King DP, Strober S, Kaplan HS (1981) Suppression of the mixed leukocyte response and of graft-vs-host disease by spleen cells following total lymphoid irradiation (TLI). J Immunol 126: 1140–1145

Knapp W, Dörken B, Rieber EP, Stein H, Gilks WR, Schmidt RE, Borne von dem AEGK (1989) Leucocyte typing IV. Oxford University Press

Kolar OJ, Hornback NB (1986) Total lymphoid irradiation in multiple sclerosis. Lancet II: 453

Koretz S, Gottlieb MS, Strober S et al. (1981) Organ transplantation on mongrel dogs using total lymphoid irradiation (TLI). Transpl Proc 13: 443–451

Kotzin BL, Strober S (1979) Reversal of NZB/NZW disease with total lymphoid irradiation. J Exp Med 150: 371–378

Kotzin BL, Strober S (1984) Total lymphoid irradiation. Clin Immunol Allergy 4: 331–358

Kotzin BL, Strober S, Engleman EG et al. (1981) Treatment of intractable rheumatoid arthritis with total lymphoid irradiation. N Engl J Med 305: 969–976

Kotzin BL, Kansas GS, Engleman EG et al. (1983) Changes in T-cell subsets in patients with rheumatoid arthritis treated with total lymphoid irradiation. Clin Immunol Immunopathol 27: 250–260

Kotzin BL, Strober S, Kansas GS, Terrell CP, Engleman EG (1984) Suppression of pokeweed mitogen stimulated immunoglobulin production. J Immunol 132: 1049–1055

Lambert LE, Paulnock DM (1987) Modulation of macrophage function by gamma-irradiation – acquisition of the primed cell intermediate stage of the macrophage tumoricidal activation pathway. J Immunol 139: 2834–2841

Langendorff H, Langendorff M, Steinbach KH, Weckesser J (1971) Vergleichende Untersuchungen zur strahlenresistenzerhöhenden Wirkung von verschiedenen bakteriellen Lipopolysacchariden. Strahlentherapie 141: 214–220

Lee SK, Woodland RT (1985) Selective effect of irradiation on responses to thymus-independent antigen. J Immunol 134: 761–764

Leitman SF, Holland PV (1985) Irradiation of blood products: indications and guidelines. Transfusion 25: 293–300

Levin B, Collins G, Waer M et al. (1985) Treatment of cadaveric renal transplant recipients with total lymphoid irradiation, antithymocyte globulin, and low-dose prednisone. Lancet II: 1321–1324

Lloyd DC (1984) An overview of radiation dosimetry by conventional cytogenetic methods. In: Eisert WG, Mendelsohn ML (eds) Biological dosimetry. Springer, Berlin Heidelberg New York, pp 3–14

Lloyd DC, Prosser JS, Lelliott DJ, Moquet JE (1982) Doses in radiation accidents investigated by chromosome aberration analysis. XII. A review of cases investigated:

1981. UK National Radiological Protection Board Report R-128

Lotzová E, Cudkowicz G (1974) Abrogation of resistance to bone marrow grafts by silica particles. J Immunol 113: 798–803

Lowenthal IW, Harris AW (1985) Activation of mouse lymphocytes inhibits induction of rapid cell death by x-irradiation. J Immunol 135: 1119–1125

Manori I, Kushilevsky A, Weinstein Y (1986) Analysis of interleukin 1 mediated radioprotection. Clin Exp Immunol 63: 526–532

McConkey DJ, Orrenius S, Jondal M (1990) Cellular signalling in programmed cell death (apoptosis) Immunol Today 11: 120–121

Mori, T, Tsoi MS, Gillis S, Santos E, Thomas ED, Storb R (1983) Cellular interactions in marrow-grafted patients. I. Impairment of cell-mediated lympholysis associated with graft vs host disease and the effect of interleukin 2. J Immunol 130: 712–715

Morrissey PJ, Charrier K, Bressler L, Alpert A (1987) The influence of IL-1 treatment on the reconstitution of the hemopoietic and immune systems following sublethal radiation. J Immunol 140: 4204–4210

Myburgh JA, Smit JA, Browde S (1984a) Total lymphoid irradiation in vascularized organ allotransplantation in primates. In: Slavin S (ed) Tolerance in bone marrow and organ transplantation. Elsevier, Amsterdam, pp 105–153

Myburgh JA, Smit JA, Stark JH, Browde S (1984b) Total lymphoid irradiation in kidney and liver transplantation in the baboon: prolonged graft survival and alterations in T cell subsets with low cumulative dose regimens. J Immunol 132: 1010–1025

Myburgh JA, Meyers AM, Botha JR, Thomson PD, Smit JA, Browde S, Lakier R (1987) Wide field low-dose total lymphoid irradiation in clinical kidney transplantation. Transpl Proc 19: 1974–1977

Najarian JS, Sutherland DER, Ferguson RM et al. (1981) Total lymphoid irradiation and kidney transplantation: a clinical experience. Transplant Proc 13: 417–424

Naparstek E, Slavin S (1988) Long-term damage to the immune system after irradiation. In: Testa NG, Gale RP (eds) Hematopoiesis. Long-term effects of chemotherapy and radiation. Marcel Dekker, New York, pp 217–239

Naeim F, Smith GS, Gale RP, and the UCLA Marrow Transplant team (1978) Morphologic aspects of bone marrow transplantation in patients with aplastic anemia. Hum Pathol 9: 295–308

Neta R, Douches S, Oppenheim JJ (1986) Interleukin 1 is a radioprotector. J Immunol 136: 2483–2485

Nossal GJV (1987) Immunology – the basic components of the immune system. N Engl J Med 316: 1320–1324

Nuesslein HG, Herbst M, Manger BJ et al. (1985) Total lymphoid irradiation in patients with refractory rheumatoid arthritis. Arthritis Rheum 28: 1205–1210

Olson GB, Bartels PH (1984) Assessment of environmental insults on lymphoid cells as detected by computer assisted morphometric techniques. In: Eisert WG, Mendelsohn ML (eds) Biological dosimetry. Springer, Berlin Heidelberg New York, pp 203–218

Olson GB, Bartels PH, Anderson RE (1982) Computer assisted morphometric analysis of radiation injury in murine lymphocytes. Anal Quant Cytol 4: 181–187

O'Reilly RJ, Collins NH, Kernan N et al. (1985) Transplantation of marrow-depleted T cells by soybean lectin agglutination and E-rosette depletion: major histocompatibility complex-related graft resistance in leukemic transplant recipients. Transpl Proc 17: 455–459

Order E (1981) Clinical radiation research in arthritis, caution, progress and hope. Int J Rad Oncol Biol Phys 7: 129–130

Paul WE (ed) (1986) Fundamental immunology. Raven, New York

Pennock JL, Reitz BA, Bieber CP et al. (1981) Survival of primates following orthotopic cardiac transplantation treated with total lymphoid irradiation and chemical immune suppression. Transplantation 32: 467–473

Pierce GF, Polmar SH, Schacter BZ, Brovall C, Hornick DL, Sorensen RU (1986) Natural cytotoxicity in immunodeficiency diseases: preservation of natural killer activity and the in vivo appearance of radioresistant killing. Human Immunol 15: 85–96

Pilepich MV, Sicard GA, Reaux SR et al. (1983) Renal graft irradiation in acute rejection. Transplantation 35: 208–211

Prosser JS (1976) Survival of human T and B lymphocytes after x-irradiation. Int J Radiat Biol 30: 459–465

Prosser JS, Moquet JE, Lloyd DC, Edwards AA (1988) Radiation induction of micronuclei in human lymphocytes. Mutat Res 199: 37–45

Ramsay NKC, Kersey JH (1984) Conditioning of bone marrow recipients with cyclophosphamide and total lymphoid irradiation. In: Slavin S (ed) Tolerance in bone marrow and organ transplantation. Elsevier, Amsterdam, pp 167–174

Reisner Y, Ben-Bassat I, Douer D, Kaploon A, Schwartz E, Ramot B (1986) Demonstration of clonable alloreactive host T cells in a primate model for bone marrow transplantation. Proc Natl Acad Sci USA 83: 4012–4015

Riggs JE, Lussier AM, Lee SK, Appel MC, Woodland RT (1988) Differential radiosensitivity among B cell subpopulations. J Immunol 141: 1799–1807

Royer HD, Reinherz EL (1987) T lymphocytes – ontogeny, function, and relevance to clinical disorders. N Engl J Med 317: 1136–1141

Rubinstein A, Radl J, Cottier H, Rossi E, Gugler E (1973) Unusual combined immunodeficiency syndrome exhibiting kappa-IgD paraproteinemia, residual gut immunity and graft-versus-host reaction after plasma infusion. Acta Paediatr Scand 62: 365–372

Rynasiewicz JJ, Sutherland DER, Kawahara K, Najarian JS (1981) Total lymphoid irradiation: critical timing and combination with cyclosporine A for immunosuppression in a rat heart allograft model. J Surg Res 30: 365–371

Sachs L, (1987) The molecular control of blood cell development. Science 238: 1374–1379

Sado T, Kamisaku H, Kubo LE (1985) Strain difference in the radiosensitivity of immunocompetent cells and its influence on the residual host-vs-graft reaction in lethally irradiated mice grafted with semiallogeneic bone marrow. J Immunol 134: 704–710

Sampson D, Levin BS, Hoppe RT et al. (1985) Preliminary observations on the use of total lymphoid irradiation, rabbit antithymocyte globulin, and low-dose prednisone in human cadaver renal transplantation. Transplant Proc 17: 1299–1303

Sanderson BJ, Morley AA (1986) Mitogenic stimulation may induce an antimutagenic repair system in human lymphocytes. Mutagenesis 1: 131–133

Sato C, Kojima K, Matzzawa T, Sairenji T, Hinuma Y (1974) Lack of recovery from radiation damage on colony forming ability and on membrane charge in a Burkitt-lymphoma cell line. J Radiat Res (Tokyo) 15: 25–31

Schacter B, Hansal S, Arno J, Levine MJ (1985) Polymorphic radiation sensitivity of human natural killer activity: possible role of DNA strand breakage. Human Immunol 14: 49–58

Schaefer UW, Beelen D (1989) Knochenmarktransplantation. Karger, Basel

Scheid W, Weber J, Traut H (1988) Chromosome aberrations induced in human lymphocytes by an x-radiation accident: results of a 4-year postirradiation analysis. Int J Radiat Biol 54: 395–402

Schrek R (1961) Qualitative and quantitative reactions of lymphocytes to x-rays. Ann NY Acad Sci 95: 839–848

Schull WJ (1984) Atomic bomb survivors: pattern of cancer risk. In: Boice JD Jr, Fraumeni JF Jr (eds) Radiation carcinogenesis: epidemiology and biological significance.. Raven, New York, pp 21–36

Schurman DJ, Hirshman P, Strober S (1981) Total lymphoid irradiation and local joint irradiation in the treatment of adjuvant arthritis. Arthritis Rheum 24: 38–44

Schwartz E, Lapidot S, Gozes D, Singer TS, Reisner Y (1987) Abrogation of bone marrow allograft resistance in mice by increased total body irradiation correlates with eradication of host clonable T cells and alloreactive cytotoxic precursors. J Immunol 138: 460–465

Sellins KS, Cohen JJ (1987) Gene induction by gamma-irradiation leads to DNA fragmentation in lymphocytes. J Immunol 139: 3199–3206

Sieber G, Zierach P, Herrmann F, Brust VJ, Ruehl H (1985) Impaired B lymphocyte reactivity in patients after radiotherapy. Int J Radiat Oncol Biol Phys 11: 777–782

Sinha AA, Lopes MT, McDevitt HO (1990) Autoimmune diseases: the failure of self tolerance. Science 248: 1380–1388

Slater J, Ngo E, Lau HS (1976) Effect of therapeutic irradiation on the immune responses. AJR 126: 313–320

Slavin S (1979) Successful treatment of autoimmune disease in (NZB/NZW) F1 female mice by using fractionated total lymphoid irradiation. Proc Natl Acad Sci USA 76: 5274–5276

Slavin S, Seidel HJ (1982) Hematopoietic activity in bone marrow chimeras prepared with total lymphoid irradiation (TLI). Exp Hematol 10: 206–216

Slavin S, Strober S, Fuks Z, Kaplan HS (1976) Long-term survival of skin allografts in mice treated with fractionated total lymphoid irradiation. Science 193: 1252–1255

Slavin S, Strober S, Fuks Z, Kaplan HS (1977a) Induction of specific tissue transplantation tolerance using fractionated total lymphoid irradiation in adult mice: long-term survival of allogeneic bone marrow and skin grafts. J Exp Med 146: 34–48

Slavin S, Strober S, Fuks Z, Kaplan HS (1977b) Use of total lymphoid irradiation in tissue transplantation in mice. Transplant Proc 9: 1001–1004

Slavin S, Reitz B, Bieber CP, Kaplan HS, Strober S (1978) Transplantation tolerance in adult rats using total lymphoid irradiation: permanent survival of skin, heart and marrow allografts. J Exp Med 147: 700–707

Slavin S, Strober S, Fuks Z, Kaplan HS (1980) Immunosuppression and organ transplantation tolerance, using total lymphoid irradiation. Diabetes 29: 121–123

Slavin S, Naparstek E, Weshler Z, Brautbar C, Rachmilewitz EA, Fuks Z (1983a) Bone marrow transplantation for severe aplastic anemia in HLA-identical siblings using total lymphoid irradiation (TLI) and cyclophosphamide. Transplant Proc 15: 668–670

Slavin S, Naparstek E, Weshler Z, Fuks Z (1983b) Total lymphoid irradiation (TLI) as part of the conditioning regimen for allogeneic bone marrow transplantation in severe aplastic anemia. In: Gale RP (ed) Recent advances in bone marrow transplantation, vol 7. UCLA Symposia on Molecular and Cellular Biology. Alan R. Liss, New York, pp 21–27

Slavin S, Or R, Weshler Z et al. (1985) The use of total lymphoid irradiation for allogeneic bone marrow transplantation in animals and man. Survey Immunol Res 4: 283–252

Slavin S, Or R, Naparstek E et al. (1986) New approaches for prevention of rejection and graft vs host disease (GVHD) in clinical bone marrow transplantation (BMT). Israel J Med Sci 22: 264–267

Smith WW, Alderman JM, Gillespie RE (1957) Hematopoietic recovery induced by bacterial lipopolysaccharide in irradiated animals. Radiat Res 7: 451

Soden M, Hassan J, Scott PL et al. (1989) Lymphoid irradiation in intractable rheumathoid arthritis. Long-term followup of patients treated with 750 rads or 2000 rads. Arthritis Rheum 32: 523–530

Sprent J, Anderson RE, Miller JFAP (1974) Radiosensitivity of T and B lymphocytes. II. Effect of irradiation on response of T cells to alloantigens. Eur J Immunol 4: 204–210

Sprent J, Gao EK, Webb SR (1990) T cell reactivity to MHC molecules: immunity versus tolerance. Science 248: 1357–1363

Starzl TE, Fung J, Venkateramman R, Todo S, Demetris AJ, Jain A (1989) FK 506 for liver, kidney, and pancreas transplantation. Lancet II: 1000–1004

Stefani S (1966) Old-tuberculin-induced radioresistance on human lymphocytes in vitro. Br J Haematol 12: 345–350

Stefani ST, Schrek R (1963) Radioprotection of human lymphocytes in vitro by phytohaemagglutinin (PHA). Radiat Res 19: 231

Strober S, Slavin S, Gottlieb M et al. (1979) Allograft tolerance after total lymphoid irradiation (TLI). Immunol Rev 46: 87–112

Strober S, Modry DL, Hoppe RT et al. (1984) Induction of specific unresponsivenes to heart allografts in mongrel dogs treated with total lymphoid irradiation and antithymocyte globulin. J Immunol 132: 1013–1019

Sutherland DER, Ferguson RM, Rynasiewicz JJ et al. (1983) Total lymphoid irradiation vs cyclosporin for retransplantation in recipients at high risk to reject renal allografts. Transplant Proc 15: 460–464

Tagliaferro, WH, Tagliaferro LG (1970) Effects of irradiation on initial and anamnestic hemolysin responses in rabbits; antigen injection before x-rays. J Immunol 104: 1364–1376

Takada A, Takada Y, Huang C, Ambrus JL (1969) Biphasic pattern of thymus regeneration after whole body irradiation. J Exp Med 129: 445–457

Takada A, Takada Y, Kim U, Ambrus JL (1971) Bone marrow, spleen and thymus regeneration pattern in mice after whole body irradiation. Radiat Res 45: 522–535

Talmadge JE, Meyers KM, Prieur PJ, Stakey JL (1980) Role of NK cells in tumor growth and metastases in beige mice. Nature 284: 622–624

Tanay A, Strober S (1984) Opposite effects of total lymphoid irradiation on T cell dependent and T cell independent antibody responses. J Immunol 132: 979–984

Tanay A, Strober S, Logue GL, Schiffman G (1984) Use of total lymphoid irradiation (TLI) in studies of the T cell dependence of autoantibody production in rheumatoid arthritis. J Immunol 132: 1036–1040

Tanay A, Field EH, Hoppe RT, Strober S (1987) Long term followup of rheumatoid arthritis patients treated with total lymphoid irradiation. Arthritis Rheum 30: 1–10

Terr AI, Moss RB, Strober S (1987) Effect of total lymphoid irradiation on IgE antibody responses in rheumatoid arthritis and systemic lupus erythematosus. J Allergy Clin Immunol 80: 798–802

Theofilopoulos AN, Balderas R, Schawler DL et al. (1980) Inhibition of T cell proliferation and SLE-like syndrome of MRL/1 mice by whole body or total lymphoid irradiation. J Immunol 125: 2137–2142

Thomas ED, Storb R, Clift RA et al. (1975) Bone marrow transplantation. N Engl J Med 292: 832–843, 895–902

Thomas ED, Clift RA, Hersman J et al. (1982) Marrow transplantation for acute nonlymphoblastic leukemia in first remission using fractionated or single-dose irradiation. Int J Radiat Oncol Biol Phys 8: 817–821

Timonen T, Ortaldo JR, Herberman RB (1981) Characteristics of human large granular lymphocytes and relationship to natural killer and K cells. J Exp Med 153: 569–582

Trentham DE, Belli JA, Anderson RI, Buckley JA, Goetzl EJ, David JR, Austen KF (1981) Clinical and immunologic effects of fractionated total lymphoid irradiation in refractory rheumatoid arthritis. N Engl J Med 305: 976–982

Troiano R, Devereux C, Oleske J et al. (1988) T cell subsets and disease progression after total lymphoid irradiation in chronic progressive multiple sclerosis. J Neurol Neurosurg Psychiatry 51: 980–983

Trowell OA (1961) Radiosensitivity of the cortical and medullary lymphocytes in the thymus. Int J Radiol Biol 4: 163–173

Trowell OA (1965) Lymphocytes. In: Willmere N (ed) Cells and tissues in culture. Academic, London, pp 95–172

Tsoi MS, Dobbs S, Brkic S, Ramberg R, Thomas ED, Storb R (1984) Cellular interactions in marrow-grafted patients. II. Normal monocyte antigen-presenting and defective T-cell-proliferative functions early after grafting and during chronic graft-versus-host disease. Transplantation 37: 556–561

van Bekkum DW, De Vries MJ (1967) Radiation chimaeras. Logos, Academic, London

van Bekkum DW, Dooren LJ, Vossen JM, Schellekens PTA (1985) Immune reconstitution of radiation chimeras. In: Van Bekkum DW, Löwenberg B (eds) Bone marrow transplantation. Marcel Dekker, New York, pp 311–350

van Bekkum DW, Löwenberg B (1985) Bone marrow transplantation. Marcel Dekker, New York

von Boehmer H, Kisielow P (1990) Self-nonself discrimination by T cells. Science 248: 1369–1373

von Melchner H, Barlett PF (1983) Mechanisms of early

allogeneic marrow graft rejection. Immunol Rev 71: 31–55

Vriesendorf HM, von Bekkum DW (1984) Susceptibility to total body irradiation. In: Broerse JJ, MacVittie TJ (eds) Response of different species to total body irradiation. Martinus Nijhoff, Boston, pp 43–57

Waer M, Vanrenterghem Y, Kianang K, van der Schueren E, Michelsen P, Vandeputte M (1984) Comparison of the immunosuppressive effect of fractionated total lymphoid irradiation (TLI) vs conventional immunosuppression (CI) in renal cadaveric allotransplantation. J Immunol 132: 1041–1048

Wald N, Conner MK (1988) Induced chromosome damage after irradiation and cytotoxic drugs. In: Testa NG, Gale RP (eds) Hematopoiesis. Long-term effects of chemotherapy and radiation. Marcel Dekker, New York, pp 159–201

Weigensberg M, Morecki S, Weiss L, Fuks Z, Slavin S (1984) Suppression of cell mediated immune responses following total lymphoid irradiation (TLI). 1. Characterization of suppressor cell of the mixed lymphocyte reaction. J Immunol 132: 971–978

Witherspoon RP, Kopecky K, Storb RF et al. (1982) Immunological recovery in 48 patients following syngeneic marrow transplantation for hematological malignancy. Transplantation 33: 143–149

Witherspoon RP, Lum LG, Storb R (1984) Immunologic reconstitution after human marrow grafting. Semin Hematol 21: 2–10

Woodruff MFA, Robson JS, Nolan B et al. (1963) Homotransplantation of kidney in patients treated by preoperative local irradiation and postoperative administration of an antimetabolite (Imuran). Report of six cases. Lancet II: 675–682

Woodruff JM, Hansen JA, Good RA, Santos GW, Slavin RE (1976) The pathology of the graft-versus-host reaction (GvHR) in adults receiving bone marrow transplants. Transplant Proc 8: 675–684

Yamada Y, Neriishi S, Ishimary T et al. (1985) Effects of atomic bomb radiation on the differentiation of B lymphocytes and on the function of concanavalin A-induced suppressor T lymphocytes. Radiat Res 101: 351–355

Zan-Bar I, Slavin S, Strober S (1978) Induction and mechanism of tolerance to bovine serum albumin after total lymphoid irradiation (TLI). J Immunol 121: 1400–1404

Zan-Bar I, Slavin S, Strober S (1979) Effect of total lymphoid irradiation (TLI) on the primary and secondary antibody response to sheep red blood cells. Cell Immunol 45: 167–174

Zarcone D, Tilden AB, Lane VG, Grossi CE (1989) Radiation sensitivity of resting and activated non-specific cytotoxic cells of T lineage and NK lineage. Blood 73: 1615–1621

Zurcher C, van Bekkum DW (1985) Pathology of radiation chimeras. In: van Bekkum DW, Löwenberg B (eds) Bone marrow transplantation. Marcel Dekker, New York, pp 213–310

6 The Nervous System:
Radiobiology and Experimental Pathology

A.J. van der Kogel

CONTENTS

6.1 Experimental Models of Radiation-Induced Injury in the Central and Peripheral Nervous System

6.1.1 Brain

6.1.1.1 Primates

Some of the most extensive studies on the acute and delayed effects of radiation on the brain have been done in rhesus monkeys, notably by HAYMAKER (1969) and CAVENESS (1980). In the studies by HAYMAKER dose–response relationships are difficult to establish because monkeys were whole body irradiated with high energy protons and an inhomogeneous dose distribution. Because of the limited penetration of the lower energy protons (32 and 55 MeV), several monkeys sur-

vived long enough for some insight to be obtained into the delayed responses of the brain. The importance of HAYMAKER's review (1969) is the consideration of the role of various cell types in acute and delayed radiation-induced lesions in the CNS. Neurons have been shown to be extraordinarily radioresistant, with doses as high as 4000 Gy required to destroy a nerve cell within 24 days in a very small irradiated volume. In larger volumes and at lower doses, death of neurons is thought to be mediated through vasculocirculatory injury. All other cell types (glial cells and vascular endothelium) were shown to be involved in the radiation-induced CNS lesions, but most of HAYMAKER's review dealt with high radiation doses. As a consequence, most observations were related to acute or relatively early reactions, and a detailed description would confuse the issue of radiation pathology in the therapeutic dose range.

Of more relevance in the present context was the evaluation of delayed radionecrosis and the recognition of specific types (HAYMAKER 1969). Three categories were discriminated:

1. *Edema necrosis.* In the acute form, tissue vacuolation occurs in the immediate vicinity of vessels and is accompanied by massive white matter necrosis. Over large areas suddenly devoid of cells, lipid–filled macrophages may become abundant. In a more chronic presentation, edema is slowly progressive and associated with severe cell injury and brain swelling, leading to the formation of large fluid-filled cystic spaces. A characteristic feature of this kind of lesion is the advanced gliosis in bordering tissue. Generally, a progressive disturbance of the blood–brain barrier is proposed to be the basis of this kind of lesion.

2. *Coagulation necrosis.* This is probably the most common type of delayed CNS injury in many species, and almost exclusively occurs in the white matter. Initially restricted to small foci, these areas seem to enlarge and then to

Professor Dr. A.J. van der Kogel, Institute of Radiotherapy, University of Nijmegen, Geert Grooteplein Zuid 32, 6525 GA Nijmegen, The Netherlands

coalesce into large areas of "coagulative necrosis." HAYMAKER assumes the main pathogenetic factor of this lesion to be "damage of vascular endothelium from long–standing blood stasis, with continued permeability disturbance." It is pointed out that vessels may appear morphologically normal but be functionally defective. It is not thought that capillary density per se is of major importance in the pathogenesis.

3. *Spongiform necrosis.* This is a multifocal lesion which does not undergo progressive enlargement. This condition may be seen in the same microscopic field as coagulation necrosis. At the basis is a rapid disintegration of tissue elements, leaving no time for a cellular reaction. It is attributed to a sudden circulatory failure.

After describing these distinct types of delayed damage, HAYMAKER arrives at one of the key issues of delayed CNS injury, namely the predilection for white matter. A differential oxygen tension is considered, but with the white matter being at a much lower O_2 tension than gray matter (ZEMAN 1966) this would predict a relative protection of the white matter. Most experimental work on this topic is done in rat spinal cord (see Sect. 6.2.7.1 for discussion). The most likely factor considered by HAYMAKER (1969) is the accumulation of edema fluid in the white matter, but this is regarded as insufficient to be the main pathogenetic factor. In a strictly vascular hypothesis, the additional factor might be the altered hemodynamics and reduced reabsorption of edema fluid. In a concluding statement, HAYMAKER arrives at the heart of the problem, still valid today: " ... it is not possible, nor is it logical, to conclude from the evidence at hand that all the damage is attributable solely to progressive vascular injury." Moreover, it is recognized that no single cell type in the CNS can be responsible for the variety of lesions observed, and that one of the problems is dosage.

With respect to dosage and specificity of lesions, a limited study by VOGEL and PICKERING (1956) is of some importance. A small group of monkeys were irradiated on the head with approximately 7–8 Gy (850 rep) of 14 MeV neutrons. This dose caused alopecia and marked induration of the skin. Over a period of 1–2 years animals were succesively killed and the brain tissue evaluated histologically. The gray matter and choroid plexuses were normal, but the white matter showed progressive demyelination, with an almost complete loss of myelin in the frontal and parietal lobes after close to 2 years. A few larger blood vessels showed some minor changes, but were generally unaffected. Although this effect is directly related to the use of neutrons, it is a demonstration of specific injury to one tissue component, myelin and the associated oligodendrocytes.

The probably most clinically relevant studies on monkey brain were done in the late 1960s and 1970s by William F. CAVENESS and co-workers. The results of studies initially done with regionally applied high single doses, and later extended to clinically relevant single and fractionated schemes on the whole brain, were reviewed by CAVENESS in 1980. In the initial experiments. 2-year-old rhesus monkeys were irradiated with a single dose of 35 Gy of 250 kV x-rays on the right occipital lobe. From 16–24 weeks, a rapidly progressive breakdown of the blood–brain barrier accompanied by extensive edema was observed. Histologically, minute focal areas of white matter necrosis occurred at 20–24 weeks, which in subsequent weeks coalesced into large areas of spongy necrosis. Also extensive vascular changes were observed.

In subsequent experiments, 2-year-old pubescent monkeys were irradiated on the whole brain with 10, 15, and 20 Gy of 20 MeV photons, a range of doses that covers the therapeutic dose range in equivalence to fractionated regimens. After a dose of 10 Gy, no abnormalities were seen during a 2-year observation period. The next higher dose of 15 Gy led to neurological changes starting at approximately 26–30 weeks. At 26 weeks, lesions were restricted to minute areas of necrosis with an empty appearance. Older lesions showed an influx of macrophages and, as a last stage, calcification. Vascular changes consisted of endothelial hyperplasia and capillary telangiectasia, in continuity with normal appearing vessels. At 1 year after 15 Gy, larger areas of coalescing necrosis were observed without much calcification. After the highest dose of 20 Gy, no animals survived beyond 26 weeks. Neurological signs started as early as 8 weeks and were rapidly progressive. Histologically, there were widely scattered focal necrotic lesions but no indication of coalescence into larger confluent areas of necrosis. The vascular lesions also included changes in the walls of small arteries. These three dose levels clearly encompassed the range of therapeutic interest, from no damage at the lowest doses to extensive early delayed injury at the highest doses.

A similar approach was taken in a fractionated series of 2 Gy per day, to total doses of 40, 60, and 80 Gy, which realistically encompasses the whole therapeutic range. No changes were seen after 40 Gy, but after 60 Gy functional changes (decreased visual evoked responses) occurred as early as 8–10 weeks. In animals killed at 26 weeks widely scattered focal necrosis was observed, with various degrees of macrophage involvement and calcification of the clearly oldest lesions. On the vascular side, capillary proliferation and telangiectasia were seen. At 52 weeks there was a clear tendency towards healing, with few small necrotic lesions but many small mineral deposits. A fractionated dose of 80 Gy was well above tolerance, with papilledema at 6–8 weeks, impairment of visual evoked responses, and overt clinical impairment of motor function from about 26 weeks. Although at 26 weeks histological findings were similar to those after 60 Gy, there was a rapid progression in the number of necrotic lesions and development of confluent areas of necrosis, without any signs of healing.

Finally, a group of 21 adult monkeys were irradiated with daily fractions of 2 Gy of 13.2 MeV photons to a total dose of 60 Gy, with alternate sides of the brain being treated on alternate days. In the studies with the 2-year-old monkeys irradiation was only applied from one side at a higher energy, which may have had radiobiological consequences because of differences in dose distributions and daily fraction size in critical subvolumes. Nevertheless, it is important to note that the changes in the aforementioned adult monkeys were less than in the young animals, with only two or three showing early papilledema. No animals showed late neurological deficits, and five of nine killed later than 24 weeks showed the characteristic minute necrotic lesions, many of them in a late mineralized phase. Vascular injury consisted of extensive capillary proliferation and telangiectasia, often without an apparent relation to the necrotic lesions.

These studies by CAVENESS and co-workers are probably the most relevant in relation to human brain tolerance and pathogenesis of delayed necrosis. In terms of dose equivalence, a single dose of 15 Gy is roughly equivalent to 60 Gy in 2 Gy fractions, which agrees with some radiobiological formalisms of CNS tolerance (see Sect. 6.2.2). Although at these dose levels no severe clinical signs were observed, most animals showed a large number of minute necrotic lesions in the white matter but without the progression into large coalescent necrotic areas seen at higher doses. However, the presence of obvious tissue damage shows that at these dose levels, which are generally accepted in the treatment of gliomas, there is a significant risk of late neurological deficits.

6.1.1.2 Dog Brain

The other large animal in which radiation-induced brain damage is systematically investigated is the beagle dog. One study (ZOOK et al. 1980) was mostly aimed at a comparison of photons and fast neutrons, and determining radiobiological effectiveness (RBE) values. With ^{60}Co photons, all animals developed encephalopathy after a dose of 90 Gy in 28 fractions, whereas none did so after a dose of 60 Gy in 28 fractions. Latencies varied from 4 to 6 months. After these high doses, the predominant histological features were hemorrhages, edema, and areas of malacia in conjunction with small vessel degeneration in primarily the white matter. Latent periods after neutrons were shorter (2–3 months), but histologically not different from photon irradiation. Unfortunately in these studies the doses used were either far above tolerance, or below it, and no observations were made on the late delayed responses.

A more detailed description of pathological changes after dog hemibrain irradiations with 4 MeV photons was given by TILLER-BORCICH et al. (1987) and FIKE et al. (1988). In the first paper single doses were given in large increments (10, 15, and 30 Gy). Pathological changes were divided into three types: (a) edema with axonal swelling and demyelination, (b) micronecrosis: well-defined focal areas of coagulation necrosis, a spongiotic border, and usually few reactive changes, and (c) macronecrosis with reactive changes (large confluent areas of coagulation necrosis, with a variable degree of infiltration with lipid-laden macrophages). No changes were seen after 10 Gy, but severe clinical signs occurred in the 15 and 30 Gy groups and most animals were killed after 5–6 months. The 30 Gy group was characterized by a generalized white matter necrosis with minimal vascular damage but extensive edema. In the 15 Gy group, killed at the same time, both micro- and macronecrosis were more extensive, which was suggested to be related to the more pronounced vascular injury. A notable difference with the whole brain studies by ZOOK et al. (1980)

is the predominance of a hemorrhagic component in those studies, after a fractionated dose roughly equivalent to the 30 Gy single dose used in the studies by Tiller-Borcich et al. (1987). In a subsequent dose–response study (Fike et al. 1988) a clinically relevant dose range was covered (11.5–17 Gy). Quantitative CT was compared with histopathological changes. In the 15 Gy and higher dose groups lethality occurred within 5–8 months, and the LD_{50} was 14.9 Gy. Using CT-low density volume as the endpoint, a similar ED_{50} of 14.6 Gy was obtained. Associated with the neurological and CT changes were coagulation necrosis, demyelination, and edema of the adjacent white matter. Some of the animals in the lower dose groups surviving at least 1 year showed more subtle CT-low density changes, consistent with a slow generalized loss or atrophy of glial cells. For these long-term changes an ED_{50} of 12.8 Gy was obtained.

6.1.1.3 Rodent Brain

The studies on rodent brain have mainly focused on pathogenesis after large single doses and large dose increments. A classical study in rodent brain employing fractionated irradiation in the therapeutic range was performed in the rabbit (Berg and Lindgren 1958). After follow-up periods of 44–52 weeks, the lesions observed were similar to those described for dog and monkey brain, with necrotic foci in the white matter as the predominant lesion. The authors stressed the interaction of glial and vascular components of injury, with the formation of "gliovascular foci." Although a direct radiation effect on glial cells was not excluded, the vascular changes were thought to be primary in the development of focal white matter necrosis.

A limited study on mouse brain was reported by Yoshii and Phillips (1982). Late vascular effects after single doses of 13–25 Gy were scored in animals killed at various time intervals, but predominantly during the 2nd year post-irradiation. A distinctive lesion was fibrinoid necrosis of the wall of larger vessels, and scoring of the incidence at approximately 60 weeks showed a shallow dose–response relation. The occurrence of focal necrosis and atrophy was associated with fibrinoid necrosis of a major artery, but a dose response was not mentioned.

The extensive work on rat brain by Hopewell and many collaborators was started in the late 1960s and is still being continued in a European collaborative project. The initial studies were performed with a limited number of large single doses (10, 20, 30 and 40 Gy x-rays), but the conclusions from those studies set the stage for an interesting hypothesis (Hopewell and Wright 1970). It was observed in normotensive animals that doses of 30 and 40 Gy produced large areas of white matter necrosis with vascular damage restricted to thalamic regions. In contrast, animals dying after 20 Gy only showed vascular damage without white matter necrosis. It was also shown that in hypertensive animals the expression of vascular-related injury was accelerated after lower doses, but not the induction of necrosis after high doses. These observations suggested the presence of two modes of injury, operating at different dose levels and affecting different tissue components. A cellular basis for these observations was also provided by observations of the depopulation of the subependymal plate, a presumed stem cell area for the replacement of neuroglia. After doses of 10 and 20 Gy this region had a normal appearance, while after 30–40 Gy the subependymal plate was almost acellular. In subsequent studies these findings were further substantiated (Cavanagh and Hopewell 1972). After doses of 2, 8, and 20 Gy, the number of mitotic cells dropped considerably within a day after irradiation, but full recovery was observed at 3 months. After a single dose of 40 Gy even at 6 months the subependymal plate was totally depleted of cells. An analysis of the fate of subpopulations of glial cells in the plate after a dose of 8 Gy showed a preferential disappearance of small dark-staining cells, regarded as the glial precursor cells (Hubbard and Hopewell 1980). These cell kinetic studies on a specific area of glial precursor cells after brain irradiation suggested a correlation with the occurrence of necrosis (Hopewell 1979). That this correlation might not be as clear as initially suggested stems from the recognition that the loss of oligodendrocytes in itself does not explain the development of massive necrosis of the white matter. It has been argued that these lesions are typically the result of infarction and edema (Blakemore and Palmer 1982), which would emphasize the importance of the vasculature as the pathological basis of most late effects in the CNS. This was also the major conclusion from a recent histological analysis of the vascular and parenchymal changes in the rat brain after single doses of 17.5–25 Gy of 250 kV x-rays (CALVO et al. 1988). Demyelination and necrosis of the white matter were only seen after doses of 22.5 Gy or higher, and not before 9 months. From scores of specific changes in blood vessels and counts of glial cells in the fimbria of the rat brain, the earliest and most predominant changes were reported in blood vessels, in close association with astrocyte enlargement, leading to the concept of a "vascular/glia unit of tissue injury." Physiological studies on vascular permeability after doses of 20 Gy or less on the rat brain did not show any alteration of the blood–brain barrier for up to 18 months after irradiation (KEYEUX et al. 1987). These studies did, however, indicate slowly progressive brain atrophy, which is similar to observations in dog brain (FIKE et al. 1988).

6.1.2 Spinal Cord

The spinal cord has been used extensively in radiobiological studies as a model for central nervous system injury. The scoring of injury in the cord is generally more straightforward, with tissue damage of any significance being directly associated with the development of paresis or paralysis. This is probably the reason why better defined dose–response relationships have been obtained for spinal cord than for brain. Also, in radiotherapeutic treatments the induction of radiation myelopathy is one of the most feared complications, providing an obvious incentive for detailed tolerance studies.

The animal species used for spinal cord studies are similar to those used for brain, and range from rodents to monkeys. Analogous to the above description of the various animal models used for brain injury, the models for spinal cord damage will be discussed and lesions compared with those observed in the brain.

6.1.2.1 Primate Spinal Cord

Little information is available on the pathology of spinal cord injury in monkeys after clinically relevant doses. An abstract on dose response for myelopathy in rhesus monkeys was published by FEIN and DI CHIRO (1974). After a dose of 15×4 Gy or 10×10 Gy on a 10 cm length of low thoracic cord, three monkeys developed a paraparesis

within 5–8 months postirradiation. An important observation concerning the pathogenesis was that angiography showed an obstruction of major radicular feeding arteries, which was compensated by collateral filling from arteries outside the irradiated area. Histology did not show evidence of ischemic infarction, but rather demyelination of all long tract systems.

A group of 30 adult monkeys were irradiated on the cervical cord with 50 MeV neutrons (13–15.5 Gy in nine fractions) or ^{60}Co γ-rays (46.2–59.4 Gy in 22 fractions) as reported by STEPHENS et al. (1983). Clinical signs of paralysis were only noted in the highest neutron dose group within 6–11 months, and histological changes consisted of extensive focal white matter necrosis (malacia) and demyelination. Vascular lesions were not common and were limited to hyaline thickening of the walls of small vessels in gray and white matter. The authors did not consider the vascular lesions to be contributory to the overall histological changes. A less severe but similar histological appearance was noted in animals from all but the lowest dose groups (neutrons and γ-rays) killed after 1–2 years. In the ^{60}Co γ-ray group, minimal to mild white matter malacia and demyelination were present in the 54 Gy and 59.4 Gy groups. Mineralized particles were seen in many of the minute focal areas of necrosis. This observation is very similar to those made by CAVENESS (1980) in monkey brain after similar doses. It is important to note that in both studies these histological changes were not accompanied by clinical signs, and that the doses were in the range of accepted tolerance levels.

6.1.2.2 Dog Spinal Cord

One of the few studies on dog spinal cord was done to evaluate the RBE of fast neutrons compared with ^{60}Co γ-rays (ZOOK et al. 1981). A 20 fraction dosage schedule similar in design to the brain study (see Sect. 6.1.1.2) covered a wide range of doses with large increments especially in the photon group. After a dose of 78.8 Gy on the cervical cord (10 cm), four out of six dogs developed paralysis within 3–4 months after irradiation. After the next lower dose of 52.5 Gy, no changes occurred during the 3- to 4-year observation period. In the neutron arm, paralysis developed in all animals of the 26 Gy and 39 Gy dose groups within 1–2 months. The gross pathology was not different for the two types of radiation; it consisted of extensive hemorrhages in both the white and the gray matter, but especially in the latter. Hemorrhagic infarcts were seen near the ventral spinal artery. Unfortunately no detailed histology was reported, but based on preliminary histopathological observations the authors commented on the unusual finding of extensive vascular lesions in the gray and to a lesser extent the white matter. Although this observation could be partly due to the high dose and the corresponding large fraction size (almost 80 Gy in 4 Gy fractions), the dose level is equivalent to the highest dose in the brain study performed by the same group (ZOOK et al. 1980). In the brain a predilection for white matter was noted, in agreement with observations in other species, including man. An ongoing study by BECK et al. (1988) may shed some light on this issue. In a pathogenesis and tolerance study, beagles were irradiated with megavoltage x-rays on the thoracic cord with an increasing number of 4 Gy fractions, up to a total dose of 76 Gy. In a preliminary report the occurrence of paralysis was noted after 2–3 months in the highest dose group, accompanied by infarcts, telangiectasia, and thromboses. In the lower dose groups no paralysis was seen within 7–8 months but a dose-related decrease in conduction velocity was measured at 4 months. The continuation of this study should show whether these more subtle changes are similar to various delayed types of injury described for dog brain by TILLER-BORCICH et al. (see Sect. 6.1.1.2).

6.1.2.3 Rat Spinal Cord

The most extensively used models of spinal cord injury are the various regions of the rat spinal cord: cervical, thoracic, lumbar, and cauda equina. One of the first studies (ASSCHER and ANSON 1962), performed in a small number of animals, is still of significance with regard to the vascular etiology of CNS radionecrosis. The cervical and upper thoracic cord of normotensive and hypertensive Wistar rats was irradiated with 15, 20, and 30 Gy of 220 kV x-rays. From the hypertensive groups, even after the lowest dose of 15 Gy, most animals died suddenly with or without ataxia after widely varying latencies of 1–8 months. The cords of these animals showed vascular lesions with fibrinoid necrosis and thrombi of the spinal arteries. None of the normotensive animals killed as controls whenever a hypertensive

rat died showed any kind of injury. Although limited in scope, this study clearly demonstrated the importance of the vasculature in the development of radiation injury in the cord at clinically relevant doses.

A number of studies at the Brookhaven National Laboratory were carried out on the rat thoracic cord with high single doses (range: 29–54 Gy), all well above the clinical range (INNES and CARSTEN 1961; ZEMAN et al. 1964; CARSTEN and ZEMAN 1966). These authors were the first to provide a detailed description of the development of delayed necrosis in the rat spinal cord. After a single dose of 35 Gy to cord segments T2-T4, paralysis developed after an average latency of 200 days (range: 166–227 days). Surprisingly, the same dose to the whole thoracic and lumbar cord showed a wider range of latencies of 150–270 days, with the same average value. A slightly lower dose of 29 Gy to the small thoracic field induced paralysis after an average latency of 248 (range: 174–309) days, suggesting an inverse relationship of dose and latent period. Microscopic changes developed in parallel with neurological deficits. The first signs of necrosis were focal, with almost simultaneous breakdown of myelin, axons, and glia, In the upper thoracic cord, a predilection was noted for anterolateral tracts, while dorsal columns became involved when massive necrosis had developed. The corticospinal tracts and the nerve roots remained well preserved. The gray matter and meninges showed very few changes. The contribution of vascular damage was tested with iodine-labeled serum albumin, which did not show up in the necrotic areas. Thus, a generalized change in vascular permeability did not occur, but foci of fibrinoid degeneration of vascular walls and erythrodiapedesis were present. The authors (ZEMAN et al. 1964) concluded that vascular lesions were unlikely to be a major contributor to white matter necrosis, possibly in contrast to brain damage in rodents.

Vascular lesions were also not very pronounced during the first 5 months after irradiation of the cervical and lumbar cords of rats with a range of single doses (1–60 Gy) (MASTAGLIA et al. 1976). An important factor to consider is that very short lengths of cord were irradiated in these studies (5 mm cervical, 10 mm lumbar), and it has been shown recently that volume is a significant variable in dose–response relationships and pathogenesis (HOPEWELL et al. 1987; HOPEWELL and van der KOGEL 1988) (see also Sect. 6.2.5). In the studies by MASTAGLIA et al. (1976) a detailed morphological analysis employing electron microscopy and nerve-teasing techniques was carried out. Myelin degeneration started with nodal widening and paranodal breakdown, followed by signs of axonal swelling and scattered disintegration of the myelin sheath. These changes occurred as early as 2 weeks postirradiation and increased with longer times and higher doses. A predilection for the ventral and superficial dorsal columns was noted. After 3 months clear signs of remyelination were observed. The importance of this study is the demonstration of early myelin-related changes even after doses as low as 5–10 Gy, providing a substrate for the clinically important Lhermitte's sign after irradiation of large parts of the spinal column such as for Hodgkins' disease. This usually transient phenomenon is associated with diffuse demyelination, which has been described as a somnolence syndrome after combined radio/chemotherapy of brain lesions. In addition, these observations show that cell depletion related events can be detected after low doses, and that threshold or tolerance dose levels are only related to gross tissue malfunction.

Differences in response of different regions of the rat spinal cord were noted by BRADLEY et al. (1977) and VAN DER KOGEL (1977a, b, 1979, 1980). In the study by BRADLEY et al., a single dose of 35 Gy was administered to three cord regions: 2 cm midthoracic (T6-T10), 3 cm thoracolumbar (T12-L3), and 3 cm cauda equina (L3-S2). As in most of the earlier studies, the dose level chosen was well above the threshold for induction of paralysis, which is about a 20 Gy single dose. Animals irradiated on the thoracolumbar field showed a wide range of times to onset of paralysis, ranging from 83–211 days. Histologically, all animals killed at 3–4.5 months showed extensive necrosis of the dorsal nerve roots, with relatively little damage in the ventral roots. Despite the high dose, most spinal cords had a normal appearance. In animals killed from about 4.5–7 months, the ventral roots also showed extensive damage. A delay in the development of ventral root necrosis compared with dorsal roots was also observed by VAN DER KOGEL (1979). After single doses in the range 22–40 Gy, equivalent degrees of nerve root necrosis developed about 1–2 months later in ventral roots. As could be expected, the occurrence of paresis correlated well with the development of ventral root necrosis, since most motor fibers are located in these roots.

In the lower lumbar and lumbosacral parts of the spinal cord, a remarkable shift in pathology occurs. In the studies on this subject (BRADLEY et al. 1977; VAN DER KOGEL and BARENDSEN 1974; VAN DER KOGEL 1979, 1983) a gradually diminishing severity of cord damage was noted when moving in the caudal direction. This was not dose related and a relative paucity of changes in the cord was even seen after single doses as high as 40 Gy. In most of the lumbar cord, at vertebral levels T12-L1, cord damage was restricted to the ventrolateral tracts close to the ventral root entry zones. At more caudal levels not only does the diameter of the cord diminish rapidly, but injury also becomes restricted to the cauda equina. Thus, after irradiation of the spine below vertebrae L1/L2, the most dominant pathological feature is nerve root necrosis (radiculopathy), which is totally in contrast to the findings in the cervical and thoracic cord. Differences in circulation do not provide an unequivocal explanation for this phenomenon. In the studies by BRADLEY et al. (1977) vascular involvement was described as an engorgement of vessels near necrotic areas, frequently accompanied by petechial hemorrhages. However, thrombosis or vessel wall changes were never detected, and spinal arteries were normal throughout the irradiated areas. The nerve root necrosis, although very like an ischemic lesion of peripheral nerves, did not show the distribution of an arterial infarction. It was concluded by BRADLEY et al. (1977) that if there was a vascular basis, it was most likely at the level of capillary obliteration.

As described in the earlier part of this section on rat spinal cord, white matter necrosis is the dominant lesion in the thoracic and cervical cord after relatively high single doses. Does this pathological characteristic remain the same at clinically relevant doses? An extensive dose–response study in combination with sequential killing to evaluate the pathogenesis was carried out by VAN DER KOGEL (review, 1983). After single doses down to approximately 20 Gy, the observed damage is basically similar to the white matter necrosis as reported by others (INNES and CARSTEN 1961) for higher doses. The distribution of the necrotic lesions seems largely random, but is influenced by cord level. Unpublished observations of this author show a predominance of dorsal tract lesions in high cervical segments, ventrolateral lesions at midcervical levels, and a further shift to dorsal lesions in the upper thoracic cord, but with a large variability. For various regions of the thoracic cord (BRADLEY et al. 1977; INNES and CARSTEN 1961) it is generally the ventrolateral white matter that is most severely affected. A selective involvement of the dorsal horn area (MYERS et al., 1986) was thought to be related to the vulnerability of this area to ischemic injury.

Undoubtedly, edema and other microcirculatory damage plays a role in the pathogenesis of white matter necrosis. With increasing doses, edema and hemorrhage become a more dominating aspect of the observed lesions (KNOWLES 1983; VAN DER KOGEL 1979, 1983) and the latency to paralysis becomes shorter. Also, after a single dose of 30 Gy to the cervical cord, vascular permeability was increased and blood flow decreased in the dorsal gray and white matter a few weeks before the occurrence of necrosis. Histologically these observations were reflected by edema and erythrodiapedesis (MYERS et al. 1987). However, whether these vascular changes are merely a component in the precipitation of the final necrotic lesion in a severely damaged glial population, or the sole dose-limiting tissue compartment, is not solved yet. A very important determinant is the radiation dose. Most of the experimental pathogenetic studies have been done with relatively high doses (single doses of 20–40 Gy) well above the therapeutic dose range. After doses below 20 Gy, changes in the blood–brain barrier permeability were not observed in the rat brain for at least 18 months after irradiation (KEYEUX et al. 1987). Also rats treated on the cervical cord with combined intrathecal ara-C and 15–22 Gy x-rays showed a generalized diffuse demyelination after 2–3 months, which several months later developed into the characteristic white matter necrosis (VAN DER KOGEL and SISSINGH 1985) (see also Sect. 6.2.9).

Another type of vascular injury, not accompanied by extensive white matter necrosis, is characterized by late degenerative changes in capillaries and larger venules. After single irradiations, this damage is seen over a narrow dose range of ~15–20 Gy. With fractionated irradiation the effective dose range becomes larger (see Sect. 6.2.1). Histologically these lesions vary from capillary proliferation and telangiectasia to massive hemorrhagic infarcts. The time of occurrence is variable but is usually later than 1 year up to the end of the life span of the rats (approximately 2 years). Animals killed near the end of their expected life span without any neurological sign often showed areas with telangiectasia and petechial hemorrhages or thrombosed vessels (VAN DER KOGEL 1979). Some of these apparently static

telangiectatic lesions may in fact be slowly progressive in longer lived species. Telangiectatic skin lesions have been shown to develop continuously over a 5- to 10-year period (TURESSON and NOTTER 1986).

6.1.2.4 Spinal Cord – Other Species

Mouse

Several investigators have studied dose–response relationships in mouse spinal cord, but detailed histology has not been reported. From the study on lumbosacral spine with x-rays and neutrons (GERACI et al. 1974) it can be tentatively concluded from photographs shown that in the lower cord regions the lumbar roots are preferentially damaged after doses of 20–25 Gy x-rays. This is similar to findings in studies on rats. The cervical and thoracic cord in mice appears unusually resistant, with single dose ED_{50} values of 50–60 Gy at 6–7 months, decreasing to 35–45 Gy at 12–18 months (GOFFINET et al. 1976; TRAVIS et al. 1982; HABERMALZ et al. 1987). Histologically the animals dying before 7 months showed white matter necrosis, and mice with paralysis at later times showed the typical late vascular injury, such as telangiectasia and focal hemorrhages (TRAVIS et al. 1982). The occurrence of two syndromes was also reported by HABERMALZ (1982, 1987) but with a large overlap between 300 and 500 days. The latter author reported hemorrhages in the gray matter to occur only after high doses and short latencies (<150 days).

Guinea Pig

The guinea pig has been used in a few studies on spinal cord. A careful histological analysis was reported by KNOWLES (1981, 1983), who showed the occurrence of white matter necrosis in the lumbar and cervical cord after single doses of 30 and 40 Gy. The distribution of the necrotic areas was mainly in the ventral columns, and the dorsal columns were only infrequently involved in combination with necrosis of other areas. Vascular injury was limited to focal fresh hemorrhages in the lumbar gray matter. The nerve roots were only damaged in a few animals irradiated on the lumbar cord (above the level of the cauda equina, which is the area showing most root injury in rats). At these dose levels in the adult guinea pig, the latency was approximately 3 months. After a dose of 20 Gy, which is close to the ED_{50} value (KNOWLES 1983), the latency times to the first neurological signs varied from 4 to 6 months but progression to full paralysis was very slow. Histological observation showed a diffuse demyelination associated with vacuolar spaces throughout the white matter. No vascular abnormalities or inflammatory response was noted in these animals, and lesions were similar in cervical and lumbar cord. In a preliminary report from a tolerance study in guinea pig spinal cord, the findings by KNOWLES were confirmed (WITHERS et al. 1987). The lumbar cord was irradiated with ^{60}Co γ-rays, and latency times to the first wave of paralyses were 2–4 months. The histological findings were characterized as diffuse demyelination.

6.1.3 Peripheral Nerves

Despite the existence of several reports on radiation-induced peripheral neuropathies in patients, experimental studies on peripheral nerves are very limited. After some early experimental work in rats it was assumed for a long time that peripheral nerves are extremely radioresistant (JANZEN and WARREN 1942). Doses used were up to 10000 R of 200 kV x-rays, but the follow-up time in those studies was only 8 weeks. In that time, a delayed radioresponsiveness was often misinterpreted as a sign of radioresistance. The effects on lumbar spinal nerve roots as described in Sect. 6.1.2.3 indicate a similar sensitivity of central and peripheral nervous tissues.

Two specific studies on the effects of x-rays on the proliferation and cell kinetics of Schwann cells in rodent peripheral nerves were reported by CAVANAGH (1968) and HASSLER (1968). In the study by HASSLER, mice were irradiated with 27.6 Gy x-rays on one hind leg, and the incorporation of ^{3}H-thymidine into the sciatic nerves was examined for up to 9 months post-irradiation. At 1, 3, and 9 months only a moderate decrease in labeled Schwann cells occurred, accompanied by slight fibrosis but no demyelination. The proliferative potential of rat sciatic Schwann cells after x-ray doses of up to 20 Gy was investigated by their response to crushing of the nerve. After doses of 10 and 20 Gy a lasting reduction in proliferative response was observed during the follow-up period of 6 months, but no demyelination or necrosis was reported to occur in this time span.

More recently, dose–response studies in peripheral nerves were performed in dogs (American foxhounds) to study their tolerance to intraoperative irradiation (KINSELLA et al. 1985). High energy electrons were administered in single doses of 20–75 Gy to the lumbosacral plexus and sciatic nerve while surgically exposed. The time to development of paresis was inversely related to dose, but even at the lowest dose of 20 Gy. three out of four dogs developed injury after 30–50 weeks. A recent preliminary report (KINSELLA et al. 1988) confirmed these findings at 20 Gy and mentioned the absence of injury after 15 Gy or lower. Histologically, the damage consisted of the loss of predominantly the large myelinated fibers, but no signs of vascular occlusion or thrombosis were noted. Extensive fibrosis was seen in the endoneurium but not the perineurium. These studies clearly showed that the tolerance to irradiation of peripheral nerves is not higher than spinal cord or brain, and that latencies after near tolerance doses may be up to a year. Of interest to the discussion of pathogenesis is the absence of vascular injury even after very large single doses.

A recent report on studies comparing intraoperative (IORT, LE COUTEUR et al. 1989) and external beam irradiation of the lumbar spinal nerves in adult beagle dogs shows a similar tolerance to IORT. At two years following IORT, an ED_{50} dose of 16.1 Gy was determined for electrophysiological signs of peripheral neuropathy. In contrast, no signs of neuropathy were seen after doses of up to 80 Gy in 30 fractions of external irradiation. The histological changes in the nerves after IORT showed some differences with the study reported by KINSELLA et al. (1988), most notably the presence of definite vascular lesions. These consisted of necrosis and hyalinization of the media of small arteries, and at higher doses also thrombosis and hemorrhage were observed. The ED_{50} for severe vessel lesions was 19.5 Gy after single dose IORT. This value only marginally decreased to 18.7 Gy when IORT was combined with 50 Gy in 25 fractions external irradiation, indicating a remarkably small effect of the fractionated irradiation. In addition, dose-response relationships were established for other lesions, such as an increase in endoneurial or perineurial fibrosis and a decrease in the axon/myelin ratio. Despite the possible differences in histological changes in the two dog studies, it is clear that the tolerance of peripheral nerves to single dose IORT is not much higher than 15 Gy.

6.1.4 Pathogenesis of Delayed Injury in the Nervous System – General Discussion

In the many pathology reports and dose–response studies in the nervous system, a variety of lesions with different latency times are described. Undoubtedly important differences exist between different species and CNS regions, but it seems worthwhile to consider the presence of a general mechanism of injury in which several variables act to modify the response. The large variability seems related to, for example, the time of observation, the irradiated volume, or the site; however, probably the most important variable is the radiation dose. In a specific region of the brain or spinal cord, a spectrum of lesions may be observed of which the components change abruptly or more gradually with changes in dose. One of the most common lesions associated with high doses, well above the threshold for lethality or paralysis, is coagulation necrosis of the white matter. In most species the latency after ED_{50}-ED_{100} doses is approximately 5–6 months, with a tendency to decrease with increasing doses. This type of injury is equivalent to the so-called early delayed CNS injury. In its most basic form, the lesion is a small punched-out area in the white matter and consists of swollen axons and loss of myelin. At the low end of the dose range, lesions may remain as scattered foci and usually become mineralized with time. After slightly higher effective doses, the individual foci rapidly expand and coalesce into larger necrotic areas. With increasing dose and a more rapid progression, severe neurological impairment and death will ensue before significant inflammatory reactions develop. Usually associated with the development of white matter necrosis is vascular edema, and it is the role of this component of vascular injury which is most controversial. In species such as the monkey and the dog widespread edema is generally reported, but this seems less pronounced in rodents such as rats and guinea pigs. In addition to the edema, a hemorrhagic component of vascular injury increases with increasing dose, and this may be involved in the shortening of the latent period.

One of the most consistent findings related to white matter necrosis is the remarkable similarity of the latent period across a widely varying range of species with different life expectancies. In analogy to other more rapidly dividing tissues it is likely that this phenomenon is related to the slow but accurately programmed turnover of one or more cell types. Since the loss of myelin is a predominant feature of the early delayed response, the oligodendrocyte is the primary cell to be considered as a potential target. A slow turnover of these cells is suggested by the results of cell kinetic studies (SCHULTZE and KORR 1981), indicating the existence of a small pool of proliferating glial cells. The presence of glial progenitor cells in the neonatal as well as the adult nervous system has been amply demonstrated (RAFF et al. 1983; FFRENCH-CONSTANT and RAFF 1986). The lack of replacement of mature oligodendrocytes lost at the normal rate of attrition leads to progressive demyelination, as demonstrated by MASTAGLIA et al. (1976) and VAN DER KOGEL (unpublished observations). A key unresolved issue in this hypothesis is whether the necrotic lesions develop primarily through a critical depletion of the oligodendroglial population, or independent of glial injury by ischemia and infarction. In the vascular compartment, endothelial and smooth muscle cells are slowly renewed as well, and it is quite possible that a depletion of these cells is of critical importance (CALVO et al. 1987).

At lower dose levels and later times, often more than a year, so-called late delayed injury may develop. When the tissue escapes the early necrotic phase, the development of chronic progressive injury may continue. At least three more or less separate types evolve from the above reviewed literature:

1. Minute focal areas of necrosis in the white matter showing various degrees of mineralization. These lesions are probably stationary remnants of the early white matter lesions, and have been described in monkey brain (CAVENESS 1980).
2. Vascular degeneration: telangiectasia, capillary proliferation, wall thickening, perivascular edema, thrombosis, petechial hemorrhages. Especially the widening of capillaries and small venules is a very consistent component of late delayed injury. In most studies, the occurrence of the chronic types of vascular damage is not related to the development of necrosis and significant neurological deficits, but its recognition and quantification is obviously an important aspect of establishing tolerance doses.
3. Glial atrophy: a generalized atrophy of nervous tissue without clear signs of vascular injury or tissue necrosis. This type of late injury has been

detected by quantitative CT scanning in dog brain after doses usually regarded as within the tolerance range (FIKE et al. 1988). Preliminary results in rat brain (KEYEUX et al. 1987) also suggest the development of tissue atrophy after relatively low doses and long follow-up times. A gradual depletion of glial cells would be hard to detect by the usual histological techniques, but these recent observations seem to warrant further investigations into the relevance of these changes.

6.2 Radiobiological Variables and Their Influence on Tolerance Doses

6.2.1 Fractionation and Overall Time

The first indications of the large influence of fractionation on tolerance doses in the CNS originated from clinical observations. From a limited number of cases with radiation myelopathy, ATKINS and TRETTER (1966) derived a slope of 0.38 on a logarithmic plot of total dose versus number of fractions (Strandqvist plot) and cautioned against the use of large fraction sizes when the spinal cord is included. A few years later PHILLIPS and BUSCHKE (1969) obtained a slope of 0.5 for number of fractions against thoracic cord tolerance, and concluded that the number of fractions and, correspondingly, the size of the dose per fraction are of importance. The first experimental data on spinal cord tolerance were reported by VAN DER KOGEL and BARENDSEN (1974). The rat lumbar cord was irradiated with up to 20 fractions of x-rays, and a double-log plot of total dose against number of fractions yielded a slope of 0.44. The underlying pathology of the lumbar cord injury was shown to be a radiculopathy (see Sect. 6.1.2.3). Higher cord regions were investigated in the rat cervical cord (VAN DER KOGEL 1977a) and in the thoracic cord (MASUDA et al. 1977), confirming the slope of 0.44 and suggesting the time factor to be negligible. The observation of different histological lesions not only in different regions but also in two types of injury in the cervical cord led to the analysis of dose–response relationships for specific endpoints (VAN DER KOGEL 1977; 1979). For three endpoints the slopes of the isoeffect curves were: lumbar radiculopathy – 0.4, cervical white matter necrosis

– 0.46, and cervical vascular damage – 0.42. The contribution of a time factor as determined by split-dose experiments was found to be insignificant during the first 6–8 weeks of treatment of the cervical/high thoracic regions (VAN DER KOGEL 1977). A lower slope of 0.35 for the lumbar endpoint was reported by WHITE and HORNSEY (1978) and later for up to 60 fractions by HORNSEY and WHITE (1980). These latter experiments were all performed in constant overall times of 6 weeks, thereby largely excluding a possible influence of a time factor. In the lumbar cord functional repopulation was shown to start at between 2 and 4 weeks (WHITE and HORNSEY 1980; VAN DER KOGEL 1979). This might explain the slightly higher slope of 0.4 obtained for lumbar cord by VAN DER KOGEL (1979), since these experiments were done with daily fractionation whereby the contribution of repopulation would increase with longer times and larger numbers of fractions.

These extensive sets of data on rat spinal cord were very consistent in their general results, showing a slope of about 0.4–0.45 for the cervical/high thoracic cord, and a tendency toward slightly lower slopes of 0.35–0.4 for the lumbar cord. Similar results were obtained in more limited fractionated exposures of the low thoracic cord in the rat (LEITH et al. 1981; MASUDA et al. 1977). Within the cervical cord the slope for threshold doses for vascular injury, which are closest to clinical tolerance doses, seems slightly lower compared with that for ED_{50} values for white matter necrosis.

The only other series of fractionated exposures of the spinal cord was performed in the mouse (HABERMALZ et al. 1987). Doses required to elicit a paralytic response in the mouse are much higher than in other species, with single dose ED_{50} values of about 40–45 Gy (GOFFINET et al. 1976; TRAVIS et al. 1982; HABERMALZ et al. 1987). The results of HABERMALZ et al. showed significantly lower slopes of isoeffect curves. A very unusual finding in these studies was the flat isoeffect curve between one and five fractions, showing no repair for large fraction sizes. From five fractions upward, slopes of Strandqvist plots varied between 0.27 and 0.30 after observation times of up to 550 days. Although the low energy of 100 kV of the used x-rays could be responsible for the decreased repair, the authors claim that irradiation with single doses or two fractions of 250 kV x-rays gave similar results compared with the lower energy x-rays.

Experimental data on fractionated irradiation of the brain from which fractionation factors can be derived are limited to a few studies. In an early study on rabbits, single doses as well as 13 and 31 daily fractions of 200 kV x-rays were administered to the right half of the brain. No functional damage was scored, but threshold doses and ED_{50} values were estimated for the induction of necrotic foci from histological evaluations (BERG and LINDGREN 1958). The average slope of the Strandqvist plots was 0.34, which was similar to curves obtained for skin reactions. In that time the fractionation effect was not yet analyzed separately from the contribution of overall time. The latter would be negligible for brain in contrast to skin, indicating a larger capacity for repair of sublethal damage in nervous tissue. These early fractionation data obtained in the rabbit were confirmed in rat brain with up to 30 fractions of 250 kV x-rays (HORNSEY et al. 1981a,b). The endpoint for brain injury is usually death of the animal, in contrast to spinal cord for which specific neurological signs can be scored. The insensitivity of this endpoint is demonstrated by the high isoeffective doses (single dose: 32 Gy). Nevertheless, the slope of the Strandqvist plot obtained by HORNSEY et al. for brain-related death is 0.38, which is similar to the values obtained for the spinal cord endpoints.

6.2.2 Isoeffect Models and Tolerance Formulas

From the previous section it can be concluded that most experimental findings clearly support the initial clinical impression of a steeper slope for myelopathy or encephalopathy compared with isoeffect curves obtained for acute injury, and various clinical isoeffect formulas have been formulated (Table 6.1). The collection of formulas clearly shows the large fractionation exponents, with small exponents for overall time added in several cases. In view of the large uncertainties in the clinical data, clearly this factor is not significantly different from zero and is negligible compared with the fractionation factor. In addition, the use of exponential time factors might only be valid in the case of slow repair which starts immediately and decays exponentially. However, most time-related recovery is thought to be due to repopulation, which even in rapidly proliferating tissues starts after a time lag. As shown above, time-related recovery in the cervical/thoracic cord does not start before 6–8 weeks; only in the

lumbar cord does this period seem to be shorter. Clinically, this would imply that for treatment periods of up to 8 weeks, it is inappropriate to use a time factor in a power-law equation for the CNS. Thus, in a generally formulated CNS equation, the total tolerated dose would be correlated with $N^{0.4-0.45}$ multiplied by a single dose equivalence value (N equals the number of fractions). For a smaller than 5% risk of late complications, the single dose value is approximately 11–13 Gy (COHEN and CREDITOR 1981; WIGG et al. 1981). The validity of these extrapolated single dose equivalence values is supported by the experimentally derived isoeffective doses for single irradiations of large animals, notably monkey and dog brain (see Sect. 6.1.1)

A power-law formalism of the above type, with an N-exponent of 0.4–0.45, seems safely applicable for doses per fraction between 2 and approximately 8 Gy. However, not only does this formula predict a rapidly falling tolerance dose with large fraction sizes; it also indicates a steep increase in tolerance when doses are decreased below 2 Gy per fraction (Fig. 6.1). This aspect is of critical clinical importance, since the use of hyperfractionated treatments (several small fractions per day) has been advocated mostly on the basis of an expected increase in late tolerance. A smaller but still significant increase in tolerance for fraction sizes below 2 Gy is predicted by the linear–quadratic (LQ) formalism. This formalism is derived from a cell survival model, in which the surviving fraction is related to a linear and squared dose term: $S \sim ad + \beta d^2$. Analogous to cells, the repair capacity of tissues is represented by the ratio α/β, for which a low value is indicative of a high repair capacity.

For tissue responses, such as the induction of paralysis after cervical or thoracic cord irradiation, α/β values can be graphically derived from a so-called Fe plot (DOUGLAS and FOWLER 1976). For a set of isoeffective doses, the inverse of the total dose is plotted against the dose per fraction. The ratio of the ordinate intercept to the slope of the curve yields the α/β value, which can be directly obtained from the plot as the negative value of the abscissa intercept. A comparison of Fe plots for human myelopathy and various rat CNS endpoints is given in Figs. 6.2 and 6.3. The human myelopathy curve is based on data collected from various centers by WIGG et al. (1981) and represents dose estimates of a complication probability of 25%–50%, which should be the

Table 6.1. Power-law formulas for CNS tolerance

Description	Formula	Reference
Clinical		
ED (effective dose)	$N^{0.38} \cdot T^{0.06}$	WARA et al. 1975
Neuret	$N^{0.44} \cdot T^{0.06}$	SHELINE et al. 1980
BTU (brain tolerance unit)	$(10.5) \cdot N^{0.45} \cdot T^{0.03}$	PEZNER and ARCHAMBEAU 1981
Brain tolerance (TD_{0-5})		
endocrine function	$(7.3) \cdot N^{0.5} \cdot T^{0.03}$	WIGG et al. 1982
large volume	$(8.6) \cdot N^{0.55}$	WIGG et al. 1981
small volume	$(12.7) \cdot N^{0.46}$	
necrosis	$(20.1) \cdot N^{0.38}$	
Thoracic cord		WIGG et al. 1981
TD_{25-50}	$(15.3) \cdot N^{0.43}$	
TD_0 (threshold)	$(13.0) \cdot N^{0.41}$	
Myelopathy (TD_5)	$(11.5) \cdot N^{0.38} \cdot T^{0.07}$	COHEN and CREDITOR 1981
Encephalopathy (TD_5)	$(7.7) \cdot N^{0.56} \cdot T^{0.03}$	COHEN and CREDITOR 1983
Experimental		
Rat brain and cord	$N^{0.38} \cdot T^{0.02}$	HORNSEY et al. 1981a,b
Rat spinal cord	$N^{0.44}$	VAN DER KOGEL 1979

best equivalent to animal ED_{50} data. From these curves it can be seen that α/β values for human and rat cervical/thoracic cord are all in the range 1.5–2.5 Gy. For three sets of data of rat low thoracic lumbar cord, α/β values are approximately 4–5 Gy, suggesting a smaller repair capacity of the lower cord regions, as was also reported by LEITH et al. (1981) (Fig. 6.4). This difference between different regions of the spinal cord could well be related to the different pathological mechanisms and target cells involved (see Sect. 6.1.2.3).

Based on the LQ model, several formulas have been proposed for the calculation of tissue tolerance with changes in fraction size. These are:

$$\text{ETD} = D_n{}^* \left[1 + d_n/(\alpha/\beta) \right] \quad \text{(BARENDSEN 1982)} \quad (1)$$

and:

$$\text{TE} = D_n{}^* \left(\alpha/\beta + d_n \right) \quad \text{(THAMES and HENDRY 1987)} \quad (2)$$

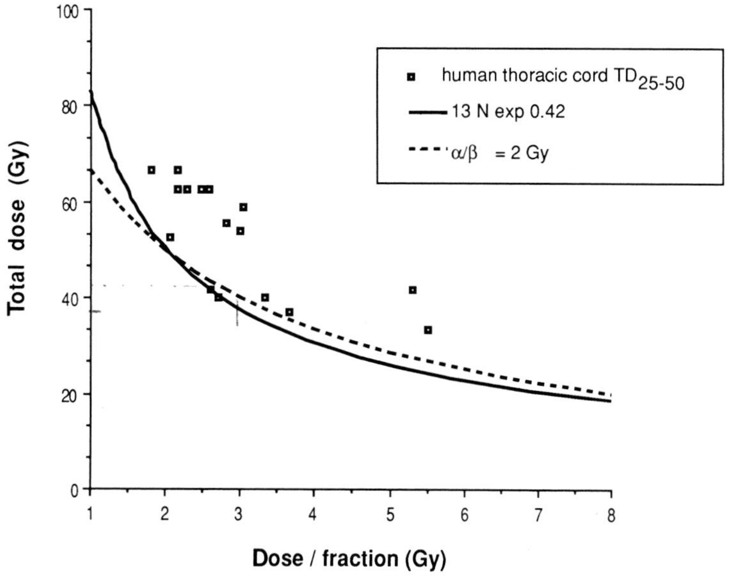

Fig. 6.1. Tolerance curves for the human spinal cord based on a reference dose of 50 Gy in 2 Gy fractions. The curves are calculated according to a power-law formalism ($D = 13.N^{0.42}$) or the linear–quadratic model with an α/β value of 2 Gy. Also plotted are dose estimates associated with a probability of 25%–50% for induction of thoracic myelopathy as collected by WIGG et al. (1981) in various radiotherapy centers. Clearly, most of these doses are well above the tolerance lines. An important difference between the two tolerance curves is the steep rise below 2 Gy per fraction predicted by the power-law formula

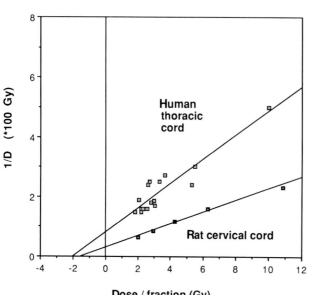

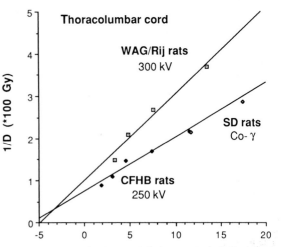

Fig. 6.4. Fe plots (as in Fig. 6.2) for paralysis (ED$_{50}$) in the low thoracic/lumbar cord in different rat strains and different types of radiation. The α/β values are approximately 5 Gy

Fig. 6.2. To derive the repair characteristics (α/β) for specific normal tissue endpoints, the inverse of the total isoeffective dose is plotted versus the dose per fraction (Fe plot). From the intercept with the abscissa, the α/β ratio can be directly obtained. The values derived for the rat cervical cord (ED$_{50}$ white matter necrosis) and the TD$_{25-50}$ estimates for human thoracic cord (WIGG et al. 1981) are not significantly different

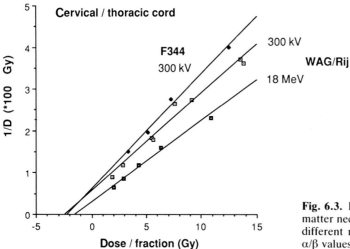

Fig. 6.3. Fe plots (as in Fig. 6.2) for paralysis due to white matter necrosis (ED$_{50}$) in the cervical/high thoracic cord in different rat strains and different types of radiation. The α/β values are 1.5–2 Gy

In these formulas D_n is the total dose in n fractions of size d_n. For a reference tolerance dose D_n at fraction size d_n. the ETD (extrapolated tolerance dose) or the TE (total effect) can be calculated assuming a value for α/β. For brain and upper spinal cord, an average α/β of 2 Gy can be used, while a value of 4–5 Gy seems more applicable for the lumbar cord. This latter value for the lumbar cord should be cautiously applied, however, since no clinical data are available to confirm its validity. When the ETD or TE is calculated for a reference schedule and relevant

Table 6.2. Repair characteristics of the spinal cord

Species (strain)	Region	Radiation	α/β (Gy)[a]	N-exp[b]	Reference
Human	Thoracic	MeV	2	0.43	WIGG et al. 1981
Mouse	T10–T13	100 kV	6.5–10	0.28	HABERMALZ et al. 1987
Rat (lumbar/low thoracic)					
CFHB	L2–L5	250 kV	4.5–5.6	0.33	HORNSEY and WHITE 1980
WAG/Rij	L2–L4	300 kV	2.5–4.7	0.42	VAN DER KOGEL 1977a
SD	T7–T12	^{60}Co γ	4.9	0.44	MASUDA et al. 1977
Rat (cervical/high thoracic)					
WAG/Rij	C5–T2	300 kV	2.4	0.43	VAN DER KOGEL 1979, 1983
	C2–T2	18 MeV	1.5	0.44	ANG et al. 1983, 1985
F344	C2–T2	300 kV	2.2	0.45	VAN DER KOGEL 1985

[a] When a range of α/β values is given, the lower value is derived by excluding fraction doses higher than 10 Gy.
[b] N-exp: exponent for fraction number in a power-law formalism.

α/β value (generally 2 Gy for CNS), total tolerated doses can be derived for changes in dose per fraction. A comparison of repair characteristics of the spinal cord for different species and regions of the cord is given in Table 6.2. In Fig. 6.1, tolerance doses predicted by the LQ formalism and a power-law equation are plotted as a function of dose per fraction, based on a tolerance dose for the spinal cord of 50 Gy in fractions of 2 Gy. These curves show that for a fraction dose of 2 Gy and above, the predicted doses are roughly equivalent for the two methods. For lower doses, the LQ-based predictions assuming an α/β of 2 Gy show a smaller but still significant increase in tolerance. These model predictions were tested experimentally by ANG et al. (1985). In a series of fractionated exposures of the rat cervical spinal cord with 18 MeV photons and doses per fraction of 2 Gy and higher, an α/β ratio of 1.5 Gy was derived based on ED_{50} values for paralysis within 7 months (Fig. 6.3). However, when fraction sizes were reduced below 2 Gy, the isoeffective doses did not show a further significant increase, in contrast to predictions based on the LQ model with an α/β ratio of 1.5 Gy. Additional experiments comparing fraction doses of 1 and 2 Gy suggested a small increase in tolerance of 10%–15% at 1 Gy per fraction (VAN DER SCHUEREN et al. 1988). Although this possible deviation from the LQ model predictions for doses below 2 Gy might have been partially due to incomplete repair between daily doses given with 4-h intervals (THAMES et al. 1988), these results show that clinical tolerance levels in hyperfractionated schedules should be only cautiously increased. Power-

law formulas as shown in Table 6.1 should definitely not be used at fraction doses below 2 Gy, since these formulas predict an even steeper increase in tolerance than the LQ-based formalisms (Fig. 6.1).

6.2.3 Dose Protraction, Repair Kinetics, and Multiple Fractions per Day

In the models and calculations discussed in the previous sections, repair of sublethal damage between daily fractions is assumed to be complete, since average intervals are 24 h. However, with the initiation of multiple daily fractionation, time between fractions can be only 3–4 h (ANG et al. 1982), and incomplete repair may result in an overestimation of tolerance doses. The occurrence of repair during continuous irradiations reduces the effectiveness, and isoeffective doses will increase with decreasing dose rate. Thus, the rate of repair is a critical factor in the calculation of dose adjustments for changes in dose rate and time intervals between fractions. Although cellular repair is a complex process involving several enzymatic reactions, for practical calculations of clinical tolerance monoexponential repair models are generally used. A detailed description of the use of an incomplete-repair model for dose calculations is beyond the scope of this chapter, and the reader is referred to a comprehensive publication (THAMES and HENDRY 1987). It suffices to introduce the parameter that characterizes the exponential repair process, the half-time ($T_{1/2}$)

or time at which half the amount of reparable damage is repaired.

Experimental studies on repair kinetics in the CNS are very limited. In a study on rat lumbar spinal cord, a continuous exposure of 8 h was compared with an acutely administered single dose, and a $T_{1/2}$ of 1.5 h was obtained (VAN DER KOGEL 1977). An identical half-time was derived from multiple daily fractionated exposures of the rat cervical cord, although a faster rate of repair was suggested with decreasing fraction size (VAN DER KOGEL and SISSINGH 1983). These findings were largely confirmed in experiments with two or four fractions and time intervals varying from 20 min to 24 h (ANG et al. 1984). Extension of this work to smaller fraction sizes and more fractions did not show a significant difference in repair kinetics over a dose range of ~2–15 Gy per fraction (ANG et al. 1987). The overall results of the experimental work on CNS repair kinetics suggest an average half-time of 1.5 h. The clinical consequences of these findings are that even at fraction sizes of ~2 Gy, time intervals between subsequent fractions have to be minimally 6–8 h to allow for complete repair. For shorter intervals the total dose has to be reduced, for which methods based on the LQ model have been published (DALE 1985; THAMES and HENDRY 1987).

6.2.4 Long-Term Regeneration and Retreatment Tolerance

As was shown in Sect. 6.2.1, the influence of total time on CNS tolerance doses is negligible during a usual treatment period of 6–8 weeks. A possible exception is the lumbar region of the spinal column, containing mostly the lower lumbosacral cord and the cauda equina. Initial split-dose experiments by WHITE and HORNSEY (1980) on rat cord (vertebral segments L3–L5) showed an increase of approximately 15% in total isoeffective dose for a 1-month interval. Later studies at 100-day intervals did not show a further increase in long-term recovery when analyzed on the basis of isoeffective doses by applying the LQ formalism (HORNSEY et al. 1982; VAN DER KOGEL 1986).

In split-dose experiments on the rat cervical cord, the earliest long-term recovery additional to Elkind repair was observed at 60–70 days and represented an increase of 15% in total isoeffective doses for the induction of early white matter

necrosis (WHITE and HORNSEY 1980; VAN DER KOGEL et al. 1982). With increasing time intervals, a plateau of ~35% rise in ETD (Sect. 6.2.2.) was reached after 4–5 months. The percent long-term recovery appeared to be similar after neutron irradiation (VAN DER KOGEL et al. 1982). When long-term recovery was analyzed for the occurrence of late vascular injury in the rat cervical cord, this appeared to start later (~3 months), but at the longest interval of 7 months the ETD was increased by as much as 65% compared with short overall times. More data for these different endpoints must be obtained for fractionated irradiations and be validated in other animal models before these experimental results can be applied in the clinic.

6.2.5 Volume

The total volume of irradiated tissue is usually assumed to play a role in the development of tissue injury. For the human spinal cord, it was suggested by BODEN in 1948 that the tolerance of a length of ≥15 cm was significantly less than that of a 5–10 cm length. Most of the cases on which these conclusions were based concerned treatment and/or dosimetric errors (such as overlapping fields) or transient myelopathies. The presented material definitely did not justify the suggestion of a large difference in tolerance for large versus small fields. Later publications on the volume effect in spinal cord tolerance (PALLIS et al. 1961; ABBATUCI et al. 1978) also suggested the presence of a moderate volume effect, but the data were insufficient to confirm the validity of any of the proposed mathematical models. These models included simple power-law formalisms that were proposed for a range of tissues, including the CNS (COHEN 1982). Other models were based on the increasing probability of normal tissue complications when larger volumes are irradiated at the same dose level (SCHULTHEISS et al. 1983). A recent extension of the probability models is the assumption of the presence of independent functional subunits in the CNS, whereby in particular the spinal cord would consist of a series of slices (WITHERS et al. 1988; YAES and KALEND 1988). The clinical consequence of these models is a continuous change in tolerance doses with changes in irradiated volume. A classical experimental study on rabbit brain seemed to support the probability models, showing a steep increase in isoeffective doses when a decreasing "slice" of brain was irradiated (BERG and LINDGREN 1963).

After irradiation of 6- or 12-mm segments of mouse spinal cord, the ED_{50} for induction of paralysis was significantly lower for the larger cord length (GOFFINET et al. 1976). Some recent data on rat spinal cord showed a steep increase in isoeffective doses for the induction of early white matter necrosis when a cord length of less than 8–10 mm was irradiated (HOPEWELL et al. 1987; VAN DER KOGEL 1987) (Fig. 6.5). For cord lengths longer than approximately 1 cm, no further decrease in isoeffective dose was noted, suggesting a discontinuous function of cord length versus isoeffective dose. In the study by HOPEWELL et al. this apparent volume effect below 1 cm seemed greatly diminished for the occurrence of late vascular injury. Thus, a possible migration of precursor cells into the small irradiated volumes may prevent the occurrence of one type of lesion (white matter necrosis), but not that of a later type due to the involvement of different target cells. These results obtained in well-characterized animal models indicate the necessity for very cautious use of any of the mathematical formalisms of volume effects. It would be especially dangerous to apply a scaling factor in translating results from small animals to man. Until data are available from large animal models, there seems no biological basis to assume a difference in the relationship between absolute volume and isoeffective dose. Thus, when comparing tissue volumes between different species, this should be done on an absolute basis without the application of scaling factors.

6.2.6 High LET Radiation

The use of fast neutrons and to a lesser extent of pions and heavy charged particles in the treatment of cancer prompted several experimental studies with these types of radiation on the CNS. Studies have been done in monkeys, dogs, and rodents to establish the relative biological effectiveness (RBE) for clinical application. This became the more urgent when studies in various organs showed higher RBE values for late effects compared with acute effects. Also, the first trials with fast neutrons on brain tumors showed the development of unusual complications such as progressive dementia (PARKER et al. 1976; SHAW et al. 1978). Histopathologically the injury to the normal brain was mostly restricted to white matter necrosis and extensive demyelination, which agreed with the early observations by VOGEL and PICKERING (1956) on monkey brain. In general, damage to nervous tissue by neutron irradiation showed a predominance of early white matter related changes, suggesting an enhanced effectiveness on glial cells and myelin.

Radiobiological studies employing the animal models described in Sect. 6.1 all showed a greatly diminished repair capacity after neutron irradiation in contrast to the (relative to other tissues) large repair capacity for x-ray induced damage. This was demonstrated by a negligible increase in isoeffective doses with decreasing fraction size (HORNSEY et al. 1981a; VAN DER KOGEL et al. 1982). When the LQ model was applied to the results obtained for rat spinal cord, α/β values for

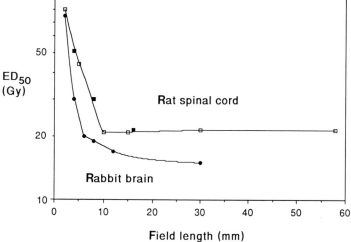

Fig. 6.5. Volume effect in the CNS. Isoeffective doses as a function of field length for rat spinal cord and rabbit brain. For rat spinal cord, ED_{50} values for paralysis due to white matter necrosis are obtained from HOPEWELL et al. (1987) (*closed symbols*) and VAN DER KOGEL (1987) (*open symbols*). For comparison, isoeffective doses reported for rabbit brain necrosis after single dose slit-field x-irradiation (BERG and LINDGREN 1963)

neutrons ranged from 20 to 50 Gy, clearly showing the absence of a fractionation effect (van der Kogel 1985). As a consequence, neutron RBE values for CNS are larger than for most other tissues and have a value of approximately 5 at x-ray doses of 2 Gy per fraction.

Besides fast neutrons the other category of high LET radiation being used clinically consists of heavy particles that deposit most of their energy in a so-called Bragg peak. Although of physical advantage for some specific tumor sites, the cost of these particles is prohibitive and in only a few centers in the world is a radiotherapy program in operation. For four fractions of carbon and neon ions the RBE for rat spinal cord was approximately 2, but extrapolation of these data to a reference x-ray dose of 2 Gy resulted in RBE values of ~5, similar to values obtained for neutrons (Leith et al. 1983). Negative pi-mesons or pions have been estimated to have a lower RBE of 1.5 or less for the rat cervical spinal cord (van der Kogel 1985).

6.2.7 Combined Modalities

6.2.7.1 Oxygen, Sensitizers, and Protectors

The oxygenation status of the CNS has been implicated as a basis for the predilection of early delayed necrosis in the white matter. It has been hypothesized that the gray matter is radiobiologically protected because of a high oxygen consumption by the neurons, resulting in a lower net tissue oxygen tension of the gray matter. However, recent studies in the rat spinal cord have shown that the three times higher oxygen consumption rate of the gray matter is compensated by a three to four times higher blood flow (Hayashi et al. 1983). The average oxygen tension in all cord segments is 17 torr in the gray matter and 15 torr in the white matter. Attempts have been made to modify the response of the spinal cord by increasing the oxygen tension. Breathing of carbogen (95% O_2 + 5% CO_2) combined with a single dose of 35 Gy x-rays did not change the degree of white matter injury but did cause more severe gray matter damage (Zeman 1966). No difference in latency was observed. After irradiation of the rat spinal cord under hyperbaric oxygen conditions, the latency was reduced for a dose of 25 Gy, but not after 35 Gy and 45 Gy (Asbell and Kramer 1971). In tolerance studies of the rat spinal cord

with fractionated irradiations, breathing of oxygen during Ethrane anesthesia did not modify ED_{50} values compared with air breathing with nembutal anesthesia (van der Kogel and Sissingh 1983).

Thus, tissue oxygenation may play a role in the CNS radiation response, but experimentally this has only been demonstrated after high single doses outside the clinical range. In a few clinical reports a sensitization of the cord by higher oxygen tensions has been suggested. In 3 of 17 patients treated for bronchogenic carcinoma under hyperbaric oxygen conditions, myelopathy developed after normally well tolerated doses (Coy and Dolman 1971). The development of myelopathy was recently shown to be significantly correlated with high blood hemoglobin concentrations (Dische et al. 1988).

The role of radioprotectors and sensitizers has received some attention. Results of the most extensive studies with the sensitizer misonidazole in the spinal cord of the mouse (Travis et al. 1982) and the rat (van der Kogel and Sissingh 1983) did not show a significant sensitization. A protective effect of WR-2721 in the rat spinal cord has been shown after single doses of 20–32 Gy, but this was only reflected by changes in latency since all animals developed paralysis at these doses (Spence et al. 1986). A modest protection of the vasculature in the rat brain by the drug gammaphos after single doses of 25 Gy has been recently demonstrated (Plotnikova et al. 1988). Since no dose–response curves near tolerance levels were obtained in these studies with protectors, the clinical relevance of these findings remains questionable.

6.2.7.2 Interactions of Radiotherapy and Chemotherapy

With respect to the interaction of chemotherapeutic agents with the radiation tolerance of the CNS, the presence of the blood–brain barrier (BBB) plays an important role. Many potentially neurotoxic drugs do not cross the barrier unless administered intrathecally or intraventricularly. Irradiation of the rat spinal cord within 30–60 min after intravenous administration of actinomycin D or vincristine (drugs which do not pass the BBB) did not show a change in ED_{50} values for early or late responses (van der Kogel, unpublished results). An early moderate increase in the BBB permeability of methotrexate has been reported for

Table 6.3. Effect of chemotherapy on the radiation response of the rat spinal cord

Drug	Route of administration[a]	Relative change in ED_{50}		Reference
		Early w.m.[b]	late vascular[c]	
Actinomycin	i.p.	0	0	VAN DER KOGEL, unpublished
Ara-C	i.v. (low dose)	0	0	VAN DER KOGEL and SISSINGH 1985
	i.p. (high dose)		−20%	MENTEN et al. 1989
	i.t. (low dose)	−30%	−20%	VAN DER KOGEL and SISSINGH 1985
AZQ	i.v.	0		ANG et al. 1986
BCNU	i.v.	0	−10%	VAN DER KOGEL, unpublished
Methotrexate	i.vent.	+10%		GEYER et al. 1988
	i.t.	+10%	+5%	VAN DER KOGEL and SISSINGH 1985
	i.v.	+10%	−20%	
Mitotane	Oral	−40%		GLICKSMAN et al. 1982
Vincristine	i.v.	0	0	VAN DER KOGEL, unpublished

[a] i.p., intraperitoneal; intravenous; i.t., intrathecal; i.vent., intraventricular.
[b] Early w.m.: early delayed white matter necrosis
[c] Late vascular: late delayed vascular injury.
The numbers associated with changes in ED_{50} are maximum values when a range of values is given in the published report.

mouse and rat brain, but only after doses of 20 Gy (GRIFFIN et al. 1977; STORM et al. 1985). Studied in cats, these early changes appeared transitory (REMLER and MARCUSSEN 1981). Late breakdown of the BBB was observed after rat brain irradiation with single doses of 20–60 Gy of heliumions (REMLER et al. 1986). Despite these indications of a BBB breakdown after CNS irradiation, no evidence has been presented to show that this phenomenon occurs after clinically relevant doses of less than 20 Gy.

Chemotherapeutic agents that have been most widely implicated in a modification of the radiation response of the CNS are methotrexate (MTX) and ara-C. As a very effective treatment of CNS localizations of acute lymphoblastic leukemia in children, the combination of CNS irradiation with intrathecal and intravenous MTX and/or ara-C has also led to the frequent observation of leukoencephalopathy and leukomyelopathy. These lesions are similar to the early delayed white matter demyelination and necrosis described in Sect. 6.1 for several animal species. Interestingly, in animal studies only ara-C has been shown to decrease significantly the tolerance of the spinal cord, while MTX may even be slightly protective when administered before irradiation (GEYER et al. 1988; VAN DER KOGEL and SISSINGH 1985). Animal studies designed to evaluate quantitatively the modifying effect of chemotherapy on the radiation tolerance of the CNS have mostly been performed in the rat spinal cord, and a review is given in Table 6.3.

References

Abbatuci JS, Delozier T, Quint R, Roussel A, Brune D (1978) Radiation myelopathy of the cervical spinal cord: time, dose and volume factors. Int J Radiat Oncol Biol Phys 4: 239–248

Ang KK, van der Schueren E, Notter G et al. (1982) Split course multiple daily fractionated radiotherapy schedule combined with misonidazole for the management of grade III and IV gliomas. Int J Radiat Oncol Biol Phys 8: 1657–1664

Ang KK, van der Kogel AJ, van der Schueren E (1983) The effect of small radiation doses on the rat spinal cord: the concept of partial tolerance. Int J Radiat Oncol Biol Phys 9: 1487–1491

Ang KK, van der Kogel AJ, van Dam J, van der Schueren E (1984) The kinetics of repair of sublethal damage in the rat cervical spinal cord during fractionated irradiations. Radiother Oncol 1: 247–253

Ang KK, van der Kogel AJ, van der Schueren E (1985) Lack of evidence for increased tolerance of rat spinal cord with decreasing fraction doses below 2 Gy. Int J Radiat Oncol Biol Phys 11: 105–110

Ang KK, van der Kogel AJ, van der Schueren E (1986) Effect of combined AZQ and radiation on the tolerance of the rat spinal cord. J Neurooncol 3: 349–352

Ang KK, Thames HD Jr, van der Kogel AJ, van der Schueren E (1987) Is the rate of repair of radiation-induced sublethal damage in rat spinal cord dependent on the size of the dose per fraction? Int J Radiat Oncol Biol Phys 13: 552–562

Asbell SO, Kramer S (1971) Oxygen effect on the production of radiation-induced myelitis in rats. Radiology 98: 678–681

Asscher AW, Anson SG (1962) Arterial hypertension and irradiation damage to the nervous system. Lancet 1343–1346

Atkins HL, Tretter P (1966) Time-dose considerations in radiation myelopathy. Acta Radiol 5: 79–93

Barendsen GW (1982) Dose-fractionation, dose-rate and

iso-effect relationships for normal tissue response. Int J Radiat Oncol Biol Phys 8: 1981–1997

Beck ER, LeCouteur RA, Powers BE, Gillette EL (1988) Pathogenesis and prediction of spinal cord irradiation damage. In: Proceedings Annual Meeting Radiation Research Society, Philadelphia, p 130

Berg NO, Lindgren M (1958) Time-dose relationship and morphology of delayed radiation lesions of the brain in rabbits. Acta Radiol [Suppl] 167: 1–118

Berg NO, Lindgren M (1963) Relationship between field size and tolerance of rabbit brain to roentgen irradiation (200 kV) via a slit-shaped field. Acta Radiol 1: 147–168

Blakemore WF, Palmer AC (1982) Delayed infarction of spinal cord white matter following x-irradiation. J Pathol 137: 273–280

Boden G (1948) Radiation myelitis of the cervical spinal cord. Br J Radiol 21: 464–469

Bradley WG, Fewings JD, Cumming WJK, Harrison RM, Faulds AJ (1977) Delayed myeloradiculopathy produced by spinal x-irradiation in the rat. J Neurol Sci 31: 63–82

Calvo W, Hopewell JW, Reinhold HS, van den Berg AP, Yeung TK (1987) Dose-dependent and time-dependent changes in the choroid plexus of the irradiated rat brain. Br J Radiol 60: 1109–1117

Calvo W, Hopewell JW, Reinhold HS, Yeung TK (1988) Time- and dose-related changes in the white matter of the rat brain after single doses of x-rays. Br J Radiol 61: 1043–1052

Carsten A, Zeman W (1966) The control of variables in radiopathological studies on mammalian nervous tissue. Int J Radiat Biol 10: 65–74

Cavanagh JB (1968) Effects of x-irradiation on the proliferation of cells in peripheral nerve during wallerian degeneration in the rat. Br J Radiol 41: 275–281

Cavanagh JB, Hopewell JW (1972) Mitotic activity in the subependymal plate of rats and the long-term consequences of x-irradiation. J Neurol Sci 15: 471–482

Caveness WF (1980) Experimental observations: delayed necrosis in normal monkey brain. In: Gilbert HA, Kagan AR (eds) Radiation damage to the nervous system. Raven, New York, pp 1–38

Cohen L (1982) The tissue volume factor in radiation oncology. Int J Radiat Oncol Biol Phys 8:1771–1774

Cohen L, Creditor M (1981) An iso-effect table for radiation tolerance of the human spinal cord. Int J Radiat Oncol Biol Phys 7: 961–966

Cohen L, Creditor M (1983) Iso-effect tables for tolerance of irradiated normal human tissues. Int J Radiat Oncol Biol Phys 9: 233–241

Coy P, Dolman CL (1971) Radiation myelopathy in relation to oxygen level. Br J Radiol 44: 705–707

Dale RG (1985) The application of the linear-quadratic dose-effect equation to fractionated and protracted radiotherapy. Br J Radiol 58: 515–528

Dische S, Warburton MF, Saunders MI (1988) Radiation myelitis and survival in the radiotherapy of lung cancer. Int J Radiat Oncol Biol Phys 15: 75–81

Douglas BG, Fowler JF (1976) The effect of multiple small doses of x-rays on skin reactions in the mouse and a basic interpretation. Radiat Res 66: 301–316

Fein JM, Di Chiro G (1974) Experimental postirradiation myelopathy. In: Annual Report of the Armed Forces Radiobiology Research Institute, Washington, p 85

Ffrench-Constant C, Raff MC (1986) Proliferating bipotential glial progenitor cells in adult rat optic nerve. Nature 319: 499–502

Fike JR, Cann CE, Turowski K, Higgins RJ, Chan ASL,

Phillips TL, Davis RL (1988) Radiation dose response of normal brain. Int J Radiat Oncol Biol Phys 14: 63–70

Geraci JP, Thrower PD, Jackson KL, Christensen GM, Parker RG, Fox MS (1974) The relative biological effectiveness of fast neutrons for spinal cord injury. Radiat Res 59: 496–503

Geyer JR, Taylor EM, Milstein JM et al. (1988) Radiation, methotrexate, and white matter necrosis: laboratory evidence for neural radioprotection with preirradiation methotrexate. Int J Radiat Oncol Biol Phys 15: 373–375

Glicksman AS, Bliven SF, Leith JT (1982) Modification of radiation damage in rat spinal cord by mitotane. Cancer Treat Rep 66: 1545–1547

Goffinet DR, Marsa GW, Brown JM (1976) The effects of single and multifraction radiation courses on the mouse spinal cord. Radiology 119: 709–713

Griffin TW, Rasey JS, Bleyer WA (1977) The effect of photon irradiation on blood-brain permeability to methotrexate in mice. Cancer 40: 1109–1111

Habermalz HJ (1982) Die Strahlenmyelopathie der Maus; Isoeffektbeziehungen und histologisches Bild nach fraktionierter Bestrahlung. Habilitationsschrift, Berlin, pp 1–62

Habermalz HJ, Valley B, Habermalz E (1987) Radiation myelopathy of the mouse spinal cord – isoeffect correlations after fractionated radiation. Strahlenther Onkol 163: 626–632

Hassler O (1968) Cellular kinetics of the peripheral nerve and striated muscle after a single dose of x-rays. Z Zellforsch 85: 62–66

Hayashi N, Green BA, Gonzalez-Carvajal M, Mora J, Veraa RP (1983) Local blood flow, oxygen tension, and oxygen consumption in the rat spinal cord. J Neurosurg 58: 516–530

Haymaker W (1969) Effects of ionizing radiation on nervous tissue. In: Bourne GH (ed) Structure and function of the nervous system, vol 3. Academic, New York, pp 441–518

Hopewell JW (1979) Late radiation damage to the central nervous system: a radiobiological interpretation. Neuropathol Appl Neurobiol 5: 329–343

Hopewell JW, van der Kogel AJ (1988) Volume effect in spinal cord. Br J Radiol 61: 973–975

Hopewell JW, Wright EA (1970) The nature of latent cerebral irradiation damage and its modification by hypertension. Br J Radiol 43: 161–167

Hopewell JW, Morris AD, Dixon-Brown A (1987) The influence of field size on the late tolerance of the rat spinal cord to single doses of x-rays. Br J Radiol 60: 1099–1108

Hornsey S, White A (1980) Isoeffect curve for radiation myelopathy. Br J Radiol 53: 168–169

Hornsey S, Morris CC, Myers R, White A (1981a) Relative biological effectiveness for damage to the central nervous system by neutrons. Int J Radiat Oncol Biol Phys 7: 185–189

Hornsey S, Morris CC, Myers R (1981b) The relationship between fractionation and total dose for x-ray induced brain damage. Int J Radiat Oncol Biol Phys 7: 393–396

Hornsey S, Myers R, Coultas PG, Rogers MA, White A (1981c) Turnover of proliferative cells in the spinal cord after x-irradiation and its relation to time-dependent repair of radiation damage. Br J Radiol 54: 1081–1085

Hornsey S, Myers R, Warren P (1982) Residual injury in the spinal cord after treatment with x-rays or neutrons. Br J Radiol 55: 516–519

Hubbard BM, Hopewell JW (1980) Quantitative changes in

the cellularity of the rat subependymal plate after x-irradiation. Cell Tissue Kinet 13: 403–413

Innes JRM, Carsten A (1961) Demyelinating or malacic myelopathy. Arch Neurol 4: 190–199

Janzen AH, Warren S (1942) Effect of roentgen rays on the peripheral nerve of the rat. Radiology 38: 333–337

Keyeux A, Ochrymowicz-Bemelmans D, Charlier AA (1987) Early and late effect on the blood brain barrier (BBB) permeability and the antipyrine (AP) distribution volumes in the irradiated rat brain. In: Fielden EM, Fowler JF, Hendry JH, Scott D (eds) Radiation research (Proceedings of the 8th International Congress of Radiation Research), vol 1. Taylor & Francis, London, p 260

Kinsella TJ, Sindelar WF, DeLuca AM et al. (1985) Tolerance of peripheral nerve to intraoperative radiotherapy (IORT): clinical and experimental studies. Int J Radiat Oncol Biol Phys 11: 1579–1585

Kinsella TJ, Sindelar WF, DeLuca AM (1988) Threshold dose for peripheral nerve injury following intraoperative radiotherapy (IORT) in a large animal model Int. J Radiat Oncol Biol Phys 15 [Suppl. I]: p. 205 (abstract)

Knowles JF (1981) The effects of single dose x-irradiation on the guinea-pig spinal cord. Int J Radiat Biol 40: 265–275

Knowles JF (1983) The radiosensitivity of the guinea-pig spinal cord to x-rays: the effect of retreatment at one year and the effect of age at the time of irradiation. Int J Radiat Biol 44: 433–442

LeCouteur RA, Gillette EL, Powers BE, Child G, McChesney SL, Ingram JT (1989) Peripheral neuropathies following experimental intraoperative radiation therapy (IORT). Int J Radiat Oncol Biol Phys 17: 583–590

Leith JT, DeWyngaert JK, Glicksman AS (1981) Radiation myelopathy in the rat: an interpretation of dose effect relationships. Int J Radiat Oncol Biol Phys 7: 1673–1677

Leith JT, Ainsworth EJ, Alpen EL (1983) Heavy-ion radiobiology: normal tissue studies. In: Lett JT Adler H (eds) Advances in radiation biology. Academic, New York, pp 191–236

Mastaglia FL, McDonald WI, Watson JV, Yogendran K (1976) Effects of x-radiation on the spinal cord: an experimental study of the morphological changes in central nerve fibres. Brain 99: 101–122

Masuda K, Reid BO, Withers HR (1977) Dose effect relationship for epilation and late effects on spinal cord in rats exposed to gamma rays. Radiology 122: 239–242

Menten J, Landuyt W, van der Kogel AJ, Ang KK, van der Schueren E (1989) Effects of high dose intraperitoneal cytosine arabinoside on the radiation tolerance of the rat spinal cord. Int J Radiat Oncol Biol Phys 17: 131–134

Myers R, Rogers MA, Hornsey S (1986) A reappraisal of the roles of glial and vascular elements in the development of white matter necrosis in irradiated rat spinal cord. Br J Cancer 53 [Suppl VII]: 221–223

Myers R, Thozer GM, Hornsey S (1987) Microvascular changes in irradiated rat spinal cord. In: Fielden EM, Fowler JF, Hendry JH, Scott D (eds) Radiation research (Proceedings of the 8th International Congress of Radiation Research), vol 1. Taylor & Francis, London, p 266

Pallis CA, Louis S, Morgan RL (1961) Radiation myelopathy. Brain 84: 460–479

Parker RG, Berry HC, Gerdes AJ, Soronen MD, Shaw CM (1976) Fast neutron beam radiotherapy of glioblastoma multiforme. AJR 127: 331–335

Pezner RD, Archambeau JO (1981) Brain tolerance unit: a method to estimate risk of radiation brain injury for various dose schedules. Int J Radiat Oncol Biol Phys 7: 397–402

Phillips TL, Buschke F (1969) Radiation tolerance of the thoracic spinal cord. AJR 105: 659–664

Plotnikova ED, Levitman MK, Shaposhnikova VV, Koshevoj JV, Eidus LK (1988) Protection of microvasculature in rat brain against late radiation injury by gammaphos. Int J Radiat Oncol Biol Phys 15: 1197–1201

Raff MC, Miller RH, Noble M (1983) A glial progenitor cell that develops in vitro into an astrocyte or an oligodendrocyte depending on the culture medium. Nature 303: 390–396

Remler M, Marcussen W (1981) The time course of early delayed blood-brain barrier changes in individual cats after ionizing radiation. Exp Neurol 73: 310–314

Remler MP, Marcussen WH, Tiller-Borsich J (1986) The late effects of radiation on the blood brain barrier. Int J Radiat Oncol Biol Phys 12: 1965–1969

Schultheiss TE, Orton CG, Peck RA (1983) Models in radiotherapy: volume effects. Med Phys 10: 410–415

Schultze B, Korr H (1981) Cell kinetic studies of different cell types in the developing and adult brain of the rat and the mouse: a review. Cell Tissue Kinet 14: 309–325

Shaw CM, Sumi SM, Alvord EC Jr, Gerdes AJ, Spence A, Parker RG (1978) Fast-neutron irradiation of glioblastoma multiforme. J Neurosurg 49: 1–12

Sheline GE, Wara WM, Smith V (1980) Therapeutic irradiation and brain injury. Int J Radiat Oncol Biol Phys 6: 1215–1228

Spence AM, Krohn KA, Edmondson SW, Steele JE, Rasey JS (1986) Radioprotection in rat spinal cord with WR-2721 following cerebral lateral intraventricular injection. Int J Radiat Oncol Biol Phys 12: 1479–1482

Stephens LC, Hussey DH, Raulston GL, Jardine JH, Gray KN, Almond PR (1983) Late effects of 50 MeV$_{d-Be}$ neutron and cobalt-60 irradiation of rhesus monkey cervical spinal cord. Int J Radiat Oncol Biol Phys 9: 859–864

Storm AJ, van der Kogel AJ, Nooter K (1985) Effect of x-irradiation on the pharmacokinetics of methotrexate in rats: alteration of the blood-brain barrier. Eur J Cancer Clin Oncol 21: 759–764

Thames HD, Hendry JH (1987) Fractionation in radiotherapy. Taylor & Francis, London

Thames HD, Ang KK, Stewart FA, van der Schueren E (1988) Does incomplete repair explain the apparent failure of the basic LQ model to predict spinal cord and kidney responses to low doses per fraction? Int J Radiat Biol 54: 13–19

Tiller-Borcich JK, Fike JR, Phillips TL, Davis RL (1987) Pathology of delayed radiation brain damage: an experimental canine model. Radiat Res 110: 161–172

Travis EL, Parkins CS, Holmes SJ, Down JD (1982) Effect of misonidazole on radiation injury to mouse spinal cord. Br J Cancer 45: 469–473

Turesson I, Notter G (1986) Dose-response and dose-latency relationships for human skin after various fractionation schedules. Br J Cancer 53 [Suppl VII]: 67–72

van der Kogel AJ (1977a) Radiation tolerance of the rat spinal cord: time-dose relationships. Radiology 122: 505–509

van der Kogel AJ (1977b) Radiation-induced nerve root degeneration and hypertrophic neuropathy in the lumbosacral spinal cord of rats: the relation with changes in aging rats. Acta Neuropathol (Berl) 39: 139–145

van der Kogel AJ (1979) Late effects of radiation on the spinal cord: dose–effect relationships and pathogenesis.

Publication of the Radiobiological Institute TNO, Rijswijk, The Netherlands

van der Kogel AJ (1980) Mechanisms of late radiation injury in the spinal cord. In: Meyn RE, Withers HR (eds) Radiation biology in cancer research. Raven, New York, pp 461–470

van der Kogel AJ (1983) The cellular basis of radiation induced damage in the CNS. In: Potten CS, Hendry JH (eds) Cytotoxic insult to tissues: effects on cell lineages. Churchill-Livingstone, Edinburgh, pp 329–352

van der Kogel AJ (1985) Chronic effects of neutrons and charged particles on spinal cord, lung, and rectum. Radiat Res 104: S208–S216

van der Kogel AJ (1986) Radiation-induced damage in the central nervous system: an interpretation of target cell responses. Br J Cancer 53: [Suppl VII]: 207–217

van der Kogel AJ (1987) Effect of volume and localization on rat spinal cord tolerance. In: Fielden EM, Fowler JF, Hendry JH, Scott D (eds) Radiation research (Proceedings of the 8th International Congress of Radiation Research), vol 1. Taylor & Francis, London, p 352

van der Kogel AJ, Barendsen GW (1974) Late effects of spinal cord irradiation with 300 KV x-rays and 15 MeV neutrons. Br J Radiol 47: 393–398

van der Kogel AJ, Sissingh HA (1983) Effect of misonidazole on the tolerance of the rat spinal cord to daily and multiple fractions per day of x-rays. Br J Radiol 56: 121–125

van der Kogel AJ, Sissingh HA (1985) Effects of intrathecal methotrexate and cytosine arabinoside on the radiation tolerance of the rat spinal cord. Radiother Oncol 4: 239–251

van der Kogel AJ, Sissingh HA, Zoetelief J (1982) Effect of x-rays and neutrons on repair and regeneration in the rat spinal cord. Int J Radiat Oncol Biol Phys 8: 2095–2097

van der Schueren E, Landuyt W, Ang KK, van der Kogel AJ (1988) From 2 Gy to 1 Gy per fraction: sparing effect in rat spinal cord? Int J Radiat Oncol Biol Phys 14: 297–300

Vogel FS, Pickering JE (1956) Demyelinization induced in the brains of monkeys by means of fast neutrons. J Exp Med 104: 435–449

Wara WM, Phillips TL, Sheline GE, Schwade JG (1975) Radiation tolerance of the spinal cord. Cancer 35: 1558–1562

White A, Hornsey S (1978) Radiation damage to the rat spinal cord: the effect of single and fractionated doses of x-rays. Br J Radiol 51: 515–523

White A, Hornsey S (1980) Time dependent repair of radiation damage in the rat spinal cord after x-rays and neutrons. Eur J Cancer 16: 957–962

Wigg DR, Koschel K, Hodgson GS (1981) Tolerance of the mature human central nervous system to photon irradiation. Br J Radiol 54: 787–798

Wigg DR, Murray RML, Koschel K (1982) Tolerance of the central nervous system to photon irradiation. Endocrine complications. Acta Radiol [Oncol] 21: 49–60

Withers HR, Mason K, Tang Q (1987) Radiation myelopathy. In: Fielden EM, Fowler JF, Hendry JH, Scott D (eds) Radiation research (Proceedings of the 8th International Congress of Radiation Research), vol 1. Taylor & Francis, London, p 236

Withers HR, Taylor JMG, Maciejewski B (1988) Treatment volume and tissue tolerance. Int J Radiat Oncol Biol Phys 14: 751–760

Yaes RJ, Kalend A (1988) Local stem cell depletion model for radiation myelitis. Int J Radiat Oncol Biol Phys 14: 1247–1259

Yoshii Y, Phillips TL (1982) Late vascular effects of whole brain x-irradiation in the mouse. Acta Neurochirur (Wien) 64: 87–102

Zeman W (1966) Oxygen effect and selectivity of radiolesions in the mammalian neuraxis. Acta Radiol [Ther] 5: 204–216

Zeman W, Carsten A, Biondo S (1964) Cytochemistry of delayed radionecrosis of the murine spinal cord. In: Haley TJ, Snider RS (eds) Response of the nervous system to ionizing radiation. Academic, New York, pp 105–126

Zook BC, Bradley EW, Casarett GW, Rogers CC (1980) Pathologic findings in canine brain irradiated with fractionated fast neutrons or photons. Radiat Res 84: 562–578

Zook BC, Bradley EW, Casarett GW, Fisher MP, Rogers CC (1981) The effects of fractionated doses of fast neutrons or photons on the canine cervical spinal cord. Radiat Res 88: 165–179

7 The Central Nervous System: Clinical Aspects

R. Sauer and L. Keilholz

CONTENTS

7.1 Introduction

Radiation damage to the central nervous system (CNS) is a consequence of deliberate therapeutic or accidental irradiation of healthy brain tissue or of the spinal cord. Radiation damage to the CNS became recognized in particular following radiation treatment of brain tumors, head and neck tumors, breast cancer, tumors of the lung, and gynecological malignancies, and after mantle field treatment of malignant lymphomas. A defined latency period between radiation exposure and the occurrence of the clinical symptomatology is typic-

Professor Dr. R. Sauer; Dr. L. Keilholz, Strahlentherapeutische Klinik und Poliklinik der Universität Erlangen-Nürnberg, Universitätsstraße 27, 8520 Erlangen, FRG

al for the various forms of radiation damage to the nervous system (NS).

Our knowledge of the pathophysiology of radiation-induced brain injuries and radiation myelopathy, of tolerance doses, of combination injuries (that is, neurotoxicity involving other noxae), and of the incidence of overall radiation damage of the NS is still incomplete. The sequelae of radiation exposure of the peripheral nerves have hardly been investigated. However, it can be stated that the NS is definitely more sensitive to ionizing radiation than appeared to be the case about 30 years ago.

In 1930, Fischer and Holfelder published the first report on radiation-induced necrosis of the brain. In 1934, Scholz pointed out that the vascular and connective tissue of the CNS can suffer damage that is qualitatively and quantitatively identical to that in other parts of the body, and also that the glial tissue reacts to radiation by producing changes comparable to those seen in connective tissue outside of the CNS. He drew a distinction between two reactions that differed both morphologically and temporally: the early reaction and the delayed reaction. While the former remained clinically silent, the delayed reaction was associated, after a symptom-free interval, with necroses that occurred preferentially in the white matter.

In 1941, Ahlbom first described the clinical symptomatology of radiation myelopathy. It was soon suspected that the tolerance of the spinal cord was less than that of the brain (Boden 1948, 1950; Franke 1963; reviews by Berlit 1987 and van der Schueren 1989).

In 1958, Lindgren made an attempt to establish the tolerance threshold of the brain on the basis of the data regarding 13 patients reported in the literature and four patients of his own with cerebral necrosis, which he entered into a double logarithmic time–dose curve introduced by Strandqvist (1944). He discovered a regression line slope of 0.26 and concluded that a minimum dose of 45–50 Gy in 30 days is capable of producing necrosis.

Since then, reports on damage to the brain and spinal cord have been increasing, and include both individual case reports and group statistics. Reviews of cases reported in the international literature are to be found in BERLIT (1987), FRANKE (1963, 1973), FRANKE and LIERSE (1978), HOLDORFF (1980a, 1980b, 1983), KRAMER and LEE (1974), LINDGREN (1958), SHELINE et al. (1980), and WIGG et al. (1981).

In more recent publications, in particular those by BERLIT (1987), FRANKE (1973), HOLDORFF (1980a), SHELINE et al. (1980), the group headed by VAN DER SCHUEREN (1989), and WIGG et al. (1981), attention has been directed towards investigating the tolerance of the CNS and additional risk factors. It has been emphasized that, apart from the total dose applied, the size of the daily fraction is of considerably greater importance for the development of acute or chronic radiation syndrome than is the duration of the treatment time.

7.2 Definitions

Radiation sequelae are defined as those injuries that occur after a typical latency period as a result of radiotherapy either alone or in combination with other physical or chemical noxae with a deleterious effect on the nervous system. These additional noxae may be operations on the nervous system, systemic or intrathecal chemotherapy, infections, or injuries induced directly by the tumor itself. Accordingly, we differentiate between radiation damage in the strict sense and combination injuries.

In general, radiation sequelae affect the irradiated volume, but they may extend beyond the irradiated region right from the beginning and involve neighboring structures.

It has become the practice to classify radiation sequelae in accordance with neuropathological findings, and to take account of the time course. Thus, a distinction is drawn between early and delayed reactions (SCHOLZ 1934; ZEMAN 1968; LIERSE and FRANKE 1970), the delayed reaction being further subdivided into an early delayed and a late delayed reaction (or late necrosis) (SCHOLZ 1934, BOELLAARD and JACOBY 1962; ZÜLCH 1963; LAMPERT and DAVIS 1964; JELLINGER 1972, 1977).

Table 7.1 shows the typical latency periods and the clinical course of the various radiation injuries to the NS.

7.2.1 Early Reaction (Acute Phase)

The early reaction appears 3–4 h after the radiation insult, or, in the case of fractionated treatment, within the first few days of treatment D. (BERG et al. 1964). If hypofractionated radiotherapy has been administered with a few high individual doses, the reaction may also manifest several days after conclusion of treatment. Neuropathological lesions to be found include intracellular and extracellular edema, inflammatory infiltration, metabolic disturbances affecting the glial cells and the neurons, and sometimes even acute radionecrosis. Depending upon their severity, these conditions may be completely reversible.

Table 7.1. Typical latency periods and clinical course of radiation injuries to the NS

	Latency	Course
1. *Acute reaction*		
Brain	Hours	Reversible within hours
Spinal cord	Hours	Often recognized; transverse lesion
Peripheral nerves	Hours/days	Often unrecognized; completely reversible
2. *Early delayed reaction*		
Brain	2–8 weeks	Reversible within 6–8 weeks
Leukoencephalopathy	2–8 weeks	In part reversible within 6–8 weeks
Hormonal disorders (hypophysial–hypothalamic axis)	9–24 months	Chronic, slow progression. Good prognosis with substitution
Psychomotor deficiency syndrome	Months to years	Progression
Spinal cord (Lhermitte's sign)	1–6 months (median 3–4 months)	Reversible within 1–5 months; chronic form rare
3. *Late delayed reaction* (late radionecrosis) Brain		
Cerebral hemisphere	9 months to 7.5 years	Progression; relatively favorable prognosis
Midline region	1–36 months	Poor prognosis; death within months
Spinal cord	4–25 months	Progression; when tetraplegia or paraplegia, death within 18 months
Peripheral nerves	4 months to 10 years	Progression

7.2.2 Early Delayed Reaction (Subacute Phase)

Several weeks or months after radiation treatment, uncharacteristic, nonlocalizable neurological symptoms may appear. In general, they are of a temporary nature and regress within a matter of weeks. BODEN (1948), DYNES and SMEDAL (1960), JONES (1964), and LAMPERT and DAVIS (1964) distinguished this early delayed reaction from late necrosis. The best-known syndrome is Lhermitte's sign in the region of the cervical and thoracic spinal cord.

Neuropathologically, focal demyelination of the white matter, perivascular lymphocyte and plasma cell infiltrations, vascular endothelial lesions, blood–brain barrier disruption, edema, circumscribed bleeding, and necroses may be observed.

7.2.2.1 Transient Radiation Myelopathy (Lhermitte's sign)

Transient radiation myelopathy (JONES 1964) manifests Clinically as dysesthesias and paresthesias in the region of the shoulder girdle and extremities, in part in the typical form of the sign named after LHERMITTE (1929). The latency period varies between 1 and 6 months (median 3–4 months) and the condition is usually completely reversible within a further 1–2 months. JONES himself interpreted transient radiation myelopathy as a symptom of a temporary demyelination of the sensory neurons. NAGASE et al. (1973) discovered vascular lesions experimentally, and PALMER (1972) detected vascular changes in two patients who died.

7.2.2.2 Leukoencephalopathy

Leukoencephalopathy is presumably a variation of the early delayed reaction (SHELINE et al. 1980). Not until the introduction of computed tomography (CT), with its ability to identify certain subclinical cerebral lesions, did it become possible to differentiate this clinical entity. The radiological signs of this condition are ventricle dilatation, widening of the subarachnoid space, hypodense areas within the brain, and intracerebral calcifications (CROSLEY et al. 1978; ENZMAN and LANE 1978; PEYLAN-RAMU et al. 1978; further literature is cited by HABERMALZ et al. 1983). Clinically,

these changes may be asymptomatic or associated with severe neurological deficits.

Neuropathologically, the findings range from noninflammatory microangiopathy with adjacent necroses and microcalcifications, through glial loss and demyelination, to severe necrotizing leukoencephalopathy with confluent demyelinated necroses within the white matter and glial and axonal degeneration (RUBINSTEIN et al. 1975; PRICE 1979).

7.2.3 Late Delayed Reaction (Late Necrosis)

The most serious of the radiation injuries to the CNS is late necrosis. This appears suddenly several months to years after conclusion of treatment, is usually irreversible, is regularly progressive, and has a very poor prognosis. The white matter is particularly affected.

HOLDORFF (1980a, 1983) pointed out that late radiation necroses in the cerebral hemispheres differ in morphology and have a higher tolerance threshold, a longer latency period, and a more favorable course – and thus prognosis – than those affecting the midline structures (optic chiasm, hypothalamus, brain stem). And so the prognosis quoad vitam of patients with hypothalamic and brain stem necroses depends less upon the radiation dose than on the vital function of the affected midline structure.

Pathogenetically, vascular injuries predominate. In addition, the glial cells reveal a direct radiation reaction, and immunological changes occur. Owing to the edema accompanying it, late necrosis presents as a space-occupying lesion (Fig. 7.1) and is often indistinguishable from a primary or recurrent tumor (SCHOLZ and HSÜ 1938; BOELLAARD and JACOBY 1962; ZÜLCH 1963; ZEMAN 1968; EYSTER et al. 1974; ZEMAN and SHIDNIA 1976; SHELINE et al. 1980).

It would appear that the early reaction, the early delayed reaction, and the late delayed reaction follow the same course throughout the CNS, although local peculiarities do occur (GODWIN-AUSTEN et al. 1975). These specific features comprise a locally varying vascular supply, differences in the development and extent of glial or fibrous scars, and the fact that the sensory pathways of the spinal cord and the pyramidal tract are particularly sensitive to radiation (PALLIS et al. 1961; FRANKE and LIERSE 1978). We do not doubt that early and delayed reactions also occur in the

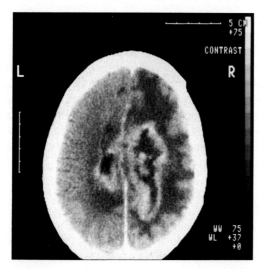

Fig. 7.1. Late necrosis in the right temporal lobe also involving the left hemisphere. The annular structures store contrast medium. Marked perifocal brain edema. Differentiation between tumor or recurrent tumor and late radionecrosis is not possible on the basis of the CT scan alone

peripheral nerves, but this situation has hardly been investigated. The lesions give rise to clinical symptoms far less frequently than has been assumed (Spiess 1970). The signs of acute reaction in particular often remain unnoticed by the patient and are submerged by the general spectrum of the other (e.g., respiratory or gastrointestinal) acute radiation reactions. As far as can be ascertained, reports in the literature deal merely with roentgenological delayed reactions in the peripheral nerves.

7.3 Incidence

7.3.1 Introductory Remarks

On the basis of the cases of late radiation necrosis reported in the international literature, it is possible to establish the necrosis doses for the brain and the spinal cord, that is, the lowest doses at which delayed reactions can occur in the brain and/or spinal cord (Berlit 1987; Boden 1948, 1950; Lindgren 1958; Pallis et al. 1961; Franke 1963; Maier et al. 1969; Jellinger and Sturm 1971; Sheline et al. 1980; Wigg et al. 1981; and others). It is not, however, possible to find unequivocal information on the incidence of early or delayed radiation reactions, either for a defined

dose range or for a defined fractionation or radiation quality. Reasons for this are as follows:

1. Most reports in the international literature are anecdotal. Usually, such important radiotherapeutic details as maximum dose in the target volume, tumor dose or maximum dose per fraction, location of the maximum dose, irradiated volume, arrangement of fields, radiation quality, and dose rate are lacking; moreover, no details are offered on the extent and nature of acute reactions. Thus, no conclusions can be drawn about the quality or appropriateness of a particular radiation treatment with fatal delayed complications.

2. Almost without exception, authors indicate the incidence of brain necrosis or radiation myelopathy without consideration of the minimum survival rate. According to Holdorff (1980b), the median latency period for brain necrosis varies between 12 and 36 months, depending upon the localization; Franke (1973) quoted 18 months for the spinal cord (some of the patients, however, were followed up for only 9 months). This means that many of the patients treated with injury-inducing radiation doses die before such radiation damage can develop. Were the patients to survive longer, such damage might in fact occur.

3. Only rarely are autopsies performed on brain tumor patients. Detailed investigations of the brain are carried out in only a very small percentage of the total number of cases. In general, however, unequivocal differential diagnosis between recurrent tumor and radiation necrosis is possible only on the basis of a postmortem examination (most important differential diagnosis: tumor progression).

4. The total number of patients in whom the brain or spinal cord was irradiated is unknown.

5. Patients receiving radiotherapy are lost to proper follow-up for a wide range of reasons. Follow-up observations are frequently incomplete and, with respect to possible radiation side-effects, incompetent. In many cases the radiotherapist is not granted the right to follow up his patients.

6. Radiation-induced complications are associated with a therapeutic accident in the mind not only of the layman but also of the radiotherapist. Although this might sometimes actually be the case, such an assumption must not be generalized to the point where side-effects of radiation are considered to represent maltreat-

ment. Even when radiation treatment is carried out extremely conscientiously, delayed complications cannot always be excluded. In this connection, it would be justified to assume that there is a not inconsiderable number of radiation injuries to the nervous system that do not come to light. ZÜLCH (1963) reported that a number of tumors of the brain, such as oligodendroglioma, spongioblastoma, glioblastoma multiforme, and various types of sarcoma, cannot be treated with curative intent without risking local necrosis. But this, of necessity, also results in damage to the surrounding brain tissue.

7.3.2 Incidence of Radiation Injuries to the Brain

From among the reports that provide information on the incidence of brain necroses as a function of total dose, treatment time, or number of fractions, we will first consider the patients reported by BODEN (1950): of 24 patients, six (25%) developed necrosis of the brain stem after prior treatment comprising small-volume irradiation of

nasopharyngeal or middleear tumors under orthovoltage conditions. The dose was 4940–5500 R applied in 13 fractions on 17 days, the dose per fraction thus being 380–425 R SHELINE et al. (1980) calculated BODEN's data in terms of MRE (megavoltage rad equivalent). According to their calculations, the dose, translated into present-day megavoltage therapy, was 5300–6540 MRE, the dose per fraction being 408–503 MRE. The NSD (nominal standard dose) according to ELLIS (1969) was 2100–2600 ret, or 1450–1780 neuret (SHELINE et al. 1980; see section FI). Table 7.2 presents a comparison of the NSD values and total doses in Gy with fractions of 1.5–2 Gy, as commonly employed today.

In 8 of 139 patients (5%) with a primary brain or hypophyseal tumor who had been treated with at least 45 Gy in daily single fractions of 1.8–2 Gy, MARKS et al. (1981) detected brain necrosis at autopsy performed after an interval of 6–55 months (median 15 months) postirradiation. Two additional cases with relevant clinical suspicion of brain necrosis were not verified by autopsy (total incidence: 10/139 = 7%). All ten patients had received a tumor dose in excess of 50 Gy (54–67.5

Table 7.2. Comparison of doses for various doses per fraction and fractions per week. The tolerance thresholds in ret[a] do not correspond with those in neuret[b]

Fractions per week		10	5	5	5	5	4	5	4
Dose per fraction (Gy)		1.2	1.5	1.8	2.0	2.5	3.0	3.0	3.5
Total dose	NSD (ret)[a] / NSD (neuret)[b]								
30 Gy		1,010	1,010	1,070	1,110	1,170	1,250	1,280	1,310a
		610	660	720	760	830	910	920	980b
35 Gy		1,110	1,110	1,190	1,230	1,300	1,380	1,410	1,450a
		660	710	780	820	900	990	1,000	1,060b
40 Gy		1,220	1,220	1,300	1,340	1,420	1,510	1,540	1,590a
		710	760	830	870	960	1,050	1,070	1,140b
45 Gy		1,310	1,310	1,400	1,450	1,530	1,630	1,670	1,720a
		750	800	880	930	1,020	1,120	1,130	1,210b
50 Gy		1,410	1,410	1,500	1,560	1,640	1,750	1,790	1,840a
		790	850	930	980	1,080	1,180	1,200	1,270b
55 Gy		1,500	1,500	1,600	1,660	1,740	1,860	1,900	1,960a
		830	890	970	1,030	1,130	1,240	1,250	1,340b
60 Gy		1,580	1,590	1,690	1,750	1,850	1,970	2,020	2,070a
		870	930	1,020	1,070	1,180	1,290	1,310	1,400b
65 Gy		1,670	1,670	1,780	1,850	1,950	2,070	2,120	2,190a
		900	970	1,060	1,120	1,230	1,350	1,360	1,450b

[a] NSD (ret) $= D \times N^{0.24} \times T^{-0.11}$.
[b] NSD (neuret) $= D \times N^{-0.44} \times T^{-0.06}$.
dashed lines $\triangleq$ tolerance threshold for doses in neuret[b]
unbroken lines $\triangleq$ tolerance threshold for doses in ret[a]

Gy) applied with a telecobalt machine. On each day of treatment only one field was irradiated. Thus, the daily maximum dose was at least 30%–35% above the indicated tumor dose of 1.8–2 Gy. One patient had received systemic BCNU treatment. The authors concluded that after ≤50 Gy/25 fractions/35 days, or ≤54 Gy/30 fractions/32 days, no radiation-induced brain damage would occur.

On the basis of a collection of published cases, Sheline et al. (1980) established a presumptive incidence for the occurrence of brain necrosis after radiation treatment of pituitary adenomas and craniopharyngiomas. They assumed that the 20 cases of brain necrosis they collected arose in a total of 5000 treated patients. They believed, however, that 5000 patients was probably a conservative estimate, since by 1978 in the University of California and the Thomas Jefferson Medical Center alone, some 1000 patients with adenomas of the pituitary had been treated without any delayed reaction occurring. Assuming that all the cases of necrosis in this pool of patients, had been reported, the incidence would be 0.4%.

Recently, more attention has been paid to the neurological functions in patients with small cell lung cancer (SCLC) who have received prophylactic brain irradiation. It was found that in 60%–70% of the long-term survivors (≥18 months), moderate to severe neurological problems or abnormalities could be seen in CT scans when, in addition to systemic chemotherapy, they had received 10 × 3 Gy whole-brain irradiation (Table 7.3).

7.3.3 Incidence of Radiation-Induced Myelopathy

According to Franke and Lierse (1978), the reported figures for radiation-induced myelitis vary between 3.3% and 14%, assuming that the spinal cord was actually within the volume irradiated.

Ahlbom (1941) reported an incidence of 2% (4/235 cases), as did Greenfield and Stark (1948) (3/180 cases). On the basis of the data provided by Dynes and Smedal (1960), an incidence of 1.25% (10/800) may be assumed. These authors had not, however, included acute and transient myelopathies. According to the review of the literature by Berlit (1987), the incidence of

Table 7.3. Risk of leukoencephalopathy induced by prophylactic brain irradiation in patients with SCLC

Dose/ fractionation	Chemotherapeutic regimen	Clinical No.	Clinical %	CT No.	CT %	References
10 × 3 Gy 10 × 2 Gy	MTX	0/16	0	8/13	70	Catane et al. (1981)
8 × 3 Gy	CCNU/MTX/VCR	–	–	4/8	50	Ellison et al. (1982)
10 × 3 Gy	CAV/VP-16	–	–	4/6	65	Craig et al. (1984)
15 × 2.4 Gy 12 × 3.0 Gy 10 × 3.5 Gy	CAV/ nitrosourea	– –	– –	8/18	44	Looper et al. (1984)
10 × 3 Gy	various	3/49	10	11/11	100	Chak et al. (1986)
10 × 3 Gy	various	3/20	12	14/20	70	Lee et al. (1986)
10 × 3 Gy	various	8/33	24	–	–	Lee et al. (1988)
10 × 3 Gy	None	6/12	50	11/12	82	Laukkanen et al. (1988)

radiation-induced myelopathy is between <1% and 10%, if no consideration is given to the survival time. With a minimum follow-up period of 1 year, the incidence rate increases to 2%–13%. The longer the minimum survival, the more likely it is that the patient will experience radiation-induced myelopathy. Thus, in the group of patients reported by REINHOLD et al. (1976), the incidence of thoracic myelopathies increased from 6.2% (19/307 patients) to 44.2% after 3 years, when account is taken of the fact that only 43 of the 307 irradiated patients survived for 30 months.

As BERLIT (1987) noted, the number of published cases of radiation myelopathy has increased considerably over the last four decades (Table 7.4). This may be due to the fact that attention was first drawn to this lesion by AHLBOM's publication in 1941. Further contributory factors are the increasing number of irradiated patients, the overall higher radiation doses now being applied, and, of course, the increase in the number of reports published by clinicians. In opposition to this we have the fact that even in the large university hospitals in Germany and Austria, very few radiation-induced myelopathies have been diagnosed over the last few years – an indication that radiation myelopathy is a very rare lesion (result of discussions at the Annual Meeting of the German Society for Vertebral Column Research, Bad Homburg, 4 December 1988).

In a carefully analyzed survey, DISCHE et al. (1988) investigated the incidence of radiation myelitis in 754 patients with carcinoma of the bronchus treated by radiotherapy. Radiomyelitis was found in 13 of 121 patients who received a spinal cord dose of >33.5 Gy given in six fractions over 17–18 days. The incidence was positively related to the hemoglobin concentration, but not to the blood pressure at the time of radiotherapy.

The cervical spinal cord is at particular risk in radiation therapy of tumors of the head and neck. This is followed by the thoracic cord, which is exposed during the treatment of bronchial, esophageal, and mediastinal tumors. The lowest incidence rate is reported to be 0.15%–1.5% following radiation treatment of Hodgkin's disease (BERLIT 1987).

In 1100 patients treated for head and neck tumors (median survival, 22 months) between January 1978 and December 1987, we ourselves did not observe a single case of cervical radiation myelopathy. In these patients, the entire cervical spinal cord was exposed to a dose of 43–48 Gy. After 40 Gy delivered at daily fractions of 2 Gy each, the fields were reduced and the spinal cord was only exposed to scatter irradiation and some direct contribution from the electron irradiation of the dorsal lymphatics; as the target dose increased to about 60 Gy, the spinal cord dose increased in 0.6 Gy fractions to 46 Gy.

In 180 patients with malignant lymphomas, we observed no chronic progressive radiation myelopathy after a median follow-up period of 60 months. Here, the entire thoracic spinal cord received a total dose of 32–34 Gy over a period of 4–5 weeks – in the first 2 weeks with fractions of 2 Gy, then in the second 2–3 weeks with fractions of 1.2 Gy. The cervical spinal cord of these patients received 26–30 Gy in daily fractions of 1.3–1.4 Gy. These data contrast with those of BERLIT (1987), who reported 12 patients (out of a total of 43) with radiation myelopathy after ≤42 Gy (in fractions of 1.4–2.0 Gy).

Finally, it is to be hoped that the work of cooperating groups in treatment studies will throw more light on the effects and side-effects of radiation treatment, and thus enable the incidence of radiation injuries to the CNS to be estimated with a greater degree of reliability.

7.4 Clinical Aspects of Radiation Damage to the Nervous System

7.4.1 Brain

The patient's complaints depend on both the extent and localization of the lesion and the phase of the radiation reaction.

7.4.1.1 Acute Reaction

In the acute phase, the tumor-associated symptoms usually decline. Uncharacteristic headaches

Table 7.4. Published cases of radiation-induced myelopathy over four decades (BERLIT 1987)

	Diagnosis established clinically (no. of patients)	Diagnosis verified by autopsy (no. of patients)
1941–1950	17	7
1951–1960	47	13
1961–1970	165	41
1971–1980	255	69

and signs of increased intracranial pressure are to be found. Somnolence, nausea, and vomiting, in contrast, are relatively rare. These symptoms may completely disappear.

It was once thought that individual doses of 2 Gy and more at the start of radiotherapy would lead to brain edema. For this reason, various institutions initiated treatment with single doses of approximately 0.5 Gy, and increased the dose daily until, after about a week, the planned individual dose had been reached. This way of proceeding is unfounded, as KRAMER et al. (1968) pointed out. In 1976, SALAZAR et al. reported that 70–80 Gy in daily fractions of 2 Gy can be applied to the whole brain without any early complications. We recommend supportive treatment with corticoids only when, with palliative intent, doses of > 2 Gy/fraction are administered to the whole brain, or in cases with marked edema of the brain tissue around the tumor.

7.4.1.2 Early Delayed Reaction

We observe this clinical picture

– After local irradiation of a brain tumor with a high, sometimes necrotizing radiation dose
– After whole-brain irradiation with a moderate radiation dose, for example, after prophylactic or therapeutic treatment for cerebral metastasis
– After low-dose irradiation of the whole brain in children to treat malignant lymphoma or acute lymphatic leukemia

The usual symptoms seen are lethargy and somnolence, sometimes augmenting the tumor-induced symptomatology. In addition nausea, vomiting, ataxia, dysphagia, horizontal nystagmus, joint pain, and a positive Romberg sign may be seen (RIDER 1963).

Early delayed reaction is rarely fatal. In general, the symptoms improve after 4 weeks and have disappeared after a further 6–8 weeks (Table 7.1). Specific treatment is not required, nor is it possible. Nevertheless, improvement can be accelerated by administering corticoids. Knowledge of these radiation reactions is very important, since neurological deficits appearing several weeks after conclusion of radiotherapy must be interpreted with caution: they need not necessarily be taken as indicative of recurrent disease, and a wait-and-see attitude should be adopted or, in some cases, a CT or an NMR investigation carried out, before treatment is changed or intensified.

As long ago as 1929, DRUCKMANN reported that 6–8 weeks after treatment, 3% of children receiving whole-brain irradiation developed marked somnolence, which persisted for 14 days. During the first 10 weeks after treatment of benign gliomas, meningiomas, and pituitary adenomas, BOLDREY and SHELINE (1967) found a number of unspecific CNS symptoms which could not be explained by the tumor itself. These tumors were most prominent in the 2nd posttreatment month and disappeared again within the following 6 weeks.

HOFFMAN et al. (1979) reported surprising findings in 51 patients with malignant gliomas. The patients had received radiotherapy with 50 Gy/6–7 weeks to the whole brain, and, in addition, a small-volume boost of 10 Gy, with subsequent BCNU treatment. Every 8 weeks they were submitted to neurological examinations. brain scintigraphy, and computed tomography, Within the first 18 weeks following radiotherapy, 25 patients deteriorated (49%), with signs of tumor progression. Seven of these (28%) improved again, however, without any form of treatment. The latency period of these transient posttherapeutic disturbances corresponds to the turnover time for myelin. The authors therefore concluded that demyelination might have been the reason for this complication of radiotherapy.

In 1973, FREEMAN et al. described a temporary somnolence accompanied by lethargy 24–56 days after prophylactic whole-brain irradiation in 28 children with acute lymphatic leukemia. The condition was mild in 39% of the cases, more marked in a further 39%, and persisted for a total of 10–38 days. The children had received whole-brain irradiation with 24 Gy/4 weeks; 21 received intrathecal methotrexate in addition, and seven irradiation of the entire spinal cord. PARKER et al. (1978) also published a prospective study of 27 children who had received 24 Gy applied to the whole brain. In 63% of these cases, the authors found a temporary somnolence syndrome; 24 of the 27 children had received intrathecal methotrexate.

Leukoencephalopathy

On the basis of our present knowledge, we would classify the cases reported by FREEMAN et al. (1973) and PARKER et al. (1978) as leukoencephalopathy, that is, a particular variety of the early delayed reaction(SHELINE et al. 1980). While the somnolence syndrome is of a temporary nature, appreciable intellectual deficits may remain, the causes of which are probably confluent demyelinating necroses and glial and axonal degeneration.

Leukoencephalopathy in Patients with Small Cell Lung Cancer After Prophylactic Cranial Irradiation

Prophylactic cranial irradiation (PCI) reduces the incidence of CNS metastases in patients with SCLC develop in 20% (all patients) to 50% (2-year survivors) CNS metastasis inspite of various chemotherapeutic procedures. Prophylactic cranial irradiation (PCI) reduces this to less than 10%. Although various randomized trials have failed to show that this effect is associated with an improvement in patient survival, PCI is routinely employed in patients who enter into complete remission on initial chemotherapy. In practical terms, therefore, PCI represents prophylactic palliation aimed at preventing overt symptoms and signs of brain metastases.

Unfortunately, a number of studies have now shown that the incidence of clinical signs of leukoencephalopathy, or findings in the CT scan or NMR image that are typical of leukoencephalopathy, is high in long-term survivors when, in addition to chemotherapy, PCI employing 8–11 fractions of 3 Gy (24–33 Gy total dose) is performed sequentially or simultaneously (Table 7.3). In 12 patients who survived for at least 2 years following PCI, LAUKKANEN et al. (1988) performed a comprehensive evaluation with respect to neuropsychological and neuroanatomical defects. CT scans revealed brain atrophy in all cases, with mild progression in those having a pretreatment baseline. Periventricular and subcortical lowdensity lesions identical with the CT signs of subcortical arteriosclerotic encephalopathy were observed in 9 of 11 cases (82%), while lacunar infarcts were seen in 6 of 11 cases (54%). Similar CT findings were reported by CRAIG et al. in 1984. None of the patients had a positive clinical dementia score, and all were capable of self-care. Half of the patients had at least one neurological abnormality attributable to the treatment, for the most part recent memory loss, subtle gait changes, and/or coordination deficits. Intellectual functioning, according to the Wechsler Adult Intelligence Scale, was of the 38th percentile. Neuropsychological performance gradings were borderline in 3 of 12 cases, and definitely impaired in seven.

In earlier studies, Cox et al. (1980) were unable to detect any clinical neurotoxic sequelae in 40 patients who had received 30–40 Gy (mainly conventional fractionation) for CNS metastases of SCLC. And although LEE et al. (1986) detected one or more CT abnormality (namely ventricular dilatation, periventricular white matter hypodensity, or parenchymal calcification) in 14 of 20 patients (70%), only 3 of 24 (12%) had neurological deficits. Likewise, LICCIARDELLO et al. (1985) observed clinical signs of neurotoxicity in only 2 of 15 long-term survivors (13%). Finally, CATANE et al. (1981) reported few or no neurological sequelae after PCI with 20–30 Gy; CT changes, however, were observed in 9 of 13 patients (70%). In a later report, LEE et al. (1988) subsequently did find more pronounced, clinically evident NS neurotoxicity in 8 of 33 cases (24%), after 10 × 3 Gy PCI. Seven of 17 patients had moderate/severe impairment in neuropsychological performance (visual–spatial processing, concentration/attention/planning ability, verbal memory), and another six showed mild impairment. In addition, neuropsychological performance impairment was discovered in six of ten patients who had no clinical evidence of neurotoxicity following PCI. JOHNSON et al. (1985) also found some degree of mental status abnormality in 9 of 15 patients.

The neurotoxic sequelae are due not only to PCI alone. JOHNSON et al. (1985), LEE et al. (1986), and FRYTAK et al. (1987) demonstrated a correlation of the severity of the neurological findings with concurrent high dose chemotherapy. Suspicion is attached to the substances methotrexate, procarbazine, etoposide, vincristine, cisplatin, and CCNU (see also Sect. 7.6.3).

In order to avoid, or at least diminish, radiation sequelae after PCI in SCLC, the following measures would appear to be indicated:

1. Deferment of PCI until after systemic chemotherapy has been completed
2. No intrathecal administration of MTX when PCI has been planned
3. Return to more conventional fractionation for elective brain irradiation, which means fractions of ≤2 Gy

Leukoencephalopathy Following Whole-Brain Irradiation in Children

The intellectual deficits occurring as late reactions to radiotherapy, which were described in the American literature in the 1970s in whole-brain irradiated children (Bamford et al. 1976; Hirsch et al. 1978, 1979; Eiser 1981; Kun et al. 1983; further literature cited in Harten et al. 1984), are difficult to establish since they are largely dependent on subjective criteria. Since most of the patients had no primary CNS involvement, and had received cranial irradiation as part of various prophylactic protocols, the effects of the treatment could be readily differentiated from tumor-induced effects. A significantly reduced intellectual performance was observed in children who had received whole-brain irradiation.

These early studies did not stand up to a critical analysis. Walther and Gutjahr (1982) established that radiation treatment of acute lymphatic leukemia (ALL) in childhood has an injurious effect on the basal psychomotor processes rather than on cognitive performance.

Harten et al. (1984) investigated 51 children who had been treated with chemotherapy and whole-brain irradiation for ALL, and who were in continuing complete remission. They compared the neurological findings with those observed in 30 children undergoing treatment for other malignant lesions. The latter had received neither CNS irradiation nor a course of methotrexate. Therapy-associated decreases in intellectual functions were not found in either of the two groups. Defects that did present were associated with previous neurological changes or with the developmental status before the disease was diagnosed. Discrete pyschomotor dysfunctions were, however, observed as a generalized slowing down. In this examination, younger children showed better results than older children, which, at least in this group, lends no support to the hypothesis that the developing brain is more vulnerable. The investigations performed by Soni et al. (1975) point in the same direction.

Whole-brain irradiation with a dose of 40–60 Gy in children does, however, lead to unequivocal functional deficiencies in long-term survivors (literature cited by Sheline et al. 1980). In 13 of 30 (43%) patients irradiated in childhood, Li et al. (1984) detected moderate to severe disorders after 5–47 years (median, 18 years). The most marked defects were to be seen in those patients who had had large, inoperable, or particularly aggressive tumors. These patients had been selected for radiation therapy, that is, they represented a negative selection. Sheline et al. (1980) cited a number of publications that reported virtually identical observations: patients with neurological

injuries prior to irradiation (due to the direct influence of the tumor or elevated intracranial pressure) show an impairment of their intellectual performance following treatment, too.

Dysfunction of the Pituitary Gland and Hypothalamus

Radiation-induced dysfunction of the hypophysial–hypothalamic system is observed following irradiation of pituitary adenomas, craniopharyngiomas, and tumors of the epipharynx, eyes, or inner ear (Buchfelder 1984; Eastman et al. 1979; Goldfine and Lawrence 1972; Richards et al. 1976; Samaan et al. 1975; Shalet et al. 1979; Sheline 1981). Although the incidence of these dysfunctions is unknown, it is certainly higher than previously considered by some clinicians. Earlier reports on a low incidence of radiation-induced hypopituitarism are not conclusive, since no adequately sensitive hormone assays have been available for investigating the hypophysial–hypothalamic system. The hormonal deficits often remain subclinical, that is, they produce no symptoms and thus are not revealed by the general clinical examination. Functional disorders present prior to radiotherapy (RT) must be distinguished from those induced by irradiation. In 65 patients who had received 40–85 Gy for treatment of malignant tumors of the nasopharynx, the paranasal sinuses, or the orbits, Samaan et al. (1975) found that between 3 and 20 years after RT the hormonal parameters revealed functional impairment of the hypothalamus in 54 patients and primary hypopituitarism in 25.

Growth hormone (HGH) production is most sensitive to radiation. Depending upon the dose, the HGH deficit appears after a latency period of between 6 and 48 months. The relevant nuclei (ventromedial and posterior) are located within the posterior hypothalamic area. They may be damaged by the expanding walls of the third ventricle, as well as by obstructive hydrocephalus or by infiltrating tumor. Low HGH values were found after insulin stimulation following RT with 25–29 Gy (Shalet 1982) and after arginine or L-dopa loading (Richards et al. 1976).

The thyroid axis is only a little less sensitive, and has been investigated predominantly in children (e.g., Richards et al. 1976; Duffner et al. 1985). Here, the latency period is greater than 9 months, and damage has been described after whole-brain irradiation with only 20–30 Gy.

Either the thyroid gland was within the irradiated field, or the pituitary gland or the hypothalamus was directly injured by radiation. Thus, primary, secondary, or tertiary hypothyroidism might result: either the T_3/T_4 values are reduced with simultaneous TSH evaluation, or the plasma levels of TSH and TRH are reduced. EASTMAN et al. (1979) investigated the function of the thyroid and adrenal axis in 47 patients with acromegaly. Following the application of 40–50 Gy, the incidence of hypopituitarism increased from 9% before RT to 19% after 10 years, while that of hypoadrenalism rose from 6% prior to RT to 30% at 5 years and 39% at 10 years.

Damage to the adrenal or gonadal axis (lack of ACTH, FSH, LH or LRH) after cranial RT is more often found in adults and adolescents than in children (ANDLER et al. 1982; COHEN and DUFFNER 1984; RICHARDS et al. 1976). In our own selective series of very large tumors (BUCHFELDER 1984), the incidence of hypopituitarism was already high even before RT (67/75 patients). In all hormonal deficiences, the number of patients requiring hormonal substitution increased with increasing observation time: hydrocortisone – 55 patients prior to and 57 patients after RT; thyroxine – 49 patients prior to and 57 after RT; sex hormones – 27 patients prior to and 38 patients after RT. Since the incidence of diabetes insipidus did not increase, it may be concluded that the posterior lobe

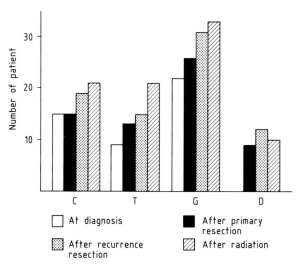

Fig. 7.2. Hormonal function in patients with pituitary adenomas at diagnosis, after primary resection, after resection of recurrent disease, and after postoperative radiation. *C*, corticotropic axis; *T*, thyrotropic axis; *G* gonadotropic axis; *D*, diabetes insipidus. (RAUHUT et al. 1986)

of the pituitary gland is less radiosensitive than the anterior lobe. Our data correspond with those reported by RAUHUT et al. (1986). In 42 patients with pituitary giant adenomas, the hypophyseal axis functions were determined by regular hormone analysis (Fig. 7.2). The thyrotropic axis was particularly subject to disturbances. At the time of the diagnosis, 15 patients had adrenal, 9 thyroid, and 22 gonadal axis disorders. Following primary adenoma resection, the hormonal function deteriorated slightly, and after the development of recurrent disease, more markedly. The situation worsened further after postoperative RT.

In conclusion, the impairment of the pituitary gland and hypothalamus by RT should be taken into account, and the hypothalamic region protected whenever possible. However, in view of the ease of hormone substitution, a small increase in the frequency and severity of anterior lobe insufficiency following RT of pituitary adenomas should not be advanced as an argument against postoperative RT when the latter is indicated.

7.4.1.3 Late Delayed Reaction

Late delayed reaction, usually radionecrosis, manifests clinically as a space-occupying lesion. On the CT scan and the NMR image, it usually cannot be distinguished from a primary or a recurrent tumor (SCHOLZ and HSÜ 1938; BOELLAARD and JACOBY 1962; ZÜLCH 1963; BERG et al. 1964; EYSTER et al. 1974; ZEMAN 1968; BURGER et al. 1979; HOLDORFF 1980b; OSTERTAG et al. 1981). Space-occupying necroses may subsequently shrink, even without operation, and revert to an atrophic state, either within the process of generalized brain atrophy (WILSON et al. 1972) or as a hypodensity usually located in the cerebral medulla (MIKHAEL 1980). A glialatrophic scar may also develop rapidly (HOLDORFF 1983). More frequently, however, progression of the symptomatology due to progressive perifocal edema is observed.

In the event of involvement of the cerebral hemispheres, local or generalized headache, signs of elevated intracranial pressure, epileptic seizures, and transient or permanent pareses are typical symptoms; more rarely, sensory deficits, aphasia, and defects of the visual field occur. According to HOLDORFF (1980b), the median latency period is 3 years (9 months to 7.5 years). It is short when irradiation is applied at high dose fractions. The prognosis is relatively favorable when the necrosis can be removed surgically from the hemisphere (Edwards and Wilson 1980).

If the necrosis has a frontobasal location, gustatory and psychomotor deficits occur, with acoustic and olfactory hallucinations and possibly also an organic psychosyndrome. The latency period is 4–42 months, with a median of 19.5 months (Shukovsky and Fletcher 1972; Holdorff 1980b).

Radiation necroses in the midline region can affect the optic chiasm, the hypothalamus, and the upper and lower brain stem. Rarely, occlusion of the major arteries, such as the internal carotid and the middle cerebral artery, may occur, The symptomatology is correspondingly variable: disturbances of vision and the visual field, endocrine deficits, psychosyndrome, epileptic seizures, signs of elevated intracranial pressure, cranial nerve deficits, a crossed sensory and motor hemiplegia symptomatology, disturbances of consciousness, ets. (for a review of the literature, see Holdorff 1980b). The latency period is 1–36 months, with a median of 12 months (Holdorff 1980b). The prognosis is poor; patients with brain stem lesions die within a few months.

7.4.2 Spinal Cord

7.4.2.1 Acute Reaction (Acute Radiomyelopathy)

The acute reaction has been described only in animal experiments (Schümmelfelder 1959); in man it has been largely ignored. The situation is different, however, in cases of an extraspinal or intraspinal space-occupying lesion that gives rise to incomplete paraplegia or threatens to do so. Under these circumstances the first fraction of radiotherapy initiated on an emergency basis may trigger a transverse lesion or complete it. The underlying cause is acute radiation edema. The latency period is only a few hours, and the condition is reversible. Therefore, in such cases radiation treatment should be carried out only after surgical decompression (laminectomy) and/ or under cortisone protection.

7.4.2.2 Early Delayed Reaction (Transitory Radiomyelopathy)

Transitory myelopathy (Jones 1964) manifests as dysesthesia and paresthesia affecting the shoulder

girdle and extremities, described as Lhermitte's sign (1929). This occurs in particular following irradiation of large sections of the spinal cord, and especially after mantle field or total nodal irradiation of malignant lymphomas. Subacute radiation myelopathy (early delayed reaction) is also observed following total CNS irradiation for medulloblastomas or ependymomas, and sometimes even after therapeutic irradiation of leukemic infiltrations of the meninges.

Jones interpreted the transient myelopathy as a sign of temporary demyelination of the sensory neurons. Nagase et al. (1973) observed lesions of the vascular walls, as did Palmer (1972), who reported vascular changes in the irradiated area in two deceased patients.

Lhermitte's sign is, characteristically, induced in the recumbent patient by flexion of the cervical spine or by having the patient lift his straight legs, that is, by longitudinal stretching of the cord or by applying tension to the spinal nerves. The latency is 1–6 months (medium 3–4 months). Usually, the symptoms regress after 1–5 months. Rarely, subacute radiation myelopathy may progress into late delayed necrosis. These clinical observations mirror experimental data, which reveal an astonishing repair capacity for sublethal injuries to the cervical cord of the rat (e.g., Ang et al. 1984; Habermalz et al. 1987).

7.4.2.3 Late Delayed Reaction (Chronic Progressive Radiation Myelopathy)

Chronic progressive radiation myelopathy is a selective late necrosis, that is, a coagulation necrosis in particular of the white matter. The necrosis is restricted to the segments directly exposed to radiation, but frequently signs of ascending and descending axonal Waller's degeneration are found. Vascular changes are observed that affect in particular the small capillaries and veins, in the form of hyalinosis and fibrosis. In the typical picture of cervical radiation myelopathy, anterior horn necroses or chromatolysis of anterior horn cells have been described. The primary pathogenetic substrate would thus appear to be vascular wall damage (cf. van der Kogel in this volume, Chap. 6).

The blood supply to the spinal cord is, cranially, via the costocervival trunk or the vertebral artery between C5 and C8, and caudally via the great radicular artery (from the aorta) between D9 and

L2. Coursing along the surface of the spinal cord are the anterior spinal artery and the paired posterior spinal arteries, which form a longitudinal anastomotic chain of the root artery branches. Those sections of the spinal cord which have a poor vascular supply are particularly susceptible to ischemic lesions (JELLINGER 1972; PISCOL 1972). These are the upper thoracic segments and the lower lumbar and sacral segments, and also the region between the anterior and posterior spinal arteries.

The theory as to primary radiation damage of nervous tissue is based on the observed discrepancy between the extent of the necrosis and the demonstrable vascular lesions. In particular it is argued that, owing to the greater vascular density in the gray matter, the extent of the necrosis ought to be greater there. Nevertheless, we tend to favor the hypothesis that myelopathy is primarily induced by vessel wall damage (cf. VAN DER KOGEL in this volume, Chap. 6).

Chronic progressive radiation myelopathy is initially subacute, a discontinuous deterioration being characteristic. In the cervical and thoracic region, the sensory nerve pathway and the pyramidal tract are first involved (DYNES and SMEDAL 1960; SINNER 1964; GLANZMANN et al. 1976; DISCHE et al. 1981). Sensory dissociation then develops, followed by spastic paresis and flaccid paresis. Cranial nerve deficiencies may also occur when the upper sections of the cervical cord are involved. The so-called partial Brown-séquard syndrome is characteristic: loss of temperature and pain sensitivity on the side contralateral to the motor defect. The worst possible eventuality is development of a complete transverse lesion. GÄNSHIRT (1978) reported that, in addition, neurological symptoms largely compatible with occlusion of the anterior spinal artery – the anterior spinal syndrome – may be observed.

In principle, delayed radiation myelopathy can arrest at any stage of its evolution, but it usually progresses gradually over months or years. At its peak, it can occasionally present as a space-occupying lesion which, in some cases, is associated with a myelographic blockage and an elevation of protein in the CSF of up to 150 mg% (DYNES and SMEDAL 1960; PALLIS et al. 1961; LECHEVALIER et al. 1973; GODWIN-AUSTEN et al. 1975; MARTINS et al. 1977; HOLDORFF 1983). Subsequently, there is a gradual development of atrophy. The latency period is at least 4 months, but chronic radiation myelopathies developing

after a period of several years have also been described. If tetraplegia or paraplegia develops, the patients die within 18 months after the onset of the initial symptoms. The cause of death are the effects of the paraplegia/tetraplegia, such as respiratory paralysis, pneumonia, sepsis, or pulmonary embolism (HOLDORFF 1983).

Chronic radiation myelopathy affecting the lumbar spine represents a special case: in the first place it is considerably less frequent than cervical or thoracic radiation myelopathy, and, secondly, flaccid paresis of the legs dominates the clinical picture, the otherwise typical pain being absent, while other sensory deficits are either not present at all or only to a very small degree. There is uncertainty as to the exact location of the lesion. While some authors trace the purely motor cauda conus syndrome that develops in these patients to an isolated injury of the anterior horn cells ('amyotrophic" form), others suspect a lesion of the lumbosacral plexus (for a review of the literature, see BERLIT 1987 and HOLDORFF 1978).

FRANKE and LIERSE (1978) collected 203 cases of radiation myelopathy from the international literature and assessed them for severity and prognosis. One hundred and twenty-two of the patients (60% of the overall number) had progressive paralysis. In one-half of these, the radionecrosis was confirmed histologically. If the patients with a transient sensory disturbance are not taken into account, 69% of the patients (122/176) died of delayed necrosis of the spinal cord (Table 7.5).

SCHULTHEISS et al. (1984, 1986) analyzed data pertaining to more than 300 cases of radiation myelopathy reported in the literature. Two hundred and twenty-five of the reports proved to be evaluable; 44% of the patients were still alive at the time of the report, 19% had died of cancer, intercurrent disease, or unknown causes, and 37%

Table 7.5. Course of radiation reactions of the spinal cord in 203 cases reported in the international literature with available irradiation data (FRANKE and LIERSE 1978)

	Temporary sensory deficits	Paresis regressive or slowly progressive; patient alive	Progressive paresis; patient dead
No. of patients	27 (15%)	54 (25%)	122 (60%)
Latent period (average)	5 months	24 months	14 months

had died of radiation myelopathy or its sequelae. The authors observed an identical latency period for cervical and thoracic lesions, while the less frequent lumbar myelopathy had a shorter latency period. The latency period decreased with increasing radiation dose. Factors that influenced patient survival were the height of the lesion up the spinal cord, the age of the patient, and the latency period. Patients with cervical myelopathy had the poorest prognosis, 70% of them dying. In contrast, the mortality for thoracic lesions was 30%. Young patients had a better prognosis than elderly patients. There was evidence of two waves of injury with different pathologies associated with different dose levels which correlate with the experimental data discussed by VAN DER KOGEL (this volume).

7.4.3 Peripheral Nerves

Radiation damage to the peripheral nerves is rare and difficult to establish. A review of the literature (SPIESS 1970; FRANKE 1973; MIKHAEL 1979; KINSELLA et al. 1980) revealed nerve damage following radiotherapy exclusively in the region of the primary tumor or in the locoregional area of tumor spread. Even with CT and modern neurophysiological examination procedures, such damage is virtually impossible to distinguish from locoregional tumor recurrence. An additional difficulty is the fact that a considerable number of the cases reported in the literature are in reality not radiation injuries to the nerves themselves but rather instances of compression of the nerves by scar tissue.

7.4.3.1 Acute Reaction

To our knowledge, acute radiation reactions of peripheral nerves have not been described as a clinical observation. Nevertheless, careful questioning of our tumor patients has revealed that they are by no means rare. We have observed such reactions after postoperative irradiation of breast cancer patients and irradiation of the pelvic region. Two or more days after the start of radiotherapy, breast cancer patients complain of lancinating pain and paresthesia affecting the inside of the upper arm and very rarely radiating into the forearm and fingers.

Following treatment of carcinoma of the urinary bladder or prostate, patients occasionally report pain and paresthesia located symmetrically in dorsal parts of the thighs. After replacing the large-volume ventrodorsal box technique by a rotation technique, the complaints usually disappear within a matter of days, only to reappear after the reintroduction of vd/dv irradiation.

7.4.3.2 Delayed Reaction

The delayed reactions of peripheral nerves manifest after an interval of several months or years as racking pain, sensory defects, and later also motor pareses and paralyses. SPIESS (1970) even reported an interval of 17 years. Among his 35 patients, he found brachial plexus lesions in the vast majority, namely 31. This was also the case in the publications cited by FRANKE (1973). The reason is to be sought not in a particularly high radiosensitivity of the brachial plexus but in two technical facts:

– The multiple-field technique used with orthovoltage therapy gave rise to noncalculable dose peaks (hot spots) in the region of the brachial plexus. In addition, the reproducibility of the field settings was completely inadequate.
– Brachial plexus lesions are found in patients with breast cancer in whom the radiation beam encounters a neurovascular bundle in the axilla that was surgically traumatized during radical dissection of lymph nodes.

Brachial plexus lesions are now rare and should no longer occur (a) when the axilla has not been radically cleared, that is, the neurovascular bundle has not been "skeletized," and (b) when the supraclavicular and infraclavicular regions are homogeneously irradiated with megavoltage techniques with a dose not exceeding 55 Gy over 6 weeks.

7.5 Diagnostic Evaluation

A detailed history and a careful neurological examination are the most informative diagnostic measures. Of importance is any information that can be provided on the situation, spread, and symptomatology of the preceding tumoral disease. The surgical report, the histological findings, and, wherever applicable, the radiation treatment plan must be studied in detail. Skeletal x-ray examinations, electroencephalography, CSF evaluation, and angiography are, in contrast, of only secondary importance. CT can also be useful, as can nuclear magnetic resonance imaging (MRI). Radiogenic edema is not limited to the irradiated region, but can, in particular in the late stage with necrosis, spread to nonirradiated regions.

The clinical diagnosis of radiation injury to the CNS is permissible only under the following conditions:

1. The relevant part of the brain or spinal cord must have been irradiated.
2. The location of the major neurological signs must correspond with that of the irradiated volume, e.g., neurological deficits of radiation myelopathy must correspond to the anatomical level of the irradiated spinal cord.
3. The radiation dose (both dose fractions and total dose) must lie within a range which would make the assumption of radiation myelopathy probable.

4. The appearance of symptoms must be preceded by a typical symptom-free latency period.
5. Other cerebral or spinal diseases must have been excluded, in particular local tumor progression and metastases.

7.5.1 Brain

The most important diagnostic aids in use today are CT, MRI, and, where indicated, angiography (for reviews see MIKHAEL 1978; DECK 1980; KINGSLEY and KENDALL 1981; DOOMS et al. 1986; CURRAN et al. 1987; CONSTINE et al. 1988).

Computed tomography provides information

Fig. 7.3a,b. Evolution of brain atrophy after partial brain irradiation in a patient with an anaplastic astrocytoma **a** CT images in January 1986 before postoperative treatment. **b** Sulcus enlargement and ventriculomegaly 2 years later

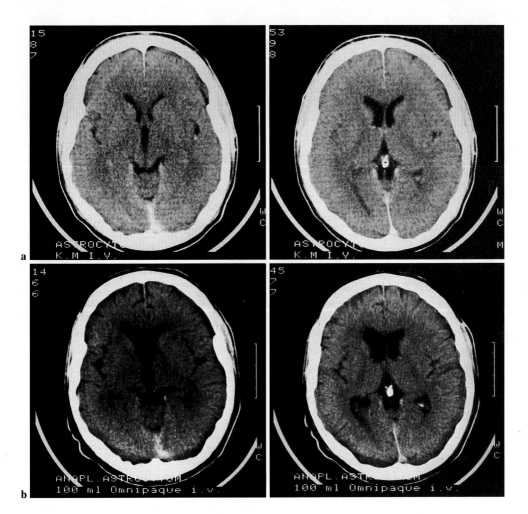

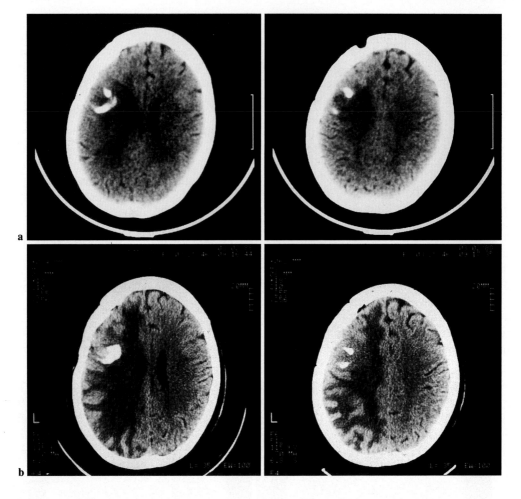

Fig. 7.4a,b. Brain necrosis in the left hemisphere after high dose irradiation. The CT scans from 1986 (**a**) and 1988 (**b**) show a constant necrotic area without any tumor but increasing edema in the irradiated hemisphere

about the character of the cerebral edema, its relationship to the irradiated volume, the width of the ventricles, possible mass displacement, posttherapeutic calcifications, hollow or annular structures, and their evolution over time (Figs. 7.3, 7.4). All of the aforementioned are roentgenological signs of delayed necrosis, which, however, may just as readily indicate the presence of recurrent tumor. Mass displacement is typical, and necrotic foci can grow for some time. Radiogenic edema is restricted to the irradiated region only in the initial phase; it can subsequently involve large portions of the nonirradiated brain tissue, too. Recurrent tumor and radiation necrosis are frequently seen simultaneously. In contrast, no CT abnormalities are associated with the delayed reaction.

With *MRI* the adverse effects of brain irradiation can be more sensitively imaged than with CT. In addition, the lesions can be visualized particularly well in the longitudinal section (Fig. 7.5). In the presence of leukoencephalopathy, discrete areas of abnormal, bright signal intensity are seen in the white matter. As signs of the late delayed reaction, confluent large foci and numerous areas of bright signal intensity may be observed in the white matter. Most such abnormalities are periventricular (DOOMS et al. 1986; CURRAN et al. 1987; CONSTINE et al. 1988). These represent signs of focal demyelination, mineralizing microangiopathies, and coagulation necrosis. At present, a correlation of MRI lesions with the neurological symptomatology is not possible, and this also applies to radiation injury and recurrent tumor.

With *angiography*, space-occupying delayed necroses present as avascular masses. Pathological blood vessels indicate a tumor, although their absence dose not exclude a poorly vascularized malignancy.

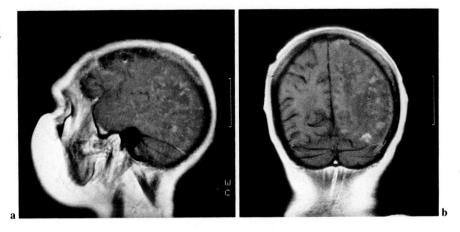

Fig. 7.5a,b. Leukoencephalopathic findings in the NMR images after irradiation of the left hemisphere: diffuse subcortical white matter injury with high signal abnormality.

In many cases, an operative biopsy is needed for definitive diagnosis and is obtained either stereotactically or via a craniotomy. The latter procedure has the advantage that, if suitably localized, the necrosis may be removed, or the brain at least decompressed.

7.5.2 Spinal Cord

The possibilities that have to be taken into account when making the differential diagnosis of radiation myelopathy are shown in Table 7.6 (BERLIT 1987), together with the necessary diagnostic procedures.

The most important differential diagnosis is metastatic spread to the spinal cord. This can be excluded with the aid of scintigraphy, CT scanning, and/or myelography. The pseudotumorous forms of radiation myelopathy might require decompression of the spinal cord; laminectomy will then rapidly clarify the situation.

A paraneoplastic myelopathy can be unequivocally differentiated clinically. It occurs only with a few types of tumor: bronchial carcinoma, cancer of the breast, and gastrointestinal cancers. The onset is abrupt with no typical latency period, is usually accompanied by a posterior cord syndrome, and is not confined to the irradiation field. In some forms of myelitis (e.g., herpes zoster) there is a direct time relationship with the primary disease. Other forms of myelitis can be detected with the aid of CSF and blood examinations.

Further diseases of the spinal cord usually can be detected clinically, by laboratory tests, or neuroradiologically, without any difficulty. Conditions that should be considered are syringomyelia, funicular myelosis, cervical myelopathy, disturbed blood supply, and traumatic injuries.

7.6 Factors Influencing Radiation Tolerance of the Nervous System

The term "tolerance dose" signifies the maximum dose which, under conditions of defined fractionation, defined treatment volume, and homogeneous dose distribution, can be tolerated by a given organ without suffering injury. Even today, tolerance doses cannot be established unequivocally, and it may be that individual parts of the NS have different radiation tolerance. Reported tolerance doses for the CNS are more or less arbitrary, and the radiotherapist tends be guided more by his subjective intuition than by experimental data. In any case, the assumption that the cerebral hemispheres are capable of tolerating higher radiation doses than the spinal cord (BODEN 1948, 1950; DYNES and SMEDAL 1960; PALLIS et al. 1961; LAMPE 1958; KRAMER and LEE 1974; FRANKE and LIERSE 1978) can no longer be considered correct.

In the brain, the midline structures are possibly more vulnerable than the cerebral hemispheres and the cerebellum (SCHOLZ and HSÜ 1938; BERG et al. 1964; HOLDORFF 1980a). In the spinal cord, the upper thoracic segments, the lower lumbar and sacral regions, and the transitional area between the anterior and posterior spinal arterial supply appear to be more susceptible to adverse effects of radiation (JELLINGER 1972; PISCOL 1972).

Despite the reservations expressed by SPIESS (1970), the most resistant part of the NS would appear to be the peripheral nerves. HAYMAKER and

Table 7.6. Differential diagnosis of radiation myelopathy (according to Berlit 1987)

Diagnosis	Distinguishing clinical features	Required diagnostic procedures
Spinal metastasis	Typical pain (radicular, press.); rapid development of transversal syndrome; often short latency period; only seen with certain primaries; often also cerebral metastases	Myelography; scintigraphy: CT scanning NMR where indicated, laminectomy
Spinal lymphomas	Frequently the first symptoms of lymphomas (85%); often brain stem lesions	Myelography; CT/NMR
Paraneoplastic myelopathy	No sharply defined sensory level; not limited to radiation field; short latency period; sudden onset; posterior cord, cerebral, and bulbar symptoms; only seen in the case of a few tumor entities (bronchogenic and gastrointestinal cancers)	CSF examination; clinical course
Spinal ischemia	Older patients and other risk factors for vascular disease; often favorable course; TID as early signs	Where indicated, angiography
Cervical myelopathy	Long history; radicular symptoms; early flaccid symptoms (arms)	Plain x-ray, myelography, EMG
Herpes zoster myelitis	Direct time relationship with skin efflorescences	CSF and serum examinations
Other forms of myelitis	Signs of inflammation (fever); meningeal symptoms	CSF and serum examinations
Funicular myelosis	Posterior cord symptoms; psychiatric and hematological symptoms	Schilling test
Angiodysgenic myelomalacia	Men are predominantly affected; only thoracolumbar; early bladder symptoms	Myelography Course
Progressive multifocal leukoencephalopathy	Only with lymphomas; always cerebral symptoms	CT
Radiation-induced neurogenic tumor	Young patients; long latency (years)	Myelography
Syringomyelia	Dysraphic stigmata; young patients; focal dissociations; sensory disturbances; early anterior horn symptoms; not limited to irradiated volume	Myelography MRI
Toxic myelopathy	Direct time relationship with intrathecal administration of cytostatics; diffuse spinal cord symptoms	CSF examination

Lindgren (1970) pointed out that the nerve endings or the terminal nerve fibers are more radiovulnerable than the peripheral nerves and nerve roots.

7.6.1 Time–Dose Relationship

7.6.1.1 Brain

Lindgren was the first person to work out the mathematics of the response of the brain to fractionation. The regression line of Fig. 7.6 indicates a dose range which is associated with a high risk of brain necrosis. The smallest dose that produced brain necroses in adults after x-ray treatment via medium-sized skin fields was between 4500 and 5000 R/30 days. Lindgren arbitrarily drew a parallel line through the lowest doses at which brain necrosis occurred; below this line, brain necroses are virtually excluded.

Zeman and Shidnia (1976) determined a tolerance threshold of 60 Gy/6 weeks which, however, according to Lindgren, would lead to a consider-

Fig. 7.6. Modified Strandqvist diagram from the original publication by LINDGREN (1958). Thirteen cases from the literature (*dots*) and four of the author's cases (*crosses*). The regression line *a* marks the time–dose range with a high risk of brain necrosis. Line *b* shows the lowest dose range at which necrosis may occur

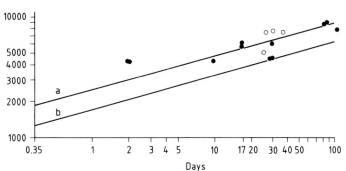

able risk of brain necrosis. On the basis of their evaluation of the literature, SHELINE et al. (1980) calculated a tolerance dose of 52 Gy/5 weeks for the brain in the case of conventional fractionation. HOLDORFF (1980a) found reports of damage to the chiasm and hypothalamus after only 45–50 Gy. ELLIS (1969) introduced the number, and thus also the size of the single fractions into the dose–time relationship. The nominal standard dose (NSD) concept, derived from irradiation of the healthy skin, takes account of the total dose (*D*) in Gy, the number of fractions (*N*), and the treatment time in days (*T*) in the following formula:

$$\text{NSD (ret)} = D \times N^{-0.24} \times T^{-0.11}$$

Table 7.2 shows the ret values for the fractionations commonly employed today, and for the usual total doses.

In the meantime, it has been established that the dose per fraction, together with the number of fractions, has a much greater influence on radiation sequelae than can be calculated by Ellis's formula. The "Ellis formula" is unsuitable for assessing the radiation risk for the CNS since it leads to overdosage (WARA et al. 1975; HARRIS and LEVENE 1976; SHELINE et al. 1980; WIGG et al. 1981). SHELINE et al. (1980) therefore modified the NSD (ret) concept to provide an NSD (neuret) concept:

$$\text{NSD (neuret)} = D \times N^{0.44} \times T^{-0.06}$$

The indices for the number of fractions and irradiation time were obtained in animal experiments on lumbar spinal cord (VAN DER KOGEL and BARENDSEN 1974; WHITE and HORNSEY 1978; VAN DER KOGEL 1979; WARA et al. 1975). They are presumably also applicable to the brain. The comparison of the NSD in ret and neuret obtained from conventional fractionation and dose shows that the tolerance figures established with the two methods are not compatible with each other (Table 7.2).

WIGG et al. (1981) collected reports in the literature on brain and spinal cord necroses, directly approached a number of radiotherapeutic centers to obtain data, and in this way arrived at further differentiated indices for *N* and *T*, as shown below for individual target organs:

Brain:	*N* 0.55 (large volume); 0.46 (small volume) *T* 0.09 (large volume) and 0.04 (small volume)
Thoracic myelitis:	*N* 0.43 *T* 0.05
Optic nerve damage:	*N* 0.33 *T* 0.000006
Brain necrosis:	*N* 0.38 *T* 0.0006

SHELINE et al. (1980) established that the total dose which may lead to brain necrosis may be surprisingly small when the overall treatment time is short, the number of fractions small, and the dose per fraction high. The regression line in Fig. 7.7 has a slope of 0.44. It marks the lowest dose at which brain necrosis has occurred. Of 80 patients with brain necroses, 26 received a total dose of ≥70 Gy. But even after ≤50 Gy, 20 patients developed brain necrosis; 17 of these had high dose fractions of between 2.5 and 37.5 Gy (85%). This stresses the importance of the dose per fraction. The highest incidence of necrosis was at about 60 Gy/30 fractions/42 days. Only four of the 80 patients with brain necroses received ≤54 ± 2 Gy with 2 Gy per fraction (see also Fig. 7.8).

HARRIS and LEVENE (1976) described a similar observation after RT of 55 patients with pituitary adenomas and craniopharyngiomas. In 27 patients who had received daily doses of ≤2 Gy, no CNS injuries were observed. Three out of 28 patients receiving fractions of 2.5–3 Gy developed a lesion of the optic nerve. One of them received a total dose of 45 Gy, and one a total dose of 50 Gy.

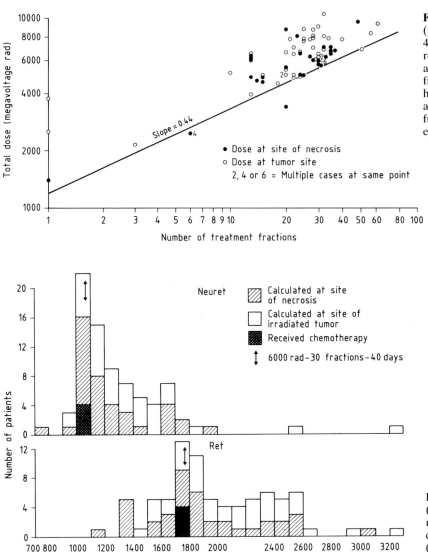

Fig. 7.7. Total dose in MER (megavoltage rad equivalent) in 40 patients with brain necrosis reported in the literature plotted against the number of individual fractions. The regression line has a slope of 0.44. Most cases are above this line. See text for further information. (Sheline et al. 1980)

Fig. 7.8. Cases of brain necrosis ($n = 79$) reported in the international literature, arranged by dose in ret (below) and neuret (above) (Sheline et al. 1980)

Similarly, Franke and Lierse (1978) and Holdorff (1980b) drew attention to the risk of applying high single doses. Marks et al. (1981) found that, at a dose of 50 Gy/25 fractions/35 days, or 54 Gy/30 fractions/42 days, no delayed radiation reaction occurred, and the risk at 60 Gy/30 fractions/42 days was greater than that at 60 Gy/35 fractions/49 days.

7.6.1.2 Spinal Cord

It is virtually impossible to define limits of tolerance for human spinal cord, despite the wealth of literature in this area. There are no comparative experimental data to show that brain and spinal cord have a different tolerance for ionizing radia-tion. van der Schueren (1989) therefore recommended setting up a worldwide register for spinal cord necroses, and a prospective register for all cases in which doses above an agreed tolerance dose are given (incidence register).

Boden (1948, 1950) indicated a tolerance threshold for the spinal cord of 35 Gy/17 days for large volumes and of 45 Gy/17 days for small volumes (Fig. 7.9). Sinner (1964) considered that 35–45 Gy/21 days, 37–48/28 days, and 41–52 Gy/43 days are equivalent to these tolerance doses. Friedmann (1954) reported a tolerance threshold of 50 Gy/50 days for the lumbar spinal cord. The frequently cited tolerance and necrosis doses indicated by Pallis et al. (1961), Franke (1963), Maier et al. (1969), and Jellinger and Sturm (1971) are shown in Fig. 7.9, published in 1978 by Franke

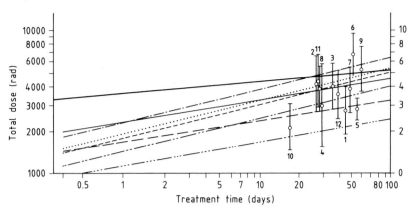

Fig. 7.9. Various regression lines for necrosis and tolerance ranges of the spinal cord as collected by FRANKE and LIERSE (1978). Bone absorption has been taken into account by applying a dose modification of 10%. ——— spinal cord "necrotic range" (FRANKE 1963); –···– spinal cord (thoracic and lumbar sections) "tolerance range" (FRANKE 1973); -- spinal cord "tolerance range" (FRANKE 1963); – · ·– spinal cord "tolerance range" for large fields (PALLIS et al. 1961); .... spinal cord "tolerance range" for small fields (PALLIS et al. 1961); --- spinal cord "tolerance range" for large fields (BODEN 1948, 1950); · – · – · – · spinal cord "tolerance range" for small fields (BODEN 1948, 1950); spinal cord (lumbar section) "necrotic range" (MAIER et al. 1969); —o— 1–12: JELLINGER and STURM 1971.

and LIERSE. FRANKE and LIERSE pointed out that the slope of the regression line becomes flatter with increasing dose cumulation and increasing degree of damage, and they considered it to be flatter than in the case of the brain. This would mean that, despite a longer treatment duration, the total dose cannot be increased appreciably before reaching the tolerance limit. ABBATUCCI et al. (1978) established that 51.1 Gy could be tolerated by the spinal cord, provided that a volume corresponding to the height of three to five vertebral bodies was not exceeded. The recommended total dose is 50 Gy/25 fractions/35 days. The secondary reference dose (5 Gy below the tolerance dose) is then 45 Gy. If the threshold is corrected with an α/β term of 2 Gy, a threshold dose of 62 Gy is obtained (VAN DER SCHUEREN 1989). The tolerance doses corrected accordingly would be 66 Gy for the doses reported by HATLEVOLL et al. (1983) and as much as 72 Gy for those reported by DISCHE et al. (1988).

It has been established that in determining a tolerance dose, fractionation is the decisive factor (VAN DER KOGEL, Chap. 6, this volume; HORNSEY and WHITE 1980): irrespective of the overall treatment time, tolerance increases with decreas-

ing dose per fraction. This is extensively discussed by VAN DER KOGEL this volume, Chap. 6). However, while substantial biological data are available for dose fractions above 2 Gy, there is still uncertainty as to the effect of dose fractions below 2 Gy.

While, in consequence of reduced radiation tolerance of the spinal cord, youth and childhood are both unfavorable prognostic factors for the incidence and evolution of radiation myelopathy, the tolerance of the individual segments of the spinal cord may differ (SCHULTHEISS et al. 1984, 1986; BERLIT 1987). Lumbar myelopathy occurs after lower doses than does thoracic myelopathy; for example in BERLIT's report myelopathy occurred after a median total dose of 43 Gy in the lumbar region, but not until after a median of 54 Gy in the thoracic region. The T1–6 region was significantly more sensitive than the lower thoracic cord (T7–12) (the median total doses at which radiation necrosis developed were 50.4 Gy and 62 Gy respectively).

In an effort to resolve the uncertainty with respect to the radiation tolerance of the human spinal cord, VAN DER SCHUEREN (personal communication, 1988) conducted a poll among several hundred radiotherapists. The majority estimated the average tolerance to be about 43 Gy with conventional fractionation, the maximum tolerance being 49.2 Gy.

7.6.1.3 Peripheral Nerves

Data on radiation reactions by the peripheral nerves are few. Most of the reports concern *brachial plexus damage* following postoperative irradiation of breast cancer patients (for a review of cases, see STOLL and ANDREWS 1966; SPIESS 1970; FRANKE 1973; MIKHAEL 1979; KINSELLA et al. 1980). The tolerance threshold has not been defined. However, with conventional fractionation it may be assumed to be 55 Gy/6 weeks.

High doses per fraction have a detrimental effect on the peripheral nerves, too. Stoll and Andrews (1966) reported that injuries to the brachial plexus occurred in 73% of patients (17/21) after the application of 55 Gy in 12 fractions. The application of 51 Gy in 11 fractions resulted in damage to the plexus in 15% of the cases. This observation was confirmed by Haymaker and Lindgren (1970). However, 55 Gy in 2 Gy fractions appears to be safe.

Westling et al. (1972) reported postoperative radiation for breast cancer with dose fractions of 4 Gy up to a total dose of 54 Gy and a subsequent boost with 10 Gy. Seventeen months later, 60% of the patients had developed injury to the plexus. After reducing the size of the supraclavicular field and changing to the megavoltage technique, the incidence dropped to 14%–16%. Finally, the authors reduced the dose per fraction to 3 Gy and the total dose to 45 Gy. Thereafter, no more plexus injuries were observed over a follow-up period of 3.5 years.

7.6.2 Radiation Quality

High LET irradiation with particles such as neutrons, pions, and heavy ions has a greater biological effect than low LET radiation such as megavoltage x-rays and electrons. The effects are not only seen in the tumor, but also as damage to normal tissue. Thus, it is possible that a tumor of the brain may be "sterilized" with neutron irradiation, at the price of severe radiation sequelae in the normal brain tissue (Boellaard and Jacoby 1962; Zeman 1964; Douglas and Castro 1984).

Hornsey et al. (1981) concluded that the neutron dose employed in all clinical brain tumor protocols was too high. Instead of a relative biological effect (RBE) of 3, as assumed by Laramore et al. (1978), Hornsey et al. determined an RBE of 5.2 for the neutron source of the Hammersmith Cyclotron (Ed = 16 MeV-Be neutrons). In view of this, they concluded that a neutron dose of 11 Gy was just tolerable for large brain volumes.

For the practical work of the therapist, it is important to note that the RBE varies even with low LET irradiation. As a guideline, we employ the clinical observations repeatedly mentioned by

Zuppiner, that the effectiveness of orthovoltage irradiation is some 15% greater than that of megavoltage photons, which, in turn, is about 10% greater that the RBE of high energy electron beams. Sheline et al. (1980), too, drew attention to the differences in the biological effect produced by orthovolt and megavolt photons.

7.6.3 Chemotherapeutic Agents

Oncological chemotherapy, applied together with, before, or after radiotherapy, may sensitize the CNS to ionizing irradiation and enhance the radiogenic reactions of the CNS. Such combination treatment modes are commonly employed in ALL, malignant lymphoma, small cell bronchiogenic carcinoma, medulloblastoma, anaplastic ependymoma, and glioblastoma. The major drugs of interest to the radiotherapist are methotrexate (MTX), vincristine, cytosine, arabinoside, L-asparaginase, and probably also BCNU/CCNU, chlorambucil, and procarbazine. Furthermore, interaction of irradiation with cytotoxic substances that are normally not found in the CSF cannot be excluded, as in tumors of the brain the particularly dense capillary endothelial structure, which in normal brain is the morphological substrate for the blood–brain barrier, is absent or present to only a limited degree (Vick et al. 1977).

The radiobiological basis for the fact that one treatment modality can render another more toxic remains to be established. The following possibilities may be considered (Bleyer and Griffin 1980):

1. Ionizing radiation and chemotherapeutic drugs may have overlapping mechanisms of neural toxicity.
2. Chemotherapeutic agents may act as radiosensitizers. Although not neurotoxic in themselves, they may enhance the sensitivity of the brain cells to ionizing radiation, or "recall" radiation-induced neurotoxicity.
3. CNS irradiation may alter the distribution kinetics of drugs in the CNS in such a manner that certain areas of the brain accumulate greater amounts of the substance

In the case of MTX in particular, the following mechanisms are under discussion:

1. Irradiation destroys the blood–brain barrier, which is otherwise impermeable to the systemically applied drug.

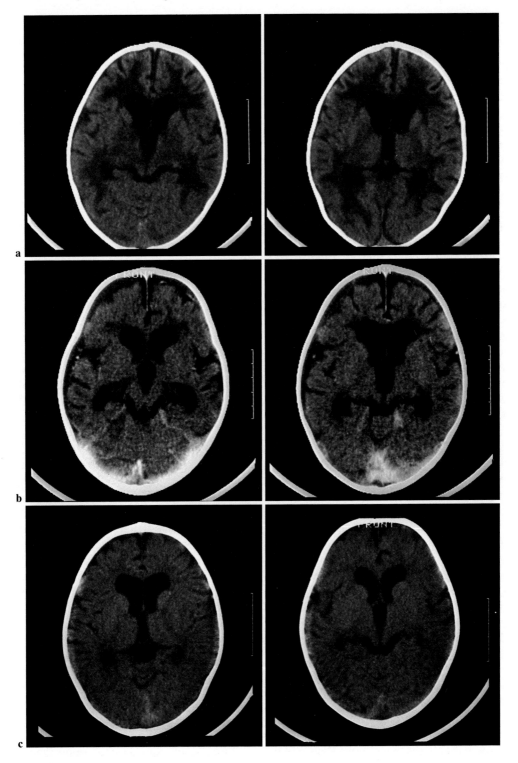

Fig. 7.10a-c. Clinical course of leukoencephalopathy in a girl with ALL. Clinical diagnosis was established in October 1985 when the girl was 4 months old. **a** Fifteen months after initial treatment with intravenous and intrathecal MTX marked leukoencephalopathy was observed. No radiotherapy was applied. The clinical diagnosis was CNS relapse. **b** The CT images obtained after the second course of MTX show more pronounced leukoencephalopathy 3 months later, with enlargement of the ventricles and sulcus. **c** In June 88 whole brain irradiation was applied. Ten months later the CT images reveal substantial recovery and disappearance of the most marked CNS damage. No adverse radiation effect occurred

2. As a result of impairment of the arachnoidal granulations or the choroid plexus, irradiation delays the production of CSF, and thus the clearance of the substance from the CNS.
3. Ionizing radiation damages the ependymal lining of the ventricular spaces, so that MTX contained within the CSF can escape from the ventricular system into the white matter.
4. The individual brain cells can accumulate more MTX than in the nonirradiated state, since radiotherapy modifies their metabolism.

Even without irradiation of the brain, MTX – like procarbazine and nitrosourea – can give rise to leukoencephalopathy (Fig. 7.10). This applies both to intravenously (Allen et al. 1980; Rosen et al. 1979; Fritsch et al. 1981) and intrathecally (Bleyer et al. 1973; Fusner et al. 1977; Bleyer and Griffin 1980) administered MTX. As far as we are aware, this syndrome has never been observed after brain irradiation with 18–25 Gy. 2–3 weeks alone.

The risk of necrotizing leukoencephalopathy in children receiving ALL therapy is greatest when all three treatment modalities are employed: intrathecal MTX, intravenous MTX, and whole-brain irradiation (Bleyer and Griffin 1980; Bleyer 1981). Three modalities employed simultaneously are more toxic than two, and the toxicity is likewise greater with two modalities than with one (Fig. 7.11). The risk may be 5% to more than 50% (Aur et al. 1978; Bleyer and Griffin 1980; Bode et al. 1980; Gutjahr and Kretzschmar 1979; Habermalz et al. 1983; Lee et al. 1986; Price and Jamieson 1975). Subclinical changes are, however, more frequent when studied by CT or MRI. Thus, Peylan-Ramu et al. (1978) found lesions in the CT scan in 8 out of 14 clinically unremarkable children. Price and Jamieson (1975) differentiated the risk with respect to both the radiation dose applied to the CNS and the amount of MTX administered. Leukoencephalopathy confirmed by autopsy never occurred at a dose below 20 Gy, while it was observed in 9 of 51 patients (17%) following administration of 20–25 Gy, in two of six patients after 25–30 Gy, and in two of three patients receiving more than 30 Gy. The incidence in the case of intravenously administered MTX was similar: 3 of 29 patients (10%) developed leukoencephalopathy after 1–200 mg, 4 of 13 (31%) after 400–600 mg, and 5 of 16 (31%) Presumably other chemotherapeutic agents also play a role in the development of treatment-

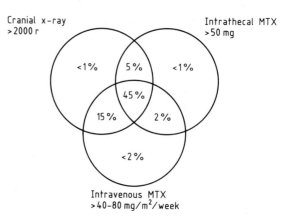

Fig. 7.11. Risk of clinical leukoencephalopathy according to the different treatment modalities for ALL in children (Bleyer and Griffen 1980)

induced brain damage. On the basis of their CT follow-up scans, Peylan-Ramu et al. (1978) suspected intrathecally applied cytosine arabinoside (ara-C) of being just such an agent. Other studies have implicated procarbazine (Lee et al. 1986), etoposide (Giever et al. 1982), LicciarDello et al. 1985), vincristine (Cassady et al. 1980; Licciardello et al. 1985), and cisplatin (Frytak et al. 1985). In patients with SCLC, there was an increase in the frequency of overall CT brain scan abnormalities ($P < 0.05$) and periventricular white matter alterations ($P < 0.05$) in a subgroup of patients who received MTX and procarbazine after whole-brain irradiation (Lee et al. 1986). The authors suspected that procarbazine possesses a synergistic neurotoxic effect when it is given with MTX after brain irradiation. Johnson et al. (1985) demonstrated a correlation of the severity of the neurological sequelae with concurrent high dose chemotherapy. Frytak et al. (1987) reported compelling evidence implicating CCNU in the pathogenesis of the problem.

In the cervical spinal cord of the rat, van der Kogel and Sissingh (1985) were able to confirm experimentally impairment of the radiation tolerance by ara-C (see also Chap. 6, this volume.)

When both chemotherapy and whole-brain irradiation are employed, the sequence of the procedures is of considerable importance: For, in general, the CNS morbidity is lower in patients in whom systemic chemotherapy is applied prior to RT than in those receiving the chemotherapy during or after RT. Account must be taken of this fact in particular in the case of drugs such as cisplatin, etoposide, MTX, actinomycin D, and the anthracyclines. It would, therefore, appear logical not to apply whole-brain irradiation until after systemic chemotherapy has been completed (BLEYER and GRIFFIN 1980; LAUKKANEN et al. 1988; BLEYER 1988; PRICE and JAMIESON 1975).

HABERMALZ et al. (1983) pointed out that in childhood in particular, CT images can be misinterpreted with respect to complications of therapy. GUTJAHR and KRETZSCHMAR (1979) had already observed the more or less typical CT abnormalities such as ventricular dilatation, widening of the subarachnoid space, and intracerebral microcalcifications, irrespective of whether the CT scan had been performed prior to or after CNS prophylaxis. HABERMALZ et al. (1983) classified the CT signs into three grades, and discovered posttreatment grade I and II abnormalities in 58% of patients. Grade I was – as the authors themselves suspected – presumably a normal variant. This means that reports in the literature on similarly high incidence rates of CT changes after CNS prophylaxis in ALL will have to be considered particularly critically. HABERMALZ et al. found a grade II abnormality in 27% of patients; a grade III abnormality was never seen. A significant correlation was observed with the duration of maintenance therapy and also with the duration of the individual dose of radiotherapy (>/<170 rd). In contrast, there was no dependence on the total radiation dose applied – at least within the range 850–2400 rd – or on the intensity of induction therapy.

7.7 Conclusions and Summary

1. The nervous system (NS) is not as radioresistant as was assumed not so long ago. Side-effects involving brain, spinal cord, and peripheral nerves must be expected after radiotherapy.
2. If injuries to the NS do occur, radiation reactions in the strict sense must be distinguished from combination radiation sequelae. The latter may be induced by surgical manipulations on the NS, systemic or intrathecal chemotherapy, infections, or damage produced by the tumor itself.
3. With respect to the time course of the radiation sequelae, early and delayed reactions are distinguished, the latter being further subdi-

vided into an early and a late delayed reaction. It looks very much as though these changes are of the same nature throughout the NS although, of course, they may present differently in different locations. Knowledge of acute radiation reactions and the early delayed reaction is of particular importance, in order not to misinterpret neurological disorders observed several weeks after completing radiotherapy as signs of failed therapy.
4. Unequivocal data on the incidence of early and delayed radiation reactions for defined dose ranges are not available in the literature. The reasons for this are that the majority of reports are anecdotal, the duration of followup is too short, brain tumor patients are only rarely submitted to autopsy, and the number of unpublished cases of radiation reactions is not known.
5. The clinical symptomatology of radiation reactions in the NS depends upon their localization and extension. Early delayed reactions are rarely fatal, and symptoms can clear completely without treatment. Leukoencephalopathy may be clinically silent, but may also manifest as somnolence, mental deficiency, disturbances of coordination, and other neuropsychological and neuroanatomical defects. The CT scan reveals ventricular dilatation, periventricular white matter hypodensity, and parenchymal calcifications.

Both in the brain and in the spinal cord, late delayed reaction may present as a space-occupying lesion which usually cannot be distinguished from recurrent tumor. But, while chronic progressive radiation myelopathy can usually be differentiated from other spinal cord lesions, in the case of brain necrosis a stereotactic or open brain biopsy may be required to clarify the diagnosis.
6. In the case of the hypophysial–hypothalamic system, growth hormone production is most sensitive to radiation. This is followed by the thyroid axis, and the adrenal and gonadal axes.
7. Radionecrosis of the cerebral hemispheres has the best prognosis, in particular when surgical removal or decompression is possible.
8. The radiosensitivity of the NS varies. It seems probable that the greatest susceptibility to radiation is to be found in the upper thoracic segments and the lower lumbar and sacral segments of the spinal cord. The latency

period of radiation sequelae is shorter in the spinal cord and midline structures of the brain than in the cerebral hemispheres, and it is even longer in the peripheral nerves.

9. The causes of radiation reactions are usually multifactorial. A high radiation dose applied over a short period via large treatment volumes and high single doses per fraction promote their development. On the other hand, at fraction sizes below 2 Gy, no further increase in the tolerance of the NS has been proven.

10. The tolerance dose for the brain, spinal cord, and peripheral nerves under clinical conditions is not known exactly. It would appear that the brain tolerates 50 Gy/25 fractions/35 days or 54 Gy/30 fractions/42 days. The threshold dose for the development of brain necroses is 60 Gy/30 fractions/42 days. The same "tolerance doses" are considered to apply to the spinal cord. However, most international radiotherapists recommend that a general tolerance dose of, on average, 43 Gy, and a maximum tolerance dose of, on average, 49 Gy should be assumed.

11. The "Ellis formula" is not suitable for estimating the radiation risk to the CNS. Its use tends to lead to an overdosage. We recommend the "neuret concept," in which greater emphasis is given to the fraction size and less to the overall treatment time. The LQ model and the neuret concept, however, are associated with the risk that the isoeffective doses for spinal cord tolerance may be overestimated for fraction sizes as small as 1 or 2 Gy.

12. Chemotherapy administered together with, prior to, or after, radiotherapy may considerably augment the radiogenic reactions of the CNS. And it is of little importance whether or not the drugs enter the CSF in the healthy brain, since in the presence of brain tumors the blood–brain barrier is impaired or even absent.

Of particular interest in this context are MTX, procarbazine, vincristine, ara-C, etoposide, L-asparaginase, cisplatin, anthracyclines, and nitrosoureas. The drug that has been most intensively studied is MTX. If whole-brain irradiation has to be combined with intrathecal or intravenous administration of MTX, the fewest side-effects are observed after sequential administration, and the MTX should be administered before irradiation of the CNS.

After combination treatment of All, high incidence rates of pathological CT changes have been reported in the literature. These reports will have to be examined critically in order to exclude the possibility of misinterpreting normal variants. To date, there have been no investigations showing the normal values for the size of the CSF spaces in childhood.

13. For the establishment of indications for radiation treatment of tumors of the brain, account should be taken not only of the radiosensitivity of the tumor but also of the life expectancy of the patient. In the case of brain tumors with a more favorable prognosis, we would recommend that the dose be kept as low as possible, since the patient will otherwise survive long enough to develop necrosis of the brain.

References

Abbatucci JS, Delozier T, Quint R, Roussel A, Brune D (1978) Radiation myelopathy of the cervical spinal cord: time, dose and volume factors. Int J Radiat Oncol Biol Phys 4: 239–248

Ahlbom HE (1941) The results of radiotherapy of hypopharyngeal cancer at Radiumhemmet, Stockholm 1930–1939. Acta Radiol 22: 155–171

Allen JC, Rosen G, Metha BM, Horten B (1980) Leucoencephalopathy following high dose i.v. methotrexate chemotherapy with leucovorin rescue. Cancer Treat Rep 64: 1261–1273

Andler W, Roosen K, Clar HE (1982) Endocrinological investigations in 68 children with brain tumors. In: Voth D, Gutjahr P, Langmaid C (eds) Tumours of the central nervous system in infancy and childhood. Springer, Berlin Heidelberg New York, pp 415–419

Aur RJA, Simone JV, Verzosa MS, Hustu HO, Pinkel DP, Barker LF (1978) Leucoencefalopatia enniños con leucemia linfocitica aguda sometido a terapeutica preventiva del sistema nervioso central. Sangre (Barc) 23: 1–12

Bamford FN, Morris-Jones P, Pearson D, Ribeiro GG, Shalet SM, Beardwell CG (1976) Residual disabilities in children treated for intracranial space-occupying lesions. Cancer 37: 1149–1151

Berg NO, Håkansson CH, Lindgren M (1964) Klinische und biologische Gesichtspunkte zur Strahlentoleranz des Hirngewebes. Radiologe 4: 194–200

Berlit P (1987) Die Strahlenmyelopathie. Klinische Analyse des Krankheitsbildes. Schriftenreihe Neurologie. Springer Berlin Heidelberg New York

Bleyer WA (1981) Neurologic sequelae of methotrexate and ionizing radiation: a new classification. Cancer Treat Rep 65 [Suppl]: 89–98

Bleyer WA (1988) Hobson's choice in the CNS radioprophylaxis of small cell lung cancer. Int J Radiat Oncol Biol Phys 15: 783–785

Bleyer WA, Griffin TW (1980) White matter necrosis, mineralizing microangiopathy, and intellectual abilities in survivors of childhood leukemia: associations with central nervous system irradiation and methotrexate therapy. In : Gilbert HA, Kagan AR (eds) Radiation damage of the nervous system. Raven New York, pp 155–174

Bleyer WA, Drake JC, Chabner BA (1973) Neurotoxicity and elevated cerebrospinal fluid methotrexate concentration in meningeal leukemia. N Engl J Med 289: 270–773

Bode U, Oliff A, Bercu BB, DiChiro G, Glaubiger DL, Poplack DC (1980) Absence of CT brain scan and endocrine abnormalities with less intensive CNS prophylaxis. Am J Pediatr Hematol Oncol 2: 21–24

Boden G (1948) Radiation myelitis of the cervical spinal cord. Br J Radiol 21: 464–469

Boden G (1950) Radiation myelitis of the brain-stem. J Fac Radiol 2: 79–94

Boellaard JW, Jacoby W (1962) Röntgenspätschäden des Gchirns. Acta Neurochir (Wien) 5: 533–564

Boldrey E, Sheline G (1967) Delayed transitory clinical manifestations after radiation treatment of intracranial tumors. Acta Radiol 5: 5–10

Buchfelder M (1984) Effekte der postoperativen Radiotherapie para- und suprasellärer Hypophysenadenome. Inaugural Dissertatic, University of Erlangen-Nürnberg

Burger PC, Mahaley MS, Dudka L, Vogel FS (1979) The morphologic effects of radiation administered therapeutically for intracranial gliomas. A postmortem study of 25 cases. Cancer 44: 1256–1272

Cassady JR, Tonnesen GL, Wolfe LC, Sallan SE (1980) Augmentation of vincristine neurotoxicity by irradiation of peripheral nerves. Cancer Treat Rep 64: 963–965

Catane R, Schwade JG, Yarr I et al. (1981) Follow-up neurological evaluation in patients with small cell lung carcinoma treated with prophylactic cranial irradiation and chemotherapy. Int J Radiat Oncol Biol Phys 7: 105–109

Chak LY, Zatz LM, Wasserstein P et al. (1986) Neurologic dysfunction in patients treated for small cell carcinoma of the lung: A clinical and radiological study. Int J Radiat Oncol Biol Phys 12: 385–389

Cohen ME, Duffner PK (1984) Brain tumors in children. Principles of diagnosis and treatment. Raven, New York

Constine LS, Konski A, Ekholm S, McDonald S, Rubin P (1988) Adverse effects of brain irradiation correlated with MR and CT imaging. Int J Radiat Oncol Biol Phys 15: 319–330

Cox JD, Komaki R, Byhardt RW, Kun LE (1980) Results of whole-brain irradiation for metastases from small cell carcinoma of the lung. Cancer Treat Rep 64: 957–961

Craig JB, Jackson DV, Moody D et al. (1984) Prospective evaluation of changes in computed cranial tomography in patients with small cell lung cancer treated with chemotherapy and prophylactic cranial irradiation. J Clin Oncol 2: 1151–1156

Crosley CJ, Rorke LB, Evans A, Nigro M (1978) Central nervous system lesions in childhood leukemia. Neurology 28: 678–685

Curran WJ, Hecht-Leavitt C, Schut L, Zimmerman RA, Nelson DF (1987) Magnetic resonance imaging of cranial radiation lesions. Int J Radiat Oncol Biol Phys 13: 1093–1098

Deck MDF (1980) Imaging techniques in the diagnosis of radiation damage to the central nervous system. In: Gilbert HA, Kagan AR (eds) Radiation damage to the nervous system. Raven New York, pp 107–127

Dische S, Martin WMC, Anderson P (1981) Radiation myelopathy in patients treated for carcinoma of bronchus using a six fraction regime of radiotherapy. Br J Radiol 54: 29–35

Dische S, Warburton MF, Saunders MJ (1988) Radiation myelitis and survival in the radiotherapy of lung cancer. Int J Radiat Oncol Biol Phys 15: 75–81

Dooms GC, Hecht S, Brant-Zawadski M, Berthiaume Y, Norman D, Newton TH (1986) Brain radiation lesions: MR imaging. Radiology 158: 149–155

Douglas BG, Castro JR (1984) Novel fractionation schemes and high linear energy transfer. In: Rosenblum ML, Wilson CB (eds) Brain tumor therapy. Prog Exp Tumor Res 28: 152–165

Druckmann A (1929) Schlafsucht als Folge der Röntgenbestrahlung. Beitrag zur Strahlenempfindlichkeit des Gehirns. Strahlentherapie 33: 382–384

Duffner PK, Cohen ME, Thomas PRM, Lansky SB (1985) The long term effects of cranial irradiation on the central nervous system. Cancer 56: 1841–1846

Dynes JB, Smedal MI (1960) Radiation myelitis. AJR 83: 78–87

Eastman RC, Gorden P, Roth J (1979) Conventional supervoltage irradiation is an effective treatment for acromegaly. J Clin Endocrinol Metab 48: 931–940

Edwards MS, Wilson CB (1980) Treatment of radiation necrosis. In: Gilbert HA, Kagan AR (eds) Radiation damage to the nervous system, Raven, New York, pp 129–143

Eiser C (1981) Psychological sequelae of brain tumours in childhood: a retrospective study. Br J Clin Psychol 20: 35–38

Ellis F (1969) Dose, time and fractionation. A clinical hypothesis. Clin Radiol 20: 1–7

Ellison N, Bernath A, Kane P, Porter P (1982) Disturbing problems of success; clinical status of long-term survivors of small cell lung cancer. Proc Am Soc Clin Oncol 1: 149

Enzman DR, Lane B (1978) Enlargement of subarachnoid spaces and lateral ventricles in pediatrie patients undergoing chemotherapy. J Pediatr 92: 535–539

Eyster EF, Nielsen SL, Sheline GE, Wilson CB (1974) Cerebral radiation necrosis simulating a brain tumor. J Neurosurg 39: 267–271

Fischer AW, Holfelder H (1930) Lokales Amyloid im Gehirn. Eine Spätfolge von Röntgenbestrahlungen. Dtsch Z Chir 227: 475–483

Franke HD (1963) Die Strahlenemplindlichkeit des menschlichen Rückenmarks. Fortschr Med 81: 345–350

Franke HD (1973) Die Strahlenemplindlichkeit des Nervensystems. In: Strahlenemplindlichkeit von Organen und Organsystemen der Säugetiere und des Menschen. Strahlenschutz in Forschung und Praxis, vol XIII. Thieme, Stuttgart, pp 172–194

Franke HD, Lierse W (1978) Strahlenbedingte Reaktionen des Gehirns und des Rückenmarks. Strahlentherapie 154: 587–598

Freeman JE, Johnston PGB, Voke JM (1973) Somnolence after prophylactic cranial irradiation in children with acute lymphoblastic leukaemia. Br Med J 4: 523–525

Friedman M (1954) Calculated risks of radiation injury of normal tissue in the treatment of cancer of the testis. Proc Second Natl Cancer Conf, New York, Am Cancer Soc, vol I, pp 390–400

Fritsch G, Urban CH, Sager D, Becker H (1981) Zur Klinik der Methotrexat-induzierten Encephalopathie. In: Hanefeld H (ed) Aktuelle Neuropädiatrie 2. Hippokrates, Stuttgart, pp 129–134

Frytak S, Earnest F, O'Neill BP, Lee RE, Creagan ET, Trautmann JC (1985) Magnetic resonance imaging for neurotoxicity in long-term survivors of carcinoma. Mayo Clin Proc 60: 803–812

Frytak S, Eagan RT, Therneau TM, Creagan ET, Richardson RL, Jett JR, Coles DT (1987) Leukoencephalopathy in patients with small cell lung cancer receiving prophylactic cranial irradiation. Proc Am Soc Clin Oncol 6: 257

Fusner J, Poplack DG, Pizzo PA, DiChiro G (1977) Leukoencephalopathy following chemotherapy for rhabdomyosarcoma: reversibility of cerebral changes demonstrated by computed tomography. J Pediatr 91: 77–79

Gänshirt H (1978) Strahlenmyelopathie. Med Welt 29: 261–264

Giever RJ, Heusinkveld RS, Manning MR, Bowden GT (1982) Enhanced radiation reaction following combination chemotherapy for small cell carcinoma of the lung, possibly secondary to VP16–213. Int J Radiat Oncol Biol Phys 8: 921–923

Glanzmann C, Aberle HG, Horst W (1976) The risk of chronic progressive radiation myelopathy. Strahlentherapie 152: 363–372

Godwin-Austen RB, Howell DA, Worthington B (1975) Observations on radiation myelopathy. Brain 98: 557–568

Goldfine ID, Lawrence AM (1972) Hypopituitarism in acromegaly. Arch Int Med 130: 720–723

Greenfield MM, Stark FM (1948) Postirradiation neuropathy. AJR 60: 617–622

Gutjahr P, Kretzschmar K (1979) Akute lymphoblastische Leukämie und maligne Non-Hodgkin-Lymphome im Kindesalter. Dtsch Med Wochenschr 104: 1068–1071

Habermalz E, Habermalz HJ, Stephani U, Henze G, Riehm H, Hanefeld F (1983) Cranial computed tomography of 64 children in continuous complete remission of leukemia I: relations to therapy modalities. Neuropediatrics 14: 144–148

Harris JR, Levene MB (1976) Visual complications following irradiation for pituitary adenomas and craniopharyngiomas. Radiology 120: 167–171

Harten G, Stephani U, Henze G, Langermann HJ, Riehm H, Hanefeld F (1984) Impairment of psychomotor skills in children after treatment of acute lymphoblastic leukemia. Eur J Pediatr 142: 189–197

Hatlevoll R, Host H, Kaalhus O (1983) Myelopathy following radiotherapy of bronchial carcinoma with large single fractions: a retrospective study. Int J Radiat Oncol Biol Phys 9: 41–44

Haymaker W, Lindgren M (1970) Nerve disturbances following exposure to ionizing radiation. In: Vinken PJ, Bruyn GE (eds) Handbook of clinical neurology, vol VII/14. American Elsevier, New York, pp 388–401

Hirsch JF, Pierre-Kahn A, Benveniste L, George B (1978) Les médulloblastomes de l'enfant. Survie et résultats fonctionnels. Neurochirurgie 24: 391–397

Hirsch JF, Reiner D, Czerichow P, Benveniste L, Pierre-Kahn A (1979) Medulloblastoma in childhood: survival and functional results. Acta Neurochir (wien) 48: 1–15

Hoffman WF, Levin VA, Wilson CB (1979) Evaluation of malignant glioma patients during the postirradiation period. J Neurosurg 50: 624–628

Holdorff B (1978) Beinplexus- und Kaudawurzelläsionen durch ionisierende Strahlen. Acta Neurol (Napoli) 5: 23–27

Holdorff B (1980a) Dose effect relationships in cervical and thoracic radiation myelopathies. Acta Radiol Oncol 19: 271–277

Holdorff B (1980b) Der Unterschied zwischen zerebralen Hemisphären- und Mittellinien-Strahlenspätnekrosen und seine Bedeutung für die Strahlentherapie. Strahlentherapie 156: 530–537

Holdorff B (1983) Strahlenschäden des Gehirns und Rückenmarks. In: Seitz D, Vogel P (eds) Hämoblastosen, zentrale Motorik, iatrogene Schäden, Myositiden. Verh Dtsch Ges Neurol, vol II. Springer, Berlin Heidelberg New York pp 158–170

Hornsey S, White A (1980) Isoeffect curve for radiation myelopathy. Br J Radiol 53: 168–169

Hornsey S, Morris CC, Myers R, White A (1981) Relative biological effectiveness for damage to the central nervous system by neutrons. Int J Radiat Oncol Biol Phys 7: 185–189

Jellinger K (1972) "Frühe" Strahlenspätschäden des menschlichen Zentralnervensystems. Verh Dtsch Ges Pathol 56: 457–463

Jellinger K (1977) Human central nervous system lesions following radiation therapy. Zentralbl Neurochir 38: 199–220

Jellinger K, Sturm KW (1971) Delayed radiation myelopathy in man. Report of 12 necropsy cases. J Neurol Sci 14: 389–408

Johnson BE, Ihde DC, Bunn PA et al. (1985) Patients with small cell lung cancer treated with combination chemotherapy with or without irradiation. Ann Intern Med 103: 430–438

Jones A (1964) Transient radiation myelopathy (with reference to Lhermitte's sign of electrical paresthesia). Br J Radiol 37: 727–744

Kingsley DPE, Kendall BE (1981) CT of the adverse effects of therapeutic radiation of the central nervous system. Am J Neuroradiol 2: 453–460

Kinsella TJ, Weichselbaum RR, Sheline GE (1980) Radiation injury of cranial and peripheral nerves. In: Gilbert HA, Kagan AR (eds) Radiation damage to the nervous system. Raven, New York, pp 145–153

Kramer S, Lee KF (1974) Complications of radiation therapy: the central nervous system. Semin Oncol 9: 75–83

Kramer S, Southard M, Mansfield CM (1968) Radiotherapy in the management of craniopharyngiomas: further experience and late results. AJR 103: 44–52

Kun LE, Mulhern RK, Crisco JJ (1983) Quality of life in children treated for brain tumors. Intellectual, emotional, and academic function. J Neurosurg 58: 1–6

Lampe I (1958) Radiation tolerance of the central nervous system. In: Buschke F (ed) Progress in radiation therapy. Grune & Stratton, New York, pp 224–236

Lampert PW, Davis RL (1964) Delayed effects of radiation on the human central nervous system. "Early" and "late" delayed reactions. Neurology 14: 912–917

Laramore GF, Griffin TW, Gerdes AJ, Parker RG (1978) Fast neutron and mixed (neutron/photon) beam teletherapy for grades III and IV astrocytomas. Cancer 42: 96–103

Laukkanen E, Klonoff H, Allan B, Graeb D, Murray N (1988) The role of prophylactic brain irradiation in limited stage small cell lung cancer: clinical, neuropsychologic, and CT sequale. Int J Radiat Oncol Biol Phys 14: 1109–1117

Lechevalier B, Humeau F, Houteville JP (1973) Myélopathies radiothérapiques hypertrophiantes. A propos de cinq observations dent une anatomoclinique. Rev Neurol (Paris) 129: 119–132

Lee JS, Umsawasdi T, Lee YY, Barkley HT Jr, Murphy

WK, Welch S, Valdivieso M (1986) Neurotoxicity in long term survivors of small cell lung cancer. Int J Radiat Oncol Biol Phys 12: 313–321

Lee JS, Sheer DE, Valdivieso M et al. (1988) Longterm effects of brain irradiation (B-XRT) and chemotherapy (chemo) on neuropsychologic performance (NP) of patients with lung cancer (ca). Proceedings of the seventy-ninth annual meeting of the AACR, vol. 29: No. 867

Lhermitte J (1929) Multiple sclerosis. The sensation of an electrical discharge as an early symptom. Arch Neurol Psych 22: 5–8

Li FP, Winston KR, Gimbrere K (1984) Follow-up of children with brain tumors. Cancer 54: 135–138

Licciardello JTW, Cersosimo RJ, Karp DD, Hoffer SM, Paquette-Tello DA, Hong WK (1985) Disturbing central nervous system complications following combination chemotherapy and prophylactic whole-brain irradiation in patients with small cell lung cancer. Cancer Treat Rep 69: 1429–1430

Lierse W, Franke HD (1970) Ultrastrukturelle Veränderungen am Gehirn des Meerschweinchens und der Ratte während der Latenzzeit der Strahlenreaktion. Fortschr Roentgenstr 112: 151–168

Lindgren M (1958) On tolerance of brain tissue and sensitivity of brain tumors to irradiation. Acta Radiol [Suppl] 170: 1–73

Looper JD, Einhorn LH, Garcia SA, Hornback NB, Vincent B, Williams SD (1984) Severe neurologic problems following successful therapy for small cell lung cancer. Proc Am Soc Clin Oncol 3: C–903

Maier JG, Perry RH, Saylor W, Sulak MN (1969) Radiation myelitis of the dorsolumbar spinal cord. Radiology 93: 153–160

Marks JE, Baglan RJ, Prassad SC, Blank WF (1981) Cerebral radionecrosis: incidence and risk in relation to dose, time, fractionation and volume. Int J Radiat Oncol Biol Phys 7: 243–252

Martins AN, Johnston JS, Henry JM, Stoffel TJ, DiChiro G (1977) Delayed radiation necrosis of the brain. J Neurosurg 47: 336–345

Mikhael MA (1978) Radiation necroses of the brain: correlation between computed tomography, pathology, and dose of radiation. J Comput Assist Tomogr 2: 71–80

Mikhael MA (1979) Delayed radiation necrosis of a spinal nerve root presenting as an intra-spinal mass. Br J Radiol 52: 905–910

Mikhael MA (1980) Dosimetric considerations in the diagnosis of radiation necrosis of the brain. In: Gilbert HA, Kagan AR (eds) Radiation damage to the nervous system. Raven, New York, pp 59–91

Nagase T, Tanaka Y, Wada T, Fujimaki T (1973) Tolerance dose of the spinal cord on radiation myelopathy. Keio J Med 22: 109–122

Ostertag CB, Weigel K, Mundinger F (1981) Computertomographische Verlaufskontrollen nach Hirntumor-Bestrahlung. In: Wannenmacher M (ed) Kombinierte chirurgische und radiologische Therapie maligner Tumoren. Urban & Schwarzenberg, Munich, pp 119–124

Pallis CA, Louis S, Morgan RL (1961) Radiation myelopathy. Brain 84: 460–479

Palmer JJ (1972) Radiation myelopathy. Brain 95: 109–122

Parker D, Malpas JS, Sandland R, Sheaff PC, Freeman JE, Paxton A (1978) Outlook following "somnolence syndrome" after prophylactie cranial irradiation. Br Med J 4: 554

Peylan-Ramu N, Poplack DG, Pizzo PA, Adornato BT, DiChiro G (1978) Abnormal CT scans of the brain in asymptomatic children with acute lymphocytic leukemia after prophylactic treatment to the central nervous system with radiation and intrathecal chemotherapy. N Engl J Med 298: 815–818

Phillips TL, Fu KK (1976) Quantification of combined radiation therapy and chemotherapy effects on critical normal tissues. Cancer 37: 1186–1200

Piscol K (1972) Die Blutversorgung des Rückenmarks und ihre klinische Relevanz. Schriftenreihe Neurologie. Springer, Berlin Heidelberg New York

Price RA (1979) Histopathology of CNS leukemia and complications of therapy. Am J Pediatr Hemat Oncol 1: 21–30

Price RA, Jamieson PA (1975) The central nervous system in childhood leukemia. II. Subacute leukoencephalopathy. Cancer 35: 306–318

Rauhut F, Clar HE, Bamberg M, Benker G, Grote W (1986) Diagnostic criteria in pituitary tumours' recurrence – combined modality of surgery and radiotherapy. Acta Neurochir (wien) 80: 73–78

Reinhold HS, Kaalen JG, Unger-Gils K (1976) Radiation myelopathy of the thoracic spinal cord. Int J Radiat Oncol Biol Phys 1: 651–657

Richards GE, Warw WM, Grumbach MM, Kaplan SL, Sheline GE, Conte FA (1976) Delayed onset of hypopituitarism: sequelae of therapeutic irradiation of central nervous system, eye, and middle ear tumors. J Pediatr 89: 553–559

Rider WD (1963) Radiation damage to the brain-a new syndrome. J Can Assoc Radiol 14: 67–69

Rosen G, Marcove RC, Caparros B, Nirenberg A, Kosloff C, Huvos AG (1979) Primary osteogenic sarcoma: the rationale for preoperative chemotherapy and delayed surgery. Cancer 43: 2163–2177

Rubinstein LJ, Herman MM, Long TF, Wilbur JR (1975) Disseminated necrotizing leukoencephalopathy; a complication of treated central nervous system leukemia and lymphoma. Cancer 35: 291–305

Salazar OM, Rubin P, McDonald JV, Feldstein ML (1976) High dose radiation therapy in the treatment of glioblastoma multiforme: a preliminary report. Int J Radiat Oncol Biol Phys 1: 717–727

Samaan NA, Bakdash MM, Caderao JB, Cangir A, Jesse RH, Ballatyne AJ (1975) Hypopituitarism after external irradiation. Evidence for both hypothalamic and pituitary origin. Ann Intern Med 83: 771–777

Scholz W (1934) Experimentelle Untersuchungen über die Einwirkung von Röntgenstrahlen auf das reife Hirn. Z Neurol Psychiatr 150: 765–785

Scholz W, Hsü YK (1938) Late damage from roentgen irradiation of the human brain. Arch Neurol Psychiatr 40: 928–936

Schultheiss TE, Higgins EM, El-Mahdi AM (1984) The latent period in clinical radiation myelopathy. Int J Radiat Oncol Biol Phys 10: 1109–1115

Schultheiss TE, Stephens LC, Peters LJ (1986) Survival in radiation myelopathy. Int J Radiat Oncol Biol Phys 12: 1765–1769

Schümmelfelder N (1959) Beitrag zur Strahlengefährdung des Rückenmarks. Zentralbl Allg Pathol 100: 360

Shalet SM (1982) Growth and hormonal status of children treated for brain tumors. Childs Brain 9: 284–293

Shalet SM, MacFarlane IA, Beardwell CG (1979) Radiation-induced hyperprolactinemia in a treated acromegaly. Clin Endocrinol 11: 169–171

Sheline GE (1981) Pituitary tumors: radiation therapy. In: Beardwell C, Robertson GL (eds) The pituitary. Butterworth, London, pp 106–139

Sheline GE, Wara WM, Smith V (1980) Therapeutic irradiation and brain injury. Int J Radiat Oncol Biol Phys 6: 1215–1228

Shukovsky LJ, Fletcher GH (1972) Retinal and optic nerve complications in a high dose irradiation technique of ethmoid sinus and nasal cavity. Radiology 104: 629–634

Sinner W (1964) Strahlenspätschäden des Rückenmarks. Strahlentherapie 125: 219–238

Soni SS, Marten GW, Pitner SE, Duenas DA, Powazek M (1975) Effects of central-nervous-system irradiation on neuropsychologic functioning of children with acute lymphocytic leukemia. N Engl J Med 293: 113–118

Spiess H (1970) Die Schädigung des Nervensystems durch ionisierende Strahlen. Ther Umsch 27: 379–386

Stoll B, Andrews JT (1966) Radiation induced peripheral neuropathy. Br Med J I: 834–837

Strandqvist M (1944) Studien über die kumulative Wirkung der Röntgenstrahlen bei Fraktionierung. Erfahrungen aus dem Radiumhemmet an 280 Haut- und Lippenkarzinomen. Acta Radiol [Suppl] 55

Szikla G, Betti O, Blond S (1979) Data on late reactions following stereotactic irradiation of gliomas. In: Szikla G (ed) Proc Inserm-Symposium on stercotactic irradiations Nr 12. Elsevier, Amsterdam, pp 167–174

van der Kogel AJ (1979) Late effects of radiation on the spinal cord. Publication of the Radiobiological Institute, TNO Rijswijk, The Netherlands, pp 118–121

van der Kogel AJ, Barendsen GW (1974) Late effects of spinal cord irradiation with 300 kV x-rays and 15 meV neutrons. Br J Radiol 47: 393–398

van der Kogel AJ, Sissingh HA (1985) Effects of intrathecal methotrexate and cytosine arabinoside on the radiation. Radiother Oncol 4: 239–251

van der Schueren E (1989) Tolerance of the central nervous system: biological basis, clinical application and legal implications. Int J Radiat Oncol Biol Phys (in press)

Vick NA, Khandekar JD, Bigner DD (1977) Chemotherapy of brain tumors. The "blood-brain barrier" is not a factor. Arch Neurol 34: 523–526

Walther B, Gutjahr P (1982) Development after treatment of cerebellar medulloblastoma in childhood. In: Voth D, Gutjahr P, Langmaid C (eds) Tumours of the central nervous system. Springer, Berlin Heidelberg New York, pp 389–398

Wara WM, Phillips TL, Sheline GE, Schwade JG (1975) Radiation tolerance of the spinal cord. Cancer 35: 1558–1562

Westling P, Svensson H, Hele P (1972) Cervical plexus lesions following postoperative radiation therapy of mammary carcinoma. Acta Radiol (Ther) 11: 209–216

White A, Hornsey S (1978) Radiation damage to the rat spinal cord: the effect of single and fractionated doses of x-rays. Br J Radiol 51: 515–523

Wigg DR, Koschel K, Hodgson GS (1981) Tolerance of the mature human central nervous system to photon irradiation. Br Radiol 54: 787–798

Wilson GH, Byfield J, Nanafee WN (1972) Atrophy following radiotherapy for central nervous system neoplasms. Acta Radiol (Ther) 11: 361–368

Zeman W (1964) Strahlenschäden des Nervensystems. Arch Psychiatr Neurol 206: 185–198

Zeman W (1968) The effects of atomic radiation. In: Minckler J (ed) Pathology of the nervous system, vol I. McGraw-Hill, New York, pp 764–839

Zeman W, Shidnia H (1976) Post-therapeutic radiation injuries of the nervous system. Reflections on their prevention. J Neurol 212: 107–115

Zülch KJ (1963) Morphologische Veränderungen an Geschwülsten nach Bestrahlung und Schädigungsmöglichkeit am normalen Hirn. Strahlentherapie 52 [Suppl]: 47–62

8 Vasculoconnective Tissue

H.S. Reinhold, J.W. Hopewell, W. Calvo, A. Keyeux, and H. Reyners

CONTENTS

8.1 Introduction

The irradiation of tissues with therapeutic doses of x-rays can result in the occurrence of acute, early, and/or late effects. This was initially recognized

H.S. Reinhold, M.D., Erasmus University and TNO Radiobiological Institute, Lange Kleiweg 151, P.O. Box 5815, 2280 GJ Rijswijk, The Netherlands

J.W. Hopewell, Ph.D., Research Institute, University of Oxford, Oxford, United Kingdom

W. Calvo, M.D., Abteilung für Klinische Physiologie, Universität Ulm, Oberer Eselsberg, 7900 Ulm, FRG

A. Keyeux, M.D., Unité de Radiobiologie, UCL, Brussels, Belgium

H. Reyners, Ph.D., Department de Radiobiologie, CEN/SCK, Mol, Belgium

before the turn of this century. While the acute and early effects of radiation manifest themselves mainly as reactions of the skin, and could be evaluated by visual inspection, the study of the origin of the late effects was, in early times, only possible through histological observations. Surprisingly, since the early observations by Gassmann (1899), Mühsam (1904), and Wolbach (1909) that the blood vessels in irradiated tissues show specific changes, a general consensus seems to have developed among radiation pathologists that blood vessels are sensitive to radiation. Later a hypothesis was proposed that blood vessels were the most likely candidate for dose-limiting late normal responses (Rubin and Casarett 1968). Of course, since the beginning of the use of x-rays either for diagnosis or therapy, the observations on radiation-induced effects in the various tissues and the multitude of changes of the blood vessels in these tissues have been repeatedly reported. The essence of the accumulated knowledge on radiopathology has recently been reviewed by Fajardo (1982).

Although histopathology, and more recently electron microscopy, remain important tools for investigations regarding the development of late radiation changes, other methods have in the last few decades contributed significantly to our understanding of the mechanisms involved and of the consequences for tissue function. These methods include physiological testing, biochemistry, and cell kinetic studies. The idea that the vascular system is the main target for radiation-induced damage to the tissues, a hypothesis mainly conceived by Rubin and Casarett (1968), has recently and rightly been challenged by Withers et al. (1980). These authors believe that radiation damage to parenchymal cells is instrumental in causing late radiation damage. However, the stroma, containing the blood vessels, and the parenchyma of the tissues are morphologically and physiologically so intimately interdependent that the damage induced to one initiates a corresponding effect on the other. This chapter will, of necessity, not deal with the effects of radiation on the various parenchymal cell types, but will concentrate upon the effects of irradiation on the vascular system and the stroma.

8.2 The Vessel Wall Lining

8.2.1 Endothelial Cell Survival

The fact that endothelial cells may be affected by irradiation has been recognized since 1899, when GASSMANN published his findings on the histology of two cases of x-ray-induced ulceration. This damage had been inflicted in one case by the diagnostic use of x-rays and in the other after an attempt, with repeated radiation doses, to treat sciatica. GASSMANN was particularly impressed by the vacuolar degeneration of the tunica intima of the arteries in the vicinity of the radiation-induced ulcer. In the following years, these findings were confirmed by many pathologists. However, experimental investigations into radiation effects on the vasculature were not performed until the late 1920s. On the basis of a series of investigations into the effects of radium irradiation on the repair of wounds of the skin of rats, TAKAHASHI (1930) concluded that newly developed capillaries were very radiosensitive. These investigations were performed using histological methods without any attempt at quantitative analysis.

With the development of radiobiological knowledge it became clear that the level of cell survival in the critical tissue component was of paramount importance for the understanding of tissue tolerance for doses in the therapeutic range. This included the determination of the parameters of cell survival of the constituents of the blood vessel walls. The first attempt directed along these lines was made by VAN DEN BRENK (1959). He performed a partially descriptive, partially quantitative investigation into the effects of radiation on the vasculature using the rabbit ear chamber. In these experiments the endpoint was the linear growth ratio of the regenerating repair blastema, which contains growing capillary sprouts. The repair rate was followed over several months, and afterwards VAN DEN BRENK concluded that "regenerating vascular endothelium, despite its wide spectrum of radiosensitivity in vivo, possesses great powers of recovery from radiation damage."

In these early experiments endothelial cell survival was probably not measured directly, but rather the combined effects of radiation-induced cell kill with subsequent recovery were assessed.

Several years later, HOPEWELL and PATTERSON (1972) again investigated the effects of radiation on the integrity of the vascular system, by evaluating the changes in the development of capillary loops after the application of free skin grafts in the upper layers of the skin of the pig. It may be appropriate at this point to discuss the requirements for an assay for assessing endothelial cell survival. A cell is being defined as surviving after irradiation if this cell is capable of producing a progeny of at least 50 daughter cells, a clone. In order to do so, especially for the endothelium, the cells must proliferate after irradiation in order to demonstrate their clonogenic potential. In an in vivo situation, this means that some form of proliferative stimulus has to be applied to the capillary bed chosen to investigate the radiation sensitivity of endothelial cells. In the case of the rabbit ear chamber experiments carried out by VAN DEN BRENK, this stimulus was the natural tendency of the vasculature of the rabbit ear to cover denuded areas by means of vascular proliferation. In the case of the pig skin experiments by HOPEWELL and PATTERSON the stimulus was the revascularization of a (surgically transposed) free skin graft. In such studies, in addition to the radiation dose, two other important parameters influence the outcome of the assay. The first is the time between irradiation and the induction of cell proliferation, i.e., the time available for additional repair. The second parameter is the time between the application of the stimulus and the moment of assay. This represents the time allotted to fully develop a colony, or its equivalent. The fact that the survival curves obtained from the studies by VAN DEN BRENK and by HOPEWELL and PATTERSON show a radioresistant endothelial cell population (Fig. 8.1, upper panel) may be explained by a combination of these two factors. The curve obtained by REINHOLD and BUISMAN (1975), plotted in the same diagram, in which the time between irradiation and assay was 32 days, also shows a tendency towards a radiation-resistant cell population. This is in line with the assumption that increased repair may take place if there is enough time between radiation and application of the proliferative stimulus.

In addition to the aforementioned approaches another group of in vivo determinations should be

Fig. 8.1. Diagram of the published survival curves for endothelium. *Upper panel: A*, ratio of growth of sprouts in the rabbit ear chamber (VAN DEN BRENK 1959); *B*, capillary loops in pig skin (HOPEWELL and PATTERSON 1972); *C*, relative vascular index in rat skin (REINHOLD and BUISMAN 1975). *Middle panel: D*, macrocolonies in the Selye pouch, rat (VAN DEN BRENK 1974b); *E*, relative vascular index in rat skin (REINHOLD and BUISMAN 1973); *F*, quantitative histology, dog cornea (FIKE and GILLETTE 1978). *Lower panel: G*, in vitro mouse kidney endothelial cells (NIAS 1974); *H*, in vitro human umbilical vein endothelial cells (DeGOWIN ET AL. 1976); *I*, in vitro bovine aorta endothelial cells (JOHNSON et al. 1982); *J*, in vitro bovine pulmonary artery endothelial cells (KWOCK et al. 1982); *K*, in vitro rabbit aorta endothelial cells (MARTIN and FISCHER 1984); *L*, in vitro pig aorta endothelial cells (PENHALIGON and LAVERICK 1985); *M*, in vitro pig brain endothelial cells (PENHALIGON and LAVERICK 1985); *N*, in vitro bovine aorta endothelial cells (RHEE and SONG 1986); *O*, in vitro human umbilical vein endothelial cells (HEI et al. 1987)

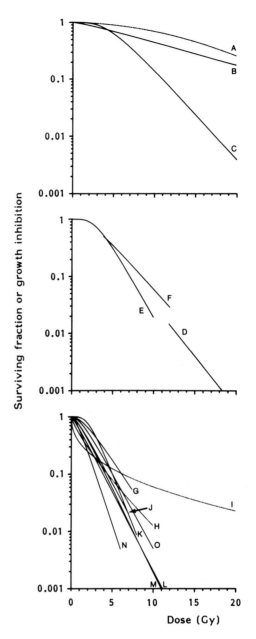

mentioned. These are shown in the middle panel of Fig. 8.1. These methods score the vascular proliferation achieved over a period of 1–2 weeks, proliferation taking place in either a capillary-free area or in an area depleted of capillaries. GILLETTE et al. (1975), FIKE and GILLETTE (1978), and FIKE et al. (1979) used the de-epithelialized cornea in the dog, VAN DEN BRENK (1974a,b) the Selye granuloma pouch of the rat skin, and REINHOLD and BUISMAN (1973) a frozen area of the rat subcutis. The assay system used by VAN DEN BRENK involved the counting of vascular macrocolonies, while the dog cornea and the rat subcutis morphometric methods employed reflected the vascular volume or surface area. In vivo, endothelial cells can be recognized as such only when they line a blood vessel. Moreover, endothelial cells tend to form tubular networks of vessels which are connected to the main vascular system of the body. This makes pure colony counting experiments impossible to perform in vivo, which explains the use of alternative endpoints for this purpose in vivo.

Nine different investigations have been published on the determination of endothelial cell survival in vitro. In many instances short-term endothelial cell cultures were used, and frequently the source of the endothelial cells were large blood vessels from which the endothelial cells were released. These vessels include the aorta or pulmonary artery of the ox, rabbit, or pig and the human umbilical vein. Mouse kidney and pig brain

have also served as a source for endothelial cells. In most of the recent investigations endothelial colonies were used as the endpoint, while in some earlier investigations a parameter derived from the fraction of control growth was used. In the two investigations in which this type of endpoint was used (DeGOWIN et at. 1976; JOHNSON et al. 1982) a survival curve that tended to flatten with increasing dose (lower panel of Fig. 8.1) was obtained. The presently accepted linear–quadratic model of cell survival predicts that curves become steeper with increasing dose whereas the multitarget theory would predict a linear increase with dose. When the two flattening curves were excluded, the average D_o value was around 1.5 Gy and the average N approximately 2.6. The various survival curves have been redrawn in the lower panel of Fig. 8.1.

Investigators who have compared the sensitivity of endothelial cells with other cell types constituting the vessel wall have concluded that the endothelial cells are the most rediosensitive (DE-GOWIN et al. 1976; JOHNSON et al. 1982; KWOCK et al. 1982; FISCHER-DZOGA et al. 1984). Therefore, there seems to be some evidence that the endothelial cell is the dose-limiting tissue component, as was suggested initially (GASSMANN 1899), and this has recently been demonstrated quantitatively in the choroid plexus of the irradiated rat brain (CALVO et al. 1987).

When considering the concept of cell survival of endothelial cells after irradiation, the question arises as to the threshold level of survival, i.e., the relative number of endothelial cells required to preserve tissue function. If it is assumed that the dose of x-rays used in the clinic is tolerated by the tissues, then it may be inferred that a dose of 30 × 2 Gy (60 Gy total dose) to the vascular system does not decrease the proportion of surviving cells to below that critical level. Illustrated in Table 8.1 are the expected levels of cell depletion as inferred from the endothelial survival data. These range from about 0.08 to less than 10^5. This difference might be explained by a slow repair process (FIELD et al. 1976), since such a process has been observed in the endothelium (VAN DEN BRENK et al. 1974a,b; REINHOLD and BUISMAN 1975) and may ameliorate considerably the eventual level of endothelial cell depletion. However, this slow repair process may not be generally applicable. In split-dose studies in pig skin, in which the incidence of ischemic dermal necrosis was used as an endpoint, no evidence of any repair other than that attributed to sublethal damage (over 24 h) was seen for interfraction intervals of 25 days (HOPEWELL et al. 1986; VAN DEN AARDWEG et al.

Table 8.1. Some published endothelial survival parameters

Author(s) and year	System	Endpoint	Survival parameters		Estimated survival after 30 × 2 Gy[a]
			N	D_o	
Assays with extended in vivo repair time					
VAN DEN BRENK 1959	Rabbit ear chamber	Ratio of growth of sprouts	–	–	–
HOPEWELL and PATTERSON 1972	Pig skin	Capillary loops	1.3	10.3	–
REINHOLD and BUISMAN 1975	Rat subcutis	Relative vascular index	6	2.73	–
In vivo assays without repair time					
VAN DEN BRENK 1974b	Rat Selye pouch	Macrocolonies	–	2.40	$<10^{-5}$
REINHOLD and BUISMAN 1975	Rat subcutis	Relative vascular index	7	1.7	0.08
FIKE and GILLETTE 1978	Dog's cornea	Quantitative histology	–	2.65	$<10^{-4}$
In vitro assays	Source of endothelial cells:				
NIAS 1974	Mouse kidney	Colony count	2.3	2	$<10^{-5}$
DeGOWIN et al. 1976	Human umbilical vein	Percentage growth	–	–	$<10^{-4}$
JOHNSON et al. 1982	Bovine aorta	Fraction of control growth	–	–	$<10^{-3}$
KWOCK et al. 1982	Bovine pulmonary artery	Colony count	1.6	1.61	$<10^{-5}$
MARTIN and FISCHER 1984	Rabbit aorta	Colony count	7	1.2	$<10^{-5}$
PENHALIGON and LAVERICK 1985	Pig aorta	Colony count	1.21	1.57	$<10^{-5}$
	Pig brain	Colony count	1.74	1.47	$<10^{-5}$
RHEE and SONG 1986	Bovine aorta	Colony count	1.9	1.01	$<10^{-5}$
HEI et al. 1987	Human umbilical vein	Colony count	2.2	1.65	$<10^{-5}$

[a] The value "$<10^{-5}$" may range from 10^{-5} to 10^{-14}.

1987). Similar findings have been made in other late-responding tissues, where vascular damage may be a contributing factor (VAN DEN AARDWEG et al. 1987). However, even if one accepts, on the basis of cell survival determinations for the endothelium, a conservative estimate of a remaining proportion of functional cells of 10^{-1}, this would still be unacceptably low for the maintenance of tissue integrity. It is difficult to envisage that even with only one in ten endothelial cells surviving that the tissue could sustain any trauma. Probably in such situations the remaining radiation-damaged endothelial cells may still be capable of one or two divisions before dying. Moreover, after irradiation, the remaining endothelial cells have been shown to be able to spread to cover a larger area of the vessel wall (NARAYAN and CLIFF 1982). It is probably because of these mechanisms that the blood vessel wall in many organs, like the CNS, is able to maintain its integrity over prolonged periods after irradiation. Abnormal proliferation of surviving endothelial cells may be the predominant factor influencing the degeneration of the capillary bed after irradiation (HOPEWELL 1974).

8.2.2 Endothelial Cell Depletion

If a radiation-sterilized cell attempts to divide, it will die either at the first or at one of the subsequent divisions. This would imply that one can expect to find, at some time after irradiation, blood vessels with a decreased number of endothelial cells, provided of course that these blood vessels remain patent. The first authors to observe a decrease in the number of endothelial cell nuclei in the endothelial lining of blood vessels were CAVENESS et al. (1974). They irradiated the right visual cortex in brains of monkeys with a single dose of 35 Gy. In the majority of animals an abrupt brain swelling developed many weeks after irradiation, and this was accompanied by neurological signs. Some monkeys were killed after the injection of Evans blue. This dye, which does not normally cross the blood–brain barrier, was shown to stain the brain tissue in irradiated areas, indicating permeability changes. Histological examination showed that the earliest recognizable change was a decrease in the number of endothelial cells in the blood vessels. CALVO et al. (1986, 1987), who have studied the choroid plexus of the rat brain, also found a decreased number of endothelial cells in the blood vessels with time

after irradiation. The degree of endothelial cell depletion was dose dependent in the dose range of 17.5–25 Gy. This was accompanied by signs of an attempt by the endothelial lining to regenerate. However, the endothelial cell density remained at about half the normal value for a period of up to a year after irradiation, which was the longest observation period. In this context it is of importance to note that the decrease in the endothelial cell density was greater, and more obviously dose related, than that of the epithelial cells covering the choroid plexus. The latter showed hardly any decrease in number.

In organs other than the central nervous system (CNS), similar observations have been made. FAJARDO and STEWART (1973) found a decreased capillary density in the irradiated rabbit heart. HIRST et al. (1979) selectively irradiated the mesentery of the mouse and analyzed, among other things, changes in the cellularity of the arterioles from histological sections. Doses of 20, 30, and 45 Gy were used and the authors observed a dose dependent depletion of endothelial cells in the arteriolar wall, the initial decrease being observed at 3–6 months. This was followed by recovery to close to normal values at 12 months. However, a second phase of endothelial cell depletion was then seen, reaching its lowest levels at 18 months, i.e., the duration of the observation period. NARAYAN and CLIFF (1982) irradiated the rabbit ear chamber with a dose of 75 Gy and followed the subsequent sequence of events for 54 days by direct and electron microscopic observations. They observed a spreading of endothelial cells in the venules, which was interpreted as an attempt to cover denuded sites. The average surface area of an irradiated venular endothelial cell increased to about three times that of the average area of an unirradiated cell. The same phenomenon did not take place in arterioles and there was no change in permeability to fluorescein-labelled albumin, as investigated by fluorescence microscopy. In the late phase the endothelium had disappeared completely from some sites, exposing the vascular basement membrane. However, there were no signs of platelet aggregation or thrombosis. Extrapolation of effects seen after such high doses to those that might occur after doses in the therapeutic range is difficult.

In quantitative morphological studies on the microvasculature of the skin (ARCHAMBEAU et al. 1984, 1985) after doses between 16 and 26 Gy, it was concluded that a second wave of skin breakdown, occurring between 36 and 70 days after irradiation in the Yorkshire pig, was the result of the loss of endothelial cells from the vessels of the papillary plexus. Over the first wave epithelial reaction of the skin the endothelial cell density had remained at control levels and it was not until 5 weeks after irradiation that increased endothelial cell pyknosis and loss of endothelial cells was observed. A parameter called the "endothelial cell separation index," which was derived on a morphometric basis and describes the length of the vessel circumference divided by the endothelial cell count, provided an arbitrary estimate of the distance between endothelial cells. With x-ray doses of more than 22 Gy to pig skin and for observation periods longer than 4–5 weeks, the separation could be increased to 16 times the normal value. This preceded dermal necrosis. There was also a continuous increase in the vessel diameter before the development of necrosis. While such changes in the relatively well vascularized papillary plexus of pig skin (YOUNG and HOPEWELL 1983) may precede ischemic dermal necrosis, they are unlikely to be the predominant cause of necrosis. This was deduced from a recent comparison of the radiation response of pig skin to β-emitters of varying energy (HOPEWELL 1986). The vessels at the level of the deep dermal plexus appeared to be the primary target; damage to this structure produced necrosis. The differential irradiation of the vessels of the papillary plexus did not induce necrosis, even at very high doses. The abnormal rate of proliferation of surviving endothelial cells in the vessels in the deep dermal plexus was thus apparently the major cause of damage, not simply endothelial cell depletion. In the rat lung (VERGARA et al. 1987), the capillary endothelium was decreased to 5%–10% of control values at 26 weeks after a dose of 30 Gy, following an initial decrease to 50%–70% at 12 weeks after irradiation.

Using morphometric techniques, a decrease in the capillary density was observed in the vasculature of the hamster cheek pouch in the first 12 weeks after irradiation with doses of ≥15 Gy (HOPEWELL et al. 1989), doses comparable with those used by ARCHAMBEAU et al. (1985) in pig skin. However, as early as 4 weeks after irradiation of the cheek pouch with a single dose of 25 Gy there was a significant reduction in the number of small arterioles, this preceding any reduction in capillary density. A reduction in capillary density has been recorded in the rat heart within 6 weeks of irradiation with 10–25 Gy (LAUK 1987) and

in the rat brain 4–12 months after a dose of 60 Gy (PLOTNIKOVA et al. 1984). Again using morphometric methods in the rabbit ear chamber system, DIMITRIEVICH et al. (1984) derived essentially similar conclusions, although the changes occurred much earlier. The capillary density was decreased 5–8 days after irradiation even with a dose of 2 Gy. The remaining vessels were, on the basis of morphometric calculations, believed to be dilated.

All these investigations indicate that, at some time after irradiation, endothelial cell depletion occurs. In some but not in all the investigations, indications of increased vascular permeability were found. Stretching of endothelial cells was also reported. In some investigations signs of attempted regeneration were encountered, with the atypical proliferation of cells leading to the occlusion of some vessels. The loss of endothelial cells may lead to a decrease in the number of endothelial cells covering the blood vessel wall. It may also be an additional cause of the direct or indirect disappearance of blood vessels. This holds particularly for the capillaries, although the primary effect may not necessarily be on these vessels. The result is a decrease in capillary density, which is a common finding. However, at this point morphometric and other methods used to evaluate radiation damage to blood vessels become difficult to interpret, because inevitably the surrounding parenchyma or stroma also becomes atrophic. In such tissues in which more factors have changed, the value of capillary density as a direct index of vascular damage is misleading.

8.2.3 Proliferation of Cells of Blood Vessel Walls

The turnover time of endothelial cells in various normal tissues and organs is slow, i.e., between 47 and 23 000 days (HOBSON and DENEKAMP 1984). The labeling index of endothelial cells in all three main types of blood vessel is low. On the basis of data compiled by HOBSON and DENEKAMP (1984), the following average labeling index for different vessel types was derived:

Arteries and arterioles	0.31%
Veins and venules	0.74%
Capillaries	0.15%

These data represent the average values calculated by HOBSON and DENEKAMP (1984), but also encompass their compilation of six sets of published results. In general, there seems to be little difference in the labeling index of the endothelial cells in various organs. However, the value for the CNS may be rather lower and that of bone somewhat higher than the average [compilation by TANNOCK and HAYASHI (1972) and REINHOLD (1974)]. The only clear exception is the value published by ADAMSON and BOWDEN (1983) for the mouse lung. Here the labeling index was 23% in unirradiated mice. This value rose to 55% 10 days after irradiation with a whole-body dose of 6.5 Gy. No explanation was offered as to the cause of these incredibly high labeling index values.

There have been some attempts to determine whether the cell proliferation rate of endothelial cells changes, or rather increases, with time after irradiation. FAJARDO and STEWART (1971) were the first to investigate this issue. At approximately 1 month after a dose of 20 Gy they observed, in the endothelium of the rabbit myocardium, that the labeling indices had increased from a normal value of 0.5% to 1.8%. However, the labeling indices had returned to a normal value of 0.2% by 3 months after irradiation. In the hamster cheek pouch a 5- to 30-fold increase in the labeling index was also observed 3–4 months after ≥20 Gy. The distribution of these labeled cells was very heterogeneous (HOPEWELL et al. 1986). Apart from the aforementioned data and the data by HIRST et al., to be discussed below, no other data are available to indicate an increase in labeling index in other organs. In investigations of cell proliferation in the rat brain (CALVO, personal communication), the proportion of labeled oligodendrocytes and endothelial cells in the cortex and corpus callosum of unirradiated animals was low (≃1%) and was unchanged in brains irradiated 15 months previously with a dose of 20 Gy. TANNOCK and HAYASHI (1972) irradiated the mouse leg with doses of 20 and 40 Gy and found no increase in the labeling index of the endothelial cells in muscle, skin, and bone over a period of 3 weeks after irradiation with 20 Gy or of 2 weeks after 40 Gy. These were relatively early times after irradiation for changes to be seen.

HIRST et al. (1980) found no significant increase in the endothelial proliferation of the mesenteric arterioles of mice at 12 and 48 weeks after doses of 20 and 45 Gy, but they did find a slight transient increase at 3 weeks. No significant change could be observed in smooth muscle cells at any time after irradiation. These authors attempted to compare the pattern of cell depletion in the arterioles with the data on cell proliferation. They concluded that the cell depletion (expressed as the relative change in endothelial cell number) came much earlier than would be expected for a slowly proliferating cell population, i.e., assuming that all the cells were cycling very slowly. The early cell depletion they found was, on the other hand, consistent with cell death resulting from proliferation of a small proportion of the cells with a shorter cycle time. In view of the fact that the repopulation of the endothelial cells between 9 and 12 months was not accompanied by a rise in the fraction of labeled cells, the authors considered the possibility that this repopulation may have originated from the migration of endothelial cells from elsewhere in the body. Two other studies are worthy of mention. One by FISCHER (1982) showed no increase in the labeling index in the rat aorta for periods as long as 15 weeks after radiation with doses between 5 and 20 Gy. The other study involved the investigation of the proliferation kinetics of the mouse bladder after irradiation (STEWART et al. 1980). It was found that a single dose of 25 Gy resulted in a compensatory proliferation of the bladder epithelium, but only from 6 months to the end of the study, at about 2 years. The labeling index of the endothelial cells in the blood vessels of the submucosa was also increased over the same period of time and this was interpreted as being secondary to the mucosa changes rather than a primary increase in endothelial cell proliferation.

In conclusion, many studies do not indicate a substantial increase in the labeling index of endothelial cells, which might be expected if doomed endothelial cells die through wear and tear and require replacement by division of neighboring endothelial cells. On the other hand, the data of FAJARDO and STEWART (1971), HOPEWELL et al. (1986), ADAMSON and BOWDEN (1983), and HIRST et al. (1980) show a trend in that direction. The latter investigators even applied with some success a cell kinetic model for the interpretation of the interaction between endothelial cell depletion and repopulation.

8.3 The Vessel Wall Structure

The blood vessel wall consists of a triple layered structure; this includes for the larger vessels an endothelial lining, the intima, a pericytic and muscular layer, the media, and an external fibroblastic layer, the adventitia. In the capillaries this architecture is reduced to a minimum and even the pericytes are often absent. Blood vessels whose diameter exceeds about 2 mm have in their walls supplying blood vessels for the nutrition of the larger blood vessel wall, the vasa vasorum.

Since the first indication of the reaction of blood vessels to irradiation (GASSMANN 1899), radiation-induced changes have been found after exposure to a variety of dose levels, in virtually all organs in all mammalian species investigated. However, no clear picture has yet emerged about specific differences. Therefore, the structural changes will be described, arranged according to the type of vessel. The sequence of development of late radiation damage is illustrated in Fig. 8.2. This figure is derived from a series of observations from human pathology.

8.3.1 Capillaries

An overview of the morphological changes induced by radiation in the capillaries of the heart, kidney, lung, striated muscle, colon, skin, brain,

and choroid plexus is given in Table 8.2. The literature mentioned in this and subsequent tables corresponds to the earliest *or* to the most important contribution on the subject. Extensive reviews on morphological blood vessel changes have been published by WARREN (1942), ZOLLINGER (1970), ZEMAN and SAMORAJSKI (1971), WHITE

Fig. 8.2. Clinical histopathology of blood vessel changes. Sequence of some typical changes after radiation therapy in capillaries, arteries, and veins. *Upper row*: No irradiation; normal, thin-walled capillary with flat endothelium. *Middle row*: About ½ year after irradiation: example of a capillary with a necrotic vessel wall of the type that may be found in scattered locations in irradiated tissue. The lumen of the capillary on the left is obliterated by fibrin. Only sporadic cell nuclei are present in the vessel wall. There are no obvious changes in the arteries and veins. *Lower row*: About 1 year after irradiation: dilated capillaries; irregular structure of the vessel wall; pyknotic endothelial nuclei. The artery shows, beside some hyalinization, a lumen that is obviously narrowed through proliferation of the intima. The figure is composed of histological sections (Prof. A.J.M. van Unnik) of the larynx of patients treated with radiation therapy (except in the upper row), followed by surgery. Illustrations by Mr. J.P. de Kler. (Modified after REINHOLD 1974)

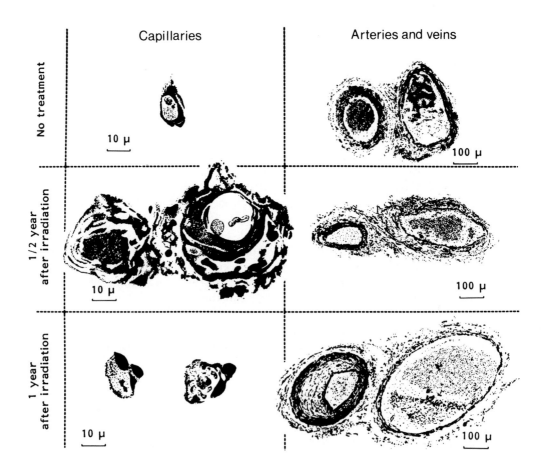

Table 8.2. Summary of the morphological changes produced by radiation in the capillaries of normal tissues

Organ, species	Radiation dose	Observations	Reference
Heart, human	10 × 2 Sabourauds	Thickening, tortuosity, abundant EC nuclei. Platelet thrombi. 2 years	SCHWEIZER 1924
Heart, human	30–98 Gy	EC proliferation in 6 of 12 cases. 6th–60th month	STEWART et al. 1967
Heart, mouse	20–40 Gy, SD	Mural thrombosis without pericardial fibrosis, 6th month	BROWN et al. 1973
Heart, rabbit	20 Gy, SD	EC swelling, reduction of lumen, 28th day; platelet thrombi, 30th day; loss of capillaries, 70th day	FAJARDO and STEWART 1973
Heart, rat	10–20 Gy. SD	Decreased capillary density. Myocardial degeneration. Little fibrosis, 1 year	TROTT 1984
Kidney, mouse	6 Gy, TBI	Premature glomerular sclerotic changes	COTTIER 1961
Kidney, human	30 Gy, FD	EC swelling, vacuolation. Nuclear pleomorphism. Obliteration of glomerular vessels, 7th month	ROSEN et al. 1964
Kidney, human	5200 R	Aneurysms in glomerulus, 4th month	ZOLLINGER 1970
Kidney, mouse	20–50 Gy, FD	Focal EC swelling and detachment from basement membrane at 1 month. Thrombosis at 9th month	FAJARDO et al. 1976
Lung, rat	20 Gy, SD	EC injury, 5th day, followed by loss of vessels	PHILLIPS 1966
Lung, mouse	6.5 Gy, TBI, SD	Focal vacuolation of EC's, 5th day. Subsequent occlusion and recanalization. Platelet thrombi, 14 day	ADAMSON and BOWDEN 1983
Lung, mouse	2000 R, SD	Edema, patchy EC enlargement, 6 h. Clusters of platelets attached to disrupted EC	MAISIN 1970
Muscle, human	3500 R	Multinucleated giant EC's 10 days after radiation	ZOLLINGER 1970
Colon. human	50–60 Gy	Telangiectasia with bizarre EC nuclei, 3 months	RUBIN and CASARETT 1968
Skin, human	50 Gy	Telangiectasia. Nuclear enlargement, 2 years	FAJARDO 1982
Skin, pig	23 Gy, SD	Abrupt EC density decrease to 50% of control, 24th day	ARCHAMBEAU et al. 1984
Ear, rabbit	10 Gy, SD	25% reduction in length, 30th day	DIMITRIEVICH and FISCHER-DZOGA 1983
Ear, rabbit	75 Gy, β-rays	Vasodilatation, loss of vasomotion within hours. Loss of vessels, 2nd week EC loss, 2nd month	NARAYAN and CLIFF 1982
Choroid plexus, rat	17.5–25 Gy, SD	Reduction in number of EC's and fibrosis, 12th week	CALVO et al. 1986

SD, single dose; FD, fractionated dose; EC, endothelial cell; TBI, total body irradiation.

(1975), and FAJARDO (1982). The most immediate change within hours is vasodilation and loss of vasomotion. One of the earliest and most constant cellular reactions in all tissues is the swelling and vacuolation of the cytoplasm of endothelial cells. Their nuclei become hyperchromatic and pyknotic or enlarged and pale and show prominent nucleoli. Bizarre and multinucleated cells have also been found within a few days, especially in the lung. Clusters of platelets attach to damaged endothelial cell sites and interrupt the blood flow in some vessels. Within a few weeks, a loss of endothelial nuclei can be observed, with a reduction in the number and length of the capillaries and occlusive changes (Fig. 8.2).

Late effects can be observed months or years after irradiation and are characterized by telangiectasia, recanalization, and proliferation of endothelial cells, alternating with long lengths of nonnucleated endothelium. Degenerative and regenerative processes become concomitant and fibrosis takes place.

8.3.2 Arteries

The structural changes in the arteries are summarized in Table 8.3. Edema of the intima and thrombosis have been found within 2 weeks and can thus be considered early effects of radiation. However, most of the morphological changes in the arteries appear much later than in the capillaries and are described as intermediate and late effects of radiation. A common finding in the irradiated arteries is myointimal proliferation causing a reduction in the size of the lumen (Fig. 8.2). Vacuolation and loss of muscle fibers can be

observed in the 3rd month. Fibroelastic proliferation of the intima and media, splitting and duplication of elastic fibers, and hyalination appear between 3 and 6 months. The eccentric accumulation of foam cells in the intima, narrowing of the lumina, and atherosclerosis are observed from the 2nd month. Depletion of endothelial cells occurs during the 3rd month, followed sometimes by an abortive recovery at around the 12th month and severe depletion by the 18th month. Stenosis, thrombosis, necrosis, and rupture of arteries are late effects that appear infrequently several years after very high doses of radiation.

Table 8.3. Summary of the morphological changes produced by radiation in the arteries of normal tissues

Organ, species	Radiation dose	Observations	Reference
Skin, human	Unknown	Segmental vacuolation and proliferation of EC's. Vacuolar degeneration and loss of muscle fibers, splitting and reduplication of elastic fibers in ulcerated skin, 3rd month	Gassman 1899
Skin, pig	23.4 Gy, SD	Focal occlusive changes	Hopewell et al. 1978
Uterus, human	40–60 Gy, FD and radium	Subendothelial foam plaques in small arteries, 1–8 months	Sheenan 1944
Ear, rabbit	25–40 Gy, SD	Atherosclerosis in hyperlipemic rabbits, 4th month	Kirkpatrick 1967
Ear, rabbit	75 Gy, β-rays SD	Loss of muscle cells. Absence of vasomotion, 4th month	Narayan and Cliff 1982
Spleen, human	40 Gy	Myointimal proliferation, 5th year	Dailey et al. 1981
Intestine, human	55 Gy	Fibrinoid changes, foam cells, hyalination, loss of muscle cells, 6th month	Berthrong and Fajardo 1981
Enteric submucosa, human	45 Gy	Arteritis and thrombosis	Fajardo 1982
Mesentery, human	50 Gy	Eccentric foam cell accumulation in intima, 60th month	Fajardo and Berthrong 1978
Mesentery, mouse	30 Gy, SD, ^{90}Sr	Depletion of EC's at 3rd month, recovery at 12th month, and severe depletion by 18th month.	Hirst et al. 1979
Aorta, human	30 Gy	Necrosis, 2.5 years	Thomas and Forbus 1959
Aorta, dog	80 Gy, FD	Fibroelastic proliferation of intima and media, 6th month	Gillette et al. 1983
Aorta, rat	25 Gy, FD	Atherosclerosis, including in coronary and pulmonary arteries, 8–15th week	Gold 1961
Coronary, human	44 Gy	Atherosclerosis, narrowing of lumen. Thrombosis, 16 month	Fajardo et al. 1968
Carotid, human	6200 R	Edema of intima. Initial thrombosis, 2nd week.	Zollinger 1970
Carotid, dog	30–225 Gy	Stenosis was rare at doses of 75 Gy (^{125}I) or 30 Gy (^{192}Ir) and increased with higher doses, 1 year	Fee et al. 1987
Carotid, rabbit	5–20 Gy	Thick plaques of lipid-laden foam cells 2 months after 10 Gy x-rays or 5 Gy neutrons in hypercholesterinemic rabbits.	Aarnoudse 1979
Femoral, mouse	10–100 Gy, SD	Dose-dependent quantitative histological changes	El-Naggar et al. 1978
Brain, human	20–60 Gy	Myointimal proliferation 2 years after 20 Gy and 6 months after 55 Gy. Fibrinoid necrosis 18 months after 60 Gy	Fajardo 1982

SD, single dose; FD, fractionated dose; EC, endothelial cell.

8.3.3 Veins

A summary of the morphological changes observed in the veins are listed in Table 8.4. Early changes can be considered to be the pyknosis and necrosis of endothelial cells and the plasmatic insudation that has been observed at 2 weeks. Focal hemorrhages have been observed very early in the brain of mice and burros, as have generalized hemorrhages in the bone marrow of rats. Other changes appear as intermediate or late effects. Veno-occlusive changes appear in the central and sublobular veins of the liver of man and dogs in the period from 1 month to 1 year after irradiation, producing luminal narrowing.

8.3.4 Observation Systems

The belief that damage to the vascular system may be instrumental in causing late radiation effects to normal tissues has prompted a number of investigators to examine the effects of radiation on the microvasculature directly, i.e., with in vivo microscopic methods. However, the accessibility of the vascular bed to microscopic examination is limited. Classical examples of observation systems are the rabbit ear chamber (VAN DEN BRENK 1959; DIMITRIEVICH et al. 1977; 1984; NARAYAN and CLIFF 1982) and the hamster cheek pouch (HOPEWELL 1980). To these may be added the mouse ear lobe (LINDOP et al. 1970) and the rat subcutis observation chamber (YAMAURA et al. 1976). The essence of such systems is that a tissue structure is obtained with an essentially two-dimensional configuration. The tissue should be thin enough for sufficient transillumination. When using observation systems, it should be possible to follow the fate of an entire vascular bed in detail for prolonged periods. However, it has not yet been possible to derive a fully comprehensive picture of the occurrence of vascular changes in such systems, although some useful information has been obtained. The reason for this is that the architecture of most of these vascular beds is not rigid enough to establish the development of changes that take place gradually over long periods.

VAN DEN BRENK (1959) used the rabbit ear chamber to study the regeneration phase of endothelium growth and observed a cessation of the growth of capillaries at the growing edge after irradiation. A fibrous barrier developed, but when

Table 8.4. Summary of the morphological changes produced by radiation in the veins and sinusoids of normal tissues

Organ, species	Radiation dose	Observations	Reference
Skin, human	15 Gy, SD, or 53.4 Gy, FD	Intimal proliferation, obliteration, 42–75 days	WINDHOLZ 1937
Subcutis, human	3400 R, FD	Pykonsis, necrosis of EC's, plasma insudation. Thrombosis, 14th day	ZOLLINGER 1970
Liver, human	30–59 Gy, FD	Veno-occlusive disease, central and sublobular veins, 31 days to 1 year	REED and COX 1966 FAJARDO and COLBY 1980
Liver, human	9.2–13.8 Gy, TBI, cyclophosphamide	Veno-occlusive disease some months after bone marrow transplantation	SHULMAN et al. 1987
Liver, dog	9.2–16 Gy, TBI, SD	Focal veno-occlusive lesions 2 months after irradiation and 125 mg/kg monocrotaline	SHULMAN et al. 1980
Liver, human	Thorotrast	Hemangioendotheliomas after several years	SILVA-HORTA 1967
Spleen, human	40 Gy, FD	Intimal proliferation, marked narrowing, 7 years	DAILEY et al. 1981
Intestine, human	1500–10000 R, FD	Sclerosis, obliteration, splitting, and duplication of elastica, 1 month to 4 years	WARREN and FRIEDMAN 1942
Brain, mice	Unspecified	Focal hemorrhages, 12 h to 66 days	OBERSTEINER 1965
Brain, burro	4.85 Gy, SD	Diffuse subarachnoid hemorrhage and perivascular cuffing, 28 h	BROWN et al. 1962
Bone marrow, rat	800 rep 15 MeV electrons	Damage to sinusoidal wall, hemorrhage, 18–30 h	FLIEDNER et al. 1955
Bone marrow, dog	2.75–6 Gy, SD	Disruption of sinusoids. Nonthrombopenic hemorrhage, 24 h	BOND et al. 1962

SD, single dose; FD, fractionated dose; EC, endothelial cell; TBI, total body irradiation.

this barrier was severed, the regeneration of the capillary bed resumed. Dimitrievich et al. (1977) demonstrated the development of repair sites in the mature microvasculature of the rabbit ear chamber after irradiation. In another study (Dimitrievich et al. 1984) the effects of radiation on such a system were investigated. The small vessels were more sensitive than the larger vessels. Similar conclusions were reached by Nayaran and Cliff (1982).

Using less artificial systems, i.e., the mouse ear lobe (Lindop et al. 1970) and the hamster cheek pouch (Hopewell 1980), a series of interesting findings were obtained. After prolonged periods, i.e., about 1 year after 25 Gy for the mouse ear lobe and after 2–3 months for the hamster cheek pouch, the arteries in both of the aforementioned vascular systems developed a pattern of constrictive changes. These were termed "sausage segments" by Lindop et al. (1970). Very recently the development of plaques in the arteries in the rat tail was observed (Hendry 1987). It seems likely that these "sausage" constrictions, which are visible as irregularly spaced narrowed sites in the image of the blood filling the arteries, are representative of endarteritis. This has frequently been observed in irradiated tissues (Mühsam 1904; Fajardo 1982). Whether or not such local strictures precede the narrowing of the larger arteries, as is seen with human arteriography, remains uncertain.

8.3.5 Telangiectasia

Very soon after x-rays were first used for therapeutic purposes, it was recognized that one of the typical late suquelae of radiation therapy was the widening of vessels, or telangiectasia (Wolbach 1909). Teleangiectases have been described in the skin, in submucosal tissues, in the kidney, and in the CNS. An example of a telangiectatic focus is illustrated in Fig. 8.3. It can be seen that the normal vasculature has been changed into a maze of coarse, widened capillaries, alternating with narrowed vessels. However, it should be realized that such areas of telangiectasia are focal. Sometimes only a single focus can be found in, for example, an entire coronal section of an irradiated rat brain. In addition, the latent period for their development is long. In the aforementioned study the average latent period after a single dose of 20 Gy was about 18 months, with a range between 12 and 24 months (Reinhold and Hopewell 1980). This is in agreement with the observation by Reyners that telangiectatic vessels, to be studied with the electron microscope, could only be found in those irradiated animals which showed signs of terminal deterioration in their condition. The clinical data reported by Turesson and Notter (1986) on the human skin after radiation treatment of carcinoma of the breast indicated an even longer latent period; the length of this period also depended on the fractionation schedule used.

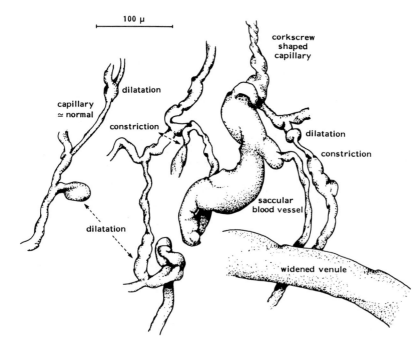

Fig. 8.3. Camera lucida drawing of blood vessel changes in the hippocampus of the brain of an adult WAG/Rij rat, 18 months after a single dose of 20 Gy. This represents a telangiectatic focus

Presently, it is not known how telangiectases develop, even though they have been observed ever since x-rays were first used. To the best of the authors' knowledge, no experiments directed towards the elucidation of their origin have been performed. This leaves us only with a description of the changes and with some hypothetical explanations. These include:

1. Weakening of the vascular envelope, or changes in the surrounding tissue, allowing an expansion of the vessels.
2. Stagnation or altered flow in certain capillaries, caused either by changes in the regulating mechanism of the microflow (spasms) or by the breakdown of downstream capillaries resulting in a ballooning of the capillaries or venules.
3. Proliferation of endothelial cells, resulting in an increased total blood vessel surface. This proliferation may be due to an accumulation of angiogenic factors, either from trapped thrombocytes or as the result of an insufficient functioning of the vascular bed.
4. Increased flow and pulse pressure in capillaries as a result of microvascular shunting, or degeneration of the regulating smooth muscle cell coating of the feeding arterioles.
5. A combination of the above-mentioned factors.

With regard to the properties of telangiectases, two recent observations may be of importance. In the first place, telangiectatic vessels in the irradiated rat brain after a dose of 20 Gy were studied with the electron microscope by REYNERS (unpublished). The following abnormalities were frequently found in animals dying with pathological changes at about 18 months after irradiation. In grossly dilated blood vessels there was extensive thickening of the basement membrane with some lamination, in the absence of any apparent endothelial cell changes. The astrocytes formed a thick layer around the vessels, showing intracellular fibers resembling those of the cytoskeleton. The reinforcement of the astrocyte attachment to the blood vessel wall indicates that reactive astrocytes appear in connection with telangiectatic vessels in the areas at risk in the irradiated rat brain. The most extensive radiation-induced changes were, therefore, apparently not in the endothelial wall but mainly in the basement membrane and the astrocytes (REYNERS, unpublished data). Secondly, in a small series of investigations with a laser-Doppler flux meter on the skin of irradiated patients, the erythrocyte flux

signal over telangiectatic spots was very high, indicating a high flux of erythrocytes in these telangiectases (REINHOLD, unpublished observations).

In conclusion, the development of telangiectases after radiation remains an intriguing phenomenon, with its dependence on fraction size and its progression with time after irradiation.

8.4 The Vascular Function

8.4.1 Endothelial Cell Function

During the last decade a number of investigations have indicated that apart from cell kill, especially of the endothelial cells, a number of other factors may influence endothelial cell function after irradiation. This applies not only to the acute changes in vessel permeability in irradiated skin, as demonstrated by local extravasation of a dye (JOLLES and HARRISON 1966), but also to other functions of the endothelial cell lining. JOLLES and HARRISON (1967) demonstrated that the extent of radiation-induced acute vascular permeability could be decreased by compounds inhibiting proteolytic enzymes. This was confirmed by EASSA and CASARETT (1973), who used ε-amino-n-caproic acid (EACA) for the same purpose.

Recently some investigations have shown that, as an acute effect of radiation, the formation or the response of substances like prostacyclin may be decreased in the endothelium. This was based on studies with the umbilical artery in vitro (ALLEN et al. 1981). On the other hand, prostacyclin production was increased in irradiated bovine aortic endothelial cells grown as a monolayer (RUBIN et al. 1985). This increase in prostacyclin production was dose dependent in bovine pulmonary artery endothelial cells (FRIEDMAN et al. 1986). The latter authors demonstrated that cultured pulmonary endothelial cells synthesize increased amounts of prostacyclin in response to direct radiation exposure, without the need for the presence of other cell types or additional serum components. This may be considered to be an early in vitro response to some kind of radiation-induced stimulus. Other endothelial cell enzymes that have been investigated are 5'-nucleotidase and alkaline phosphatase. VEGT et al. (1985) investigated a number of biochemical changes that take place 1–2 days after a single dose of 20 Gy to cultured endothelial cells isolated from the veins of the human umbilical cord. It appeared that the enzyme 5'-nucleotidase, which is located on the surface of the endothelial cells, was especially increased after irradiation. This would imply a possible inhibition of platelet aggregation and the irradiation therefore does not induce thrombosis because of this effect on 5'-nucleotidase. On the other hand, there is evidence that as a late effect in vivo, that irradiated rat lung may produce increased amounts of prostacyclins. This could be interpreted as an attempt to counteract the long-term effects of radiation-induced hypoperfusion (Ts'AO et al., 1983a). This finding contrasts with an observation by SINZINGER and FIRBAS (1985), who showed that (stimulated) prostacyclin formation was decreased in abdominal aortic segments from the rabbit after irradiation, when compared with unirradiated controls.

Many of these investigations have not included a quantitative analysis of the number of surviving endothelial cells in the various systems. Therefore it is difficult to state whether the reported changes are due to changes in the function of the individual endothelial cells, or, for example, to endothelial cell depletion, possibly compensated for by stretching of the endothelial cytoplasm. Evidence for the latter was obtained by Ts'AO and WARD (1985), who observed that radiation-induced cell loss from a monolayer was compensated for by hypertrophy of surviving cells to preserve the continuity of the monolayer. Using the rat lung as a model, the same group of workers used a series of markers to study radiation effects on the pulmonary vascular system. These included prostacyclin (Ts'AO et al. 1983a), angiotensin-converting enzyme (WARD et al. 1983), plasminogen activator (Ts'AO and WARD 1985), and thromboxane (WARD et al. 1987b). It appeared that the dose–response relationships for these various markers was not identical. The protective effect of treatment with D-penicillamine was lacking for some of the markers, i.e., for angiotensin-converting enzyme and for plasminogen activator (WARD et al. 1987a,b). This can be taken as an indication that other factors (i.e., a decrease in the production of cell products) besides endothelial cell kill may play a role in the development of late radiation damage (WARD et al. 1985).

Recently, a highly interesting observation was made by LAUK (1987). She observed that the alkaline phosphatase activity of capillary endothelial cells in the rat heart showed foci with absence of enzyme activity after doses of 10–25 Gy in otherwise normal looking capillaries. This preceded myocardial degeneration in these foci. This process seemed to be independent of clonogenic cell kill. The appearance of foci of multiple, confluent capillaries with abnormal enzyme activity is presently difficult to explain and intensive further research is required.

An additional important point is the observation that the activity of the fibrinolytic enzymes may be decreased after irradiation (GERBER et al. 1977; HENDERSON et al. 1983). GERBER et al. found this effect in the rat lung, while HENDERSON et al. investigated the livers of dogs. An extensive loss of fibrinolytic activity was found after irradiation, even though loss of the endothelium was not a prominent finding. Therefore, the loss of vascular fibrinolytic activity could not be explained by a loss of the endothelium. This finding rather pointed towards an inhibition of the production of the fibrinolysis-initiating enzyme, i.e., plasminogen activator, which is in keeping with the finding of Ts'AO and WARD (1985) that plasminogen activator was decreased in irradiated rat lung and in cultured aortic endothelial cells. This would support the hypothesis proposed by LAW (1981) that the vascular system may become leaky during the intermediate phase after irradiation, resulting in extravasation of fibrinogen and of clotting factors, and the formation of fibrin in the interstitium. If this fibrin is not removed, it may lead to fibroblast accumulation and the synthesis of collagen. The fact that one of the functions of endothelial cells is the release of plasminogen activator (Ts'AO and WARD 1985) and that this release is specifically inhibited by irradiation (Ts'AO and WARD 1985) provides further support for the hypothesis proposed by LAW (1981). It would imply that fibrin, once it is deposited in the tissues, remains in place due to a depletion of endothelial cells and because the surviving endothelial cells are incapable of releasing sufficient plasminogen activator. However, no explanation has yet been offered as to the cause of the leaky vascular barrier, unless one assumes that temporary defects develop when doomed endothelial cells attempt division and die, leaving a deficient vascular barrier before the defect is repaired.

8.4.2 Blood Flow and Permeability; General Principles

For nonexchange blood vessels, the concept of flow is adequately related to blood pressure and vascular resistance. For exchanging vessels in the microcirculation the blood flow is controlled by the capacity of a substance (acting as an indicator) to leave or to enter the blood by crossing, without any significant restriction, the vascular wall and to disperse in an infinite extravascular space. However, the extractability of a suitable flow indicator for a given organ or tissue is far from homogeneous along the entire vasculature. This fact suggests the existence of parallel vascular networks with different flow properties, which implies that the "*total blood flow*" is not necessarily identical to the "*effective nutritional blood flow*." The nutritional blood flow can be regarded as that fraction of the total input of blood which is associated with nonrestricted exchange of a substance (indicator) between the blood and the extravascular space; it concerns the vascular circuit with a high extraction capacity. Its complement can be termed the "*non-nutritional blood flow*," which could be related to anatomical shunting by arteriovenous anastomosis and capillary bypasses with significantly little extraction capacity. However, the fact that changes in total blood flow are not always associated with a proportional shift in exchange can also be explained by "functional shunting." Such functional shunting occurs in situations with increased flow rates. According to this blood flow concept, the only plausible alternatives regulating the relative importance of nutritional and nonnutritional blood flow in an organ would be either a redistribution of blood flow (anatomical shunting) or a change in the permeability of the capillary wall (functional shunting). These considerations emphasize that in order to understand the effects of radiation on the microcirculation in an organ, as a whole, several closely related aspects need to be taken into consideration, namely the vascular permeability, the total flow, and the nutritional blood flow.

8.4.3 Vascular Wall Permeability

The exchange between the blood and the medium in direct contact with the tissues is controlled by a selectively permeable barrier. The anatomical substrate of this barrier is the capillary wall, and primarily the endothelium, which has specific properties in different organs. Several reports (Table 8.5) support the view that early and late increases in the vascular permeability are observed after irradiation in the majority of organs. Increases in permeability were mainly demonstrated by the presence, in the extravascular space, of an increasing amount of intravascular material (dye bound to plasma proteins or

Table 8.5. Effects of irradiation on vascular permeability in various organs

Organ	Species	Single doses (Gy)	Method	Permeability	Times of onset[a] (days after irr.)		Refs.
Skin (ear)	Rabbit	80	^{125}I-albumin	Increased	1–4	12–?	A, J
Skin (flank)	Rabbit	10	Pontamine sky blue	Increased	2–3	10–17	B, J
Skin (ear)	Rat	20	^{125}I-albumin	Increased	1–7	7–35	C
Skin (ear)	Rat	40	^{125}I-albumin	Increased	1–4	4–?	C
Skin (thorax)	Rat	18–25	^{125}I-albumin	Increased	1–4	9–?	D
Lung (both)	Mouse	20	Horseradish peroxidase	Increased	1–7	160–200	E
Lung (right)	Mouse	20–25	^{131}I-albumin	Increased	56–120	170–330	F
Lung (both)	Rat	18–25	^{125}I-albumin	Increased	1–4	14–30	D
Heart	Rat	18–25	^{125}I-albumin	Increased	1–2	14–26	D
Whole brain	Monkey	20	Trypan blue	Increased	3 (killed)		G, K
Whole brain	Monkey	20	^{14}C-α-aminoisobutyric acid	Increased	3 (killed)		H
Whole brain	Rat	20	Evans blue	No leakage	At any time		I

[a] The two columns relate to early and late increases in vascular permeability.

A, Mount and Bruce 1964; B, Eassa and Casarett 1973; C. Law and Thomlinson 1978; D, Evans et al. 1986; E, Maisin et al. 1973; F, Law 1985; G, Clemente and Holst 1954; H, Caveness 1980; I, Keyeux et al. 1987; J, Dunjic. 1974b; K, Keyeux 1974b.

proteins labeled with radioisotopes) after irradiation. However, abnormal accumulations of proteins in the extravascular space may be due to an increase in the hydrostatic pressure in the microvessels, to cellular damage in the endothelial barrier, and/or to impaired removal by the lymphatic drainage. Concerning the latter mechanism, there is some agreement on the absence of modification in the lymphatic drainage after irradiation with doses as high as 80 Gy (JOVANOVIC 1974). However, some transient changes were, observed in human skin (WELLS 1963) and pig skin (MORTIMER et al. 1985/1986). The alternative mechanisms may both be relevant to the radiation response at different times and after different doses, depending on the tissue studied.

The vascular response of the blood microcirculation to radiation has been most extensively studied in the skin. Numerous data suggest that early changes represent a secondary inflammatory reaction of the dermal vasculature to the radiation-induced epidermal damage (DUNJIC 1974b; LAW 1981; HOPEWELL 1983). The release of endogenous substances like histamine and 5-hydroxytryptamine may initiate vasodilatation, local hydrostatic pressure increases, and the separation of endothelial cells at their boundaries. The consequence is early modification of the oncotic equilibrium due to the transfer of proteins into the extravascular space. It is admitted that this mechanism does not account for the later phase of increase which may result in various organs from cell endothelial damage. The loss of endothelial cells leads to an enlargement of the diameter of intracellular and intercellular pores, activation of pinocytosis for a number of macromolecules, and release of lysosomal enzymes from dying cells. The action of lysosomal enzymes is well demonstrated by the redution, to a certain extent, in the degree and duration of the delayed increase in the capillary permeability in the irradiated skin after administration of EACA an agent which blocks lysosomal activation and antagonizes the activity of proteases as well as histamine (EASSA and CASARETT 1973). This effect was not observed with a pure antihistaminic drug (DUNJIC 1974b).

According to these arguments, the delayed increase in vascular permeability is mainly related to radiation-induced endothelial cell death (LAW 1981). Therefore, the biphasic change in the permeability of the vascular wall after irradiation is due to, on the one hand, the combined effects of mediators released as a reaction to direct injury and from dying endothelial cells and, on the other, endothelial cell depletion.

The effect of radiation on the permeability of the blood–brain barrier, in contrast to that on other organs, is obviously dependent on the species (Table 8.5). Early and late radiation-induced alterations of the blood–brain barrier demonstrated by the leakage of dye found in the monkey and dog were not found in the rat at any time after irradiation (KEYEUX et al. 1987). The large diameter of the albumin-dye complex (70 Å) used in KEYEUX et al.'s study was not responsible for this finding, since a smaller water-soluble molecule like pertechnetate (5 Å) did not reveal any leakage of the vascular wall in any part of the brain. As emphasized in the introduction, the relative distribution of blood flow between the nutritional and nonnutritional components depends on the vascular permeability. With this in mind the rat would appear a particularly suitable animal for the study of blood flow changes in the brain after therapeutic doses of radiation becuase the influence of this additional factor, permeability changes, does not affect the measurement procedure.

8.4.4 Total and Nutritional Blood Flow

Blood flow is decreased in many organs after irradiation (Table 8.6). However, this general conclusion does not take into account the likely existence of several phases in the vascular response, as for example in the skin and brain, and the type of flow which is measured. Both of these points are of particular importance for the understanding of apparently opposite effects reported in the brain. In a few experiments the blood flow measurements represent blood velocity recording in major vessels (e.g., the internal carotid arteries) and are therefore closely related to the total blood flow (CHAPMAN and YOUNG 1968). However, as for permeability evaluation, the majority of the methods used for measuring blood flow are based on the behavior of a radioactive indicator introduced into the irradiated area. There are three methods which are related to specific principles of tracer kinetics: the "indicator blood dilution" method for the measurement of total blood flow and blood volume, and the "indicator tissue saturation" and "indicator tissue clearance" methods, both of which are used for the measurement of nutritional blood flow.

Table 8.6. Effects of irradiation on blood flow in various organs

Organ	Species	Single doses (Gy)	Method	Blood flow	Times of onset (days after irr.)	Refs.
Brain (Occ)	Monkey	35	^{14}C-AP	nCBF decreased	200–280	A
Brain (whole)	Rat	20	^{125}I-IAP	nCBF decreased	84	B
Brain (whole)	Rat	20	^{125}I-IAP	nCBF decreased	250	B
Brain (whole)	Rat	20	^{99m}Tc-pertech.	TCBF decreased	170	C
Brain (whole)	Rat	15 and 20	^{99m}Tc-pertech.	TCBF decreased	500	C, D, L
Brain (whole)	Rat	20	^{131}I-IAP	nCBF decreased	500	C, M
Skin (plantar)	Rat	20	^{99m}Tc-pertech.	Decreased	280	D, J
Skin (plantar)	Pig	20.7–23.4	^{99m}Tc-pertech.	Increased	6	E
Skin (plantar)	Pig	20.7–23.4	^{99m}Tc-pertech.	Decreased	80 and 700	E
Skin (tail)	Mouse	30	^{133}Xe	No change	100–450	F, J
Skin (chest)	Mouse	15	^{86}Rb	No change	10–360	G, J
Lung (right)	Rat	15	^{131}I-MAI	Decreased	14–230	D, K
Lung (right)	Mouse	15	^{86}Rb	Decreased	80–160	G, K
Liver	Rat	15	^{198}Au colloids	Decreased	15 and 50	D, K
Liver	Mouse	15	^{86}Rb	No change	10–360	G, K
Kidney (both)	Rat	40	PAH	Decreased	28–?	H, K
Kidney (one)	Dog	5 and 10	^{131}I-hippuran	Decreased	140–200	I, K
Kidney (both)	Mouse	11–19	^{86}Rb	Decreased	60–360	G, K
Kidney (both)	Pig	8.8–12.6	^{131}I-hippuran	Decreased	28–?	N

Occ, occipital lobe; AP, antipyrine; IAP, iodoantipyrine; MAI, albumin macoraggregate; PAH, sodium para-aminohippurate; nCBF, nutritional cerebral blood flow; TCBF, total cerebral blood flow

A, Tanaka et al. 1975; B, Moustafa and Hopewell 1980; C, Keyeux et al. 1983; D, Keyeux et al. 1971; E, Moustafa and Hopewell 1979; F, de Ruiter and van Putten 1975; G, Glastein 1973; H, Smith and Boss 1957; I, Gup et al. 1962; J, Dunjic 1974b; K, Dunjic 1974a; L, Keyeux 1974b; M, Keyeux and Ochrymowicz-Bemelmans 1978; N, Robbins and Hopewell 1988.

8.4.5 Changes in Circulation Parameters in Various Organs

8.4.5.1 Brain

The indicator blood dilution method, using ^{99m}Tc-pertechnetate, has been applied for the evaluation of changes in total cerebral blood flow (TCBF) and total cerebral volume (CBV) after irradiation of the brain (20 Gy) in rats (Fig. 8.4). The results showed that TCBF was depressed and CBV increased 6 months after exposure. This result was reversed 6 months later, an effect that was enhanced 18 months after irradiation. On the other hand the indicator tissue saturation method, with ^{131}I-iodoantipyrine, used for the evaluation of the nutritional cerebral blood flow (nCBF), showed changes that paralleled those in the CBV. The nCBF was significantly decreased at 12 and 18 months after irradiation (Keyeux et al. 1983). Both of these changes strongly support the pre-

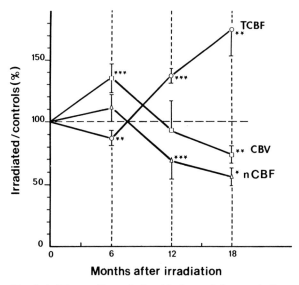

Fig. 8.4. Time–effect relationship for radioisotope indices evaluating the total cerebral blood flow (*TCBF*), the total cerebral blood volume (*CBV*), and the nutritional cerebral blood flow (*nCBF*) after 20 Gy x-rays to the brain of the adult rat. *$P < 0.05$; **$P < 0.01$; ***$P < 0.001$

sence of late alterations in the capillary network after radiation. In this context, the increase in TCBF appears to represent luxury perfusion which could be interpreted as a response of the cerebral blood vessels to tissue hypoxia. The discrepancy in the literature concerning radiation effects on the cerebral blood flow results from a lack of distinction between the different blood flow components.

8.4.5.2 Skin

The blood flow in the skin is highly regulated and, particularly in species without fur or having lost hair due to radiation, depends more on thermoregulation than on nutritional requirements. This is the likely reason why large variations in blood flow are observed in normal skin. The resulting poor reproducibility of the data obtained with skin blood flow measurements of any type makes it difficult to demonstrate radiation-induced changes unless conditions are carefully standardized. The removal of a locally injected radioactive indicator from the skin has been used by a number of investigators to measure blood flow in irradiated skin, and both increases and decreases as well as the absence of any effect have been reported (Table 8.6). The most widely reported pattern of skin response to radiation doses in the therapeutic range comprises an early increase (0–6 weeks) followed by a decrease (6–12 weeks) and then either a progressive restoration or the persistence of the decrease 1 year after irradiation. Some investigators who found no change in the resting blood flow showed that the hyperemic response normally observed after releasing a temporary occlusion was reduced (DE RUITER and VAN PUTTEN 1975). This means that the radiation-induced reduction in the vascular capacity makes the blood flow insufficient in a situation of high requirement, such as exists after trauma or surgery (YOUNG and HOPEWELL 1983).

8.4.5.3 Lung

Only a few studies (Table 8.5) have demonstrated the modification of lung vascular permeability. Following radiation doses of at least 7 Gy, there is an early and progressive increase in the extravascular albumin content in the lung. These changes occur concomitantly with a reduction in the pulmonary blood volume (LAW 1985). Using the embolization of ^{131}I-macroaggregated serum albumin and scintigraphic methods the pulmonary capillary perfusion was shown to be transiently depressed after 10 Gy and persistently depressed after 12.5–15 Gy (KEYEUX et al. 1971). The absence of recovery after 12.5–15 Gy was not confirmed by a study using the ^{86}Rb extraction method (GLATSTEIN 1973). However, the two approaches are not equivalent: the former is only influenced by the number of open microvessels in the pulmonary circulation while the latter is influenced by the total mass of cells and evaluates both the pulmonary and the bronchial circulation. Taking these considerations into account, the discrepancy between the radiation responses measured by these blood flow methods could reflect a difference in radiosensitivity between the pulmonary and the bronchial microcirculation. Unfortunately, this hypothesis cannot be confirmed because data on radiation effects on the bronchial circulation alone are not available.

8.4.5.4 Liver

Of the total hepatic blood flow, 85% is normally supplied by the portal vein and 15% by the hepatic artery. In addition to the difference in the origin of the blood, the endothelial cells of the walls of the associated capillary networks are also different. The blood flow in the irradiated liver has been evaluated almost exclusively by the uptake of radioactive colloids by Kupffer cells (DUNJIC 1974a). Unfortunately, this method does not allow discrimination between the two components of hepatic blood flow. With this limitation in mind, the majority of the studies show a two-phase reduction in hepatic blood flow for radiation doses between 5 and 20 Gy (KEYEUX et al. 1971; DUNJIC 1974a). It seems that the reduction in flow which occurs between 1 and 40 days after exposure cannot be explained by a reduction in the capacity of the Kupffer cells to trap colloids or by hepatocyte dysfunction. The fact that heparin prevents, or reduces, the early modification in hepatic blood flow suggests that the radiation injury to the liver is mainly confined to the endothelial cells (KINZIE et al. 1972). The second phase of reduction in blood flow starts at about 2 months after exposure and is progressively associated with fibrosis of the liver parenchyma. This could be the ultimate consequence of alterations in the endothelial cell (LAW 1981). However, no changes in ^{86}Rb extraction were observed in the liver until 1 year after irradiation (KEYEUX et al. 1971). This fact underlines the complexity of the radiation response, which also depends upon the functional organization of the liver parenchymal cells.

8.4.5.5 Kidneys

The kidneys receive 20% of the cardiac output. This blood flow is far in excess of the metabolic need (nutritional blood flow) of the kidneys, but its maintenance within narrow limits is critical to their normal function (functional blood flow). The functional blood flow is thus the main component of the total renal blood flow. The total blood flow may be evaluated using the ^{86}Rb extraction method. Following local irradiation of both kidneys with doses of 5–40 Gy a progressive dose- and time-dependent reduction in blood flow was observed.

The functional fraction of the renal blood flow is that which supplies the renal secretory tissue and is also termed the "effective renal plasma flow" (ERPF). ERPF may be estimated by measuring the clearance of para-aminohippuric acid (PAH) or ^{131}I-hippurate. Although simple and easy to perform, this technique has the disadvantage of being limited by the secretory capacity of the kidney tubules. Any reduction of this capacity will result in an apparent reduction in ERPF. Despite this important limitation, several authors have attributed the observed decline in PAH plasma clearance to a reduction in functional renal blood flow. This reduction in blood flow is time and dose dependent. It has been observed as late as 5–7 months after exposure to 5 and 10 Gy in rats (GUP et al. 1962), between 4 and 8 weeks after 8.8–12.6 Gy in pigs (ROBBINS and HOPEWELL 1988), and as early as 28 days after a single dose of 40 Gy in rats (SMITH and BOSS 1957). A similar reduction was observed when the total renal blood flow was measured by the ^{86}Rb extraction technique (GLATSTEIN 1973). Such similarity underlines the predominant influence of the functional blood flow in the response of total renal blood flow to radiation. Although the functional renal blood flow is an essential factor in producing the "renogram" pattern, it is generally admitted that no single renal function can be derived from a renogram without extensive analysis (DUNJIC 1974a). However, the results obtained with renography are concordant with those reported

above. Therefore, the conclusion is that function changes parallel the decline in blood flow in the irradiated kidney.

8.4.6 Conclusions on the Radiation-Induced Changes in Blood Flow and Permeability

Both vascular permeability and blood flow are modified after therapeutic doses of radiation. The variations in radiation-induced changes in permeability are dependent not only on the organ and thus on the structure of the endothelium but also on the animal species. For instance, ischemic necrosis may develop in the skin of pigs and man, but not in rodents, where the vascular supply is different (HOPEWELL 1986). The organization and regulation of flow in the brain and the cardiac and skeletal muscles contrasts markedly with the largely nonnutritional blood flow in the skin, the lungs, the liver, and the kidneys. The nonnutritional blood flow in these tissues is mainly devoted to specific functions and is much higher than the nutritional blood flow requirement. Unfortunately, a clear-cut evaluation of the separate effect of radiation on each component of flow is not possible for these organs. However, the fact that after irradiation a loss of function parallels the reduction in vascularization (KEYEUX 1971; DUNJIC 1974a), which results in tissue fibrosis in some tissues rather than in necrosis, strongly suggests that the functional component of blood flow is more responsive than the nutritional component. On the other hand, delayed radiation necrosis in the brain occurs as a consequence of a radiation-induced reduction in the nutritional blood flow, which is the most important component of the cerebral blood flow. The fact that myocardial infarctions have been described several months after irradiation (KEYEUX et al. 1974a; STEWART and FAJARDO 1984) leads to a similar conclusion. These considerations suggest that the consequences of the radiation-induced changes in the microcirculation are far from uniform and depend on the main physiological purpose of the capillary network of the specific organ or tissue.

8.5 The Extravascular Components

Connective tissue is present in all organs and tissues, though its composition and structure vary.

Its biochemistry under normal conditions and after irradiation has recently been reviewed by ALTMAN and GERBER (1983), and the reader is referred to this article for biochemical details. An increase in connective tissue elements can be observed morphologically in most irradiated organs but only in a few organs have determinations pertaining to changes in the collagen content been carried out. This is because not every tissue is suitable for the biochemical determination of collagen. Most investigations have been performed on lung tissue, although some have been carried out on other tissues, such as granulation tissue (RANTANEN 1973; VAN DEN BRENK 1974a,b) or skin (ULLRICH and CASARETT 1977).

In the investigations by ULLRICH and CASARETT the thigh skin of the rat was used. The local radiation treatment induced an early increase in the rate of extravasation of iodine-labelled albumen. There was also an increase in collagen 6–9 months after irradiation as measured by the hydroxyproline content. However, this increase occurred not only in the irradiated area but also in the contralateral shielded thigh. When the authors pretreated the animals with cobra venom, which has the effect of depleting the body of complement, this abolished the changes that developed in the contralateral region and reduced the late development of collagen after 20 Gy.

RANTANEN (1973) examined the effects of irradiation on the development of subcutaneous granulation tissue, which was induced by embedding viscose cellulose sponge into rats. After implantation a number of reactive phases occurred. A phase of mobilization and migration of cells was followed by a phase of proliferation, which in turn was followed by collagen synthesis. Finally, after 1 month, there was a phase of involution. Irradiation with a dose of 10 Gy in the various phases resulted in different effects. Exposure at the phase of proliferation and at the phase of collagen synthesis produced an excessive accumulation of insoluble collagen, in spite of decreased cellularity in the irradiated tissue. RANTANEN (1973) suggested that irradiation resulted in inhibition of collagenolysis and that this then caused an accumulation of insoluble collagen, which might eventually lead to fibrosis. However, it should be borne in mind that the sequence of events in irradiated, reactive granuloma tissue is not necessarily the same as that which takes place during the development of late radiation fibrosis in tissue, like the lung. There has been some speculation that radiation fibrosis

results indirectly from plasma proteins leaking out from the vessels, either during the acute radiation reaction or during the latent period, in which radiation-sterilized cells undergo division and die, leaving a denuded site. However, recently investigations by WALKLIN and LAW (1986) and LAW et al. (1986) on the rate of biosynthesis of protocollagen as well as on changes in the albumin distribution space of the rat lung have indicated that there is probably no causal relationship between the exudation of vascular protein and the increase in collagen biosynthesis. In this context it is important to note that MILLER et al. (1986) found a dose dependent increase in type I collagen levels in the irradiated mouse lung, which occurred concomitantly with fibrosis. In addition, GERBER et al. (1977) observed a decrease in fibrinolytic activity in the rat lung over prolonged periods after hemithoracic irradiation with a dose of 10 Gy. However, as pointed out by ALTMAN and GERBER (1983), the pathways leading to radiation fibrosis are not yet clear: radiation effects on the integrity of the vascular system may be primarily responsible, but direct effects on connective tissue or fibroblasts cannot be ruled out. The recent findings by MARTIN et al. (1986) point in the latter direction. In these studies, the growth potential, in vitro, of fibroblasts isolated from irradiated pig muscle was compared with that of fibroblasts isolated from surgically wounded muscle. The results showed that the growth potential of cells taken from the irradiated sites 5–6 months after irradiation far exceeded that of fibroblasts from surgically wounded sites. This seems to indicate that fibroblasts in irradiated areas are apparently more vital than in control sites! The irradiation in these experiments comprised a single dose of 30–40 Gy, which is rather high when compared with fractionated doses in man.

8.6 Some Additional Methods of Measuring Vascular Viability

Another way of investigating radiation-induced damage to the connective tissue of the stroma is by applying some kind of stimulus for vascular proliferation, and measuring the increase in the time taken to reach a given level of effect. Such experiments can never measure the amount of cell sterilization, but they can be used to investigate indirectly factors like the influence of fraction size or overall time intervals on the vascular response. Examples of such determinations are the investigations on the tumor bed effect (TBE) (Hewitt and Blake 1968; Begg and Terry 1984; Camplejohn and Penhaligon 1985; Milas et al. 1987) or the efficiency of repair of bone fractures (Hayashi and Suit 1971). The latter authors estimated the dose required to inhibit callus formation in 50% of animals (CID_{50}). The CID_{50} increased significantly with the number of fractions, but not with the time interval between two fractions. While the effect of fraction number, or fraction size, was as might be expected, i.e., the fractionation exponent was about 0.3, the factor "time" was not important, with an exponent of only 0.024. This is somewhat surprising in a model system where extensive endothelial cell proliferation occurs, given that other investigators working with capillary-sprouting assays (van den Brenk 1974a,b; Reinhold and Buisman 1975) have found a strong capacity for repair, amounting to one or two decades in systems which approximate to cell survival, when the interval between irradiation and proliferation was delayed for a number of weeks. This apparent discrepancy has not yet been explained, but it may be related to differences between clonogenic and subclonogenic proliferation.

The other stimulus for vascular proliferation, i.e., the TBE, seemed to have an optimal effective dose of between 5 and 10 Gy; little increase in effect was achieved by increasing the dose further (Hewitt and Blake 1968). Begg and Terry (1984) used the TBE to investigate the stromal/vascular sensitivity to fractionated irradiation. Their data indicated a fractionation exponent of 0.25 and an α/β value of 6.2 Gy. These data show that the TBE can be used for fractionation studies, although the α/β value obtained was rather high compared with the value of 2–3 Gy which is usually associated with late responding tissues. Using this system, with overall times ranging from 1 to 11 days, no effect attributable to slow repair or to repopulation could be demonstrated. In addition, Camplejohn and Penhaligon (1985) pointed out that tumors growing in preirradiated sites have different cell kinetics and necrotic volumes, and that one should be cautious about using the TBE for tumor growth studies. Finally, Milas et al. (1987) showed that the prolonged tumor growth rate with the TBE gradually decreased in the months following irradiation.

Studies with the TBE consist typically of irradiation of the tumor bed, followed after some time by inoculation with tumor cells obtained from tumor cell suspensions. However, few investigators seem aware that cell suspensions obtained from tumors inevitably contain unirradiated endothelial cells from the donor's tumor vascular system. No information is available on the behavior of such unirradiated endothelial cells in irradiated sites, but the possibility should be considered that their proliferation may cause bias in the results obtained with these methods.

8.7 Conclusions

There can be little doubt that the vascular system is very sensitive to radiation. This holds true not only for morphological criteria but also for the functional changes in the vascular system. Which cell type of the vascular wall is the most sensitive to radiation has not yet been completely clarified, but all investigations which have compared cell survival after irradiation have indicated that the endothelial cell is more sensitive than the other cells. This in itself does not prove that the endothelial cell is the dose-limiting cell in radiation therapy, or even that the blood vessel system is the dose-limiting tissue component. Recently, it has been demonstrated in the irradiated rat brain (Reyners, unpublished data) that in telangiectasia the vessels are still lined with endothelium and that the basement membrane, as well as the adjacent astrocytes, also shows many abnormalities. This could be taken to indicate a complex interaction between blood vessels and their environment.

Thus, the question of which element represents the dose-limiting tissue component has, as yet, not been resolved. It is very likely that the blood vessel system plays a key role in the development of late radiation sequelae (Hopewell 1987), but the exact mode of its impact remains to be elucidated.

Acknowledgments. The authors wish to thank Dr. J.J. Michiels (Dept. of Hematology, Erasmus University, Rotterdam) for his invaluable comments. This work forms part of the collaborative programme of the European Late Effects Project Group and was partly supported by the Radiation Protection Programme of the Commission of the European Communities, Contract No. BI6-D-099-D.

References

Aarnoudse MW (1979) Vessel wall damage by x-rays and 15 MeV neutrons. An experimental study. Groningen University, The Netherlands

Adamson IYR and Bowden DH (1983) Endothelial injury and repair in radiation-induced pulmonary fibrosis. Am. J. Pathol. 112: 224–230

Allen JB, Sagerman RH and Stuart MJ (1981) Irradiation decreases vascular prostacyclin formation with no concomitant effect on platelet thromboxane production. The Lancet 1193–1196

Altman KI, Gerber GB (1983) The effect of ionizing radiations on connective tissue. Adv Radiat Biol 10: 237–304

Archambeau JO, Ines A, Fajardo LF (1984) Response of swine skin microvasculature to acute single exposures of x-rays: quantification of endothelial changes. Radiat Res 98: 37–51

Archambeau JO, Ines A, Fajardo LF, (1985) Correlation of the dermal microvasculature morphology with the epidermal and the endothelial population changes produced by single x-ray fractions of 1649, 2231 and 2619 rad in swine. Int J Radiat Oncol Biol Phys 11: 1639–1646

Begg AC, Terry NHA (1984) The sensitivity of normal stroma to fractionated radiotherapy measured by a tumour growth rate assay. Radiother Oncol 2: 333–341

Berthrong M, Fajardo LF (1981) Radiation injury in surgical pathology. Part II. Alimentary tract. Am J Surg Pathol 5: 153–178

Bond VP, Fliedner TM, Usenik E, Upton LI, (1962) Early bone marrow hemorrhage in the irradiated dog. Arch Pathol 73: 13–29

Brown DG, Sasmore DP, Jones LP, (1962) Acute central nervous system syndrome of burros. In: Haley, TJ, Snyder RS (eds) Response of the nervous system to ionizing radiation. Academic, New York, pp 503–511

Brown JM, Fajardo LF, Stewart JR (1973) Mural thrombosis of the heart induced by radiation. Arch Pathol 96: 1–4

Calvo W, Hopewell JW, Reinhold HS, Yeung TK, (1986) Radiation induced damage in the choroid plexus of the rat brain: a histological evaluation. Neuropathol Appl Neurobiol 12: 47–61

Calvo W, Hopewell JW, Reinhold HS, Van den Berg AP, Yeung TK (1987) Dose-dependent and time-dependent changes in the choroid plexus of the irradiated rat brain. Br J Radiol 60: 1109–1117

Camplejohn RS, Penhaligon M (1985) The tumour bed effect: a cell kinetic and histological investigation of tumours growing in irradiated mouse skin. Br J Radiol 58: 443–451

Caveness WF (1980) Experimental observations: delayed necrosis in normal monkey brain. In: Gilbert HA, Kagan AR (eds) Radiation damage to the nervous system: a delayed therapeutic hazard. Raven, New York, pp 1–38

Caveness WF, Tanaka A, Hess KH, Kemper TL, Tso MOM, Zimmerman LE (1974) Delayed brain swelling and functional derangement after x-irradiation of the right visual cortex in the Macaca mulatta. Radiat Res 57: 104–120

Chapman PH, Young RJ (1968) Effect of cobalt-60 gamma irradiation on blood pressure and cerebral blood flow in the Macaca mulatta. Radiat Res 35: 75–85

Clemente CD, Holst EA (1954) Pathological changes in neurons, neurologia and blood-brain barrier induced by x-irradiation of heads of monkeys. Arch Neurol Psychiatry 71: 66–79

Cottier H (1961) Strahlenbedingte Lebensverkürzung. Springer Berlin Heidelberg New York

Dailey MO, Coleman CN, Fajardo LF (1981) Splenic injury caused by therapeutic irradiation. Am J Surg Pathol 5: 325–331

DeGowin RL, Lewis LJ, Mason RE, Borke MK, Hoak JC (1976) Radiation-induced inhibition of human endothelial cells replicating in culture. Radiat Res 68: 244–250

de Ruiter J, van Putten LM (1975) Measurement of blood flow in the mouse tail after irradiation. Radiat Res 61: 427–438

Dimitrievich GS, Fischer-Dzoga K (1983) Effects of x-ray dose fractionation on the microvasculature in vivo. In: Broerse JJ, Barendsen GW, Kal HB, van de Kogel AJ (eds) Radiation research. Proceedings of the 7th International Congress of Radiation Research. Martinus Nijhoff, Publ. The Hague

Dimitrievich GS, Hausladen SL, Kuchnir FT, Griem ML (1977) Radiation damage and subendothelial repair to rabbit ear chamber microvasculature. Radiat Res 69: 276–292

Dimitrievich GS, Fischer-Dzoga K, Griem ML (1984) Radiosensitivity of vascular tissue. I. Differential radiosensitivity of capillaries: a quantitative in vivo study. Radiat Res 99: 511–535

Dunjic A (1974a) The influence of radiation on blood vessels and circulation. Blood flow and permeability in liver, kidney and lung. Curr Top Radiat Res Q 10: 109–134

Dunjic A (1974b) The influence of radiation on blood vessels and circulation. Blood flow and permeability in irradiated skin. Curr Top Radiat Res Q 10: 151–169

Eassa E -HM, Casarett GW, (1973) Effect of ε-amino-n-caproic acid (EACA) on radiation-induced increase in capillary permeability. Radiology 106: 679–688

El-Naggar AM El-Baz LM, Carsten AL, Chanana AJ, Cronkite EP (1978) Radiation-induced damage to blood vessels: a study of dose-effect relationship with time after x-irradiation. Int J Radiat Biol 34: 359–366

Evans ML, Graham MM, Mahler PA, Rasey JS (1986) Changes in vascular permeability following thorax irradiation in the rat. Radiat Res 107: 262–271

Fajardo LF (1982) Pathology of radiation injury. Masson, New York

Fajardo LF, Berthrong M (1978) Radiation injury in surgical pathology. Part I. Am J Surg Pathol 2: 159–199

Fajardo LF, Berthrong M (1988) Vascular lesions following radiation. Pathol Annu 23: 297–330

Fajardo LF, Colby TV (1980) Pathogenesis of venoocclusive liver disease after radiation. Arch Pathol Lab Med 104: 584–588

Fajardo LF, Stewart JR (1971) Capillary injury preceding radiation-induced myocardial fibrosis. Radiology 101: 429–433

Fajardo LF, Stewart JR (1973) Pathogenesis of radiation-induced myocardial fibrosis. Lab Invest 29: 244–257

Fajardo LF, Stewart JR, Cohn KE (1968) Morphology of radiation-induced heart disease. Arch Pathol 86: 512–519

Fajardo LF, Brown JM, Glatstein E (1976) Glomerular and juxtaglomerular lesions in radiation nephropathy. Radiat Res 68: 177–183

Fee WE, Goffinet DR, Fajardo LF, Guthaner D, Handen C (1987) Safety of [125]iodine and [192]iridium implants to the canine carotid artery. Acta Otolaryngol (Stockh) 103: 514–518

Field SB, Hornsey S, Kutsutani Y (1976) Effects of fractionated irradiation on mouse lung and a phenomenon of slow repair. Br J Radiol 49: 700–707

Fike JR, Gillette EL (1978) ^{60}Co gamma and negative Pi meson irradiation of microvasculature. Int J Radiat Oncol Biol Phys 4: 825–828

Fike JR, Gillette EL, Clow DJ (1979) Repair of sublethal radiation damage by capillaries. Int J Radiat Oncol Biol Phys 5: 339–342

Fischer JJ (1982) Proliferation of rat aortic endothelial cells following x-irradiation. Radiat Res 92: 405–410

Fischer-Dzoga K, Dimitrievich GS, Griem ML (1984) Radiosensitivity of vascular tissue. II. Differential radiosensitivity of aortic cells in vitro. Radiat Res 99: 536–546

Fliedner TM, Sandkühler S, Stodtmeister R (1955) Die Knochenmarkstruktur bei Ratten nach Bestrahlung mit schnellen Elektronen. Z Zellfors 43: 195–205

Friedman M, Ryan US, Davenport WC, Chaney EL, strickland EL, Kwock L (1986) Reversible alterations in cultured pulmonary artery endothelial cell monolayer morphology and albumin permeability induced by ionizing radiation. J Cell Physiol 129: 237–249

Gassmann A (1899) Zur Histologie der Roentgenulcera. Fortschr Roentgenstr 2: 199–207

Gerber GB (1979) The role of connective tissue in late effects of radiation. In: Okada S, Imamura M, Terashima T, Yamaguchi H (eds) Radiation research. Proceedings of the 6th International Congress of Radiation Research, JARR (Japanese Association for Radiation Research). Tokyo, pp 669–705

Gerber GB, Dancewicx AM, Bessemans B, Casale G (1977) Biochemistry of late effects in rat lung after hemithoracic irradiation. Acta Radioy Ther Phys Biol 16: 447–455

Gillette EL, Maurer GD, Severin GA (1975) Endothelial repair of radiation damage following beta irradiation. Radiology 116: 175–177

Gillette EL, Hoopes PJ, Withrow SJ (1983) Aortic changes following intraoperative electron or fractionated x-irradiation. D3–15. In: Broerse JJ, Barendsen GW, Kal HB, van de Kogel AJ (eds) Radiation research. Proceedings of the 7th International Congress of Radiation Research. Martinus Nijhoff, The Hague

Glatstein E (1973) Alteration in rubidium-86 extraction in normal mouse tissues after irradiation. An estimate of long-term blood flow changes in kidneys, lung, liver, skin and muscle. Radiat Res 53: 88–101

Gold H (1961) Production of arteriosclerosis in the rat. Arch Pathol 71: 268–273

Gup AK, Schlegel JU, Caldwell I, Schlosser J (1962) Effects of irradiation on renal function. J Urol 97: 36–39

Hayashi S, Suit HD (1971) Effect of fractionation of radiation dose on callus formation at site of fracture. Radiology 101: 181–186

Hei TK, Marchese MJ, Hall EJ (1987) Radiosensitivity and sublethal damage repair in human umbilical cord vein endothelial cells. Int J Radiat Oncol Biol Phys 13: 879–884

Henderson BW, Bicher HI, Johnson RJ (1983) Loss of vascular fibrinolytic activity following irradiation of the liver. An aspect of late radiation damage. Radiat Res 95: 646–652

Hendry JH (1987) Lack of differential sparing of late ischaemic atrophy and early epidermal healing after

dose-fractionating of mouse tails down to 2.2 Gy per fraction. Radiat Ther Oncol 8: 153–160

Hewitt HB, Blake ER (1968) The growth of transplanted murine tumours in pre-irradiated sites. Br J Cancer 12: 808–824

Hirst DG, Denekamp J, Travis EL (1979) The response of mesenteric blood vessels to irradiation. Radiat Res 77: 259–275

Hirst DG, Denekamp J, Hobson B (1980) Proliferation studies of the endothelial and smooth muscle cells of the mouse mesentery after irradiation. Cell Tissue Kinet 13: 91–104

Hobson B, Denekamp J (1984) Endothelial proliferation in tumours and normal tissues: continuous labelling studies. Br J Cancer 49: 405–413

Hopewell JW (1974) The late vascular effects of radiation. Br. J Radiol 47: 157–158

Hopewell JW (1979) Late radiation damage to the central nervous system: a radiobiological interpretation. Neuropathol Appl Neurobiol 5: 329–343

Hopewell JW (1980) The importance of vascular damage in the development of late radiation effects in normal tissues. In: Meyn RE, Withers HR (eds) Radiation biology in cancer research. Raven, New York, pp 449–459

Hopewell JW (1983) Radiation effects on vascular tissue. In: Potten CS, Hendry JH (eds) Cytotoxic insult to tissue. Churchill Livingstone, Edinburgh, pp 228–257

Hopewell JW (1986) Mechanisms of the action of radiation on skin and underlying tissues. In: Radiation damage to skin. Br J Radiol [Suppl] 19: 39–47

Hopewell JW (1987) The role of the vasculature in normal tissue responses. In: Fielden EM, Fowler JF, Hendry JH, Scott D (eds) Proceedings of the 8th International Congress of Radiation Research. Taylor and Francis, London, pp 789–794

Hopewell JW, Patterson TJS (1972) The effect of previous x-irradiation on the revascularization of free skin grafts in the pig (abstr). Biorheology 9: 45

Hopewell JW, Foster JL, Gunn Y (1978) Role of vascular damage in the development of late radiation effects in the skin. In: Late biological effects of ionizing radiation. IAEA, Vienna 1: 483–492

Hopewell JW, Campling D, Calvo W, Reinhold HS, Wilkinson JH, Yeung TK (1986) Vascular irradiation damage: its cellular basis and likely consequences. Br J Cancer 53 [Suppl VII]: 181–191

Hopewell JW, Calvo W, Reinhold HS (1989) Radiation effects on blood vessels: role in normal tissue damage In: Steel GG, Adams GE and Horwich A (eds) The biological basis of radiotherapy. 2nd Edition Eds. Elsevier (Amsterdam) pp 101–113

Johnson LK, Longenecker JP, Fajardo LF (1982) Differential radiation response of cultured endothelial cells and smooth myocytes. Anal Quant Cytol 4: 188–198

Jolles B, Harrison RG (1966) Enzymic processes and vascular changes in the skin radiation reaction. Br J Radiol 39: 12–18

Jolles B, Harrison RG (1967) Enzymic processes in vascular permeability and fragility changes in the skin radiation reaction. Bibl Anat 9: 482–487

Jovanovic D (1974) The influence of radiation on blood vessels and circulation. Lymphatics. Curr Top Radiat Res Q 10: 85–97

Keyeux A (1974a) The influence of radiation on blood vessels and circulation: functional response of heart and major vessels. Curr Top Radiat Res Q 10: 98–108

Keyeux A (1974b) The influence of radiation on blood vessels and circulation. Blood flow and permeability in the central nervous system. Curr Top Radiat Res Q 10: 135–150

Keyeux A, Ochrymowicz-Bemelmans D (1978) Late response of the cerebral circulation to x-irradiation of the brain in the rat. In: Late biological effects of ionizing radiation. IAEA, Vienna 2: 251–260

Keyeux A, Dunjic A, Royer E, Jovanovic D, van de Merckt J (1971) Late functional and circulatory changes in rats after local irradiation. Int J Radiat Biol 20: 7–25

Keyeux A, Reinhold HS, Hopewell JH, Gerber GB, Reyners H, Calvo W (1983) Sequence of events in the development of late irradiation changes in the rat brain. Nr. C2–08. In: Broerse JJ, Barendsen GW, Kal HB, van der Kogel AJ Radiation research. Proceedings of the 7th International Congress of Radiation Research. Martinus Nijhoff, The Hague

Keyeux A, Ochrymowicz-Bemelmans D, Charlier AA (1987) Early and late effect on the blood-brain barrier permeability and the antipyrine distribution volumes in the irradiated rat brain. Radiation research. In: Fielden EM, Fowler JF, Hendry JH, Scott D (eds) Proceedings of the 8th International Congress on Radiation Research, vol. 1. Taylor and Francis, London, E22–7p

Kinzie J, Studer RK, Perez B, Potchen EJ (1972) Noncytokinetic radiation injury: anticoagulants as radioprotective agents in experimental radiation hepatitis. Science 175: 1481–1483

Kirkpatrick JB (1967) Pathogenesis of foam cell lesions of irradiated arteries. Am J Pathol 50: 291–309

Kwock L, Douglas WH, Lin PS, Bauer WE, Fanburg BL (1982) Endothelial cell damage after γ-irradiation in vitro: impaired uptake of α-aminoisobutyric acid. Annu Rev Respir Dis 125: 95–99

Lauk S (1987) Endothelial alkaline phosphatase activity loss as an early stage in the development of radiation-induced heart disease in rats. Radiat Res 110: 118–128

Law MP (1981) Radiation-induced vascular injury and its relation to late effects in normal tissues. Adv Radiat Biol 9: 37–73

Law MP (1985) Vascular permeability and late radiation fibrosis in mouse lung. Radiat Res 103: 60–76

Law MP, Thomlinson RH (1978) Vascular permeability in the ears of rats after x–irradiation. Br J Radiol 51: 895–904

Law MP, Ahier RG, Coultas PG (1986) The role of vascular injury in the radiation response of mouse lung. Br J Cancer 53 [Suppl VII]: 327–329

Lindop PJ, Jones A, Bakowska A (1970) The effect of 14-MeV electrons on the blood vessels of the mouse earlobe. Proceedings of the NCIAEC Carmel Symposium on time and dose relationship in radiation biology as applied to radiotherapy. BNL 50203, pp 174–180.

Maisin JR (1970) The ultrastructure of the lung of mice exposed to a supralethal dose of ionizing radiation on the thorax. Radiat Res 44: 545–564

Maisin JR, Oledzka-Slotwinska H, Lambiet-Collier M (1973) Ultrastructure of lung parenchyma and permeability changes of the blood air barrier after a local exposure of mice to 2000 R of x-rays. Adv Radiat Res Biol Med 3: 1347–1360

Martin DG, Fischer JJ (1984) Radiation sensitivity of cultured rabbit aortic endothelial cells. Int J Radiat Oncol Biol Phys 10: 1903–1906

Martin M, Remy J, Daburon F (1986) In vitro growth potential of fibroblasts isolated from pigs with radiation-induced fibrosis. Int J Radiat Biol 49: 821–828

Milas L, Hunter N, Peters LJ (1987) The tumor bed effect; dependence of tumor take, growth rate, and metastasis on the time interval between irradiation and tumor cell transplantation. Int J Radiat Oncol Biol Phys 13: 379–383

Miller G, Siemann D, Scott P, Dawson D, Muldrew K, Trépanier P, McGann L (1986) A semiquantitative probe for radiation-induced normal tissue damage at the molecular level. Radiat Res 105: 76–83

Mortimer PS, Simmonds RH, Rezvani MS, Hopewell JW, Ryan TJ (1985/1986) Lymph flow clearance changes in pig skin after a single dose of x-rays. CRC Normal Tissue Radiobiology Research Group (Univ. of Oxford), Annual Report, pp 33–34

Mount D, Bruce WR (1964) Local plasma volume and vascular permeability of rabbit skin after irradiation. Radiat Res 23: 430–445

Moustafa HF, Hopewell JW (1979) Blood flow clearance changes in pig skin after single doses. Br J Radiol 52: 138–144

Moustafa HF, Hopewell JW (1980) Late functional changes in the vasculature of the rat brain after local x-irradiation. Br J Radiol 53: 21–25

Mühsam R (1904) Ueber Dermatitis der Hand nach Roentgenbestrahlung (Fingeramputation). Archiv. für Klin. Chirurgie, Bd. 74/2: 434–453

Narayan K, Cliff WJ (1982) Morphology of irradiated microvasculature: a combined in vivo and electron-microscopic study. Am J Pathol 106: 47–62

Nias AHW (1974) The clinical significance of cell survival curves. In: Friedman M (ed) Biological and clinical basis of radiosensitivity. Thomas, Springfield, pp 156–169

Obersteiner H (1965) The effect of ionizing radiation on the nervous system. Adv Biol Med Phys 10: 1–9

Penhaligon M, Laverick M (1985) Radiation response of endothelial cells in vitro. Br J Radiol 58: 913–914

Phillips TL (1966) An ultrastructural study of the development of radiation injury in the lung. Radiology 87: 49–54

Plotnikova ED, Levitman MK, Shaposhnikova VV, Koshevoy JV, and Eidus LK (1984) Protection of microcirculation in rat brain against large radiation injury by gammaphos. Int J Radiat Oncol Biol Phys 10: 365–368

Rantanen J (1973) Radiation injury of connective tissue. Acta Radiol Supplementum 330

Reed GB, Cox AJ (1966) The human liver after radiation injury. A form of veno-occlusive disease. Am J Pathol 48: 597–612

Reinhold HS (1974) Structural changes in blood vessels. Curr Top Radiat Res Q 10: 58–74

Reinhold HS, Buisman GH (1973) Radiosensitivity of capillary endothelium. Br J Radiol 46: 54–57

Reinhold HS, Buisman GH (1975) Repair of radiation damage to capillary endothelium. Br J Radiol 48: 727–731

Reinhold HS, Hopewell JW (1980) Late changes in the architecture of blood vessels of the rat brain after irradiation. Br J Radiol 53: 693–696

Rhee JG, Song CW (1986) The clonogenic response of bovine aortic endothelial; cells in culture to radiation. Radiat Res 106: 182–189

Robbins MEC, Hopewell JW (1988) Effects of single doses of x-rays on renal function in the pig after the irradiation of both kidneys. Radiother Oncol 11: 253–262

Rosen S, Swerdlow MA, Muerche RC, Pirani CL (1964)

Radiation nephritis: light and electron microscopic observations. Am J Clin Pathol 41: 487–502

Rubin DB, Drab EA, Ts'ao C-H, Gardner D, Ward WF (1985) Prostacyclin synthesis in irradiated endothelial cells cultured from bovine aorta. The American Physiological Society, pp 592–597

Rubin P, Casarett GW (1968) Clinical radiation pathology, vols. I and II. W.B. Saunders, Philadelphia

Schweizer E (1924) Über spezifische Röntgenschädigungen des Herzmuskels. Strahlentherapie 18: 812–828

Sheehan JF (1944) Foam cell plaques in intima of irradiated small arteries. Arch Pathol 37: 297–308

Shulman HM, McDonald GB, Matthews D, Doney KC, Kopecky KJ, Gauvreau JM, Thomas ED (1980) An analysis of hepatic veno-occlusive disease and centrilobular hepatic degeneration following bone marrow transplantation. Gastroenterology 79: 1178–1191

Shulman HM, Luk K, Deeg HJ, Shuman WB, Storb R (1987) Induction of hepatic veno-occlusive disease in dogs. Am J Pathol 126: 114–125

Silva-Horta J (1967) Late effects of thorotrast on the liver and spleen and their efferent lymph nodes. Ann NY Acad Sci 145: 676–699

Sinzinger H, Firbas W (1985) Irradiation depresses prostacyclin generation upon stimulation with the platelet-derived growth factor. Br J Radiol 58: 1023–1026

Smith LH, Boss WR (1957) Effects of x-irradiation on renal function of rats. Am J Physiol 188: 367–370

Stewart FA, Denekamp J, Hirst DG (1980) Proliferation kinetics of the mouse bladder after irradiation. Cell Tissue Kinet 13: 75–89

Stewart JR, Fajardo LF (1984) Radiation-induced heart disease: an update. Prog Cardiovasc Dis XXVII: 173–194

Stewart JR, Cohn KE, Fajardo LF, Hanock EW, Kaplan HS (1967) Radiation-induced heart disease. A study of 25 patients. Radiology 89: 302–310

Takahashi T (1930) The action of radium upon the formation of blood capillaries and connective tissue. Br J Radiol 3: 439–445

Tanaka A, Ueno H, Yamashita Y, Caveness WF (1975) Regional cerebral blood flow in delayed brain swelling following x-irradiation of the right occipital lobe in the monkey. Brain Res 96: 233–246

Tannock IF, Hayashi S (1972) The proliferation of capillary endothelial cells. Cancer Res 32: 77–82

Thomas E, Forbus WD (1959) Irradiation injury to the aorta and the lung. Arch Pathol 67: 256–263

Trott KR (1984) Chronic damage after radiation therapy: challenge to radiation biology. Int J Radiat Oncol Biol Phys 10: 907–913

Ts'ao CH, Ward WF (1985) Plasminogen activator activity in lung and alveolar macrophages of rats exposed to graded single doses of gamma rays to the right hemothorax. Radiat Res 103: 393–402

Ts'ao CH, Ward WF, Port CD (1983a) Radiation injury in rat lung. I. Prostacyclin (PGI$_2$) production, arterial perfusion, and ultrastructure. Radiat Res 96: 284–293

Ts'ao CH, Ward WF, Port CD (1983b) Radiation injury in rat lung. III. Plasminogen activator and fibrinolytic inhibitor activities. Radiat Res 96: 301–308

Turesson I, Notter G (1986) The predictive value of skin teleangiectasia for late radiation effects in different normal tissue. Int J Radiat Oncol Biol Phys 12: 603–609

Ullrich RL, Casarett GW (1977) Interrelationship between the early inflammatory response and subsequent fibrosis after radiation exposure. Radiat Res 72: 107–121 Academic, New York

van den Aardweg GJMJ, Hopewell JW, Simmonds RH (1987) Repair and necrosis in the epithelial and vascular connective tissues of pig skin after irradiation. Radiother Oncol 10: 73–82

van den Brenk HAS (1959) The effect of ionizing radiation on capillary sprouting and vascular remodelling in the regenerating repair blastema observed in the rabbit ear chamber. AJR 81: 859–884

van den Brenk HAS (1972) Macro-colony assay for measurement of reparative angiogenesis after x-irradiation. Int J Radiat Biol 21: 607–611

van den Brenk HAS, Orton C, Stone M, Kelly H (1974a) Effects of x-radiation on growth and function of the repair blastema (granulation tissue). I. Wound contraction. Int J Radiat Biol 25: 1–19

van den Brenk HAS, Sharpington C, Orton C, Stone M (1974b) Effects of x-radiation on growth and function of the repair blastema (granulation tissue). II. Measurements of angiogenesis in the Selye pouch in the rat. Int J Radiat Biol 25: 277–289

Vegt GB, Wassenaar AM, Kawilarang-de Haas EWM, Schütte PP, van der Linden M, Di Bon-de Ruijter M, Boon A (1985) Radiation induced changes in the cell membrane of cultured human endothelial cells. Radiat Res 104: 317–328

Vergara JA, UR, Thet LA (1987) Changes in lung morphology and cell number in radiation pneumonitis and fibrosis: a quantitative ultrastructural study. Int J Radiat Oncol Biol Phys 13: 723–732

Walklin CM, Law MP (1986) Biosynthesis of collagen in the lung of the mouse after x-irradiation. Br J Cancer 53 [Suppl VII]: 368–370

Ward WF, Solliday NH, Molteni A, Port CD (1983) Radiation injury in rat lung. II. Angiotensin-convering enzyme activity. Radiat Res 96: 294–300

Ward WF, Molteni A, Solliday NH, Jones GE (1985) The relationship between endothelial dysfunction and collagen accumulation in irradiated rat lung. Int J Radiat Oncol Biol Phys 11: 1985–1990

Ward WF, Molteni A, Ts'ao CH, Solliday NH (1987a) Functional responses of the pulmonary endothelium to thoracic irradiation in rats: differential modification by D-penicillamine. Int J Radiat Oncol Biol Phys 13: 1505–1513

Ward WF, Molteni A, Ts'ao CH, Solliday NH (1987b) Pulmonary endothelial dysfunction induced by unilateral as compared to bilateral thoracic irradiation in rats. Radiat Res 111: 101–106

Warren S (1942) Effects of radiation on normal tissues. VI. Effects of radiation on the cardiovascular system. Arch Pathol 34: 1070–1079

Warren S, Friedman NB (1942) Pathology and pathologic diagnosis of radiation lesions in the gastro-intestinal tract. Am J Pathol 18: 499–514

Wells FR (1963) The lymphatic vessels in radiodermatitis: a clinical and experimental study. Br J Plast Surg 16: 243–256

White DC (1975) An atlas of radiation histopathology. Technical Information Center, Office of Public Affairs, U.S. Energy Research and Development Administration

Windholz F (1937) Zur Kennis der Blutgefässveränderungen im Röntgenbestrahlten Gewebe. Strahlentherapie 59: 662–670

Withers HR, Peters LJ, Kogelnik HS (1980) The pathobiology of late effects of irradiation. In: Meyn RE, Withers

HR (eds) Radiation Biology in Cancer Research. Raven, New York, pp 439–448

Wolbach SB (1909) The pathological histology of chronic x-ray dermatitis and early x-ray carcinoma. J Med Res 21: 415–449

Yamaura H, Yamada K, Matsuzawa T (1976) Radiation effect on the proliferating capillaries in rat transparent chambers. Int J Radiat Biol 30: 179–187

Young CMA, Hopewell JW (1983) The effect of preoperative x-irradiation on the survival and blood flow of pedicle skin flaps in the pig. Int J Radiat Oncol Biol Phys 9: 865–870

Zeman W, Samorajski T (1971) Effects of irradiation in the nervous system. In: Berdjis CC (ed) Pathology of irradiation. Williams and Wilkins, Baltimore, pp 213–277

Zollinger HU (1970) Die Strahlenvasculopathie. Path Eur 5: 145–163

9 Effects of Radiation on the Eye and Ocular Adnexa

CONTENTS

9.1 Introduction

The effects of irradiation on the tissues of the eye and orbit have been studied intensively ever since Roentgen's discovery of x-rays. CHALUPECKY (1897) investigated in animal experiments the effect of x-rays on the cells and tissues of the eye, especially the structures of the anterior segment. BIRCH-HIRSCHFELD (1904) demonstrated that the ocular tissues are highly radiosensitive. AMMAN (1906) was the first to report the development of radiation-induced cataract. Thereafter, numerous publications focused on the problem of radiation cataractogenesis. Other tissues such as the optic nerve and retina were studied to a lesser degree (RUBIN and CASARETT 1968).

The severity of late injury from orthovoltage irradiation, and the sensitivity of the lens to cataract formation, led many ophthalmologists and radiation oncologists to employ this treatment very reluctantly. Despite improvements in treatment techniques, especially due to better precision in planning and dose delivery, radiation therapy to the eye is often rejected because cancer of the eye is not common and except in the few specialized ophthalmological centers in the world the techniques to minimize the late effects of irradiation are not well known. Modern radiotherapy of ocular tumors should only be performed in the few specialized centers which guarantee the close cooperation of ophthalmologists, pediatricians, radiation oncologists, medical physicists, imaging specialists, and plastic surgeons.

In this chapter the effects of radiation upon each of the ocular structures are analyzed according to the different types of radiation treatment, i.e., external beam and plaque therapy, for neoplasms in and around the eye and orbit.

9.2 Lids, Tarsus, and Meibomian Glands

The eyelids react to radiation therapy similar to the skin elsewhere in the body, with erythema followed by dry and moist desquamation. Erythema can be observed after 20–40 Gy[1] and moist desquamation after 50–60 Gy during a course of daily irradiation for basal cell carcinoma of the lids over 6 weeks. Healing usually starts some weeks later, leaving no significant scars or lid deformations. Concomitant bacterial or viral infection of the outer eye during irradiation, or radiation doses in excess of 60 Gy, may lead to severe scarring of the eyelid resulting in ectropion or entropion.

In the case of radiotherapy of tumors of the eyelid, permanent epilation of the eyelashes is observed after a radiation dose in excess of 30 Gy in 3 weeks. Radiation therapy may be used for epilation in patients with trichiasis, to avoid corneal ulceration and perforation.

W. ALBERTI, Priv.-Doz. Dr., Klinik für Strahlentherapie und Nuklearmedizin, Alfried-Krupp-Krankenhaus, Alfried-Krupp-Straße 21, 4300 Essen 1, FRG

[1] The dose quoted refers to radiotherapy with five fractions of 2 Gy per week unless otherwise stated (xf/yw).

The tarsus, the fibrocartilaginous plate in the lids, is quite resistant to irradiation. Late atrophy of the tarsus may occur and does not produce functional impairment.

Little is known about the radiation tolerance of the meibomian glands. Findings in rabbit eyelids indicate that these glands tolerate a dose of 40 Gy (13f/4w) (Hartzler et al. 1984).

9.3 Lacrimal Apparatus

The production of tears and mucus which ensures the physical environment needed for a clear cornea is located in the accessory lacrimal glands of the superior conjunctival fornix and in the upper lid. The major lacrimal gland lies lateral to and above the outer canthus. In planning radiotherapy shielding should be considered for the lateral upper lid and for the lacrimal gland since the remaining glands can lubricate the eye sufficiently, if only part of the lacrimal tissue is damaged. The majority of patients tolerate doses in the range of 30–40 Gy to the entire orbit without developing severe symptoms of a dry eye (Parsons et al. 1983). Atrophy of the lacrimal gland may occur with doses of 50–60 Gy (Merriam et al. 1972). With the same doses, the puncta and canaliculi of the lacrimal ducts will frequently be obliterated and result in tearing which, however, usually does not require treatment.

9.4 Conjunctiva

Damage to the conjunctiva may be a problem in patients with tumors around the eye which must be irradiated using high doses of β-radiation or external beam therapy.

Conjunctival glands are responsible for the production of tears and mucus ensuring an optimal corneal environment. Chronic inflammation in the conjunctiva with damage to its accessory lacrimal glands leads to a depleted precorneal tear film. Drying, scarring, and vascularization can produce lid shortage, corneal opacification, or damage by the abrasive effects of lashes.

Conjunctivitis may develop during radiation therapy with doses in the range of 50 Gy and may be associated with infections, including bacteria, viruses, and other organisms. Responding well to local steroids and antibiotics, conjunctivitis is usually transient. The damage to deeper layers of the conjunctiva, subconjunctival tissues, and tarsus is often followed by scar formation and subsequent contracture. Such scarring is seldom seen with doses lower than 60 Gy (Haik et al. 1986). Keratinization of the conjunctival epithelium has been observed after β-irradiation with 50–100 Gy (Merriam 1956).

Symblepharon may result from denudation of the epithelium in the palpebral and bulbar conjunctiva with subsequent adhesions of the lids to the globe and scarring lids (entropium). This complication has been described only after 80–100 Gy, which is rarely used in treatment (Merriam et al. 1972). Such patients should undergo surgery although this is not always successful.

9.5 Cornea

If the cornea cannot be shielded adequately during treatment, various early and late effects may occur. Punctate keratitis may develop during radiation therapy with doses of 30–50 Gy in 4–5 weeks (Merriam et al. 1972) or 20 Gy in about 8 days (Perrers-Taylor et al. 1965) (neither author cited fractionation). Punctate keratitis is characterized by multiple small defects in the corneal epithelium. Symptoms include irritation of the eye with tearing. In general, this superficial keratitis heals within some weeks or months after radiation therapy. Local antibiotics and corticosteroids can help in this situation. Proper coating of the conjunctival shields with paraffin, or other material, to protect the cornea and palpebral conjunctiva is important (Merriam et al. 1972).

Corneal ulceration, usually preceded by punctate keratitis and edema, has been reported to occur with doses exceeding 60 Gy (Merriam et al. 1972). Corneal ulcers may result in various degrees of scarring with subsequent visual impairment, but in addition corneal perforation following severe, prolonged ulceration has been described after doses of 60 Gy. Perforation can lead to endophthalmitis and loss of sight or of the eye.

Keratinization is a late effect which has been observed after 50 Gy (Merriam et al. 1972) and can become quite severe with higher doses. Secondary corneal vascularization or lipid infiltration usually has been observed after β-irradiation with a ^{90}Sr applicator giving a dose of 200–300 Gy

(MERRIAM 1955, 1956). Keratinization, vascular-ization, and lipid deposits can result in severe visual loss several years after therapy.

9.6 Sclera

The sclera is resistant to radiation but damage to the sclera has been reported after high dose brachytherapy of choroidal melanoma or pterygia. Very high doses, up to 1000 Gy to the posterior sclera, from ^{106}Ru/^{106}Rh plaques caused necrosis in animal experiments (LOMMATZSCH 1968) and in patients (LOMMATZSCH 1973). Yet after irradiation with a ^{90}Sr plaque giving single doses of 20–52 Gy following excision of a pterygium scleral ulceration with a significant risk of infective endophthalmitis has been described (TARR and CONSTABLE 1981). The latter authors suggested that the absence of tissue over the affected sclera, and severe changes in the adjacent conjunctiva, may potentiate scleral ulceration.

Deep scleral ulcerations should be repaired with a scleral patch graft to prevent the endoph-thalmitis which may occur. Thinning of the sclera, often observed in the area of high dose plaque treatment, does not require any treatment.

9.7 Iris

Acute iritis can occur with doses of 70–80 Gy delivered to the anterior segment of the eye (ELLSWORTH 1969; MERRIAM 1955, 1956). Local-ized iris atrophy after β-irradiation of pterygia is asymptomatic. It was observed in both eyes of one patient treated with 45 Gy over 3 consecutive days as a late complication 9 years after pterygium treatment with a ^{90}Sr plaque (TARR and CONST-ABLE 1981). If inflammatory cells close the filtra-tion angle, this can lead to the development of iris neovascularization (rubeosis iridis) and subse-quent glaucoma.

9.8 Lens

The cataractogenic potential of ionizing radiation was recognized as long ago as the beginning of this century. A cataract is defined by the loss of normal transparency. Vision is impaired depending on location, size, and density of the lens opacity. The degree of opacity varies from only a small station-ary cataract, with little or no visual impairment, to a progressive cataract, resulting in loss of vision.

Cataract development is a complex process that may be affected by different risk factors such as age, diabetes mellitus, familial predisposition, ultraviolet and microwave radiation, and drugs (LESKE and SPERDUTO 1983). These factors must be considered when evaluating data on the occurr-ence of radiation-induced cataracts.

The severity and latency of radiation cataract are dose dependent. The latent period between irradiation and cataract formation decreases as the dose increases. The lens is more susceptible to radiation cataractogenesis in younger than in older people. Fractionation reduces the risk and delays the onset of cataract formation (RUBIN and CASARETT 1968). This is confirmed by the clinical data of several authors as analyzed by MERRIAM et al. (1972). The time of onset of cataract ranged from 6 months to many years, with an approxi-mate average of 2–3 years. In the series of MERRIAM and FOCHT (1956) there were only two stationary opacities at a dose to the lens of 2 Gy in a large number of patients. The lowest dose at which a progressive cataract was observed was 5 Gy. Eight out of 14 patients developed progressive cataract after doses between 5 Gy and 8.2 Gy. Patients in this study were divided into three groups: (a) those receiving a single dose, (b) those receiving multiple doses over periods of 3 weeks to 3 months, and (c) those receiving multiple doses over periods greater than 3 months. The minimum cataractogenic dose for each group was 2 Gy, 4 Gy, and 5.5 Gy, respectively. In the first group very few patients developed a stationary cataract. The maximum dose not producing an opacity in the three groups was 2 Gy, 10 Gy, and 10.5 Gy (MERRIAM 1956).

Posterior lens cataracts of varying severity were diagnosed in 25 of 38 eyes irradiated for retinob-lastoma (EGBERT et al. 1978). Therapy was admi-nistered through one or two lateral fields to the whole retina. The dose to the retina ranged from 35 to 60 Gy but the dose to the lens is difficult to assess in these reports.

DEEG (1984) reported 277 patients conditioned with total body irradiation for bone marrow transplantation. Follow-up ranged from 2 to 13 years. One hundred and five patients were given 10 Gy in a single dose, and 76 patients received

12–15 Gy in fractions of 2–4 Gy over 6–7 days. Posterior capsular cataract was observed in 86 patients beginning 1 year after treatment. After single doses patients developed cataracts four times more frequently than after fractionated irradiation.

Schipper et al. (1985) reported 39 children with retinoblastoma (73 affected eyes) treated with a precise megavoltage irradiation technique (Schipper 1983). Forty-five Gy was given to the retina in 15 fractions delivered three times per week. Eighteen eyes developed a clinically detectable cataract; in five of them the lens was aspirated. Cataracts developed exclusively in those lenses where more than 1 mm of the posterior lens was included in the treatment field. The likelihood and the degree of cataract formation were only related to the dose absorbed by the germinative zone of the lens epithelium. The minimum cataractogenic dose found in this series was 8 Gy in 15 fractions. These cataracts did not impair vision. When the dose to the germinative zone of the lens epithelium increased from 8 to 25 Gy, the severity of cataract also increased.

These clinical findings agree with experimental studies of the dose–response relationship for cataracts in rabbits treated with fractionated irradiation and the same accurate irradiation technique (Schipper and Rutgers 1983).

When treating the entire orbit of children with orbital rhabdomyosarcoma, decreased vision was the most common functional problem. In most patients this complication was related to cataract formation, which occurred in 90% of the eyes (36/40) (Heyn et al. 1986). Cataracts were seen with estimated lens doses ranging from <10 Gy to >50 Gy. The latency of onset varied from 1 year and 2 months to 4 years after completion of radiotherapy. Eight children in these series had cataract surgery and useful vision was attained.

McCormick et al. (1988) compared a lens-sparing technique with a modified lateral beam technique in retinoblastoma for local control and side-effects. The lens-sparing technique included an anterior electron beam with a contact lens mounted lead shield, combined with a lateral field. The lateral beam technique was used with lateral electrons and superior and inferior lateral oblique split beam wedged photons. The estimated dose to the lens with the lens-sparing technique was less than 30% of the prescription dose, i.e., approximately 11.5–15 Gy. Six cataracts developed in 97 eyes treated, and all of these were associated with the lens-sparing technique. Mean follow-up of all patients was 33 months. Because positioning of the lens block and the setup of the irradiation field are not reproducible, these specifications on the lens dose are useless. The large number of cataracts simply reflects the insufficiency of the applied radiation technique.

Parsons et al. (1983) made some recommendations on indications for and various approaches to cataract surgery and ensuing rehabilitation. If a cataract impairs vision, the lens should not be removed when the fellow eye has good vision. If extraction is performed, visual rehabilitation can be obtained using a contact lens but it may not be tolerated well if the eye is dry after radiotherapy. Before cataract extraction, retinal function should be evaluated with electroretinography and transscleral visual evoked response. The presence of retinopathy makes the restoration of vision unlikely. In all patients with cataracts, lens implants should be considered.

Augsburger and Shields (1985) studied patients with posterior uveal malignant melanoma treated with ^{60}Co plaque therapy, who underwent extraction of mature cataracts. The study showed that neovascular glaucoma developed as a late complication only in those eyes in which the advanced cataract was not removed (five of six eyes with cataract). Cataract surgery did not improve the visual function of the irradiated eye compared with the nonoperated group of patients. There was no significant difference in terms of tumor characteristics, tumor–related complications, radiation parameters, visual acuity during the follow-up, and observation period. The major reasons for the poor final visual acuity in six eyes included neovascular glaucoma (five eyes) and radiation retinopathy and/or optic neuropathy (one eye).

9.9 Retina

Radiation retinopathy was first described by Stallard (1933) following radon seed implantation for treatment of retinoblastoma. Retinopathy after external beam and brachytherapy has been well documented in a large number of reports (Perrers-Taylor et al. 1965; Stallard 1966; McFaul and Bedford 1970; Bedford et al. 1970; Hayreh 1970; De Schryver et al. 1971; Merriam et al. 1972; Shukovsky and Fletcher 1972; Char et al. 1977; Wara et al. 1979; Brown et al. 1982;

LOMMATZSCH 1983; PARSONS et al. 1983; THOMPSON et al. 1983; KINYOUN et al. 1984; NOBLE and KUPERSMITH 1984; FOERSTER et al. 1986; GRAGOUDAS et al. 1987).

Radiation retinopathy is characterized by microaneurysms of the capillaries, "cotton-wool spots," intraretinal hemorrhages, and leakage of the retinal vessels with hard exudates (CIBIS et al. 1955; PERRERS-TAYLOR et al. 1965; CHEE 1968; HAYREH 1970; HARRIS and LEVENE 1976) (Figs. 9.1–9.3). Progressive occlusion of small retinal vessels with secondary ischemia and edema can be observed subsequently. Chronic changes include vitreous hemorrhage, retinal detachment, and optic nerve atrophy with blindness.

BEDFORD et al. (1970) observed a special susceptibility of the retinal vessels near the optic disk following ^{60}Co plaque therapy. SHUKOVSKY and FLETCHER (1972) noted that the fovea centralis, the most avascular part of the retina with a preponderance of small vessels, is probably the area most sensitive to vascular injury.

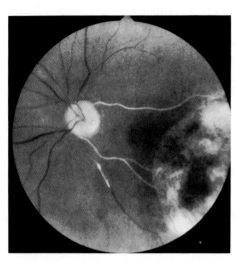

Fig.9.1. Vascular occlusion of retinal vessels of a 61-year-old female patient after ruthenium therapy

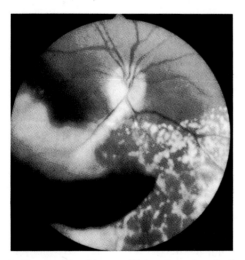

Fig.9.2. Fundus of a 36-year-old female patient harboring a uveal melanoma in the lower temporal quadrant. The patient developed preretinal hemorrhages and extensive lipid exudates 15 months after ruthenium therapy

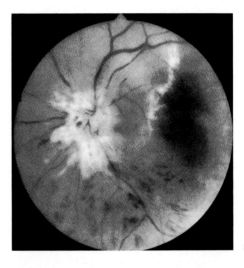

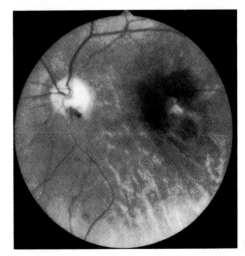

Fig.9.3.a Radiation retinopathy in a 60-year-old patient 11 months after ruthenium plaque therapy of a uveal melanoma of 40° diameter in the temporal quadrant with cotton-wool spots, hemorrhages, and extensive edema and lipid exudates in the area adjacent to the tumor (FOERSTER et al. 1986). **b** The same patient as in **a** 1 year later showing atrophic changes of retinal pigment epithelium, choriocapillaris, and optic nerve

In most cases radiation retinopathy occurs 1/2 to 3 years after high dose radiation therapy (Merriam et al. 1972; Brown et al. 1982). During this interval, visual acuity frequently remains normal; then over a period of several months vision progressively deteriorates (Parsons et al. 1983). There is a wide range in the clinical severity of retinopathy, from little impairment to complete loss of vision. Pain occurs only if neovascular glaucoma is present at the same time.

The addition of chemotherapy may potentiate radiation retinopathy (Chan and Shukovsky 1976; Fishman et al. 1976; Brown et al. 1982). These authors reported that eyes treated with combined radio- and chemotherapy had a higher risk of developing blindness than eyes receiving radiotherapy alone. In addition, the latency period for development of injury was shorter in the combined treatment group (Chan and Shukovsky 1976).

The fundoscopic and fluorescein angiographic appearance of radiation retinopathy is similar to that of diabetic and hypertensive retinopathy (Hayreh 1970). These retinal vascular diseases can potentiate the effect of radiation therapy on retinal vessels, as shown by Brown et al. (1981) and Dhir et al. (1982).

Fluorescein angiography discloses abnormalities of the retinal circulation, including areas of capillary nonperfusion, macular edema, vessel leakage, microaneurysms, and telangiectasia (Howard 1966; Chee 1968; Hayreh 1970) (Fig. 9.4).

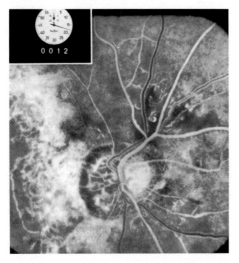

Fig.9.4. Temporal optic atrophy 7 months after ruthenium therapy in a 45-year-old patient with a uveal melanoma of 40° diameter in the macula with capillary nonperfusion without exudation

Several authors state that radiation optic neuropathy is a consequence of radiation retinopathy (McFaul and Bedford 1970; Merriam et al. 1972; Shukovsky and Fletcher 1972). This assumption is supported by the fluorescein angiographic studies of Chee (1968) and Hayreh (1970), who found pathological changes in the capillaries and arterioles initially and later on in the larger arteries with subsequent damage in the retina and fasciculus opticus. The frequency and extent of retinopathy depends on total dose, fractionation, dose rate, beam energy, and radiation field arrangement. The latent period before retinopathy varies from report to report over a wide range between 1 month (Char et al. 1977) and 15 years (Chaudhuri et al. 1981). Usually radiation retinopathy occurs within 3 years after treatment (Brown et al. 1982). A shortening of latency was not observed with increased radiation dose.

Data about the threshold dose of retinal damage vary. With doses of 15–21 Gy in 8 days to 27–31 Gy in 24 days, Perrers-Taylor et al. (1965) noted retinal changes in 20% (24/119) of their patients with a latent period of 2–4 years; there was no reported loss in visual acuity. Complications increase significantly as doses increase to 50 Gy. Shukovsky and Fletcher (1972) reported that 7 of 15 patients developed retinal damage 2–3.5 years after irradiation exceeding 68 Gy in 6 weeks (or a NSD of 2000 rets). Chan and Shukovsky (1976) reported that 2 of 22 patients treated with 60 Gy for carcinoma of the paranasal sinus developed blindness. According to Merriam et al. (1972), 30–35 Gy is the threshold dose for the production of retinal changes. With doses of 70–80 Gy, 85% of the eyes will show retinopathy within several months. Ellsworth (1977) showed that some vascular damage occurred in 10% of cases treated with 35 Gy, 66% with 45 Gy, and 100% with 80 Gy. These observations include children up to 3 years old with retinoblastoma irradiated with dose fractions of 3 Gy.

Schipper et al. (1985) reported a series of 54 patients with retinoblastoma treated with 45 Gy (15f/5w). They observed retinal vascular necrosis in three patients, 8 months (two patients) and 24 months after irradiation. All three eyes retained useful vision.

Histologically the affected retinal vessels have thickened hyalinized walls, and the lumen may be partly or completely obliterated (Howard 1966; Egbert et al. 1980). In addition, shrinkage of choroidal vessels, inner retinal layer atrophy

(PERRERS-TAYLOR et al. 1965), and narrowing of central retinal and ciliary arteries (EGBERT et al. 1980) have been observed. Histological examination of the proximal fasciculus opticus after radiotherapy demonstrates that radiogenic vascular obliteration and perivasculitis are significant, especially in the region of the lamina cribrosa (RIEDEL et al. 1983), resulting in impaired vascular nutrition of the retina.

THOMPSON et al. (1983) reported on patients with posterior nasal space carcinoma treated with 60–70 Gy and daily fractionation over 7–30 weeks. Often the posterior parts of the eye were within the treatment volume and exposed to 60–65 Gy. Radiation retinopathy occurred in seven of ten survivors; five of the affected patients lost vision as a result of vascular damage.

DE SCHRYVER et al. (1971) reported on 30 survivors 7–30 years after irradiation for nasopharyngeal carcinoma. They noted mild retinal changes in 18 patients (estimated eye exposure 13–35 Gy, delivered in 3–6 weeks) with none of them having visual loss from retinopathy.

The significance of fractionation for the development of radiation retinopathy has been stressed by several authors (HARRIS and LEVENE 1076; ARISTIZABAL et al. 1977; PARSONS et al. 1983).

PARSONS et al. (1983) analyzed daily dose fractionation regimens in patients with tumors in and around the eye. In patients with retinal injury producing visual loss, they found an increasing risk of injury with total doses greater than 50 Gy. Below this dose only one severe retinopathy occurred; however, this patient received additional chemotherapy. The analysis of injury-risk vs. time–dose factors was difficult because of the four patients receiving doses in the 50–55 Gy range, three of whom were treated with either chemotherapy (one) or large daily fractions of approximately 3 Gy (two). Almost all of the patients receiving doses in the range of 60 Gy (1.7–2.0 Gy fractions) developed severe retinal injury. The authors concluded that fraction size is the most important factor in producing retinal and optic nerve damage and recommended daily fractions no larger than 2 Gy. So, too, did HARRIS and LEVENE (1976), ARISTIZABAL et al. (1977), WARA et al. (1979), and NAKISSA et al. (1983), who emphasized that the incidence of vascular damage apparently increases with increased fraction size.

KINYOUN et al. (1984) reported that ten fractions of 4 Gy, to a total dose of 40 Gy in 2 weeks, in patients with Graves' ophthalmopathy caused severe retinopathy; three of the four treated patients developed blindness.

There is little information on the successful treatment of the neovascularization frequently associated with radiation retinopathy. CHAUDHURI et al. (1981) reported successful treatment of optic disk and retinal new vessels in a case of radiation retinopathy with argon laser photo-coagulation; the follow-up was 4 months. PARSONS et al. (1983) used laser photocoagulation in one of their irradiated patients; the neovascularization had not progressed 3 years following treatment. In the series of THOMPSON et al. (1983), one patient was treated by argon laser panretinal ablation with a regression of new vessels and cessation of recurring vitreous hemorrhage.

No promising treatment exists for progressive severe retinal damage, which results in progressive deterioration of vision and eventual blindness.

The spontaneous resolution of microvascular abnormalities described by NOBLE and KUPERSMITH (1984) in a 34-year-old patient with bilateral radiation retinopathy is unique. This patient received 45 Gy after subtotal removal of a pituitary adenoma. The fractionation was not reported.

Experimental studies on the effect of radiation on the retina in monkeys, dogs, cats, rabbits, minipigs, rats, and mice have been performed during recent decades (POPPE 1942; BROWN et al. 1955; CIBIS et al. 1955; CIBIS and BROWN 1955; DONEGAN 1956; NOELL 1962; CAVAGGIONT et al. 1969; GRAGOUDAS et al. 1979; IRVINE et al. 1981; LOMMATZSCH et al. 1986; IRVINE and WOOD 1987; ALBERTI et al. 1989). They largely confirm and corroborate the conclusions drawn from the clinical reports described here. An excellent review of the effects of radiation on the retina in experimental animals is given by MERRIAM et al. (1972).

9.10 Optic Nerve

Radiation optic neuropathy (RON) may develop in patients receiving high doses of irradiation for malignant neoplasms in and about the optic nerve and anterior visual pathway. Optic neuropathy can cause acute bilateral or unilateral loss of vision ranging from mild to severe. Following radiation therapy of pituitary adenoma, optic neuropathy is actually part of a more extensive delayed radionecrosis of the central nervous system. This severe complication can also occur following radiation therapy for craniopharyngiomas (Ghatek and White 1969; Harris and Levene 1976; Aristizabal et al. 1977; Martins et al. 1977) or for other tumors (Shukovsky and Fletcher 1972; Ross et al. 1973; Fitzgerald et al. 1981; Parsons et al. 1983; Nakissa et al. 1983). A number of investigators have reported optic nerve injuries after local plaque therapy or external beam irradiation of intraocular malignancies (Cassady et al. 1969; McFaul 1977; Ellsworth 1977; Egbert et al. 1978, 1980; Brown et al. 1982; Shields et al. 1982; Lommatzsch 1983; Foerster et al. 1986; Gragoudas et al. 1987).

The clinical characteristics of radiation-induced anterior optic neuropathy have been described by several authors (Shukovsky and Fletcher 1972; Brown et al. 1982; Parsons et al. 1983; Kline et al. 1985). According to Parsons et al. (1983), two types of RON can be differentiated clinically: (a) injury at the distal end of the nerve, which produces an ischemic neuropathy with disk pallor, edema, and hemorrhages on or around the disk; (b) more proximal injury, producing retrobulbar optic neuropathy without detectable disk edema or hemorrhage. Visual loss occurs suddenly and may be complete or partial with progression over a period of several months. Visual acuity is often reported as "finger counting" or "light perception" vs "no light perception" (McFaul 1977). Visual loss generally was found in one eye and is acute in onset. If both eyes were within the target volume, vision in the fellow eye could deteriorate at the same time or weeks to months later.

After ^{60}Co plaque therapy and external beam irradiation of ocular tumors RON presents with acute signs including disk swelling, peripapillary hard exudates, hemorrhages, and subretinal fluid. "Cotton-wool spots" are often observed (Brown et al. 1982). Most of these eyes also show the typical fluorescein angiographic signs of nerve head ischemia with retinal capillary nonperfusion areas. RON is most often associated with retinopathy, but can sometimes be found alone.

The diagnosis of RON requires careful ophthalmoscopic and radiographic examination. According to Kline et al. (1985) diagnostic criteria include: (a) acute visual loss (monocular or binocular), (b) visual field defects indicating optic nerve or chiasmal dysfunction, (c) absence of optic disk edema, (d) onset usually within 3 years of therapy (peak: 1–1½ years), and (e) no computed tomographic evidence of visual pathway compression. The diagnosis of RON requires high resolution CT scanning with 1.5–2 mm sections and axial and coronal scans. Cerebral redionecrosis appears on CT as an area of decreased attenuation within white matter (Mikhael 1979).

Latency periods from the completion of radiotherapy until the development of RON vary from several months to many years. They seem to be shorter after ^{60}Co plaque treatment (12 months) than after external beam irradiation (19 months) (Brown et al. 1982), probably due to the higher doses delivered with plaque therapy (mean dose: 125 Gy vs 55 Gy). Doses ranged from 35 to 230 Gy in the plaque treated cases, while patients with external beam therapy received 36–70 Gy. The time of development of RON ranged from 3 to 22 months in the former group and from 5 to 36 months in the latter group. Excluding one patient with diabetes mellitus, the lowest dose at which retinopathy occurred was 95 Gy in the plaque group and 36 Gy in the external beam group (fractions not reported). Since doses of about 100 Gy or more are used in the plaque treatment of choroidal melanomas, the lowest dose at which retinopathy should be expected may be lower. In this series with visual loss, predominantly secondary to RON, some eyes experienced improvement in visual acuity several months after the onset of disk swelling. However, improvement of vision is unusual in patients with visual loss caused by RON. Kline et al. (1985) reported four cases with RON and visual loss developing within 3 years after irradiation with doses from 46 to 63.4 Gy in 25–47 fractions. All patients underwent surgery for pituitary adenoma prior to receiving radiation to the perisellar region. In these patients optic nerve deficits are often present and they probably have an increased risk of radiation injury.

In the series of Egbert et al. (1978), one of 28 children irradiated for bilateral retinoblastoma with 47 Gy in 5 weeks (midplane dose) received an additional 49 Gy in 5 weeks for recurrent disease in one eye. Sixteen and 17 years later, respectively, vision decreased in both eyes to light perception only. It was assumed that this patient had an ischemic insult to the optic nerves as a result of late radiation damage.

Abramson et al. (1982) noted a 24.4% incidence of enucleations (22/104) due for radiation complications after a second or third course of external beam therapy for retinoblastoma with total accumulated doses ranging from 54 to 165

Gy. Seventy patients were given chemotherapy as well. In 90 patients treatment failed because of progressive tumor, enucleation, or death. Tumor control was achieved in 14 eyes, all but two belonging to groups I, II, or III according to Reese classification at the time of the second course of irradiation. The main reason so few eyes were lost to irradiation complications (vascular necrosis, i.e., RON) is that so many were lost to uncontrollable disease. Had more of the eyes been salvaged, the majority of eyes would have been lost to complications.

HARRIS and LEVENE (1976) noted optic nerve damage in 5 of 28 patients (18%) with sinus carcinoma using 2.5 Gy or more per fraction, compared with no radiation damage in 27 patients at the rate of 2 Gy per day (total dose: 42–70 Gy). In the series of ARISTIZABAL et al. (1977), 22% of all patients with pituitary adenomas treated with 2.5 Gy fractions developed optic nerve damage, as against 12.5% with 2 Gy fractions to the same total dose of 50 Gy.

PARSONS et al. (1983) gave an account of 12 eyes with RON in 74 patients treated for tumors of the orbit and paranasal sinuses (51) or nasopharynx (17), or for retinoblastoma (6). Sixty to 73 Gy with 1.65–1.9 Gy per fraction produced injuries in 8% (2/24) of long-term survivors. Following daily doses of ≥1.95 Gy, the risk of RON within the same dose range increased to 41% (7/17). Therefore, these authors recommended that the daily dose to the optic nerves should not exceed 1.8–1.9 Gy when the total dose is ≥60 Gy. Portals should be reduced after 50 Gy to cover only a short segment of the optic nerves.

The significance of fractionation is demonstrated through observations by KINYOUN et al. (1984), who observed RON in four patients treated for Graves' ophthalmopathy. A review of the radiotherapy records indicated that three of these patients received daily doses of 4 Gy to a total dose of 40 Gy in 2 weeks. This exceeds the recommended maximum fraction size of 2 Gy (HARRIS and LEVENE 1976) and the generally accepted upper total dose limit of 35 Gy to avoid retinal injury (DUKE-ELDER 1972). SHUKOVSKY and FLETCHER (1972) reported 3 of 30 patients with visual loss due to RON who were irradiated for ethmoid sinus and nasal cavity tumors. These patients received about 70–75 Gy in 34–41 days (fractions not reported). Latency periods to RON were 33, 37, and 42 months.

Optic nerve injury after plaque therapy is related to the energy of the nuclide, the applied dose, the dose rate, and the site and size of the tumor. $^{106}Ru/^{106}Rh$ plaque radiotherapy for posterior uveal malignant melanoma resulted in complete atrophy of the optic nerve in 9.8% (13/132) of treated patients, whereas 3.8% (5/132) had partial atrophy (LOMMATZSCH 1983). Mean follow-up after irradiation was 5.4 years, with a range from 6 months to 16 years. FOERSTER et al. (1986) reported complications from local β-irradiation ($^{106}Ru/^{106}Rh$) of uveal melanomas. Optic neuropathy was observed in 4.1% (12/295) after a mean follow-up period of 1.3 years (maximum follow-up: 5 years). In all cases, tumors were located within 20° adjacent to the optic nerve head. According to the authors no statistically significant relationship could be found between RON and the delivered dose.

Long-term results of 128 proton beam irradiated uveal melanomas showed only two patients developing RON and one patient, radiation papillopathy (GRAGOUDAS et al. 1987). In 22 eyes (17%) radiation vasculopathy which involved the macula occurred. Since optic nerve injury is assumed to be the result of vascular injury, patients with retinopathy may eventually develop RON with longer follow-up than in this series (median: 5.4 years; range: 2.7–10.5 years). In the majority of cases, the total dose delivered to the tumor and to a 1.5 mm margin around the tumor was 70 cobalt Gy equivalent (CGE) in five fractions over 7–10 days (63.6 proton Gy × 1.1 relative biological effectiveness = 70 CGE). Forty-three percent of the tumors were located less than 3 mm from the fovea and/or the optic nerve. Radiation dose in the optic nerve and latency period in patients with RON were not specified (GRAGOUDAS et al. 1987).

FISHMAN et al. (1976) and MARGILETH et al. (1977) noted optic nerve atrophy in patients receiving systemic or intrathecal chemotherapy along with prophylactic cranial irradiation (24 Gy), although the dose of radiation was below that which would be expected to produce neurotoxicity.

CHAN and SHUKOVSKY (1976) reported more frequent loss of vision when 5-FU was given in conjunction with irradiation than when radiation therapy was administered alone. In addition, patients receiving whole eye irradiation with 5-FU developed cataracts, corneal lesions, and chronic conjunctivitis significantly more often.

The exact pathogenesis of delayed radionecrosis of the optic nerve is unknown. Most investigators believe that retinal vascular damage causes subsequent optic neuropathy. A causal relationship is difficult to prove because retinal injury and RON can occur simultaneously after irradiation within the same dose range.

There has until now been no effective treatment for visual loss following RON. GUY and SCHATZ (1986) reported on four patients with RON treated with hyperbaric oxygen therapy initiated within several days after deterioration of vision. In one patient there was an episode of amaurosis fugax, normal vision returning after the second hyperbaric treatment (follow-up: 9 months). In another patient both eyes developed visual loss; light perception was retained in one eye and there was an improvement of 20/200 in the fellow eye. In two other patients decreased visual acuity did not change. The authors recommended that hyperbaric oxygen therapy be offered to patients with visual loss within 2 weeks after the event. In this context it should be mentioned that BROWN et al. (1982) observed that visual acuity in some eyes with decreased vision due to RON improved over a period of several months. Attempts to improve visual function were also made with high dose corticosteroids, but to no avail (KLINE et al. 1985). In general, treatment of delayed radionecrosis of the anterior visual pathway is unsuccessful.

9.11 Orbit

Orbital and facial deformity is a well known late effect in children treated for retinoblastoma (REESE et al. 1949; ELLSWORTH 1969). This complication is caused by growth retardation of the irradiated lateral wall of the orbit. In patients with retinoblastoma formerly treated with an additional nasal field a saddle-nose deformity was observed. Facial deformation was a severe problem with orthovoltage irradiation due to a high absorbed dose in the bone. With megavoltage radiotherapy and doses of 40–50 Gy in 4–5 weeks malformations of the face are minimal. According to our experiences, preenucleation irradiation of large choroidal melanomas with 20 Gy (5f/1w) may produce atrophy of orbital soft tissue, making a good prosthetic fit difficult or even impossible.

9.12 Radiation-Induced Malignancies

The occurrence of secondary malignant neoplasms in survivors of retinoblastoma has been reported in many case reports and series (REESE et al. 1949; FORREST 1961; SOLOWAY 1966; SAGERMAN et al. 1969; JENSEN and MILLER 1971; SHAH et al.1974; ABRAMSON et al. 1976, 1984; MEADOWS et al. 1980, 1985; SCHLIENGER et al. 1985; DRAPER et al. 1986; ALBERTI and HALAMA 1987; MESSMER et al. 1987; KOTEN et al. 1988; SMITH et al. 1989). Since more than 98% of those patients who develop secondary nonocular tumors have bilateral disease (ABRAMSON et al. 1984), which is usually treated with radiation, these tumors have frequently been attributed to radiation. However, one-third to one-half of these patients develop tumors outside the irradiation field (ABRAMSON et al. 1984; SCHLIENGER et al. 1985; DRAPER et al. 1986; ALBERTI and HALAMA 1987; SMITH et al. 1989) or without irradiation (JENSEN and MILLER 1971; SCHIMKE et al. 1974; LENNOX et al. 1975; ABRAMSON et al. 1979; ALBERTI and HALAMA 1987; MESSMER et al. 1987).

The majority of secondary malignant tumors are osteosarcomas and occur in patients with bilateral retinoblastoma, i.e., heritable disease. Modern molecular genetic techniques have demonstrated similar deletions of DNA sequences for retinoblastoma, osteosarcoma, and possibly other mesenchymal tumors at the retinoblastoma locus (band q14 on chromosome 13). The genetic link between these tumors is probably responsible for the high risk of osteosarcomas or other sarcomas in patients with heritable retinoblastoma. Therefore, it is difficult to substantiate the role of radiation or chemotherapy in the induction of nonocular cancer.

SAGERMAN et al. (1969) described a dose – response relationship demonstrating an increased risk of secondary malignant tumors with increasing doses of radiation. This was confirmed by the data of ALBERTI and HALAMA (1987), who found a higher risk in patients treated with 55 Gy and more than in those treated with lesser doses. ABRAMSON et al. (1984) studied 688 survivors of hereditary retinoblastoma. They concluded that a second or third course of betatron irradiation did not increase the incidence of secondary cancer. The role of chemotherapy was not analyzed. SCHIPPER and ALBERTI (1985) reported 102 patients with bilateral retinoblastoma irradiated in Essen between 1959 and 1972, with a follow-up of at least 10 years. Seventy-two of these patients received orthovoltage therapy alone and the remaining 30 received additional chemotherapy with alkylating agents. The incidence of radiogenic secondary tumors (i.e., within the irradiation field) was 4% (3/72) in those with orthovoltage therapy alone and 20% (6/30) in those who received chemotherapy as well.

DRAPER et al. (1986) reported 882 patients with retinoblastoma, 90 of whom received cyclophosphamide. They found that the addition of chemotherapy increased the risk of secondary malignancies (within and outside the irradiation field) significantly.

The cumulative risk at 10, 20, and 30 years was 6%, 19%, and 38%, respectively, in the study of SMITH et al. (1989) and 20%, 50%, and 90%, respectively, in the series of ABRAMSON et al. (1984). DRAPER et al. (1986) reported a cumulative risk of 4.3% at 12 years and 8.4% at 18 years. KOTEN et al. (1988) reported an 11% incidence at 35 years in heritable disease. Life table analysis of our data demonstrates a 47.5% incidence in the high dose orthovoltage group (>55 Gy) and a 5% incidence in the low dose group (<55 Gy) after 16 years (ALBERTI and HALAMA 1987).

In the future, more patients with retinoblastoma will probably die from secondary cancer rather than from metastatic disease. Careful treatment planning, sophisticated radiation techniques, limitation of the radiation dose, and the employment of additional ophthalmological methods such as photocoagulation and cryotherapy or of hyperthermia may reduce the risk of secondary tumors. Because there seems no evidence that chemotherapy is of benefit in the treatment of retinoblastoma, its use should be restricted to patients with metastatic disease. The occurrence of nonocular malignancies, after long latent periods, must be considered in the management of retinoblastoma.

9.13 Effect of Combined Hyperthermia and Radiation Therapy

It is reasonable to assume that, with suitable techniques, choroidal melanomas can be heated more successfully than malignancies encountered elsewhere in the body. Various thermoradiotherapy applicators have been developed to treat choroidal melanoma. For an episcleral approach,

a hyperthermia source (4.8 GHz microwave antenna) was incorporated at the base of a ^{125}I scleral plaque by FINGER et al. (1985).

Clinical experience with hyperthermia in retinoblastoma and choroidal melanoma is limited (COLEMAN et al. 1986; SCHIPPER and LAGENDIJK 1986; RIEDEL et al. 1987; FINGER et al. 1989; SCHIPPER et al., in press). There is a large clinical series including 26 patients with recurrent or advanced retinoblastoma and two monocular patients with choroidal melanoma treated with microwave-induced hyperthermia and external beam therapy (SCHIPPER et al., in press). Although the first patients were treated in 1981, knowledge of late effects is sparse because enucleation was required for most stage 5A tumors. The rate of cataract formation was not increased in the eyes receiving combined hyperthermia and irradiation compared with radiation therapy alone. Hyperthermia had to be discontinued in three patients after either two (one patient) or three (two patients) heat treatments because of a small thermal burn, probably due to a hot spot opposite the stripline. One patient with a choroidal melanoma and one with a retinoblastoma had follow-ups of 37 and 55 months, respectively; no significant damage to the lens, retina, or optic nerve was noted.

Thermoradiotherapy was used by FINGER et al. (1989) in 18 patients with medium and large choroidal melanomas according to the technique described above (FINGER et al. 1985). Tumors were treated with 48-88 Gy at the apex and 46°-52.5°C at the base for 45 min in one session. No evidence of damage to normal ocular structures outside the target volume was noted at a mean observation time of 13.3 months (range 1-29 months).

In experimental investigations, no enhancement of radiation damage was observed in rabbit eyes treated with additional hyperthermia below 45°C (SCHIPPER et al., in press). At temperatures between 45°C and 46°C a subcapsular posterior pole lens cataract appeared. At temperatures above 46°C, iris-lens adhesions, severe hemorrhages, and mature cataracts occurred. Additionally, in two rabbits with healthy eyes and 13 rabbits with Greene melanoma transplanted to the anterior chamber of both eyes, the effect of radiotherapy alone or radiotherapy combined with hyperthermia was examined. Both eyes were irradiated simultaneously to a total dose of 36, 45, or 54 Gy (three fractions of 3 Gy per week) with an accurate megavoltage technique (Schipper 1983). After combined treatment, careful ophthalmoscopic examination demonstrated no enhancement of radiation damage compared with radiation therapy alone.

Alberti et al. (1988) studied ocular late effects in minipigs (Göttingen breed) with and without fractionated external beam therapy (40 Gy, 16f/4w). Hyperthermia at 43°C for 30 min was applied twice weekly. No radiation retinopathy or radiation-induced neuropathy was observed with ophthalmoscopy and fluorescein angiography until 24 months after combined treatment. Two eyes could be examined by light and electron microscopy 6 months after hyperthermia alone. Changes noted in the retina and optic nerve included alteration in several retinal layers, particularly the photoreceptor cell layer, and myelin sheaths and axolemma. The pathological changes were similar to those obtained after fractionated radiotherapy alone (40 Gy, 16f/4w).

Acknowledgments. I am grateful to Dr. Robert Sagerman, Syracuse, N.Y., for his advice and for reviewing the manuscript. I thank Dr. M.H. Foerster, Essen, for allowing me to include fundus photographs (Figs. 9.1–9.4) from his publication: Foerster MH, Bornfeld N, Schulz U, Wessing A, Meyer-Schwickerath G (1986) Graefes Arch Clin Exp Ophthalmol 224: 336–340.

References

Abramson DH, Ellsworth RM, Zimmerman LE (1974) Nonocular cancer in radiotherapy for retinoblastoma. Am Surg 40: 485–490

Abramson DH, Ronner HJ, Ellsworth RM (1979) Second tumors in nonirradiated bilateral retinoblastoma. Am J Ophthalmol 87: 624–627

Abramson Dh, Ellworth RM, Zimmerman LE (1976) Nonocular cancer in retinoblastoma survivors. Trans Am Acad Ophthal Otolaryng 87: 624–627

Abramson DH, Ellsworth RM, Rosenblatt M, Tretter P, Jereb B, Kitchin D (1982) Retreatment of retinoblastoma with external beam irradiation. Arch Ophthalmol 100: 1257–1260

Abramson DH, Ellsworth RM, Kitchin D, Tung G (1984) Second nonocular tumors in retinoblastoma survivors. Are they radiation-induced? Ophthalmology 91: 1351–1355

Alberti W, Halama J (1987) Tumoren des Auges und der Orbita. In: Scherer E (ed) Strahlentherapie, Radiologische Onkologie. Springer, Berlin Heidelberg New York, pp 412–467

Alberti W, Adametz KP, El-Hifnawi E, Bornfeld N, Foerster MH (1988) Preliminary results after hyperthermia of minipig eyes with and without external beam

therapy. In: Sugahara T, Saito M (eds) Hyperthermic oncology, 1, 1988, summary papers. Taylor & Francis, London, pp 100–102

Amman E (1906) Zur Wirkung der Röntgenstrahlen auf das menschliche Auge. Korrespondenz-Blatt für Schweizer Ärzte 15

Aristizabal S, Caldwell WL, Avita J (1977) The relationship of time-dose fractionation factors of complications in the treatment of pituitary tumors by irradiation. Int J Radiat Oncol Biol Phys 2: 667–673

Augsburger JJ, Shields JA (1985) Cataract surgery following cobalt-60 plaque. Radiotherapy for posterior uveal malignant melanoma. Ophthalmology 92: 815–822

Bedford MA, Bedotto C, MacFaul PA (1970) Radiation retinopathy after the application of a cobalt plaque. Br J Ophthalmol 54: 505–509

Birch-Hirschfeld A (1904) Die Wirkung der Röntgen- und Radiumstrahlen auf das Auge. Graefes Arch Ophthalmol 59: 229–310

Blodi FC (1958) The late effects of x-radiation on the cornea. Trans Am Ophthalmol Soc 56: 413

Blodi FC (1960) The effects of experimental x-radiation on the cornea. Arch Ophthalmol 63: 44–53.

Brown CD, Cibis PA, Pickering JE (1955) Radiation studies on the monkey eyes. Arch Ophthalmol 59: 249–256

Brown GC, Shields JA, Sanborn G, Augsburger JJ, Savino PJ, Schatz NJ (1981) Radiation retinopathy. Ophthalmology 43: 144–151

Brown GC, Shields JA, Sanborn G, Augsburger JJ, Savino PJ, Schatz NJ (1982) Radiation optic neuropathy. Ophthalmology 89: 1489–1493

Cassady JR, Sagerman RH, Tretter P, Ellsworth RM (1969) Radiation therapy in retinoblastoma. Radiology 93: 405–409

Cavaggioni A, Peracchia G, Rosati G (1969) Electrical activity of the ganglion cells in irradiated retinas. Radiat Res 39: 658

Chalupecky H (1897) Über die Wirkung der Röntgenstrahlen auf das Auge und die Haut. Zentralbl Augenheilkd 21: 234

Chan RC, Shukovsky LJ (1976) Effects of irradiation on the eye. Radiology 120: 673–675

Char DH, Lonn LI, Margolis LW (1977) Complications of cobalt plaque therapy of choroidal melanomas. Am J Ophthalmol 84: 536–540

Chaudhuri PR, Austin DJ, Rosenthal AR (1981) Treatment of radiation retinopathy. Br J Ophthalmol 65: 623–625

Chee PHY (1968) Radiation retinopathy. Am J Ophthalmol 66: 860

Cibis PA, Brown DVL (1955) Retinal changes following ionizing radiation. Am J Ophthalmol 40: 84–88

Cibis PA, Noell WK, Eichel B (1955) Ocular effects produced by high intensity x-radiation. Arch Ophthalmol 53: 651

Coleman DJ, Lizzi FL, Burgess SEP (1986) Ultrasonic hyperthermia and radiation in the management of intaocular malignant melanoma. Am J Ophthalmol 101: 635–642

Deeg HJ (1984) Bone marrow transplantation: a review of delayed complications. Br J Haematol 57: 185–208

De Schryver A, Wachtmeister L, Baryd I (1971) Ophthalmologic observations on long-term survivors after radiotherapy for nasopharyngeal tumours. Acta Radiol 10: 193–209

Dhir SP, Joshi AV, Banerjee AK (1982) Radiation

retinopathy in diabetes mellitus. Acta Radiol Oncol 21: 111–113

Donegan J (1956) Ocular effects of body ^{60}Co irradiation. Am J Ophthalmol 42: 309

Draper GJ, Sanders BM, Kingston JE (1986) Second primary neoplasms in patients with retinoblastoma. Br J Cancer 53: 661–671

Duke-Elder S (1972) System of ophthalmology, vol 14, part 2: Injuries; nonmechanical injuries. CV Mosby, St. Louis, 985–999

Egbert PR, Donaldson SS, Moazed K, Rosenthal R (1978) Visual results and ocular complications following radiotherapy for retinoblastoma. Arch Ophthalmol 96: 1826–1830

Egbert PR, Fajardo LF, Donaldson SS, Moazed K (1980) Posterior ocular abnormalities after irradiation for retinoblastoma: a histopathological study. Br J Ophthalmol 64: 660–665

Ellsworth RM (1969) The practical management of retinoblastoma. Trans Am Ophthalmol Soc 67: 462–534

Ellsworth RM (1977) Retinoblastoma. Mod Probl Ophthalmol 18: 94–199

Finger PT, Packer S, Svitra PP, Paglione RW, Chess J, Albert S (1984) Hyperthermic treatment of intraocular tumors. Arch Ophthalmol 102: 1477–1481

Finger PT, Packer S, Svitra PP, Paglione RW, Anderson LL, Kim JH, Jakobiec FA (1985) Thermoradiotherapy for intraocular tumors. Arch Ophthalmol 103: 1574–1578

Finger PT, Packer S, Svitra PP, Paglione RW, Gatz JF, Ho TK, Bosworth JL (1989) Thermoradiotherapy of choroidal melanoma. Ophthalmology 96: 1384–1388

Fishman ML, Bean SC, Cogan DG (1976) Optic atrophy following prophylactic chemotherapy and cranial radiation for acute lymphocytic leukemia. Am J Ophthalmol 82: 571–576

Fitzgerald CR, Enoch JM, Temme LA (1981) Radiation therapy in and about the retina, optic nerve and anterior visual pathway; psychophysical assessment. Arch Ophthalmol 99: 611–623

Foerster MH, Bornfeld N, Schulz U, Wessing A, Meyer-Schwickerath G (1986) Complications of local beta radiation of uveal melanomas. Graefes Arch Clin Exp Ophthalmol 224: 336–340

Forrest AW (1961) Tumors following radiation about the eye. Trans Am Acad Ophthalmol Otolaryngol 65: 694

Ghatak NR, White BE (1969) Delayed radiation necrosis of the hypothalamus. Arch Neurol 21: 425–430

Gragoudas ES, Zakow NZ, Albert DM (1979) Long-term observations of proton-irradiation monkey eyes. Arch Ophthalmol 97: 2184–2191

Gragoudas ES, Seddon JM, Egan K et al. (1987) Long-term results of proton beam irradiated uvea melanomas. Ophthalmology 94: 349–353

Guy J, Schatz NJ (1986) Hyperbaric oxygen in the treatment of radiation induced optic neuropathy. Ophthalmology 93: 1083–1088

Haik BG, Jereb B, Smith ME, Ellsworth RM, McCormick B (1986) Radiation and chemotherapy of parameningeal rhabdomyosarcoma involving the orbit. Ophthalmology 93: 1001–1009

Harris JR, Levene MB (1976) Visual complications following irradiation for pituitary adenomas and craniopharyngiomas. Radiology 120: 167–171

Hartzler J, Neldner KH, Forstot L (1984) x-ray epilation for the treatment of trichiasis. Arch Dermatol 120: 620–624

Hayreh SS (1970) Post radiation therapy. A fluorescence fundus angiographic study. Br J Ophthalmol 54: 705–714

Heyn R, Ragab A, Raney B et al. (1986) Late effects of therapy in orbital rhabdomyosarcoma in children. Cancer 57: 1738–1743

Howard GM (1966) Ocular effects of radiation and photocoagulation. Arch Ophthalmol 76: 7

Irvine AR, Wood IS (1987) Radiation retinopathy as an experimental model for ischemic proliferative retinopathy and rubeosis iridis. Am J Ophthalmol 103: 790–797

Irvine AR, Alvarado JA, Wara WM, Morris BW, Wood IS (1981) Radiation retinopathy: an experimental model for the ischemic proliferative retinopathies. Trans Am Ophthalmol 79: 103–122

Jensen RD, Miller RW (1971) Retinoblastoma: epidemiology characteristics. N Engl J Med 285: 307–311

Kinyoun JL, Kalina RE, Brower SA, Mills RP, Johnson RH (1984) Radiation retinopathy after orbital irradiation for Graves' ophthalmopathy. Arch Ophthalmol 102:1473–1476

Kline LB, Kim JY, Ceballos R (1985) Radiation optic neuropathy. Ophthalmology 92: 1118–1126

Koten JW, der Kindren DJ, Otter WD (1988) Editorial reply. N Engl J Med 318: 581–582

Lennox EL, Draper GJ, Sanders BM (1975) Retinoblastoma: a study of natural history and prognosis of 268 cases. Br Med J 3: 731–734

Leske MC, Sperduto RD (1983) The epidemiology of senile cataracts: a review. Am J Epidemiol 118: 152–165

Lommatzsch P (1968) Morphologische und funktionelle Veränderungen des Kaninchenauges nach Einwirkung von Betastrahlen auf den dorsalen Bulbusabschnitt. Graefes Arch Klin Exp Ophthalmol 176: 100–125

Lommatzsch P (1973) Experiences in the treatment of malignant melanoma of the choroid with 106Ru/106Rh beta ray applicators. Trans Ophthalmol Soc UK 93: 119–132

Lommatzsch P (1983) β-Irradiation of choroidal melanoma with 106Ru/106Rh applicators. Arch Ophthalmol 101: 713–717

Lommatzsch P, Weise B, Ballin R (1986) Ein Beitrag zur Optimierung der Bestrahlungszeit bei der Behandlung des malignen Melanoms der Aderhaut mit β-Applikatoren (106Ru/106Rh). Klin Monatsbl Augenheilkd 189: 133–140

Margileth DA, Poplack DG, Pizzo PA, Leventhal BG, (1977) Blindness during remission in two patients with acute lymphoblastic leukemia. Cancer 39: 58

Martins AN, Johnston JS, Henry JM (1977) Delayed radiation necrosis of the brain. J Neurosurg 47: 336–345

McCormick B, Ellsworth R, Abramson D, Haik B, Tome M, Grbowski E, LoSasso T (1988) Radiation therapy for retinoblastoma: comparison of results with lens-sparing versus lateral beam techniques. Int J Radiat Oncol Biol Phys 15: 567–574

McFaul PA (1977) Local radiotherapy in the treatment of malignant melanoma of the choroid. Trans Ophthalmol Soc UK 97: 421–427

McFaul PA, Bedford MA (1970) Ocular complications after therapeutic irradiation. Br J Ophthalmol 54: 237–247

Meadows AT, Strong LC, Li FP et al. (1980) Bone sarcomas as a second malignant neoplasm in children: influence of radiation and genetic predisposition. Cancer 46: 532–538

Meadows AT, Baum E, Fossati-Bellami F et al. (1985)

Second malignant neoplasms in children: an update from the late effects study group. J Clin Oncol 3: 532–538

Merriam GR (1955) Late effects of β-radiation on the eye. AMA Arch Ophthalmol 53: 708–717

Merriam GR (1956) A clinical study of radiation cataracts. Trans Am Ophthalmol Soc 54: 611–653

Merriam GR, Focht EF (1962) A clinical and experimental study of the effect of single and divided doses of radiation on cataract production. Trans Am Ophthalmol Soc 60: 35–52

Merriam GR, Szechter A, Focht EF (1972) The effects of ionizing radiations on the eye. Front Radiat Ther Oncol 6: 346–385

Messmer EP, Richter HJ, Höpping W, Havers W, Alberti W (1987) Nichtokulärer, maligner Zweittumor nach Spontanheilung eines Retinoblastoms. Klin Monatsbl Augenheilkd 19: 299–303

Mikhael MA (1979) Radiation necrosis of the brain: correlation between patterns on computed tomography and dose of radiation. J Comput Assist Tomogr 3: 241–249

Nakissa N, Rubin P, Strohl R, Keys H (1983) Ocular and orbital complications following radiation therapy of paranasal sinus malignancies and review of literature. Cancer 51: 980–986

Noble KG, Kupersmith MJ (1984) Retinal vascular remodelling in radiation retinopathy. Br J Ophthalmol 68: 475–478

Noell WK (1962) x-Irradiation studies on mammalian retina. In: Haley Snider (eds) Response of the nervous system to ionizing radiation. Academic, New York

Parsons JT, Fitzgerald CR, Hood CI, Ellingwood KE, Bova FJ, Million RR (1983) The effects of irradiation on the eye and optic nerve. Int J Oncol Biol Phys 9: 609–612

Perrers-Taylor M, Brinkley D, Reynolds T (1965) Choroido-retinal damage as a complication of radiotherapy. Acta Radiol 3: 431–440

Poppe E (1942) Experimental investigations of the effects of roentgen rays on the eye. Thesis, Oslo

Reese AB, Merriam GR, Martin HE (1949) Treatment of bilateral retinoblastoma by irradiation and surgery. Am J Ophthalmol 32: 175

Riedel KG, Stefani FH, Kampik A (1983) Histopathologische Veränderungen im proximalen Fascikulus optikus nach therapeutischer Bestrahlung. Fortschr Ophthalmol 80: 48–52

Riedel KG, Svitra PP, Seddon JM et al. (1985) Proton beam irradiation and hyperthermia. Effects on experimental choroidal melanoma. Arch Ophthalmol 103: 1862–1869

Riedel KG, Schaal GS, Svitra PP, Albert DM, Finger PT, Packer S (1987) Ocular changes following combined microwave hyperthermia and beta-irradiation in rabbit eyes. Invest Ophthalmol Vis Sci 28: 59

Ross HS, Rosenberg S, Friedman AH (1973) Delayed radiation necrosis of the optic nerve. Am J Ophthalmol 76: 683–686

Rubin PH, Casarett GW (1968) Organs of special sense: the eye and the ear. In: Rubin PH, Casarett GW (eds) Clinical radiation pathology. WB Sauders, Philadelphia, pp 662–719

Sagerman RH, Cassady JR, Tretter P, Ellsworth RM (1969) Radiation induced neoplasia following external beam therapy for children with retinoblastoma. AJR 105: 529–535

Schimke RN, Lowman JT, Cowan GAB (1974) Retinoblastoma and osteogenic sarcoma in siblings. Cancer 34: 2077–2079

Schipper J (1983) An accurate and simple method for megavoltage irradiation therapy of retinoblastoma. Radiother Oncol 1: 31–41

Schipper J, Alberti W (1985) Letter to the editor. Ophthalmology 92: 60a–62a

Schipper J, Lagendijk JJW (1986) The treatment of retinoblastoma by fractionated radiotherapy combined with hyperthermia. In: Anghileri LJ, Robert J (eds) Hyperthermia in cancer treatment. CRC Press, Boca Raton, Fl, pp 79–87

Schipper J, Rutgers DH (1983) The dose-response relationship for cataracts arising after fractionated irradiation of the entire posterior portion of the lens of the rabbit. Proceedings of the 7th International Congress of Radiation Research, July 1983, Amsterdam, C 2–12

Schipper J, Tan KEWP, van Peperzeel HA (1985) Treatment of retinoblastoma by precision megavoltage radiation therapy. Radiother Oncol 3: 117–132

Schipper J, Lagendijk JJW, Tan KEWP (in press) Hyperthermia in the treatment of intraocular tumors, in particular retinoblastoma. In: Alberti W, Sagerman RH (eds) Radiotherapy of intraocular and orbital tumors. Springer, Heidelberg, Berlin, New York

Schlienger P, Calle R, Haye C, Vilcoq JR (1985) Sarcomes osseux et tumeurs malignes de la retine. Bull Cancer 72: 16–24

Shan IC, Arlen M, Miller T (1974) Osteogenic sarcoma developing after radiotherapy for retinoblastoma. Ann Surg 40: 485–490

Shields JA, Augsburger JJ, Brady LW, Day IL Cobalt plaque therapy for posterior uveal melanomas. Ophthalmology 89: 1201–1207

Shukovsky LJ, Fletcher GH (1972) Retinal and optic nerve complications in a high dose irradiation technique of ethmoid sinus and nasal cavity. Radiology 104: 629–634

Smith LM, Donaldson SS, Egbert PR, Link MP, Bagshaw MA (1989) Aggressive management of second primary tumors in survivors of hereditary retinoblastoma. Int J Radiat Oncol Biol Phys 17: 499–505

Soloway HB (1966) Radiation induced neoplasms following curative therapy for retinoblastoma. Cancer 19: 1984–1988

Stallard HB (1933) Radient energy as (a) a pathogenic, (b) a therapeutic agent in ophthalmic disorders. Br J Ophthalmol, Monograph Supplement 6

Stallard HB (1966) Radiotherapy for malignant melanoma of the choroid. Br J Ophthalmol 50: 147–155

Tarr KH, Constable IJ (1981) Radiation damage after pterygium treatment. Aust J Ophthalmol 9: 97–101

Thompson GM, Migdal CS, Whittle RJM (1983) Radiation retinopathy following treatment of posterior nasal space carcinoma. Br J Ophthalmol 67: 609–614

Wara WM, Irvine AR, Neger RE, Howes EL, Phillips TL (1979) Radiation retinopathy. Int J Radiat Oncol Biol Phys 5: 81–83

10 Oral Cavity and Salivary Glands

K.K. Ang, L.C. Stephens, and T.E. Schultheiss

CONTENTS

10.1 Introduction

Radiation therapy plays an essential role in the management of patients with head and neck cancers. Radiotherapy is the preferred single modality

K.K. Ang, M.D., Ph.D., Professor, Division of Radiotherapy, The University of Texas, M.D. Anderson Cancer Center Houston, TX 77030, USA

L.C. Stephens, D.V.M., Ph.D., Associate Professor, Division of Veterinary Medicine and Surgery, The University of Texas, M.D. Anderson Cancer Center Houston, TX 77030, USA

T.E. Schultheiss, Ph.D., Associate Professor, Division of Radiotherapy, The University of Texas, M.D. Anderson Cancer Center Houston, TX 77030, USA

treatment for the majority of patients with small lesions (e.g., T_1 and T_2 tumors) since it is as effective as surgery in the local eradication of the neoplastic disease but, in general, produces less functional impairment and less cosmetic deformity. Combinations of surgery and radiation therapy are recommended for patients with advanced locoregional disease. The rationale behind combined treatment is that surgical resection of gross tumor eliminates the most common cause of radiotherapeutic failure, whereas radiotherapy is more efficient at sterilizing microscopic tumor beyond the margins of the surgical resection. Unfortunately, radiation doses required in these clinical settings do induce transient normal tissue injuries, functional deficits, and occasionally, persistent complications. The scope of this chapter is to review the various major side-effects associated with head and neck radiotherapy. To facilitate the discussion, we shall first describe some basic concepts and also the terminology used throughout this chapter.

Operationally, morbidities associated with irradiation of normal tissues are divided into acute and late effects depending on their time of manifestation relative to radiation treatment. Acute reactions by definition occur mostly during a course of fractionated irradiation or soon thereafter, and, in most cases, can be attributed to mitotic-linked reproductive killing of stem cells in rapidly proliferating tissues, e.g., mucous membranes of the aerodigestive tracts. Recently, however, another mode of cell killing not linked to the cellular reproductive activity, termed 'interphase' cell killing, was found to underlie the pathogenesis of a bothersome side-effect associated with radiotherapy of the head and neck area, namely xerostomia (El Mofty and Kahn 1981; Sholley et al. 1974; Sodicoff et al. 1974; Stephens et al. 1986a,c,d).

Late radiation sequelae have their onset months or even years after therapy has been completed. The exact mechanism of most late injuries is incompletely understood. Since tissues that manifest late radiation reactions generally have less well defined proliferative compartments, it is more difficult to ascribe late injury to death of a single cell type in a given organ. Therefore for most slowly proliferative late-reacting normal tissues it has not been established whether the final injury results predominantly from damage to the parenchymal or to stromal elements of the tissues, or more likely, to a combination of damage to both components (HOPEWELL 1980; VAN DER KOGEL 1980; WITHERS et al. 1980). In certain circumstances, however, late normal tissue injury may occur as a consequence of severe epithelial denudation rather than direct radiation injury to the late-responding tissues. This type of injury is termed "consequential late effect" (PETERS et al. 1988). Examples of this type of morbidity in the head and neck area include soft tissue necrosis resulting from chronic mucosal ulcers, and tooth decay leading to osteonecrosis following irradiation of oral cavity and salivary gland. The fractionation characteristics of consequential late effects are, by definition, the same as those for acute reactions.

The difference in the time of manifestation of radiation injury in various tissues (acute vs late effects) has an important clinical implication. In a conventionally fractionated course of radiotherapy, acute reactions usually manifest themselves during treatment, which allows for therapeutic modifications to be made in the event that they are excessive. If, however, the overall treatment time is drastically reduced, the acute tissular reactions may not reach the maximal intensity before completion of treatment. This precludes the opportunity to adjust treatment to the severity of side-effects. Obviously, since late effects never occur before completion of radiotherapy, therapeutic decisions can be made only on a probability basis. For these reasons, it is important to understand the factors that determine the tolerance of acute- and late-responding tissues and the mode and extent of interaction between various treatment modalities.

10.2 Mucous Membrane

10.2.1 Anatomy

The oral cavity consists of an outer portion, the vestibule, and an inner larger portion, the mouth cavity proper. The vestibule communicates with the exterior superiorly and inferiorly through the lips. It is bounded laterally by the cheeks and internally by the gums and teeth. It receives the secretions of the parotid gland from the opening of Stensen's duct alongside the second upper molar. The mouth cavity proper communicates with the pharynx. It is bounded laterally and ventrally by the alveolar arches and teeth. The roof of the mouth cavity is the hard and soft palates while the greater part of the floor is formed by the tongue. Secretions from the submandibular and sublingual salivary glands enter the mouth cavity proper on the ventral surface of the tongue.

The vestibule and mouth cavity proper are lined by mucous membrane that is covered by nonkeratinizing, stratified squamous epithelium. The lack of cornification, under normal conditions, and a somewhat higher rate of cell renewal distinguish the epithelium of the oral mucosa from that of the skin. Senescent surface cells of the mucosa, without becoming cornified, slough off into the fluids of the mouth. Secretions from the major and minor salivary glands prevent drying of the mucous membranes.

Beneath the epithelium of the mucosa is the lamina propria, a relationship that is the counterpart of dermis to epidermis. It consists of collagen and elastic fibers with numerous blood vessels, abundant innervation with sensory nerve branches, and dispersed minor salivary glands. A submucosa of variable depth is present in the cheek and soft palate areas, but it is essentially absent in such regions as the hard palate and alveolar ridge. The lamina propria covering the alveolar ridge, i.e., gums, is composed of dense fibrous connective tissue that is closely connected to the periosteum of the alveolar processes surrounding necks of the teeth. The mucous membrane of the gum is very smooth and highly vascular, but it lacks the rich nerve innervation of the other locations. Around the teeth this membrane sends numerous fine papillae and is reflected into the alveoli, where it is continuous with the periosteal membrane lining this cavity.

The tongue is a mass of interlacing bundles of skeletal muscle that is largely encased by mucous membrane. The epithelium of the underside is smooth and relatively thin, whereas the dorsal surface consists of thickened and rough epithelium that forms numerous papillary projections and depressions, which are taste buds.

10.2.2 Significance

Mucous membranes are rapidly proliferating tissues and hence manifest radiation injury early. Since the advent of skin-sparing megavoltage radiotherapy equipment, the acute mucous membrane reactions of the upper aerodigestive tracts have limited the pace by which radiation treatment can be delivered. Acute radiation-induced side-effects on mucous membranes result from reproductive killing of stem cells in the basal layer of the epithelium. Death of these cells has no instantaneous clinical consequence, but the physiological loss of cells in the superficial layers of the epithelium by wear and tear is not rectified. This causes, after a lag period, determined by cytokinetics and radiation dose, mucosal denudation. This denudation triggers the stem cells surviving radiation insult into accelerated proliferation in attempts to offset this induced cell depletion and to repopulate the tissue. The magnitude and length of denudation depend on numerous factors such as time–dose fractionation factors of radiation treatment and presence of radiation response modifiers. The available clinical and experimental data on these various subjects will be summarized in a systematic fashion.

10.2.3 Morphology of Irradiated Oral Mucosa

Although the macroscopic changes are quite familiar, biopsy of the oral mucosa to examine the histology of the acute changes is rarely done. Therefore, only generalities can be made from limited observations on human and animal material.

Shortly following commencement of fractionated irradiation, dividing cells in the basal layer of the stratified squamous epithelium undergo degeneration and necrosis. The lamina propria and submucosa become edematous and contain infiltrations of neutrophils. Capillaries may be dilated and the endothelium swollen. These cause an observable erythema. Minor salivary glands, which are mainly of the mucous variety, may show some distention of ducts and acini filled with secretions, but necrotic cells are only rarely observed. Oral lymphoid tissue, such as Waldeyer's ring, contains numerous dead cells and abundant nuclear debris (FAJARDO 1982). Atypical fibroblasts may appear in the submucosa during the acute phase but are more commonly seen

later. Approximately 2–4 weeks into a 6- to 7-week course of fractionated irradiation, erosion and desquamation of mucosal epithelium occur. The denuded surface becomes covered with a pseudomembrane of fibrin, cell debris, and leukocytes. Regeneration and repopulation of the epithelium are usually completed within a month of the end of a 6- to 7-week course of radiotherapy, although the epithelium remains thin and, sometimes, more pale than before irradiation. Microscopically, there is atrophy of the basal layers of the stratified squamous epithelium and it may show parakeratosis. At this stage the major histological lesions in the oral mucosa, uncomplicated by infection, are chronic progressive changes in the supportive tissue. There is fibrosis of the lamina propria and submucosa. As part of the repair process following ulceration, these tissues may be replaced by granulation tissue. Some capillaries are telangiectatic, and arterioles can have thick, hyaline walls. Fibrosis invests blood vessels, nerves, skeletal muscle fibers of the tongue, and lobules of minor salivary gland. Although the mucous acini do not show remarkable acute alterations, at later stages the acini may be atrophic and a relatively common finding is squamous metaplasia of the ducts (FRIEDMAN and HALL 1950).

Related to the progressive scarring and vascular compromise, the oral mucosa remains susceptible to even minor trauma. Potentially serious chronic ulceration may develop even months following irradiation. With certainty, some of the persistent oral mucosal changes are related to other complications of irradiation of the area, namely xerostomia, dental caries, and osteoradionecrosis (BAKER 1982; BERTHONG 1986; FAJARDO 1982; WHITE 1975).

10.2.4 Clinical Data on Radiation Response of Mucous Membrane

10.2.4.1 Pattern of Radiation-Induced Mucosal Reactions

Characteristics of the response of mucous membranes of the head and neck area to ionizing radiation were first reported by COUTARD in the early 1930s (COUTARD 1932, 1934). Although treatments were given with orthovoltage apparatus, the fractionation schedule used was not uniform, and dosimetry was not very accurate, essential clinical experience was gained. In a group of patients with squamous epitheliomas of the hypopharynx and larynx treated with a radiotherapy schedule delivering 45 H (i.e., Holzknecht Unit; 1 H corresponds to approximately 1 Gy) from one side of the neck and 15 H from the other side over an area of $\sim$ 50 cm^2 and in an overall time of 14 days, COUTARD observed that the "radioepithelitis of the mucosa" (defined as denudation of the epithelium followed by the formation of plates of false membrane) occurs 14 days after commencement of irradiation and lasts for about 2 weeks.

In addition, in the same group of patients, COUTARD also observed that the time of manifestation and duration of mucositis varied with the overall time of radiation treatment. When 60 H (45 H to one side and 15 H to the contralateral side) was given in 10 days instead of 14 days, mucous membrane denudation occurred 10 days after commencement of irradiation and lasted about 4 weeks. On the other hand, when 60 H was delivered in 18 days, mucosal denudation did not occur until day 18 and lasted only for approximately 1 week. These data indicate the importance of stem cell proliferation in determining the radiation response of rapidly turning-over tissues.

Furthermore, in reviewing the data from a large group of patients treated for various head and neck cancers, COUTARD observed that besides small variations in the time of appearance and the duration of mucositis among different individuals irradiated under similar conditions, there was a difference in the timing and course of mucosal reactions over different segments of the mucous membrane of the upper aerodigestive tracts. In general, when 60 H was delivered in 14 days, mucosal denudation appeared first at the junction of the pillars of fauces and the uvula, on approximately day 13 after the beginning of irradiation, followed by breakdown of the mucous membranes of the hypopharynx, vallecula, and floor of the mouth on days 14–15, of the cheek and hard palate on day 16, and of the laryngeal surface of the epiglottis and interarytenoid space on day 18. The vocal cords and dorsum of the tongue did not become covered by false membrane until the 20th–22nd day after commencement of fractionated irradiation, and usually only after high doses. The difference in the pattern of mucosal reactions between various segments of the upper airway and digestive mucous membrane may reflect a slight difference in the radiosensitivity of the mucosal

stem cells or the cell turnover rate of the tissues, or both. No direct clinical data, however, are as yet available.

10.2.4.2 Time, Dose, and Fractionation Factors

FLETCHER and colleagues (1962) were the first to document meticulously the features of mucous membrane reactions associated with megavoltage radiation treatment of cancers of the oral cavity and oropharynx with a range of fractionation schedules. These investigators observed, for example, that when a total dose of $\sim$ 55 Gy (6000 rads) was given in 4–4½ weeks (i.e., $\sim$ 13.8 Gy per week, $\sim$ 2.75 Gy per fraction) to the mucous membrane of the oropharynx, all patients developed a confluent mucosal denudation starting at the end of the 2nd week of treatment; mucositis reached its peak in the middle of the 3rd week and usually subsided from the 5th to the 8th week. When the same total dose was delivered in 5–5½ weeks (i.e., $\sim$ 11 Gy per week, $\sim$ 2.2 Gy per fraction) some patients developed confluent mucositis whereas the majority only experienced spotted mucosal denudation lasting for $\sim$ 4 weeks. Upon further protraction of the overall duration of treatment to 6–6½ weeks ($\sim$ 9.20 Gy per week, $\sim$ 1.83 Gy per fraction) the mucosal reactions ranged from marked erythema to small islands of denuded mucous membrane. The mucositis usually subsided completely by the 8th–10th week after the beginning of treatment.

These data again clearly demonstrate sparing of mucous membrane injury by fractionation and protraction of radiation treatment. Since lengthening of overall duration of radiotherapy is associated with reduction of the size of the dose per fraction, the decrease in the intensity of mucosal reactions is the result of two independent mechanisms, i.e., the sparing effect and stem cell regeneration during the course of treatment. It is not possible with these data to dissociate the relative contribution of these two underlying processes because the duration of treatment and the size of dose per fraction were changed simultaneously.

The magnitude of sparing of mucous membrane injury by stem cell repopulation, however, can be approximated from the results of recent trials on altered fractionation schedules. In an attempt to improve the local control rate, PERACCHIA and SALTI (1981) used a condensed accelerated fractionation schedule to treat patients with advanced head and neck cancers. In their study, patients were given three fractions of 2 Gy on each treatment day, separated by an interval of 4 h, to a total dose of about 50 Gy in 1½ weeks. This schedule was found to produce much more severe acute mucosal injury than that of a standard fractionation regimen delivering 70 Gy in 35 fractions over a total time of 7 weeks. Of the 22 patients treated with the condensed accelerated fractionation schedule, 12 developed severe consequential late complications such as soft tissue necrosis and fistula. This finding indicates that stem cell regeneration during the last 5½ weeks of the course of a standard 7-week fractionation regimen accounts for approximately 20 Gy worth of sparing of mucosal injury, assuming a 4-h interfraction interval is sufficient to allow cellular repair processes to approach completion after a 2 Gy dose. Thus, during the continuous 7-week course of conventional daily irradiation the mucous membrane of the upper aerodigestive tracts rectifies more than 25% of the cytocidal effect of the total radiation dose by increasing the rate of stem cell proliferation. In other words, the regenerative response of mucosal stem cells neutralizes on average the effect of 0.4 Gy of radiation each day.

The results of the EORTC trial (van den Bogaert et al. 1985) and several pilot studies conducted at the University of Leuven (van der Schueren et al. 1983) demonstrated that the extent by which stem cell proliferation accelerates within a given overall duration of treatment also varies with the pattern of fractionation. In the EORTC study, patients were given three fractions of 1.6 Gy on each treatment day, 3–4 h apart, to a dose of 48 Gy in 2 weeks. At this point therapy was interrupted to allow mucositis to subside, and following a 3–4 week rest, treatment was continued with the same fractionation schedule to deliver a total dose of 70 Gy in 6–7 weeks. All patients developed severe confluent mucosal denudation around day 13 after commencement of the first portion of radiation treatment, But healing started from day 22 and was completed during the rest of the treatment break period. Approximately half the patients experienced mild mucosal breakdown (spotted mucositis) of short duration following the second course of treatment, with the other half having only erythema during this period. It was concluded that the intensity of mucosal denudation induced by this experimental fractionation schedule was similar to that of conventional daily irradiation (70 Gy in 35 frac-

tions given once daily from Monday to Friday during 7 weeks), but the total duration of confluent mucositis was shorter in the split-course accelerated regimen. This phenomenon suggests that mucosal stem cells regenerate more efficiently during the treatment-free period between two series of intensive irradiation than during the continuous course of conventional daily fractions.

This view is substantiated by the results of pilot studies at the University of Leuven. In one study, three series of irradiation were given with two treatment break periods of 2 weeks each. In each series a dose of 22.4 Gy was administered in 4 days by giving three fractions of 1.6 Gy per day. In this way, 67.2 Gy is given in an overall time of 7 weeks. It was observed that this schedule induced three repetitive mucosal reaction waves with nearly complete healing between the reaction periods. No cumulative effect was observed. The average mucosal reaction induced by this fractionation schedule was clearly less than for conventional treatment or the radiation regimen used in the EORTC trial. Approximately two-thirds of the patients developed confluent mucosal denudation of short duration, whereas the remaining individuals experienced only spotted mucositis or less. In the subsequent pilot study, radiation therapy was further fragmented into four short series, separated each time by 13 days. Each series consisted of four fractions of 2 Gy per day, 3 h apart, during 2 days (16 Gy total). This resulted in a dose of 64 Gy in 32 fractions over 6½ weeks. Most patients had only spotted mucositis. These results demonstrated that within an overall treatment time of 6–7 weeks the magnitude of stem cell regeneration during treatment is determined, to some extent, by the distribution of dose fractions. When therapy is given in intensive courses of multiple irradiations per day alternating with rest periods, peracute stem cell regeneration increases with increasing total length of treatment breaks. Unfortunately, the available clinical data are insufficient to allow quantitation of the difference in the magnitude of regenerative response during various fractionation schedules. The same limitation applies for quantitation of sparing of mucosal injury by changes in dose per fraction. These two determinants of radiation response, however, have been studied extensively in animal models (see further).

10.2.4.3 Combination of Chemotherapy and Radiotherapy

During the last few years, there has been an explosive increase in the number of studies assessing the effects of adding chemotherapy to radiation in the treatment of patients with locally advanced squamous cell carcinoma of the head and neck. Unfortunately, it is not possible to evaluate correctly the mucosal toxicity of most of the combined treatments because the majority of studies were single-arm trials that involved selection of patients, and the number of patients treated was small or the mucosal reactions were not recorded or reported in detail. Therefore, we will review only those clinical trials that randomized 50 patients or more to receive radiotherapy alone versus radiotherapy combined with chemotherapy and carefully recorded the treatment toxicity. We will restrict our discussion to mucosal reactions and their consequences. The materials are divided into two groups according to timing of drug administration relative to radiation treatment: concurrent or sequential chemotherapy.

Radiation and Concurrent Chemotherapy

Table 10.1 summarizes the results of clinical trials assessing the effects of radiotherapy with concurrent chemotherapy. In four studies radiation was combined with one cytotoxic drug. One trial combined radiation with a regimen containing seven drugs, and the other series employed the strategy of concurrent chemotherapy followed by adjuvant chemotherapy.

In summary, all of the drugs tested so far increased mucous membrane injury when administered concurrently with radiation treatment. It is not possible, however, to estimate from the clinical data the extent by which the radiation reactions were enhanced by the various drugs (i.e., the dose-modifying factor). Nor is it possible to clarify the underlying mechanism of enhancement of mucosal response.

Sequential Chemotherapy and Radiotherapy

Table 10.2 summarizes the data of four phase III studies. All four trials randomized patients to receive radiotherapy alone or radiotherapy preceded by methotrexate. As shown in Table 10.2, the dose, frequency, and route of drug administration varied among the studies. The general impression is that low daily doses of methotrexate (<20 mg/day) did not increase the mucosal response to subsequent radiation treatment. High doses of methotrexate, i.e., ≥ 60 mg/m^2 preceding radiation, however, did increase the mucositis.

Since the drug was not administered concurrently with radiation, the potentiation of mucous

Table 10.1. Randomized studies comparing radiotherapy alone with concurrent chemotherapy and radiation for advanced head and neck cancers

Authors	No. of pts.	Type of CTH	Mucosal reactions
STEFANI et al. (1971)	126	Hydroxyurea, p.o., 80 mg/kg, 2x/wk	Increase in intensity and duration of mucositis
GOLLIN et al. (1972) Lo et al. (1976)	151	5-FU, i.v., 10 mg/kg on days 1, 2, and 3, 5 mg/kg on day 4 and then 3x/wk	Many patients had to be hospitalized because of acute mucositis
CACHIN et al. (1977)	186	Bleomycin, i.m. or i.v., 15 mg, 2x/wk for 5 wks	Increased incidence of severe mucositis and weight loss
VERMUND et al. (1985)	222	Bleomycin, i.m., 5 mg/day during RT	Increased acute side-effects
FU et al. (1987)	104	Bleomycin, i.v., 5 U, 2x-wk during RT; bleomycin, 15 U and MTX, 25 mg/m^2, i.v., weekly × 16 after RT	Significantly worse radiation mucositis
BEZWODA et al. (1979)	58	Combination of Adria, BLM, MTX, 5-FU, HU, and 6-MP	Increased incidence of buccal mucosa ulcerations

Adria, Adriamycin; BLM, bleomycin; 5-FU, fluorouracil; HU, hydroxyurea; 6-MP, 6-mercaptopurine; MTX, methotrexate; RT, radiation therapy; CTH, chemotherapy.

Table 10.2. Randomized studies comparing radiotherapy alone with chemotherapy followed by radiotherapy for advanced head and neck cancers

Authors	No. of pts.	Type of CTH	Mucosal reactions
KNOWLTON et al. (1975)	96	MTX, i.v., 0.2 mg/kg/ day × 5 or 240 mg/m² on days 1, 5, and 9 followed by leucovorin rescue	Increased mucosal reactions in the high dose MTX group
FAZEKAS et al. (1980)	638	MTX, i.v., 25 mg every 3rd day × 5 without leucovorin rescue	Inconclusive
ARCANGELI et al. (1983)	142	MTX, i.a., 3–5 mg/day × 25–40	No increase in mucosal reactions
TAYLOR et al. (1985)	95	MTX, i.m. 60 mg/m² × 4 90 mg/m² × 4 120 mg/m² × 4 Leucovorin rescue	Increased mucosal reactions

MTX, methotrexate.

membrane injury is thought to be the result of additive killing of mucosal stem cells. The relative extent of cell killing by each modality is unknown.

Numerous studies testing the antitumor effect and toxicity of a variety of cytotoxic agents or combination of drugs administered prior to definitive radiation are ongoing. Detailed reports are awaited with interest.

10.2.5 Animal Studies

Clinical data on radiation-induced reactions of the mucous membrane of the upper aerodigestive tract have been collected from patients undergoing radiotherapy for head and neck cancers. There has been some variation in the fractionation schedules used by different schools, and more recently a variety of experimental regimens have been investigated. However, each type of radiation therapy scheme aimed to deliver biological doses in the proximity of "maximal tolerance" of normal tissues surrounding the neoplastic disease in order to achieve the highest tumor control probability with an acceptable treatment-related morbidity. So the range of the doses delivered within each type of fractionation regimen has been small and dose–response curves for radiation mucositis are not available. In addition, as pointed out earlier, modification of clinical regimens frequently involved simultaneous alterations in several parameters, e.g., fraction size and treatment time.

Consequently, it is not possible to assess quantitatively the contribution of various factors in determining the radiation response of mucous membrane from the clinical information. For these reasons one has to rely on animal studies for quantitative information.

10.2.5.1 Models

Mouse Lip Mucosa Model

A murine model for studying oral mucosal reactions to radiation has been developed in the Gray laboratory and the University of Leuven (PARKINS et al. 1983; XU et al. 1984). In this model, the lip/ snout of mice was exposed to ionizing radiation, and the reactions of the mucosa were scored five or six times a week for a period of 3–4 weeks according to an arbitrary scale as follows:

Erythema/desquamation
1. slight reddening
2. severe reddening
3. focal desquamation
4. exudation covering ≤ 50% of the area
5. exudation covering > 50% of the area

Edema
1. slight swelling
2. severe swelling

Maximal total score = 7

It was observed that after a single exposure to γ rays from a cobalt source with doses ranging from 18 to 22.5 Gy, mucosal reactions started at day 7. The intensity of mucositis increased progressively to reach a maximum at days 11–12, upon which healing ensued until mucous membranes regained their normal appearance at about days 20–21 (Fig. 10.1). Animals developing exudation of more than 50% of the lip mucosa and severe edema were killed since fluid and food intake was compromised.

The average mucosal reactions were than calculated by averaging the scores between days 8 and 17 from the time of irradiation. Dose–response curves were obtained by plotting the average mucosal reactions on the ordinate versus total doses on the abscissa. This procedure was repeated for different fractionation schedules to produce a series of dose–response curves. From these curves the doses required to induce a given level of mucosal reactions, i.e., the isoeffective doses, with various fractionation schedules was derived. Subsequently, a variety of isoeffect curves were constructed by plotting the isoeffective doses against the number of fractions, the size of dose per fraction, or the overall treatment time. The dose–response curve and isoeffect curve variables were then used to quantitate the parameters of fractionation effect, magnitude of regenerative response, dose-modifying factors of chemotherapeutic agents, etc.

Mouse Tongue Epithelium Model

The mouse tongue epithelium model was developed in Munich (MOSES et al. 1984). The lower side of the mouse tongue was exposed to low energy x-rays (29 kV), and the induced changes were scored systematically. After doses of 15 Gy and more, ulcerative lesions developed on day 9, reached a maximum intensity on days 10 and 11, and subsided on day 14. The radiation dose–response curve was constructed using a quantal endpoint, i.e., plotting the percentage of animals developing an ulcer versus the radiation dose. The isoeffect curve was obtained using the same procedure as described in the mouse lip mucosa model.

10.2.5.2 Response of Oral Mucosa to Fractionated Irradiation

Kinetics of Cellular Repair

Repair kinetics have been studied using both short fractionation intervals (ANG et al. 1985) and changes in dose rate (SCALLIET et al. 1987). In the split-dose experiments, two equal doses were given with interfraction intervals of 1, 2, 3, and 24 h. Repair was efficient, having a half-time (T1/2) of approximately 1 h. Operationally, repair of lesions induced by a dose as large as 10 Gy could be considered complete in 4 h.

Five dose rates (i.e., 642, 76.8, 14.1, 2.9, and 1.5 Gy h^{-1}) have been assessed in the low dose rate experiments. The T1/2 estimated according to the method of DALE (1985) was ~ 0.8 h.

The possible effect of fraction size on the rate of repair was investigated by first giving a fixed small dose (e.g., 5 Gy) followed, after various intervals, by larger graded second doses or by first giving a fixed large dose (e.g., 10 Gy) followed by smaller second doses. A trend toward faster repair after small fraction sizes was found. The half-times for repair were found to be 0.9 h and 1.2 h for 5–6 Gy and 10 Gy fractions, respectively.

Magnitude of Cellular Repair

The extent of sparing of mucous membrane damage by repair processes occurring at the cellular level during the intervals between treatment sessions is determined, as in other tissues, by measuring the magnitude of increase in the total doses required to produce a given effect when radiation is delivered in progressively smaller doses per fraction (i.e., in increasing numbers of fractions). In order to eliminate, or at least minimize, the confounding effect of stem cell regeneration during fractionated irradiation in this rapidly turning-over tissue, the overall time of treatment has to be limited to at most 4 days. Hence, the maximum number of fractions that could be delivered with a sufficient interfraction interval (i.e., 4 h) to allow repair processes to approach completion is 24. This makes assessment of tissue response to fraction sizes of 2 Gy or less impossible since more than 24 irradiations would have to be delivered in order to induce scorable mucous membrane reactions. This dilemma was circumvented by the application of the concept of partial tolerance, established and validated in the rat spinal cord model (ANG et al. 1983).

The basic approach with the concept of partial tolerance is to deliver radiation treatments in two portions. The first portion is given with various fractionation schedules to produce a given level of subclinical tissue injury. These treatment regimens are then followed by a constant top-up dose(s) in order to produce observable lesions. This allows a substantial reduction in the number of fractions.

Using the partial tolerance concept, it was possible to design a large series of fractionation experiments on mouse lip mucosa covering fraction sizes from 10 Gy down to 1.2 Gy (ANG et al. 1987). The data showed that decreasing the dose per fraction progressively from 10 Gy down to 2 Gy resulted in a progressive sparing of mucous membrane, that is, a successive increase in the isoeffective dose. The ratio of the parameters of the linear–quadratic model for dose response, α/β, derived from the reciprocal-dose plot (Fe plot) of the data was 5.8 Gy.

The results of a preliminary study on mouse tongue epithelium exposed to a single dose or fractionated irradiation (up to ten fractions) covering fractions sizes between 2 and 11 Gy revealed an α/β value of 6.7 Gy (DORR and KUMMERMEHR, personal communication). These α/β values are smaller than those of other rapidly proliferating tissues such as colon, esophagus, jejunum, skin, spleen, and testis, which range from 8 to 13.2 Gy (COUGLAS and FOWLER 1976; FOWLER et al. 1974; HORNSEY et al. 1975; THAMES et al. 1980; TUCKER and THAMES 1983; WITHERS 1975; WITHERS et al. 1975).

The mouse lip mucosa data (ANG et al. 1987) also demonstrated that there was no additional increase in total isoeffective doses when the dose per fraction was decreased from 2 to 1.5 Gy or even to as low as 1.2 Gy. This is in accordance with the data obtained by DUTREIX et al. (1973) in human skin, but in disagreement with those for mouse foot skin showing that sparing by fractionation persists down to 1 Gy per fraction (DOUGLAS and FOWLER 1976; JOINER et al. 1986). The existing data are thus controversial with regard to the adequacy of the linear–quadratic model in estimating the gain in tissue tolerance to radiation given in repeated doses of less than 2 Gy.

10.2.5.3 Proliferative Response of Mucous Membrane to Radiation Insult

Regenerative response of mucosal stem cells during fractionated irradiation has been measured both in lip mucosa (ANG et al. 1985) and in tongue epithelium (DORR and KUMMERMEHR, personal communication).

Two series of experiments were carried out in mouse lip mucosa. The first study assessed the time of onset of repopulation and the subsequent kinetics of stem cell proliferation. This was accomplished by progressively increasing the interfraction interval of split-dose experiments from 1 day to up to 10 days. The data showed that repopulation starts within 3 days following the first dose and, after onset, the rate of proliferation tends to rise exponentially. The second study was designed to quantify the relative contribution of protraction and distribution of irradiations as a function of time to the gain in mucosal tolerance. For this purpose ten fractions were delivered in the following three schedules: (a) 3 days (three irradiations a day, 4 h apart), (b) 11 days (daily fractions excluding weekend), or (c) two short courses, each consisting of five fractions given in 1.5 days separated by a rest period of 8 days, with an overall time of 11 days. The respective isoeffective doses of these three schedules are 33.2 Gy, 46.8 Gy, and 51 Gy. These data demonstrate a large influence of repopulation on the radiation tolerance of this rapidly turning-over tissue. Between days 3 and 11 of continuous daily irradiation stem cell proliferation accounts for recovery of 13.6 Gy, i.e., 29% of the total irradiation dose. In addition, delivering the treatment in two short courses separated by a rest period leads to a supplemental recovery of 4.2 Gy. The recovery in excess of that resulting from treatment protraction was attributed to a faster repopulation during the treatment-free period than during continuous daily irradiation.

DORR and KUMMERMEHR (personal communication) have elaborated on the proliferation kinetics of mouse tongue epithelium during irradiation. The aim was to determine the rate of repopulation during each week of a 3-week treatment. They found that repopulation is first delayed, but after 1 week mounts to a rate proportional to the damage inflicted. The rate of regeneration increases during the 2nd week.

10.2.5.4 Combination of Chemotherapy and Radiotherapy

There has been a strong trend to treat patients who have advanced head and neck cancers with combinations of chemotherapy and radiation. Unfortunately, because of the paucity of data on the mechanisms and magnitude of interaction between various cytotoxic drugs and radiation, the majority of clinical studies have been designed on a trial and error basis, simply adding active agents to radiotherapy. Some such pragmatically designed combined schedules have led to therapeutic disaster, owing to an increased normal tissue toxicity without beneficial impact on the tumor control probability (see clinical data on chemotherapy). For this reason, the Leuven group initiated a series of experimental studies aimed at gaining insight into and providing quantitative data on drug–radiation interaction in mouse lip mucosa. It is hoped that the results from animal studies could promote a more rational design of clinical studies.

Combination of Bleomycin and Radiation

The influence of the dose, timing, sequence, and mode of drug administration on the response of mouse lip mucosa to a single dose of irradiation was first studied (FENG et al. 1986). It was found that bleomycin administered concurrently with irradiation increased the mucosal reaction. Maximal enhancement occurred when the drug was given 2 h prior to irradiation and the magnitude of intensification was drug-dose dependent between 5 and 60 mg/kg.

The effect of bleomycin on the mucosal response to fractionated irradiation was assessed in the subsequent set of experiments (VANUYTSEL et al. 1986). Animals received radiation treatment given in 2, 4, 10, and 20 exposures with or without bleomycin administered at a dose of 40 mg/kg in a continuous subcutaneous infusion over 7 days. It was found that, except for two fractions, the absolute dose reduction values increased progressively with increasing number of fractions (or decreasing size of dose per fraction). Thus, concurrent administration of bleomycin significantly reduces the tolerance of lip mucosa to fractionated irradiation. For example, the drug reduces the isoeffective dose of irradiation given in 20 exposures by a factor of ∼ 1.8. This finding is consistent with the limited clinical experience and observations in mouse skin (MOLIN et al. 1981) and intestine (PHILLIPS et al. 1979).

The investigators thought that the observed effects of the drug could be explained by assuming two different modes of action for bleomycin. The first process is a direct cell kill by bleomycin accounting for a parallel shift of the dose–response curve as was demonstrated in single-dose experiments. The second presumed mode of action is modification of the shoulder region of the cell survival curve, by virtue of its radiomimetic effect, resulting in less pronounced tissue sparing by dose fractionation.

Combination of 5-Fluorouracil and Radiation

The possible interaction of 5-fluorouracil (5-FU) and irradiation was studied in the lip mucosa model. Special attention was paid to the mode of drug administration, i.e., bolus injection (intraperitoneally) or continuous subcutaneous infusion for 7 days (LEER et al. 1987). But single-dose and fractionation experiments with or without 5-FU showed that this drug did not amplify the radiation response of lip mucosa.

Combination of Cis-dichlorodiammine Platinum (Cis-DDP) and Radiation

LANDUYT et al. (1986) studied the radiation response of mouse lip mucosa to a single radiation exposure and fractionated irradiation with or without Cis-DDP. It was found that Cis-DDP given in various schedules did not alter the sensitivity of the lip mucosa to a single radiation exposure. Cis-DDP ($1.2–1.6$ mg/kg^{-1}) given 30 min before each of the five radiation fractions resulted even in a slight reduction of the lip mucosal reactions. This was attributed to a partial synchronization of mucosal stem cells during treatment. Split-dose experiments with or without Cis-DDP revealed that this drug did not interfere with the cellular repair processes or the kinetics of stem cell regeneration.

10.3 Salivary Glands

10.3.1 Anatomy

Major salivary glands, in contrast to minor salivary glands, are discrete masses of glandular tissue that communicate with the oral cavity by way of a duct system. The three major salivary glands, the parotid, submandibular, and sublingual glands, are paired and occupy relatively large, bilaterally symmetrical locations. The parotid is the largest. It is located superficially on the side of the face beneath the ear between the zygomatic arch and the angle of the mandible. The parotid is the main source of stimulated saliva and is exclusively composed of serous secretory acini. The second largest major salivary gland is the submandibular. It is located in a fossa at the medial angle of the mandible. It is the major source of resting or unstimulated saliva. The sublingual is the smallest of the three major salivary glands. It is situated beneath the mucous membrane of the floor of the mouth on each side of the lingual frenulum. The submandibular and sublingual glands are mixed salivary glands composed of both serous and mucous acini. However, serous acini predominate in the submandibular gland whereas the sublingual gland contains mainly mucous acini. The major salivary glands produce 70%–80% of saliva during both resting and stimulated conditions. The remainder of oral secretions are produced by minor salivary glands. The minor salivary glands are dispersed throughout the mucosa of the palate, lips, cheeks, tongue, and tonsils. They are predominantly mucus secreting.

10.3.2 Significance

Transient dysfunction of the salivary glands can occur following total body irradiation with doses of approximately 10 Gy in patients being prepared for bone marrow transplantation (DEEG 1983). However, the major concern for permanent radiation injury of the major salivary glands is in patients with cancer of the head and neck who are treated with definitive radiotherapy. One or more of the major salivary glands are frequently in close proximity to primary tumors of the head and neck region and to the pathways for lymphatic spread of these tumors. Therefore, it is frequently impossible to avoid inclusion of all or part of these tissues in radiation treatment fields. The most common distressing side-effects of head and neck radiotherapy result, directly or indirectly, from radiation injury to the major salivary glands (DREIZEN et al. 1977; ENEROTH et al. 1971; MOSSMAN and SCHEER 1977; PARSONS 1984).

10.3.3 Clinical Manifestations of Salivary Gland Irradiation

10.3.3.1 Acute Physical Changes

Irradiation of the major salivary glands can produce an acute clinical syndrome of swelling, tenderness, and pain of one or more of the glands. These symptoms are more frequently associated with the submandibular gland than the parotid, although it may be similarly affected (PARSONS 1984). Dryness of the mouth (xerostomia), difficulty in swallowing (dysphagia), and hyperamylasemia develop. These early reactions can occur within 12 h after the first radiation treatment but more commonly are encountered during the 1st or 2nd week of standard fractionated radiotherapy (KASHIMA et al. 1965; PARSONS 1984; SHANNON et al. 1978). The acute syndrome usually subsides spontaneously within days of development despite permanent alteration in the volume and physical properties of the saliva. Accompanying the acute physical changes are the subjective complaints of loss of taste (ageusia) or decreased taste sensitivity (hypogeusia), unusual taste sensations (dysgeusia), and diminished appetite.

10.3.3.2 Xerostomia

The most consistent manifestation of salivary gland irradiation is xerostomia. A certain amount of subjectivity determines what constitutes adequate oral moisture. As a result, the complaints of the patient regarding oral changes and discomfort may not always correlate with the actual amounts of saliva loss and alteration. Although some patients experience subjective improvement of xerostomia several years after treatment, objective recovery of salivary flow is not usually demonstrated (PARSONS 1984). The degree to which irradiation of the salivary glands reduces the quantity of saliva may be influenced by several objective factors such as inherent salivary gland activity, age, and sex.

There is great variation in the saliva flow rate between different individuals. ENEROTH et al. (1972) postulated that the salivary glands of patients with inherently high initial flow rates were less affected by radiation than the salivary glands of patients with low initial flow rates. Young patients seemed to be more likely to recover salivary flow than older individuals. MIRA et al. (1981) noted that males had roughly twice the salivary output of females and found that salivary flow rate exponentially declined after irradiation of the salivary glands independent of the initial flow rate. A particular dose of radiation reduced salivary secretion not by the same amount, but by the same fraction. So in their exponential decay model, patients with high initial flow rates took more radiation dose than those with low initial flow rates before saliva flow reached unacceptable low levels.

Reductions in saliva flow and amount have been attributed to decreased water content of saliva from irradiated salivary glands (DREIZEN et al. 1976). The electrolytes sodium, chloride, calcium, and magnesium become more concentrated (BEN-ARYEH et al. 1975; DREIZEN et al. 1976). The viscosity of the saliva is further increased by a greater proportion of mucinous material relative to the loss of watery, serous secretions (SHANNON et al. 1978). The pH of saliva decreases after irradiation of the salivary glands because of lowered levels of bicarbonate (DREIZEN et al. 1976; SHANNON et al. 1978) and loss of serous secretions, which normally buffer acids produced by bacterial flora (SHAW 1987). Reductions in saliva protein secretion rates have been observed following salivary gland irradiation (MOSSMAN et al. 1981; and BROWN et al. 1976). An important protein in saliva is secretory immunoglobulin (SIgA), which is produced by plasma cells in the stroma and regional lymphoid tissues. MARKS and associates (1981) found that increasing doses of radiation to the parotid gland resulted in progressive reduction of saliva SIgA.

10.3.3.3 Side-Effects Secondary to Xerostomia
Dental Caries

Dental caries is a chronic infectious disease caused by agents of the indigenous oral flora (SHAW 1987). Although early investigators attributed dental decay to direct radiation injury of teeth, it is now accepted that the deterioration of the teeth

following irradiation is secondary to xerostomia (DALY 1980; FRANK et al. 1965; PARSONS 1984). The reduced amount of saliva and its increased viscosity is less effective in removing particulate matter from the mouth. Diminished secretory antibodies and the lowered pH favor the growth of cariogenic bacteria and yeast (BROWN et al. 1975; KUTEN et al. 1986; MARKS et al. 1981; RICE and GILL 1979). Dental caries result from the dissolution of enamel and dentin by acids produced by metabolism of food residues by these organisms that colonize tooth surfaces in the altered oral environment (SHAW 1987).

Taste Dysfunction

Patients with greater pretreatment taste acuity seem to experience the most rapid loss of taste following irradiation of the oral cavity (CONGER 1973). Taste dysfunction can alter digestion because of impaired stimulation of digestive enzyme secretion, decreased gastric contractions, and reduced intestinal motility (SCHIFFMAN 1983). These factors may compromise the overall health of the patient and impair the recovery of radiation injury (CHENCHARICK and MOSSMAN 1983; MOSSMAN et al. 1982). Even though hypogeusia and dysgeusia are common, it is difficult to determine the relative contributions of direct radiation damage to taste buds and secondary damage to taste buds caused by xerostomia since salivary glands and taste buds are frequently irradiated simultaneously (SHATZMAN and MOSSMAN 1982). Some studies have shown that dysfunction of the salivary glands precedes impairment of taste, and the presence of saliva is believed to play an important role in the maintenance of normal taste acuity (KUTEN et al. 1986; MOSSMAN 1983; MOSSMAN et al. 1982). Furthermore, the shapes of the dose–response curves for salivary dysfunction and taste impairment are different, which suggests different patterns of radiation damage in salivary and gustatory tissues (MOSSMAN 1983). Clinically, the salivary glands appear to have a greater sensitivity to radiation damage than the gustatory tissue (KUTEN et al. 1986). As much as a 60% reduction in saliva flow can occur during the 1st week of radiotherapy (MOSSMAN and HENKIN 1978; SHANNON et al. 1978), whereas impaired taste acuity is manifested approximately 3 weeks after initiation of radiotherapy (MOSSMAN and HENKIN 1978; MOSSMAN et al. 1982). Permanent alteration of saliva suggests that recovery of the salivary glands from radiation injury is limited (CHENG et al. 1981; MIRA et al. 1981. MOSSMAN et al. 1982). In spite of this fact, recovery of taste acuity usually occurs within 60–120 days after the completion of radiotherapy; taste impairment was attributed to reversible damage of taste cell microvilli instead of taste cell death (CONGER 1973).

10.3.4 Volume and Dose

The volume of salivary tissue that is irradiated correlates directly with the severity of the oral complications (CHENG et al. 1981; KUTEN et al. 1986; MIRA et al. 1981). This is particularly true for parotid glands since they are the largest of the major salivary glands, the main source of alkaline, serous secretions, and the most sensitive to radiation injury (CHENG et al. 1981; MIRA et al. 1981; SHANNON et al. 1978; STEPHENS et al. 1986a,c; TSUJII 1985). If more than half of both parotid glands is irradiated, along with the rest of the other major salivary glands, significant xerostomia usually results (PARSONS 1984). Irradiation of submandibular and sublingual glands while sparing most parotid tissue rarely causes problems even though submandibular and sublingual glands are the major sources of unstimulated saliva (MIRA et al. 1981; SHANNON et al. 1978).

It has been stated that it is not possible to define specifically a critical radiation dose to the parotid glands that gives pathologically low secretion (ENEROTH et al. 1972).

Radiation doses to all major salivary glands that result in permanent xerostomia have been reported to vary from 4.5 to 40.5 Gy (SHANNON 1978; WESTCOTT et al. 1978). The wide range of tolerance is likely due to the variation in individual pretreatment saliva flow rate. MIRA et al. (1981) found that radiation doses of 35–40 Gy to most salivary tissue produced drastic reduction of whole saliva flow in patients with initially high flow rates, whereas doses of only 5–15 Gy resulted in minimal flow in patients with initially low flow rates. In general, however, a total dose of 40–60 Gy given in fractionated treatments was found to produce complete cessation of salivary secretion in about 80% of the individuals, and 60 Gy or more caused complete dryness in all patients (MARKS et al. 1981). One group suggested that split-course irradiation might allow salivary tissue to recover (MIRA et al. 1981) but others failed to see a sparing effect from this approach (PARSONS 1984).

10.3.5 Morphology of Irradiated Human Salivary Glands

The rapid clinical response of salivary glands to radiation indicates that morphological studies shortly following irradiation might provide insight into the mechanisms of injury. However, legitimate concern for delayed wound healing discourages salivary biopsy to study the early morphological alterations. As a result, information on the acute changes is limited. The fact that late clinical side-effects are largely due to persistence of the acute alterations makes it difficult to define a specific time of demarcation for examination of acute and chronic lesions (WHITE 1975). After the initial sharp reduction of salivary gland secretion, the rate of progression becomes slower with increasing time after irradiation.

KASHIMA et al. (1965) compared the acute lesions in parotid and submandibular glands 24–48 h after exposure to single doses of up to 20 Gy. Both glands contained acute inflammation but the acinar lesions were more extensive in the purely serous parotid glands. In the mixed serous–mucous submandibular glands, the serous acinar cells exhibited degeneration and necrosis whereas mucous cells were unaltered. Although there may be absolute increases in mucous secretion by major salivary glands and perhaps even minor salivary glands in response to radiation, increased viscosity of saliva is influenced by diminution or lack of serous dilution of mucinous secretions (BAKER 1982; BERTHONG 1986). The rapid loss of the secretory acini is in harmony with the early occurrence of xerostomia, and the acute inflammatory reaction can account for the pain and swelling experienced by many patients. A lowered proportion of alkaline, serous secretions contributes to lowering of the pH of the mouth because of the enduring acidic, mucinous secretions.

Although loss of serous acini occurs very quickly, early gross atrophy of the salivary glands may be concealed by swelling caused by the inflammatory reaction (ENEROTH et al. 1971). After irradiation is completed and the inflammation subsides, the salivary glands clinically exhibit atrophy or, in the case of the submandibular gland, firm to hard enlargement that may mimic neoplastic involvement (EVANS and ACKERMAN 1954; BERTHONG 1986). Microscopically, the principal features of the chronic changes are atrophy and loss of serous acini, fibrosis, and chronic inflammation. In mixed serous–mucous submandibular and sublingual glands, serous acinar loss is greater than mucous acinar loss (ACKERMAN 1972; FAJARDO 1982; KASHIMA et al. 1965; WHITE 1975). Serous acinar destruction is often focal and remaining mucous cells can be hyperplastic and even atypical (BERTHONG 1986; FRIEDMAN and HALL 1950). The duct system is increased in prominence relative to the loss of acinar tissue, and duct epithelium commonly shows loss of polarity, atypical large nuclei, and squamous metaplasia (EVANS and ACKERMAN 1954; FRIENDMAN and HALL 1950; HARWOOD et al. 1973). The cytological abnormalities of epithelial and stromal cells help to distinguish salivary gland atrophy caused by irradiation from that resulting from salivary duct obstruction (EVANS and ACKERMAN 1954; HARWOOD et al. 1973). One study found intralobular fat along with fibrosis in irradiated salivary glands, while those with obstructed ducts had only fibrosis (HARWOOD et al. 1973). In irradiated, atrophic salivary glands there are highly variable diffuse infiltrations and focal accumulations of lymphocytes and plasma cells (HARWOOD et al. 1973). Vascular changes of hyalin thickening of arterioles, telangiectasia, arterial intimal proliferation, and endothelial cell enlargement are likewise inconsistent changes of variable severity (ACKERMAN 1972; HARWOOD et al. 1973).

Two studies, 24–48 h following irradiation of the major salivary glands with single doses of 7.25–20 Gy, correlated rises in serum amylase values with morphological observations of destruction of salivary acini (KASHIMA et al. 1965; VAN DEN BRENK et al. 1969a). One of the studies showed that amylase reaches a peak level 24–36 h after single-dose salivary gland irradiation but then declines to preirradiation values over a subsequent 24- to 48-h period (KASHIMA et al..1965). Serial assays in patients receiving daily fractions of 2 Gy showed maximal rises of serum amylase within 4 or 5 days; the degree of hyperamylasemia was related quantitatively to the amount of salivary tissue that was irradiated (BECCIOLINI et al. 1984). The transient nature of hyperamylasemia implies that serous cell lysis occurs suddenly rather than lasting for a protracted peiod or time. This specific serum biochemical change taken with the persistence of diminished parotid saliva after the 1st week of radiotherapy suggests that early serous cell injury may be most significant in the pathogenesis of chronic xerostomia. Salivary amylase is produced by serous cells but not by mucous cells; therefore, elevation of serum levels of amylase (hyperamylasemia) is specific for lysis or, at least, increased permeability of serous cells (BECCIOLINI et al. 1984; KASHIMA et al. 1965; KORSRUD and BRANDTZAEG 1982).

10.3.6 Observations in Rodents

Most of the experimental studies of radiation injury in salivary glands have been carried out in rodents. In one early experiment, major salivary glands of rats were examined histologically at intervals of 1 h to 1 year following localized x-irradiation of the head with a wide range of radiation doses (CHERRY and GLUCKSMANN 1959). It was found that all doses damaged acini more than ducts and the parotid glands exhibited the most extensive collapse, degeneration, and necrosis of acinar cells. With doses of more than 3000 R, little regeneration or repair of serous acini in parotid glands was detected, whereas mucous secretion persisted in submandibular glands. With doses of less than 3000 R, the loss of acini was less in parotid glands and by 7 months no radiation injury could be detected (CHERRY and GLUCKSMANN 1959). Additional light microscopic and histochemical studies of irradiated rat salivary glands confirmed that the parotid was the most radiosensitive of the three major salivary glands (ELZAY et al. 1969; GREENSPAN et al. 1964; VAN DER BRENK et al. 1969b). After single doses of 40 Gy, serous acini of parotid glands showed histochemical changes as quickly as 8 h and focal acinar cell necrosis at 24 h.

Although some investigators were unable to detect rises of serum amylase after radiation of rat salivary glands (VAN DER BRENK et al. 1969a), others found a positive correlation between phases of morphological responses with levels of amylase in the tissue and saliva (PHILLIPS 1970) or in vitro acinar cell function (BODNER et al. 1984). Severe necrosis of serous acini was observed between 24 h and 4 days. Amylase activity in the tissue declined

---

Fig. 10.1a–d. Progression of acinar alterations and inflammation in parotid glands of monkeys irradiated with 7.5 Gy. **a** Nonirradiated: Serous cell cytoplasmic granularity and location, shape, size, and staining of nuclei are uniform. **b** Three hours: Serous cells exhibit swelling and variability of granularity, and some nuclei are pyknotic. Neutrophils fill vessels. **c** Six hours: Increased variability of serous cell granularity and nuclei. Neutrophils among acini. **d** Twenty-four hours: Necrosis of whole acini. Neutrophils infiltrate acini in the necrotic area. (STEPHENS et al. 1986c) HE, ×250

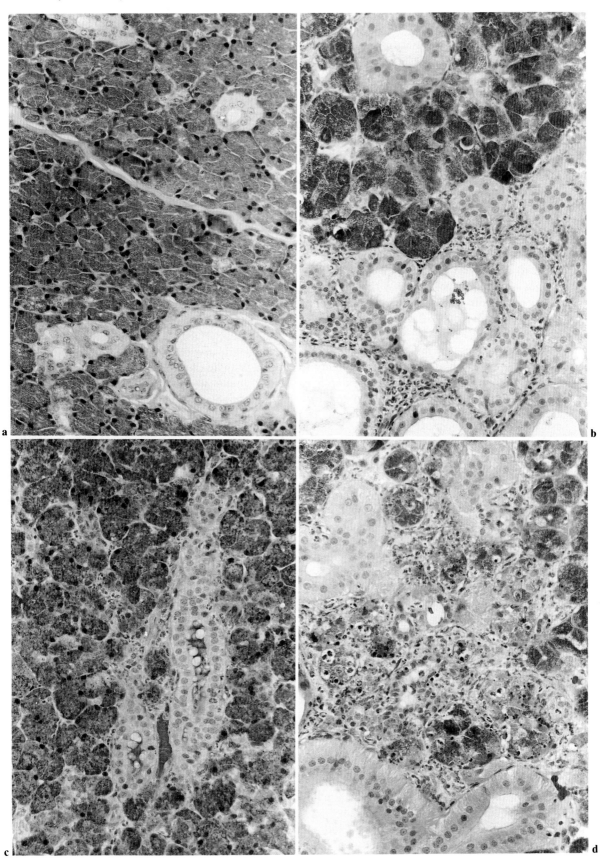

to only 20% of control values at day 4 after irradiation. A return to near normal morphology and a rise in amylase levels to about 35% above control levels at day 16 after irradiation were thought to reflect a reparative phase, whereas by day 42 there was a secondary phase of atrophy and diminished amylase activity to about 50% of control levels (PHILLIPS 1970). Reduced parotid saliva secretion during the 1st week after irradiation is due to acinar loss rather than loss of function because rat parotid cells that survive irradiation remain able to produce amylase in vitro (BODNER et al. 1984).

Studies of radiation injury in rat parotid glands using electron microscopy showed significant alteration of serous acinar cells as early as 3 h after exposure to 16 Gy (PRATT and SODICOFF 1972). Additional study demonstrated that the extent of damage varied with dose and that acinar cell destruction was maximal by 2 days (Sholley et al. 1974; Sodicoff et al. 1974). The lack of significant ultrastructural lesions in the microvasculature, even after a dose as high as 64 Gy, caused them to conclude that microvascular impairment did not contribute to early acinar cell injury in the rat parotid gland (SHOLLEY et al. 1974).

10.3.7 Observations in Nonhuman Primates

The findings in rodents have been corroborated and expanded upon by the use of rhesus monkeys. The anatomy, the physiology, and, perhaps, the radiosensitivity of rhesus major salivary glands more closely resemble those of humans than do those of rodents (STEPHENS et al. 1986b). Submandibular and sublingual salivary glands of rhesus monkeys that received orthovoltage irradiation of 44.25–46.50 Gy given in daily fractions of 1.95–3.1 Gy were examined by light microscopy at 10, 20, 30, or 60 days after irradiation (BOWERS et al. 1981). The serous cells of the submandibular glands showed vacuolation, degeneration, and necrosis to a greater extent than the mucous cells in the same glands.

Our morphological study of irradiated parotid and submandibular salivary glands of rhesus monkeys addressed the evolution of the early radiation injury by examining biopsies of these glands within 1–72 h of irradiation with single photon doses of 2.5–15 Gy (STEPHENS et al. 1986a,c,d). Degeneration and apoptosis of serous cells in both parotid and submandibular glands

were consistently observed, as early as 1 h after irradiation. Although the number of dead serous cells increased with time through 72 h, most of the injury had been clearly expressed by 24 h. The extent of acute serous cell damage increased with dose of radiation. Parotid and submandibular glands exposed to doses of 2.5 and 5 Gy had widely scattered apoptosis of individual serous cells, but no mucous cells were altered. The glands treated with 7.5 or 10 Gy had, in addition to extensive piecemeal death of serous cells, occasional loss of entire serous acini (Figs. 10.1, 10.2). The remaining serous cells were swollen and exhibited marked variability in granule size and number. Although damage to serous cells was extensive, death of mucous cells was only rarely observed. Extensive destruction of serous acini was seen in salivary glands irradiated with doses of 12.5 or 15 Gy. Complete loss of all serous cells comprising multiple acini occurred in many lobules of the glands. Scattered mucous cells were dead in some acini after these higher doses. With all of the doses, the destruction of the acinar tissue was accompanied by neutrophilic inflammation.

Further study of the irradiated primate salivary glands at 16–22 weeks and 40 weeks after irradiation revealed that the extent of atrophy was comparable at the two times (Figs. 10.3, 10.4). Reduction of serous acini in parotid glands was proportional to radiation dose (Fig. 10.5). A dose of 15 Gy caused loss of acini to approach 100% (STEPHENS et al. 1986a). It was suggested that the ability of the acinar cells, especially serous acinar cells, to regenerate after the acute injury was limited. Similar study of rhesus salivary glands treated with 10.2 Gy given in six fractions showed that fractionation provided little sparing from late atrophy (STEPHENS et al. 1986a). These observations in primates appear to be consistent with what is observed in human patients. However, researchers using rats showed that fractionated 64 Gy

Fig. 10.2a-d. Progression of acinar alterations and inflammation in submandibular glands of monkeys irradiated with 10 Gy. **a** Nonirradiated: Serous acini are more plentiful than mucous acini. Serous cells have uniform granularity. **b** Three hours: Serous cells are smaller, and granularity is variable. Neutrophils fill vessels. **c** Six hours: Increased variability of serous cell granules and nuclei. Pyknosis of some serous cell nuclei. Neutrophils among acini. **d** Twenty-four hours: Selective necrosis of serous cells. Edema and neutrophils infiltrating acini. (STEPHENS et al. 1986d) HE, ×250

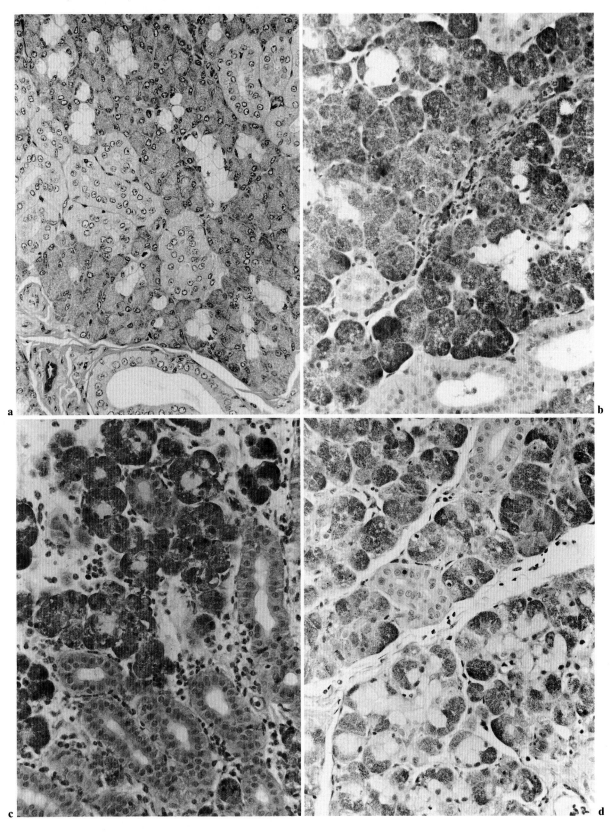

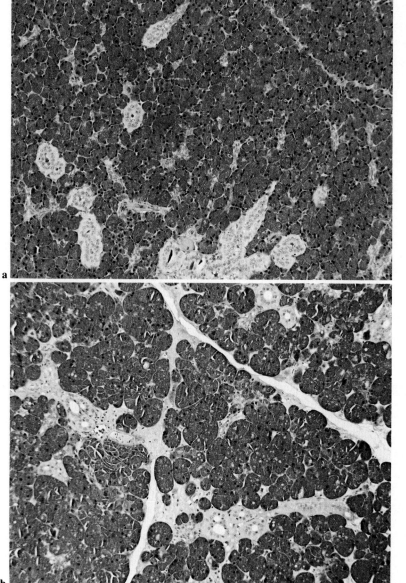

a

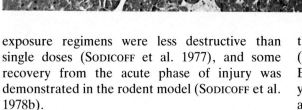

b

Fig. 10.3a-c. Atrophy of irradiated parotid glands. **a** Nonirradiated for comparison of lobule size and amount of stroma. **b** With a dose of 7.5 Gy 20 weeks after irradiation. Lobule size is reduced, and periductal and interlobular connective tissue is increased. **c** With a dose of 15 Gy 20 weeks after irradiation. Marked reduction in lobule size and number of acini. Abundant sclerosis. (STEPHENS et al. 1986c) HE, ×100

exposure regimens were less destructive than single doses (SODICOFF et al. 1977), and some recovery from the acute phase of injury was demonstrated in the rodent model (SODICOFF et al. 1978b).

10.3.8 Interpretation of the Radiation Response of Salivary Glands

Salivary acinar cells are highly specialized epithelial cells that exhibit distinctive morphological and biological characteristics. Based upon rodent data,

these secretory cells have life spans of 40–65 days (CHERRY and GLUCKSMANN 1959; FAJARDO 1982; BERTHONG 1986). Autoradiographic studies of young rat salivary glands have shown labeling at 1 h of 0.5% acinar cells. One week after x-irradiation of 4–8 Gy, insignificant increases in mitotic activity occurred, but a dose of 12 Gy caused mitosis to decrease and sometimes become nil (VAN DEN BRENK et al. 1969b). Administration of isoproteronol can cause hypertrophy and hyperplasia of salivary acinar cells (KLEIN and HARRINGTON 1977; NOVI and BASERGA 1971). However, studies of salivary gland embryogenesis and

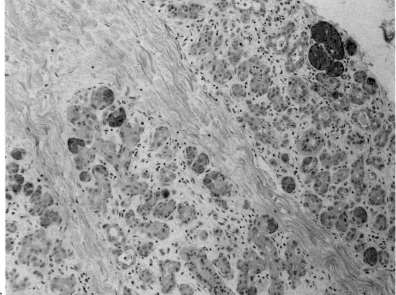

Fig. 10.3c

histiogenesis of salivary gland neoplasms strongly indicate that most acinar development, repair, and replenishment is achieved by replication of terminal duct epithelial cells rather than by division of acinar cells themselves (Batsakis 1979, 1980; Eversole 1971). Mitotic figures are rarely seen in acini of adult salivary glands so the majority of the cells might be regarded as out of an active cell cycle or in interphase. Nonetheless, the potential for division causes them to be classified as postmitotic-reverting cells (Casarett 1980; Rubin and Casarett 1968). In terms of radiosensitivity, this category of cells is expected to show only low to moderate susceptibility to direct radiation injury and exhibit responses relatively slowly (Casarett 1980; Rubin and Casarett 1968).

Proponents of the relative radioresistance of postmitotic-reverting cells attribute both the early and the late damage of salivary tissue to vascular injury and inflammation (Rubin and Casarett 1968). However, the rapid clinical response and histopathological observations of human salivary glands within 1 or 2 days of irradiation show necrosis of the acinar cells with no visible vascular lesions (Kashima et al. 1965; van den Brenk et al. 1969a). These observations and more recent studies of irradiated salivary tissue from patients led to the conclusion that direct acinar cell injury is an inescapable explanation for the early injury (Fajardo 1982). Furthermore, limited clinical improvement from the acute deficits, especially of

serous secretions, indicates persistence and limited recovery from the early atrophy. In addition to lack of regeneration of surviving acinar cells, some late atrophy and eventual fibrosis likely result from concomitant injury to vascular connective tissue that progresses more slowly (Fajardo 1982).

The rodent and primate studies support the concept of acute direct radiation injury of salivary secretory cells. In rodents, primates, and man, serous cells exhibit the greatest sensitivity and show dramatic acute morphological changes typical of cell death. However, the mechanism or subcellular target responsible for the rapid demise after irradiation of these highly specialized cells remains unknown. There appears to be a consensus that death of salivary acinar cells is not linked to mitosis. Hence, acute death of these cells is an interphase rather than reproductive type death (El-Mofty and Kahn 1981; Sholley et al. 1974; Sodicoff et al. 1974; Stephens et al. 1986a,c,d). Apoptosis, also known as shrinkage necrosis and necrobiosis, is a term used to designate this mode of cellular self-destruction (Kerr and Searle 1980). Cells that die by either apotosis or necrosis share the classical histological features of nuclear pyknosis, karyorrhexis, or karyolysis along with increased cytoplasmic eosinophilia. However, it was suggested that the processes are distinguished by the fact that irradiation of susceptible nondividing cells triggers the rapid, active cellular self-destruction of apoptosis rather than the slower

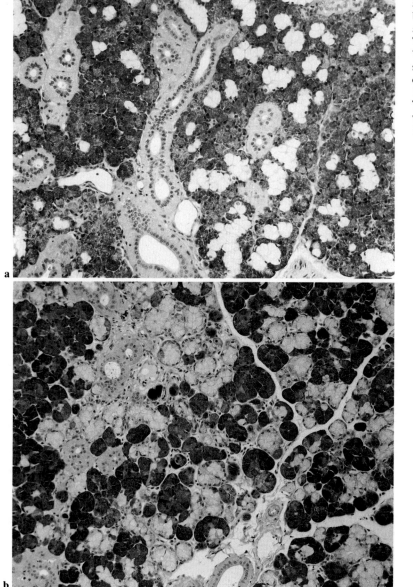

Fig. 10.4a-c. Atrophy of irradiated submandibular glands. **a** Nonirradiated for comparison of relative numbers of serous and mucous acini along with amount of stroma. **b** Twenty weeks after irradiation with 7.5 Gy. There are reductions in the size and number of serous acini. **c** Twenty weeks after irradiation with 15 Gy. Marked reduction of acini. The increased stroma is infiltrated with lymphoid cells. (STEPHENS et al. 1986d) HE, ×100

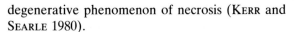

degenerative phenomenon of necrosis (KERR and SEARLE 1980).

PRATT and SODICOFF (1972) considered the possibility of primary nuclear damage as the cause of the self-destruction of parotid acinar cells. However, glandular cells are believed to be resistant to direct DNA damage (FARBER and BASERGA 1969; LIEBERMAN 1972). Most attention to the mechanism of injury to glandular cells has focused upon radiation-induced damage of membranes, release of lysosomal or secretory enzymes, or both processes occurring in some related or unrelated

fashions. The release of proteolytic enzymes is an appealing proposal that could explain why serous cells are more radiosensitive than mucous cells: serous cells contain these enzymes but mucous cells do not (BECCIOLINI et al. 1984; KORSRUD and BRANDTZAEG 1982; SHACKLEFORD and KLAPPER 1962; SHEAR 1972). However, release of lysosomal enzymes is believed to be a manifestation of cell death, rather than its cause (EL-MOFTY and KAHN 1981; TRUMP et al. 1980). Nonetheless, there is evidence that degranulated serous cells are less radiosensitive than when fully granulated. The

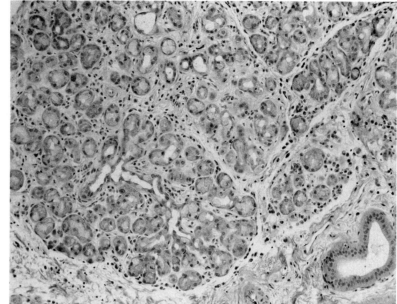

Fig. 10.4. c

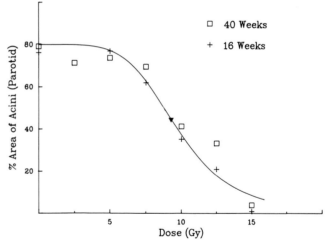

Fig. 10.5. Percent of acini in parotid sections plotted as a function of dose. Data from biopsies taken 16 and 40 weeks postirradiation are shown. The *solid curve* represents a logistic function fit to the data, weighted in proportion to the area of the section. The *inverted triangle* is the datum obtained from 6 × 1.7 Gy fractionations placed on the solid curve at the location corresponding to the percent atrophy observed. The abscissa of this point is at 9.3 Gy. (STEPHENS et al. 1986a)

common property of producing degranulation of rat parotid serous cells has been proposed as the mechanism for favorable dose–response modification by isoproterenol and WR-2721 (SODICOFF et al. 1978a,b, 1979). These compounds might further protect the cells by stimulating the normally nondividing cells into the S phase (CONGER et al. 1985). It was further suggested that isoproterenol might afford radioprotection by increasing intracellular levels of cAMP and glutathione in the parotid gland (CONGER et al. 1985).

The rapid development of intracellular edema in parotid acinar cells has been taken as an indication of disturbance of the cell membrane (EL-MOFTY and KAHN 1981). Production of free radicals resulting in peroxidation of membrane lipids was proposed as the mechanism for membrane injury, which could allow intracellular accumulation of potentially damaging ions like calcium or potassium (EL-MOFTY and KAHN 1981; VAN DEN BRENK et al. 1969a). A study of rat submandibular glands explained the differing radiosensitivity of serous and mucous cells by correlating the production of free radicals with redox reactions by metals (Zn, Mn, Fe) contained in serous granules but absent from mucous granules (ABOK et al. 1984).

In conclusion, the acute clinical response of the salivary glands is attributed to the rapid death of the specialized serous secretory cells. Although the mode of interphase cell death can be defined as apoptosis, the subcellular mechanism for this unexpected radiation response has not been characterized. Therefore, one can hope that better understanding of the mechanism of radiation injury of serous cells might reveal ways to protect these tissues and thereby ameliorate the source of significant oral side-effects in patients receiving radiotherapy for head and neck cancer. In another context, the exquisite radiosensitivity of serous cells can be a sensitive detector of radiation exposure in unplanned circumstances like space travel, reactor accidents, or nuclear war.

10.4 Bones of the Oral Cavity

10.4.1 Anatomy

The major bones susceptible to complications of head and neck radiotherapy are those that bear teeth, i.e., the mandible, maxilla, and premaxilla. All bones seem rigid and unchanging, but in fact, bone is an actively metabolizing tissue that is constantly being reworked and remodeled and is dependent on an adequate blood supply. The oral bones have thin plates of compact bone enclosing medullary spaces bridged by spongy bone. These bones have an alveolar part that has hollow sockets in the spongy bone that vary in size and depth according to the teeth they contain. In old age, the size of the alveolar portion is reduced, especially if the teeth are lost.

Compact and spongy bones have the same cell types and intercellular substances but they differ somewhat in arrangement and density. The cells of bone are mesenchymal cells derived from either the hematopoietic or stromal cell populations. Osteoclasts, which resorb bone from endosteal surfaces, are phagocytes derived from the hematopoietic system. Osteoblasts and osteocytes are derived from stromal cells. Both hematopoietic and stromal compartments contain stem cells that divide into differentiated cells and additional stem cells. With rare exceptions, the differentiated cells do not divide. The bone-forming cells are the osteoblasts. These cells produce and mineralize the bone matrix or osteoid. Osteoid is mainly composed of collagen and a solid mineral phase of hydroxyapatite crystals. The life span of osteoblasts is probably only a few days, whereas the small proportion of osteoblasts that become buried in osteoid become osteocytes, which are known to survive for decades in humans.

10.4.2 Significance

Radiation osteonecrosis in the head and neck may arise from several pathological processes. Although radiation alone can sometimes be the sole causative factor in this injury, more frequently extrinsic factors such as dentition, post-irradiation tooth extraction, loss of salivary gland function, prior bone (mandibular) surgery, and tumor proximity are associated with osteonecrosis. Similarly the morbidity of radiation osteonecrosis has a broad range. It frequently heals spontaneously with conservative management, but it can be contributory to death from cachexia or septicemia. Because of multiple causative factors and the range of morbidities (giving rise to inconsistent definitions of this injury), dose–response functions are difficult to obtain.

The incidence of radiation-induced osteonecrosis of the mandible in curative radiotherapy could be as high as 30%. Even higher rates are observed for certain subsets of patients. However, in addition to the many extrinsic factors that contribute to this injury (and to the variations in incidence), the reported incidence is also greatly influenced by the operational definition of osteonecrosis used in the study.

10.4.3 Morphology and Pathogenesis of Osteonecrosis

Radiologically, the mildest mandibular reaction is described by patchy demineralization, cortical thickening, and alterations in the trabecular pattern (DOLEZAL et al. 1982). Advanced lesions are osteolytic, with evidence of sclerosis and periosteal changes of osteomyelitis (DOLEZAL et al. 1982; BAKER 1983). Radiological changes trail the disease process (BAKER 1983). Histologically, the radiation effects are characterized by loss of osteocytes, osteoblasts, and cementoblasts and a decrease in vasculature and hematopoietic marrow. Various amounts of fibrosis in the marrow have been observed along with new bone proliferation (ROHRER et al. 1979).

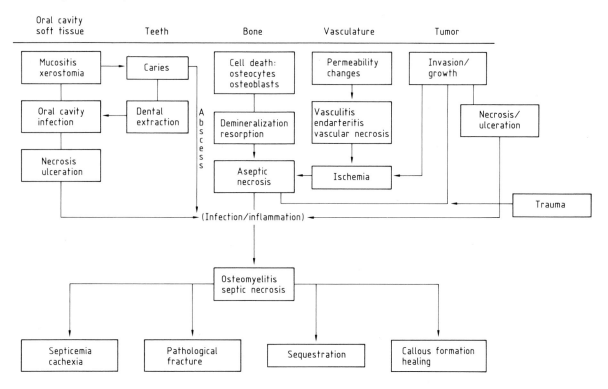

Oral cavity soft tissue | Teeth | Bone | Vasculature | Tumor

Fig. 10.6. Pathways leading to radiation osteonecrosis of the mandible

Only the relatively advanced radiation lesions in the mandible become clinically apparent. Minimal changes characteristic of bony atrophy match the mild radiological findings listed above. As osteolysis increases, the more advanced but asymptomatic stage of aseptic osteomyelitis may be reached. The symptomatic stage of septic osteonecrosis or osteomyelitis usually occurs as a result of trauma due to surgery, tooth extraction, poor dental hygiene, tumor growth, or a level of vascular damage that also leads to extensive soft tissue breakdown. Even at this level of tissue damage, 25%–50% of the lesions can be successfully treated by conservative measures alone (EPSTEIN et al. 1987; MURRAY et al. 1980b).

Fig. 10.6 illustrates the pathways that may lead to aseptic and/or septic osteonecrosis (osteomyelitis). This figure illustrates that, in addition to a direct effect on bone parenchyma, clinical radiation-induced bone lesions can be at least partially attributable to effects on teeth, oral cavity tissues, blood vessels, tumor, and other trauma. Furthermore, these lesions may heal spontaneously or after conservative or aggressive treatment. In some cases they may never heal, even leading to septicemia, cachexia, and death.

10.4.4 Clinical Data

10.4.4.1 Photon Treatment

The various degrees of morbidity lead to different definitions of radiation osteonecrosis and reporting of different incidences. Furthermore, it is also clear from Fig. 10.6 that eliminating any of the possible pathways will alter the incidence of clinical lesions.

Because the mandible experiences a greater exposure to trauma and has a less redundant vascular supply, it exhibits a far greater frequency of osteonecrosis than other bones irradiated in cancers of the head and neck. MORRISH et al. (1981) reported that only 1 of 22 of their cases of osteonecrosis occurred in the maxilla.

Even though reported rates vary, the incidence of osteonecrosis does appear to be dose dependent. With high energy photons, the "threshold" for occurrence is between 60 and 65 Gy, depending upon factors such as dentition and the author's definition of osteonecrosis (MORRISH et al. 1981; BEUMER et al. 1972; MURRAY et al. 1980b). BEDWINEK et al. (1976) showed a correlation between spontaneous osteonecrosis (unrelated to dental extraction) and dose. At between 50 and 60 Gy to the mandible they observed no necrosis in 29 patients; there were two cases in 111 patients treated with mandibular doses of 60–70 Gy, and ten cases in 111 patients who received 70–80 Gy. However, there was also a correlation between T stage and the rate of osteonecrosis, and it is certainly possible that tumor size or treatment volume accounts partially for the dose effect. MORRISH et al. (1981) reported no osteonecroses in patients who received less than 65 Gy to the bone, but among patients who received more than 75 Gy, 85% of the dentulous and 50% of the edentulous patients developed osteonecrosis. Interestingly, they found no correlation with T stage. Most authors find that dentate patients are at higher risk than edentulous patients, because of the possibilities of caries and trauma from tooth extraction (BEUMER et al. 1982; MORRISH et al. 1981). However, the routine extraction of healthy teeth prior to radiation is not recommended (EPSTEIN et al. 1987). It has been reported that extractions following radiation treatment carry a greater risk than extraction prior to radiation. However, EPSTEIN et al. (1987) reported only a 1.7% (absolute) higher incidence (7.1% vs 5.4%) in patients with postradiation extractions.

MURRAY et al. (1980a) found only three significant factors in determining the risk of osteonecrosis: dose, proximity of tumor to bone, and dental status. If the patient is in all high risk categories, his risk is increased 18-fold compared to a patient in all low risk categories. In 82 patients surviving 2 years after treatment with conventional fractionation for squamous cell carcinoma of the tonsillar fossa, WONG et al. (in press) observed mandibular necroses requiring resection in six patients who received a dose to the primary of more than 67 Gy. Of these six, two had stage T_1 or T_2 disease and four stage T_3 or T_4 disease. It is not possible to determine whether the increased incidence for T_3 and T_4 tumors is a result of tumor proximity or larger treatment volume.

10.4.4.2 Neutron Treatment

COHEN et al. (in press) have reported on 268 patients treated at Fermilab with neutrons alone for cancer of the head and neck. Treatment was generally given in 12 fractions over a 4-week period. Tumor doses ranged from 15 to 27 Gy. Among other complications they observed 17 cases of bone or cartilage necrosis.

In this study, osteonecrosis of the mandible after neutron irradiation did not exhibit features demonstrably different from those observed after photon treatments. Slightly more than half of these necroses occurred after dental extractions or secondary to tumor growth. Only one was asymptomatic. The latent period varied from 4 to 54 months but was often determined by dental treatment. There were no necroses of the maxilla.

Randomized trials comparing photon irradiation with neutron irradiation have not found a difference in the incidence of osteonecrosis for approximately equivalent tumoricidal doses (DUNCAN et al. 1987).

10.4.4.3 Volume Factor

In a study of 174 radiotherapy patients with squamous cell carcinoma of the base of the tongue, SPANOS et al. (1976) did not demonstrate an increase in the frequency of mandibular necrosis with field sizes above 40 cm^2. (Only one patient had fields smaller than 40 cm^2.) However, when classified according to whether the field size was larger or smaller than 90 cm^2, the authors found that only one out of nine cases with mandibular necrosis resulting from treatment with smaller fields required resection, as against five of six with necrosis resulting from treatment with larger fields. Thus, it appears that larger volumes result in greater morbidity but not necessarily in greater probability of injury.

10.4.5 Experimental Findings

As with most other radiation injuries, both vasculature damage and direct damage to parenchyma occur. The direct damage occurs only within the radiation field. However, progressive necrosis can spread outside the irradiated region. The following effects were observed by ROHRER et al. (1979)

on rhesus monkeys given 45 Gy in ten daily fractions and observed at 1 week, 3 months, and 6 months: In the outer lamellar and haversian bone, osteocytes were lost at all three observation times. No loss of osteocytes was noted in medullary bone or outside the radiation field. Bony proliferation was found in the irradiated region of the marrow after 3 months. There was a loss of vessels throughout the periosteum, and arterioles and arteries in the marrow were narrowed and sometimes occluded. Under light microscopy, there was no apparent change in capillaries. A brisk reaction of the oral mucosa was observed starting about the last day of treatment and lasting about 2 weeks. As is usually the case, the radiation changes in the human are more variable, are more dependent on vascular injury, and have a greater inflammatory component than is observed in experiments with animals.

JARDINE et al. (1975) treated the jaws of ten rhesus monkeys to a neutron dose of 22 Gy in 13 fractions over 6 1/2 weeks. Acutely, mild erythema without mucositis was noted. Oromucosal necrosis was seen in all but two of the animals. All cases with soft tissue necrosis progressed to mandibular exposure, but no bone necrosis was noted. The animals were followed for 18 months or until sacrifice because of impending death related to radiation morbidity.

10.4.6 Treatment

The treatment of osteonecrosis of the mandible depends upon the extent of the lesion, the presence or absence of infection, and the oral hygiene of the patient. Aggressive surgery is recommended only for advanced lesions. After removal of necrotic bone and soft tissue as well as fibrotic soft tissues, coverage by nonirradiated flap aids in the restoration of vascularity to the irradiated region, without which the necrosis will progress (BAKER 1983). Conservative management of smaller lesions should include strict oral hygiene and removal of bony irritants while awaiting bone sequestration. Although most investigators recommend against postradiation dental extractions, close attention to wound healing and oral hygiene has reduced the rate of significant osteonecrosis in these patients (EPSTEIN et al. 1987).

Treatment with hyperbaric oxygen to enhance the revascularization has been shown to be efficacious both in the treatment of osteonecrosis and in the prevention of osteonecrosis in patients at risk (MARX 1983; MAINOUS and HART 1975). It has been suggested that hyperbaric oxygen is the treatment of choice for the more severe stages of osteonecrosis (BAKER 1983).

10.5 Summary

Radiation therapy is an effective treatment for the majority of cancers of the upper aerodigestive tracts, but it is associated with some morbidity. The features of the most significant side-effects are discussed in this chapter. These are mucosal reactions, salivary gland dysfunction and its consequences, and osteonecrosis of facial bone. Each of these normal tissue reactions has a rather unique pathogenesis and has an important impact on the desired ultimate treatment outcome, i.e., disease- and complication-free survival of patients.

Radiation-induced mucosal reactions result from reproductive death of the epithelial stem cells. Acute mucositis limits the pace by which radiation treatment can be delivered. However, protraction of radiotherapy, in general, allows more opportunity for tumor clonogens to proliferate and hence reduce the tumor control probability. Intensive clinical and experimental studies during the last decade have provided detailed insight into the repair and regeneration kinetics of mucous membranes and some information on the combined drug–radiation effects on this tissue. This is leading to the design of new fractionation strategies that will hopefully improve the tumor control rate. Some of the strategies are being tested.

The response of salivary glands to ionizing radiation is unique in the sense that the mode of cell injury in this tissue differs from that of the surrounding normal tissues. It is apparent now that serous acinar cells undergo interphase cell death after irradiation. This finding stimulates investigations aiming to pinpoint the underlying mechanism of cell injury. It is also hoped that measures could be developed to protect selectively salivary gland from radiation damage. Success in preventing xerostomia would be a big step forward in the management of patients with head and neck cancers.

Analysis of the data of patients treated for head and neck cancers in different institutions has identified various factors contributing to the pathogenesis of osteonecrosis of the mandible. Elimination of some of the factors such as poor dentition and oral hygiene has already reduced the complication rate. Better understanding of the radiation biology of bone may further reduce the incidence of osteonecrosis.

Acknowledgment. This investigation was supported in part by grants CA06294 and CA16672 awarded by the National Cancer Institute, U.S. Department of Health Human Services.

References

Abok K, Brunk U, Jung B, Ericsson J (1984) Morphologic and histochemical studies on the differing radiosensitivity of ductular and acinar cells of the rat submandibular gland. Virchows Arch [B] 45: 443–460

Ackerman LV (1972) The pathology of radiation effect of normal and neoplastic tissue. AJR 114: 447–459

Ang KK, van der Kogel AJ, van der Schueren E (1983) The effect of small radiation doses on the rat spinal cord: the concept of partial tolerance. Int J Radiat Oncol Biol Phys 9: 1487–1491

Ang KK, Xu FX, Landuyt W, van der Schueren E (1985) The kinetics and capacity of repair of sublethal damage in mouse lip mucosa during fractionated irradiations. Int J Radiat Oncol Biol Phys 11: 1977–1983

Ang KK, Landuyt W, Xu FX, Vanuytsel L, van der Schuren E (1987) The effect of small radiation doses per fractionation on mouse lip mucosa assessed using the concept of partial tolerance. Radiother Oncol 8: 79–86

Arcangeli G, Nervi C, Righini R, Creton G, Mirri MA, Guerra A (1983) Combined radiation and drugs: the effect of intra-arterial chemotherapy followed by radiotherapy in head and neck cancer. Radiother Oncol 1: 101–107

Baker DG (1982) The radiobiological basis for tissue reactions in the oral cavity following therapeutic x-irradiation. Arch Otolaryngol 108: 21–24

Baker SR (1983) Management of osteoradionecrosis of the mandible with myocutaneous flaps. J Surg Oncol 24: 282–289

Batsakis JG (1979) Tumors of the major salivary glands. In: Tumors of the head and neck, 2nd edn. Williams & Wilkins, Baltimore, pp 1–75

Batsakis JG (1980) Salivary gland neoplasia: an outcome of modified morphogenesis and cytodifferentiation. Oral Surg 49: 229–232

Becciolini A, Giannardi G, Cionini L, Porciani S, Fallai C, Pirtoli L (1984) Plasma amylase activity as a biochemical indicator of radiation injury to salivary glands. Acta Radiol [Oncol] 23: 9–13

Bedwinek JM, Leonard MD, Shukovsky LJ, Fletcher GH, Daley TE (1976) Osteonecrosis in patients treated with definitive radiotherapy for squamous cell carcinomas of the oral cavity and naso- and oropharynx. Radiology 119: 665–667

Ben-Aryeh H, Gutman D, Szargel R, Laufer D (1975) Effects of irradiation on saliva in cancer patients. Int J Oral Surg 4: 205–210

Berthong M (1986) Pathologic changes secondary to radiation. World J Surg 10: 155–170

Beumer J III, Silverman S Jr, Benak SB Jr (1972) Hard and soft tissue necroses following radiation therapy for oral cancer. J Prosthet Dent 27: 640–644

Bezwoda WR, de Moor NG, Derman DP (1979) Treatment of advanced head and neck cancer by means of radiation therapy plus chemotherapy. A randomized trial. Med Pediatr Oncol 6: 353–358

Bodner L, Kuyatt BL, Hand AR, Baum BJ (1984) Rat parotid cell function in vitro following x-irradiation in vivo. Radiat Res 97: 386–395

Bowers DE, Connors NA, Cannon MS (1981) Irradiated salivary glands in the rhesus monkey. J Med Primatol 10: 228–239

Brown LR, Dreizen S, Handler S, Johnston DA (1975) Effect of radiation-induced xerostomia on human oral microflora. J Dental Res 54: 740–750

Brown LR, Dreizen S, Rider L, Johnston D (1976) The effect of radiation-induced xerostomia on saliva and serum lysozyme and immunoglobin levels. Oral Surg Oral Med Oral Pathol 41: 83–92

Cachin Y, Jortay A, Sancho H, Eschwege F, Madelain M, Desaulty A, Gerard P (1977) Preliminary results of a randomized EORTC study comparing radiotherapy and concomitant bleomycin to radiotherapy alone in epidermoid carcinomas of the oropharynx. Eur J Cancer 13: 1389–1395

Casarett GW (1980) Major digestive and endocrine glands. In: Radiation histopathology. CRC, Boca Raton, pp 51–73

Chencharick JD, Mossman KL (1983) Nutritional consequences of the radiotherapy of head and neck cancer. Cancer 51: 811–815

Cheng VST, Downs J, Herbert D, Aramany M (1981) The function of the parotid gland following radiation therapy for head and neck cancer. Int J Radiat Oncol Biol Phys 7: 253–258

Cherry CP, Glucksmann A (1959) Injury and repair following irradiation of salivary glands in male rats. Br J Radiol 32: 596–608

Cohen L, Schultheiss TE, Hendrickson FR, Mansell J, Saroja KR, Lennox A (in press) Normal tissue reactions and complications following high-energy neutron beam therapy. Int J Radiat Oncol Biol Phys

Conger AD (1973) Loss and recovery of taste acuity in patients irradiated to the oral cavity. Radiat Res 53: 338–347

Conger AD, Sodicoff M, Samel A (1985) Comparison of cAMP with other radioprotectors against chronic damage to the rat parotid gland. Radiat Res 102: 99–105

Coutard H (1932) Roentgen therapy of epitheliomas of the tonsillar region, hypopharynx, and larynx from 1920 to 1926. Am J Roentgenol Radium Ther 28: 313–331

Coutard H (1934) Principles of x-ray therapy of malignant diseases. Lancet II: 1–8

Dale RG (1985) The application of the linear-quadratic dose effect equation to fractionated and protracted radiotherapy. Br J Radiol 58: 515–528

Daly TE (1980) Dental care in the irradiated patient. In: Fletcher GH (ed) Textbook of radiotherapy, 3rd edn. Lea & Febiger, Philadelphia, pp 229–237

Deeg HJ (1983) Acute and delayed toxicities of total body irradiation. Int J Radiat Oncol Biol Phys 9: 1933–1939

Dolezal RF, Baker SR, Krause CJ (1982) Treatment of the patient with extensive osteoradionecrosis of the mandible. Arch Otolaryngol 108: 179–183

Douglas BG, Fowler JF (1976) The effect of multiple small doses of x-rays on skin reactions in the mouse and a basic interpretation. Radiat Res 66: 401–426

Dreizen S, Brown LR, Handler S, Levy BM (1976) Radiation-induced xerostomia in cancer patients. Cancer 38: 273–278

Dreizen S, Daly TE, Drane JB (1977) Oral complications of cancer radiotherapy. Postgrad Med J 61: 85–92

Duncan W, Orr JA, Arnott SJ, Jack WJL, Kerr GR, Williams JR (1987) Fast neutron therapy for squamous cell carcinoma in the head and neck region: results of a randomized trial. Int J Radiat Oncol Biol Phys 13: 171–178

Dutreix J, Wambersie A, Bounik C (1973) Cellular recovery in human skin reactions: application to dose fraction number, overall time relationship in radiotherapy. Eur J Cancer 9: 159–167

El-Mofty SK, Kahn AJ (1981) Early membrane injury in lethally irradiated salivary gland cells. Int J Radiat Biol 39: 55–62

Elzay RP, Levitt SH, Sweeney WT (1969) Histologic effect of fractionated doses of selectively applied megavoltage irradiation on the major salivary glands of the albino rat. Radiology 93: 146–152

Eneroth CM, Henrikson CO, Jakobsson PA (1971) The effect of irradiation in high doses on parotid glands. Acta Otolaryngol 71: 349–356

Eneroth CM, Henrikson CO, Jakobsson PA (1972) Effect of fractionated radiotherapy on salivary gland function. Cancer 30: 1147–1153

Epstein JB, Giuseppe R, Wong FLW, Spinelli J, Stevenson-Moore P (1987) Osteonecrosis: study of relationship of dental extractions of patients receiving radiotherapy. Head Neck Surg 10: 48–54

Evans JG, Ackerman LV (1954) Irradiated and obstructed submaxillary salivary glands simulating cervical lymph node metastasis. Radiology 62: 550–555

Eversole LR (1971) Histogenic classification of salivary gland neoplasms. Arch Pathol 92: 433–443

Fajardo LF (1982) Salivary glands and pancreas. In: Pathology of radiation injury. Masson, New York, pp 77–87

Farber E, Baserga R (1969) Differential effects of hydroxyurea on survival of proliferating cells in vivo. Cancer Res 29: 136–139

Fazekas JT, Sommer C, Kramer S (1980) Adjuvant intravenous methotrexate or definitive radiotherapy alone for advanced squamous cancers of the oral cavity, oropharynx, supraglottic larynx or hypopharynx. Concluding report of an RTOG randomized trial on 638 patients. Int J Radiat Oncol Biol Phys 6: 533–541

Feng Y, Vanuytsel L, Landuyt W, Ang KK, van der Schueren E (1986) The combined effect of bleomycin and irradiation on mouse lip mucosa. I: Influence of timing, sequence and mode of drug administration with single dose irradiation. Radiother Oncol 6: 143–151

Fletcher GH, Maccomb WS, Ballantyne AJ (1962) Radiation therapy in the management of cancer of the oral cavity and oropharynx. Charles C. Thomas, Springfield, Ill.

Fowler JF, Denekamp J, Delapeyre C, Harris SR, Sheldon PW (1974) Skin reactions in mice after multifraction x-irradiation. Int J Radiat Biol 25: 213–223

Frank RM, Herdly J, Philippe E (1965) Acquired dental defects and salivary gland lesions after irradiation for carcinoma. J Am Dent Assoc 7: 868–883

Friedman M, Hall JW (1950) Radiation-induced squamous cell metaplasia and hyperplasia of the normal mucous glands of the oral cavity. Radiology 55: 848–851

Fu KK, Phillips TL, Silverberg IJ et al. (1987) Combined radiotherapy and chemotherapy with bleomycin and methotrexate for advanced inoperable head and neck cancer: update of a Northern California Oncology Group randomized trial. J Clin Oncol 5: 1410–1418

Gollin FF, Ansfield FJ, Brandenburg JH et al. (1972) Combined therapy in advanced head and neck cancer: a randomized study. AJR 114: 83–88

Greenspan JS, Melamed MR, Pearse AGE (1964) Early histochemical changes in irradiated salivary glands and lymph nodes of the rat. J Pathol Bacteriol 88: 439–453

Harwood TR, Staley CJ, Yokoo H (1973) Histopathology of irradiated and obstructed submandibular salivary glands. Arch Pathol 96: 189–191

Hopewell JW (1980) The importance of vascular damage in the development of late radiation effects in normal tissues. In: Meyn RE, Withers HR (eds) Radiation biology in cancer research. Raven, New York, pp 449–459

Hornsey S, Kutsutani Y, Field SB (1975) Damage to mouse lung with fractionated neutrons and x-rays. Radiology 116: 171–174

Jardine JH, Hussey DH, Boyd DD, Raulston GL, Davidson TJ (1975) Acute and late effects of 16-and 50-MeVd → Be neutrons on the oral mucosa of rhesus monkeys. Radiology 117: 185–191

Joiner MC, Denekamp J, Maughan RL (1986) The use of 'top up' experiments to investigate the effect of very small dosage per fraction in mouse skin. Int J Radiat Biol 49: 565–580

Kashima HK, Kirkham WB, Andrews JR (1965) Postirradiation sialadenitis: a study of the clinical features, histopathologic changes and serum enzyme variations following irradiation of human salivary glands. AJR 94: 271–291

Kerr JFR, Searle J (1980) Apoptosis: its nature and kinetic role. In: Meyn RE, Withers HR (eds) Radiation biology in cancer research. Raven, New York, pp 367–384

Klein RM, Harringon DB (1977) Isoproterenol and G2 acinar cells in the developing rat parotid gland. J Dent Res 56: 177–180

Knowlton AH, Percarpio B, Bobrow S, Fischer JJ (1975) Methotrexate and radiation therapy in the treatment of advanced head and neck tumors. Radiology 116: 709–712

Korsrud FR, Brandtzaeg P (1982) Characterization of epithelial elements in human major salivary glands by functional markers. J Histochem Cytochem 30: 657–666

Kuten A, Ben-Aryeh H, Berdicevsky I, Ore L, Szargel R, Gutman D, Robinson E (1986) Oral side effects of head and neck irradiation: correlation between clinical manifestations and laboratory data. Int J Radiat Oncol Biol Phys 12: 401–405

Landuyt W, Ang KK, van der Schuren D (1986) Combinations of single doses and fractionated treatments of cis-dichlorodiammine platinum (II) and irradiation: effect on mouse lip mucosa. Br J Cancer 54: 579–586

Leer JWH, Landuyt W, van der Schueren E (1987) Irradiation of murine lip mucosa in combination with 5-fluorouracil, administered by single dose injection or continuous infusion. Radiother Oncol 10: 31–37

Lieberman MW (1972) DNA metabolism, cell death, and cancer chemotherapy. In: Farber E (ed) The pathology of transcription and translation. Marcel Dekker, New York, pp 37–53

Lo TC, Wiley AL, Ansfield FJ (1976) Combined radiation therapy and 5-fluorouracil for advanced squamous cell carcinoma of the oral cavity and oropharyns. AJR 125: 229–235

Mainous EG, Hart GB (1975) Osteoradionecrosis of the mandible. Arch Otolaryngol 101: 173–177

Marks JE, Davis CC, Gottsman VL, Purdy JE, Lee F (1981) The effects of radiation on parotid salivary function. Int J Radiat Oncol Biol Phys 7: 1013–1019

Marx RE (1983) Osteoradionecrosis: a new concept of its pathophysiology. Oral Maxillofac Surg 47: 283–288

Mira JG, Westcott WB, Starcke EN, Shannon JL (1981) Some factors influencing salivary function when treating with radiotherapy. Int J Radiat Oncol Biol Phys 7: 535–541

Molin J, Sogaard PE, Overgaard J (1981) Experimental studies on the radiation-modifying effect of bleomycin in malignant and normal mouse tissue in vivo. Cancer Treat Rep 65: 583–589

Morrish RB Jr, Chan E, Silverman S Jr, Meyer J, Fu KK, Greenspan D (1981) Osteonecrosis in patients irradiated for head and neck carcinoma. Cancer 47: 1980–1983

Moses R, Kummermehr J, Pfeifer H (1984) Radiation response of the mouse tongue epithelium. Annual Report of the Gesellschaft fur Strahlen- und Umweltforschung, Munich, pp 103–113

Mossman KL (1983) Quantitative radiation dose-response relationships for normal tissues in man. II. Response of the salivary glands during radiotherapy. Radiat Res 95: 392–398

Mossman KL, Henkin RI (1978) Radiation-induced changes in taste acuity in cancer patients. Int J Radiat Oncol Biol Phys 4: 663–670

Mossman KL, Scheer A (1977) Some complications of the radiotherapy of head and neck cancer. Ear Nose Throat J 56: 145–149

Mossman KL, Shatzman AR, Chencharick JD (1981) Effects of radiotherapy on human parotid saliva. Radiat Res 88: 403–412

Mossman K, Shatzman AR, Chencharick JD (1982) Long-term effects of radiotherapy on taste and salivary function in man. Int J Radiat Oncol Biol Phys 8: 991–997

Murray CG, Herson J, Daly TE, Zimmerman S (1980a) Radiation necrosis of the mandible: a 10 year study. Part I. Factors influencing the onset of necrosis. Int J Radiat Oncol Biol Phys 6: 543–548

Murray CG, Herson J, Daly TE, Zimmerman S (1980b) Radiation necrosis of the mandible: a 10 year study. Part II. Dental factors; onset, duration and management of necrosis. Int J Radiat Oncol Biol Phys 6: 549–553

Novi AM, Baserga R (1971) Association of hypertrophy and DNA synthesis in mouse salivary glands after chronic administation of isoproterenol. Am J Pathol 62: 295–308

Parkins CS, Fowler JF, Yu S (1983) A murine model of lip epidermal/mucosal reactions to x-irradiation. Radiother Oncol 1: 159–166

Parsons JT (1984) The effect of radiation on normal tissues of the head and neck. In: Million RR, Cassisi NJ (eds) Management of head and neck cancer. JB Lippincott, Philadelphia, pp 173–207

Peracchia G, Salti C (1981) Radiotherapy with twice-a-day fractionation in a short overall time. Int J Radiat Oncol Biol Phys 7: 99–104

Peters LJ, Ang KK, Thames HD (1988) Accelerated Fractionation in the treatment of head and neck cancer: a critical comparison of different strategies. Acta Radiol 27: 185–194

Phillips RM (1970) x-ray-induced changes in function and structure of the rat parotid gland. J Oral Surg 28: 432–437

Phillips TL, Ross GY, Goldstein LS, Begg AC (1979) The interaction of radiation and bleomycin in intestinal crypt cells. Int J Radiat Oncol Biol Phys 5: 1509–1512

Pratt NE, Sodicoff M (1972) Ultrastructural injury following x-irradiation of rat parotid gland acinar cells. Arch Oral Biol 17: 1177–1186

Rice DH, Gill G (1979) The effect of irradiation upon the bacterial flora in patients with head and neck cancer. Laryngoscope 89: 1839–1841

Rohrer MD, Kim Y, Fayos JV (1979) The effect of cobalt-60 irradiation on monkey mandibles. Oral Surg 48: 424–440

Rubin P, Casarett GW (1968) Major digestive glands: salivary gland, liver, biliary tree, and pancreas. In: Rubin P, Casarett GW (eds) Clinical radiation pathology, vol I. WB Saunders, Philadelphia, pp 241–292

Scalliet P, Landuyt W, van der Schueren K (1987) Effect of decreasing the dose rate of irradiation on the mouse lip mucosa. Comparison with fractionated irradiations. Radiother Oncol 10: 39–47

Schiffman SS (1983) Taste and smell in disease. N Engl J Med 308: 1275–1279

Shackleford JM, Klapper CE (1962) Structure and carbohydrate histochemistry of mammalian salivary glands. Am J Anat 111: 25–48

Shannon IL (1978) Management of head and neck irradiated patients. In: Zelles T (ed) Advances in physiological science, saliva and salivation. Pergamon, New York, pp 313–322

Shannon IL, Trodahl JN, Starcke EN (1978) Radiosensitivity of the human parotid gland. Proc Soc Exp Biol Med 157: 50–53

Shatzman AR, Mossman KL (1982) Radiation effects on bovine taste bud membrane. Radiat Res 92: 353–358

Shaw JH (1987) Causes and control of dental caries. N Engl J Med 317: 996–1004

Shear M (1972) Substrate film technique for the histochemical demonstration of amylase and protease in salivary glands. J Dent Res (Suppl) 51: 368–380

Sholley MM, Sodicoff M, Pratt NE (1974) Early radiation injury in the rat parotid gland. Lab Invest 31: 340–354

Sodicoff M, Pratt NE, Sholley MM (1974) Ultrastructural radiation injury of rat parotid gland: a histopathologic dose-response study. Radiat Res 58: 196–208

Sodicoff M, Pratt NE, Trepper P, Sholley MM, Hoffenberg S (1977) Effects of x-irradiation and the resultant inanition on amylase content of the rat parotid gland. Arch Oral Biol 22: 261–267

Sodicoff M, Conger AD, Pratt NE, Trepper P (1978a) Radioprotection by WR-2721 against long-term chronic damage to the rat parotid gland. Radiat Res 76: 172–179

Sodicoff M, Conger AD, Trepper P, Pratt NE (1978b) Short-term radioprotective effects of WR-2721 on the rat parotid glands. Radiat Res 75: 317–326

Sodicoff M, Conger AD, Pratt NE (1979) Isoproterenol in comparison to WR-2721 as a chemoradioprotector of the rat parotid gland. Invest Radiol 14: 166–170

Spanos WJ, Shukovsky LJ, Fletcher GH (1976) Time, dose, and tumor volume relationships in the irradiation of squamous cell carcinomas of the base of the tongue. Cancer 37: 2591–2599

Stefani S, Eells RW, Abbate J (1971) Hydroxyurea and radiotherapy in advanced head and neck cancer. Radiology 101: 391–396

Stephens LC, Ang KK, Schultheiss TE, King GK, Brock WA, Peters LJ (1986a) Target cell and mode of radiation injury in rhesus salivary glands. Raiother Oncol 7: 165–174

Stephens LC, King GK, Ang KK, Schultheiss TE, Peters LJ (1986b) Surgical and micropscopic anatomy of parotid and submandibular salivary glands of rhesus monkeys (*Macaca mulatta*). J Med Primatol 15: 105–119

Stephens LC, King GK, Peters LJ, Ang KK, Schultheiss TE, Jardine JH (1986c) Acute and late radiation injury in rhesus monkey parotid glands: evidence of interphase cell death. Am J Pathol 124: 469–478

Stephens LC, King GK, Peters LJ, Ang KK, Schultheiss TE, Jardine JH (1986d) Unique radiosensitivity of serous cells in rhesus monkey submandibular glands. Am J Pathol 124: 479–487

Taylor SG IV, Applebaum E, Showel JL et al. (1985) A randomized trial of adjuvant chemotherapy in head and neck cancer. J Clin Oncol 3: 672–679

Thames HD Jr, Withers HR, Fletcher GH (1980) Test of equal effect per fraction and estimation of initial clonogen number in microcolony assays of survival after fractionated irradiation. Br J Radiol 53: 1071–1077

Trump BF, McDowell EM, Arstila AU (1980) Cellular reaction to injury. In: Hill RB, LaVia MF (eds) Principles of pathobiology, 3rd edn. Oxford University Press, New York, pp 20–111

Tsujii H (1985) Quantitative dose-response analysis of salivary function following radiotherapy using sequential ri-sialography. Int J Radiat Oncol Biol Phys 11: 1603–1612

Tucker SL, Thames HD Jr (1983) Flexure dose: the low-dose limit of effective fractionation. Int J Radiat Oncol Biol Phys 9: 1373–1383

van den Bogaert W, van der Schueren E, Tongelen CV, Horiot JC, Chaplain G, Arcangeli G, Gonzalez Svoboda V (1985) Late results of multiple fractions per day (MFD) with misonidazole in advanced cancer of the head and neck. A pilot study of the EORTC radiotherapy group. Radiother Oncol 3: 139–144

van den Brenk HAS, Hurley RA, Gomez C, Richter W (1969a) Serum amylase as a measure of salivary gland radiation damage. Br J Radiol 42: 688–700

van den Brenk HAS, Sparrow N, Moore V (1969b) Effect or x-irradiation on salivary gland growth in the rat. I. Effect of single doses on post-natal differentiation and growth of acinar and duct components. Int J Radiat Biol 16: 241–266

van der Kogel AJ (1980) Mechanisms of late radiation injury in the spinal cord. In Meyn RE, Withers HR (eds) Radiation biology in cancer research. Raven, New York, pp 461–470

van der Schueren E, van den Bogaert W, Ang KK (1983) Radiotherapy with muliple fractions per day (MFD). In: Peckham M, Adams G, Steel G (eds) Biological basis of radiotherapy. Elsevier Science, Amsterdam, pp 195–210

Vanuytsel L, Feng Y, Landuyt W, Leer JW, van der Schueren E (1986) The combined effect of bleomycin and irradiation on mouse lip mucosa. 2. Influence on accumulation and repair of sublethal damage during fractionated irradiation. Radiother Oncol 6: 267–273

Vermund H, Kaalhus O, Winther F (1985) Bleomycin and radiation therapy in squamous cell carcinoma of the upper ailodigestive tract. A phase III clinical trial. Int J Radiat Oncol Biol Phys 11: 1877–1886

Westcott WB, Mira JG, Starke EN, Shannon IL, Thornby JI (1978) Alterations in whole saliva flow rate induced by fractionated radiotherapy. AJR 130: 145–149

White DC (1975) Mouth, pharynx, and salivary glands. In: An atlas of radiation histopathology. ERDA Technical Information Center, Oak Ridge, Tenn, pp 126–134

Withers HR (1975) Isoeffect curves for various proliferative tissues in experimental animals. In: Proceedings of the Conferences on Time-Dose Relationship in Clinical Radiotherapy. Medicine Printing and Publishing, Madison, pp 30–38

Withers HR, Chu AM, Reid BO, Hussey DH (1975) Response of mouse jejunum to multifraction radiation. Int J Radiat Oncol Phys 1: 41–52

Withers HR, Peters LJ, Kogelnik HD (1980) The pathobiology of late effects of irradiation. In: Meyn RE, Withers HR (eds) Radiation biology in cancer research. Raven, New York, pp 439–448

Wong CS, Ang KK, Fletcher GH, Thames HD, Peters LJ, Byers RM, Oswald MJ (in press) Definitive radiotherapy for squamous cell carcinoma of the tonsillar fossa. Int J Radiat Oncol Biol Phys

Xu FX, van der Schueren E, Ang KK (1984) Acute reaction of lip mucosa of mice to fractionated irradiation. Radiother Oncol 1: 369–374

11 Radiation Effects on Abdominal Organs

K.-R. Trott and T. Herrmann

CONTENTS

11.1 Introduction

The abdominal organs are all rather radiosensitive, which has limited the use of radiotherapy in the treatment of the most common abdominal cancers. Even though the pathogenesis of the acute and chronic complications after irradiation

K.-R. Trott, Professor Dr., Department of Radiation Biology, Medical College of St. Bartholomew's Hospital, University of London, Charterhouse Square, London ECIM 6BQ, UK

T. Herrmann, Doz. Dr. Sc. med., Medizinische Akademie "Carl Gustav Carus", Klinik für Radiologie, Abteilung für Strahlentherapie, Fetscherstraße 74, 0-8019 Dresden, FRG

of the various abdominal organs is essentially similar, the clinical and pathomorphological manifestations of radiation injury are very different and relate to differences in the structure and the function of the organs. Therefore, radiation effects on the stomach, bowel, liver, and pancreas are described in separate sections. As the literature is extensive (especially that regarding radiation effects on the intestines), we have been selective in discussing only those aspects of radiation injury which we regard as most relevant to clinical radiotherapy.

11.2 Radiation Effects on the Stomach

Although gastric cancer is among the most common types of cancer in man, and the results of surgical treatment are poor, radiotherapy does not have any significant place in its treatment. Clinical experience regarding the radiation response of the human stomach has derived mostly from patients who have received radiotherapy for other malignancies but whose treatment field has included a large part of the noninvolved stomach. The most informative source has been a group of patients receiving 50 Gy to their para-aortic lymph nodes (Hamilton 1947).

11.2.1 Clinical Radiation Response

Acute gastric radiation effects are registered if, with fractionated radiotherapy, a dose of 20 Gy to the stomach is exceeded. They increase in severity with ongoing radiotherapy. Patients complain of epigastric pain, nausea, loss of appetite, and vomiting, similar to patients suffering from other forms of acute gastritis. Symptoms reach their peak at the end of the treatment course and usually decrease rapidly thereafter. The clinical and gastroscopic diagnosis is that of acute gastritis.

If the corpus and the fundal region of the stomach are in the primary field, decreased acidity of the gastric juice is a typical sign (BRUEGEL 1917). RICKETTS et al. (1948) demonstrated a dose dependence of the incidence and severity of the suppression of hydrochloric acid production but not of its duration. These observations formed the basis for treatment of peptic ulcers by radiotherapy (LENK 1926). PALMER and TEMPLETON (1939) reported a pronounced decrease in hydrochloric acid production at the end of a course of radiotherapy with 15–20 Gy in 2–3 weeks; this decrease progressed during the subsequent months and usually lasted for more than a year. FINDLEY (1974) measured a decrease in hydrochloric acid production to 30% of pretreatment levels 11 months after a dose of 15 Gy, and to less than 60% after 30 months. BERDOV et al. (1988) recorded a significant reduction in the secretion of gastric juice after stimulation in patients given 20 Gy to the stomach before surgery for gastric cancer.

Low dose radiotherapy has been extensively used to treat peptic ulcers. CARPENDER et al. (1956) looked into the long-term side-effects of this treatment but, at doses below 20 Gy, they were unable to find any significant late injury or increased rate of gastric cancer.

Severe radiation injury of the stomach with ulceration and perforation may, however, occur months or even years after radiotherapy with doses of 40 Gy or more. According to HAMILTON (1947), clinical symptoms and pain from a radiation-induced ulcer of the stomach are less dependent on meals than are those of the typical peptic ulcer. The most commonly mentioned symptoms of patients developing chronic gastric radiation injury are loss of appetite, weight loss, and epigastric cramps (RUBIN and CASARETT 1968; HAMILTON 1947).

The radiographic presentation of a radiation-induced gastric ulcer is similar to that of a peptic ulcer. It is usually found at the dorsal wall of the antrum and the small curvature (ELLINGER 1957). On fluoroscopic investigation the pronounced decrease in peristalsis is obvious; investigation of the gastric juice may reveal decreased acidity if the corpus and the fundus have received significant radiation doses. Due to differences in the position of the stomach in relation to the treatment field in para-aortic lymph node radiotherapy, the results of investigations into the acidity of the gastric juice 2–18 months later are very variable, ranging from hypoacidity to hyperacidity even in those cases in which a radiation-induced gastric ulcer has been suspected (BRICK 1947).

Treatment of radiation-induced gastric ulcers is very difficult and may require subtotal gastrectomy(ROSWIT et al. 1972). All patients from the series of the Walter Reed Hospital described in detail by HAMILTON (1947) had to be treated surgically as pain, vomiting, and hemorrhage could not be controlled by conservative measures. At surgery, the stomach appeared edematous with a .rigid thickened wall and was pale, indicating decreased blood perfusion. Since the compromised vascularization of the stomach and of the irradiated bowel loops is liable to result in the breakdown of anastomoses, BOWERS and BRICK (1947) strongly advised against performing a Billroth I operation in these cases.

Besides the radiation ulcer, chronic atrophic gastritis may develop late after radiotherapy. In most cases of upper abdominal radiotherapy it is only the antrum which receives the full tumor dose. Therefore, chronic changes are usually found there and changes in acid secretion are rare. RUBIN and CASARETT (1968) did not observe any impairment of vitamin B_{12} resorption in patients who developed chronic atrophic gastritis after total stomach irradiation with total doses up to 20 Gy or irradiation of the antrum only with doses up to 45 Gy, in contrast to the classical picture of chronic atrophic gastritis. LAYER et al (1986) described a patient who developed gastric paresis with failure of gastric emptying without endoscopic or radiological evidence of mechanical obstruction within a few months after 40 Gy to the

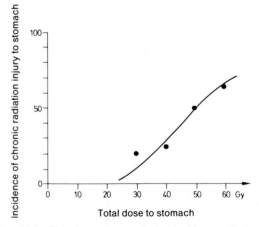

Fig. 11.1. The dependence of the incidence of chronic radiation injury to the stomach on radiation dose (data from FRIEDMAN in RUBIN and CASARETT 1968)

para-aortic lymph nodes; the condition was successfully treated by the cholinergic drug carbachol. The pathophysiological mechanisms of this functional radiation response remain obscure but some form of autonomous dysregulation of neuromuscular synapses seems to be involved in this and other radiation responses of the stomach, as has also been described in the animal experiments of BREITER et al. (1989).

The incidence of radiation ulcers of the stomach increases with radiation dose. The threshold dose appears to be 40 Gy in 20 fractions over 4 weeks (RUBIN and CASARETT 1968). FRIEDMAN (1942) analyzed the experience of the Walter Reed Hospital: 15 out of 61 patients who had received a dose of 45–54 Gy to their stomach developed a radiation ulcer, as did 7 out of 22 who had received 55–64 Gy. All types of significant chronic radiation damage taken together showed the dose dependence plotted in Fig. 11.1.

11.2.2 Histopathology

Serial biopsies were performed by DOIG et al. (1951) and GOLDGRABER et al. (1954) during and after radiotherapy in patients treated with doses up to 15–20 Gy for gastric ulcer. The gastric mucosa has a rapid cell turnover, yet differences are great between different regions within the organ (BERTHRONG and Fajardo 1981). The turnover rate of the various gastric glands, however, is much slower. The complete renewal of the convoluted glands may take up to 1 year.

GOLDGRABER et al. (1954) studied serial biopsies in three patients treated with ten daily doses of 1.6 Gy for gastric ulcer. As soon as 8 days after the start of treatment, pyknotic cells (both parietal and chief cells) were observed at the base of the glandular tubules. This was followed, towards the end of radiotherapy, by deepening of the pits. The neck cells proliferated and grew down into the tubules to replace necrotic cells. At the peak of the reaction, 2–3 weeks after radiotherapy, the normal architecture was disorganized, as evidenced by markedly altered surface epithelium, deepened pits, active neck cell proliferation, loss of glandular substance, distortion and degeneration of some of the remaining glands, and chronic inflammatory infiltration of the edematous interstitial tissue. Regeneration and reversion to an almost normal mucosa occurred within a few weeks. According to DOIG et al. (1951), results of gastric juice analysis correlated well with histological changes in the gastric mucosa (Fig. 11.2).

Histopathological studies after higher radiation doses are rare and restricted to patients operated on because of severe symptoms from chronic radiation ulcer. BERTHRONG and FAJARDO (1981) described the surgical specimen of a patient who had a gastrectomy 8 months after 55 Gy because of a radiation ulcer which could not be adequately managed by conservative measures. The mucosa

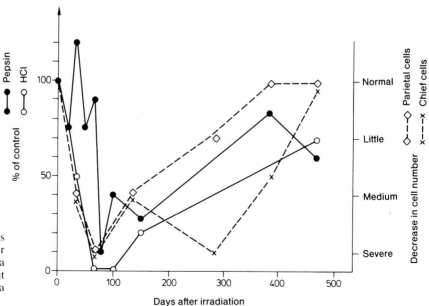

Fig. 11.2. The relative changes in gastric secretion and cellular changes in the gastric mucosa after radiotherapy of a patient suffering from peptic ulcer (data from DOIG et al. 1951)

was moderately atrophic and showed a pronounced inflammatory response. Parietal cells were markedly reduced; the chief cells were better preserved but many glands were dilated. The muscularis mucosae was distorted by fibrosis and the submucosa was edematous with thick bundles of homogenized collagen, telangiectases with bizarre endothelial cells, atypical fibroblasts, and hyalinized arterioles. The muscularis showed focal and sometimes severe interstitial fibrosis. The penetrating ulcer differed from the usual gastric peptic ulcer only in the atypism of the reactive fibroblasts at its base, the bizarre endothelial cells of the granulation tissue, and perhaps the extent of the intimal fibrosis in arteries at a considerable distance from the ulcer crater (FAJARDO 1982).

11.2.3 Pathogenesis

The clinical and histopathological changes during the acute and the chronic phase after local irradiation of the stomach may be adequately explained by the general model of radiation damage pathogenesis, acute effects being mainly due to disturbance of proliferation of critical parenchymal cells and chronic effects developing primarily in the vascular connective tissue. Necrosis and ulceration are usually due to secondary injury to the atrophic and poorly perfused tissue. At present no good explanation can be given for the persistent decrease in gastric secretion long after the mucosa has regenerated, or for the alterations in gastric motility which are seen during the acute phase with high single doses. In mice a decreased rate of gastric emptying has been demonstrated just a few hours after upper abdominal irradiation, (SWIFT et al. 1955). In patients, however, gastric emptying is faster after radiotherapy of large abdominal fields (NEUMEISTER 1973). These changes are probably influenced by alterations to the autonomic nerve system rather than resulting from direct injury to the gastric mucosa or gastric wall.

The histopathological changes of the stomach during the chronic phase are remarkably similar to those observed in the small bowel and the large bowel and stress the importance of vascular changes and of secondary atrophy and their interaction with parenchymal injury. In addition, functional and structural changes in the smooth muscles of the organ, the muscularis mucosae, and the muscularis proper are likely to be of primary

importance, although little is known about the pathogenesis of these effects.

11.2.4 Animal Models

Several experiments have been performed in rabbits, dogs, rats, and mice to study the effects of local irradiation on the stomach. Histological changes and the rate of gastric emptying have been studied (reviewed by NEUMEISTER 1973) but until recently these studies were rather phenomenological and not designed to study dose and fractionation effects in a quantitative way.

Local irradiation of the stomach with a single dose of 15 Gy leads to an acute, perforating gastric ulcer in rabbits within 2–6 weeks. Histologically this ulcer is similar to peptic ulcers in man (ENGELSTAD 1938). After about 12 Gy HAOT (1965) observed mucosal erosions but no ulcerations; after 15 Gy all rabbits developed an ulcer with 20% perforating into the peritoneum. As early as 1 week after irradiation severe edema of the gastric wall was observed. After 10 days superficial erosions were seen; these progressed to deep ulcerations within a few days, the ulcerations being surrounded by progressive wall fibrosis. In surviving animals, regeneration started after 4 weeks and was complete after 8 weeks. In dogs, 20 daily fractions of 3 Gy produced an acute,

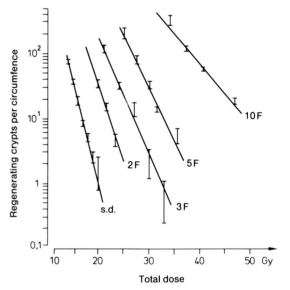

Fig. 11.3. The dependence of the number of regenerating mucosal crypts per stomach circumference on radiation dose given as a single dose (*s.d.*) or with two, three, five, or ten daily fractions (data from CHEN and WITHERS 1972)

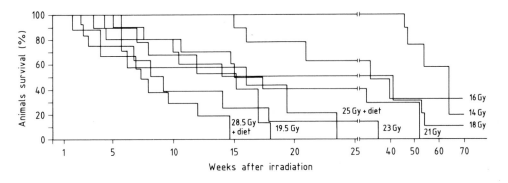

Fig. 11.4. Survival curves of rats locally irradiated to the stomach (data from Breiter et al. 1989). Animals irradiated with 25 or 28.5 Gy were fed a fully resorbable diet to help them survive the acute radiation gastritis

perforating gastric ulcer very soon after irradiation (Hueper and Carvajal-Forero 1944).

Chen and Withers (1972) developed a clonal assay for the radiation response of the gastric mucosa of mice. The stomach was surgically exposed and given single or fractionated doses of radiation. Ten days later the gastric mucosa was severely damaged; however, regenerating foci could be observed within the degenerating glandular necks and were assumed to represent clones arising from surviving mucosal stem cells. With increasing radiation dose their number decreased exponentially, the D_0 being about 1.4 Gy (Fig. 11.3). From the fractionation experiment it was concluded that each gland contained about 70

stem cells (or gland-rescuing units). The extrapolation number of the stem cell survival curve appeared to be high (n being about 100).

Recently, Breiter et al. (1989) developed a rodent model for chronic radiation effects in the stomach. Stomach irradiation was planned according to radiographs taken after a barium meal, and single doses were given to the stomach region, excluding other critical organs as far as possible. Three waves of lethality or severe symptoms occurred in these animals, each representing a different pathological syndrome in the stomach (Fig. 11.4). An erosive and ulcerative gastritis developed within 2–3 weeks after single doses in excess of 25 Gy. Doses between 16 and 25 Gy caused gastroparesis with severely delayed stomach emptying after a latency of several months. The incidence of gastroparesis showed a steep dependence on radiation dose (Fig. 11.5). Its pathogenesis remains obscure at present. After latency times in excess of 7 months functional gastric fibrosis associated with cystic infiltrations penetrating into the muscular wall of the stomach were observed after doses between 14 and 20 Gy. The dose dependence of the late radiation injury of the stomach was not as well defined as that of the subacute/subchronic gastric dilatation. However, it may be concluded that, in correspondence with the complexity of the functional and structural organization of the stomach, radiation injury to different target cell populations may result in different pathogenetic routes to functional gastric obstruction and to radiation ulcers which, histologically, have been observed in all three stages of the radiation injury to the rat stomach.

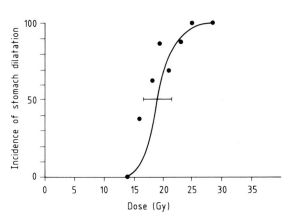

Fig. 11.5. The dependence on radiation dose of the incidence of stomach dilatation 20–25 weeks after irradiation (data from Breiter et al. 1989)

11.2.5 Fractionation Effects on Radiation Injury

The only experimental data on the effect of dose fractionation on the stomach have been reported by Chen and Withers (1972) based on their clonal assay for mucosal stem cells (Fig. 11.3). These results demonstrate a very marked fractionation effect. The slope in the Strandqvist plot of log total dose versus log number of fractions is 0.44; the α/β value may be estimated at about 2 Gy. These values are consistent with a fair amount of split dose recovery and fast repopulation of surviving stem cells, with a doubling time of 44 h (which may be but one reason for the α/β value being unusually low for an acute effect). No other data are available, either from clinical observations or from animal experiments, that permit estimation of the effects of dose fractionation on the various chronic injuries to the stomach.

11.3 Radiation Effects on the Bowels

11.3.1 Clinical Radiation Response

Acute radiation responses of the bowels are frequent side-effects of radiotherapy of abdominal tumors, especially those of the uterus, the ovaries, the kidneys, the prostate, the bladder, and the para-aortic lymph nodes. Between 50% and 70% of all patients treated for carcinoma of the uterus by Neumeister (1973) complained of diarrhea, which is the most obvious sign of acute radiation injury to the bowels, while all patients receiving radiotherapy to their para-aortic lymph nodes as part of the treatment of testicular cancer had diarrhea. Yet it is the chronic radiation injury to the bowels with intestinal obstruction and perforation rather than the transient acute reactions which limits the tolerated radiation dose and thus, frequently, the prospect of cure. Acute and chronic side-effects on the bowels during and after radiotherapy are better documented than those in any other internal organ. However, due to the relatively infrequent use of radiotherapy for tumors to the upper abdomen and the high frequency of radiotherapy of cancer of the uterus, about 90% of all chronic rectosigmoid radiation injuries (Craig and Buie 1949) and the majority of chronic radiation injuries to the terminal ileum and descending colon are observed after radiotherapy of uterine cancer (Senn and Lund-sgaard-Hansen 1956). After postoperative radiotherapy of cancer of the kidney, chronic radiation injury of the flexure of the colon may be observed (Rübe and Seegelken 1974).

Clinical symptoms of intestinal radiation injury depend very much on which part of the bowels has been affected. The acute consequence of radiation exposure of the small bowel is diarrhea, which may start at any time during the course of radiotherapy but usually does so in the 2nd or 3rd week (Neumeister 1973). This is often accompanied by cramps and pain. During the last third of the radiotherapy course to the true pelvis the symptoms of acute proctitis are usually reported by the patient, i.e., pain, frequent defecation of soft, even watery stools, a sensation of incomplete evacuation, and sometimes painful cramps of the sphincter muscles (tenesmus).

The passage of feces is usually faster during the acute reaction. Neumeister (1973) studied the passage of a barium meal in 30 patients at the end of abdominal radiotherapy and found a significant increase in the passage rate in 23 patients, confirming some older published studies. These acute reactions of the small bowel are often accompanied by disturbances of absorption, e.g., of fatty acids (Reeves et al. 1959; Goodrich and Hickman 1962), carbohydrates (Nrumeister 1973), glucose, and amino acids (Thomson et al. 1986).

The most extensive, systematic study on functional changes in the bowels during fractionated radiotherapy with daily fractions of 2 Gy up to 45–55 Gy was performed in Florence on more than 100 patients and summarized by Becciolini (1987). Tests included mucosal biopsies, radiological determinations of transit times, assays of blood, urine, and feces for the absorbed quantities of substances administered orally (such as various carbohydrates, oleic acid, and vitamin B_{12}), and assessment of changes in gastric, biliary, and pancreatic secretion and in the bacterial flora. The observed functional changes were correlated with histopathological findings. The most significant effects associated with acute abdominal distress were an increase in stool weight, an increase in discharge frequency, and a decrease in the absorption of carbohydrates. The relatively greater reduction of sucrose absorption compared with that of glucose halfway through and at the end of radiotherapy was related to a reduction in the activity of brush border enzymes. Minor changes occurred in the absorption of proteins, of amino acids, and of oleic acids and in the secretion of biliary and pancreatic juices. Remarkably little effect on the permeability of the intestinal mucosa was recorded.

In most patients, the acute intestinal side-effects subside within 2–3 weeks after the end of radiotherapy. However, in the months following irradiation a substantial number of patients develop or continue to suffer diarrhea or (after pelvic irradiation) fecal incontinence which may be very distressing (MEERWALDT 1984). Severe chronic side-effects of the small intestine may suddenly become manifest after several months, sometimes even showing the clinical picture of an acute abdomen. More often, they progress slowly, causing progressive but unspecific distress. Severe chronic radiation injury of the ileum and colon may occur without any preceding severe reaction in the acute phase (SENN and LUNDGAARD-HANSEN 1956).

The clinical picture of severe chronic radiation injury of the small bowel was clearly described by GRAUDINNS (1969) in 15 patients he had observed himself. Constipation and abdominal pain were the dominant symptoms. Of the 15 patients, nine had to have emergency surgery, six because of ileus and three because of peritonitis after perforation. Among the 50 patients described by MORGENSTERN et al. (1977) the indication for surgery was obstructive ileus in 37; the next most frequent indications were fistulas, ulcerations, and perforation. In 12 of the 15 cases of GRAUDINNS (1969) latency between radiotherapy and manifestation of the life-threatening radiation injury of the small bowel was less than 2 years.

Less dramatic is the chronic radiation injury of the small bowel which develops into a malabsorption syndrome with pernicious anemia and steatorrhea (DUNCAN and LEONHARD 1965). In radiographic investigations, partial obstruction and persisting stenosis are usually described. It is often difficult to differentiate this picture from that of a malignant tumor (WILEY and SUGARBAKER 1950). If surgery is performed, extensive adhesions make it very difficult to get a clear picture of the extent of injury, which may be multifocal. SENN and LUNDSGAARD-HANSEN (1956) described the injured bowel which, at surgery, is characterized by a thickened and whitish serosa, often showing telangiectases and sluggish or missing peristalsis.

The clinical symptoms of chronic radiation injury of the colon are localized pain, constipation, and flatulence. Radiography may show a circumscribed stenosis with a narrow lumen, poorly defined mucosal structure, and rigid intestinal walls. Differential diagnosis from colonic cancer may be very difficult (RÜBE and SEEGELKEN 1974).

Treatment of chronic radiation injury to the bowel is, if at all possible, by generous surgical resection of the affected parts and end-to-end anastomosis. Based on their experience in more than 50 cases, MORGENSTERN et al. (1977) emphasized the high frequency of postoperative complications like perforation, abscesses, and fistulas. Postoperative lethality is about 25% (KOSLOWSKI and NEUGEBAUER 1984). Therefore MORGENSTERN et al. (1977) warned against too generous indication for surgery and advocated conservative treatment. KOSLOWSKI and NEUGEBAUER (1984) advised performing a colostomy as an emergency measure in all severely ill patients and deferring more radical and definitive surgery until the general condition of the patient has improved enough to permit evaluation of the prospects of such high risk surgery. In 51 patients referred for treatment of late radiation injury to the large bowel, KOSLOWSKI and NEUGEBAUER (1984) performed 32 emergency colostomies. In more than 20% a second operation became necessary, usually because of breakdown of anastomoses and dehiscence. CRAM et al. (1977) emphasized that success with resection and anastomosis depends crucially upon securing proximal and distal resection margins free from radiation damage. Yet reliable identification of the full extent of the involved segment is difficult, especially when one considers that the changes are progressive over a long time. Proximal diverting colostomy is therefore recommended as the only treatment, especially for those patients in whom surgical intervention is required early in the course of the pathological process.

Severe subacute and chronic radiation injury to the intestines is a relatively infrequent but usually life-threatening complication of abdominal radiotherapy. The most extensive study on the frequency of chronic bowel injury after para-aortic lymph node radiotherapy is that from the Walter Reed Hospital (ROSWIT et al. 1972).

For small bowel complications, fixation of small bowel loops by preceding surgery is the most important risk factor. According to POWEL-SMITH (1965) each previous abdominal surgical intervention increases the risk of chronic radiation injury to the small bowel after abdominal radiotherapy by a factor of 2–3. This is assumed to be due to the fact that those regions of the small bowel which are fixed to the peritoneal wall by adhesions receive the full target dose, whereas the free small bowel will change position during the long course of fractionated radiotherapy so that different parts of the small bowel receive the fraction dose at each subsequent session (HEYDE and SCHMERMUND 1953; GAUWERKY 1949). Except for abdominal surgery at any time before radiotherapy, no risk factors for the intraperitoneal portion of the bowels could be determined (MORGENSTERN et al. 1977).

In contrast to chronic radiation injury of the intraperitoneal gut, injuries developing in the retroperitoneal rectosigmoid are usually associated with hemorrhage at their first presentation 6–12 months after radiotherapy (CRAIG and BUIE 1949; KOTTMEIER and GRAY 1961), as well as cramps and mucinous discharge, suggesting the diagnosis of radiation proctitis, usually after radiotherapy for uterine cancer. If the sigmoid is involved, too, diarrhea may prevail. At rectoscopic examination, one usually sees an inflamed, atrophic mucosa and telangiectases with focal hemorrhage. If ulcerations occur they are usually located on the anterior rectal wall opposite the posterior vaginal fornix (RUBIN and CASARETT 1968). In contrast to the treatment of chronic radiation injury of intraperitoneal gut, that of chronic radiation proctitis is usually conservative (SENN and LUNDSGAARD-HANSEN 1956). Secondary complications of radiation proctitis are ulcerations, fibrotic stenosis, and rectovaginal fistulas.

Data on the incidence of chronic radiation injury of the gut depend very much on the criteria used for classification and may vary between 1% and 19% for the same type of treatment (NEUMEISTER 1973). The widely accepted classification by GRAY and KOTTMEIER (1957) of radiation injury to the retroperitoneal gut distinguishes between three grades:

1. Subjective symptoms without objective changes
2. Ulceration, stenosis, and hemorrhage which can be treated conservatively
3. Ulcerations, stenosis, and hemorrhage which have to be treated surgically

Recently, the RTOG and the EORTC jointly proposed a scoring system for acute and late radiation morbidity of the gut which should, in future, be employed whenever applicable (Table 11.1).

KOTTMEIER and GRAY (1961) reported the dose dependence of the incidence of late grade II and III rectal complications, which increased from 5% at 50 Gy to 20% at 80 Gy. The dose–response curve reported by CROOK et al. (1987) for all grades of severity of rectal complications rose from 10% at 60 Gy or less to 50% at over 85 Gy cumulated dose (Fig. 11.6).

The most precise method for diagnosing radiation proctitis is endoscopy. GEHRIG et al. (1987) investigated 155 patients 1–6 years after radiotherapy for uterine cancer and found endoscopic evidence of radiation proctitis in 33%. Except for radiation dose, no other factor like surgery, hypertension, or diabetes had any significant influence on the prevalence of radiation proctitis. The incidence of endoscopically diagnosed radiation proctitis was 0% at 40 Gy, 20% at 60 Gy, and 50% at 90 Gy and was thus similar to the clinically derived dose–response curve of Fig. 11.6.

DEN HARTOG JAGER et al. (1985) described the rectoscopic findings in 90 patients 3 months to 8 years after radiotherapy for gynecological or bladder cancer. The most characteristic endoscopic finding was telangiectasia (in 49/90 patients) which consisted of small convoluted arteries and dilated mucosal and submucosal capillaries. Rec-

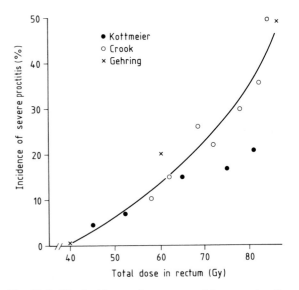

Fig. 11.6. The incidence of severe proctitis on total radiation dose to the rectum in patients treated for gynecological cancers [data from KOTTMEIER and GRAY 1961 (●), CROOK et al. 1987 (○), and GEHRIG et al. 1987 (x)]

Table 11.1. Acute and late radiation morbidity scoring criteria (RTOG/EORTC)[a]

Organ/tissue	0	Grade 1	Grade 2	Grade 3	Grade 4
Acute radiation morbidity scoring criteria					
Upper GI	No change	Anorexia with ≤5% weight loss from pretreatment baseline; nausea not requiring antiemetics; abdominal discomfort not requiring parasympatholytic drugs or analgesics	Anorexia with ≤15% weight loss from pretreatment baseline; nausea and/or vomiting requiring antiemetics; abdominal pain requiring analgesics	Anorexia with >15% weight loss from pretreatment baseline, requiring nasogastric tube or parenteral support; vomiting requiring nasogastric tube or parenteral support; abdominal pain severe despite medication; hematemesis or melena; abdominal distention (flat plate radiograph demonstrates distended bowel loops)	Ileus, subacute or acute obstruction, perforation, GI bleeding requiring transfusion; abdominal pain requiring tube decompression or bowel diversion
Lower GI including pelvis	No change	Increased frequency or change in quality of bowel habits not requiring medication; rectal discomfort not requiring analgesics	Diarrhea requiring parasympatholytic drugs; mucous discharge not necessitating sanitary pads; rectal or abdominal pain requiring analgesics	Diarrhea requiring parenteral support; severe mucous or blood discharge necessitating sanitary pads; abdominal distention (flat plate radiograph demonstrates distended bowel loops)	Acute or subacute obstruction, fistula or perforation, GI bleeding requiring transfusion; abdominal pain or tenesmus requiring tube decompression or bowel diversion
Late radiation morbidity scoring criteria					
Small/large intestine	None	Mild diarrhea; mild cramping; bowel movement 5 times daily; slight rectal discharge or bleeding	Moderate diarrhea and colic; bowel movement > 5 times daily; excessive rectal mucus or intermittent bleeding	Obstruction or bleeding requiring surgery	Necrosis; perforation; fistula
Liver	None	Mild lassitude; nausea dyspepsia; slightly abnormal liver function	Moderate symptoms; some abnormal liver function tests; serum albumin normal	Disabling hepatic insufficiency; liver function tests grossly abnormal; low albumin; edema or ascites	Necrosis; hepatic coma or encephalopathy

[a] Grade 5: Death directly related to radiation effect.

ognition of telangiectasia may vary with time as its detection may be difficult if there is edema or inflammation. The mucosa appears either pale with an opaque glossy aspect due to submucosal edema or reddish with erythematous patches, friability, and hypervascularity. Luminal narrowing due to edema with diminished distensibility or fibrosis was registered in 80% of the patients.

FRIEDMAN (quoted in RUBIN and CASARETT 1968) reported the dependence on radiation dose of the incidence of severe chronic radiation injury of the colon (Fig. 11.7), which rose from 3/40 at accumulated doses below 54 Gy to 16/57 (30%) at doses between 60 and 64 Gy. Both dose–response curves (Figs. 11.6, 11.7) are surprisingly steep if one considers the heterogeneity of fields, treatment conditions, etc. Increasing the dose by 20% above tolerance increases the incidence of late

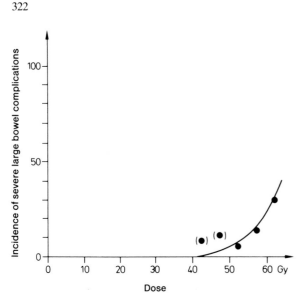

Fig. 11.7. The dependence of severe complications of the large bowel on radiation dose in patients treated for testicular cancer (data from Friedman in Rubin and Casarett 1968)

complications both in the rectum and in the colon by about 20%.

Besides dose, the spatial distribution of dose is of special importance for the incidence and severity of intestinal complications. Crook et al. (1987) analyzed the relationship of the dose distribution associated with different techniques of low dose rate intracavitary radiotherapy of cancer of the cervix to the pattern, frequency, and severity of intestinal complications and confirmed the usefulness of the recommendations for dose and volume specification for reporting intracavitary radiotherapy in gynecology (ICRU 1985). They showed a clear interdependence of treatment volume, defined as the volume included in the 60 Gy isodose, and the cumulated mean rectal dose for the risk of moderate and severe rectal complications.

After radiotherapy of bladder cancer, Edwards (1968) did not observe a clear correlation between the incidence of severe bowel injury and dose or treatment volume. In this and other similar studies, however, dose and volume specification is virtually impossible due to the motility of the bowels. This also has to be taken into account when ranking the radiosensitivities of the various parts of the intestinal tract. Yet most radiotherapists would agree with Friedman's statement that the radiosensitivity of the intestinal

tract decreases between the stomach and the rectum. According to his experience, after a mean dose of 50 Gy the risk of severe chronic radiation injury in the stomach is 50%, in the small bowel 35%, in the colon 20%, and in the rectum about 5%.

11.3.2 Histopathology

Morphological changes in the mucosa of patients during radiotherapy were rarely observed except for some systematic studies like those described by Becciolini (1987). Mucosal changes in radiotherapy patients are very similar to those recorded in numerous animal experiments. After high single doses, pyknosis and karyorrhexis are seen within a few hours, predominantly in the proliferative zones of the crypts. Depression of cell proliferation and continuing loss of postmitotic mucosal cells lead to epithelial denudation within a week. With fractionated radiotherapy, the number and size of crypts decrease, reaching a plateau when total dose approaches 40 Gy (Becciolini 1987). During this phase, infiltration of the lamina propria by inflammatory cells is marked but may be very variable. Due to the high capacity for regeneration, extensive epithelial denudation is very rare during fractionated radiotherapy although some focal erosions may occur (Berthrong and Fajardo 1981; Cronkite and Fliedner 1972). Usually, mucosal recovery is complete within 1 month after termination of radiotherapy.

Wiernik and Plant (1970) performed repeated jejunal biopsies in a group of patients treated with postoperative radiotherapy for carcinoma of the stomach. The most reliable criterion for assessing the acute radiation effect on the jejunal mucosa was the number of cells per crypt or per villus. After 5 Gy, mitoses disappeared for several days and the number of goblet cells increased. Within 1 week, the number of epithelial cells per crypt decreased to half. When radiotherapy was continued with three fractions of 3.5 Gy per week the structure of the mucosa became completely disorganized after a total dose of 40 Gy. Yet rapid and overshooting regeneration occurred immediately after termination of radiotherapy. Mitoses were more frequent than before irradiation, the villi were broad and irregular, and the crypts were often branched and irregular. This hyperplastic response of the irradiated intestinal mucosa disappeared only slowly and could be observed in some patients even several months after radiotherapy.

The histopathological appearance of the chronic radiation effects in the irradiated small bowels is very variable and is primarily dependent on the interval to irradiation (BERTHRONG and FAJARDO 1981). After short intervals, edema, fibrinous peritonitis, and other inflammatory reactions are observed, whereas after longer intervals fibrotic and hyaline changes predominate. The peritoneal surface of the gut loses the usual cover of fat, and the wall appears thickened and indurated. The mucosal surface may show superficial erosions, and rarely deep ulcers. The histopathological appearance of the mucosal epithelium is very variable; villi are broad, and focal erosions are surrounded by acute inflammatory infiltrations of the lamina propria. The lymphatic plaques in the intestinal wall are usually atrophic. Telangiectases may be numerous in the lamina propria, and the muscularis mucosae may be enlarged. The most severe changes are usually found in the submucosa, the loose connective tissue being replaced by hyaline or fibrotic tissues. Fibroblasts with grossly abnormal nuclei may be conspicuous. Capillaries are dilated, appearing like lymph sinusoids. In arteries and arterioles, thickening of the intima and hyalinization of the vessel wall are typical signs of chronic radiation damage. Scarring may be seen in the muscularis proper. Subserosal fibrosis and fibrinous exudate on the serosal surface may be observed even late after irradiation, indicating the progressive formation of gut-related peritoneal adhesions.

In the rectum, the acute histopathological changes have been documented by GELFAND et al. (1968), who studied serial biopsies in 11 patients during radiotherapy up to 20 Gy. Abnormal cells were seen in the crypts and the number of goblet cells decreased. Small abscesses occurred containing eosinophilic granulocytes. One month after termination of radiotherapy, the mucosa appeared normal again. In the submucosa, edema and eosinophilic infiltration may be seen (BERTHRONG and FAJARDO 1981). In the chronic phase, the mucosa is usually atrophic. The most impressive histological feature of chronic radiation injury to the colorectal gut is colitis cystica profunda, which, however, is not very common (BERTHRONG and FAJARDO 1981; BLACK and ACKERMANN 1965). The mucosa infiltrates into the muscular layer and forms glandular structures covered by Paneth cells. The chronic changes in the colon are similar to those in the small intestine. The connective tissue is edematous and is progressively replaced by hyaline, eosiniphilic material. The terminal picture of hyaline fibrosis, telangiectasia, and dilated lymph vessels with grossly abnormal endothelial cells takes about 6 months to develop. The clinical picture of intestinal obstruction is usually correlated with extensive submucosal fibrosis. Vascular changes are similar to those in other organs and may play an important role in the development or progression of chronic radiation injury in the bowels.

11.3.3 Pathogenesis

Acute intestinal effects of abdominal irradiation are primarily caused by direct radiation action on the mucosal parenchyma, i.e., the killing of proliferating cells and the sterilization of stem cells (HENDRY et al. 1983). The pathogenesis thus corresponds to the general concept of radiation effects on steady state tissues with a well-defined turnover time (CRONKITE and FLIEDNER 1972). Clinical signs and symptoms develop when, after the postmitotic differentiating cells have exhausted their physiological life span, the decreased supply of new cells leads to acute mucosal hypoplasia with decreased intestinal surface and focal denudation. In accordance with this general concept of pathogenesis, the latency to clinical manifestation of radiation injury is closely related to the tissue turnover time: the small bowel responds earlier than the large bowel, and mice respond earlier than man (FLIEDNER and CRONKITE 1972). By holding mice in germ-free conditions, the turnover time of the intestinal mucosa is prolonged and consequently so is the latency to intestinal radiation injury (MATSUZAWA and WILSON 1965).

The development of diarrhea as the most typical sign of acute intestinal radiation injury does not require mucosal denudation and occurs with intact mucosal cover but, due to shrinkage of villi, reduced intestinal surface area. Various factors associated with bacterial flora, intestinal contents like bile acids, the autonomous nerve system, etc. play an important role in determining the objective and subjective severity of the acute diarrhea in the second half of abdominal radiotherapy. These have been discussed extensively by Neumeister (1973). Especially bile and pancreatic secretions in the lumen appear to enhance radiation-induced small bowel injury in experimental animals (Mulholland et al. 1984). Radiation-induced changes in the duodenal papilla have been demonstrated in the mouse, leading to a loss of sphincter function which might result in permanent flow of pancreatic juice into the duodenum. Thus, the pathogenesis of diarrhea appears to be complex. Neumeister (1973) stressed the importance of alterations in the intestinal bacterial flora, which often is already abnormal at the start of radiotherapy. Studies by Meerwaldt (1984) pointed to the importance of bile acid reabsorption by the injured ileum and increased loss with the feces, which correlates well with fecal weight and frequency of bowel movement. In the individual patient, however, the serum concentration of bile acids did not correlate very closely with stool frequency, which suggests that more than one factor plays a role in the pathogenesis of diarrhea.

Mucosal changes in subacute and chronic radiation injury to the intestines appear to be secondary to primary radiation effects on other tissue components in the intestinal wall, primarily secondary to vascular injury. In the large bowel of mice, Dewit et al. (1987) concluded from semiquantitative histological scoring of various changes in the intestinal wall up to 180 days after irradiation with tolerated radiation doses or with doses leading to late rectal obstruction that the most important effect is the development of submucosal edema progressing to submucosal fibrosis, transforming the rectum into a rigid tube. Submucosal fibrosis and perirectal adhesions finally lead to progressive narrowing of the rectal lumen. Ito et al. (1986) showed that the increase in hydroxyproline content more than 1 year after irradiation correlated with morphological fibrosis, which, however, appeared to be due to parenchymal atrophy rather than to accumulation of new collagen as the hydroxyproline content per unit bowel length remained constant. Also in late radiation injury of the small bowel, Hauer Jensen et al. (1986) did not measure any increased amount of hydroxyproline in the irradiated segment.

The morphologically apparent fibrosis, which may be due to atrophy or to an increase in fibrous tissue, results in reduced compliance of the rectum, as has been measured in patients by Varma et al. (1985) and in mice by Martin (1988).

In rats, Trott et al. (1986) stressed the importance of tissue breakdown leading to deep ulceration with infiltration and destruction of the muscular layer for the development of clinical rectal obstruction. By modifying the amount and the texture of feces they demonstrated that the primary radiation effect is on the microcirculation in the mucosa and submucosa, leading to progressive atrophy of the mucosa and perivascular fibrosis. Additional injury, caused by hard feces (Trott et al. 1986), by pancreatic secretions (Hauer Jensen et al. 1986), or by chemotherapy may then lead to acute tissue necrosis and deep ulceration. Healing of deep ulceration will result in the histopathological picture of colitis cystica profunda (Hubmann 1982; Trott et al. 1986). The important role of the reduced microcirculation in the bowel wall for the pathogenesis of chronic radiation injury was also demonstrated in a microangiographic study of colectomy specimens from patients treated surgically for radiation-induced bowel disease (Carr et al. 1984). A highly significant diffuse reduction in vascular volume and marked alterations in vascular architecture were observed. Experiments in mice by Dewit and Oussoren (1987) showed a significant reduction in vascular volume in the irradiated rectal wall long before submucosal fibrosis became manifest.

11.3.4 Animal Models

After total body irradiation, the mean survival time of rodents decreases with increasing dose to reach a plateau between 10 and 100 Gy (Cronkite and Fliedner 1972). This constancy of survival time is related to the turnover time of the small bowel mucosa, which is shorter than that of other steady state tissues and which, therefore, determines the latency to death at radiation doses which severely damage all acutely responding tissues in the body (Quastler 1956). Over a small dose range, survival for the 1st week after total body irradiation depends strongly on radiation dose. Determination of the LD$_{50/5}$ i.e., the mean lethal dose within 5 days, is the most simple criterion of radiation effects on small bowel mucosa and has been used to study various radiobiological problems (e.g., Hornsey and Alper 1966).

Withers developed two methods to measure the survival of individual mucosal stem cells after irradiation, counting regenerating foci either macroscopically (Withers and Elkind 1968) or microscopically in the jejunum (WITHERS and ELKIND 1970) or the colon (WITHERS and MASON 1974) after most of the proliferating cells and the majority of the stem cells had been sterilized by high doses of radiation. Above a certain threshold dose needed to reduce the mean number of stem cells per regenerating unit (i.e., crypt) to 1, any further increase in radiation dose leads to an exponential decrease in the number of regenerating crypts per bowel circumference which can be easily determined in histological sections of the jejunum removed 3–4 days after irradiation or of the colon removed 7–10 days after irradiation. Dose–response curves are well defined over slightly more than a factor of 10 of stem cell survival. The value of this animal model goes far beyond studying the radiation response of those cells which are ultimately responsible for the development of the acute intestinal radiation syndrome. It is among the most reliable and sensitive in vivo models of cell survival and has been used extensively to study the influence of modifying factors like fractionation, protraction, and drug–radiation interactions on clonogenic cell survival.

Only recently, attempts to develop relevant animal models for chronic intestinal radiation injury have been successful – in the small bowel those by GERACI et al. (1974), HAUER JENSEN et al. (1983), and DEWIT and OUSSOREN (1987), and in the large bowel those by HUBMANN (1981), KISZEL et al. (1984), and TERRY et al. (1983).

GERACI et al. (1974) irradiated a single eventrated loop of jejunum of mice with single or fractionated radiation doses and, after relocation and closure of the abdomen, observed the development of small bowel stenosis which occurred after a mean latency time of 30–40 days. Its incidence showed a sharp dependence on dose; the mean lethal dose was 22.5 Gy (Fig. 11.8). A similar technique was used by HAUER JENSEN et al. (1983) in rats. A 10 cm long intestinal segment was irradiated with single doses. Death occurred between 8 and 44 weeks after irradiation; the mean lethal dose was 22 Gy. Systematic histological analysis using a scoring system for acute mucosal and late vascular connective tissue changes was performed and evidence was presented for interactions between acute mucosal injury and late stromal effects in the development of the functional endpoint. Yet, no postmortem analysis into the actual causes of fatal small bowel stenosis was reported. The technique has recently been improved to allow repeated irradiation without

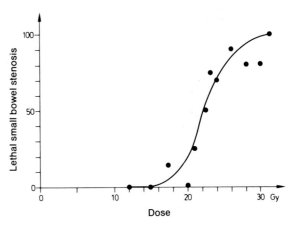

Fig. 11.8. The dependence of the incidence of lethal small bowel stenosis on the radiation dose after local single dose irradiation of an exteriorized small bowel loop in rats (data from GERACI et al. 1974)

repeated surgery by transposing a duodenal loop into the scrotum of orchiectomized rats (HAUER JENSEN et al. 1988).

A less invasive method for studying chronic radiation injury to the small bowel of mice was developed by DEWIT and OUSSOREN (1987). Mice were given 14 daily fractions of 3 Gy through a partial abdominal radiation field. Whereas up to 3 months after irradiation no effects could be observed at postmortem, 6 months later small bowel fibrosis, adhesions, submucosal edema, and mucosal atrophy were obvious. The existence of degenerative changes in the blood vessels and reduced blood perfusion suggested that the observed chronic radiation effects in the small bowel were secondary to vascular injury. As a consequence of reduced blood perfusion in the mucosa and submucosa, partial hypoxia may develop, making the regenerated mucosa more resistant to subsequent irradiation; this is especially marked 6 months after a single dose of 11.5 Gy to the abdomen of mice (REYNAUD and TRAVIS 1984).

PECK and GIBBS (1987) achieved localized irradiation of a defined part of the jejunum by surgically fixing it to the anterior abdominal wall and, 4 weeks later, lifting the abdominal wall together with the fixed jejunum to irradiate the gut. At various times after irradiation the irradiated small bowel was removed and its mechanical properties were tested. Both extensibility and stiffness changed after irradiation and could serve as a measure for radiation fibrosis of small bowel.

McBride et al. (1989) developed yet another model for chronic radiation enteropathy in mice by quantitating the amount of gut-associated peritoneal adhesions after total abdominal irradiation with single doses between 13.5 and 17.3 Gy. Whereas the severity of adhesions was very variable and did not depend on radiation dose, the incidence increased with time in a dose-dependent fashion.

Colorectal radiation injury has been studied after external irradiation to the pelvis of mice (Terry et al. 1983) or of a more localized field in rats (Hubmann 1981). Hubmann developed a model for chronic radiation injury in the rat rectosigmoid by irradiating a well-defined length of the sigmoid and registering the clinical consequences which developed after a latency of 2–7 months with typical signs of rectal obstruction. Further studies by Kiszel et al. (1984) demonstrated that rectal obstruction was always correlated with the development of a circular deep ulcer. Rectoscopic studies by Breiter et al. (1988) and Tekieh and Trott (1988) demonstrated that the acute mucosal injury healed completely before the first signs of secondary tissue breakdown could be observed, which gradually progressed to deep ulceration encompassing the whole bowel circumference.

The incidence of large bowel stenosis increased steeply with radiation dose (Fig. 11.9). The mean effective dose showed a pronounced dependence on the treated volume. Reducing the length of irradiated bowel from 50 to 10 mm increased the tolerance dose by a factor of 2 (Kiszel et al. 1985).

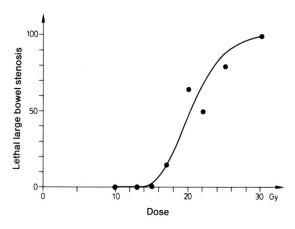

Fig. 11.9. The dependence of lethal large bowel stenosis on radiation dose after local single dose irradiation to the rectosigmoid in rats (data from Kiszel et al. 1984)

Terry et al. (1983) observed various clinical consequences in mice after whole pelvis irradiation with doses between 10 and 30 Gy. In contrast to the rat model, there was no sharp demarcation between early and late phases of injury. In addition to lethality, fecal deformation appeared to be a useful indicator of progressive rectal fibrosis developing about 6 months after irradiation. Rectal stenosis had a mean latency of 20–25 weeks and showed a steep dose–response relationship similar to the rat rectum (Dewit et al. 1987). As in the rat, rectal obstruction was associated with the development of deep ulceration and pronounced submucosal fibrosis and edema.

11.3.5 Fractionation Effects on Radiation Injury

Both acute and chronic radiation effects on the bowels depend very much on dose fractionation and dose rate. Clinical data, however, are sparse. For acute effects, animal experiments have been performed either in the mouse using the crypt colony assay to study more general problems of stem cell response to fractionation and dose rate or, more recently, in dogs in connection with research into optimal conditioning schedules for bone marrow transplantation.

Dose fractionation effects on mouse jejunal crypt stem cells were studied by Withers and Elkind (1970) and the dependence of split-dose recovery on dose per fraction and interval between fractions was reported. The data are consistent with an α/β value of 7.1 Gy. The dose-rate effect on the same system was investigated by Fu et al. (1975). Huczkowski and Trott (1984, 1987) and Dale et al. (1988) performed a systematic study on the relationship between the dose-rate effect and the fractionation effect for different dose rates as both are presumed to be due to the same cellular mechanism, i.e., repair of sublethal radiation damage. The fractionation response to high dose rate γ-rays (Fig. 11.10) could be described with an α/β value of 13 Gy and a half-time of recovery of slightly less than 30 min. As the actual dose rate of the fractions decreased, more sublethal injury was repaired even during irradiation and the α/β value increased (Fig. 11.11). Further analysis of these data revealed that repair rate depended on dose rate, repair being faster during very low dose rate irradiation than between fractions or during intermediate dose rate irradia-

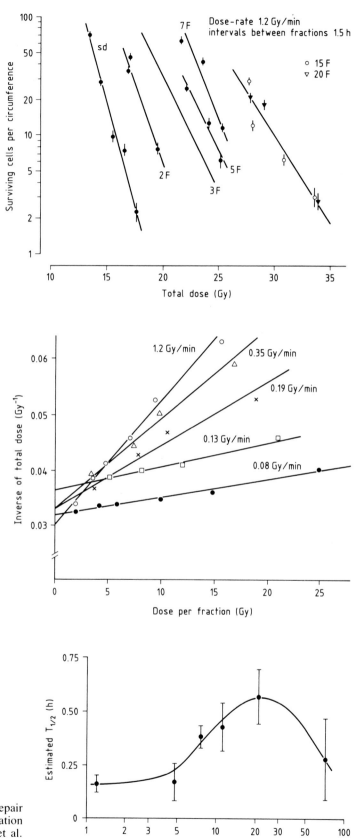

Fig. 11.10. Survival curves of jejunal crypt stem cells after single or multiple doses of γ-rays at high dose rate (data from HUCZKOWSKI and TROTT 1984)

Fig. 11.11. The dependence of the inverse of total dose to yield ten surviving crypt stem cells on the dose per fraction after fractionated irradiation given at different dose rates (data from HUCZKOWSKI and TROTT 1987)

Fig. 11.12. The dependence of the estimated repair half time $T_{1/2}$ on the actual dose rate of irradiation of jejunal crypt stem cells (data from DALE et al. 1988)

tion (Fig. 11.12). Repopulation after the first dose does not become significant before 12–18 but then proceeds with a doubling time of about 8 h (Withers and Elkind 1970; Blott and Trott 1989). Studies on the colonic mucosa resulted in an α/β value of 8.4 Gy, a repair half-time of about 45 min, and a repopulation doubling time of about 24 h.

Kolb et al. (1979) studied the influence of dose rate and dose fractionation on intestinal morbidity in total body irradiation of dogs treated with syngeneic bone marrow transplantation. By varying the dose rate and the overall treatment times, Kolb et al. (1979) were able to separate two repair processes: By decreasing the dose rate from 0.5 to 0.05 Gy/min, the LD_{50} increased from 12 to 24 Gy, yet no further increase in tolerance could be achieved by reducing the dose rate even further to 0.005 Gy/min, indicating that repair of sublethal radiation injury during irradiation at 0.05 Gy/min was already nearly complete. However, dose fractionation with intervals of 48 h between three fractions each given at 0.05 Gy/min led to a further increase in tolerance due to rapid repopulation of surviving mucosal stem cells.

Clinical data suggested that chronic radiation injury to the bowels depends even more on dose fractionation than does acute radiation injury. When Singh et al. (1978) and Browde and DeMohr (1982) treated patients with carcinoma of the cervix with one fraction per week instead of five fractions per week, keeping overall time constant and correcting total dose using the NSD formula, no increased acute intestinal effects were observed, but there was a pronounced increase in the incidence of severe late intestinal complications. This observation is consistent with a greater dependence of chronic radiation effects in the bowels on the dose per fraction as compared with acute effects.

Of particular concern to clinical radiotherapy are the problems connected with the move in intracavitary radiotherapy of cancer of the uterus from low dose rate (less than 0.05 Gy/min) to high dose rate (more than 1 Gy/min) afterloading radiotherapy. In various large series of patients rectal complication rates were actually lower in patients treated with the high dose rate afterloading method if the number of applications was doubled and the total dose reduced by 30%–40% (Glaser 1988; Cikaric 1988; Uzel et al. 1988). Giving the same external beam radiotherapy to both groups of patients, the rate of severe rectal

complications was 22% after three fractions of 15–20 Gy at a dose rate of less than 0.05 Gy/min and only 2% after six fractions of 6–7 Gy given at a dose rate of more than 1 Gy/min (Glaser 1988). These favorable results of high dose rate afterloading therapy are only partly due to adequate modification of dose per fraction and fraction number. Improved precision in dose delivery might be another important factor.

Experimental data on the fractionation effect on the chronic radiation injury of the bowels suggest a lower α/β value than for acute effects, but a higher value than for other late-responding tissues. In the mouse rectum, the late LD_{50} data of Terry and Denekamp (1984) are consistent with an α/β value of 3–5 Gy. Kiszel et al. (1984), Breiter and Trott (1986), and Hauer Jensen et al. (1986), however, demonstrated a strong dependence of the fractionation effect not only on dose per fraction but also on overall treatment time, which they ascribed to the fact that at short overall treatment times mucosal reactions may interact with the developing chronic reaction. At short overall treatment times less sparing is observed by reducing the dose per fraction and an α/β value of 10 Gy may be estimated. Yet if by prolongation of interfraction intervals the development of acute mucositis is prevented, lower α/β values are estimated (Breiter and Trott 1986). The data of Geraci et al. (1977) on late injury to the small bowel do not fit the linear–quadratic formula well enough to define an α/β value, but from the two to five fractions data a value similar to that calculated from the mouse colorectal data can be deduced. Kiszel et al.

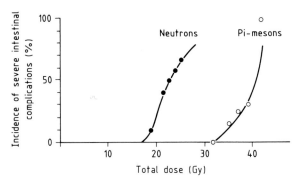

Fig. 11.13. The dependence of the incidence of severe intestinal complications after radiotherapy of abdominal cancers with fast neutrons (data from Battermann et al. 1981) and pi-mesons (data from Greiner and Blattmann 1987), both given in 16–20 fractions

(1985) irradiated the sigmoid colon of rats with an afterloading technique and showed a marked increase in chronic rectal tolerance with decreasing dose rate. These data are consistent with an α/β value of 6 Gy.

11.3.6 Radiation Effects with High LET Radiations

BATTERMANN et al. (1981) reported a very high rate of severe chronic bowel injury after fast neutron radiotherapy of abdominal cancers. Their incidence rose sharply as the total dose was increased beyond 18 Gy, to reach 50% at about 22 Gy, whereas acute reactions were not enhanced during fast neutron radiotherapy (Fig. 11.13). A similarly steep dose–response curve of severe chronic bowel complications was described by GREINER and BLATTMANN (1987) for pion radiotherapy of bladder cancer (Fig. 11.13). At a total dose of 37 Gy or less, one of 18 patients developed chronic bowel complications, whereas after 38 Gy or more 10 of 15 patients developed severe and sometimes even fatal bowel complications after a mean latency time of 12 months. These data are consistent with the experimental observations of GERACI et al. (1977), who observed a much greater neutron RBE for chronic radiation injury in the small bowel than for acute radiation injury, and with those of TERRY and DENEKAMP (1984) in the mouse rectum and BREITER et al. (1986) in the rat colon. For chronic radiation injury after fast neutron radiotherapy the maximal RBE at very low doses per fraction can be estimated to be between 7 and 13.

11.3.7 Radiotherapy–Chemotherapy Interactions

Extensive clinical experience has demonstrated that acute intestinal reactions may be increased by simultaneous chemotherapy and radiotherapy (PHILLIPS 1980). A similar enhancement of the acute response of crypt stem cell survival was also found in various experimental studies (e.g., PHILLIPS and FU 1976; SCHENKEN et al. 1976; DETHLEFSEN and RILEY 1979; VON DER MAASE 1984, 1986). The significance of these phenomenological investigations is, however, limited by the fact that, usually, single drug and radiation doses were combined in various sequences. Few data have

been published on the effects of chemotherapeutic agents on the acute response to fractionated irradiation. DEWIT et al. (1985) demonstrated that cisplatin and fractionated irradiation had mainly independent effects on the survival of jejunal stem cells, although some impairment of split-dose recovery was suggested by the increase in the α/β value from 13 to 20 Gy. On the other hand, BLOTT and TROTT (1989) did not observe any effect of actinomycin D on either the amount or the kinetics of repair or of repopulation in jejunal stem cells, just independent toxicity.

An increase in the incidence of delayed intestinal complications has been reported especially in the sequential combination of radiotherapy and 5-fluorouracil in the treatment of colorectal carcinomas (DANJOUX and CATTON 1979). Experimental studies in the rat model demonstrated that simultaneous treatment with fluorouracil was less toxic than fluorouracil treatment several weeks after irradiation, i.e., during the period of rapid regeneration of the acute mucosal reaction and developing mucosal atrophy (TROTT 1986). Cisplatin, on the other hand, did not enhance the chronic response of the mouse rectum to radiation (DEWIT et al. 1987).

11.4 Radiation Effects on the Liver

Until recently the liver was classified as a radioresistant organ (ZOLLINGER 1960), although WARREN and FRIEDMAN (1942) and ELLINGER (1957) had already questioned the supposed radioresistance of the liver in their textbooks.

Morphological investigations into the effects of radiation on the liver were published by ZOLLINGER (1960) and BRAUN (1963). After radiation doses used in radiotherapy they described some changes which, however, were very discrete, as is typical for any postmitotic cell. The most prominent feature was mitochondrial swelling. The majority of the reported effects on the liver in experimental animals were those after total body irradiation, comprising histological changes and functional changes in the metabolism of glycogen and fatty acids. However, these are likely to be secondary reactions of the liver to the massive alterations in other organs of the body after total body irradiation rather than direct radiation effects on the liver itself. These effects of total body irradiation on the liver have been well summarized by Braun (1963) and Cottier (1961).

Homogeneous irradiation of the entire liver in patients was possible only after megavoltage radiation was introduced into clinical radiotherapy and, consequently, the first report on a new type of liver disease developing in radiotherapy patients and called radiation hepatitis appeared soon after megavoltage radiotherapy became widely available. Today we know that the liver is among the most radiosensitive organs in man. In a number of treatment plans large proportions of the liver receive the full target dose; this is especially so in the treatment of pancreatic cancer, carcinoma of the right kidney, carcinoma of the ovaries, lymphomas, and other systemic malignancies.

Ogata et al. (1963) were the first to describe vascular changes in the liver of three patients who died 20, 50, and 100 days after radiotherapy for lung cancer in the right basal lobe. The most obvious changes were seen in the small branches of the hepatic vein. Endothelial cells were missing, the subintimal argyrophilic fibers were thickened, and the vessel lumen was blocked. They concluded that the primary effect of radiation on the liver was on its vascular system and that any injury to the parenchymal cells in the liver was secondary to vascular damage.

11.4.1 Clinical Radiation Response

Ingold et al. (1965) published the most comprehensive investigation into radiation hepatitis in radiotherapy patients. In 40 patients with disseminated carcinoma of the ovary and spread to the peritoneal cavity or with various lymphomas, the entire liver was given fractionated radiation doses between 13 and 51 Gy. Immediate tolerance was surprisingly good. Except for some transient nausea, vomiting, and diarrhea, no acute hepatic side-effects occurred during radiotherapy. However, 2–6 weeks after the end of radiotherapy, first clinical signs were observed, consisting of a rapid increase in body weight and distention of the abdomen. The authors described this condition as radiation hepatitis, in analogy to radiation nephritis or radiation pneumonitis, without invoking any sort of inflammatory reaction of the liver to radiation. Clinical investigations revealed ascites and liver enlargement. Most tests for liver function and serum enzymes were pathological. Serum

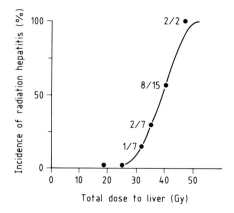

Fig. 11.14. The dependence of radiation hepatitis on radiation dose to the liver in the series of Ingold et al. (1965)

alkaline phosphatase levels were the most reliable indicator of radiation hepatitis. Of the 40 patients, 13 developed radiation hepatitis as diagnosed by clinical investigation or by high levels of serum alkaline phosphatase. The incidence showed a clear dose dependence (Fig. 11.14), increasing from 0% at 25 Gy to 100% at 45 Gy. Of the 13 patients with radiation hepatitis, three died from disseminated tumor soon after radiotherapy while three others died from liver failure; two of the latter patients had received doses in excess of 45 Gy. Seven patients survived, but two of them had pathological results of biochemical liver function tests and, on clinical investigation, an enlarged liver long after radiotherapy. Five patients showed complete recovery. Treatment of these patients consisted of unspecific therapy for liver failure, especially dietary measures, salt restriction, diuretics against ascites, and bed rest. No steroids were given.

Several less comprehensive reports on the clinical features, on the results of clinical investigations using nuclear medicine techniques, computerized tomography, and nuclear magnetic resonance imaging, and on pathohistological findings were published after this pioneering publication. The older publications were well summarized by Marcial et al. (1977). They concluded that, at doses per fraction of 2 Gy, total doses of 30 Gy may lead to hepatic injury in some patients. The severity of clinical symptoms depends on the fraction of total liver irradiated (Austin-Seymour et al. 1986). Latency was consistently described as being between 2 and 6 weeks. In addition to the symptoms described by Ingold et al. (1965), other investigators reported shortness of breath, icterus, and pleural effusions in some cases. Radionuclide scans showed loss of isotope accumulation in the irradiated liver, indicating functional deficits in Kupffer cells. Computerized tomography is useful in the diagnosis of radiation hepatitis (KOLBENSTVEDT and KJOLSETH 1980; JEFFREY et al. 1980; SONODA et al. 1983; UNGER et al. 1987; SPARENBERG et al. 1988), especially if it affects only a part of the liver. Radiation hepatitis appears as a sharply demarcated region of lower attenuation and decreased perfusion in the portal venous phase of CT angiography. In magnetic resonance imaging, radiation hepatitis appears to have a high signal on the T2 weighted image and increased water content as determined by proton spectroscopic imaging methods (UNGER et al. 1987).

Radiation hepatitis is a severe and often fatal disease. Prognosis depends predominantly on the irradiated volume (AUSTIN-SEYMOUR et al. 1986), on the functional reserve of the unirradiated part of the liver, and, thus, on additional damaging factors like alcohol and drugs (KUN and CAMITTA 1978). As mentioned above, of the 13 cases described by INGOLD et al. (1965), three proved fatal owing to hepatic failure, while of the 11 cases described by AUSTIN-SEYMOUR et al. (1986), one was fatal. WHARTON et al. (1973) described eight cases of acute radiation hepatitis, five of them fatal, among 25 patients who were given 24–29 Gy to the liver using the moving strip technique for ovarian carcinoma. Some of the fatal cases were also treated with L-phenylalanine mustard during the phase of radiation hepatitis for suspected tumor progression which may have aggravated hepatic failure. In addition to the eight cases of acute radiation hepatitis, WHARTON et al. (1973) described six further cases of subacute hepatic radiation injury developing later, up to 24 weeks after radiotherapy. Two of the six patients developing delayed radiation hepatitis died. Comparing the cases of WHARTON et al. and those of INGOLD, one recognizes the lower tolerance dose in the former group. According to Fig. 1.14, a 25% incidence of severe radiation hepatitis has to be expected at a total dose of about 35 Gy, yet WHARTON et al. (1973) observed such an incidence at 25 Gy. Differences in the treatment technique, including differences in dose fractionation, may be responsible. The lower tolerance of the liver to the moving strip technique is also apparent in one case of fatal radiation hepatitis described by SCHACTER

et al. (1986) after a dose of 22 Gy and one case described by FEIGEN et al. (1983) after 22.5 Gy.

TEFFT et al. (1970) reported on 115 children who received radiotherapy to the liver as part of integrated treatment for Wilms' tumors and other retroperitoneal malignancies. All patients had chemotherapy, too; 108 of them had actinomycin D. In 91 patients, only the right liver lobe or the left liver lobe was given a medial dose of 30 Gy. In 19 patients, however, the entire liver received about 25 Gy. Five patients had radiotherapy after partial hepatectomy. In the latter group, the most severe and fatal complications were recorded. Five cases of radiation hepatitis were diagnosed clinically after radiotherapy of the right lobe only. A good correlation was observed between serum alkaline phosphatase level and nuclear medical tests and the degree of thrombopenia, all three being suitable criteria for the diagnosis of radiation hepatitis.

Among the cases of TEFFT et al. (1970), no correlation of the results of liver function tests with radiation dose or with irradiated volume was found. Yet it has to be noted that any of the commonly used liver function tests becomes pathological only if more than 75% of the liver tissue fails. This is the reason why, in clinical radiotherapy, where part of the liver is often in the treatment field, radiation hepatitis is a rare complication. However, the techniques of nuclear medicine, computerized tomography, and nuclear magnetic resonance allow the detection of functional deficits in smaller parts of the liver which receive high radiation doses. Focal deficits in the function of both the reticuloendothelial system and the liver parenchyma can be clearly diagnosed.

The first nuclear medicine studies on radiation injury of the liver were reported by USSELMAN (1965), JOHNSON et al. (1967), and CONCANNON et al. (1967). Between 6 and 8 weeks after partial liver irradiation with 40–55 Gy, complete suppression of the function of the RES in the treated liver volume was observed; however, complete recovery was seen after 3–6 months. KUROHARA et al. (1967) performed repeated isotope scans of the liver in 39 patients after radiotherapy to part of their liver–in 31 of them postoperative radiotherapy to the para-aortic lymph nodes with 40–52 Gy for testicular cancer. No patient showed any clinical or biochemical signs of liver injury. The functional defects detected by radiogold colloid scans were more pronounced than those detected

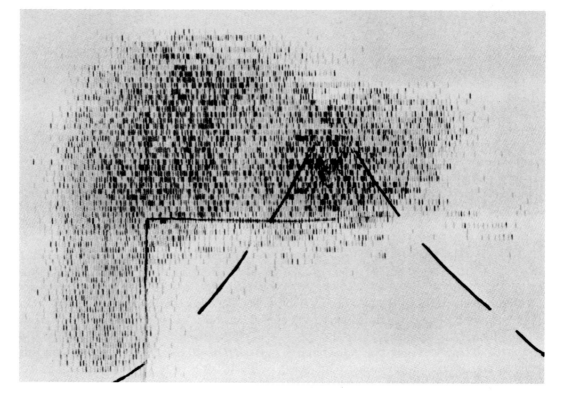

Fig. 11.15. Liver scan with gold-labeled colloid taken 6 weeks after radiotherapy for adenocarcinoma of the right kidney. The margins of the treatment field are marked

by the bengal rose scan although the time pattern of the changes was similar with both methods. Even during radiotherapy a decrease in liver function was discernible after accumulated doses of 20–30 Gy. Maximal depression occurred soon after termination of radiotherapy (Fig. 11.15). Recovery was slow and some pathological results were observed even 5 years after radiotherapy. BRASE et al. (1972) studied 38 patients for 2 years after radiotherapy to para-aortic lymph nodes with 40–45 Gy for malignant lymphoma. No effect was seen halfway through radiotherapy, but a pronounced decrease in the function of the reticulum was observed at the end of radiotherapy in all patients. According to the ratio of impulse counts over the irradiated compared with the unirradiated liver, functional impairment was graded into five stages, with stage III being a significant decrease in impulse density and stage IV patchy accumulation of radioisotopes only (Fig. 11.16). As described by KUROHARA previously, the I-Bromsulphalein test for liver parenchymal func-

tion showed less damage after radiotherapy than the radiogold test, which led BRASE et al. (1972) to conclude that liver cells are less radiosensitive than the reticular cells. However, the pathogenesis and pathophysiology of radiation hepatitis is too complex to allow such simple interpretations. Recovery was complete after 2 years but it took longer in patients with larger volumes of liver in the radiation field and in those who received higher doses.

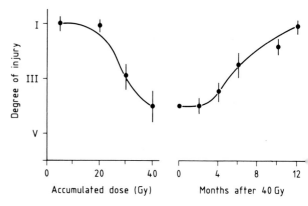

Fig. 11.16. The changes in the degree of radiation injury to the liver as quantitated by liver scan with gold-labeled colloid, its increase with increasing accumulated radiation dose, and its recovery with time after the end of treatment (data from BRASE et al. 1972)

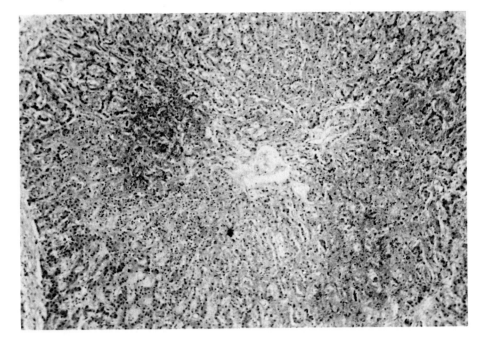

Fig. 11.17. Histological changes in the pig liver 5 months after 6 × 5 Gy local irradiation. Severely congested and hyperemic sinusoids, perivascular fibrosis of the central vein, severe atrophy of hepatocytes

Prophylaxis and treatment of radiation hepatitis have been attempted by giving anticoagulant drugs (LIGHTDALE et al. 1979), unspecific liver diet (INGOLD et al, 1965), and even by performing a portocaval shunt surgically (FEIGEN et al. 1983); however, treatment success is difficult to assess.

AUSTIN-SEYMOUR et al. (1986) performed a systematic investigation into the influence of irradiated volume on the clinical symptoms of radiation hepatitis. Treatment of 11 patients with heavy particles for inoperable pancreatic cancer was carefully planned with CT scans which allowed precise determination of the portion of the liver in the treatment field and the dose distribution in the entire liver. One patient developed histologically proven radiation hepatitis 5 weeks after therapy. The authors concluded that 30% of the liver may tolerate 30–35 Gy if the remainder of the liver does not receive more than 18 Gy. Daily doses should not exceed 2 Gy.

11.4.2 Histopathology

Early histopathological changes in the liver represent veno-occlusive disease, while late histopathological changes comprise periportal fibrosis. The histopathological findings of the Stanford cases of acute radiation hepatitis presented by INGOLD et al. (1965) were described in great detail by REED

and Cox (1966). Gross morphology of the liver consistently showed severe congestion of the liver with edema and hyperemia but always limited to the irradiated part of the liver – as has also been emphasized by TEFFT et al. (1970). Histologically, hyperemia is the most obvious early sign after liver irradiation (Fig. 11.17).

The most severe changes were seen in the small branches of the hepatic vein, the histological picture being similar to that of other diseases causing congestion of the central liver veins, e.g., Budd-Chiari syndrome. No inflammatory response was observed. DJAKOVA et al. (1985) investigated 15 patients who had received 20 Gy in five daily fractions before surgery for stomach cancer and found dilatation of the central veins and sinusoids, edema of perivascular connective tissue, and pressure atrophy of hepatocytes.

Liver cell atrophy increased as the interval between irradiation and biopsy or autopsy became longer (REED and Cox 1966); however, 4 months after irradiation, central veins as well as liver cells showed definite signs of recovery.

In the early phase, no real central venous thrombosis was found. The earliest changes in the

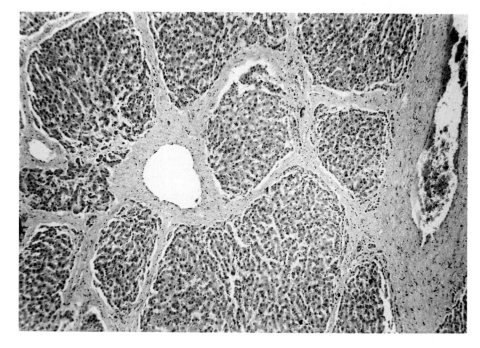

Fig. 11.18. Histological changes in the pig liver 7 months after 6 × 4.75 Gy local irradiation. Massive periportal fibrosis

lumen of central veins were collagen fibers which contained a large amount of packed erythrocytes. Hemosiderin, being a typical sign of thrombosis, was not detected. Only the small branches of the hepatic vein were affected by the venous occlusion process. Subintimal fibrosis was another early sign and was followed later by fibrin deposition in the vessel lumen finally leading to complete vessel occlusion. Its rapid organization leads to the appearance of fibrous nodules in the center of hepatic lobules; however, recanalization may also occur rapidly and is obvious after about 100 days. Other liver vessels always looked normal. Changes in the small portal vessels and the hepatic artery were minimal and very different from those in the hepatic vein. During the acute phase, the general structure of the lobules was still intact; this was in particular true of the peripheral regions of the lobules as well as the portal vessels and bile ducts.

By means of electron microscopy, FAJARDO and COLBY (1980) demonstrated the presence of a fibrin mesh in the central veins of 11 patients suffering from veno-occlusive disease. In contrast light microscopy showed intraluminal fibrin in only 2 of the 11 patients. They suggested that this fibrin mesh was secondary to endothelial cell injury. Red blood cells may be trapped in the mesh, which probably acts as the primer for the development of collagen fibers.

Much less is known about the delayed, chronic injury in the irradiated liver, which appears more variable. It is mostly associated with parenchymal atrophy in the center of the lobules and mild dilatation of the sinusoids. Frequently, the wall of the central veins is thickened (KAPLAN and BAGSHAW 1968) and, side to side, a completely organized occlusion and signs of recanalization may be found. The most characteristic feature of the chronic phase is periportal fibrosis surrounding the portal vein and the bile ducts (Fig. 11.18). Even if pronounced histological changes suggesting lobular atrophy are present, functional deficiencies are not necessarily observed: they depend mainly on the irradiated volume (LEWIN and MILLIS 1973).

11.4.3 Pathogenesis

At present, quite a number of questions regarding the sequence of events leading to acute or chronic radiation injury of the liver are still open. In part this may be due to the fact that, so far, no animal models have been available which reproduce the type of radiation injury in the human liver sufficiently well and in a reproducible and quantifiable way.

Summarizing the present state of knowledge, it appears that the first alterations take place in the walls of the central veins, leading to endothelial cell injury (not necessarily endothelial cell death) and the formation of the intraluminal fibrin mesh.

Ectatic changes in the portal veins which were demonstrated by microangiographic techniques in rabbits by BRASE et al. (1974) lead to decreased blood flow, which may further facilitate the trapping of red blood cells (but not of platelets) in the fibrin mesh (FAJARDO and COLBY 1980). In this way, the central veins gradually accumulate fibrinoid, edematous structures which spread in a centrifugal way to the periphery of the hepatic lobules. DJAKOVA et al. (1985) explain the atrophy of the hepatocytes as a consequence of increased pressure from the dilated and congested sinusoids, although atrophy may also be caused by nutrient deficiency due to impaired blood flow. The typical features of veno-occlusive disease of the liver are associated with severe functional deficits. The latter are, in principle, reversible if the patient survives the acute phase, and occluded central veins may be recanalized. However, others may be organized into fibrous tissue.

The sequence of changes follows a rather fixed time pattern in patients; therefore the changes after irradiation with doses above a threshold dose depend more on the interval to irradiation than on radiation dose to the liver (REED and COX 1966; TEFFT et al. 1970).

Late changes apparently develop independently from the acute changes. Fibrosis is mainly located near the portal vein and the bile ducts in the trigone of Glisson. The typical structure of the liver architecture may disappear in the chronic phase, yet the enormous capacity of the remaining, undamaged parts of the liver to compensate partial losses of liver tissue may allow normal liver function to continue.

11.4.4 Animal Models

No adequate animal model for radiation hepatitis has been developed, so far. Only in pigs does local irradiation with doses similar to those currently used in radiotherapy (five fractions of 6 Gy in 1 week) produce syndromes similar to those of veno-occlusive disease and late periportal fibrosis seen in patients (TROTT and HERRMANN 1988) (Figs. 11.17, 11.18). No dose–response relation-

ship data are yet available in this model, though.

A few radiobiological experiments studied the response to irradiation of the rodent liver after partial hepatectomy. Removal of a large proportion of the liver by surgical resection or by toxic agents recruits the remaining liver cells into synchronous proliferation KELLY et al. (1956) studied the effect of radiation on recruitment, while FABRIKANT (1967) investigated its effect on the time course of the wave of liver cell proliferation. COGGLE (1968) used the partially hepatectomized liver as a model to investigate the relative radiosensitivities of G_0 cells in their resting phase or after stimulation into proliferation by scoring abnormal metaphase figures. These studies do not bear any relation to the pathogenesis of radiation hepatitis but represent models to investigate more fundamental radiobiological questions.

GERACI et al. (1985) combined high dose liver irradiation with partial hepatectomy in rats and produced a fulminant radiation hepatitis with massive ascites and hepatic failure after a mean latency of only 2 weeks. Radiation doses between 17 and 30 Gy were given to the surgically exposed liver, immediately followed by resection of two-thirds of the liver. Lethality increased steeply with increasing dose, LD_{50} being 24 Gy (Fig. 11.19).

Massive ascites developing 8 days after irradiation and severe impairment of liver function as assessed by rose bengal clearance suggested liver failure to be the main cause of death; this was substantiated by histological findings of severe distortion of liver structure, coagulation necrosis, enlarged hepatocytes, and many other signs of

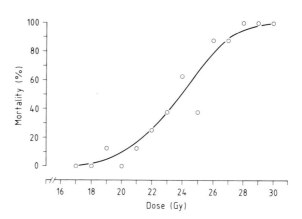

Fig. 11.19. The dependence of fatal liver failure on radiation dose after single dose total liver irradiation followed by partial hepatectomy in rats. (data from GERACI et al. 1985)

acute liver injury. No signs of veno-occlusive disease were observed. In animals irradiated with 30 Gy no functional or histological changes in the liver were observed if partial hepatectomy was not performed to reduce the functional reserve of the liver and to stimulate proliferation and thus promote early manifestation of radiation damage.

The most detailed study on the time course of radiation injury in the liver of rats was published by HEBARD et al. (1980). After a single dose of 80 (!) Gy to the left liver lobe, morphometric analysis of the histopathological changes was performed at regular intervals (Fig. 11.20). Over a period of 9 months, the relative weight of the irradiated lobe decreased to 60%, which was entirely due to loss of hepatocytes. In contrast to most other studies, HEBARD et al. (1980) observed an early inflammatory response up to the 12th week, with massive infiltration of small lymphocytes and plasma cells. After 4 weeks, periportal fibrosis was already discernible, increasing up to the 16th week. A second wave of radiation injury started after the 16th week, with progressive changes in the central veins characterized by concentric lamellations and compromise of their lumen leading to localized portal hypertension, decreased blood perfusion, and secondary late parenchymal injury. The histological changes observed in the early phase in this study were quite different from those in pigs and patients. GERACI et al. (1980) used this model to study the RBE of fast neutrons. Histological changes, hydroxyproline content, and uptake of bengal rose were quantitated 4 months and 12

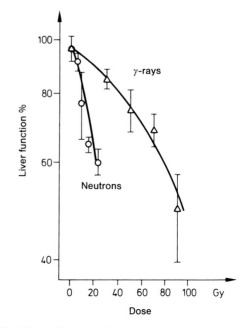

Fig. 11.21. The dose dependence of the decrease in liver function as determined by the uptake of bengal rose in rat livers after single doses of γ-rays or neutrons(data from GERACI et al. 1980)

months after local irradiation of the left liver lobe. Perivascular fibrosis developed primarily in the periportal fields and led to progressive atrophy of liver parenchyma. Whereas 4 months after irradiation no functional deficit could be detected, 12 months after irradiation uptake of bengal rose decreased progressively with increasing dose according to some sort of shoulder curve (Fig. 11.21). The decreased uptake of bengal rose in the irradiated lobe was mainly related to the decreased number of hepatocytes rather than to functional deficits in the hepatocytes. Conversely, 1 year after irradiation, the relative hydroxyproline content increased, indicating progressive periportal fibrosis. The RBE of neutrons with a mean energy of 8 MeV was determined with this model. Even at a neutron dose of 10 Gy, RBE was well above 3.

The microangiographic study on the radiation effects on the irradiated rabbit liver by BRASE et al. (1974) demonstrated rather early changes in vascular morphology after single doses of 5–30 Gy to the liver. Serial x-ray pictures were taken at 4 s intervals after rapid injection of 10 ml contrast medium into the mesenteric vein. As early as 1 week after doses above 10 Gy, definite changes in the structure of the portal vascular system were

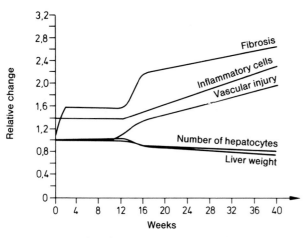

Fig. 11.20. The time course of histological changes as determined in morphometric analysis of rat livers irradiated with a single dose of 80 Gy (data from HEBARD et al. 1980)

obvious, such as irregularities in vessel diameter, interruption of vessel continuity, decreased capillary density, and sluggish blood flow. Four months after 10 Gy, a normal angiogram was recorded, yet after doses above 12 Gy persistent vascular irregularities, including focal loss of capillaries and very narrow lumina of major vessels, were recorded. Despite these pronounced vascular changes and extensive edema in histological sections, the typical histological picture of radiation hepatitis was not observed in these rabbits. BICHER et al. (1976) studied the microcirculation in the liver of dogs before and 2 weeks after a dose of 46 Gy given in 23 fractions in 35 days. The most sensitive indicator for radiation injury to the microcirculation was an early increase in reoxygenation time which correlates well with the microangiographic findings of BRASE et al. (1974). Thus morphological and functional changes in the microcirculation of the liver are the earliest demonstrable forms of radiation injury, yet their relationship to the development of early and late radiation-induced liver disease remains to be elucidated.

Investigations of liver function in animals after local liver irradiation are scarce, the most extensive being those by BIRZLE and FRANZIUS (1965) and BIRZLE et al. (1970) in rabbits. Within 24 h after doses between 5 and 20 Gy, dose-dependent decreases in the elimination of Bromsulphalein and N-acetyl-paraaminophenol were recorded which, however, recovered within a few days. BRASE et al. (1973) investigated the accumulation of radiogold colloid and of I-Bromsulphalein in rabbit livers locally irradiated with 5–20 Gy (Fig. 11.22). Whereas after 10 Gy, effects were barely significant, after 12 Gy a transient decrease in liver function was recorded which recovered to normal within 6 weeks. A single dose of 16 Gy to the rabbit liver was lethal within 3–4 weeks.

Recently, methods have been developed to study the clonogenic potential of individual hepatocytes and their radiosensitivity. JIRTLE et al. (1981) irradiated the livers of donor animals (rats) in vivo, prepared a single cell suspension, and injected different cell numbers into the interscapular fat pad of recipient animals which had undergone partial hepatectomy 1 h beforehand. Brown nodules developed at the transplantation site over a period of up to 3 months; upon histological examination these nodules showed cords and clusters of hepatocytes surrounded by fibrovascular connective tissue and even some bile ducts. There was active DNA synthesis in the hepato-

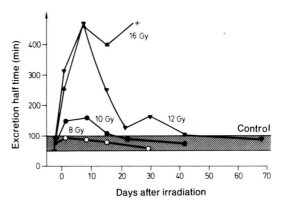

Fig. 11.22. Changes in the hepatic excretion of Bromsulphalein after single dose irradiation of the rabbit liver (data from BRASE et al. 1973)

cytes. Electron microscopy and enzyme histochemistry proved that colony-forming cells were indeed hepatocytes. Twenty days after transplantation, distinct colonies could be identified, the take rate increasing with increasing inoculum size and the 50% take inoculum size increasing with increasing radiation dose. The dose–response curve constructed with this endpoint dilution assay had a D_0 of about 2.5 Gy.

This technique also works well in mice. FISHER and HENDRY (1988) and FISHER et al. (1988) have reported on the dependence of clonogenic survival on dose fractionation and on the interval between irradiation and assay for clonogenicity. Single dose survival curves were characterized by an extrapolation number of 1.6 and a D_0 of 2.4 Gy; however, as the interval between irradiation and cell isolation increased, cells became increasingly radioresistant (after just 1 day this increase was already nearly 40%) Eleven months later resistance had increased more than threefold. This increase was assumed to be due to a slow intracellular repair phenomenon, as there is no significant proliferative response in the liver to irradiation.

11.4.5 Dependence of Radiation Effects on Dose Fractionation and the Combination with Chemotherapy

Few experimental and clinical data are available for analysis of the fractionation effect, the most important relating to comparison of liver tolerance after open field whole abdominal radiotherapy and moving strip radiotherapy. No patient developed any clinical sign of liver injury after eight fractions of 2.25 Gy using the moving strip technique (Perez et al. 1978), while 8 of 25 patients developed severe radiation hepatitis after eight fractions of 3.5 Gy using the moving strip technique (Wharton et al. 1973; Delclos et al. 1963) Of 40 patients, 13 developed radiation hepatitis after open field irradiation of the liver with doses between 25 and 40 Gy given in fraction doses of 1–2 Gy (Fig. 11.14). Ignoring other differences in irradiation techniques and volumes, one may relate these differences in dose and incidence to differences in fractionation. In the Strandqvist plot, a slope of greater than 0.4 results from this comparison and a very low α/β value close to 0 Gy is estimated. This very pronounced repair capacity of the liver was also observed in experiments studying clonogenic survival of hepatocytes using the quantitative transplantation assay (Fisher and Hendry 1988). Varying the dose per fraction between 1 and 8 Gy and performing the assess-

ment 1 day later, they derived an α/β value of less than 2 Gy (Fig. 11.23). This low α/β value did not change as the interval between fractionated irradiation and assay was prolonged up to 10 months, which suggested that this very pronounced repair capacity of hepatocytes is not related to prolonged stay in the resting state, but also is not related to the slow repair mentioned above or to the shoulder size of the single dose–response curve (*n* being only 1.6!).

A 25% incidence of veno-occlusive disease has been observed after total body irradiation with 10 Gy followed by bone marrow transplantation (Fajardo and Colby 1980; McDonald et al. 1984) and has usually been related to the additional effects of chemotherapy and graft-versus-host disease. However, since extrapolation of the above-mentioned data arrives at a single effective dose of about 10 Gy, it is equally conceivable that irradiation is the most important contributor to the development of veno-occlusive disease after total body irradiation and bone marrow transplantation (Trott and Herrmann 1988).

Kun and Camitta (1978) reported on one case of fatal radiation hepatitis occurring after liver irradiation with 17 fractions of 1.4 Gy after previous chemotherapy with 275 mg/m^2 adriamycin and one case of reversible radiation hepatitis after liver irradiation with 23 fractions of 1.1 Gy after previous chemotherapy with 180 mg/m^2 adriamycin, suggesting a pronounced decrease in liver tolerance after remarkably low doses of this drug. No other information on the influence of chemotherapy on the radiosensitivity of the liver has been published so far.

11.5 Radiation Effects on the Pancreas

The pancreas receives the full tumor dose in any radiotherapy of para-aortic lymph nodes. Its clinical consequences, however, and the functional and morphological response to irradiation, have not been studied properly so far. Some older observations in patients and experimental animals have been summarized by Friedman (1942). This lack of information on the radiation effects in the pancreas may be due to difficulties in examining the pancreas in patients and, even more so, in experimental animals but also to the unspecific and insidious nature of clinical consequences of

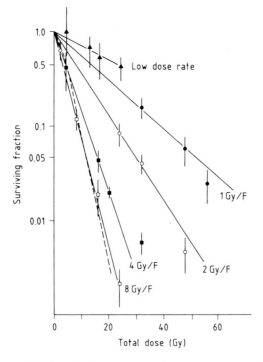

Fig. 11.23. Survival curves of hepatic clonogens assayed 24 h after single dose (*dolted line*), fractionated or continuous irradiation: dose per fraction was 1, 2, 4, or 8 Gy. Triangles represent continuous irradiation at a dose rate of 0.03 Gy/h (Data from Fisher and Hendry 1988)

any acute or chronic injury to the pancreas. Thus, the role of radiation injury to the pancreas in the development of acute and chronic gastrointestinal syndromes after abdominal radiotherapy is poorly understood.

11.5.1 Clinical Radiation Response

Pancreatic function in patients after radiotherapy of the upper abdomen has been studied in only a small number of patients. BECCIOLINI et al. (1987) analyzed the duodenal juice after a standardized test meal in patients after 50 Gy in 25 fractions but did not measure any significant changes in the activity of trypsin or amylase. They concluded that radiation effects on the pancreas did not contribute to the transient acute malabsorption syndrome in irradiated patients. Yet MITCHELL et al. (1979) described two patients who suffered from severe malabsorption syndrome which they attributed to radiation-induced pancreatitis. STEGLICH (1988) studied 27 patients during and after upper abdominal radiotherapy and compared them with 42 patients with pelvic radiotherapy (Fig. 11.24) Serum lipase activity increased in patients directly irradiated to their pancreas but also in patients after pelvic radiotherapy, although to a lesser degree. There was no clear correlation between gastrointestinal symptoms and the rise in enzyme activities. Moreover, maximal enzyme activities i serum occurred during the 1st week of radiother apy, in contrast to the subjective symptoms of the gastrointestinal syndrome, which reach their max-

imum in the 3rd and 4th weeks of fractionated radiotherapy. Thus, although changes in the function of the pancreas can be demonstrated during upper abdominal radiotherapy, we cannot, at present, evaluate their clinical significance for the general picture of acute and chronic side-effects in the epigastric region.

11.5.2 Histopathology

The most extensive study on histopathological changes after local irradiation of the pancreas has been that by VOLK et al. (1966). In 23 dogs the surgically exposed pancreas was given a single dose of 50–90 (!) Gy, and histological changes were registered up to 21 days after irradiation. Whereas light microscopy did not show any pronounced changes (only after 21 days were some fibrotic reactions seen between the acini and the follicles), electron microscopy revealed irradiation to have dramatic effects. Cytoplasmic lesions in the acinar cells 5–8 days after irradiation and a reduction in the number and size of zymogen granules are the submicroscopic signs of acute injury to the exocrine pancreas. They correspond to a decrease in enzyme activities in the pancreatic tissue. The same authors (WELLMANN et al. 1966) also reported on chronic pancreatic injury in these animals for up to 1 year. They distinguished between three phases of histopathological changes in the irradiated pancreas: The degenerative phase lasted from 1 week to the 3rd month after irradiation and was followed by a recovery phase between 3 and 6 months after irradiation. Normalization of the submicroscopic pattern of acinar cell injury occurred between 6 and 9 months. However, despite the morphological restitution of the exocrine pancreas, a progressive decrease in serum lipase activity was recorded which did not reach a plateau even after 9 months.

ARCHAMBEAU et al. (1966) observed progressive interstitial fibrosis in the pancreas of dogs after upper abdominal irradiation with 45–50 Gy in 20 fractions, which was accompanied by a decrease in serum amylase activity at 5 months after irradiation.

KOVACS (1976) studied the pancreas of rats for up to 150 days after 16 daily fractions to a total dose of 80 Gy. In the acute phase, necrobiotic areas were surrounded by intact gland tissue. The necrobiotic areas were interpreted as secondary

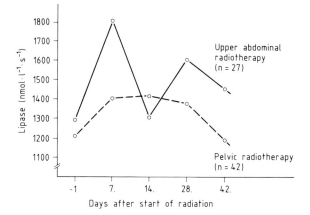

Fig. 11.24. Changes in the activity of serum lipase during radiotherapy of upper abdominal fields or pelvic fields (data from STEGLICH 1988)

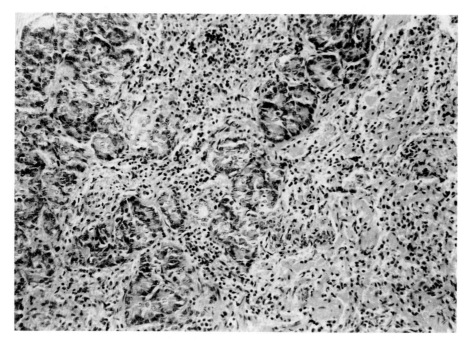

Fig. 11.25. Histological changes 6 months after irradiation of the pig pancreas with 6 × 5 Gy. Severe pancreatic fibrosis

injury caused by pancreatic enzymes released from functioning acini, and it was suggested that alteration of the membrane permeability of the pancreatic ducts is the primary radiation effect on the pancreas which lays the pancreatic tissue open to the attack of pancreatic enzymes. The lesions to the arteriolar vessels which were seen shortly after irradiation increased during the chronic phase and led to progressive fibrosis (Fig. 11.25), which, however, in these experiments never involved the entire pancreatic tissue.

The only histopathological study on human pancreatic tissue was reported by Magyar et al. (1980). Autopsy specimens were investigated from eight patients who had received upper abdominal radiotherapy (including the pancreas) 1 day to 6 years before death. Histopathological findings were compared with those in patients who had received radiotherapy not encompassing the pancreas and were classified into early, intermediate, and late changes (Table 11.2). It is interesting to note that despite the presence of marked histopathological changes, there were no obvious clinical signs of pancreas-related digestive failure. Like Volk et al. (1966), the authors observed hyalinization of individual islands of Langerhans, which, however, did not lead to any clinical

symptoms of diabetes. Zook et al. (1983) compared histological changes in dogs after fractionated irradiation with photons or 15 MeV neutrons, total photon doses ranging from 30 to 67.5 Gy. Like Archambeau (1966), they observed progressive interstitial fibrosis and, especially, severe degenerative changes in the small arterial vessels. After several months, periductal fibrosis was also very obvious.

In dogs, radiation-induced damage to the pancreas has also been documented after total body irradiation conditioning the animals for bone marrow transplantation. Between 40 and 90 days after three fractions of 6 Gy total body irradiation followed by cryopreserved autologous bone marrow transplantation, Michel et al. (1986) observed a pronounced reduction in exocrine pancreatic tissue with extra- and intralobular fibrosis.

In summary, histopathological studies have revealed severe radiation lesions in the exocrine pancreas which, due to the large reserve capacity of the organ, only rarely lead to clinical symptoms. Radiation injury to the vessels and fibrosis appear earlier than in other tissues, which has been explained by additional injury from the digestive enzymes produced in the organ and released into the interstitial tissue as membranes become leaky after irradiation. Even in those areas which do not show any light microscopic changes, severe alterations may be seen in the electron microscope.

Table 11.2. Changes in the pancreas produced by irradiation

Early	Intermediate	Late
Necrosis and fibrinoid degeneration of arterioles, and small and middle size arteries	Fibrinoid necrosis and hyaline thickening of the arterioles and small and middle size arteries	Hyaline thickening of the walls and narrowing of the lumen of arterioles and small and middle size arteries
Interstitial edema	Fibrosis of the interstitium	Marked fibrosis of the interstitium
	Infiltration of interstitium by chronic inflammatory cells. Scattered foci of necrosis and acute inflammatory reaction	
Swelling and degenerative changes of the secretory cells	Atrophy of the exocrine glands	Atrophy and reduction in the number of exocrine glands
Necrosis and loss of epithelial lining of the small excretory ducts		Periductal fibrosis
		Enlargement and hyalinization of the islets of Langerhans

11.5.3 Pathogenesis

No systematic studies have been published on the pathogenesis of pancreatic radiation injury. The most relevant data are those of VOLK et al. (1966), from serial investigations performed on dogs between 30 min and 9 months after irradiation. The primary lesion appears to be in the acinar cell system of the pancreas. Later partial regeneration of the acinar cells was observed, while there was some late gradual degeneration of Langerhans' islands by about 20%. This may be related to the slowly progressive vascular lesions and interstitial and periductal fibrosis (MAGYAR et al. 1980; KONERMANN et al. 1979). The early development of interstitial fibrosis may be due to a precipitating effect of pancreatic enzymes leaking into the tissue stroma. This mechanism is similar to that proposed by HAUER JENSEN et al. (1985) for the pathogenesis of interstitial fibrosis in the bowel wall.

11.5.4 Animal Models

Most experiments in rodents and dogs were performed to study functional changes of the exocrine or the endocrine glands in the pancreas after local irradiation. The earliest studies were reported in 1926 by ORNDORFF et al. and by FISHER et al. Several later publications reported experiments on different animals determining serum activities of pancreatic enzymes or the amount of pancreatic juice in the pancreatic duct after local irradiation with high single doses (e.g., RAUCH and STENSTROM 1952). HEINKEL and BERGENTHAL (1963) recorded decreased lipase activity only a few days after local irradiation of rat pancreas with single doses between 10 and 50 Gy, whereas in dogs WELLMANN et al. (1966) did not observe decreased serum lipase activity until 3–4 months had elapsed.

In summary, studies in experimental animals after local irradiation of the pancreas have generally shown, initially, a transient increase in the secretion of pancreatic juice and an increase in serum enzyme activity which is followed later by a gradual decrease to below normal levels at longer follow-up times. The results of different studies differ considerably due to differences in irradiation technique and assay methods for pancreatic enzymes in tissue or serum. No animal model has been developed which could be used to study the incidence of clinically relevant pancreatic radiation damage as a function of dose, fractionation, or combined treatment. One major obstacle is insufficient understanding of the contribution of radiation injury of the pancreas to the complex side-effects appearing early and late after upper abdominal radiotherapy.

11.5.5 Fractionation Effects on Radiation Injury

No systematic studies on the effects of dose fractionation on pancreatic radiation injury have been published. The only study with local fractionated irradiation has been performed by PIERONI et al. (1976). Six dogs received six fractions of 4 Gy and the response of the pancreas to stimulating drugs was studied by collecting the pancreatic juice with a tube surgically fixed in the pancreatic duct. After initial hypersecretion, a progressive decrease in pancreatic function, reaching 10% of normal values after 3 months, was observed. No comparison was made with other doses or other fractionation schedules. In any case, these studies demonstrate the marked radiosensitivity of the pancreas in dogs.

Clinical experience shows better subjective tolerance to radiotherapy which includes the pancreas if the doses per fraction are reduced, yet it is not known whether this is due to decreased pancreatic injury. Since the pancreas enjoys a central position in the digestive functions of the intestines and since some experimental data have documented severe functional deficits and morphological injury at longer follow-up after moderate radiation doses given locally to the pancreas, systematic studies on the dose and fractionation response of the pancreas and its significance for clinical side-effects are urgently needed.

References

Archambeau J, Griem M, Harper P (1966) The effects of 250 kV x-rays on the dog's pancreas: morphological and functional changes. Radiat Res 28: 243–256

Austin-Seymour MM, Chen GTY, Castro JR, Saunders WM, Pitluck S, Woodruff KH, Kessler M (1986) Dose volume histogram analysis of liver radiation tolerance. Int J Radiat Oncol Biol Phys 12: 31–35

Battermann JJ, Hart GAM, Breur K (1981) Dose-effect relations for tumour control and complication rate after fast neutron therapy for pelvic tumours. Br J Radiol 54: 899–904

Becciolini A (1987) Relative radiosensitivities of the small and large intestine. Advances in radiation biology, vol 12. Academic, New York, pp 83–128

Berdov BA, Wedzizewa TB, Bassalyk LS (1988) Der funktionelle Status gastrinproduzierender Zellen bei Patienten mit Magenkarzinom unter lokaler Bestrahlung. Radiobiol Radiother (Berl) 29: 187–192

Berthrong M, Fajardo LF (1981) Radiation injury in surgical pathology. II. Alimentary tract. Am J Surg Pathol 5: 153–178

Bicher HI, Ashbrook DW, Harris DR, Dalrymple GV (1976) Changes in platelet and microcirculation function induced by ionizing radiation to the liver. Int J Radiat Oncol Biol Phys 1: 679–685

Birzle H, Franzius E (1965) Über die funktionelle Strahlenempfindlichkeit der Leber. Strahlentherapie 126: 119–131

Birzle H, Beek K, Nusselt I (1970) Die Wirkung gezielter Röntgentiefenbetrahlung der Leber auf deren Entgiftungsleistung durch Paarung mit Glucuronsäure beim Kaninchen. Strahlentherapie 139: 347–353

Black WC, Ackermann LV (1965) Carcinoma of the large intestine as a late complication of pelvic radiotherapy. Clin Radiol 16: 278–281

Black WC, Gomez LS, Yuhas JM, Kligermann MM (1980) Quantitation of the late effects of x-radiation on the large intestine. Cancer 45: 444–451

Blott P, Trott K-R (1989) The effect of actinomycin D on split dose recovery and repopulation in jejunal crypt cells in vivo. Radiother Oncol 15: 73–78

Bowers RF, Brick JB (1947) Surgery in radiation in injury of the stomach. Surgery 22: 20–40

Brase A. Bockslaff H, Kaufmann M (1972) Szintigraphische Befunde der Leber nach Teilbestrahlung mit Kobalt 60. Strahlentherapie 143: 41–47

Brase A, Bockslaff H, Heindl H, Järivinen S (1973) Tierexperimentelle Funktionsuntersuchungen mit Radionukliden an der Leber nach gezielter Co-60 Bestrahlung. Strahlentherapie 146: 198–207

Brase A, Bockslaff H. Emminger E (1974) Angiographische Untersuchungen der portalen Lebergefäße bei Kaninchen nach Strahleninsult. Strahlentherapie 147: 278–289

Braun H (1963) Leber. In: Scherer E, Stender HS (eds) Strahlenpathologie der Zelle. Thieme, Stuttgart

Breiter N, Trott K-R (1986) Chronic radiation damage in the rectum of the rat after protracted fractionated irradiation. Radiother Oncol 7: 155–163

Breiter N, Kneschaurek P, Burger G, Huczkowski J, Trott K-R (1986) The r.b.e. of fast fission neutrons (2MeV) for chronic radiation damage of the large bowel of rats after single dose and fractionated irradiation. Int J Radiat Biol 49: 1031–1038

Breiter N, Sassy T, Trott K-R, Unsold E (1988) Die endoskopische Verlaufskontrolle und deren histologische Korrelation des chronischen Strahlenschadens am Enddarm der Ratte. Strahlentherapie 164: 674–680

Breiter N, Trott K-R, Sassy T (1989) Effects of x-irradiation on the stomach of the rat. Int J Radiat Oncol Biol Phys 17: 779–784

Brick IB (1947) The effect of large dosages of irradiation on gastric acidity. N Engl J Med 237: 48–51

Browde S, de Mohr N (1982) Non-standard fractionation schemes in the treatment of advanced carcinoma of the uterine cervix and advanced head and neck cancer. In: Nervi C, Fletcher GH (eds) The biological and clinical basis of radioresistance. Thomas, Springfield

Bruegel C (1917) Die Beeinflussung des Magenchemismus durch Röntgenstrahlen. Münch Med Wochenschr 64: 379–382

Carpender JWJ, Levin E, Clapman LB, Miller RE (1956) Radiation in the therapy of peptic ulcer. AJR 75: 374–379

Carr ND, Pullen BR, Hasleton PS, Schofield PF (1984) Microvascular studies in human radiation bowel disease. Gut 25: 448–454

Chen KY, Withers HR (1972) Survival characteristics of stem cells of gastric mucosa subjected to localized gamma irradiation. Int J Radiat Biol 21: 521–534

Cikaric S (1988) Radiation therapy of cervical carcinoma using either HDR or LDR afterloading: comparison of 5-year results and complications. In: Vahrson H, Rauthe G (eds) High dose rate afterloading in the treatment of cancer of the uterus, breast and rectum. Urban & Schwarzenberg, Munich

Coggle JE (1968) Effect of cell cycle on recovery from radiation damage in the mouse liver. Nature 217: 180–182

Concannon JP, Edelmann A, Rich JC, Kunkel G (1967) Localized "radiation hepatitis" as demonstrated by scintillation scanning. Radiology 89: 136–139

Cottier H (1961) Strahlenbedingte Lebensverkürzung. Springer, Berlin Heidelberg New York

Craig MS, Buie LA (1949) Factitial (irradiation) proctitis. A clinicopathological study of 200 cases. Surgery 25: 472–487

Cram RE, Pearlman NW, Jochimsen PR (1977) Surgical management of complications of radiation-injured gut. Am J Surg 133: 551–553

Cronkite EP, Fliedner TM (1972) The radiation syndromes. In: Hug O, Zuppinger A (eds) Strahlenbiologie 3. Springer, Berlin Heidelberg New York (Handbuch der Medizinischen Radiologie vol II/3)

Crook JM, Esche BA, Chaplain G, Isturiz J, Sentenac I, Horiot JC (1987) Dose-volume analysis and the prevention of radiation sequelae in cervical cancer. Radiother Oncol 8: 321–332

Dale RG, Huczkowski J, Trott K-R (1988) Possible dose rate dependence of recovery kinetics as deduced from a preliminary analysis of fractionated irradiations at varying dose rates. Br J Radiol 61: 153–157

Danjoux CE, Catton GE (1979) Delayed complications in colorectal carcinoma treated by combination radiotherapy and 5-fluorouracil – Eastern Cooperative Oncology Group Pilot Study. Int J Radiat Oncol Biol Phys 5: 311–315

Delclos L, Braun EJ, Herrera JR, Sanpiere VC, van Rosenbeek E (1963) Whole abdominal irradiation with Co-60 moving strip technic. Radiology 81: 632–641

den Hartog Jager FCA, van Haastert M, Battermann JJ, Tytgat GNJ (1985) The endoscopic spectrum of late radiation damage of the rectosigmoid colon, Endoscopy 17: 214–217

Dethlefsen LA, Riley RM (1979) The effects of adriamycin and x-irradiation on the murine duodenum. Int J Radiat Oncol Biol Phys 5: 507–513

Dettmer CA, Kramer S, Driscoll DH, Aponte GE (1968) A comparison of the chronic effects of irradiation upon the normal, damaged, and regenerating rat liver. Radiology 91: 993–997

Dewit L, Oussoren Y (1987) Late effects in the mouse small intestine after a clinically relevant multifractionated radiation treatment. Radiat Res 110: 372–384

Dewit L, Begg AC, Kohler Y, Stewart FA, Bartelink H (1985) Influence of cis-diamminedichloroplatinum (II) on mouse duodenal crypt stem cell survival after multifraction x-ray treatment. Int J Radiat Oncol Biol Phys 11: 1809–1816

Dewit L, Oussoren Y, Bartelink H (1987) Early and late damage in the mouse rectum after irradiation and cisdiamminedichloroplatinum. Radiother Oncol 8: 57–70

Djakova AM, Stefani NV, Zagrebin VM, Senokosov NI, Berdov BA (1985) Postradiogene Effekte im Lebergewebe von Patienten mit Magenkarzinomen nach der Radiosensibilisation mit Metronidazol. Radiobiol Radiother (Berl) 26: 343–350

Doig RK, Funder JF, Weiden S (1951) Serial gastric biopsy studies in a case of duodenal ulcer treated by deep x-ray therapy. Med J Aust 38: 828–830

Duncan W, Leonard JC (1965) The malabsorption syndrome following radiotherapy. Q J Med 34: 319–329

Edwards DN (1968) Complications following megavoltage radiation for carcinoma of the bladder. Clin Radiol 19: 27–33

Ellinger F (1957) Medical radiation biology, Thomas, Springfield

Engelstad RB (1938) The effect of roentgen on the stomach in rabbits. AJR 40: 243–263

Fabrikant JI (1967) Cell proliferation in the regenerating liver of continuously irradiated mice. Br J Radiol 40: 487–495

Fajardo LP (1982) Pathology or radiation injury. Masson, New York

Fajardo LF, Berthrong M (1981) Radiation injury in surgical pathology.III. Am J Surg Pathol 5: 279–296

Fajardo LF, Colby TV (1980) Pathogenesis of veno-occlusive liver disease after radiation. Arch Pathol Lab Med 104: 584–588

Feigen M, Lavrin L, Mameghan H, Peters L (1983) Radiation hepatitis following moving strip radiotherapy. Int J Radiat Oncol Biol Phys 9: 397–399

Findley JM, Newaisky GA, Sircus W, McManus JPA (1974) Role of gastric irradiation in management of peptic ulceration and esophagitis. Br Med J 3: 769–771

Fisher DR, Hendry JH (1988) Dose fractionation and hepatocyte clonogens: $\alpha/\beta = 1$–2 Gy, and β decreases with increasing delay before assay. Radiat Res 113: 51–57

Fisher DR, Hendry JH, Scott D (1988) Long-term repair in vivo of colony forming ability and chromosomal injury in x-irradiated mouse hepatocytes. Radiat Res 113: 40–50

Fisher NF, Groot JT, Bachem A (1926) The effects of x-rays on the pancreas. Am J Physiol 76: 299–305

Friedman NB (1942) Effects of radiation on the gastrointestinal tract, including the salivary glands, the liver and the pancreas. Arch Pathol 34: 749–787

Fu KK, Phillips TL, Kane LJ, Smith V (1975) Tumor and normal tissue response to irradiation in vivo: variation with decreasing dose rates. Radiology 114: 709–716

Gauwerky F (1949) Die Komplikationen bei der Radiumbehandlung der Kollumkarzinome und ihre Bedeutung für den Behandlungserfolg. Strahlentherapie 80: 51–70

Gehrig J, Hacki WH, Schulthess HK Reinisch E, Kunz J, Stamm B (1987) Strahlenproktitis nach gynaekologischer Radiotherapie: eine endoskopische Studie. Schweiz Med Wochenschr 117: 1326–1332

Gelfand MD, Tepper M, Katz LA, Binder HJ, Yesner R, Floch MH (1968) Acute irradiation proctitis in man. Development of eosinophilic crypt abscesses. Gastroenterology 54: 401–411

Geraci JP. Jackson KL, Christensen GM, Parker RG, Fox MS, Thrower PD (1974) The relative biological effectiveness of cyclotron fast neutrons for early and late damage to the small intestine of the mouse. Eur J Cancer 10: 99–102

Geraci JP, Jackson KL, Christensen GM, Thrower PD, Weyer BJ (1977) Acute and late damage in the mouse small intestine following multiple fractionations of neutrons or x-rays. Int J Radiat Oncol Biol Phys 2: 693–696

Geraci JP, Jackson KL, Thrower PD, Mariano MS (1980) Relative biological effectiveness of cyclotron fast neutrons for late hepatic injury in rats. Radiat Res 82: 570–578

Geraci JP, Jackson KL, Mariam MS, Leitch JM (1985) Hepatic injury after whole-liver irradiation in the rat. Radiat Res 101: 508–518

Glaser FH (1988) Comparison of HDR afterloading with 192 Ir vs. conventional radium therapy in cervix cancer: 5-year results and complications. In: Vahrson H, Rauthe G (eds) High dose rate afterloading in the treatment of cancer of the uterus, breast and rectum. Urban & Schwarzenberg, Munich

Goldgraber MB, Rubin CE, Palmer WL, Dobson RL, Massey BW (1954) The early gastric response to irradiation. A serial biopsy study. Gastroenterology 27: 1–20

Goodrich JK, Hickmann BT (1962) Oleic acid I^{131} intestinal absorption in pelvic Co^{60} irradiation. AJR 87: 69–75

Graudinns J (1969) Über Strahlenspätschäden am Dünndarm. Langenbecks Arch Chir 324: 120–130

Gray MJ, Kottmeier HL (1957) Rectal and bladder injuries following radium therapy for carcinoma of the cervix at the Radiumhemmet. Am J Obstet Gynecol 74: 1294–1303

Greiner R, Blattmann H (1987) Strahlentherapic mit negativen Pi-Mesonen. In: K.Z. Winkel (ed.) Wirkungssteigerung der Strahlentherapic maligner Tumoren Springer Berlin

Hamilton E (1978) Cell proliferation and ageing in mouse colon. Repopulation after repeated x-ray injury in young and old mice. Cell Tissue Kinet 11: 423–431

Hamilton FE (1947) Gastric ulcer following radiation. Arch Surg 55: 394–399

Haot J (1965) Contribution à l'étude de l'ulcere radiologique de l'estomac. Rev Belg Pathol Med Exp 31: 203–225

Hauer Jensen M, Sauer T, Devik F, Vygaard K (1983) Late changes following single dose roentgen irradiation of rat small intestine. Acta Radiol [Oncol] 22: 299–304

Hauer Jensen M, Sauer T, Berstad T, Nygaard K (1985) Influence of pancreatic secretion on late radiation enteropathy in the rat. Acta Radiol [Oncol] 24: 555–560

Hauer Jensen M, Sauer T, Sletten K, Reitan JB, Nygaard K (1986) Value of hydroxyproline measurements in the assessment of late radiation enteropathy. Acta Radiol [Oncol] 25: 137–142

Hauer Jensen M, Poulakos L, Osborne JW (1988) Effects of accelerated fractionation on radiation injury of the small intestine: a new rat model. Int J Radial Oncol Biol Phys 14: 1205–1212

Hebard DW, Jackson KL, Christensen GM (1980) The chronological development of late radiation injury in the liver of the rat. Radiat Res 81: 441–454

Heinkel K, Bergenthal B (1963) Blutamylase- und -lipasegehalt bei Röntgenbestrahlung der Pankreasgegend. Strahlentherapie 121: 154–159

Hendry JH, Potten CS, Roberts NP (1983) The gastrointestinal syndrome and mucosal clonogenic cells; relationships between target cell sensitivities, LD$_{50}$ and cell survival and their modification by antobiotics. Radiat Res 96: 100–112

Heyde W, Schmermund HJ (1953) Zur Vermeidung von Darmschäden bei der intravaginalen Bestrahlung des Kollumkarzinoms. Geburtshilfe Frauenheilkd 13: 392–401

Hornsey S, Alper T (1966) Unexpected dose-rate effect in the killing of mice by radiation. Nature 210: 212–213

Hubmann FH (1981) Effect of x-irradiation on the rectum of the rat. Br J Radiol 54: 250–254

Hubmann FH (1982) Proctitis cystica profunda and radiation fibrosis in the rectum of the female Wistar rat after x-irradiation: a histopathological study. J Pathol 138: 193–204

Huczkowski J, Trott K-R (1984) Dose fractionation effects in low dose rate irradiation of jejunal crypt stem cells. Int J Radiat Biol 46: 293–298

Huczkowski J, Trott K-R (1987) Jejunal crypt stem-cell survival after fractionated gamma irradiation performed at different dose rates. Int J Radiat Biol 51: 131–137

Hueper WC, Carvajal-Forero J de (1944) The effect of repeated irradiation of the gastric region with small doses of roentgen rays upon the stomach and blood of dogs. AJR 52: 529–534

Ingold JA, Reed GB, Kaplan HS, Bagshaw MA (1965) Radiation hepatitis. AJR 93: 200–208

International Commission on Radiation Units and Measurements (ICRU) (1985) Dose and volume specification for reporting intracavitary therapy in gynecology. ICRU report 38, Bethesda, Md.

Ito H, Meistrich ML, Barkley HT, Thames HD, Milas L (1986) Protection of acute and late radiation damage of the gastrointestinal tract by WR-2721. Int J Radiat Oncol Biol Phys 12: 211–219

Jeffrey RB, Moss AA, Quivey JM, Fedevle MP, Wara WM (1980) CT of radiation-induced hepatic injury. AJR 135: 445–448

Jirtle RL, Michalopoulos G, McLain JR, Crowley J (1981) Transplantation system for determining the clonogenic survival of parenchymal hepatocytes exposed to ionizing radiation. Cancer Res 41: 3512–3518

Johnson PM, Grossman FM, Atkins HL (1967) Radiation induced hepatic injury, its detection by scintillation scanning. AJR 99: 453–462

Kaplan HS, Bagshaw MA (1968) Radiation hepatitis: possible prevention by combined isotopic and internal radiation therapy. Radiology 91: 1214–1220

Kelly LS, Hirsch JD, Beach G, Palmer W (1956) The time function of P^{32} incorporation into DNA of regenerating liver; the effect of irradiation. Cancer Res 16: 117–121

Kinzie J, Studer RK, Perez B, Potchen EJ (1972) Noncytokinetic radiation injury: anticoagulants as radioprotective agents in experimental radiation hepatitis. Science 175: 1481–1483

Kiszel Z, Spiethoff A, Trott K-R (1984) Large bowel stenosis in rats after fractionated local irradiation. Radiother Oncol 2: 247–254

Kiszel Z, Spiethoff A, Trott K-R (1985) Chronische Strahlenfolgen am Enddarm der Ratte nach intracavitärer Bestrahlung mit unterschiedlicher Dosisleistung. Strahlentherapie 161: 348–353

Kolb JJ, Rieder I, Bodenberger B, Netzel B, Schaffer E, Kolb H, Thierfelder S (1979) Dose rate and dose fractionation studies in total body irradiation of dogs. Pathol Biol (Paris) 27: 370–372

Kolbenstvedt A, Kjolseth I (1980) Postirradiation changes of the liver demonstrated by computer tomography. Radiology 135: 391–196

Konermann G, Petersen KG, Slanina J, Blachnitzky EO, Kraft C (1979) Zur Funktion und Histologie der Langerhanschen Inseln der Maus nach fraktionierter Telekobaltbestrahlung mit Tumordosen. Strahlentherapie 155: 856–863

Koslowski L, Neugebauer W (1984) Chirurgie der Strahlenfolgen am Magen–Darm-Trakt. In: Lemperle, G, Koslowski L (eds) Chirurgie der Strahlenfolgen. Urban & Schwarzenberg, Munich

Kottmeier HL, Gray MJ (1961) Rectal and bladder injuries in relation to radiation dosage in carcinoma of the cervix. A 5 year follow-up. Am J Obstet Gynecol 82: 74–82

Kovacs L (1976) Histologische Untersuchungen von Pankreasveränderungen verursacht durch experimentelle, fraktionierte, lokale Bestrahlung. Strahlentherapie 152: 455–468

Kun LE, Camitta BM (1978) Hepatopathy following irradiation and adriamycin. Cancer 42: 81–84

Kurohara SS, Swensson NL, Usselmann JA. George FW (1967) Response and recovery of liver to radiation as demonstrated by photoscan. Radiology 89: 129–135

Layer P, Demol P, Hotz J, Goebell H (1986) Gastroparesis after radiation. Successful treatment with carbachol. Dig Dis Sci 31: 1377–1380

Lenk R (1926) Die Röntgentherapie der Erkrankungen des Verdauungstraktes. In: Meyer H (ed) Lehrbuch der Strahlentherapie, vol III. Urban & Schwarzenberg, Berlin pp 451–486

Lewin K. Millis RR (1973) Human radiation hepatitis. A morphologic study with emphasis on the late changes. Arch Pathol 96: 21–26

Lightdale CJ, Wasser J, Coleman M, Brower M, Tefft M, Pasmantier M (1979) Anticoagulation and high dose liver irradiation: a preliminary report. Cancer 43: 174–181

Magyar E, Talerman A, Treurniet E (1980) Radiation pancreatitis: a necropsy study. Acta Med Acad Scient Hung 37: 183–190

Marciàl VA, Santiago EA, Lanaro EA et al. (1977) Radiation-induced liver damage. In: Radiobiological research and radiotherapy, vol II. International Atomic Agency, Wien

Matsuzawa T, Wilson R (1965) The intestinal mucosa of germfree mice after whole body x-irradiation with 3 kiloroentgens. Radiat Res 25: 15–24

Martin SG, Murray JC, Voinovic B, Orchard RA (1988) A new method for the investigation of radiation-induced colorectal damage in the mouse (abstr). Br J Radiol 61: 879–880

McBride WH, Mason KA, Davis C, Withers HR (1988) Adhesion formation in experimental chronic radiation enteropathy. Int J Radiat Oncol Biol Phys 16: 737–743

McDonald GB, Sharma P, Matthews DE, Shulman HH, Thomas FD (1984) Veno-occlusive disease of the liver after bone marrow transplantation: diagnosis, incidence and predisposing factors. Hepatology 4: 116–122

Meerwaldt JH (1984) Post-irradiation diarrhea. A study of its mechanism after pelvic irradiation. Diss MD, University of Rotterdam

Michel C, Calvo W, Raghavachar A, Fliedner TM (1986) Histochemical studies on the effects of lethal total body x-irradiation on the pancreas of dogs rescued by autologous bone marrow transplantation. Cell Mol Biol 32: 519–526

Mitchell CJ, Simpson FG, Davision AM, Losowsky MS (1979) Radiation pancreatitis: a clinical entity? Digestion 19: 131–136

Morgenstern L, Thompson R, Friedman NB (1977) The modern enigma of radiation enteropathy: sequelae and solutions. Am J Surg 134: 166–172

Mulholland MW, Levitt SH, Song CW, Potish RA, Delaney JP (1984) The role of luminal contents in radiation enteritis. Cancer 54: 2396–2402

Neumeister K (1973) Die Strahlenreaktionen des Gastrointestinaltraktes. Thieme, Leipzig

Ogata K, Hizawa K, Yoshida M, Kitamuro T, Akagi G, Kagawa K, Fukuda F (1963) Hepatic injury following irradiation – a morphologic study. Tokushima J Exp Med 9: 240–251

Orndorff BH, Farrell JI, Ivy AC (1926) Studies on the effect of roentgen rays on glandular activity. V. The effect of roentgen rays on external pancreatic secretion. AJR 16: 349–355

Palmer WL, Templeton F (1939) The effect of radiation therapy on gastric secretion. JAMA 112: 1420–1434

Peck JW, Gibbs FA (1987) Assay of premorbid murine jejunal fibrosis based on mechanical changes after x-irradiation and hyperthermia. Radiat Res 112: 525–543

Perez CA, Korba A, Zivnuska F. Prasad S, Katzenstein AL (1978) ^{60}Co moving strip technique in the management of carcinoma of ovary: analysis of tumor control and morbidity. Int J Radiat Oncol Biol Phys 4: 379–388

Phillips TL (1980) Tissue toxicity of radiation-drug interactions. In: Sokol GH, Maickel RP (eds) Radiation-drug interactions in the treatment of cancer. Wiley, New York

Phillips TL, Fu KK (1976) Quantification of combined radiation therapy and chemotherapy effects on critical normal tissues. Cancer 37: 1186–1200

Pieroni PL, Rudick J, Adler M, Nacchiero M, Ryback BJ, Perlberg HJ, Dreiling DA (1976) Effect of irradiation on the canine exocrine pancreas. Ann Surg 184: 610–614

Powel-Smith C (1965) Factors influencing the incidence of radiation injury in cancer of the cervix. J Assoc Canad Radiol 16: 132–137

Quastler H (1956) The nature of intestinal radiation death. Radiat Res 4: 303–320

Rauch RF, Stenstrom KW (1952) Effects of x-radiation on pancreatic function in dogs. Gastroenterology 20: 595–603

Reed GS, Cox AJ (1966) The human liver alter radiation injury. Am J Pathol 48: 597–611

Reeves RJ, Cavanaugh PJ, Sharpe KW, Thorne WA, Winkler C, Sanders AP (1959) Fat absorption from human gastrointestinal tract in patients undergoing radiation therapy. Radiology 73: 398–401

Reeves RJ, Sanders AP, Isley JK, Sharpe KW, Baylin GJ (1965) Fat absorption studies and small bowel x-ray studies in patients undergoing Co^{60} teletherapy and or radium application. AJR 94: 848–851

Reynaud A, Travis EL (1984) Late effects of irradiation in mouse jejunum. Int J Radiat Biol 46: 125–134

Ricketts WE, Palmer WL, Kirner JB, Hamann A (1948) Radiation therapy in peptic ulcer. An analysis of results. Gastroenterology 11: 789–806

Roswit B, Malsky SJ, Reid CB (1972) Radiation tolerance of the gastrointestinal tract. Front Radiat Ther Oncol 6: 160–181

Rübe W, Seegelken K (1974) Dickdarmstenosen nach Bestrahlung von Nierentumoren. Strahlentherapie 147: 63–68

Rubin P, Casarett GW (1968) Clinical radiation pathology. Saunders, Philadelphia

Schacter L, Crum E, Spitzer T, Maksem J, Diwan V, Kolli S (1986) Fatal radiation hepatitis: a case report and review of the literature. Gynecol Oncol 24: 373–380

Schenken LL, Burholt DR, Hagemann RF, Lesher S (1976) The modification of gastrointestinal tolerance and responses to abdominal irradiation by chemotherapeutic agents. Radiology 120: 417–420

Senn A, Lundsgaard-Hansen P (1956) Diagnose und Therapie der Bestrahlungsschäden am Gastrointestinaltrakt. Schweiz Med Wochenschr 86: 1015–1020

Singh K (1978) Two regimes with the same TDF but differing morbidity used in the treatment of stage III carcinoma of the cervix. Br J Radiol 51: 357–362

Sonoda T, Reynolds RD, Galey WT (1983) The computerized tomographic appearance of patchy liver congestion due to irradiation. Comput Radiol 7: 135–140

Sparenberg A, Hamm B, Ernst H (1988) Postaktinische fokale Leberlaesionen. Strahlentherapie Onkol 164: 289–291

Steglich R (1988) Untersuchungen der Serumlipasen als Indikator einer radiogenen Pankreasaffektion. Diss MD, Med. Akad. Dresden

Swift MN, Taketa ST, Bond VP (1955) Delayed gastric emptying in rats after whole and partial body irradiation. Am J Physiol 182: 479

Takahashi T (1964) A study on preoperative and postoperative telecobalt therapy in gastric cancer. Three year results of Co[60] irradiation following palliative gastric resection. Nippon Acta Radiol 24: 129–132

Tefft M, Mitus A, Das L, Vawter GF, Filler RM (1970) Irradiation of the liver in children: review of experience in the acute and chronic phases, and in the intact normal and partially resected. AJR 108: 365–385

Tekieh S, Trott K-R (1988) Direct observation of the progression of acute radiation injury to chronic radiation ulcer in the rectum of rats (abstr). Br J Radiol 61: 880

Terry NHA, Denekamp J (1984) RBE values and repair characteristics for colorectal injury after 137 Cs gammarays and neutron irradiation. 2. Fractionation up to 10 doses. Br J Radiol 57: 617–629

Terry NHA, Denekamp J, Maughan RL (1983) RBE values for colorectal injury after caesium 137 gamma-ray and neutron irradiation. 1. Single doses. Br J Radiol 56: 257–265

Thomson ABR, Keelan M, Cheeseman Cl, Walker K (1986) Fractionated low doses of abdominal irradiation alters jejunal uptake of nutrients. Int J Radiat Oncol Biol Phys 12: 917–925

Trott K-R (1986) Radiation-chemotherapy interactions. Int J Radiat Oncol Biol Phys 12: 1409–1413

Trott K-R, Herrmann T (1988) Radiation injury to abdominal organs. Br J Radiol [Suppl] 22: 30–32

Trott K-R, Breiter N, Spiethoff A (1986) Experimental studies on the pathogenesis of the chronic radiation ulcer of the large bowel in rats. Int J Radiat Oncol Biol Phys 12: 1637–1643

Unger EC Lee JKT Weyman PU (1987) CT and MR imaging of radiation hepatitis. J Comput Assist Tomogr 11: 264–268

Usselman JA (1965) Liver scanning in the assessment of liver damage from therapeutic external irradiation. J Nuel Med 6: 353–364

Uzel R. Okkan S, Tore G, Koca S (1988) Results and complications of HDR intracavitary radiotherapy compared with conventional dose rate in carcinoma of the cervix. In: Vahrson H, Rauthe G (eds) High dose rate afterloading in the treatment of cancer of the uterus, breast and rectum. Urban & Schwarzenberg, Munich

Varma GF, Smith AN, Busuttil, A (1985) Correlation of clinical and manometric abnormalities of rectal function following chronic radiation injury. Brit J Surg 72: 875–878

Volk BW, Wellmann KF, Lewitan A (1966) The effect of irradiation on the fine struture and enzymes of the dog pancreas. I. Short term studies. Am J Pathol 48: 721–753

von der Maase H (1984) Interactions of radiation and 5-fluorouracil, cyclophosphamide or methotrexate in intestinal crypt cells. Int J Radiat Oncol Biol Phys 10: 77–86

von der Maase H (1986) Interaction of radiation and adriamycin, bleomycin, mitomycin C or cis-diamminedichloroplatinum in intestinal crypt cells. Br J Cancer 49: 779–786

Warren SH, Friedman NP (1942) Pathology and pathological diagnosis of radiation lesions in the gastrointestinal tract. Am J Pathol 18: 499

Wellmann KF, Volk BW, Lewitan A (1966) The effect of irradiation on the fine structure and enzyme content of the dog pancreas. II. Long term studies. Lab Invest 15: 1007–1023

Wharton JT, Delclos L, Gallager S, Smith JP (1973) Radiation hepatitis induced by abdominal irradiation with the cobalt-60 moving strip technique AJR 117: 73–80

Wiernik G, Plant M (1970) Radiation effects on the human intestinal mucosa. Curr Top Radiat Res 7: 327–368

Wiley HM, Sugarbaker ED (1950) Roentgenotherapeutic changes in the small intestine. Surgical aspects. Cancer 3: 629–640

Withers HR, Elkind MM (1968) Radiosensitivity and fractionation response of crypt cells of mouse jejunum. Radiat Res 38: 598–613

Withers HR, Elkind MM (1970) Microcolony survival assay for cells of mouse intestinal mucosa exposed to radiation. Int J Radiat Biol 17: 261–267

Withers HR, Mason KA (1974) The kinetics recovery in irradiated colonic mucosa of the mouse. Cancer 34: 896–904

Zollinger HU (1960) Radiohistologie und Radiohistopathologie. In: Roulet F (ed) Strahlung und Wetter. Springer, Berlin Heidelberg New York (Handbuch der Pathologie, vol X/1, p 127)

Zook BC, Bradley FW, Casarett GW, Rogers CC (1983) Pathologic effects of fractionated fast neutrons or photons on the pancreas, pylorus and duodenum of dogs. Int J Radiat Oncol Biol Phys 9: 1493–1504

12 Heart

S. Schultz-Hector

CONTENTS

Most of the available clinical data on late effects of thoracic radiotherapy on the heart refer to pericarditis. However, with treatment techniques which are considered standard today, pericarditis should be a rare event and with increasing cure rates very late effects on cardiac function or on coronary arteries should become more important. But, while pericarditis is a relatively specific symptom that can easily be attributed to irradiation, impaired ventricular function, conduction defects, and coronary artery disease are very unspecific symptoms. They can rarely be attributed to a single cause in the individual patient and can only be investigated in large studies where matched groups of irradiated and unirradiated patients are compared. Therefore, analysis of the published clinical observations will overemphasize the clinical importance of radiation-induced pericarditis in comparison to effects on coronary arteries and myocardium.

12.1 Clinical Features of Radiation-Induced Heart Disease

Radiation-induced heart disease occurs only in a few malignanacies as a late side-effect of treatment. In Table 12.1 a total of 422 cases of radiation-induced heart disease, compiled from all the references mentioned in the following, are analyzed for the primary tumor that was treated. Of these patients, 73% had undergone radiation therapy for mediastinal Hodgkin's disease, where a large portion of the heart receives at least the tumor dose. Because of the high cure rate of Hodgkin's disease and the young age of many of the patients, very late side-effects of therapy are of particular importance in this group of patients. Therefore not only most of the case reports but also most of the clinical studies investigating radiation-induced heart disease refer to mantle treatment for Hodgkin's disease. About 11% of the cases of heart disease occurred following postoperative radiation therapy for breast cancer, and about 15% following radiation therapy for lung cancer; very few cases were reported following other diseases such as oesophageal cancer or seminoma.

COHN, STEWART, and co-workers (COHN et al. 1967; STEWART and FAJARDO 1971a,b) were the first to give a detailed report on the incidence and clinical course of radiation-induced heart disease, their data being based on 318 Hodgkin and 201 breast cancer patients. They found that radiation can damage each of the different layers of the

SUSANNE SCHULTZ-HECTOR Dr. med., Institut für Strahlenbiologie der Gesellschaft für Strahlen- und Umweltforschung mbH, Ingolstädter Landstraße 1, 8042 Neuherberg, FRG.

heart, leading to a wide spectrum of clinical symptoms typical for the affected anatomical structures rather than of radiation induction.

Table 12.1. Cases of radiation-induced heart disease, subdivided according to primary tumor

Malignant disease	No.	%
Hodgkin's disease	307	73
Breast cancer	47	11
Lung cancer	63	15
Others	5	1

12.1.1 Pericardium

Transient, asymptomatic pericardial effusions diagnosed on routine chest x-rays or at echocardiography are the mildest form of pericardial reaction. PIERCE et al. (1969) observed that one-third of asymptomatic pericardial effusions completely clear away within 2–5 months. Large effusions cause symptoms of cardiac tamponade with Kussmaul's sign, pulsus paradoxus, and dyspnea. If effusions do not clear away spontaneously they are sometimes treated successfully by aspiration of pericardial fluid. However, persistent effusions often recur after aspiration or occur as a concomitant symptom of pericardial constriction which cannot be improved by aspiration alone. Therefore pericardectomy or at least pericardial fenestration is often necessary, and it has been suggested that surgery should be carried out early, before the condition of the patient deteriorates and the risk of thoracic surgery increases (KAGAN et al. 1969). Pericardial disease can also present with typical symptoms of acute pericarditis such as acute chest pain, cough, dyspnea, friction rub, and fever. In most instances these subside spontaneously or after treatment with anti-inflammatory agents, but there are some cases where acute pericarditis progresses to chronic pericardial constriction. Constrictive pericarditis with or without pericardial effusions is the most severe, life-threatening form of pericardial disease. It is progressive and often requires surgical treatment. In 6 of 35 cases, pericardectomy or pericardial fenestration did improve but symptoms of constriction were not resolved; five of the patients died from cardiac failure. The clinical courses of 179 patients with pericardial disease, as

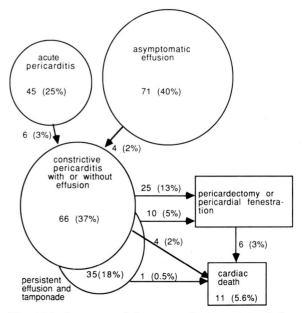

Fig. 12.1. Summary of the types of symptoms and the clinical course of 179 cases of radiation-induced pericarditis. Compiled from all reported references

described in case reports or clinical studies, are summarized in Fig. 12.1 (ALI et al. 1976; BYHARDT et al. 1975; CARMEL and KAPLAN 1976; COHN et al. 1967; COLTART et al. 1985; GHEORGIADE et al. 1986; GOTTDIENER et al. 1983; GREEN et al. 1977; GREENWOOD et al. 1974; HAAS 1969; KURTZ et al. 1981; LAWSON et al. 1972; MACLEOD et al. 1969; MARKS et al. 1973; MASLAND et al. 1968; MILL et al. 1984; MORTON et al. 1973; PIERCE et al. 1969; POHJOLA-SINTONEN et al. 1987; VAN RENTERGHEM et al. 1985; ROWLAND and MURTHY 1986; SCOTT and THOMAS 1978; STEINBERG 1967; THAR and MILLION 1980). In 40% pericardial disease presented first as asymptomatic effusion, and in 25% as acute pericarditis. Thirty-seven percent of the patients developed constrictive pericarditis, which was accompanied by chronic pericardial effusions and tamponade in nearly half of the cases. Constrictive pericarditis required surgical treatment in 18% of the patients. A total of 11 patients (5.6%) were reported to have died with or from severe pericardial disease. The reported observation may not always have been at the final stage of pericardial disease and the number of patients progressing from asymptomatic effusions to symptomatic disease may have been underestimated. If not given in the case reports, the dose to the anterior pericardium was estimated from the midplane dose and the treatment technique. Since many of the patients included in Fig. 12.1 were treated with techniques no longer in use, the average radiation dose to the anterior heart surface of 51 ± 7 Gy is considerably higher than the dose given to the heart with current radiation techniques. Therefore very severe forms of pericardial reaction may be less common today.

The incidence of pericarditis observed in several clinical studies on late effects of mantle treatment for Hodgkin's disease is summarized in Fig. 12.2 (APPLEFELD and WIERNIK 1983; BYHARDT et al. 1975; CARMEL and KAPLAN 1976; COLTART et al. 1985; GOTTDIENER et al. 1983; GREENWOOD et al. 1974; MILL et al. 1984; PIERCE et al. 1969; STEWART and FAJARDO (1971a,b). Since the anterior pericardium receives the highest radiation dose, the incidence of pericarditis in each study is plotted against the dose or dose range at 2–3 cm depth. The risk of pericarditis appears to be very low at doses of less than 35 Gy and rises steeply to more than 50% at around 60 Gy. Figure 12.2 is only a rough estimate of the dose–effect relationship, because the data included are not entirely comparable. In each of the studies the diagnostic criteria defining radiation-induced pericardial disease were different. PIERCE et al. (1969) and BYHARDT et al. (1975) carried out frequent chest x-rays 6–18 and 18–30 months, respectively, after treatment, recording radiological evidence of pericardial effusion irrespective of clinical symptoms. STEWART et al. (1971), CARMEL et al. (1976), COLTART et al. (1985), MILL et al. (1984), and GREENWOOD et al. (1974) retrospectively reviewed medical records for diagnosis of symptomatic radiation-induced pericarditis. GOTTDIENER et al. (1983) and APPLEFELD and WIERNIK (1983) carried out a retrospective cardiological evaluation, on patients who had received radiation therapy at a wide range of latency times of 2.5–25 years previously. Thus the incidences quoted in Fig. 12.2 refer not only to different clinical symptoms but also to different time periods after radiation.

The tumor doses were around 39–40 Gy in all studies. The dose distribution across the thorax, however, was very variable, depending on the quality of radiation, the SSD, and the relative weighting of anterior and posterior fields. Even assuming optimal treatment conditions (photons of nominal energy 10 MeV, 150 cm SSD), the dose to the anterior heart surface in a very thin patient with a chest of an anterior-posterior separation of 14 cm and the anterior pericardium located at about 2 cm depth would be nearly 10% lower than

in a patient with a chest diameter of 30 cm and the anterior pericardium at about 4 cm depth. In view of the steep dose–response curve for the risk of pericarditis shown in Fig. 12.2, such variations may still result in a significant risk of pericarditis in individual patients.

With echocardiography a much more sensitive method for the detection of asymptomatic pericardial disease has become available. Small pericardial fluid volumes down to the physiological range of 16–30 ml can be recorded (HOROWITZ et al. 1974), whereas in the chest x-ray significant enlargement of the heart shadow can be discovered only when at least 250–500 ml have accumulated. Thus IKÄHEIMO et al. (1985) detected by echocardiography small pericardial effusions in 33% of a group of breast cancer patients examined 6 months after postoperative radiation therapy, although no changes were observed in the chest radiographs. Similarly, MORGAN et al. (1985) reported a small pericardial effusion in 2 of 25 Hodgkin patients with a normal cardiac silhouette in the chest radiographs. Moreover the pericardial diameter can be determined precisely by echocardiography. This technique was used in a retrospective study and a high incidence of pericardial thickening (42.9%) was observed at a median of 7.5 years after radiotherapy (GREEN et al. 1987). A relatively wide range of radiation doses (22–44 Gy) to the anterior pericardium had been given. GREEN et al. (1987) found that the incidence of pericardial thickening was lower after latency times of less than 72 months than after longer latency times, suggesting a progression with post-irradiation time. However, clinical symptoms or other echocardiographic findings of constriction, such as reduced ventricular dimensions, were not present. Although the clinical significance of such minimal pericardial disease is not known, it is remindful of the fact that the incidences given in Fig. 12.2 refer to rather gross abnormalities and that asymptomatic changes that may possibly aggravate cardiac diseases of other causes are much more frequent.

12.1.2 Myocardium

As long ago as 1960 CATTERALL and EVANS described a high incidence of T wave changes in the ECG (mainly flattening or inversion of the

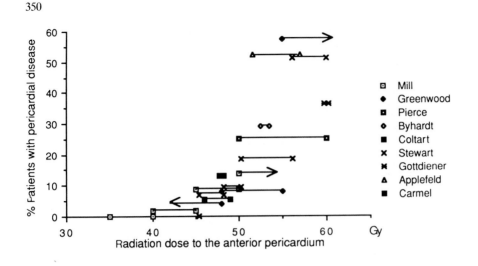

Fig. 12.2. Incidence of pericarditis as a function of total radiation dose to the anterior pericardium in patients with Hodgkin's disease

wave) within 4 months after conclusion of thoracic radiation therapy. The changes lasted for 9 months and were completely resolved by 1 year after treatment. This finding was confirmed in several studies (Biller et al. 1979; Larsson et al. 1976; Heider et al. 1982; Fröhlich et al. 1984) in which patients were examined during or shortly after thoracic radiation therapy. A variety of ECG abnormalities were observed, but T wave changes were the only feature present in all of these studies. Strender et al. (1986) showed in a 10-year follow-up study that early T wave changes at 6 months posttreatment are not correlated with any later ECG changes. Sinus tachycardia was observed by Biller et al. (1979) immediately after postoperative radiotherapy for breast cancer as well as by Sapiro et al. (1978) following radiotherapy for esophageal cancer. Sapiro et al. (1978) found that tachycardia resolved immediately after conclusion of treatment with less than 40 Gy, but persisted for 3–7 months when more than 40 Gy had been delivered to part of the heart. In conclusion, early functional changes may be caused by radiation therapy to the heart, but their pathogenetic significance for later symptomatic heart disease is not evident.

In a number of case reports patients with severe conduction defects, such as right or left bundle branch blocks or atrioventricular (AV) blocks, have been described. In 13 patients the clinical history and the details of radiation therapy have been reported (Ali et al. 1976; Cohen et al. 1981;

Kereiakes et al. 1983; Pohjola-Sintonen et al. 1987; Rubin et al. 1973; Töttermann et al. 1983; Tzivoni et al. 1977; Velebit et al 1986). Eleven were treated for Hodgkin's disease and two for lung cancer, receiving doses of 29 to 67 Gy (median 41 Gy) to the mediastinum. Conduction defects developed after a latency time of 6–23 years. At that time the patients were between 12 and 63 years old. Ten patients were younger than 35 years and had no other disease that could account for conduction defects. Right bundle branch blocks were most frequent and were observed in eight patients. Six patients presented with AV blocks from grade I to complete AV blocks, and one patient presented with a bifascicular block. In seven patients conduction defects were accompanied by pericardial effusions. The predominance of right bundle branch blocks may be due to a higher radiation dose in that area. The study of Pohjola-Sintonen et al. (1987) is the only one in which conduction defects were described as a frequent and important finding after mediastinal irradiation. They carried out an extensive cardiological evaluation of 28 patients who had received mantle field treatment for Hodgkin's disease 5–12 years previously and found conduction defects in four (14%) patients. In nine patients radiotherapy was given 10 years or more before examination, which is a much longer follow-up time than in most other clinical studies.

12.1.3 Changes in Ventricular Function

With radionuclide angiography, ventricular function can be assessed noninvasively in asymptomatic patients. Gottdiener et al. (1983) evaluated 25 patients at 5–15 years after radiation therapy and found a decrease in left ventricular dimension in 50% and a decreased ventricular ejection fraction in 33% of them. However, high radiation doses of about 40 Gy to the posterior and 60 Gy to the anterior heart surface had been given, and 16% of the patients suffered from clinical symptoms of pericarditis or cardiac failure. APPLEFELD and WIERNIK (1983) examined patients irradiated with a similar radiation dose and technique at 3–14 years after treatment. They observed severe pericardial reaction (23% constrictive pericarditis) but reported a reduced left ventricular ejection fraction in only 17 patients. However, their technique of radionuclide angiography and exercise routine as well as their definition of normal values may have been different from that in GOTTDIENER et al.'s study. Cardiac catheterization, revealing an inappropriate increase in right heart diastolic pressure during fluid challenge in 29% of patients, indicates a higher incidence of reduction in ventricular function.

GOMEZ et al. (1983) and MORGAN et al. (1985) detected a significant impairment of cardiac function in Hodgkin patients who had not experienced cardiac symptoms at any time during an observation period of 2.5–20 years after mantle field irradiation. Patients had received 30–36 Gy to the midheart with little dose variation across the heart.

The results of functional studies are summarized in Fig. 12.3. The incidence of a reduced left ventricular ejection fraction is plotted as a function of the approximate radiation dose or dose range to the heart. The dose variation across the heart in GOTTDIENER et al.'s (1983) and APPLEFELD

and WIERNIK's (1983) study was taken into account by quoting the dose range from the posterior to the anterior heart surface. From APPLEFELD and WIERNIK's (1983) data the incidence of abnormal hemodynamic response to fluid challenge was included. Although neither the measurement procedures nor the definition of abnormality were exactly the same in different studies, Fig. 12.3 suggests a correlation between the incidence of reduced cardiac function and radiation dose to the heart.

GREEN et al. (1987) described a group of young patients, aged 11–27 years, with echocardiographically normal or even increased left ventricular ejection fraction at 1.5–15 years after mediastinal irradiation for Hodgkin's disease. This can be explained by the lower radiation dose of 20.3–39.8 Gy given with little variation across the thorax, by the lower sensitivity of echocardiography in comparison to radionuclide angiography, or by the young age of the patients, which precluded interaction of radiation-induced and spontaneous heart disease.

GOMEZ et al. (1983) analyzed ventricular function with respect to the heart volume included in the treatment beam. Patients were divided into three groups according to treatment field size. Separate analysis of these groups showed a decrease in the average left ventricular ejection fraction with increasing field size. It was 50% when 20%–50% of the heart volume was irradiated and was reduced to 43% with more than 60% of the heart volume in the treatment field. The incidence of abnormal left ventricular ejection fractions increased with increasing field size, but this was not statistically significant.

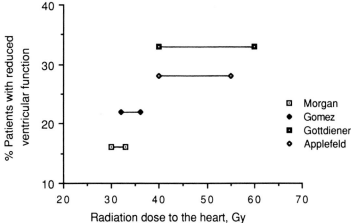

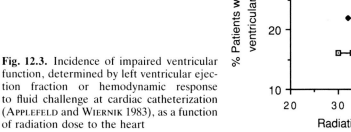

Fig. 12.3. Incidence of impaired ventricular function, determined by left ventricular ejection fraction or hemodynamic response to fluid challenge at cardiac catheterization (APPLEFELD and WIERNIK 1983), as a function of radiation dose to the heart

As in these retrospective studies cardiac evaluation was carried out once in each patient, at arbitrary latency times after treatment, they provide no information about the time course of functional changes. Ikäheimo et al.'s (1985) finding of normal left ventricular ejection fractions at 1 year after treatment for Hodgkin's disease using a mantle field suggests that it starts to decrease between 1 and 3 years after treatment.

12.1.4 Coronary Artery Disease

There are 32 case reports describing young patients (under 42 years) with myocardial infarctions that appeared to be due to previous heart irradiation because few or no other risk factors for coronary artery disease were found (Ali et al. 1976; Alibelli et al. 1978; Angelini et al. 1985; Audebert et al. 1982; Dollinger et al. 1966; Dunsmore et al. 1986; Fournial et al. 1979; Fraumeni et al. 1967; Hamilton and Reed 1978; Huff and Sanders 1972; Iqbal et al. 1977; Leong et al. 1979; McReynolds et al. 1976; Miller et al. 1983; Nigond et al. 1987; Pucheu et al. 1986; Prentice 1965; Rasmussen et al. 1978; Rodgers 1976; Tenet et al. 1986; Töttermann et al. 1983; Tracy et al. 1974; Yahalom et al. 1983). Radiation doses to the mediastinum were between 29 and 50 Gy. In one case (Iqbal et al. 1977) two courses of irradiation of 38 and 68 Gy were given, but angina pectoris started before the second treatment. The average latency until onset of coronary artery disease was 5.5 years; the distribution of latency times is shown in Fig. 12.4. Fifteen patients died from acute myocardial infarction and four from cardiac failure preceded by severe angina pectoris. Six patients survived myocardial infarction; four had a bypass operation. Of seven patients living with angina pectoris at the time of observation, three had undergone bypass surgery. Although each of these cases appears to be unusual, it can only be speculated whether or not coronary artery disease was caused by radiation therapy. If there was any systematic difference between irradiated and other young patients with myocardial infarction, this would suggest a different pathogenesis. Therefore some patient characteristics of these case reports will be compared with the results of two studies investigating myocardial infarction in patients of less than 40 years of age. Uhl and Farrell (1983) described

coronary risk factors and clinical findings, whereas Virmani et al. (1983) carried out an autopsy study in young patients who have died from myocardial infarction.

Uhl and Farrell (1983) observed only one nonirradiated patient without any risk factor out of a total of 160. Comparing patients with myocardial infarcts aged more or less than 40 years, Uhl and Farrell (1983) concluded that a high incidence (61%) of hyperlipidemia was typical for young patients whereas smoking and other risk factors were about equally frequent in young and old patients. In 16 of 32 irradiated patients no coronary risk factors were found. Of 16 irradiated patients who had coronary risk factors, 13 (81%) were smokers and only six (37.5%) had hyperlipidemia. This does not support experimental findings (Gold 1962; Tiamson et al. 1970; Lee et al. 1971) of a synergistic effect of hypercholesterinemia and heart irradiation, but it suggests some difference between myocardial infarctions occurring spontaneously and after radiation. In order to find out whether coronary artery disease after heart irradiation occurs in typical localizations, different from those in nonirradiated patients, angiographic and autopsy results are compared in Table 12.2. Of the 32 irradiated patients only the 16 without any other risk factors were included. One of them had a normal coronary angiogram. In ten (63%) one vessel was severely narrowed or occluded; in four (25%) patients two vessels were affected, and in one, three vessels. Diagnosis was made either by angiography or at autopsy. In the two control studies, the percentage of patients with only one or no vessel narrowed was much lower (34% and 44% respectively). In Table 12.3 the localization of stenosis in 16 irradiated patients

Table 12.2. Comparison of the number of stenosed coronary arteries in patients with heart irradiation and patients with spontaneous coronary artery disease

No. of stenosed vessels	Irradiated patients; case reports; angiography or autopsy ($n = 16$)	Not irradiated; Uhl and Farrell 1983; angiography ($n = 81$)	Not irradiated; Virmani et al. 1983; autopsy ($n = 48$)
0	6%	11%	0%
1	63%	23%	44%
2	25%	35%	40%
3	6%	31%	16%

Table 12.3. Types and combinations of the four major coronary arteries narrowed in irradiated and unirradiated patients

Coronary artery involved	Irradiated; case reports ($n = 16$)	Not irradiated; VIRMANI et al. 1983 ($n = 48$)
Left anterior descending	37.5%	35%
Left circumflex	6%	4%
Left main stem	13%	4%
Left anterior descending and left circumflex	6%	6%
Left anterior descending and right main stem	13%	25%

is compared with the autopsy results in unirradiated patients reported by VIRMANI et al. (1983). The two most frequent patterns of stenosis are the left anterior descending coronary artery with 37.5% in irradiated and 35% in nonirradiated patients and a combination of the left anterior descending and the right main stem in 13% and 25% respectively.

In spite of the large number of case reports in which coronary artery disease has been attributed to previous thoracic radiotherapy, these data do not give very strong evidence of the importance of heart irradiation as a cause of coronary artery disease.

Several clinical studies have been carried out to compare the incidence of coronary artery disease in groups of patients with previous mediastinal irradiation and in unirradiated control groups.

BOIVIN and HUTCHISON (1982) analyzed the death certificates of 935 Hodgkin patients with and 277 without mantle irradiation. The ratio of observed incidence of coronary artery disease to expected incidence according to the criteria of the American Heart Association was 2.1:1 in patients with radiotherapy versus 1.5:1 without. This difference was not statistically significant. However, 667 of the study patients had died within 0–4 years after radiation therapy and only 62 were more than 10 years at risk. The results of the following studies suggest that this observation time was too short to observe a significant effect.

ANNEST et al. (1983) found no case of recorded coronary artery disease in 44 Hodgkin patients who survived mediastinal irradiation for less than 10 years, yet five out of 29 (18%) patients who survived longer either died from myocardial infarction or had coronary bypass surgery. According to the criteria of the American Heart Association the expected risk for coronary artery disease in this group was only 4.9%.

In a study on the benefit of postoperative irradiation in breast cancer, HOST et al. (1986) reported lethal myocardial infarction in 10 out of 170 (5.9%) irradiated patients versus 0.5% in the control group. The internal mammary lymph nodes had been irradiated to 50–60 Gy 10–20 years previously.

These very long latency times are confirmed by BLITZER et al.'s study (1987) on postoperative irradiation in breast cancer patients. Death certificates of 916 irradiated patients and 573 control patients were analyzed for cardiac death, presumably mostly due to coronary artery disease (HUTCHISON, oral communication, 1987). At 10 years after treatment the death rate of irradiated patients rose significantly above that in the control group, and at 20 years a death rate excess of 10% after right-sided and 12% after left-sided irradiation was observed.

In summary, heart irradiation appears to be a risk factor for coronary artery disease at 10 years or more after treatment. Case reports provide no evidence that this risk is particularly enhanced by hyperlipidemia. In young irradiated patients there is more often only one artery narrowed than in unirradiated patients. Since coronary artery disease following irradiation does not have any specific clinical characteristics, it is not possible clinically to attribute disease in an individual patient to previous heart irradiation.

12.1.5 Distribution of Latency Times of Clinical Symptoms

Pericarditis, conduction defects, and coronary heart disease each have a different range of latency times after irradiation of the heart. Fig. 12.4 shows the cumulative percentage of patients developing symptoms with postirradiation time. Most of the cases of pericarditis occur within 2 years after radiation therapy, whereas only 50% of cases with coronary heart disease were observed within 5 years and 50% of conduction defects within 11 years. The incidence of coronary heart disease and conduction defects increases nearly linearly with postirradiation time. Figure 12.4 summarizes the data from all case reports on pericarditis quoted in Fig. 12.1. For coronary

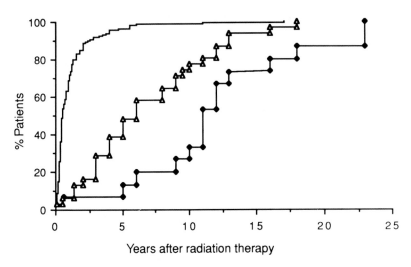

Fig. 12.4. Cumulative latency time until onset of symptoms of radiation-induced pericarditis, coronary heart disease, or conduction defects (•, pericarditis; △, coronary artery disease; ◆, conduction defects). Compiled from all reported references

heart disease and conduction defects the latency times given in the 32 and 13 case reports quoted above are included, assuming that each of these cases was caused by radiation.

12.2 Histopathology

Since radiation-induced heart disease is rarely lethal and since in patients dying from extracardiac causes a histological evaluation of the heart is not routinely done, there are few relevant autopsy reports. Most of those that are available describe patients who received higher radiation doses to the heart than are considered acceptable today. Therefore the following may not represent the exact anatomical correlate of the above-described clinical symptoms.

FAJARDO et al. (1968) gave a detailed description of nine necropsy and seven pericardectomy specimens from patients who had received between 30 and 98 Gy (mean 57 Gy) to the heart at 6–84 months (mean 30 months) before examination. The patients were between 13 and 68 (mean 39) years old. Fourteen of the patients had pericardial effusions either at necropsy or in their clinical history. When the fluid was examined it was a sterile, serosanguinous exudate with many lymphocytes but free of malignant cells. In all instances pericardium and endocardium were thickened up to 0.5 cm. Collagen was replacing adipose tissue and in most cases fibrinous exudate, a large number of fibroblasts, and fibrous adhesions were seen. Proliferating capillaries were

always present, and hemorrhage and hemosiderin deposition were frequently observed. Especially when adhesions between peri- and epicardium were present, mesothelial cells were swollen and prominent. In all nine necropsy cases the myocardium showed areas of diffuse interstitial fibrosis where individual myocardial fibers were surrounded and separated from each other by bands of collagen, as demonstrated in Fig. 12.5. The severity as well as the extent and location of fibrosis varied widely. In FAJARDO et al.'s (1968) study myocardial necrosis was seen only in one case, as the result of a myocardial infarction. This was also the only case in which severe coronary atherosclerosis was observed. Endothelial cell proliferation was found in 6 out of 12 patients in whom large, medium, and small vessels could be examined. However, no systematic evaluation of coronary arteries was carried out.

BROSIUS et al. (1981) studied the hearts of 16 young patients (less than 35 years, mean age 26) who had received mean radiation doses of 56 Gy to the anterior heart and 39 Gy to the posterior heart at 5–144 months (mean 55) before autopsy. In contrast to FAJARDO et al.'s study, ten patients had been treated with chemotherapy, including doxorubicin in three cases. The pericardial and myocardial changes were very similar to FAJARDO et al.'s observations, but in addition BROSIUS et al. found fibrosis and thickening of cardiac valves in 13 of the 16 patients. The four major coronary arteries were examined systematically in each patient. Ten age-matched patients with malignant diseases who had received chemotherapy similar to or more intensive than that in the study patients

Fig. 12.5. Severe interstitial myocardial fibrosis in the heart of a patient 7 years after treatment for Hodgkin's disease, with a radiation dose to the whole heart of 55 Gy. (FAJARDO et al. 1968) Gomori's trichrome stain, ×200 Copyright 1968, American Medical Association

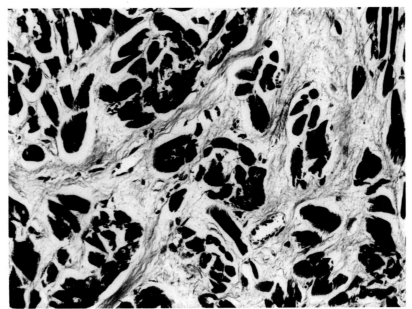

but no thoracic radiotherapy served as a control group. In six patients one or more major coronary arteries (in most cases, three or four) were narrowed by more than 75%. Of a total of 64 coronary arteries from 16 study patients, 16 (25%) were narrowed by more than 75%, in comparison to one narrowed coronary artery out of 40 taken from ten control patients. The narrowing was mainly caused by intimal fibrosis, with some intra- and extracellular lipid or calcific deposits; the internal elastic membrane was often disrupted. These changes were not different from typical atherosclerosis in unirradiated patients. However, a loss of medial smooth muscle cells was noticed in the irradiated group that was only very rarely observed in the control group. Thus BROSIUS et al.'s observations support the clinical studies suggesting an increased coronary risk after heart irradiation. The average latency time between irradiation and examination was 55 months, as compared with 30 months in FAJARDO et al.'s study. The risk of clinically manifest coronary artery disease increases with postirradiation time and significantly exceeds control levels only at 5–10 years after treatment (ANNEST et al. 1983; HOST et al. 1986). Therefore the shorter latency time may explain why vascular changes were rarely found in FAJARDO et al.'s study (1968).

In case reports on histological changes after heart irradiation very similar observations were described (STROOBANDT et al. 1975; SCHNEIDER and EDWARDS 1979; SCULLY et al. 1978; RUBIN et al. 1973; COHEN et al. 1981). Besides interstitial fibrosis, vacuolation and degeneration of myocytes were observed. Coronary arteries were not specially examined, but no gross changes were noted. The patient described by COHEN et al. (1981) had died with a second and intermittent third degree heart block. Severe vacuolar degeneration and necrosis of myocytes as well as fibrosis were found in the approaches of the AV node as the obvious morphological correlate of clinical symptoms.

In several species of laboratory animals heart failure was caused by heart irradiation and studied histologically. In rabbits (FAJARDO and STEWART 1970), rats (LAUK et al. 1985), and dogs (GAVIN and GILLETTE 1982; McCHESNEY et al. 1988b) peri- or epicardial thickening and fibrosis are typical findings that are very similar in all three species. Often they are accompanied by pericardial effusions, and occasionally by fibrous adhesions between epi- and pericardium. In rabbit heart a single dose of 20 Gy resulted in diffuse interstitial fibrosis. Bundles of muscle fibers or individual fibers were separated from each other by collagen and there was probably a loss of myocytes. These changes occurred in patches and were observed at 70–120 days after 20 Gy. Most of the animals had sterile, serosanguinous effusions at the time of sacrifice. In two different rat strains focal myocardial degeneration and necrosis without any significant increase in interstitial connective tissue were

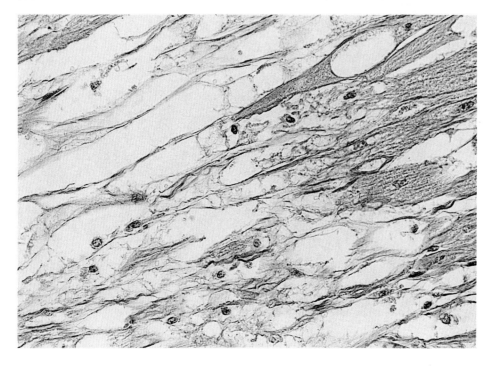

Fig. 12.6. Area of severe myocardial degeneration in a rat heart 30 weeks after 20 Gy, showing that mostly only empty sarcolemmal sheaths are left, while the few remaining muscle fibers show large vacuoles. HE ×300

seen in all animals that were killed because of radiation-induced heart failure. Muscle fibers were more or less severely vacuolated and sometimes only the sarcolemmal sheaths were left (Fig. 12.6). The foci were distributed randomly throughout the myocardium. Vascular damage, such as arterial wall thickening by smooth muscle cell or intima proliferation or thrombi, was mostly found within areas of degeneration. Dogs were examined at 1 year following fractionated irradiation by McCHESNEY et al. (1988b). After 4 × 9 or 4 × 11 Gy there was only very mild focal myocardial degeneration characterized by fiber swelling and changes in staining. Only after 4 × 13 Gy were cytoplasmic vacuolation and replacement fibrosis seen. Occasionally small arteries were narrowed or occluded by intimal thickening. In all dose groups the ventricular weights were below control levels. However, the dogs had not shown any clinical signs of heart disease at the time of sacrifice.

12.3 Pathogenesis and Pathophysiology

In patients, clinical symptoms of radiation-induced heart disease develop over a wide range of latency times. A follow-up study that is carried out over a long enough period to correlate different effects in one group of patients to find out the sequence of pathogenetic events is not practicable. Clinical observations can only be roughly classified according to their time course:

1. T wave changes in the ECG have been recorded within only 6–12 months after radiation only and disappear later. They have not been correlated with more serious late effects and their importance is therefore not known.
2. Effusive pericarditis occurs between 1 and 2 years after irradiation and resolves spontaneously in most cases. Later than 2 years after treatment the risk of developing pericarditis decreases.
3. Clinical symptoms and functional abnormalities involving the myocardium are observed very long after radiotherapy and their incidence increases with time after irradiation. Myocardial injury develops progressively, with an increasing risk of causing clinical symptoms or aggravating other cardiovascular diseases.

Experimental findings can be divided into similar phases:

1. Early changes which occur immediately after treatment and are completely reversible
2. Pericardial disease
3. Late myocardial changes that develop progressively and finally cause heart failure

MAEDA et al. (1980) and NOVI (1969) both described electron microscopic changes in the hearts of rabbits and rats within hours after 3000 and 500 R respectively. In both studies the most conspicuous changes in myocytes were seen in mitochondria. After just 1 h, mitochondria were swollen and vacuolated. This was still the case at 6 months following 3000 R, but resolution occurred within 30 days after 500 R. In addition NOVI (1969) and FAJARDO and STEWART (1971) described a reversible, focal accumulation of glycogen granules in myocytes. Light microscopically FAJARDO and STEWART (1973) saw inflammatory infiltration of all tissue layers ("pancarditis"), which completely resolved within 48 h.

12.3.1 Pericardium

Pericarditis was observed in most animal species studied systematically. In dogs the probability of developing pericardial effusions was highest 3 months after treatment with 4 × 11 or 4 × 13 Gy, and most of the effusions cleared away later (McCHESNEY et al. 1988a). In Wistar rats pericardial and pleural effusions started to form 3–4 months after single doses of 20 Gy or more. The clinical condition of animals that had received 25 Gy or more deteriorated quickly after the development of effusions. Following 20 Gy most of the effusions cleared away and massive pleural effusions only recurred at the time when heart failure developed in the individual animal (LAUK et al. 1985). In contrast, Sprague-Dawley rats did not develop "early" effusive pericarditis. Pleural effusions developed only when clinical heart failure was imminent (LAUK 1986).

12.3.2 Myocardium

The sequence of morphological changes leading to myocardial degeneration is well described and the major steps are quite similar for different species of laboratory animals.

MORGENROTH et al. (1967) were the first to suggest capillary endothelial cells as the primary target for radiation damage in the heart. In an electron microscopic study the sequential changes in endothelial and myocardial cells in the hearts of rats irradiated locally with 3000 R were very carefully described. Endothelial cell swelling was observed 16 days after treatment. At 26 days the capillaries were narrowed by increased endothelial swelling and by cytoplasmic projections into the lumen. By day 44 some capillaries were occluded and myocytes started to show vacuoles. Seventy-two days was the longest observation period in this study. By then vacuolation of myocytes was increased while capillary damage was unchanged. The authors concluded that myocardial degeneration is secondary to radiation damage to endothelial cells. This was later confirmed by FAJARDO and STEWART (1971, 1973) in a similar study in rabbits. Using a light microscope FAJARDO and STEWART (1970) observed that myocardial degeneration and fibrosis developed after 70 days. At the same time the number of capillaries appeared to be reduced. Endothelial cell degeneration had disappeared by 49 days, but the reduction of capillary density was still present at 99 and 134 days (FAJARDO and STEWART 1971).

Morphometric assessment of percentage vascular component in the ventricles gave contradictory results in dogs after single-dose or fractionated irradiation (GAVIN and GILLETTE 1982; GILLETTE et al. 1985; McCHESNEY et al. 1988b). In rats (LAUK 1987), endothelial cells were identified by their alkaline phosphatase activity and the capillary density was found to decrease continually, starting at about 1 month after 20 Gy, whereas myocardial damage is not observed before 70 days. Thus severe rarefaction of the capillary network is present before any other morphological changes or clinical symptoms are observed. In rabbits (FAJARDO and STEWART 1973) and rats (LAUK and TROTT 1990) the ^{3}H-thymidine labeling index of capillary endothelial cells was increased threefold at 20–30 days after 20 Gy, indicating stimulated endothelial proliferation. The normal turnover time of capillary endothelial cells is at least 120 days and probably much longer and is therefore not related to expression of radiation damage in capillaries (LAUK and TROTT 1990). It is not known by what stimulus endothelial proliferation is initiated at 20–30 days after treatment, but it appears to precipitate early endothelial cell loss and capillary

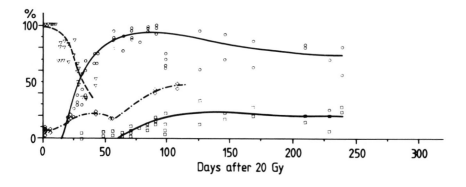

Fig. 12.7. Time course of morphological changes following irradiation with 20 Gy in the rat heart. ○, percentage section area where alkaline phosphatase activity was lost; □, percentage section area of myocardial degeneration and necrosis; ▽, volume density of capillaries plotted as percentage of normal values; ◇, percentage of capillary endothelial cells labeled by ³H-thymidine autoradiography (×10)

rarefaction. In rats the change in microvascular anatomy was accompanied by loss of alkaline phosphatase activity from surviving capillary endothelial cells (LAUK 1987). Enzyme loss occurred simultaneously with rarefaction of capillaries in defined, randomly distributed areas of the myocardium. When areas of myocardial degeneration developed, they were always situated within areas of enzyme loss and were smaller than those areas. The time course of these events following a single dose of 20 Gy is summarized in Fig. 12.7. The extent of both types of capillary damage, i.e., rarefaction and enzyme loss, was dose dependent. After a sublethal radiation dose to the heart of 15 Gy there was structural and functional recovery of the capillary network at 300–400 days. Comparison of two strains of rat (LAUK 1986; YEUNG et al. 1989) showed that the sequence of events was identical in both strains, but that the length of latency periods to histological changes was strain specific and correlated to latency times of clinical heart failure.

The final morphological expression of radiation damage is focal myocardial degeneration, which has been described above. The predominance of fibrosis observed by FAJARDO and STEWART (1970) in rabbits was not seen in rats or dogs. In an electron microscopic study in rabbits that had received 10 or 13 Gy to the heart, KHAN (1973) described myofibrillolysis and collapse of muscle fibers with intact sarcolemmal membranes as early

as 49 days posttreatment, followed by progressive interstitial fibrosis. In whole thorax irradiated mice, total heart hydroxyproline was unchanged for 8 months after 8–16 Gy, while hydroxyproline synthesis was decreasing (MURRAY and PARKINS 1988), but the animals did not show myocardial degeneration by that time either. These two observations both suggest that development of fibrosis is secondary to myocardial degeneration and is highly species dependent.

12.3.3 Functional Changes

Functional changes resulting from myocardial radiation damage show much more interspecies variation than the underlying morphology. The reported experimental findings cannot be condensed into one logical sequence of events.

In dogs treated with fractionated irradiation of 4 × 11 or 4 × 13 Gy, the heart rate at rest was found to increase at 3 months and was still elevated after 1 year, when the experiment was terminated. At that time cardiac function was still compensated, but animals were not followed up any longer. The left ventricular ejection fraction was reduced at 1 and 3 months after treatment, but recovered later. Since heart rate was still increased, it means that cardiac output in these dogs must have been increased from 6 months postirradiation onwards (MCCHESNEY et al. 1988a).

In Sprague-Dawley rats cardiac output was found to decrease continually after single doses of heart irradiation. Following doses of >20 Gy this was significant at 4 months postirradiation, while following 20 Gy it was significant at 6 months postirradiation. The sequential morphological and functional changes were compared in Sprague-Dawley and Wistar rats after single doses of 20 and 17.5 Gy respectively (YEUNG et al. 1989). The doses had been chosen so as to cause identical histological changes in myocardium and capillary network as well as identical survival times in both strains. Ventricular blood flow was kept approximately constant in spite of the capillary rarefaction in both strains. This was achieved in Sprague-Dawley rats by increasing the percentage of cardiac output distributed to the heart while cardiac output was decreasing. In Wistar rats cardiac output increased between 70 and 100 days postirradiation and the percentage of cardiac output distributed to the heart did not change after irradiation. In Wistar rats the number of α- and β-adrenergic receptors has been found to increase above control levels between 50 and 200 days after 15 or 20 Gy (LAUK et al. 1989). Since adrenergic receptors mediate inotropism as well as chronotropism, this is likely to result in an increased cardiac output. Noninvasive examination of cardiac function in non-anaesthetized animals showed that the breathing rate in Wistar rats started to increase at about 75 days after 20 Gy. The recovery time of pre-exercise heart rate was prolonged after a standardized exercise challenge from 120 days onwards after 20 Gy and at 180 days after 15 and 17.5 Gy (GEIST et al. 1990). These changes can be explained by a reduced functional reserve capacity of the myocardium and are compatible with an increased number of adrenergic receptors.

12.3.4 Coronary Arteries

Narrowing or occlusion of coronary artery branches was occasionally seen in dogs after fractionated irradiation with 4 × 11 or 4 × 13 Gy (McCHESNEY et al. 1988b). SENDEROFF et al. (1961) reported that heart irradiation with 13–27 Gy given 4–6 days prior to coronary artery ligation in dogs resulted in smaller areas of myocardial infarction compared with nonirradiated animals at 4 and 6 months after treatment. In rats vascular changes were only seen within areas of severe myocardial degeneration and were considered to be secondary to necrosis (LAUK et al. 1985). However, longer observation times after sublethal doses and in animals presenting with other risk factors might give different results. Experiments in rats (GOLD 1962), rabbits (AMROMIN et al. 1964; TIAMSON et al. 1970), and pigs (LEE

et al. 1971) suggested a synergistic effect of irradiation and high cholesterol diet on coronary arteries.

12.4 Experimental Models

Early experiments started from the hypothesis of pronounced cardiac radioresistance that was first suggested by experiments of SABRAZÈS and RIVIERE (1897) and LEACH and SUGIURA (1941, 1942). Very high single doses of 8000–20 000 R were given to the hearts of dogs and were found to be lethal within 24–28 days (STONE et al. 1964; PHILLIPS et al. 1964).

STEWART et al. (1968) and FAJARDO and STEWART (1970) were the first to investigate dose–effect relationships in animals treated with clinically relevant radiation doses. Rabbits were given local heart irradiation and were killed when they developed severe pericarditis or at 120 or 202 days after treatment. The incidence of effusive pericarditis observed within 80–202 days after irradiation showed a steep dose dependence (Fig. 12.8).

The heart is surrounded by radiosensitive organs such as lung, esophagus, and spinal cord. In order to avoid side-effects, radiation has to be delivered very precisely to the heart, shielding spinal cord and esophagus and as much lung as possible. This is the more important the longer the observation period is and requires individual treatment planning for each animal (GAVIN and GILLETTE 1982; YEUNG and HOPEWELL 1985; LAUK et al. 1985).

12.4.1 Pericardium

GAVIN and GILLETTE (1982) irradiated the heart in dogs and observed pericardial effusions with cardiac tamponade within 180 days in all animals treated with more than 15 Gy (Fig. 12.8). Although experimental designs were different with respect to follow-up periods, Fig. 12.8 shows that the effective dose range is very similar for rabbits and dogs. Own data in rats are included in Fig. 12.8 and fit well into this picture.

360 S. Schultz-Hector

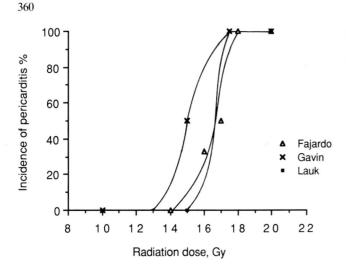

Fig. 12.8. Incidence of pericarditis as a function of radiation dose in rabbits (Fajardo and Stewart 1970; Gavin and Gillette 1982; Lauk et al. 1985)

12.4.2 Myocardium

In contrast to the large number of papers describing radiation-induced myocardial damage, only a few attempts have been made to develop animal models suitable for quantitative comparison of different treatment modalities. A quantal or quantitative endpoint, characterizing severity of disease in the individual, needs to be defined. Pathogenetic studies, however, have shown that radiation-induced heart disease progresses over the whole life span of the individual animal. Modification of radiation dose or treatment schedule may therefore affect not only the maximal severity of disease but also the time course of the sequence of events finally leading to heart failure. If the rate of progression is dose dependent, measurement at different latency times will yield different dose–

effect relationships. However, extension of the follow-up period throughout the animal's lifetime is not always practicable.

In dogs a number of histological and physiological parameters were quantified at constant latency times of 3 and 6 months after different fractionation schedules (Gillette et al. 1985). At 6 months the interstitial connective tissue component was found to be increased with radiation dose up to a certain dose level and to be decreased paradoxically at a still higher radiation dose (Fig. 12.9). Since a qualitatively different effect on connective tissue of low and of high doses of radiation is unlikely, this observation may be explained by a wave-like time course of interstitial reaction. In a later experiment by the same group (McChesney et al. 1988b) a similar time course of an increase followed by a return to normal values

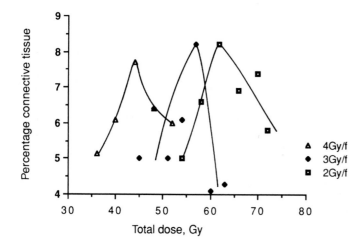

Fig. 12.9. Variation in percentage of connective tissue in the right and left ventricles 6 months after irradiation, according to total irradiation dose. Variable numbers of 2 Gy, 3 Gy, and 4 Gy fractions were given. (After Gillette et al. 1985)

Fig. 12.10. Mean survival times and standard errors after single dose and fractionated irradiation in Wistar rats (after LAUK et al. 1987)

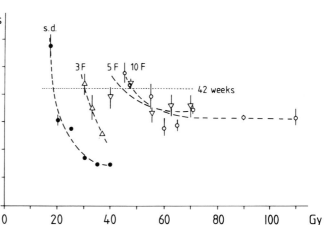

was found for ventricular weights; the increase was interpreted as being due to early, reversible interstitial edema and might well be related to growth of connective tissue. This example shows that knowledge of the underlying time course of parameters may be important for interpretation of quantitative data. In the study by GILLETTE et al. (1985) the diastolic thickness of the posterior left ventricular wall was determined by echocardiography at 3 and 6 months following irradiation. It was found to increase with radiation dose, but the dose–effect relationships, i.e., the α/β ratios, determined for the two time points differed from each other. Thus there is experimental evidence for dose dependence of the time course and progression rate of radiation-induced changes in the heart. For a quantitative comparison of different treatment schedules or modalities, time must consequently be taken into account.

In rat experiments the animals were therefore observed until development of clinical signs of heart failure. In Wistar rats heart failure is accompanied by effusive pericarditis after higher radiation doses, but after 20 and 17.5 Gy pericardial effusions were transient and the animals developed congestive heart failure mainly due to myocardial radiation damage. Following single-dose as well as fractionated irradiation, mean latency times until development of congestive heart failure decreased with increasing radiation dose for a certain dose range. When radiation doses were increased further, survival times reached a minimal plateau (Fig. 12.10). This minimal survival time was lower for single doses than for fractionated irradiation. Pathological and histological findings suggested that early deaths

after high single doses are due to acute pericarditis, whereas deaths in dose-dependent regions of survival time curves are due to radiation-induced myocardial failure. Therefore a survival time of 42 weeks was chosen as isoeffect for comparison.

The disadvantage of this approach is that deaths at different times may be due to different types of damage and may therefore not be comparable. For comparison of treatment modalities that necessarily involve different pathogenetic mechanisms such as chemotherapy and irradiation, assessment of latency times alone would not be a suitable experimental design.

In conclusion, the quality of damage as well as its time course has to be determined for a biologically meaningful quantitative comparison of different treatments. Attempts to quantify one variable alone are not satisfactory experimental models for radiation-induced heart disease. On the other hand any quantitative comparison of treatment groups cannot easily take two variables into account.

12.5 Fractionation Response of Radiation-Induced Heart Disease

As shown in Fig. 12.2, a wide range of incidences of pericarditis has been reported for patients receiving between 50 and 60 Gy to the anterior heart surface. For studies where enough information on radiation techniques was given, the doses per fraction were calculated or estimated. In most studies only one port was treated per day. The dose per fraction to the anterior heart surface is

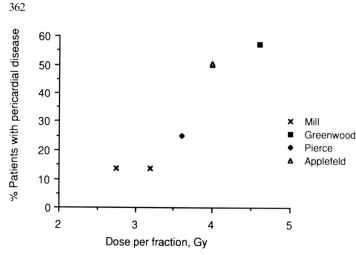

Fig. 12.11. Variation of incidence of pericarditis with dose per fraction to the anterior heart surface through the anterior treatment port. Total doses at 2 cm depth were 50–60 Gy

much higher through the anterior than through the posterior field. Therefore the incidence of pericarditis is plotted in Fig. 12.11 against the dose per fraction to the anterior heart surface which was delivered through the anterior field. The incidence of pericarditis appears to increase with the dose per fraction for similar total doses to the anterior pericardium. This is confirmed in a study by COSSET et al. (1988). They reported an increase in the incidence of pericarditis from 0% to 9% after the dose per fraction to the thorax midplane was increased from 2.5 to 3 Gy while all other treatment parameters were kept constant. The total tumor dose was 39–41 Gy, and the total dose to the anterior heart surface can be estimated as 43–44 Gy. Comparison with the data in Fig. 12.2 shows 9% to be an unusually high incidence of pericarditis for this range of total doses, which can only be explained by the high dose per fraction. In the two treatment groups doses per fraction to the anterior heart surface through the anterior field were approximately 3 and 4 Gy respectively. MARKS et al. (1973) reported on a group of 95 patients, 28 of whom received tumor doses of 45–50 Gy, and found not a single case of pericarditis. The total dose to the anterior heart surface in this subgroup was 49–55 Gy. For this dose range incidences of pericarditis of 10%–29% have been reported by other authors (Fig. 12.2). Yet MARKS et al. (1973) had treated both the anterior and the posterior field daily with 1.5–2 Gy to the thorax midplane. Thus the highest possible dose per fraction to the anterior heart surface in their study was only 2.2 Gy. Assuming α/β ratios of either 1 or 3 Gy, total doses to the anterior heart surface were calculated to be equivalent to a treatment giving 2 Gy per fraction

of megavoltage irradiation to the midthorax through equally weighted anterior and posterior fields. In Fig. 12.12 the incidence of pericarditis is plotted against the corrected total doses and compared with actual observations of pericarditis after radiotherapy given at 2 Gy per fraction to the pericardium. The observed dose–effect curve lies between the calculated curves for patients treated with different doses per fraction, assuming an α/β ratio of 1 or 3 Gy.

Thus there is consistent clinical evidence that the dose per fraction to the heart has a considerable impact on the risk of radiation-induced heart disease, and particularly pericarditis. For myocardial damage this is further confirmed by experimental studies. The experimental models used for these studies (GILLETTE et al. 1985; LAUK et al. 1987) have been discussed above. GILLETTE et al. (1985) measured the severity of histological or echocardiographic changes at arbitrarily defined latency times after fractionated irradiation. LAUK et al. (1987) chose the average latency time until development of symptoms of heart failure as a parameter. In both experiments a marked sparing effect of fractionation was found, yielding α/β ratios between 1 and 5 Gy.

12.6 Volume Effect

Following radiotherapy to the chest wall for breast cancer the incidence of pericarditis is lower than in Hodgkin patients, although radiation doses to tumor and heart are higher. STEWART and FAJARDO (1971 a + b) observed pericardial disease in 4% of breast cancer patients versus 6.8% of Hodgkin

Fig. 12.12. Incidence of pericarditis with corrected and uncorrected total doses. *a* and *c*: Corrected total doses equivalent to therapy with megavoltage giving 2 Gy per fraction to the thorax midplane, treating one field per day and assuming an α/β ratio of 1 Gy (*a*) or 3 Gy (*c*) respectively. *b*: Uncorrected total radiation dose to the anterior heart surface given in 2 Gy fractions to the thorax midplane (*circled symbols*)

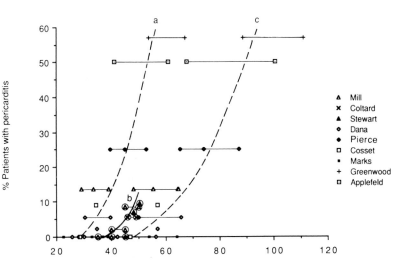

Corrected total dose to anterior pericardium

Fig. 12.13. Incidence of pericarditis or of cardiac death as a function of the heart volume irradiated. Total radiation dose to the thorax midplane was 40–45 Gy (Mill et al. 1984; Carmel and Kaplan 1976; Blitzer et al. 1987), except in breast cancer patients treated by Stewart and Fajardo (1971), who received 50–60 Gy to the tumor. In Blitzer et al.'s study (1987) the incidences given represent "excess cardiac death"

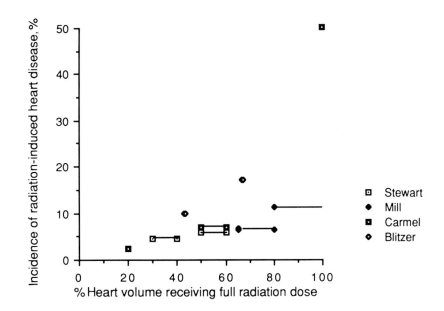

patients, while tumor radiation doses ranged from 50 to 60 Gy and 40 to 50 Gy respectively. Since treatment fields for breast cancer include only 30%–40% of the heart volume compared with 50%–60% for Hodgkin's disease, this observation suggests a correlation of the irradiated heart volume and the incidence of pericarditis. This was confirmed by Mill et al. (1984) and Carmel and Kaplan (1976), who analyzed the incidence of pericarditis separately for different field sizes. Carmel and Kaplan (1976) reviewed the medical records of 377 Hodgkin patients treated in Stanford to a total midthorax dose of 40 Gy. In 14 patients the whole pericardium was irradiated with more than 30 Gy, in 119 patients the lateral

pericardium was shielded by lung blocks, and in 79 patients a subcarinal block was added after 25–30 Gy. The incidence of pericarditis in these three groups was 50%, 7%, and 2.5% respectively. In Fig. 12.13 the incidence of pericarditis is plotted against the fraction of heart volume included in the treatment beam. Blitzer et al. (1987) calculated the increased risk of cardiac death for patients receiving radiation therapy for breast cancer in comparison to patients treated by surgery and chemotherapy alone. Comparing patients with right- and left-sided irradiation, they found a significant difference in the risk of cardiac death. Although the authors did not specify the type of heart disease, the data are included in Fig. 12.13.

12.7 Modification of the Effect of Radiation on the Heart

12.7.1 Interaction with Preexisting Heart Disease

Except for pericarditis, the clinical symptoms of heart disease following radiation therapy are non-specific. Heart diseases are one of the most common causes of death and usually there are multiple etiological factors involved. Therefore findings such as a decrease in left ventricular function and coronary artery disease can very rarely be attributed to a single cause in the individual patient. Often several noxious factors are needed to result in clinical symptoms. It is therefore difficult to assess the pathogenetic importance of previous radiotherapy in the individual case of heart disease. Although there are no clinical data on the interaction of spontaneous heart diseases and heart irradiation, radiation is likely to contribute to the cardiac risk.

In spontaneously hypertensive rats it was shown that the latency time of radiation-induced heart failure is shorter in males, which are more severely hypertensive than females (LAUK and TROTT 1988).

12.7.2 Interaction with Chemotherapy

Adriamycin is known to be cardiotoxic by itself and is frequently used as a chemotherapeutic agent in Hodgkin's disease, breast cancer, and small cell lung cancer. Adriamycin may induce acute, transient changes of cardiac function within 24 h of administration as well as chronic cardiomyopathy. Chronic injury presents shortly after termination of chemotherapy as progressive myocardial failure and has a high rate of mortality within a few weeks. The incidence of chronic cardiomyopathy is dependent on the Adriamycin dose (VON HOFF et al. 1979). A total dose of 450 mg/m^2 is generally recommended as the maximal cumulative Adriamycin dose.

In patients receiving high cumulative Adriamycin doses of 450–550 mg/m^2, PRAGA et al. (1979) and GILLADOGA et al. (1975) observed a four- to fivefold increase in the incidence of Adriamycin-induced cardiomyopathy if mediastinal radiotherapy has been given previously.

BILLINGHAM et al. (1977) and BRISTOW et al. (1981) examined myocardial biopsies taken by cardiac catheterization at the end of Adriamycin treatment and described typical vacuolation of myocytes, which increased in severity with Adriamycin dose. Patients who had undergone mediastinal radiotherapy 6 months to 14 years earlier had more severe vacuolation and in addition showed interstitial fibrosis (Fig. 12.14).

MORGAN et al. (1981) measured left ventricular ejection fractions during chemotherapy, prior to each dose of Adriamycin. The incidence of subnormal left ventricular ejection fraction was significantly increased in patients who had received radiotherapy for lung cancer within 6 months before chemotherapy. In breast cancer patients who were irradiated at least 12 months before chemotherapy, ventricular function was not different from that in nonirradiated patients. However, no follow-up studies to assess the prognostic significance of these early changes were carried out. These clinical observations suggest that previous mediastinal radiotherapy makes patients slightly more susceptible to Adriamycin cardiotoxicity.

LE CHEVALIER et al. (1988) found pericardial effusions in 50% of patients after treatment for lung cancer with 45 Gy to the thorax and chemotherapy including a total of 240–320 mg/m^2 Adriamycin. According to the results of studies on radiation therapy alone (Fig. 12.2), pericarditis would have been expected in less than 5% of the patients. Thus simultaneous Adriamycin therapy appears to increase considerably the risk of radiation-induced pericarditis, too.

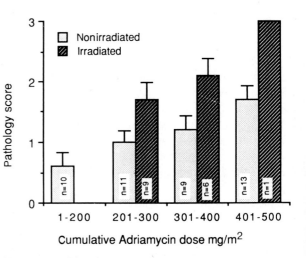

Fig. 12.14. Comparison of pathology scores in cardiac biopsies from nonirradiated and irradiated patients for different ranges of cumulative Adriamycin doses (after BILLINGHAM 1979)

In two recent studies (LaMonte et al. 1986; Santoro et al. 1987) the late effects of combined modality treatment including low doses of Adriamycin were investigated. LaMonte et al. (1986) evaluated cardiac function by ECG, echocardiography, and radionuclide angiography at 15.5–69.5 months after mediastinal irradiation with 20–45 Gy followed by a combination of MOPP and ABVD. Total Adriamycin doses of 86–229 mg/m^2 were given. One out of 20 patients developed congestive heart failure 15 months after treatment, with a left ventricular ejection fraction of 37%. Later autopsy confirmed the diagnosis of Adriamycin-induced cardiomyopathy. The rest of the patients were considered to have normal ventricular function, although four of them showed slight abnormalities of left ventricular ejection fraction at rest or during exertion. Santoro et al. (1987) compared late side-effects of MOPP and ABVD combined with mediastinal radiotherapy for Hodgkin's disease. Groups of 114 and 118 patients had been given 35 Gy to the mediastinum accompanied by either ABVD (including 245 mg/m^2 Adriamycin) or MOPP. Within a median follow-up time of 84 months one patient from the ABVD group died from pericarditis and one from congestive heart failure, whereas no cardiac death was recorded in the MOPP group. However, this difference was not statistically significant. In both studies the cardiac risk of combined low dose radiotherapy and Adriamycin treatment was considered to be low.

No suitable animal model is available for studying the combined effect of Adriamycin and heart irradiation. In rabbits and rats (Eltringham et al. 1975; Fajardo et al. 1976; Kimler et al. 1984) Adriamycin is not only cardiotoxic but also causes a severe nephrotic syndrome which is not observed in humans and which may be lethal. Histological studies in the hearts of rats suffering from nephrotic syndrome caused by other drugs such as puromycin aminonucleoside show changes identical to those observed after Adriamycin treatment (van der Vijgh et al. 1987; van Velzen et al. 1986). In these animal species cardiac changes after Adriamycin may be caused directly by the drug or they may be secondary to kidney damage.

Acknowledgment. Professor K-R Trott initiated my interest in radiation effects on the heart, beginning with my doctoral thesis in 1983, and has supported it ever since. Without his guidance and stimulation this work would not have been possible. H. Trappmann helped to analyze clinical case reports.

References

Ali MK, Khalil LM, Fuller LM et al. (1976) Radiation-related myocardial injury; management of two cases. Cancer 38: 1941–1946

Alibelli MJ, Marco J, Fournial G, Sabatie JB, Dardenne P (1978) Insuffisance coronarienne sévère chez une jeune femme, après radiothérapie médiastinale. Arch Mal Coeur 71: 1311–1317

Amromin GD, Gildenhorn HL, Solomon RD, Nadkarni BB, Jacobs ML (1964) The synergism of x-irradiation and cholesterol-fat feeding on the development of coronary artery lesions. J Atheroscler Res 4: 325–334

Angelini A, Benciciolini P, Thiene G (1985) Radiation-induced coronary atherosclerosis and sudden death in a teenager. Int J Cardiol 9: 371–373

Annest LS, Anderson RP, Li W, Hafermann MD (1983) Coronary artery disease following mediastinal radiation therapy. J Thorac Cardiovasc Surg 85: 257–263

Applefeld MM, Wiernik PH (1983) Cardiac disease after radiation therapy for Hodgkin's disease: analysis of 48 patients. Am J Cardiol 51: 1679–1681

Audebert AA, Cussac A, Krulik M, Lecomte D, Lab JP, Berton JL, Graisely B, Debray J (1982) Études de coronaropathies post-radiques. Une observation. Ann Med Interne (Paris) 133: 269–271

Biller H, Kop EA, Prignitz R (1979) EKG-Veränderungen nach postoperativer Bestrahlung von Mammakarzinom-Patientinnen. Strahlentherapie 155: 541–548

Billingham ME (1979) Endomyocardial changes in anthracycline-treated patients with and without irradiation. Front Radiat Ther Oncol 13: 67–81

Billingham ME, Bristow MR, Glatstein E, Mason JW, Masek MA, Daniels JR (1977) Adriamycin cardiotoxicity: endomyocardial biopsy evidence of enhancement by irradiation. Am J Surg Pathol 1: 17–23

Blitzer PH, Hutchison GB, Salenius SA, Hsieh C-C (1987) Increased incidence of cardiac deaths long after irradiation of the heart. Radiation Research Society, 35th Annual Meeting, Feb 1987

Boivin JF, Hutchison GB (1982) Coronary artery mortality after irradiation for Hodgkin's disease. Cancer 49: 2470–2475

Botti RE, Driscol TE, Pearson OH, Smith JC (1968) Radiation myocardial fibrosis simulating constrictive pericarditis. Cancer 22: 1254–1261

Bristow MR, Mason JW, Billingham ME, Daniels JR (1978) Doxorubicin cardiomyopathy: evaluation by phonocardiography, endomyocardial biopsy, and cardiac catheterization. Ann Intern Med 88: 168–175

Brosius FC, Waller BF, Roberts WL (1981) Analysis of 16 young (aged 15–33 years) necropsy patients who received over 3500 rads to the heart. Am J Med 70: 519–530

Burns RJ, Bar-Shlomo B-Z, Druck MN, Herman JG, Gilbert BW, Perrault DJ, McLaughlin PR (1983) Detection of radiation cardiomyopathy by gated radionuclide angiography. Am J Med 74: 297–302

Byhardt R, Brace K, Ruckdeschel J, Chang P, Martin R, Wiernik P (1975) Dose and treatment factors in radiation-related pericardial effusion associated with the mantle technique for Hodgkin's disease. Cancer 35: 795–802

Carmel RJ, Kaplan HS (1976) Mantle irradiation in Hodgkin's disease: an analysis of technique, tumour eradication and complications. Cancer 37: 2813–2825

Catterall M, Evans W (1960) Myocardial injury from therapeutic irradiation. Br Heart J 22: 168–174

Cohen S, Bharati S, Glass J, Lev M (1981) Radiotherapy as a cause of complete atrioventricular block in Hodgkin's disease. An electrophysiological pathological correlation. Arch Intern Med 141: 676–679

Cohn KE, Stewart JR, Fajardo LF, Hancock EW (1967) Heart disease following radiation. Medicine 46: 281–298

Coltart RS, Thom CH, Roberts JT (1985) Severe constrictive pericarditis after single 16 MEV anterior mantle irradiation for Hodgkin's disease. Lancet I: 488–489

Cosset JM, Henry-Amar, Girinski T, Malaise E, Dupouy N, Dutreix J (1988) Late toxicity of radiotherapy in Hodgkin's disease. The role of fraction size. Acta Oncol 27: 123–129

Dana M, Colombel P, Bayle-Weisgerber C, Teillet F, Desprez-Curely JP, Bernard J (1978) Les péricardites après irradiation du médiastin par grands champs pour la maladie de Hodgkin. J Radiol Electrol 59: 335–341

Dollinger MR, Lavine DM, Foye LV (1966) Myocardial infarction due to postirradiation fibrosis of the coronary arteries. JAMA 195: 316–319

Dunsmore LD, LoPonte MA, Dunsmore RA (1986) Radiation-induced coronary artery disease. J Am Coll Cardiol 8: 239–244

Eltringham JR, Fajardo LF, Stewart JR (1975) Adriamycin cardiomyopathy: enhanced cardiac damage in rabbits with combined drug and cardiac irradiation. Radiology 115: 471–472

Fajardo LF, Stewart JR (1970) Experimental radiation-induced heart disease. Am J Pathol 59: 299–316

Fajardo LF, Stewart JR (1971) Capillary injury preceding radiation-induced myocardial fibrosis. Radiology 101: 429–433

Fajardo LF, Stewart JR (1973) Pathogenesis of radiation-induced myocardial fibrosis. Lab Invest 29: 244–257

Fajardo LF, Steward JR, Cohn KE (1968) Morphology of radiation-induced heart disease. Arch Pathol 86: 512–519

Fajardo LF, Eltringham JR, Stewart JR (1976) Combined cardiotoxicity of adriamycin and x-irradiation. Lab Invest 34: 86–96

Fournial G, Alibelli MJ, Berthoumieu F, Marco J (1979) Complications cardiovasculaires de la radiothérapie médiastinale. A propos de deux observations. Ann Cardiol Ageiol (Paris) 28: 167–172

Fraumeni JF, Herweg JC, Kissante JM (1967) Panaortitis complicating Hodgkin's disease. Ann Intern Med 67: 1242–1247

Fröhlich D, Adler K, Neumeister K, Uhlmann B (1984) Elektrokardiographische Befunde bei Strahlentherapie im Thoraxbereich. Radiobiol Radiother 25: 99–106

Gavin PR, Gillette EL (1982) Radiation response of the canine cardiovascular system. Radiat Res 90: 489–500

Geist BJ, Trott K-R, Lauk S (1990) Physiologic consequences of local heart irradiation in rats. Int J Radiat Oncol Biol Phys 18: 1107–1113

Gheorgiade M, Cheek BH, Chakko SC (1986) Isolated right heart tamponade following mediastinal irradiation. Am Heart J 112: 167–169

Gilladoga AC, Corazon M, Tan CC, Wollner N, Murphy ML (1975) Cardiotoxicity of adriamycin (NSC-123127) in children. Cancer Chemother Rep part 3 vol 6: 209–214

Gillette EL, McChesney SL, Hoopes PJ (1985) Isoeffect curves for radiation-induced cardiomyopathy in the dog. Int J Radiat Oncol Biol Phys 11: 2091–2097

Gold H (1962) Atherosclerosis in the rat. Effect of x-ray and a high fat diet. Proc Soc Exp Biol Med 111: 593–595

Gomez GA, Park JJ, Panahon AM et al. (1983) Heart size and function after radiation therapy to the mediastinum in patients with Hodgkin's disease. Cancer Treat Rep 67: 1099–1103

Gottdiener JS, Katin MJ, Borer JS, Bacharach SL, Green MV (1983) Late cardiac effects of therapeutic mediastinal irradiation. Assessment by echocardiography and radionuclide angiography. N Engl J Med 308: 569–588

Green B, Zornoza J, Ricks JP (1977) Eccentric pericardial effusion after radiation therapy of left breast carcinoma. AJR 128: 27–30

Green DM, Gingell RL, Pearce J, Panahon AM, Ghoarah J (1987) The effect of mediastinal irradiation on cardiac function of patients treated during childhood and adolescence for Hodgkin's disease. J Clin Oncol 5: 239–245

Greenwood RD, Rosenthal A, Cassady R, Jaffe N, Nadas AS (1974) Constrictive pericarditis in childhood due to mediastinal irradiation. Circulation 50: 1033–1039

Haas JM (1969) Symptomatic constrictive pericarditis developing 45 years after radiation therapy to the mediastinum. Am Heart J 77: 89–95

Hamilton DV, Reed PI (1978) Myocardial infarction following radiotherapy for Hodgkin's disease. Br J Clin Pract 32: 181

Heider KM, Drobny H, Salewski D et al. (1982) Kardiale Veränderungen nach supradiaphragmaler Mantelfeldbestrahlung. Radiobiol Radiother 23: 517–525

Host H, Brennhovd IO, Loeb M (1986) Postoperative radiotherapy in breast cancer – long-term results from the Oslo study. Int J Radiat Oncol Biol Phys 12: 727–732

Huff H, Sanders EM (1972) Coronary artery occlusion after radiation. N Engl J Med 286: 780

Ikäheimo MJ, Niemelä MM, Linnaluoto MM, Jakobsson MJT, Takkunen JT, Taskinen PJ (1985) Early cardiac changes related to radiation therapy. Am J Cardiol 56: 943–946

Iqbal SM, Hanson EL, Gensini GG (1977) Bypass graft for coronary artery stenosis following radiation therapy. Chest 71: 664–666

Kagan AR, Morton DL, Hafermann MD, Johnson RE (1969) Evaluation and management of radiation-induced pericardial effusion. Radiology 92: 632–634

Kereiakes DJ, Morady F, Ports TA (1983) High-degree atrioventricular block after radiation therapy. Am J Cardiol 51: 1233–1234

Khan MY (1973) Radiation-induced cardiomyopathy. Am J Pathol 73: 131–146

Kimler BF, Mansfield CM, Svoboda DJ, Cox GG (1984) Ultrastructural evidence of cardiac damage resulting from thoracic irradiation and anthracyclines in rat. Int J Radiat Oncol Biol Phys 10: 1465–1469

Kurtz B, Maisch B, Voß A-C (1981) Zur Ätiologie des Perikardergusses nach Strahlentherapie des Morbus Hodgkin. Strahlentherapie 157: 571–575

LaMonte CS, Yeh SDJ, Straus DJ (1986) Long-term follow-up of cardiac function in patients with Hodgkin's disease treated with mediastinal irradiation and combination chemotherapy including doxorubicin. Cancer Treat Rep 70: 439–444

Larsson L-E, Lindahl J, Unsgaard B (1976) Effects on the cardiovascular system of irradiation for malignant lymphoma. Acta Radiol Ther Phys Biol 15: 529–540

Lauk S (1986) Strain differences in the radiation response of the rat heart. Radiother Oncol 5: 333–335

Lauk S (1987) Endothelial alkaline phosphatase activity loss as an early stage in the development of radiation-induced heart disease in rats. Radiat Res 110: 118–128

Lauk S, Trott K-R (1988) Radiation induced heart disease in hypertensive rats. Int J Radiat Oncol Biol Phys 14: 109–114

Lauk S, Kiszel Z, Buschmann J, Trott K-R (1985) Radiation induced heart disease in rats. Int J Radiat Oncol Biol Phys 11: 801–808

Lauk S, Rüth S, Trott K-R (1987) The effects of dose-fractionation on radiation-induced heart disease in rats. Radiother Oncol 8: 363–367

Lauk S, Böhm M, Feiler G, Geist BJ, Erdmann E. (1989) Increased number of cardiac adrenergic receptors following local heart irradiation. Rad Res 119: 157–165

Lauk S, Trott K-R (1990) Endothelial cell proliferation in the rat heart following local heart irradiation. Int J Radiat Biol 57: 1017–1030

Lawson RAM, Ross WM, Gold RG, Blesovsky A, Barnsley WC (1972) Postradiation pericarditis. Report on four more cases with special reference to bronchogenic carcinoma. J Thorac Cardiovasc Surg 63: 841–847

Leach JE, Sugiura K (1941) The effect of high voltage roentgen rays on the heart of adult rats. AJR 45: 414–425

Leach JE, Sugiura K (1942) Late effects of high voltage roentgen rays on the heart of adult rats. AJR 48: 81–87

Le Chevalier T, Arriagada R, de Thé H et al. (1988) Combination of chemotherapy and radiotherapy in limited small cell lung carcinoma: results of alternating schedule in 109 patients. NCI Monogr 6: 335–338

Lee KT, Jarmolych J, Kim DN, Grant C, Krasney JA, Thomas WA, Bruno AM (1971) Production of advanced coronary atherosclerosis, myocardial infarction and "sudden death" in swine. Exp Mol Pathol 15: 170–190

Leong ASY, Forbes JI, Ruzic T (1979) Radiation related coronary artery disease in Hodgkin's disease. Aust NZ J Med 9: 423–425

MacLeod CA, Schwartz H, Linton DB (1969) Constrictive pericarditis following irradiation therapy. JAMA 24: 2281–2282

Maeda S (1980) Pathology of experimental radiation Pancarditis. I Observation on radiation-induced heart injuries following a single dose of x-ray irradiation to rabbit heart with special reference to its pathogenesis. Acta Pathol Jpn 30: 59–78

Marks RD, Agarwal SK, Constable WC (1973) Radiation-induced pericarditis in Hodgkin's disease. Acta Radiol Ther Phys Biol 12: 305–312

Martin RG, Ruckdeschel JC, Chang C, Byhardt R, Bouchard RJ, Wiernik PH (1975) Radiation-related pericarditis. Am J Cardiol 35: 216–220

Masland DS, Rotz CT, Harris JH (1968) Postradiation pericarditis with chronic pericardial effusion. Ann Intern Med 69: 97–102

McChesney SL, Gillette EL, Orton EC (1988a) Canine cardiomyopathy after whole heart and partial lung irradiation. Int J Radiat Oncol Biol Phys 14: 1169–1174

McChesney SL, Gillette EL, Powers BE (1988b) Radiation-induced cardiomyopathy in the dog. Radiat Res 113: 120–132

McReynolds RA, Gold GL, Roberts WC (1976) Coronary heart disease after mediastinal irradiation for Hodgkin's disease. Am J Med 60: 39–45

Mill WB, Baglan RJ, Kurichety P, Prasad S, Lee JY, Moller R (1984) Symptomatic radiation-induced pericarditis in Hodgkin's disease. Int J Radiat Oncol Biol Phys 10: 2061–2065

Miller DD, Waters DD, Dangoisse V, David P-R (1983) Symptomatic coronary artery spasm following radiotherapy for Hodgkin's disease. Chest 83: 284–285

Morgan GW, Mcliveen BM, Freedman A, Murray IPC (1981) Radionuclide ejection fraction in doxorubicin cardiotoxicity. Cancer Treat Rep 65: 629–638

Morgan GW, Freeman AP, McLean RG, Jarvie BH, Giles RW (1985) Late cardiac, thyroid and pulmonary sequelae of mantle radiotherapy for Hodgkin's disease. Int J Radiat Oncol Biol Phys 11: 1925–1931

Morgenroth K, Junge-Hülsing G, Hauss WH (1967) Über Veränderungen am Rattenherzen nach gezielter Röntgenbestrahlung. Strahlentherapie 133: 610–620

Morton DL, Glancy DL, Joseph WL, Adkins PC (1973) Management of patients with radiation-induced pericarditis with effusion: a note on the development of aortic regurgitation in two of them. Chest 64: 291–297

Muggia FM, Cassileth PA (1968) Constrictive pericarditis following radiation therapy. Am J Med 44: 116–123

Murray JC, Parkins CS (1988) Collagen synthesis in CBA mouse heart after total thoracic irradiation. Radiother Oncol 13: 137–143

Nigond J, Bertinchant JB, Tailland M, Bosc E, Grolleau-Raoux R (1987) Les coronaropathies post-radiques. Présentation de 7 cas et revue de la littérature. Ann Cardiol Angeiol (Paris) 36: 399–403

Novi AM (1969) Effects of low irradiation doses on the ultrastructure of the rat myocardium. Virchows Arch [B] 2: 24–31

Phillips SJ, Reid AJ, Rugh R (1964) Electrocardiographic and pathological changes after x-irradiation in dogs. Am J Heart 68: 524–533

Pierce RH, Haferman MD, Kagan AR (1969) Changes in the transverse cardiac diameter following irradiation for Hodgkin's disease. Radiology 93: 619–624

Pohjola-Sintonen, Tötterman K-J, Salmo M, Siltanen P (1987) Late cardiac effects of mediastinal radiotherapy in patients with Hodgkin's disease. Cancer 60: 31–37

Praga C, Beretta G, Vigo PL et al. (1979) Adriamycin cardiotoxicity: a survey of 1273 patients. Cancer Treat Rep 63: 827–834

Prentice RTW (1965) Myocardial infarction following radiation. Lancet 62: 643–644

Pucheu A, Thomas D, Dobrinski G et al. (1986) Les sténoses coronaires postradiothérapiques. Etude clinique de 5 cas et revue de la litterature. Arch Mal Coeur 79: 1609–1615

Rasmussen S, Dossing M, Walbom-Jorgenson S (1978) Coronary heart disease – a possible risk in megavoltage therapy? Acta Med Scand 203: 237–239

Rodgers DL (1976) Precocious myocardial infarction after radiation treatment for Hodgkin's disease. Chest 70: 675–677

Rowland KM, Murthy A (1986) Hodgkin's disease. Long-term effects of therapy. Med Ped Oncol 14: 88–96

Rubin E, Camara J, Grayzel D, Zak FG (1973) Radiation-induced cardiac fibrosis. Am J Med 34: 71–75

Sabrazès J, Rivière P (1897) Recherches sur l'action biologique des rayons X. CR Acad Sci 124: 979

Santoro A, Bonadonna G, Valagussa P et al. (1987) Long-term results of combined chemotherapy-radiotherapy approach in Hodgkin's disease: superiority of ABVD plus radiotherapy versus MOPP plus radiotherapy. J Clin Oncol 5: 27–37

Săpiro IB, Asdapov BA (1978) Die röntgenfunktionelle. Beurteilung des Herzens bei der Strahlentherapie des Osophaguskarzinoms. Radiobiol Radiother 2: 109–116

Schneider JS, Edwards JE (1979) Irradiation-induced pericarditis. Chest 75: 560–564

Scott DL, Thomas RD (1978) Late onset of constrictive pericarditis after thoracic radiotherapy. Br Med J 11: 341–342

Scully RE, Galdabini JJ, McNeely BU (1978) Case records of the Massachusetts General Hospital. Case 20–1978. N Engl J Med 298: 1184–1192

Senderoff E, Kaneko M, Beck RA, Baronofsky ID (1961) The effects of cardiac irradiation upon the normal canine heart. AJR 86: 740–751

Steinberg I (1967) Effusive-constrictive pericarditis. Am J Cardiol 19: 434–439

Stewart JR, Fajardo LF (1971a) Dose response in human and experimental radiation-induced heart disease. Radiology 99: 403–408

Stewart JR, Fajardo LF (1971b) Radiation-induced heart disease. Clinical and experimental aspects. Radiol Clin North Am 9: 511–531

Stewart JR, Fajardo LF, Cohn KE, Page V (1968) Experimental radiation-induced heart disease in rabbits. Radiology 91: 814–817

Stone HL, Bishop VS, Guyton AC (1964) Progressive changes in cardiovascular function after unilateral heart irradiation. Am J Physiol 206: 289–293

Strender LE, Lindahl J, Larsson LE (1986) Incidence of heart disease and functional significance of changes in the electrocardiogram 10 years after radiotherapy for breast cancer. Cancer 57: 929–934

Stroobandt R, Knieriem H-J, de Wolf L, Joossens JV (1975) Radiation-induced heart disease. Acta Cardiol 30: 383–392

Tenet W, Missri J, Hager D (1986) Radiation-induced stenosis of the left main coronary artery. Cathet Cardiovasc Diagn 12: 169–171

Thar T, Million RR (1980) Complications of radiation treatment of Hodgkin's disease. Semin Oncol 7: 174–183

Tiamson E, Fritz KE, Campana H, Anzola E, Zgoda A, Daoud AS (1970) Studies in rabbits of cellular mechanisms accounting for enhancement of diet-induced atherosclerosis by x-irradiation. Exp Mol Pathol 12: 175–184

Töttermann KJ, Pesonen E, Siltanen P (1983) Radiation-related chronic heart disease. Chest 83: 875–878

Tracy GP, Brown DE, Johnson LW, Gottlieb AJ (1974) Radiation-induced coronary artery disease. JAMA 228: 1660–1662

Tzivoni D, Ratzkowski E, Biran S, Brook J, Stern S (1977) Complete heart block following therapeutic irradiation of the left side of the chest. Cest 71: 231–234

Uhl GS, Farrell PW (1983) Myocardial infarction in young adults: risk factors and natural history. Am Heart J 105: 548–553

van der Vijgh WJF, van Velzen D, van der Poort JSEM, Schlüper HMM, Mross K, Feijen J, Pinedo HM (1987) Morphometric study of myocardial changes during puromycin aminonucleoside induced nephropathy in rats. Anticancer Res 7: 1111–1116

van Renterghem D, Hamers J, de Schryver A, Pauwels R, van der Straeten M (1985) Chylothorax after mantle field irradiation for Hodgkin's disease. Respiration 48: 188–189

van Velzen D, Alons CL, Veldhuizen RW (1986) Morphometric study of myocardial changes in adriamycin cardiomyopathy of the rat. J Lab Clin Med 108: 319–320

Velebit V, von Segesser L, Gabathuler J, Jornod J, Faidutti B (1986) Right ventricular outflow obstruction after radiation therapy. J Thorac Cardiovasc Surg 92: 153–161

Virmani R, Robinowitz M, McAllister HA (1983) Coronary heart disease in 48 autopsy patients 30 years old and younger. Arch Pathol Lab Med 107: 535–540

von Hoff DD, Layard MW, Basa P, Davis HL, von Hoff AL, Rozencweig M, Muggia FM (1979) Risk factors for doxorubicin-induced congestive heart failure. Ann Intern Med 91: 710–717

Yahalom J, Hasin Y, Fuks Z (1983) Acute myocardial infarction with normal coronary arteriogram after mantle field radiation for Hodgkin's disease. Cancer 53: 637–641

Yeung TK, Hopewell JW (1985) Effects of single doses of irradiation on cardiac function in the rat. Radiother Oncol 3: 339–345

Yeung TK, Lauk S, Simmonds RH, Hopewell JW, Trott K-R (1989) Morphological and functional changes in the rat heart after x-irradiation: strain differences. Radiat Res 119: 489–499

13 Radiation Injury of the Lung: Experimental Studies, Observations After Radiotherapy and Total Body Irradiation Prior to Bone Marrow Transplantation

M. Molls and D. van Beuningen

CONTENTS

13.1 Introduction

The history of radiation research shows that clinical problems give rise to experimental studies and that, in turn, radiobiological findings contribute to the improvement of radiotherapeutic procedures. As long ago as 1922 Groover et al. (1922) and Hines (1922) described the clinical features of radiation-induced pneumonitis and fibrosis of the alveolar wall. Wintz (1923) paid special attention to the complications related to pneumonitis after radiotherapy for bronchial and

M. Molls, Priv.-Doz., Dr.med., Oberarzt, Radiologisches Zentrum, Universitätsklinikum Essen, Hufelandstraße 55, 4300 Essen 1, FRG

D. van Beuningen, Professor Dr., Oberfeldarzt, Akademie des Sanitats- und Gesundkeitswesens der Bundeswehr, Neuherbergstraße 11, 8000 München 45, FRG

mammary carcinoma. The clinical observation that the lung is a critical tissue in radiotherapy of organs of the chest wall or within the thorax led to intensive experimental investigations. At a relatively early stage the chronology of the pathological alterations was studied in rabbits (Englestad 1940). An excellent and fundamental review of injuries contributing to lung morbidity and organ dysfunction was published by Rubin and Casarett (1968). They updated not only experimental findings but also knowledge on histopathological alterations observed in irradiated human lung.

Morbidity of the lung is a major and often lethal complication after radiochemotherapy and subsequent bone marrow transplantation (BMT) (Deeg et al. 1988). It has been reported that the incidence of interstitial pneumonitis (IP) ranges up to about 50% after this therapeutic procedure, performed mainly in patients with leukemia (Storb 1983; Bamberg et al. 1986). Although IP is not always related to total body irradiation (TBI) alone, the observations after BMT have clearly underlined the high radiosensitivity of the lung. Once the risk of TBI was recognized, further radiobiological studies followed. The current experimental investigations aim in particular at achieving a better understanding of the mechanisms involved in the development of radiation pneumonitis.

It has been pointed out that more than 40 cell types are found in the lung, and most of them are considered to be relatively radioresistant (Coggle et al. 1986). However, the lung is unable to tolerate large doses of radiation since the organ as a whole has little regenerative capacity (Coggle et al. 1986). Ionizing radiation causes immediate damage at the biochemical, subcellular, and cellular levels, but the gross tissue injury associated with organ dysfunction is delayed (Rubin and Casarett 1968; Molls and van Beuningen 1985; Coggle et al. 1986). It is well known that the degree of functional disturbances, such as impaired ventilation and gas diffusion, is dependent on the total dose, the fractionation schedule, the dose rate, and the irradiated volume of the lung (RUBIN and CASARETT 1968).

The first part of this review concentrates on experimental morphological, biochemical, and physiological findings. The radiobiological observations help to clarify the complex development of clinically apparent pneumonitis and lung fibrosis. In discussing clinical data, special emphasis is given to lung morbidity after TBI prior to BMT. The significance of the combined action of irradiation and chemotherapeutic substances is stressed, as are possible treatments of pneumonitis.

13.2 Experimental Investigations

13.2.1 Morphological Studies

The alveoli are lined by an epithelium which consists of very thin (0.2 μm), membrane-like cells (type I pneumocytes) and thicker, round-shaped cells (type II pneumocytes). The cells rest on a basement membrane. Under the epithelium and the basement membrane lies a network of capillaries. In the interstitium between the alveolar epithelium and the capillaries, reticular and elastic fibers as well as mesenchymal and inflammatory cells are found. The diffusion distance between the capillaries and the air space of alveoli is 0.5–2.5 μm (LEONHARDT 1981; MOLLS and VAN BEUNINGEN 1985; COGGLE et al. 1986; TRAVIS 1987).

The type II pneumocytes represent the stem cell population for type I pneumocytes. They synthesize, store, and secrete the phospholipid and protein components of surfactant (ADAMSON and BOWDEN 1977; EVANS et al. 1973, 1976; TRAVIS 1987). During expiration surfactant prevents the collapse of the alveoli and thus atelectasis. Furthermore, lack of surfactant which balances hydrostatic and osmotic pressures leads to transudation of serum proteins and blood into the alveoli (PATTLE 1963; VAN DEN BRENK 1971).

The pathomorphological effects in the irradiated lung have been reviewed by several authors (RUBIN and CASARETT 1968; VAN DEN BRENK 1971; GROSS 1977b; CASARETT 1980; MOLLS and VAN BEUNINGEN 1985; COGGLE et al. 1986; TRAVIS 1987). There are three main phases of radiation response which are characterized by typical alterations. These are summarized in Table 13.1 and are outlined below.

13.2.1.1 Early Phase–Latent Period of Pneumonitis

During the 1st month after x-irradiation with single doses between 10 and 20 Gy, light microscopy does not reveal the typical inflammatory alterations of acute pneumonitis. MAISIN (1970, 1974) used electron microscopy to study the very early alterations. Several hours after a dose of 20 Gy, ultrastructural injuries were observed in type I and II pneumocytes and in endothelial cells of

Table 13.1. Morphological alterations in the irradiated lung as observed in animals and humans

Early phase, 1st month: latent peroid of pneumonitis	Intermediate phase, 3rd week up to several months: acute pneumonitis	Late phase, about 6th month and later: fibrosis
Ultrastructural lesions of type I and II pneumocytes and endothelium: a) Alterations of membranes and cell organelles b) Sloughing of type I pneumocytes c) Irregularities of lamellar bodies in type II pneumocytes d) Sloughing of endothelial cells, swelling, and obstruction of capillaries Interstitial edema Fibrin exudation into alveoli Release of surfactant Decrease in macrophages	Further decrease in type I cells Hyperplasia and increased number of type II cells Obstruction of capillaries due to platelets, collagen, and fibrin-reduced permeability of capillaries Increase of leukocytes, plasma cells, macrophages, fibroblasts Increase of collagenic and elastic fibers Increasing thickening of alveolar septa; alveolar space becomes smaller	Loss of capillaries; capillaries filled with collagenic fibers Alveolar septa 3–6 times thicker than normal Alveolar space small or absent Generalized fibrosis

mouse lungs. The changes included dilatation of the endoplasmic reticulum and mitochondria as well as disruption of plasma membranes. Polymorphic cell nuclei showed condensation of the chromatin. The lamellar bodies of type II cells, which store the phospholipid and protein components of surfactant, were enlarged and irregular. Permeability of the capillaries was increased, probably due to membrane changes. Interstitial edema occurred. Hypertrophy and vacuolation of the cytoplasm of endothelial cells led to obstruction and swelling of the capillaries.

PHILLIPS (1966) and PHILLIPS and MARGOLIS (1974) reported that the earliest damage in rat lung was endothelial injury at 24 h after a dose of 24 Gy. Interestingly, alterations of the epithelium or basement membrane were not observed. The investigations of ADAMSON et al. (1970) suggested that the onset of ultrastructural effects is dose dependent. Degeneration of the endothelium leading to distention and blockage of rat lung capillaries was observed within 2 and 5 days after 11 and 6.5 Gy respectively. In experiments by MOOSSAVI et al. (1977) interstitial edema due to increased capillary permeability was observed 14 days after one-lung x-irradiation of dogs. Doses between 2 and 8 Gy caused minimal damage to capillaries and endothelium. In contrast the alterations were pronounced when single doses of 24–32 Gy were given.

PENNEY and RUBIN (1977) irradiated mice with single and fractionated doses of 10, 20, and 30 Gy x-rays. On electron microscopy they found an increase in microvilli projecting into the capillary lumen, which might have impaired blood flow and contributed to aggregation of thrombocytes. According to these authors the primary and most marked alterations are those of type II and to a lesser extent of type I pneumonocytes associated with edema, fibrin deposition, and invasion of histiocytes within 24 h. Ultrastructural alterations of type II pneumocytes, which occur relatively early after irradiation, had already been reported by GOLDENBERG et al. (1968) and FAULKNER and CONNOLLY (1973). PENNEY and RUBIN (1977) observed a decrease in lamellar bodies beginning at 1 h after irradiation. At 24 h this decrease was marked whereas 7 days later the number of lamellar bodies was increased. Between 3 and 4 weeks after irradiation type II cells showed severe ultrastructural damage of mitochondria and intracellular membrane systems as well as sloughing into the alveolar lumina. Damage to type II cells,

edema, and invasion of histiocytes were comparatively more pronounced after fractionated irradiation. Damage to type I pneumocytes was less impressive. A loss of integrity of intracelluear organelles was only occasionally found at 24 h after irradiation. Areas of denuded basement membranes did not occur, although edema of alveolar walls was observed (PENNEY and RUBIN 1977).

In contrast, ADAMSON et al. (1970) found, in an ultrastructural study of mouse and rat, focal swelling, necrosis, and sloughing of type I pneumocytes followed by a denuded basement membrane. The effect was maximal at 10 and 14 days after irradiation of the whole body with doses of 11 and 6.5 Gy respectively or at 14 days after 30 Gy to the hemithorax. Damage of type II cells was not observed. Furthermore there was no proliferation of type II pneumocytes as occurs after exposure to oxygen and nitrogen dioxide.

In the hamster lung all alveolar cell types developed progressive ultrastructural changes within 14 days after irradiation. A very efficient regenerative hyperplastic response of type II cells was observed. Denudation of basement membrane did not occur (MADRAZO et al. 1973).

13.2.1.2 Intermediate Phase–Acute Pneumonitis

As stated by COGGLE et al. (1986), the early ultrastructural changes are consistent with reports of early proteinosis and early variations in capillary permeability and perfusion. The latter biochemical and physiological alterations, which are described in more detail in the following chapters, include an increased leakage of serum proteins into the alveolar space (HENDERSON et al. 1978; GROSS 1980a; AHIER et al. 1984), deposition of fibrin-rich serum proteins on the alveolar surfaces (VAN DEN BRENK 1971), formation of hyaline membranes (PHILLIPS and MARGOLIS 1972; PENNEY and RUBIN 1977; LEROY et al. 1966), a transiently increased pulmonary diffusion capacity for carbon monoxide (TEATES 1968), increased pulmonary capillary perfusion (FREEDMAN et al. 1974), but also very early transitory reductions in perfusion (FREEDMAN et al. 1974; KORSOWER et al. 1971).

It is generally recognized that the major cellular, vascular, and pathophysiological alterations occur at about 2–6 months postirradiation, during the clinical period of life-threatening acute pneumonitis. Morphologically, acute pneumonitis is characterized by thickening of the alveolar septa, edema of the interstitium and exudation into air spaces, infiltration of inflammatory cells, alterations of the capillaries, and reaction of the pneumocytes.

The two cell populations with the most active proliferation in the lung are type II pneumocytes and alveolar macrophages. As radiation preferentially kills proliferating cells, both these cell populations have been considered to be comparatively radiosensitive. Postirradiation DNA labeling indices of type II pneumocytes have been investigated by several authors. In considering the results, one has to be aware that they can be misleading, as precise studies of cell kinetics in a system with labeling indices as low as about 0.4% are difficult (COGGLE et al. 1986). When the thorax of mice was irradiated with doses of 2.5 and 10 Gy the labeling index of type II cells initially decreased at day 7. Three months after irradiation the value was 5 times higher than in unirradiated animals (PEEL 1979). Also in the experiments of COULTAS et al. (1981) proliferation of type II cells decreased for the first 6 days after irradiation with 10 Gy of x-rays or 7.7 Gy of neutrons. Up to 3–5 weeks after irradiation a gradual increase above control values was observed.

MEYER and co-workers developed a method to study the radiosensitivity of the presumed stem cells (MEYER et al. 1980; MEYER and ULLRICH 1981). The response was studied after stimulation of division of type II cells with the antioxidant butylated hydroxytoluene (BHT). BHT selectively kills type I pneumocytes, which arise from type II cells. D_0 values for the proliferation fraction of type II cells were 1.2 Gy of x-rays and 0.6 Gy of neutrons when the BHT stimulus was given immediately after irradiation. Irradiating with x-rays after BHT treatment, the D_0 values increased to 3.6 Gy at day 2 and 5.8 Gy at day 14 after BHT. Comparing day 0 with day 2 no change was observed after irradiation with neutrons. At day 14 post-BHT, D_0 was 3.45 Gy. COGGLE et al. (1986) pointed out that the split-dose studies showed the capability of short-term (1–2 days) and longer term (several weeks) recovery of type II pneumocytes and that the latter phenomenon might be the cellular basis of slow repair (FIELD and HORNSEY 1977).

From the above-described experiments it can be concluded that repopulation of type II cells is a slow and prolonged mechanism which compensates for cell death and aims at achieving histological integrity of lung tissue after irradiation.

Obviously the loss of type II pneumocytes depends on radiation dose. After a single dose of 20 Gy in mice the loss increased with increasing time as observed by electron microscopy. The investigation was performed over a period of 6 months after x-ray exposure (TRAVIS et al. 1977). Fractionated irradiation with 5×4 Gy produced a comparatively small loss whereas after 10×2 Gy cell loss could not be observed.

In addition to repopulation a further compensatory mechanism seems to be hyperplasia of type II pneumocytes. In dogs hyperplasia was found after relatively high single doses (24–32 Gy) at about 7 and 11 weeks after irradiation (MOOSAVI et al. 1977). Hyperplasia of murine type II cells had previously been reported by MAISIN (1970). It is suggested that hyperplasia is associated with an increase in surfactant-containing lamellar bodies. Such an increase has been described by PENNEY et al. (1981) and MOOSAVI et al. (1977).

COGGLE et al. (1986) pointed out that there is a particular interest in the postirradiation kinetics of alveolar macrophages due to their clearance function after inhalation of radioactive particles. Furthermore a radiation-induced depression of macrophages would also be critical after TBI prior to BMT as this could increase the risk of fatal lung infections. The results which have been reported after external irradiation (photons, neutrons) are conflicting. Both suppression of function and resistance to radiation have been observed in macrophages (BRENNAN and AINSWORTH 1977; KIM et al. 1976; GODLESKI and BRAIN 1976; SCHMIDTKE and DIXON 1971, 1973; GROSS and BALIS 1978). In mice the reduced rate of pulmonary clearance has been assumed to be due to the direct radiation effect on alveolar macrophages. Both short-lived β-emitters ($^{144}CeO_2$) and long-lived α-emitters ($^{239}PuO_2$) produced a reduction in clearance of inhaled bacteria (*Staphylococcus aureus*) (LUNDGREN and HAHN 1979).

The decrease in and recovery of alveolar macrophages has been determined in the endobronchial lavage fluid. Using this direct method the lowest number of macrophages was found at about 4 days after thorax irradiation of mice with doses of 2, 5, and 10 Gy. Depletion was more pronounced after the higher doses. When compared with 2 Gy, 5 and 10 Gy were followed by a longer lasting depression. Recovery occurred at about 7 weeks after x-ray exposure. At 8–10 weeks even an overshoot of the number of macrophages was observed (PEEL and COGGLE 1980; COGGLE et al. 1986). After inhalation of the x-emitter $^{239}Pu\,O_2$ an acute decrease in the number of murine alveolar macrophages was followed by a sustained depression in the case of high lung burdens (MOORES et al. 1986). As stated in previous review articles, the depletion in all these studies was dose dependent and sensitive to fractionation, which suggests that there exists a radiosensitive, proliferating pool of intrapulmonary macrophages or precursor cells (GROSS 1977a; COGGLE et al. 1986). The cell kinetic studies of TARLING and COGGLE (1982a–c) and LIN et al. (1982a) support the idea of proliferating subpopulations of pulmonary macrophages. It has been reported that the D_0 value obtained from survival curves of mouse and hamster alveolar macrophages was about 2 Gy (LIN et al. 1982b). This figure might characterize the radiosensitivity of dividing lung macrophages.

Considering the alveolus as a whole, thickening of the alveolar wall is a very important alteration during the acute phase of pneumonitis. JENNINGS and ARDEN (1961, 1962) observed in rats that this effect was in particular due to an accumulation of reticular fibrils and sustained infiltration by mononuclear cells. Alveolar septa of mice showed an increase in fibroblasts and other cellular elements (TRAVIS 1980a). After x-irradiation with doses of 12 and 14 Gy the effects were most prominent at about 36 weeks. The spatial distribution of septal alterations within the histological cross-section was of slight or moderate density after these doses. The mortality of mice receiving 14 Gy was 50% at 36 weeks postradiation.

Vascular injuries developing during the early and acute phase of pneumonitis and, most significantly, relatively late after irradiation are characterized by lesions of the capillary walls, by obstruction of vessels due to aggregation of platelets, collagen, and fibrin, and by reduced permeability of capillaries (RUBIN and CASARETT 1968; GROSS 1977b; COGGLE et al. 1986). It has also been suggested that death of irradiated endothelial cells when entering mitosis plays a significant role in the development of vascular damage. In the lung of young, growing mice the doubling time of endothelial cells was 8 weeks or longer (TANNOCK and HAYASHI 1972). In the regenerating lung the endothelium showed a mitotic activity comparable to that of type II pneumocytes (ADAMSON and BOWDEN 1974). The turnover time of endothelial cells in nongrowing organs is long and takes months to years (LAW 1981). Based on these latter observations one can explain why significant vascular damage in the lung occurs comparatively late after irradiation (COGGLE et al. 1986).

13.2.1.3 Late Phase – Pulmonary Fibrosis

Between 8 and 15 months after irradiation of mice, electron microscopic studies revealed thickened alveolar walls which showed pronounced sclerosis and accumulations of hyalin. The lumina of many capillaries were obliterated by collagenic fibers. Cell debris and fibrin were present in the alveolar spaces. The number of inflammatory cells was low (MAISIN 1970). The phase of fibrosis in rats was characterized by alveolar walls which were 3–6 times thicker than normal. Interestingly, in many alveolar septa a dislocation of the capillaries was observed so that they were located sufficiently near to the air spaces. In these studies the septa showed a considerable number of mononuclear cells (JENNINGS and ARDEN 1961).

The investigations of TRAVIS (1980a) in mice yielded a threshold dose of 13 Gy for late fibrotic changes. This dose was somewhat higher than the threshold dose for early and intermediate alterations, namely 11 Gy. This observation supports the assumption that at least a moderate inflammatory reaction can resolve and leave little or no histopathologically detectable change, except perhaps for subtle vascular changes (CASARETT 1980). Considering the time sequence of fibrotic changes, the late effects developed earlier after 19 Gy than after 13 Gy (TRAVIS 1980a). It has also been reported that severe fibrosis occurs more frequently in female rats than in males (KUROHARA and CASARETT 1972).

The term "fibrotic" is a morphological one and describes an increase in connective tissue fibers in the histological slide. However, the changes leading and related to pulmonary fibrosis are very complex (RENNARD et al. 1982). They comprise biochemical alterations of connective tissue metabolism and disturbances of the lung physiology. These effects are described in the following sections.

13.2.2 Biochemical Alterations (Surfactant, Proteins, Collagen, Glycosaminoglycans, etc.)

Surfactant is a substance which alters the surface tension and prevents the collapse of alveoli at the end of expiration. By reduction of surface tension reinflation is facilitated. A further important function of surfactant is to maintain the balance of hydrostatic and osmotic pressure between the air space of the alveoli and the interstitium. In this way an outward flow of fluid from the capillaries into alveoli is inhibited. Alterations in the function of surfactant are followed by edema, atelectasis, and septal fibrosis (Pattle 1963; van den Brenk 1971).

Surfactant is a mixture of phospholipids in the liquid film covering the alveolar surface. It contains phosphatidylcholine and unsaturated phospholipids. Additionally, in the liquid film mucopolysaccharides and mucoproteins are found. Surfactant is produced by type II pneumocytes and is stored in the lamellar bodies of these cells (Faulkner and Connolly 1973; Travis et al. 1977; Moosavi et al. 1977).

Morphologically, after irradiation loss of lamellar bodies, recovery and subsequent lamellar body hyperplasia are observed (Jennings and Arden 1962; Penney and Rubin 1977; Penney et al. 1982b; Rubin et al. 1986). The reaction concerning lamellar bodies and surfactant occurs very soon after irradiation (Gross 1981; Keane et al. 1981; Rubin et al. 1980, 1983,1986; Shapiro et al. 1984). Rubin et al. (1980) have demonstrated that increase in surfactant in the alveoli is one of the early detectable changes following lung irradiation. In the investigations of Ahier et al. (1985) alveolar surfactant increased after x-irradiation and neutrons in a biphasic pattern. The early phase, beginning within hours of irradiation, probably resulted from an early loss of lamellar bodies which are extruded from type II cells into the alveolar space (Shapiro et al. 1984). However, the peak levels of alveolar surfactant recovered by lung lavage occurred at about 3 weeks after irradiation. The lipid composition showed no alteration (Ahier et al. 1985). At this time unsaturated phosphatidylcholine, which is the major component of surfactant, was also increased in lung tissue (Ahier et al. 1985).

Thrombropulos and Thomas (1970) measured an increased incorporation of radioactive labeled palmitate into the lipids within the initial weeks after irradiation. Coultas et al. (1987) studied turnover and synthesis rates of surfactant following thoracic irradiation of mice with 10 Gy x-rays. At between 2 and 6 weeks, when levels of surfactant in the alveoli showed the highest increase, there was a reduction in the rate of radioactivity loss from ^{3}H-choline labeled unsatured phosphatidylcholine from the lung. This observation indicated a reduced turnover of surfactant. The authors discussed that the reduced number of macrophages recovered from alveolar lavage between about 2 and 6 weeks after irradia-

tion might have been a reason for the longer turnover times of surfactant. Furthermore, the results suggested that at between 2 and 3 weeks after irradiation, removal and degradation of surfactant almost ceased but that synthesis continued normally. However, by 3 weeks postirradiation, surfactant synthesis was obviously increased by a factor of about 2 as concluded from ^{3}H-choline incorporation into unsatured phosphatidylcholine. It was pointed out that the stimulated surfactant production that occurs from about 3 weeks onwards suggests an additional active response to radiation by the type II pneumocytes.

Starting the investigation several days after irradiation, Gross (1978b) found an increasing phosphatidylcholine content up to 12 weeks after irradiation in mice. The synthesis rate remained unchanged. At 12 weeks the values returned to control levels. In considering such discrepancies between phospholipid amount and synthesis rate, the following mechanisms have to be discussed. The type II pneumocyte differentiates to the type I pneumocyte (Adamson et al. 1970; Maisin 1970). Only type II pneumocytes contain large amounts of phosphatidylcholine. On the other hand macrophages remove phospholipids from the alveolar surface. After irradiation the number of macrophages is reduced and phosphatidylcholine might be accumulated. Thus besides synthesis and degradation (biochemical processes), changes in the different cell populations also play a role.

Rubin and colleagues (1986) found no biphasic course of surfactant. They studied biochemically surfactant and ultrastructurally type II pneumocytes (Penney and Rubin 1977; Penney et al. 1981, 1982a,b; Rubin et al. 1980, 1983, 1986; Shapiro et al. 1981, 1984). One hour after 10–30 Gy the number of lamellar bodies of type II pneumocytes decreased. At the same time surfactant phospholipids increased markedly in the alveolar space. The increase in phospholipids in the alveolar lavage was accompanied by a decrease in phospholipids in the lung tissue. Thus the type II pneumocyte seems to be a highly radiosensitive cell that expresses radiation damage very early. On the other hand there is evidence that type II pneumocytes can recover within the 1st month after exposure as lamellar bodies showed hyperplasia. The latter finding might mean that synthesis is increased but secretion of surfactant is decreased.

Rubin et al. (1980, 1983) reported on observations which provided evidence that in mice alveolar surfactant release uncovered hours to days after irradiation may be an early biochemical marker that predicts for subsequent pneumonitis radiation injury. The increases in surfactant (at 7 and/or 28 days postradiation) and lethality were of comparable steepness over the dose range of about 12–15 Gy. However, doubt has been cast on this hypothesis (Down et al. 1988). It has been pointed out that while neutron irradiation is between 1.5 and 2 times as efficient as x-rays in causing radiation pneumonitis, these two qualities of radiation have closely similar effects on surfactant levels in CFLP mice (Fowler et al. 1982; Phillips et al. 1974; Ahier et al. 1985). Furthermore, when Rubin et al. (1986) studied surfactant levels in different mouse strains and rabbits, clear differences were found to exist between the mouse strains. For instance in LAF1 and C3H mice the increase in surfactant was observed at very different times. In rabbits the threshold for lethality was higher by a factor of about 2.5 when compared with that for surfactant release (Rubin et al. 1986). In reply to the critique of Down et al. (1988), Rubin (1988) agreed that the mechanism for surfactant release which is controlled by a β-adrenergic mechanism may be different from the mechanism for death of type II cells. However, it was pointed out that with the development of a radioimmunoassay specific for the apoprotein of surfactant the bronchoalveolar lavage assays have become more reproducible and accurate than the original phospholipid assays based upon detection of unsaturated phosphatidylcholine. In addition it was reported that the more recent rabbit data were more consistent with the mouse dose–response curves, in which the surfactant threshold more closely preceded lethality (Rubin 1988).

With regard to surfactant and lung function there exist some interesting older publications. Naimark et al. (1970) observed a decrease in phosphatidylcholine in lungs of rats at 4 months after irradiation and palmitate incorporation into the lung lipids was diminished. In parallel, a decreased compliance was found. However, this latter effect had already been observed 2 months prior to the biochemical alterations. In experiments by Gross (1978a) the decreased level of phosphatidylglycerol and phosphatidylethanolamine could not explain the reduced elasticity of the lung as the biochemical effect was only moderately pronounced.

Said et al. (1965) and Smith et al. (1963) assumed that besides the phospholipids other components such as fibrinogen can change the properties of surface tension in the alveolar film. A high amount of serum protein in the alveolar lavage fluid was found at about 4 weeks after irradiation of mice (Ahier et al. 1984). After doses of <10 Gy proteinosis resolved by 6 weeks, while after 15 Gy it persisted into the phase of pneumonitis. Gross (1978a) found large amounts of protein in the lavage material of lungs of mice after irradiation. He identified this partly as fibrinogen. A direct correlation existed between the protein content and increase in surface tension. Gross (1978a) suggested that surfactant is inactivated by forming a complex with a protein component. This might explain the discrepancy between the relatively slight decrease in phospholipids and the strong decline in compliance which is described above.

A large number of biochemical investigations have been performed with the aim of clarifying the process of radiation-induced lung fibrosis. Whole-body plethysmography (Travis 1979; Travis et al. 1980), studies with the radioprotective agent WR-2721 (Travis and Fowler 1982; Down et al. 1984; Miller et al. 1986a), work with a special strain of mice (Down et al. 1982; Down and Steel 1983), lung mortality dose–response curves (Siemann et al. 1982), fractionation experiments (Travis and Down 1981), and histological investigations (Travis and Down 1981; Travis et al. 1980) have provided some experimental evidence that a dissociation exists between early pneumonitis and late fibrotic changes. However, biochemical changes do not, in general, show clear demarcations between the two phases of injury (Coggle et al. 1986).

In mice lung weight was measured up to 18 weeks after irradiation by Sharplin and Franko (1982). In other studies lung density was investigated by computed tomography (Miller et al. 1986a; van Dyk and Hill 1983). There are cases in which an increase in lung weight or density correlates with an increase in hydroxyproline content (Dubrawsky et al. 1978, 1981). The amino acid hydroxyproline is found only in collagen and elastin. An absolute or relative increase in both appears to result in fibrosis.

There is considerable controversy about the nature of lung fibrosis induced by ionizing radiation. Biochemical studies disagree about the increased collagen content. Especially the significance of de novo synthesis of collagen and the relative increase due to depletion of lung parenchyma has to be further clarified (see below).

Tombropoulos and Thomas (1970) observed an increase in hydroxyproline in collagen and elastin after irradiation of rat lungs with 8 Gy. The maxima occurred at day 4 and day 8, respectively. The values decreased to control levels at day 8 and day 14, respectively. However, the study was performed only up to day 30 after irradiation. Obviously the effects were temporary. Dancewicz et al. (1976) found a decrease in hydroxyproline after 30 Gy during the acute phase; thereafter hydroxyproline increased.

In detailed studies Pickrell and colleagues investigated collagen metabolism in irradiated lungs Pickrell et al. 1975a,b, 1976a,b, 1978; Pickrell 1981; Pickrell and Mauderly 1981). In Syrian hamsters they found increased proline incorporation into collagen 14 weeks after doses of 40–60 Gy. It was suggested that collagen was newly synthesized. However, the content of collagen was only increased 7 weeks afterwards. The reason for this long latency period is not clear. At later time points proline incorporation was normal.

Law et al. (1976) found an increased hydroxyproline content per gram dry weight after 20–40 Gy. The increase took place between the 24th and 36th weeks after irradiation. No further changes were observed up to the 48th week. However, the hydroxyproline content per lung and the dry weight per lung decreased. This could mean that catabolism of collagen was inhibited and that there was no de novo synthesis of collagen. On the other hand histology showed that a large deposition of collagen took place (Law et al. 1976).

In several investigations the increase in collagen was dose dependent. Changes occurred earlier after higher doses than after lower doses (Law et al. 1976). Dubrawsky et al. (1978) found in rats a dose-dependent increase in collagen concentration as a result of reduction in total lung weight. Ward et al. (1983, 1985) observed a dose-dependent increase in collagen after doses between 10 and 30 Gy. Coggle et al. (1986) exposed the thorax of mice to x-ray doses of between 5 and 15 Gy. The collagen content was significantly elevated after 15 Gy. Travis et al. (1985) measured hydroxyproline content per lung and found only a poor correlation between dose and collagen accumulation.

Walklin and co-workers irradiated the whole thorax of mice and measured the ratio of type I (coarse fibered) to type III (meshwork) collagen and the activity of prolyl-4-hydroxylase and protein disulfide isomerase in irradiated mouse lung (Walklin and Law 1986; Walklin et al. 1987). Synthesis of procollagen was increased at 2 months after 5, 7.5, and 9 Gy. The maximal increase was observed 6–7 months after a dose of 9 Gy. The data indicate increased intracellular biosynthesis of procollagen during that time. Fibrosis was not observed. The discrepancy between synthesis and accumulation of collagen could not be explained by increased extracellular degradation, as x-irradiation had no influence on collagenase activity. On the other hand Pickrell et al. (1975a) found biosynthesis as well as degradation of collagen in Syrian hamster lungs. Changes in the ratio of different collagen types have been reported by Seyer et al. (1981), Reiser and Last (1981), and Kirk et al. (1983). It has been suggested that changes in enzyme activities may represent alterations in the balance of collagen types and an overall increase in the rate of collagen synthesis. The data of Walklin et al. (1987) did not confirm this assumption and led to the conclusion that the fibrotic changes are due to an increased procollagen synthesis.

Murray and Parkins (1987) measured collagen and protein synthesis in CBA mice. The ^{3}H-proline incorporation into collagen decreased 2 months after irradiation with doses between 8 and 16 Gy. It recovered at 4 months after treatment. Six months after irradiation the collagen synthesis rate increased in a dose-dependent fashion; after 14 Gy the synthesis rate was 4.6 times higher than in the control group. Yet, net accumulation of collagen was seen much later than the increase in synthesis rate. The authors found a slight increase in the ratio of type I to type III collagen. It is suggested that the turnover of newly synthesized collagen increases while the concentration of mature collagen is unchanged. This may explain the discrepancy between the increased synthesis rate and the lack of histological observation of fibrosis.

As yet it is unclear whether the accumulation of collagen is preceded by an increased breakdown and then by an increased biosynthesis as can be concluded from the experiments of Pickrell et al. (1975a, b, 1978). Murray and Parkins (1987), on the other hand, postulated an overall increase in collagen metabolism, which may lead to an increase as well as a decrease in lung collagen. There may be a balance of synthesis and breakdown.

Both might be accelerated at similar times. Increase or loss of collagen may depend on radiation dose and/or radiation fractionation.

In conclusion, collagen metabolism is affected by ionizing radiation. The experimental results are conflicting. The time course of collagen deposition seems to differ from species to species (GROSS 1977b). It also depends on mouse strain and radiation dose (DOWN and STEEL 1983; TRAVIS 1980a). For mice a threshold dose for fibrosis was reported which is 13–15 Gy at about 24 weeks after treatment (LAW 1985; TRAVIS 1980a). In contrast, MILLER et al. (1986b) and PENNEY et al. (1986) demonstrated fibrosis at a year or later after doses as low as 5 Gy. WALKLIN et al. (1987) found no histological signs of lung fibrosis 1 year after 5 Gy, but foci of septal fibrosis were observed later than 24 weeks after 10 Gy. PHILLIPS (1966) observed an effect 2–3 months after 20 Gy in rats. The changes were progressive up to 1 year (PHILLIPS and MARGOLIS 1974). In mice the effect seems to occur later. MAISIN (1970) found deposition of collagen not before 8 months postradiation. LAW et al. (1976) obtained comparable results.

With regard to collagen synthesis rate, it is not clear whether a decreasing synthesis rate is due to a depletion or inhibition of collagen-producing cells. It is not yet possible to identify the target cells in lung, because many cell types are able to synthesize collagen (RENNARD et al. 1982). Increased collagen biosynthesis may be due to increased intracellular enzyme activity or to stimulated proliferation of collagen-producing cells (WAHL 1985). An increased labeling index was found after x-irradiation. This could mean that lung fibroblasts are stimulated to proliferate (ADAMSON and BOWDEN 1983). Differences in radiosensitivity and proliferation of such cells could be responsible for the species-specific reactions. As long as these cells are not identified in more detail or cannot be isolated, a clear understanding of the biochemical changes cannot be obtained.

Collagen content has been stated in various ways: per whole lung, per mg protein, per gram dry weight, per gram wet weight. It is arguable which is the most appropriate way when describing radiation effects on collagen metabolism. Another problem arises with the measurement of protein synthesis rate in vivo based upon the incorporation of radioactive labeled amino acids (PETERKOVSKY and PROCKOP 1962; LAURENT et al. 1978; LAURENT 1982). It is not known to what extent the specific activity of the free pool is changed after irradiation. Consequently the results should be considered with caution. To diminish this problem high levels of unlabeled precursors have been used, but it is possible that these high concentrations affect synthesis rates. Studies from HILDEBRAN et al. (1981) and BAICH et al. (1980) showed that the protein and collagen synthesis rates are apparently not influenced by changes in proline concentrations. However, it is not known whether the endogeneous hydroxyproline pool remains unchanged after irradiation.

Another insight into the mechanisms involved in the development of lung fibrosis comes from investigation of glycosaminoglycans (GAG). These are complex, long-chain polyanionic polysaccharides. They are a component of the amorphous ground substances of all connective tissues. The GAG content in a normal lung is less than 0.5% of dry weight and the synthesis rate is very low. Therefore it is very difficult to study the GAG metabolism. KARLINSKY (1982) measured GAG concentration in hamster lung after bleomycin treatment. The total amount of GAG was elevated in fibrotic lung but the relative distribution of all GAG subtypes remained unchanged. DROZDZ et al. (1981) found an increase in total GAG content after a single dose of 5 Gy in rat lungs, an increase in hyaluronic acid, and a decrease in heparin. It seems that GAG increased before changes in collagen content occurred. Research into GAG metabolism and radiation-induced changes could be a new and interesting way to study mechanisms which lead to radiation fibrosis, because it is obvious that irradiation produces severe disturbances in GAG metabolism.

The interaction between cells and extracellular matrix are of increasing interest with regard to the pathogenesis of fibrosis. PENNEY and ROSENKRANS (1984) and ROSENKRANS and PENNEY (1985, 1986) found a dose-dependent decrease in proteoglycans in alveolar as well as in capillary basal lamina relatively early after irradiation. Later a replacement was observed, during which proteoglycans increased. An increase was also found for laminin and fibronectin (ROSENKRANS and PENNEY 1987). It is suggested that loss of matrix components is followed by recruitment of fibroblasts through the secretion of fibronectin (RENNARD et al. 1981) and alveolar macrophage derived growth factor from activated macrophages and neutrophils (BITTERMANN et al. 1982). Fibronectin has chemotactic and fibrinogenic activities and acts on fibroblasts.

Both fibronectin and the mentioned growth factor may have an influence on fibrillogenesis.

Several other biochemical studies have been performed after experimental irradiation. Koc-mierska-Grodzka and Gerber (1974) observed an increase in β-glucuronidase. Oledzka-Slotvinska and Maisin (1970) found changes in mucopolysaccharides. Fibrinolysis was increased after irradiation (Fleming et al. 1962). Caulet et al. (1970) reported on a decrease in alkaline and an increase in acid phosphatase as well as an increase in β-glucuronidase at the time when collagen deposition started.

Dancewicz et al. (1976) studied various enzyme activities. During the first, exudative phase lysosome enzymes such as acid phosphatase and cathepsin were increased. But 2 weeks after irradiation cathepsin decreased. It is possible that this decrease correlates with macrophage depletion (Moayer and Riley 1969). In the fibrotic phase cathepsin and β-glucuronidase increased again.

Furthermore, Dancewicz et al. (1976) observed a temporary increase in serotonin after irradiation. The authors suggest that this finding is related to changes in vascular permeability. At later times the serotonin level increased again. Concomitantly mast cell infiltration of the lung was found. Dancewicz et al. (1976) also found reduced fibrinolytic activity. It was assumed that this was related to fibrin deposition in the alveoli and capillaries. Similar findings were reported by Fleming et al. (1962). Immunological effects have also been observed (Mancini et al. 1965; Kumar et al. 1985). Lissner et al. (1966) concluded from findings after unilateral lung irradiation in rabbits that autoimmunological mechanisms are responsible for development of lung fibrosis.

There are many discrepancies and ambiguities in biochemical data. Nevertheless, one can summarize that radiation-induced decrease in surfactant leads to severe functional disturbancies. These are followed by development of fibrosis. Two mechanisms are responsible for mechanical changes of respiration: increase in surface power and changes in the composition of lung parenchyma. Both factors can be measured by biochemical methods, but not in a satisfactory way.

13.2.3 Physiological Changes

The histological and biochemical changes result in alterations of lung function which have been studied with physiological methods. Sweany et al. (1959) irradiated the thorax of dogs with single x-ray doses between about 10 and 29 Gy or fractionated doses of 30–48 Gy with weekly doses of 2 or 3 Gy. The static compliance of the whole thorax, of the thoracic wall, and of the lung was measured, as were the functional residual capacity, the diffusion capacity, and the arterial and venous pressure of the lung vessels. Early after irradiation histopathological changes were observed. However, lung function remained unchanged. Clear effects on functional parameters were found 20 weeks after irradiation. The pressure in pulmonary vessels increased 24 weeks after irradiation. This was found just at the time when fibrosis, cellular infiltration, obstruction of vessel diameter, etc. occurred. The morphological alterations were considered to be responsible for the disturbed gas exchange and the subsequent decrease in arterial oxygen tension. Moss and Haddy (1960) found a decrease in compliance 4 weeks after irradiation of rats. The effect was less severe when the animals were irradiated under high oxygen pressure. Interestingly, hyperplasia of adrenal glands was seen under these conditions. The authors assumed that lung damage was decreased by increased corticoid production.

Teates (1965) irradiated the hemithorax of dogs with a total dose of about 45 Gy in 23–27 days. Lung function was measured up to 21 weeks after irradiation. The measured parameters were inspiration volume, oxygen uptake, carbon dioxide release, diffusion capacity, and compliance. Starting at 6 weeks after irradiation the values for all parameters decreased continuously. Teates (1965) found a high interindividual variability for morphological tissue reaction as well as for functional parameters. Generally, compliance and pulmonary blood flow decreased. From the ratio of oxygen uptake to carbon dioxide release he concluded that no alveolocapillary block existed. A disproportion between ventilation and perfusion or decreased alveolar ventilation seemed to be the reason for the reduced diffusion capacity. However, these studies also showed that overall lung function (irradiated plus nonirradiated) was not impaired. This is an indication of the good compensatory potential of nonirradiated lung tissue. Rüfer et al. (1973) measured pressure–

volume relationships in the isolated rat lung up to 14 weeks after irradiation. Morphological changes appeared relatively early but functional disturbances of respiration were not observed until later. They assumed that surfactant, which was reduced after the 14th week following irradiation, played a dominant role: functional disturbances were prevented by a sufficient concentration of surfactant before that time.

TRAVIS et al. (1979) studied the function of mouse lung by a plethysmographic method. They measured respiratory frequency and amplitude. After a threshold dose of 11 Gy the frequency increased and the amplitude decreased. Both effects occurred before onset of fibrosis in the 16th week after irradiation.

The functional, plethysmographic method is comparatively sensitive, because changes are seen after relatively low radiation doses. The method is noninvasive and quantitative. However, interpretation of the amplitude signal is difficult due to the complexity of lung alterations. The signal reflects changes in ventilation, lung volume, respiratory flow volume, and resistance of respiratory flow. All these parameters can be changed simultaneously.

SHRIVASTAVA et al. (1974) irradiated both lungs of mice similar to the experiments of TRAVIS et al. (1979). They found a decrease in compliance 6 weeks after irradiation with 15 Gy. Also in these studies functional changes preceded histological collagen deposition. Inflammation, edema, pleural effusion, and focal atelectasis were detected earlier. Doses lower than 15 Gy had no influence on the pressure–volume relationship.

FINE et al. (1979) irradiated the upper pulmonary lobe of baboons. Doses ranged between 30 and 40 Gy. Twenty-four weeks after irradiation the pressure–volume relationship was not changed in comparison to the control group. Elastin content per gram dry weight was increased in the upper lobe as well as in the nonirradiated lower lobe. However, the dry weight of the upper lobe was decreased and other constituents such as cellular elements had diminished, and the elastin increase may have been relative. The lower lobe, in contrast, showed hypertrophy; therefore the elastin and also the collagen content were absolutely higher. From these data the authors concluded that the accumulation of connective tissue does not lead to changes in the pressure–volume relationship, when it occurs in non-unfolded parts of lung or as a result of compensatory lung growth.

Thus alterations in the pressure–volume relationship have to be considered critically, especially when lung irradiation is inhomogeneous or the reactions of different parts of the lungs differ.

GROSS (1978a) studied the elasticity of thorax wall, lung tissue, and alveolar surface. Four weeks after irradiation he found a decrease in the compliance of the whole lung after 24 Gy, given in two fractions. The thoracic wall was less involved (GROSS 1978a; SHRIVASTAVA et al. 1974; SWEANY et al. 1959). The decrease in compliance is mainly due to changes in lung tissue. GROSS (1978a) found a decrease in alveolar surface elasticity during the pneumonitis phase, 4 months after irradiation; the elasticity of the thoracic wall and of the lung parenchyma remained unchanged. Between the 2nd and the 12th week after irradiation no changes in the alveolar surface compliance were observed. (GROSS 1978b).

The studies show that irradiation causes alterations of lung function. As yet it is unclear how the described histological changes, especially those of capillaries, are related to the functional alterations during radiation pneumonitis. Generally it can be assumed that a decrease in compliance of the alveolar surface increases the respiratory work. This is followed by a disturbed balance between ventilation and perfusion and leads to an impaired gas exchange resulting in the typical signs of radiation pneumonitis. Functional changes observed later than 20 weeks after irradiation are assumed to be due to radiation fibrosis.

13.2.4 Mechanisms in the Development of Radiation Pneumonitis

As stated by COGGLE et al. (1986), the pathogenesis of radiation pneumonitis remains a puzzle of cause and effect. Obviously, alterations or lesions of the alveolar epithelium as well as of capillaries play an important role.

According to RUBIN and CASARETT (1968) the injury of the vascular network is the predominant event in the development of radiation pneumonitis. Swelling of endothelium, congestion, thrombosis, increased vascular permeability, edema, fibrin exudation, diapedesis, and activation of fibroblasts are considered to be the characteristic effects. Furthermore they reported that these alterations are associated with or followed by destruction and obliteration of blood vessels and sclerosis of connective tissue. Finally, localized atelectasis, compensatory emphysema, secondary infection, and more fibrosis may occur. There are several further publications which support the idea that in principle the damage is vascular, with sloughing of dead and dying endothelial cells followed by capillary leakage into the interstitium and onto the alveolar surface (PHILLIPS 1966; GROSS 1980a; MAISIN 1970; JENNINGS and ARDEN 1962; PHILLIPS et al. 1962).

In contrast VAN DEN BRENK (1971) assumed that damage to the epithelial cells is of the highest importance. He suggested that radiation-induced impairment of cell proliferation leads to progressive depopulation of alveolar cells, which is followed by a lack of surfactant, exudative alterations, atelectasis, and a nonspecific inflammatory response as a consequence of alveolar cell death. Reticuloendothelial cells present in the lung and derived from the blood were supposed to be involved in the inflammatory reaction. With progressing fibrosis the fine network of elastic fibers is replaced by collagenic cicatrization. In parallel, rarefaction of blood vessels occurs.

Considering the alveolar epithelium as the primary target, it is not only death and dysfunction of type II pneumocytes with seriously altered levels of surfactant (VAN DEN BRENK 1968; RUBIN et al. 1980; NAIMARK et al. 1970; GROSS 1978b) which may be the decisive event. Other investigations suggest that necrosis and sloughing of type I cells, leaving denuded basement membranes and alveolar debris, are the fundamental alteration (MAISIN 1970; GROSS 1981; ADAMSON et al. 1970). The extent of final injury may also depend on hyperplasia and differentiation of type II cells which repair the radiation-induced damage of the alveolar epithelial layer (GROSS 1981). Finally there are publications pointing out the important role of lymphocytes (BENNET et al. 1969) and the immune system (MADRAZO et al. 1973). A final conclusion with regard to the predominant mechanism in the development of radiation pneumonitis cannot be drawn at present.

13.2.5 Radiation Pneumonitis: Dose-Effect Relationship, Fractionation, Dose Rate, and Recovery

A direct assay of target cell response has not been developed. Therefore it is difficult to define a representative endpoint which allows a dose–effect relationship for radiation-induced lung dam-

age to be established. PHILLIPS and MARGOLIS (1972) observed that mice died from pulmonary injury at 80–180 days after irradiation of the thorax. In a number of studies the $LD_{50/80-180}$ is determined. The dose required to kill 50% of animals between 80 and 180 days after irradiation is used as a measure of radiation response of the lung. In general, the $LD_{50/180}$ value ranges from 10–14 Gy for a single acute x-ray dose. It varies with species and strain (WARA et al. 1973; FIELD et al. 1976; COGGLE et al. 1986; TRAVIS 1987).

Fractionated application of the total radiation dose is the common way by which sparing of normal tissues is achieved in clinical radiotherapy. The lung shows greater sparing from dose fractionation than do more rapidly proliferating tissues (DUTREIX et al. 1979; VEGESNA et al. 1985). When a dose of 10 Gy is given in four fractions to the lungs of mice or rats the frequency of pneumonitis is reduced to the level seen after a single dose of 5.7 or 7.2 Gy respectively (WARA et al. 1973; DUTREIX and WAMBERSIE 1975).

Different formalistic models adjust total doses to achieve equivalent tissue effects (isoeffects) with change in fractionation pattern. WARA et al. (1973) studied the $LD_{50/80-180}$ in mice after fractionated irradiation with up to 20 fractions. Applying the formalism introduced by ELLIS (1969, 1971), WARA et al. (1973) determined the exponents for N (number of fractions) and T (overall treatment time) as 0.38 and 0.06 respectively.

Comparable figures were found by FIELD et al. (1976). Using the LD_{50} (between 40 and 180 days) after irradiation of the thorax of mice as a measure of lung damage, the exponent for N was 0.39 when x-irradiation was given in eight fractions. In the case of 8–30 fractions it was 0.25. The exponent for T was 0.07 and was independent of the number of fractions. In pigs various clinical and physiological parameters were used to determine isoeffective doses. The radiogenic lung reaction was adequately described by a similar relation: $D \sim N^{0.32} \cdot T^{0.05}$ (HERRMANN et al. 1986a,b). The finding that the LD_{50} increases with increasing treatment time (FIELD and HORNSEY 1977) is somewhat unexpected. FIELD et al. (1976) argued that repopulation cannot be the reason for sparing with increasing time because lung is a very slowly proliferating tissue. As shown in Fig. 13.1, the $LD_{50/180}$ value increased with increasing time intervals between fractions. The most dramatic changes occurred over the first few hours after the first x-ray treatment due to repair of sublethal

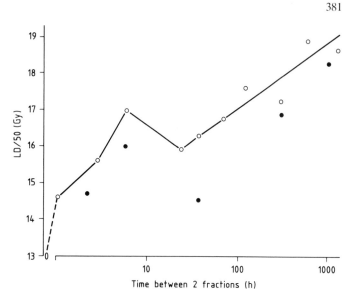

Fig. 13.1. The $LD_{50/80-180}$ (Gy) as a function of the time interval between two fractions of x-rays. At the time point 0 a single dose of 13 Gy was given. Time is plotted on a logarithmic scale. (Data from FIELD 1977; FIELD et al. 1976)

damage. For time intervals greater than 6 h the increase in $LD_{50/180}$ was less, about 0.08 Gy per day, up to 28 days (FIELD AND HORNSEY 1974; FIELD 1977). This latter phenomenon was considered to be a process of "slow repair."

In the case of neutron irradiation the LD_{50} increased when a dose was split into two fractions. However, there was no significant difference when the number of fractions was increased to 15 and given in the same overall treatment time (FIELD et al. 1976). In conclusion, for neutron irradiation there is much reduced repair and no evidence of the "slow repair" component (FIELD 1977). Repair factors for neutrons were also small in the experiments of PARKINS et al. (1985) and PARKINS and FOWLER (1985). FIELD et al. (1977) reported that the RBE for a 7.8 Gy single neutron dose is 1.5. In the investigations of PARKINS et al. (1985) the RBE was approximately 1.8 at a single neutron dose of 6 Gy and increased to approximately 5 at the lowest dose per fraction measured. High RBE values (>4) have also been observed with fractionated neutron irradiation in beagles (ALDERSON et al. 1979; BRADLEY et al. 1977). In pigs, for fractionated 6.2 MeV neutrons the RBE value was about 4 (HERRMANN et al. 1986b). Comparable to the above-described observations of Field (1977), extension of the overall treatment time in pigs did not result in an important increase in ED_{50} level (HERRMANN et al. 1986b).

Using the lethality and breathing rate assay, PARKINS and FOWLER (1985) studied the fractionation response with low doses per fraction down to 1.1 Gy x-rays and 0.18 Gy of 3 MeV neutrons.

Similar to the data of VEGESNA et al. (1985), the results indicated that further significant sparing of x-ray-induced lung damage could be observed when the size of the dose per fraction was reduced from 1.6 Gy to approximately 1.1 Gy per fraction, even for two fractions per day with a 6-h interval. Both pneumonitis and fibrosis could be spared by this procedure. However, no such repair was seen with fractionated fast neutrons. Furthermore it was pointed out that there is still an experimental gap to be filled between the administered doses per fraction of 1.1 Gy and the predicted continuing extra repair down to about 0.3 Gy per fraction.

With regard to the number of fractions per day (2.75 or 3 Gy per fraction, 1.8 Gy/min), a loss of repair for pneumonitis in mice was not clearly demonstrated at up to ten fractions of x-rays, although the possibility of such a loss having occurred could not be excluded. There was no suggestion of a loss of repair for fibrosis after the same number of fractions (TRAVIS et al. 1983a). Also in these experiments the repair capacity was tested by lethality and breathing rate.

These results, like those of all other fractionation studies published since 1985, can be described using the linearquadratic formalism, with the fractionation sensitivity given by the α/β dose. Table 13.2 lists α/β values derived from animal experiments and clinical analyses of pneumonitis and lung fibrosis responses.

Several authors have reported α/β ratios for lung tissue (TRAVIS et al. 1985, 1987a,b; VEGESNA et al. 1985; PARKINS et al. 1985). Summarizing experimental data, WITHERS (1987) reported on

Table 13.2. α/β ratios and repair halftimes for lung damage

	α/β	Repair halftime: T½	Author
Mouse		0.76 h (trend toward shorter halftime with large fraction sizes)	Travis et al. (1987a)
Mouse		0.8–1.2h	Parkins et al. 1988)
Mouse	3.74 Gy	0.84 h	Down et al. (1986)
Mouse	4.0 Gy	0.75 h	Vegesna et al. (1989)
Mouse	3.7 Gy, analysis of data from Travis et al. (1987a)		Thames et al. (1989)
Mouse	3.7 Gy, analysis of data from Vegesna et al. (1985)		Thames et al. (1989)
Mouse	2.5–4.0 Gy, analysis of data from Parkins et al. (1985)		Tucker and Travis (1990)
Mouse	5.5 Gy, analysis of data from Field et al. (1976)		Tucker and Travis (1990)
Mouse	3.7 Gy, analysis of data from Wara et al. (1973)		Tucker and Travis (1990)
Mouse	about 3.0 Gy (ignoring a time factor)		Fowler (1990)
Rat	3.5 Gy (pneumonitis) 2.3 Gy (fibrosis)	0.95 h (pneumonitis) 1.13 h (fibrosis)	van Rongen et al. (1990)
Rat	2.7 Gy (ignoring a time factor)		van Dyk et al. (1990)
Pig	3.7 Gy		Herrmann et al. (1986a, 1987)
Animals	5.0 ± 1.0 Gy (acute damage) 2.0 Gy (late damage)	Analysis of data from the literature, including a factor for overall treatment time	van Dyk et al. (1989)
Human	3.3 ± 1.5 Gy		van Dyk et al. (1989)

values ranging from 2.5 to 4.5 Gy. Thames and Hendry (1987) gave values between 2.1 and 4.3 (LD$_{50}$/pneumonitis). In relatively large animals such as pigs the α/β ratio was 3.7 (Herrmann et al. 1986a). Parkins et al. (1985) obtained an α/β ratio of 3 Gy after irradiation with x-rays. In contrast, after application of neutrons (3 MeV, Van de Graaff accelerator) the values were 30–40 Gy. Travis et al. (1987b) found a ratio of 28 Gy in the case of irradiation with neon ions.

The effect of protracted irradiation of the lung has been studied by inhalation of radioactive nuclides in dogs. A relatively brief exposure to the β-emitter ^{90}Y caused death at between 30 and 200 days in 50% of the animals after a cumulative dose of about 100 Gy. In the case of protracted exposure to the β-emitter ^{90}Sr the animals died at between 180 and 450 days after a cumulative dose

of about 560 Gy (McClellan et al. 1976). Similar data were reported for acute death from pneumonitis and fibrosis in dogs that had inhaled the α-emitter ^{239}PuO$_2$ (Park et al. 1972). In these experiments it was clearly shown that the protracted exposure to irradiation is beneficial with regard to survival. The sparing effect of low dose rate irradiation has been observed in a number of x-irradiation experiments. Hill (1983) and Lopez Cardozo et al. (1985) determined the LD$_{50}$ at 180 days after thoracic irradiation. A decrease in the dose rate led to an increase in the LD$_{50}$. For dose rates of 1.1 Gy/min (mice) and 0.8 Gy/min (rats) the LD$_{50}$ values were 11 and 13.3 Gy, whereas for 0.08 Gy/min they were 20 Gy and 22.7 Gy respectively. An effect of dose rate was also found when lung function was tested by measuring carbon monoxide uptake (Depledge and Barrett

1982). The impairment of lung function increased with increasing dose rate over the range 0.02–1 Gy/min. Recently DOWN et al. (1986) provided evidence for much less dose sparing with 0.05 Gy/min than with a conventional fractionated schedule of 2 Gy per fraction. Only at dose rates as low as 0.02 Gy/min was single protracted irradiation comparable to fractionation in allowing sublethal repair. Comparable observations have been reported by TARBELL et al. (1987). Further details concerning the significance of dose rate in lung irradiation will be discussed in Sect. 13.4.

13.3 The Lung as a Critical Organ in Conventional Radiotherapy, Alone and in Combination with Chemotherapy

The evaluation of histopathological alterations in the irradiated human lung can be complicated by secondary effects such as infections, sequelae of heart and circulatory diseases, and postmortem artifacts. JENNINGS and ARDEN (1962) investigated the influence of dose and time on the development of radiation pneumonitis. Especially the following effects were registered: edema, blood stasis, atelectasis, fibrin exudation into alveoli, epithelial alterations, fibrillar thickening and cellular infiltration of alveolar walls, fibrosis, and proliferative alterations of blood vessels. However, the observations concerning edema, blood stasis, and atelectasis did not differ between irradiated and unirradiated lungs. In 165 cases a few or all of the above-described histopathological changes occurred. The time intervals between irradiation and autopsy ranged between <30 days and >5 years. The applied irradiation techniques were the typical ones in the USA for the period 1950–1956.

Forty-one percent of the lungs showed fibrinous membranes. These were most frequent and pronounced at 6–24 months after irradiation with doses >20 Gy. Generally, they could be observed from 30 days to 5 years after irradiation.

Three types of proliferative alterations of the connective tissue were prominent. Increases in the cell number in the alveolar septa, in particular of histiocytes and fibroblasts, occurred in 16% of the cases, especially after doses of 20–50 Gy. Twenty-seven percent of the lungs showed fibrillar deposits in the alveolar septa. These were most frequent after doses >30 Gy and when the time interval after irradiation was longer than 6 months. Fibro-

sis of septa was found at a frequency of 42%. Surprisingly in a few cases fibrosis was already observed at 30 days after irradiation. However, the incidence of fibrosis was relatively high when the time intervals were 6 months or longer. Although the lungs were investigated very carefully, proliferative alterations of the blood vessels such as obliterations were found in only 14%.

Reviewing the literature, GROSS (1977b) concluded that microscopic studies of lungs of patients who died 4–12 weeks after radiotherapy revealed changes of all irradiated lung structures. Several groups described atypical, hypertrophic, and desquamated alveolar epithelial cells (WARREN and SPENCER 1940; JENNINGS and ARDEN 1962; BENNET et al. 1969; MARGOLIS and PHILLIPS 1969). Thrombi of small arterial vessels, as well as blood congestion, were related to vascular injury (JACOBSEN 1940; MARGOLIS and PHILLIPS 1969). Furthermore edema and alterations of the intima and media concurrent with an increased number of lipid-containing, subintimal macrophages were observed (BENNET et al. 1969). Several studies reported on fibrin-like deposits in the alveoli, hyaline membranes, and early thickening of the alveolar septa due to edema, infiltration of mononuclear cells, and accumulations of connective tissue material (WARREN and SPENCER 1940; JENNINGS and ARDEN 1962; MARGOLIS and PHILLIPS 1969; BENNET et al. 1969). Six months and later after irradiation thickening of alveolar walls, fibrosis, and in some cases a decrease in vascular supply were the typical histological alterations. Although the histopathological studies in humans have been less systematic than experimental investigations, the findings underline the common features of response after irradiation of the lung.

Pneumonitis can be a very serious clinical event, especially after irradiation of a large volume of the lung. However, if it is mild it may subside spontaneously (CASARETT 1980). On the other hand, severe reactions in parts of the lung may progress so that fibrosis develops. Clinical characteristics of pneumonitis are acute violent cough and shortness of breath; striation, mottling, and cloudiness constitute the x-ray picture (Fig. 13.2) (EICHHORN et al. 1983). The development of clinical signs of pneumonitis depends significantly on the total radiation dose, the fractionation schedule, and the irradiated volume of the lung (RUBIN and CASARETT 1968; PHILLIPS and MARGOLIS 1972; MOLLS et al. 1986). The time sequence of the pulmonary alterations is given in Table 13.1.

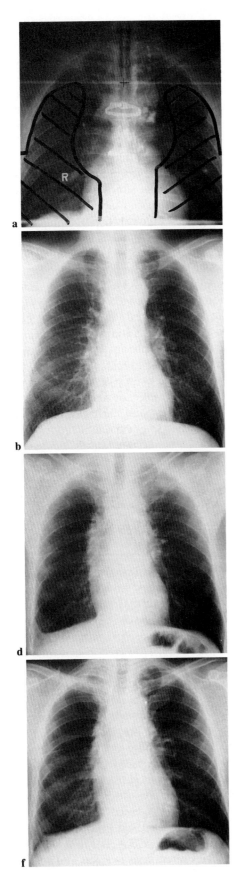

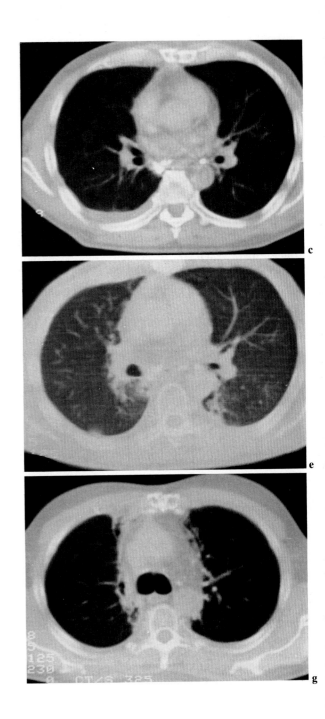

Fig. 13.2a-g. Radiographs and CT-scans of a 59 years old patient with a low malignant non-Hodgkin lymphoma of the mediastinum. **a** Tumor resection by thoracotomy and subsequent mantle-field irradiation. The total dose was 36 Gy, 5x2 Gy per week. **b, c** The first radiographic and computertomographic control reveals no pathological alteration at 4 weeks after completion of radiotherapy **d, e** six months after irradiation radiographic signs of pneumonitis were observed in the paramediastinal region of the radiation field as well as a small pleural effusion in the right co-stodiaphragmatic recessus. **f, g** Eighteen months after irradiation pneumonitis has developed into fibrosis

With regard to the radiosensitivity of the human lung, there are clinical observations after single-dose and fractionated irradiation, either of the whole lung or of parts of it. We will outline some fundamental aspects which are of practical importance in the case of conventionally fractionated irradiation. Data obtained after half and in particular total body irradiation prior to bone marrow transplantation are discussed in the following section.

A recent study in adults has generated a dose–response relationship between radiation-induced pulmonary damage and the estimated single-dose representation of fractionated radiotherapy schedules. MAH et al. (1987) measured the increase in lung density within the irradiated volume by computed tomography. Fifty-four patients with various malignancies of the thorax completed the prospective study. A 50% incidence of pulmonary damage was found for 1000 ± 40 ED (estimated single dose) units, which corresponds to 33 Gy in 15 fractions over 19 days (2.2 Gy per fraction). A lung dose of 24.7 Gy in 15 daily fractions yielded a comparatively low incidence of only 5%. NEWTON and SPITTLE (1969) treated adults with pulmonary metastases by irradiation of the total thorax with doses of 20 or 25 Gy given at daily fractions of 1.5 Gy. Survival of patients ranged between 1 and 85 months (mean: 15 months). No early or late pulmonary complications were observed, whereas in seven patients who received 30 Gy at daily fractions of 3 Gy, radiotherapy resulted in an unacceptable incidence of radiation pneumonitis. After lung irradiation of patients with macroscopic or suspected subclinical metastases with a dose of 20 Gy given in ten fractions, no radiation pneumonitis occurred (BREUR et al. 1978; COX 1972). According to PHILLIPS and MARGOLIS (1972), the dose that will cause clinical pneumonitis in 5% of patients is about 26 Gy in 20 fractions.

It is well known that morphological pulmonary alterations are observed even if only a part of the thorax is irradiated (JENNINGS and ARDEN 1962; CARMEL and KAPLAN 1976; GROSS 1977b). The frequency of radiographically detected lung alterations after treatment for breast cancer is relatively high. Doses to the chest wall of 35–60 Gy yielded lung alterations in 6%–90% of patients (HERRMANN and MOLLS, in press). Recently it was reported that almost every one of 263 patients had radiographic evidence of apical pulmonary fibrosis but that only 12% had symptomatic pneumonitis

(LEVITT and PEREZ 1987). Thus, the clinical expression of radiation injury of a comparatively small lung volume is uncommon due to the anatomical and functional reserve. Obviously the lung can tolerate relatively high doses when only part of the organ is irradiated.

This can also be concluded from the clinical experience in Hodgkin's disease. KAPLAN (1972) reported radiation-induced lung morbidity in only 6% of the patients who were treated with mantle field technique (6 MeV linear accelerator). Yet, a high rate of radiographic pneumonitis and fibrosis was observed in the patients studied in Freiburg (SLANINA 1977; SLANINA et al. 1977, 1982), although without severe functional alterations. Chest x-rays were taken in 119 patients during mantle field irradiation with a 4 MeV linear accelerator (extended field satellite technique and tumor doses of 40–46 Gy) and at routine follow-up examinations (SLANINA et al. 1982). On average, onset of pneumonitis was observed 12 weeks after the start of radiotherapy. After 15 weeks a florid pneumonitis and after 20 weeks a florid pneumonitis with initial signs of shrinkage occurred. After 5–9 months (average: 34 weeks) the pulmonary reaction terminated in stable paramediastinal lung fibrosis (Fig. 13.2). SLANINA and co-workers also observed that in no case did radiomorphological pneumonitis heal completely; rather, each case of pneumonitis developed into fibrosis. Grading the radioreaction, slight pneumonitis was found in 44% of cases, moderate pneumonitis in 29%, and severe pneumonitis in 16%. Clinical symptoms were observed only among those patients with a radiographically moderate or severe reaction. In a further group of patients, who had been treated earlier with telecobalt or orthovolt x-rays, the radiographic alterations were comparable with those described above. As regards functional alterations, slight and moderate restrictive disturbances of ventilation were found in 68%, impairment of oxygen diffusion in 18%, and obstructive disturbances of ventilation in 7%. Severe functional changes were not observed. Interestingly, oxygen diffusion was impaired to a significantly greater extent among smokers than among non-smokers (SLANINA et al. 1977; SLANINA 1977).

The highest lung doses are applied when radiotherapy is performed for lung cancer. The figures in the literature concerning the frequency of lung complications range between 0% and 75% for doses of 40–70 Gy. This demonstrates the different opinions of radiotherapists with regard to the severity of radiation-induced lung reactions (HERRMANN and MOLLS, in press). It also underlines that in the case of fractionated irradiation of a partial lung volume, relatively high doses can be given. Recently KOGA et al. (1988) reported that severe radiation pneumonitis was more often observed in elderly (70 years or more) patients with lung cancer than in younger ones (<70 years). In both age groups pneumonitis occurred earlier when the field size was 90 cm^2 or more. About one-third of the patients also received chemotherapy.

It has been pointed out that secondary complications are usually of greater clinical significance (COGGLE et al. 1986). In large areas of fibrosis, cystic or bronchiectatic alterations can be found. Furthermore, pleural effusion, spontaneous pneumothorax, and even bronchial obstruction as a consequence of tumor collapse have been reported (PHILLIPS and WYATT 1980). The main sequelae of radiation-induced fibrosis arise from shrinkage of lung volume. A shift of the mediastinum towards the irradiated side together with a deviation of the trachea may occur, as may pulmonary hypertension (PHILLIPS and WYATT 1980; PAGANI and LIBSHITZ 1982). The fact that fibrosed lung is prone to infection is also of importance. Such infection may exacerbate cardiac problems arising from pulmonary vascular damage, and in extreme cases right heart failure may develop (STONE et al. 1956).

Radiation therapists often encounter the problem of having to treat lung cancer patients with borderline lung function. In surgery the use of quantitative lung perfusion scanning has been demonstrated to be helpful for determining a patient's ability to undergo resection of lung (KANAREK 1983). Quantitative perfusion lung scanning and forced expiratory volume have also been used to predict pulmonary function following lung irradiation (RUBENSTEIN et al. 1988). From the serial follow-up observations it was concluded that such determinations can be of value in formulating a treatment plan for patients with significantly impaired pulmonary function.

There is a further important practical aspect in radiotherapy of thoracic organs. Frequently irradiation is performed after, concomitant with, or prior to chemotherapy. It is well known that some cytotoxic drugs alone may cause acute and late pulmonary toxicity. Summaries have been given by ROSENOW (1972), PHILLIPS et al. (1975), WEISS

and MUGGIA (1980), RUBIN (1984), and SCHEULEN (1987). Concerning the combination of radiotherapy and chemotherapy, a number of experimental and clinical studies have been dedicated to combined effects on the lung. Table 13.3 lists some of the most important chemotherapeutic substances and shows to what extent they may increase radia-

Table 13.3. Summary of experimental studies which provide evidence for drug-induced enhancement of lung morbidity[a]

Drug	Endpoint	Enhancement for drug given			Reference[b]
		Before	With	After	
Cyclo-phosphamide	Lethality		+++		1
	Lethality		+++		2
	Function	++	+++	++	3
Cisplatin	Lethality		−		2
	Function	−	−	−	4
	Function		−		2
Methotrexate	Lethality	−			1
	Lethality		−		2
	Function	+	−	−	4
	Function		−		2
Hydroxyurea	Lethality		−		5
Vincristine	Lethality		+		5
	Function	+	+	+	4
Actinomycin	Lethality	+	+++	−	5
	Lethality	−			1
	Function	−	+		4
Adriamycin	Lethality		+++		6
	Lethality	++			1
	Lethality		++	+	7
	Lethality		+++		2
	Function	−	+++	++	4
	Function		+++		2
Bleomycin	Lethality		−		5
	Lethality	++			1
	Lethality		++		2
	Function	++	++	++	4
	Function		+++		2
Mitomycin C	Lethality		+++		2
	Function		+++		2
BCNU	Lethality		−		5
5-Fluorouracil	Lethality		−		2
	Function		−		2

[a] The extent to which the drug increased the damage over that produced by irradiation alone is indicated by approximate dose enhancement factors (DEF): +++ DEF above 1.4; ++ DEF 1.2–1.4 + DEF up to about 1.2; − no effect. Before: 7–28 days before irradiation. After: 7–28 days after irradiation.
[b] References: 1, STEEL et al. 1979; 2, VAN DER MAASE et al. 1986; 3, COLLIS and STEEL 1983; 4, COLLIS 1981; 5, PHILLIPS et al. 1975; 6, REDPATH et al. 1978; 7, REDPATH et al. 1981 (from STEEL 1988, with modifications).

tion damage of the lung under experimental conditions. Obviously the combination with cisplatin has only a slight effect on the radiation response of the lung. We have irradiated the whole lung of sarcoma patients with lung metastases with a dose of 12 Gy given at a fractionation of 2×0.8 Gy per day. Thereafter the dose to a small volume (macroscopic metastasis) was increased to 50–65 Gy (5×2 Gy per week). During the 1st week of whole lung irradiation we also gave cisplatin (5×20 mg/m^2) and ifosfamide (3×50 mg). No serious pulmonary complications in this cisplatin-containing regimen were observed (ZAMBOGLOU et al. 1988). Cyclophosphamide and methotrexate are substances used in bone marrow transplantation. Special aspects related to the combination of these drugs with total body irradiation are discussed in the following section.

Treatment of small cell lung cancer, in which chemotherapy is given in combination with radiotherapy, is a paradigmatic situation. The combination of bleomycin + CTX + VCR + ADRIA with chest radiotherapy led to pulmonary fibrosis in 38% of patients and was fatal in 23% (EINHORN et al. 1976). However, irradiation with a regimen in which bleomycin was lacking (CTX + ADRIA + VCR) also resulted in pneumonitis in 37% of patients; about 50% of these cases were fatal (17% of the whole group) (JOHNSON et al. 1978). Interestingly, concurrent treatment for 6–9 weeks had the highest toxicity (25%–50% treatment-related toxic deaths, mostly from pulmonary injury), whereas toxic deaths were less frequent (about 10%) when concurrent treatment was performed for only 3 weeks (CATANE et al. 1981). A further reduction in pulmonary toxicity (so that only about 3% of patients were affected) apparently could be achieved when the same cytotoxic substances were applied sequentially with radiotherapy or concomitantly for only 10 days (CHOI and CAREY 1976; MOORE et al. 1978).

In conclusion, when radiotherapy to the chest is performed the lung is the dose-limiting organ. The combination of irradiation with chemotherapy may increase the risk of lung damage. At a dose of about 40 Gy given with conventional fractionation, morphological alterations of the lung can be expected in about 50% of the treated volumes (HERRMANN and MOLLS, in press). In most cases serious clinical symptoms will not arise if the irradiated lung volume is relatively small, i.e., less than 20% of total lung volume. After regimes which involve one-third to one-half of one lung,

pneumonitis with nonproductive cough, spiking fever, shortness of breath, and even respiratory distress will occur in about 10% of patients (COGGLE et al. 1986). In patients with borderline lung function the use of lung function tests can be helpful for deciding on a treatment plan. At least prior to radiotherapy the ratio between irradiated and unirradiated lung volume has to be assessed. The unirradiated part must be able to compensate for damage in the irradiated volume and guarantee sufficient lung function (HERRMANN and MOLLS, in press).

13.4 Interstitial Pneumonitis After Half and Total Body Irradiation Administered Prior to Bone Marrow Transplantation

The doses given in TBI prior to BMT damage not only the hematopoietic system but also other organs. While changes in lung function, such as transient restrictive ventilatory defect and prolonged disturbance of gas transfer, are of secondary importance, the development of interstitial pneumonitis (IP) may become a life-threatening event (DEPLEDGE et al. 1983; BARRETT et al. 1987; WEINER et al. 1986; DEEG et al. 1988). Therefore the lung has been considered to be the most important treatment-limiting organ in TBI followed by BMT.

There are large differences in the clinical practice of TBI between institutions. Total lung doses range between about 5 and 13 Gy. TBI is given as single-dose or fractionated irradiation. Schedules with one fraction per day differ from those with several daily fractions. The dose rate may be rather low (<0.06 Gy/min) or high (0.1–0.5 Gy/min) (BARRETT 1982a, b; SHANK et al. 1983; BAMBERG et al. 1986; MOLLS et al. 1987; QUAST 1987; DEEG et al. 1986, 1988; COSSET et al. 1989).

Treatment techniques (beams, fields, treatment conditions) as well as TBI dosimetry (dosimetry in the patient, heterogeneity correction, dose precision) vary considerably (VAN DYK 1987; QUAST 1986a, b, 1987). One of the most difficult problems in the planning of TBI is the determination of the dose to the lung (DUTREIX and BROERSE 1982; VAN DYK 1983, 1985; GLAESER 1986). Prior to TBI, CT scans might be helpful with regard to dosimetric calculations for the lung (GEISE and McCULLOUGH 1977; SONTAG et al. 1977; McCULLOUGH 1978.

Rosenblum et al. 1978, 1980; Lagrange et al. 1987; Mah and van Dyk 1988).

The above-mentioned differences in clinical practice, the uncertainties in the estimation of lung dose (about ± 15%), and differences in other factors contributing to lung morbidity (chemotherapeutic regimen, graft versus host disease prophylaxis, conditions of gnotobiotic care, patient selection, etc.) make it difficult to compare the currently used TBI procedures with regard to their risk of inducing pneumonitis. In the following, we describe some important features of TBI-related IP and try to delineate the critical points which have to be considered when aiming to achieve reduction of radiation-induced toxicity of the lung.

The median time from transplantation to onset of IP was nearly 2 months in a large group of 932 patients (Weiner et al. 1986), and thus shorter than after local thorax irradiation. The interstitial inflammatory alteration of the lung is associated with hypoxemia, air hunger, and shortness of breath. In addition to severe dyspnea, cough and fever may be further clinical symptoms. A chest radiograph shows interstitial markings which can be localized or, more frequently, diffuse (Deeg et al. 1988).

With CT densitometry increases in lung density were observed prior to the onset of respiratory changes. Since these CT findings could be correlated with the clinical course it has been suggested that CT lung densitometry should be used for prediction of lung complications before onset of clinical symptoms (El-Khatib et al. 1989).

Total body irradiation is a significant etiological factor in the pathogenesis of IP after BMT. However, there are also other influences which play an important role and which in principle are able to cause lung morbidity. These include chemical substances (cyclophosphamide, busulfan, methotrexate) and infections [Pneumocystis carinii, Legionella, Chlamydia trachomatis; cytomegalovirus (cmv), herpes simplex virus, varicella zoster virus]. The most frequent infectious agents are CMV and Pneumocystis carinii, in that order. The former may account for almost half the cases of IP observed after BMT. The large number of patients in whom no infectious agent can be detected are classified as having idiopathic IP. It is thought that these cases are directly due to irradiation and possibly to chemotherapy (Barrett 1982a,b; Deeg 1983; Buckner et al. 1984; Lopez Cardozo and Hagenbeek 1985; Lopez Cardozo et al. 1985; Molls et al. 1986; Deeg et al. 1988).

The frequency of IP increases steeply within a very short dose range (Rubin 1984). Fundamental data indicating the critical dose range have been obtained after half body irradiation. Upper half body irradiation of 150 patients (TBI was administered in a small number of patients) with large single doses at a dose rate of 0.5–4.0 Gy/min yielded a dose–effect curve which showed a threshold for radiation pneumonitis at about 7.5 Gy, with a 5% actuarial incidence at approximately 8.2 Gy. An incidence of 50% and 90% was observed at 9.3 and 10.6 Gy respectively (Fig. 13.3). The time of onset of the clinical radiation pneumonitis syndrome was between 1 and 7 months. Radiation was given mainly to relieve pain of advanced cancer using the upper half body irradiation technique. Patients with significant previous and subsequent lung irradiation, previous lung disease, or tumor in the lung were excluded from the study (Fryer et al. 1978; van Dyk et al. 1981). The quantitative data were in good agreement with a previous estimation of the incidence of radiation pneumonitis after half body irradiation (Salazar et al. 1978).

These data provide a basis for estimation of the quantitative influence of the total dose on the risk of IP after TBI prior to BTM. However, no generally accepted dose–effect relationship for TBI has yet been established. Sloane et al. (1983) found no relationship between lung doses of 9.1–13 Gy and the incidence of IP. In a large multicenter study (69 centers) of the International Bone Marrow Transplant Registry (932 patients) no dose–response effect of irradiation was observed within the range 5.6–12.8 Gy. Adjusting for the number of fractions and dose rate did not alter this conclusion (Weiner et al. 1986). As described above, the TBI methods and the procedures related to BMT differed between the different centers. This may have obscured a dose–response relationship. However, Keane and colleagues (1981) published a dose–effect curve for idiopathic IP obtained by evaluation of the data of several TBI centers using different single doses (Fig. 13.3). The dose rates varied between 0.028 and 0.5 Gy/min. Although the dose–effect curve is based on preliminary data, a comparison with the dose–effect curve obtained after upper half body irradiation (van Dyk et al. 1981, see Fig. 13.3) is interesting. In TBI the critical dose range shifts to the right. This can be explained by the sparing effect of the comparatively lower dose rates in TBI.

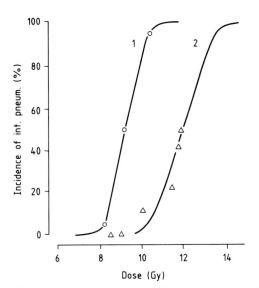

Fig. 13.3. The incidence of interstitial pneumonitis after single-dose irradiation at a high dose rate of 0.5–4.0 Gy/min (*1*, VAN DYK et al. 1981) and a low dose rate of 0.028–0.15 Gy/min (*2*, KEANE et al. 1981). The patients received upper half body irradiation for palliation (1) or total body irradiation prior to bone marrow transplantation (2). See text for further details

One possibility to reduce the incidence of life-threatening IP in TBI is the specific reduction of the total lung dose without compromising treatment results by reducing overall body dose. Shielding of the lung by the patient's arms or by standardized or individualized shieldings for reduction of the lung dose is performed by many institutions (QUAST et al. 1986; QUAST 1987; Molls et al. 1987). Another possibility to decrease the risk of IP is to perform TBI with a relatively low total dose. At the Princess Margaret Hospital TBI was given with a single dose of 5.5–6.2 Gy to the whole body and the lung. The dose rate was relatively high: 0.5 Gy/min. Using this technique the frequency of idiopathic IP was somewhat lower than 10% (KEANE et al. 1981; RIDER and MESSNER 1983).

An effect of dose rate on the risk of IP was observed in the study of the International Bone Marrow Transplant Registry, in which, as mentioned above, the data of 932 patients were analyzed retrospectively (WEINER et al. 1986). The disease was considered to be idiopathic in 50% of the 268 patients who developed IP. In patients given methotrexate after transplantation for prevention of graft-versus-host disease the risk of developing IP increased with increasing dose rate. The IP frequencies were 5%, 20%, 25%, and 30% at dose rates of 0.02–0.029, 0.03–0.039,

0.04–0.049, and 0.05–0.059 Gy/min respectively. At 0.06–0.099 and 0.10–0.108 Gy/min the IP rate showed a plateau, at 35%. In principle, the data are in agreement with previous findings. BARRETT et al. (1983) observed a very low incidence of IP (10%, 5% lethal) in 107 patients with acute leukemia. Except in a group of 16 patients in whom a study of escalating doses of TBI (up to 13 Gy) was undertaken, lung doses were between 9.5 and 10.5 Gy (single dose irradiation) given at a dose rate of only 0.025 Gy/min. It was postulated that lowering the dose rate of TBI to below 0.05 Gy/min will shift the threshold for significant IP to 11–12 Gy (BARRETT et al. 1983).

The relative significance of the instantaneous (constant) and the average dose rate over the whole irradiation period is not exactly known. One study compared ^{60}Co TBI at a constant dose rate of 0.047–0.063 Gy/min with that of a sweeping beam technique using a linear accelerator. Because the field size permitted only one-third of the patient to be exposed at a given time, TBI was achieved by having the beam sweep over the patient with an average interval of 30 s per sweep and the prescribed dose was delivered over a period of 140–150 min as a series of small dose fractions. The average dose rate to the whole body was 0.06–0.065 Gy/min but the instantaneous dose rates in any segment were 0.21–0.235 Gy/min. All patients (22 patients, 11 patients per group) received 9 Gy TBI in a single fraction. The case fatality rate for IP appeared to be greater with the sweeping beam technique, suggesting that the instantaneous dose rate during irradiation was the critical factor.

In an experimental investigation this observation could not be confirmed (LEHNERT 1985). The thorax of mice was irradiated using ^{60}Co rays adjusted to give an instantaneous dose rate of 0.06 or 0.25 Gy/min. An intermittent beam was achieved by switching the cobalt unit on and off, the exposure time being 2.0 min, giving an average dose rate of 0.06 Gy/min. The response to intermittent irradiation with an average dose rate of 0.06 Gy/min did not differ from that to irradiation with an instantaneous dose rate of 0.06 Gy/min.

Fractionated TBI was compared with low dose-rate TBI in a mathematical model based on an extension to the linear-qua-dratic formalism and affected by a number of variables. The results suggested that with regard to sparing of the lung, extremely low dose rates leading to a very long overall duration of TBI might be required for equivalence to conventionally fractionated schedules (O'DONOGHUE 1986).

However, the multicenter study of the International Bone Marrow Transplant Registry (WEINER et al. 1986) yielded no evidence that fractionated irradiation reduced the risk of IP within the range of applied doses and in the schedules tested. The possible benefit of fractionation might have been obscured by the large variations in the TBI techniques of the 69 centers involved. As judged by the publications of the Seattle group, the incidence of IP seems to be lower when up to eight equal fractions to a total dose of 12–15 Gy are delivered as compared with a single dose of 10 Gy (THOMAS et al. 1982; MEYERS et al. 1983; DEEG et al. 1986, 1988). In a randomized trial 53 patients with nonlymphoblastic leukemia in first remission were given either six fractions of 2 Gy in 3 days ($n = 26$) or a single dose of 10 Gy ($n = 27$) (THOMAS et al. 1982; DEEG et al. 1986). After single-dose irradiation the incidence of IP was 7/27 (two idiopathic), after fractionation only 4/26 (one idiopathic). In a further investigation a large group of patients ($n = 614$) was retrospectively analyzed (MEYERS et al. 1983). Out of 299 patients who received single-dose TBI, 44% developed IP (13% idiopathic). In contrast, after fractionation the incidence of IP among 315 patients was 29% (5% idiopathic). A large number of nonrandomized studies with smaller numbers of patients concluded that fractionation is beneficial when compared with single-dose TBI (ROHLOFF et al. 1987, 1988; HÜBENER et al. 1987; EHNINGER et al. 1987; MOLLS et al. 1987; PINO et al. 1982; VITALE et al. 1983; BLUME et al. 1987; SHANK et al. 1983; COSSET et al. 1989).

13.4.1 Factors Contributing to the TBI-Related Risk of Interstitial Pneumonitis

In addition to TBI, infections, chemotherapy, and other risk factors may contribute to the development of IP. The extent to which these components interact with TBI is not exactly known (BAMBERG et al. 1986; MOLLS et al. 1986). Risk factors for which a contribution to IP is proven or discussed are shown in Table 13.4. Most of them have been reviewed in more detail by DEEG et al. (1988).

Table 13.4 shows that some of the risk factors, such as seropositivity for CMV, transfusion of CMV-positive blood products, and omission of trimethoprim/sulfamethoxazole prophylaxis, are

associated especially with infectious IP (CMV, Pneumocytis carinii). Other factors may be critical with regard to any etiological cause of IP [primary disease, increasing patient age, allogeneic graft, gnotobiotic care, graft-versus-host disease (GVHD), GVHD prophylaxis with methotrexate; controversial: performance rating, interval from diagnosis to transplant]. The risk of TBI-related IP may be increased especially by prior radiotherapy to the chest wall, increasing patient age, GHVD prophylaxis with methotrexate, and gnotobiotic care (WEINER et al. 1986; BEELEN et al. 1988; DEEG et al. 1988; MOLLS et al. 1990). It also has to be stressed that some noncytotoxic agents (analgesics, endocrine substances, antibiotics, inhalants, neuroactive and vasoactive agents, miscellaneous) may contribute to pulmonary disease (ROSENOW 1972). Furthermore, pollutants and different lung affections may come into play (MOLLS et al. 1986). If it is true that several factors are involved in the complex development of IP, it cannot be excluded that even a nonchemotherapeutic drug or other influences with a low toxic potential may exert the decisive effect which causes an "imbalance" in the biological system and leads inevitably to fatal IP.

Frequently TBI is given together with high dose cyclophosphamide. Cyclophosphamide-induced lung damage in man has been reviewed in detail (GINSBERG and COMIS 1982). It has also been reported that cyclophosphamide can sensitize the lung to radiotherapy (TRASK et al. 1985). In an experimental BMT model in rats the influence of cyclophosphamide on mortality was different in high dose rate (0.8 Gy/min) and low dose rate (0.05 Gy/min) experiments. Lung damage ($LD_{50/180}$) after high dose rate irradiation (8–18 Gy) was not significantly altered by the addition of cyclophosphamide (100 mg/kg) 1 day prior to irradiation. In contrast, cyclophosphamide (100 mg/kg) 1 day prior to low dose rate irradiation (16–24 Gy) caused an enhancement of radiation damage with a decrease in the $LD_{50/180}$ by a factor of 1.07. When the cyclophosphamide dose was split into two doses of 50 mg/kg given on 2 consecutive days prior to irradiation, the enhancement was no longer significant.

An interesting aspect of the lung toxicity of the combination of TBI and cyclophosphamide is the effect of timing. In mice cyclophosphamide (100 mg/kg) was given at various times from 28 days before to 28 days after thoracic irradiation (13.7 Gy). Although increased lung damage (ventilation rate, mortality) was seen at all times, the extent

Table 13.4. Risk factors for which a contribution to IP has been proven or discussed (according to DEEG et al. 1988)

Etiological factors		Additional risk factors
TBI:	Total lung dose Fractionation Dose rate	Prior radiotherapy Methotrexate — GVHD prophylaxis
Infection:	CMV *Pneumocystis carinii* Others	Primary disease Performance rating Increasing patient age Interval from diagnosis to transplant
Chemotherapy:	Cyclophosphamide Busulfan Methotrexate	Gnotobiotic care Seropositivity for CMV Transfusion of CMV-positive blood products GVHD Allogeneic graft Omission of trimethoprim/sulfamethoxazole prophylaxis Miscellaneous drugs (see text) Pollutants Lung affections not related to BMT

showed marked variation depending on the time interval (COLLIS and STEEL 1983). Maximal enhancement occurred after cyclophosphamide application at 24 h before or simultaneously with irradiation. A minimal response was observed when the drug was given 12 h before or after x-ray exposure. From these results it was concluded that it may be prudent for the clinician to avoid close time intervals between cytotoxic drugs and irradiation, unless a specific time-related therapeutic gain can be exploited. Clinical schedules give cyclophosphamide over a period of several days before TBI but the sequence of agents has also been reversed without obvious worsening of results (MOLLS et al. 1990; for review: DEEG et al. 1988).

13.5 The Difficulty in Treating Radiation-Induced Pulmonary Injury

Some experimental but also clinical investigations suggest that corticosteroids may reduce the morbidity and mortality of radiation-induced pneumonitis (RUBIN and CASARETT 1968; PHILLIPS et al. 1975; FRYER et al. 1978; PARRIS et al. 1979; GROSS 1980b; GROSS et al. 1988). In irradiated mice

corticosteroids stimulated surfactant production, which prevented abnormalities in pulmonary mechanics and alveolar fluid surface tension (GROSS 1980). Also a corticosteroid-induced augmentation of the enhanced reproductive activity of irradiated type II cells has been described (GROSS and NARINE 1988). These data suggest that the beneficial effect of corticosteroids may be due to improvement of the physiological state of the alveolar surface as well as maintenance of the population of alveolar epithelial cells (GROSS and NARINE 1988).

Clinically, in a relatively large number of patients with the symptoms of pneumonitis application of steroids were found to have no protective effect. However, their withdrawal precipitated the radiation pneumonitis syndrome in a small number of cases (FREYER et al. 1978). In a patient undergoing radiation therapy for recurrent, metastatic breast cancer, a mixture of propoxyphene and acetaminophen was given for intercurrent viral infection. Discontinuation of therapy with this medication coincided with the appearance of pneumonitis, reminiscent of steroid withdrawal (HALPERN et al. 1985). In patients in whom symptoms of pneumonitis are mild and infections have been ruled out, treatment is not required. If, however, symptoms worsen, a course of corticosteroids has been recommended (MYERS and KINSELLA 1985). Conclusive proof of efficacy of steroids is nevertheless lacking. This is also true in the case of idiopathic IP after TBI prior to BMT (DEEG et al. 1988).

Since disturbance of surfactant release appears to be an important pathogenetic mechanism in radiation-induced lung morbidity, the substitution of this phospholipid should be considered. The feasibility of tracheal or bronchial instillation of surfactant of human and bovine but also synthetic origin has been shown especially in pediatric clinical studies. After application of surfactant in premature infants with hyaline membrane disease an improvement in oxygenation and alveolar gas diffusion was observed (FUJIWARA et al. 1980; KWONG et al. 1985; GITLIN et al. 1987; SPEER et al. 1988). Preclinical and clinical studies could clarify the role of surfactant substitution in therapy for radiation pneumonitis.

With regard to lung fibrosis, drugs with anti-inflammatory properties are of potential protective value. Bleomycin-induced collagen accumulation in rat lungs has been inhibited by glucocorticoids and indomethacin (STERLING et al. 1982;

THRALL et al. 1979). In the same experimental model L-3, 4-dehydroproline was able to prevent collagen synthesis (KELLEY et al. 1980). Further experimental inhibitors of bleomycin-induced lung fibrosis were D-penicillamine, β-aminobenzoic acid, and β-aminoproprionitrile (OTSUKA et al. 1977; ZUCKERMAN et al. 1980). WARD et al. (1983, 1984, 1987) found that D-penicillamine ameliorated endothelial damage and hydroxyproline (collagen) accumulation in irradiated rat lung. This substance should be considered for careful clinical testing in those rare cases in which pulmonary fibrosis associated with severe functional changes develops after radiotherapy.

Recently it has been reported that inhibitors of the angiotensin converting enzyme (ACE) decrease radiation-induced pulmonary endothelial dysfunction and pulmonary fibrosis in rats (WARD et al. 1988, 1989). Four markers of endothelial function were monitored: ACE activity, plasminogen activator, and prostacyclin and thromboxane production. The ACE inhibitors captopril and CL242817 ameliorated pulmonary endothelial dysfunction. After application of CL242817 radiation-induced pulmonary fibrosis assessed by lung hydroxyproline content was clearly reduced (WARD et al. 1989).

Another interesting concept relates to platelet-derived growth factor (PDGF), which is an important mediator in the process of cicatrization. In patients with idiopathic pulmonary fibrosis the accumulation of mesenchymal cells in the alveolar walls has been explained by the observation of increased secretion of PDGF-like molecules by macrophages of the respiratory tract (MARTINET et al. 1987). PDGF-like proteins may contribute to alveolar epithelial injury, alveolar septal collapse, and incorporation of intraluminal exudates into alveolar septae that are characteristic of idiopathic pulmonary fibrosis (KATZENSTEIN 1985; DEUEL and SENIOR 1987). One may speculate that specific antagonists might be developed for therapeutic use to block the development of radiation-induced pulmonary injury.

Prophylaxis of lung morbidity can be achieved by chemical radiation protectors. A protective effect of N-acetylcysteine inhalation on the tolerance of thoracic irradiation in mice has been reported (TARBELL et al. 1986). A radioprotective effect of WR-2721 in the mouse lung was studied using breathing rate and lethality measurements (TRAVIS and DE LUCA 1985; TRAVIS et al. 1985). The substance protected better against late func-

tional pulmonary changes and late deaths than against earlier changes in the same assays (protection factors: 1.6 and 1.5 vs 1.4 and 1.3). There was no loss of protection as the dose per fraction was decreased from 15 Gy to approximately 5 Gy per fraction. Furthermore it was also shown that WR-2721 protected endothelial cells and type II cells in mouse lung after single doses of x-rays. Endothelial cell function was assayed by ACE and type II cell function by phosphatidylcholine and total protein present in lavage fluid (protection factors: 1.2) (TRAVIS et al. 1987c). Studies in progress should establish the role of radioprotectors in clinical practice.

References

Adamson IYR, Bowden DH (1974) The type 2 cell as progenitor of alveolar epithelial regeneration. Lab Invest 30: 35–42

Adamson IYR, Bowden DH (1975) Deviation of type 1 epithelium from type 2 cells in the developing rat lung. Lab Invest 32: 736–745

Adamson IYR, Bowden DH (1977) Origin of ciliated alveolar epithelial cells in bleomycin-induced lung injury. Am J Pathol 87: 569–575

Adamson IYR, Bowden DH (1983) Endothelial injury and repair in radiation induced pulmonary fibrosis. Am J Pathol 112: 224–230

Adamson IYR, Bowden DH, Wyatt JP (1970) A pathway to pulmonary fibrosis: an ultrastructural study of mouse and rat following radiation to the whole body and hemithorax. Am J Pathol 58: 481–498

Ahier RG, Anderson RL, Coultas PG (1984) Response of mouse lung to irradiation. J Eur Soc Ther Radiol Oncol 3: 61–68

Ahier RG, Anderson RL, Coultas PG (1985) Responses of mouse lung to irradiation. I. Alterations in alveolar surfactant after neutrons and x-rays. Radiother Oncol 3: 61–68

Alblas A, van Furth R (1979) Origin, kinetics and characteristics of pulmonary macrophages in the normal steady state. J Exp Med 149: 1504

Alderson PP, Bradley EW, Mendenhall KG, Vieras F, Siegel BA, Sloan GE, Rogers CC (1979) Radionuclide evaluation of pulmonary function following hemithorax irradiation of normal dogs with Co-60 or fast neutrons. Radiology 130: 425

Altmann HW, Hunstein W, Stutz E (1961) Über Lungenveränderungen und Lungentumoren nach Bestrahlung mit radioaktiven Strontium (^{90}Sr). Beitr Pathol Aust Allg Pathol 124: 145–175

Anderson RL, Ahier RG, Coultas PG (1985) Responses of mouse lung to irradiation. 2. Levels of alveolar protein in lung lavage fluid following neutrons or x-rays. Radiother Oncol 4: 167–174

Archer VE, Saccomanno G, Jones JH (1974) Frequency of different histologic types of bronchogenic carcinoma as related to radiation exposure. Cancer 34: 2956–2060

Archer VE, Gilliam JD, Wagoner JK (1976) Respiratory disease mortality among uranium miners. Ann NY Acad Sci 271: 280–293

Baich A, Chen P, Cummings S (1980) Effect of proline on synthesis of collagen by cells in culture. Physiol Chem Phys 12: 63–67

Bamberg M, Beelen DW, Mahmoud HK, Molls M, Schaefer KW (1986) The incidence of interstitial pneumonitis: comparison of total body irradiation schedules for allogeneic bone marrow transplantation. Strahlenther Onkol 162: 218–222

Barrett A (1982a) Clinical aspects of total body irradiation. J Eur Radiother 4: 159–164

Barrett A (1982b) Total body irradiation before bone marrow transplantation: a review. Clin Radiol 33: 131–135

Barrett A (1983) Systemic radiotherapy. In: Steel GG, Adams GE, Peckham MJ (eds) The biological basis of radiotherapy. Elsevier, Amsterdam, pp 249–259

Barrett A, Depledge MH (1982) Total-body irradiation – some factors affecting outcome. Exp Hematol [Suppl] 10: 56–63

Barrett A, Depledge MH, Powles RL (1983) Interstitial pneumonitis following bone marrow transplantation after low dose rate total body irradiation. Int J Radiat Oncol Biol Phys 9: 1029–1033

Barrett A, Nicholls J, Gibson B (1987) Late effects of total body irradiation. Radiother Oncol 131–135

Bässler R, Buchwald W (1966) I. Lungenfibrose nach Röntgenbestrahlung: Radiologie, Klinik und Untersuchungen zur Pathomorphogenese. Radiologie 6: 95–103

Bate D, Guttman RJ (1957) Changes in lung and pleura following two-million-volt therapy for carcinoma of the breast. Radiologie 69: 372–382

Bauer EA, Cooper TW, Huang JS, Altman J, Deuel TF (1985) Stimulation of in vitro human skin collagenase expression by platelet-derived growth factor. Proc Natl Acad Sci USA 82: 4132–4136

Beelen DW, Quabeck K, Graeven U, Sayer HG, Schaefer UW, Schmidt CG (1988) Influence of treatment -related factors on the results of allogeneic marrow transplantation for leukemia. J Cancer Res Clin Oncol 114 [Suppl]: 144

Beir II (1972) National Research Council, Advisory Committee on the Biological Effects of Ionizing Radiation, National Academy of Sciences, Washington, DC

Bellet-Barthas M, Barthelemy L, Bellet M (1980) Effects of ^{60}Co radiation on the rabbit lung surfactant system. Int J Radiat Oncol Biol Phys 6: 1169–1177

Bennet DE, Million RR, Acherman LV (1969) Bilateral radiation pneumonitis, a complication of the radiotherapy of bronchogenic carcinoma. Cancer 23: 1001–1018

Bertalanffy FD, Leblond CP (1953) The continuous renewal of the two types of alveolar cells in the lung of the rat. Anat Rec 115: 515–536

Bittermann PB, Rennard SI, Hunninghake GW, Crystal RG (1982) Human alveolar macrophage growth factor for fibroblasts: regulation and partial characterization. J Clin Invest 70: 806–822

Blum RH, Carter SK, Agre K (1973) A clinical review of bleomycin – a new neoplastic agent. Cancer 31: 903–914

Blume KG, Forman SJ, Snyder DS et al. (1987) Allogeneic bone marrow transplantation for acute lymphoblastic leukemia during first complete remission. Transplantation 43: 389–392

Bowden DH, Adamson IYR (1972) The pulmonary interstitial cell as immediate precursor of the alveolar macrophage. Am J Pathol 68: 521–546

Bowden DH, Grantham WG, Thomas CE (1966) Cellular morphogenesis of the alveolar surface lining. Fed Proc 25: 603

Bowden DH, Davies E, Wyatt JP (1968) Cytodynamics of pulmonary alveolar cells in the mouse. Arch Pathol 86: 667–670

Bowden DH, Adamson IYR, Grantham WG, Wyatt JP (1969) Origin of the lung macrophage. Arch Pathol 88: 540

Bradley EW, Alderson PO, Sloan EG, Mendenhall KG, Rogers CC (1977) The effect of fractionated fast neutrons or photons on the canine lung. Int J Radiat Oncol Biol Phys 2 [Suppl 2]: 166

Brennan PC, Ainsworth EJ (1977) Early and late effects of fission-neutron or gamma irradiation on the clearance of bacteria from the lungs of B6 CF$_1$ mice. In: Sanders CL, Schneider RP, Dagle GE, Ragan HA (eds) Pulmonary macrophage and epithelial cells. ERDA Symp. Series, No 43. Springfield, VA, pp 552–565

Breur K, Cohen P, Schweisguth O, Hart AMM (1978) Irradiation of the lungs as an adjuvant therapy in the treatment of osteosarcomas of the limbs. Eur J Cancer 14: 461–471

Brown RF (1956) Effects of cortisone on the radiation reaction of the rat lung. AJR 75: 796–806

Bublitz G (1972) Morphologische und biochemische Untersuchungen über das Verhalten des Bindegewebes bei strahlenbedingter Lungenfibrose. In: Bargemann W, Doerr W (eds) Normale und Pathologische Anatomie, no 26. Thieme, Stuttgart, p 89

Buckner CD, Meyers JD, Springmeyer SC et al. (1984) Pulmonary complications of marrow transplantation. Review of Seattle Experiences. Exp Hematol 12 [Suppl 15]: 1–5

Carmel RJ, Kaplan HS (1976) Mantle irradiation in Hodgkin's disease. An analysis of technique, tumor eradication and complications. Cancer 37: 2813–2825

Casarett GW (1980) Radiation histopathology, CRC Press, Boca Raton, FL

Catane R, Lichter A, Lee YJ et al. (1981) Small cell lung cancer: analysis of treatment factors contributing to prolonged survival. Cancer 48: 1936–1943

Caulet T, Adnet JJ, Legay G, Gnonet JL (1970) Leions tardives du poumon de rat, apres irradiation generale. Observations histochimiques et ultrastructurales. Int J Radiat Biol 17: 269–276

Cember H, Watson JA (1958) Carcinogenic effects of strontium-90 beads implanted in the lungs of rats. Ann Ind Hyg Assoc J 19: 36–42

Chameaud J, Perraud R, Lafuma J, Masse R, Pradel J (1974) Lesions and lung cancer induced in rats by inhaled radon-222 at various equilibriums with radon daughters. In: Karbe E, Park JF (eds) Experimental lung cancer: carcinogenesis and bioassays. Springer, Berlin Heidelberg New York, pp 411–421

Choi CH, Carey RW (1976) Small cell anaplastic carcinoma of the lung. Reappraisal of current managenent. Cancer 37: 2651–2657

Chu FCH, Phillips R, Nickson JJ (1955) Pneumonitis following radiation therapy of cancer of the breast by tangential technic. Radiology 64: 642–653

Clapp NK, Darden EB, Jernigan MC (1973) Relative effects of whole-body sublethal doses of 60 MeV protons and 300 kVp x-rays on disease incidences in RF mice. Radiat Res 57: 158–186

Coggle JE, Tarling JD (1982) Cell kinetics of pulmonary alveolar macrophage in the mouse. Cell Tissue Kinet

Coggle JE, Lambert BE, Moore SR (1986) Radiation

effects in the lung. Environ Health Perspect 70: 261–291

Collis CH (1981) The response of the lung to ionizing radiation and cytotoxic drugs. M.D. Thesis. University of Cambridge

Collis CH (1982) A kinetic model for the pathogenesis of radiation lung damage. Int J Radiat Biol 42: 253–263

Collis CH, Steel GG (1982) Dose-dependence of the time of appearance of lung damage in mice given thoracic irradiation. Int J Radiat Biol 42: 245–252

Collis CH, Steel GG (1983) Lung damage in mice from cyclophosphamide and thoracic irradiation: the effects of timing. Int J Radiat Oncol Biol Phys 9: 685–689

Cosset JM, Shank B (1989) Reply to: TBI schedules prior to bone marrow transplantation: requirements for comparison (letter to the Editor). Radiother Oncol 15: 211–212

Cosset IM, Baume D, Pico JL, Shank B, Girinski T, Benhamou E, Briot E, Malaise E, Hayat M, Dutreix J (1989) Single dose versus hyperfractionated total body irradiation before allogeneic bone marrow transplantation: a non-randomized comparative study of 54 patients at the Institut Gustave-Roussy. Radiother Oncol 15: 151–160

Cottier H (1966) Phänomenologie der Strahlenwirkungen auf Organe und Organsyteme. I. Histopathologie der Wirkung ionisierender Strahlen auf höhere Organismen (Tier und Menschen). In: Zuppinger A (ed) Handbuch der Medizinischen Radiologie; Strahlenbiologie, Vol II/2. Springer, Berlin Heidelberg New York, p 35

Coultas PG, Ahier RG, Field SB (1981) Effects of neutron and x-irradiation on cell proliferation in mouse lung. Radiat Res 85: 516–528

Coultas PG, Ahier RG, Anderson RL (1987) Altered turnover and synthesis rates of lung surfactant following thoracic irradiation. Int J Radiat Oncol Biol Phys 13: 233–237

Cox JD (1972) Total pulmonary irradiation for metastases from testicular carcinoma. Radiology 105: 163–167

Cross FT, Palmer RF, Filipy R E, Dagle GE, Stuart BO (1982) Carcinogenic effects of radon daughters, uranium ore dust and cigarette smoke in beagle dogs. Health Phys 42: 33–52

Dancewicz AM, Mazanowska A, Gerber GB (1976) Late biochemical changes in the rat lung after hemithoracic irradiation. Radiat Res 67: 482–490

Darden EB, Cosgrove GE, Upton AC (1967) Late somatic effects in female RF/Un mice irradiated with single doses of 14 MeV fast neutrons. Int J Radiat Biol 12: 435–452

Deeg HJ (1983) Acute and delayed toxicities of total body irradiation. Int J Radiat Oncol Biol Phys 9: 1933–1939

Deeg HJ, Sullivan KM, Buckner CD et al. (1986) Marrow transplantation for acute non lymphoblastic leukemia in first remission: toxicity and long-term follow-up of patients conditioned with single dose or fractionated total body irradiation. Bone Marrow Transplant 1: 151–157

Deeg HJ, Klingemann H-G, Phillips GL (1988) A guide to bone marrow transplantation. Springer, Berlin Heidelberg New York, p 120

Depledge MG, Barrett A (1982) Dose rate dependence of lung damage after total body irradiation in mice. Int J Radiat Biol 41: 325–334

Depledge MH, Barrett A, Powles RL (1983) Lung function after bone marrow grafting. Int J Radiat Oncol Biol Phys 9: 145–151

Deuel TF, Senior RM (1987) Growth factors in fibrotic diseases. N Engl J Med 317: 236–237

de Villiers AJ, Gross P (1966) Morphological changes induced in the lungs of hamsters and rats by external radiation (x-rays). Cancer 19: 1399–1410

Down JD, Steel GG (1983) The expression of early and late damage after thoracic irradiation: a comparison between CBA and C57Bl mice. Radiat Res 96: 603–610

Down JD, Husband JE, Nicholas D, Steel GG (1982) The independent expression of early and late damage in the lungs of mice after external irradiation. Br J Radiol 55: 943

Down JD, Collis CH, Jeffrey PK, Steel GG (1983) The effects of anaesthetics and misonidazole on the development of radiation-induced lung damage in mice. Int Radiat Oncol Biol Phys 9: 221–226

Down JD, Laurent GJ, McAnulty RJ, Steel GG (1984) Oxygen-dependent protection of radiation lung damage in mice by WR2721. Int J Radiat Biol 46: 597–607

Down JD, Easton DF, Steel GG (1986) Repair in the mouse lung during low dose rate irradiation. Radiother Oncol 6: 29–42

Down, JD, Coultas PG, Field SB (1988) Is surfactant release a reliable predictor of radiation pneumonites? Int J Radiat Oncol Biol Phys 19: 211–212

Drozdz M, Kucharz E, Glowacki A, Sylka J (1981) Effect of irradiation on glycosaminoglycans content in rat tissue. Arch Immunol Ther Exp 29: 515–519

Dubrawsky C, Dubravsky NB, Withers HR (1978) The effects of colchicine on the accumulation of hydroxyproline and on lung compliance after irradiation. Radiat Res 73: 111–120

Dubrawsky C, Dubravsky NB, Jampolis S, Mason K, Hunter N, Withers HR (1981) Long-term effects of pulmonary damage in mice on lung weight, compliance, hydroxyproline content and formation of metastases. Br J Radiol 54: 1075–1080

Dutreix A, Broerse JJ (1982) Summary of round table discussion on physical aspects of total body irradiation. J Eur Radiother 3: 165–173

Dutreix J, Wambersie A (1975) Cell survival curves deduced from non-quantitative reaction of skin, interstitial mucosa and lung. In: Alper T (ed) Cell survival after low dose of radiation. John Wiley, Bristol, pp 335–341

Dutreix J, Wambersie A, Bounik C (1973) Cellular recovery in human skin reaction: application to chose, fraction number, overall time relationship in radiotherapy. Eur J Cancer 9: 159–167

Dutreix J, Wambersie A, Coiretta M, Biosserie G (1979) Time factors in total body irradiation. Pathol Biol (Paris) 27: 365-369

Dutreix J, Gluckmann E, Brule JM (1982) Biological problems of total body irradiation. J Eur Radiother 4: 165–173

Ehninger G, Einsele H, Dopfer R, Waller HD (1987) The role of total body irradiation in conditioning adults for bone marrow transplantation. Strahlenther Onkol 163: 210–211

Eichhorn H-J, Hüttner J, Dallüge K-H, Welker K (1983) Preliminary report on "one-time" and high dose irradiation of the upper and lower half-body in patients with small cell lung cancer. Int J Radiat Oncol Biol Phys 9: 1459–1465

Einhorn L, Kranse M, Hornback N et al. (1976) Enhanced pulmonary toxicity with bleomycin and radiotherapy in oat cell lung cancer. Cancer 37: 2414–2416

El-Khatib EE, Sharplin J, Battista JJ (1983) The density of mouse lung in vivo following x-irradiation. Int Radiat Oncol Biol Phys 9: 853–858

El-Khatib EE, Freeman CR, Rybka WB, Lehnert S, Podgorsak E (1989) The use of CT densitometry to predict lung toxicity in bone marrow transplant patients. Int J Radiat Oncol Biol Phys 16: 85–94

Elkind MM, Sutton H (1959) x-ray damage and recovery in mammalian cells in culture. Nature 184: 1293

Ellis F (1969) Time dose and fractionation: a clinical hypothesis. Clin Radiol 20: 1–8

Ellis F (1971) Nominal standard dose and the ret. Br J Radiol 44: 101

Emirgil C, Heinemann HO (1961) Effects of irradiation of chest on pulmonary function in man. J Appl Physiol 16: 331–338

Engelbrecht FM, Thiart BF, Classens A (1960) Fibrosis and collagen in rats' lungs produced by radioactive mine dust. Am J Occup Hyg 2: 257–266

Engelstad RB (1940) Pulmonary lesion after roentgen and radium irradiation. AJR 43: 676–681

Engermann RL, Pfaffenbach D, Davis MD (1967) Cell turnover in capillaries. Lab Invest 17: 738–743

Evans JC (1960) Time-dose relationship of radiation; fibrosis of lung. Radiology 74: 104

Evans MJ, Bils RF (1969) Identification of cells labelled with tritiated thymidine in the pulmonary alveolar walls of the mouse. Am Rev Respir Dis 100: 372–378

Evans MJ, Hackney JD (1972) Cell proliferation in lungs of mice exposed to elevated concentrations of oxygen. Aerosp Med 6: 620–622

Evans MJ, Cabral CJ, Stephens RJ, Freeman G (1973) Renewal of alveolar epithelium in the rat following exposure to NO_2. Am J Pathol 70: 175–198

Evans MJ, Johnson CV, Stephens RJ, Freeman G (1976) Cell renewal in the lungs of rats exposed to low levels of ozone. Exp Morph Pathol 24: 70–83

Farrell P, Zachmann R (1973) Induction of choline phosphotransferase and lecithin synthesis in the foetal lung by corticosteroids. Science 179: 297

Faulkner CS, Connolly KS (1973) The ultrastructure of ^{60}Co radiation pneumonitis in rats. Lab Invest 28: 545–553

Field SB, (1972) the Ellis formula for x-rays and fast neutrons. Br J Radiol 45: 315–317

Field SB (1977) Early and late normal tissue damage after fast neutrons. Int J Radiat Biol Phys 3: 203–210

Field SB, Hornsey S (1974) Damage to mouse lung with neutrons and x-rays. Eur J Cancer 10: 621–627

Field SB, Hornsey S (1975) The response of mouse skin and lung to fractionated x-rays. In: Alper T (ed) Cell survival after low doses of radiation. Wiley, New York, p 362

Field SB, Hornsey S (1977) Slow repair after x-rays and fast neutrons. Br J Radiol 50: 600–601

Field SB, Hornsey S, Kutsutani Y (1976) Effects of fractionated on mouse lung and a phenomenon of slow repair. Brit J Radiol 49: 700–707

Fine R, McCullough B, Collins JF, Johanson EG (1979) Lung elasticity in regional and diffuse pulmonary fibrosis. J Appl Physiol 47: 138–144

Fleming WH, Szakacs JE, King ER (1962) The effects of gamma radiation on the fibrinolytic system of dog lung and its modification by certain drugs: relationship to radiation pneumonitis and hyaline membrane formation in lung. J Nucl Med 3: 341–351

Fowler JF (1984) Review: total doses in fractionated radiotherapy-implications of new radiobiological data. Int J Radiat Biol 2: 103–120

Fowler JF (1989) Review article: the linear–quadratic

formula and progress in fractionated radiotherapy. Br J Radiol 62: 679–694

Fowler JF (1990) Radiation-induced lung damage: dose-time fractionation considerations (Letter to the Editor). Radiother Oncol 18: 184–187

Fowler JF, Parkins CS, Denekamp J, Terry NHA, Maughan RL, Travis EL (1982) Early and late effects in mouse lung and rectum. Int J Radiat Oncol Biol Phys 8: 2089–2093

Fowler JF, Travis EL (1978) The radiation pneumonitis syndrome in half-body therapy. Int J Radiat Oncol Biol Phys 4: 1111–1113

Freedman GS, Sken B, Cofgren SB, Kligerman MM (1974) Radiation-induced changes in pulmonary perfusion. Radiology 112: 435–437

Fryer CJ H, Fitzpatrick PJ, Ridge WD, Doon P (1978) Radiation Pneumonitis experience following a large single dose of radiation. Int J Radiat Oncol Biol Phys 4: 931–936

Fujiwara T, Maeta H, Chida S, Morita T, Watabe Y, Abe T (1980) Artificial surfactant therapy in hyaline-membrane disease. Lancet I: 55–59

Furth J, Lorenz E (1954) Carcinogenesis by ionizing radiation. In: tollaender A (ed) Radiation biology, vol I. McGraw-Hill, New York, pp 1145–1201

Furth J, Upton AC, Kimball AW (1958) Late pathological effects of atomic detonation and their pathogenesis. Radiat Res [Suppl I] 243–264

Geise RA, McCullough EC (1977) The use of CT scanners in megavoltage photon beam therapy. Radiology 124: 141–147

Ginsberg SJ, Comis RL (1982) The pulmonary toxicity of antineoplastic agents. Semin Oncol 9: 34–51

Gitlin JD, Soll RF, Parad RB, Horbar JD, Feldmann HA, Lucey JF, Taeusch HW (1987) Randomized controlled trial of exogenous surfactant for the treatment of hyaline membrane disease. Pediatrics 79: 31–37

Glaeser L (1986) Influence of lung tissue on the dose distribution of high energy photon beams, review. Strahlentherapie Onkol 162: 266–270

Godleski JJ, Brain JD (1976) The origin of alveolar macrophages in mouse radiation chimaeras. J Exp Med 136: 630–643

Golde DW, Byers LA, Finley TN (1974) Proliferative capacity of human alveolar macrophage. Nature 247: 373

Goldenberg VE, Warren S, Chute R, Besen M (1968) Radiation pneumonitis in single and parabiotic rats. I. Short term effects of supralethal total body irradiation. Lab Invest 18: 215–226

Goldmann JM, Gale PG, Horowitz MH et al. (1988) Bone marrow transplantation for chronic myelogenous leukemia in chronic phase. Increased risk for relapse associated with T-cell depletion. Ann Intern Med 108: 806–814

Groover TA, Christie AC, Merrit EA (1922) Observations on the use of the cooper filter in the roentgen treatment of deep-seat malignancies. South Med J 15: 440–444

Gross NJ (1977a) Alveolar macrophage number: an index of the effect of radiation on the lung. Radiat Res 72: 325–332

Gross NJ (1977b) Pulmonary effects of radiation therapy. Ann Intern Med 86: 81–92

Gross NJ (1978a) Experimental radiation pneumonitis: changes in physiology of the alveolar surface. J Lab Clin Med 92: 991–1001

Gross NJ (1978b) Early physiologic and biochemical effects

of thoracic x-irradiation on the pulmonary surfactant system. J Lab Clin Med: 537–544

Gross NJ (1979) Experimental radiation pneumonitis. III. Phospholipid studies on the lungs. J Lab Clin Med 93: 627–637

Gross NJ (1980a) Experimental radiation pneumonitis. IV. Leakage of circulatory proteins onto the alveolar surface. J Lab Clin Med 95: 19–31

Gross NJ (1980b) Radiation pneumonitis in mice. Some effects of corticosteroids on mortality and pulmonary physiology. J Clin Invest 66: 504–510

Gross NJ (1981) The pathogenesis-induced lung damage. Lung 159: 115–125

Gross NJ, Balis JV (1978) Functional, biochemical and morphological changes in alveolar macrophages following thoracic irradiation. Lab Invest 39: 381–389

Gross NJ, Narine KR (1988) Experimental radiation pneumonitis, corticosteroids increase the replicative activity of alveolar type 2 cells. Radiat Res 115: 543–549

Gross NJ, Narine KR, Wade R (1988) Protective effects of corticosteroids on radiation pneumonitis in mice. Radiat Res 113: 112–119

Gross P, Pfitzer EA, Watson J (1969) Experimental carcinogenesis. Bronchial intramural adenocarcinomas in rats from x-ray irradiations of the chest. Cancer 23: 1046–1060

Hale G, Waldmann H (1988) Campath-1 for prevention of graft versus host disease and graft rejection. Summary of results from a multicenter study. Bone Marrow Transplant 3 [Suppl 1]: 11–14

Halpern J, Baerwald H, Johnson R, Takita H, Ambrus JL (1985) Propoxyphene and acetaminophen mixture (Darvocet) related radiation induced pneumonitis. Arch Intern Med 145: 1509–1510

Ham JM (1976) Report of the Royal Commission on the Health and Safety of Workers in Mines. Ministry of the Attorney General, Province of Ontario, Toronto

Hedlund LW, Vock P, Effmann EL, Lischko MM, Putman CE (1984) Hydrostatic pulmonary edema. An analysis of lung a density changes by computed tomography. Invest Radiol 19: 254–262

Hellmann S, Kligerman MM, von Essen CF, Scibetta MP (1964) Sequelae of radical radiotherapy of carcinoma of the lung. Radiology 82: 1055–1061

Henderson RF, Muggenburg BA, Manderley JL, Tuttle WA (1978) Early damage indicators in the lung. II. Time sequence of protein accumulation and lipid loss in the airways of beagle dogs with beta irradiation of the lung. Radiat Res 76: 145–158

Herrmann T, Molls M (1990) Effekte nach Bestrahlung der Respirationsorgane. In: Neumeister, Streffer, Yarmomenko (eds) Strahlenbiologische Grundlagen der klinischen Radiologie. VEB Georg Thieme, Leipzig

Herrmann T, Voigtmann L, Knorr A, Lorenz J, Johanssen U (1986a) The time-dose relationship for radiation-induced lung damage in pigs. Radiother Oncol 5: 127–135

Herrmann T, Voigtmann L, Knorr A, Lorenz J, Johanssen U, Welker K (1986b) Fractionated lung irradiation in young pigs with 6.2 MeV neutrons and cobalt-60. Radiother Oncol 7: 69–75

Herrmann T, Voigtmann L, Knorr A, Lorenz J (1987) Zum Reparaturverhalten der Lunge – experimentelle und klinische Ergebnisse. Stralenther Onkol 163: 370–377

Hildebran JN, Airhart J, Stirewalt WS, Low RB (1981) Prolyl-tRNA-based rates of protein and collagen synthesis in human lung fibroblasts. Biochem J 198: 249–258

Hill RP (1983) Reponse of mouse lung to irradiation at different dose rates. Int J Radiat Oncol Biol Phys 9: 1043–1047

Hines LE (1922) Fibrosis of the lung following roentgen-ray treatment for tumor. JAMA 79: 720–722

Hirst DG, Denekamp J, Hobson B (1980) Proliferation studies of the endothelial and smooth muscle cells of the mouse mesentery after irradiation. Cell Tissue Kinet 13: 91–104

Horacek JV, Placek JV, Seve J (1977) Histologic types of bronchogenic cancer in relation to different conditions of radiation exposure. Cancer 40: 832–835

Hubener K-H, Schmidt B, steidle B (1987) Clinical results of bone marrow transplantation in Tübingen after total body irradiation from the radiotherapeutical view. Strahlenther Onkol 163: 214–216

Jacobsen VC (1940) The deleterious effects of deep roentgen irradiation on lung structure and function. AJR 4: 235–249

Jaeger P, Foullon X, Granier M, Hainot J, Josipovici JJ, Kermarec J, Allard P (1983) Les risques de la radiotherapie thoracique. Medicine et Armees 1: 21–25

Jennings FL, Arden A (1961) Development of experimental radiation pneumonitis. Arch Pathol 71: 437–446

Jennings FL, Arden A (1962) Development of radiation pneumonitis. Time and dose factors. Arch Pathol 74: 351–360

Johnson RE, Breston HD, Kent C (1978) "Total" therapy for small cell carcinoma of the lung. Am Thorac Surg 25: 509–515

Kanarek DJ (1983) Assessment of pulmonary function in lung cancer. In: Choi NC, Grillo HC (eds) Thoracic oncology. Raven, New York, pp 103–113

Kapanci Y, Weibel ER, Kaplan HP, Robinson FR (1969) Pathogenesis and reversibility of the pulmonary lesions of oxygen toxicity in monkeys. II. Ultrastructural and morphometric studies. Lab Invest 20: 101–118

Kaplan HS (1972) Hodgkin's disease. Harvard University Press, Cambridge

Kaplan HS, Stewart JR (1973) Complications of intensive megavoltage radiotherapy for Hodgkin's disease. Natl Cancer Inst Monogr 36: 439–444

Karlinsky JB (1982) Glycosaminoglycans in emphysematous and fibrotic hamster lung. Am Rev Respir Dis 125: 85–88

Katzenstein A-LA (1985) Pathogenesis of "fibrosis" in interstitial pneumonia: an electron microscopic study. Hum Pathol 16: 1015–1024

Keane TJ, van Dyk J (1989) TBI schedules prior to bone marrow transplantation: requirements for comparison (Letter to the Editor). Radiother Oncol 15: 207–209

Keane TJ, van Dyke J, Rider WD (1981) Idiopathic interstitial pneumonia following bone marrow transplantation: the relationship with total body irradiation. Int J Radiat Oncol Biol Phys 7: 1365–1370

Kehrer JP, Witschi H (1980) In vivo collagen accumulation in an experimental model of pulmonary fibrosis. Exp Lung Res 1: 259–270

Kelley J, Newman RA, Evans JN (1980) Bleomycin-induced pulmonary fibrosis in the rat. Prevention with an inhibitor of collagen synthesis. J Lab Clin Med 96: 954–964

Kilburn KH (1974) Functional morphology of the distal lung. Int Rev Cytol 37: 153–174

Kim M, Goldstein E, Levis JP, Lippert W, Warshauer D (1976) Murine pulmonary alveolar macrophages: rates of bacterial ingestion, inactivation and destruction. J Infect Dis 133: 310–320

Kim TH, Rybka WB, Lehnert S, Podgorsak EB, Freeman CR (1985) Interstitial pneumonitis following total body irradiation for bone marrow transplantation using two different dose rates. Int J Radiat Oncol Biol Phys 11: 1285–1291

Kirk, JME, Heard BE, Kerr I, Turner-Warwick M, Laurent GJ (1983) Quantitation of types I and III collagen in biopsy lung samples from patients with cryptogenic fibrosing alveolitis. Coll Relat Res 4: 169–182

Kocmierska-Grodzka, Gerber GB (1974) Lysosomal enzymes in organs of irradiated rats. Strahlenther Onkol 147: 271–277

Koga K, Kusumoto S, Watanabe K, Nishikawa K, Harada K, Ebihara H (1988) Age factor relevant to the development of radiation induced pneumonitis in radiotherapy of lung cancer. Int J Radiat Oncol Biol Phys 14: 367–371

Korr H, Schultze B, Maurer W (1975) Autoradiographic investigations of glial proliferation in the brain of adult mice. II. Cycle time and mode of proliferation of neuroglia and endothelial cells. J Comp Neurol 160: 477–490

Korsower TS, Skovron MC, Ghossein NA, Goldman HS (1971) Acute changes in pulmonary arterial perfusion following irradiation. Radiology 100: 691–693

Kozubek S, Vodvarka P (1984) Late effects of fractionated irradiation of normal tissue. Neoplasma 31: 203–212

Kumar RK, Watkins StG, Lykke AWJ (1985) Pulmonary responses to bleomycin-induced injury: an immunomorphologic and electron microscopic study. Exp Pathol 28: 33–43

Kurohara SS, Casarett GW (1972) Effects of single thoracic x-ray exposure in rats. Radiat Res 52: 262–290

Kwong MS, Egan EA, Notter RH, Shapiro DL (1985) Doubleblind clinical-trial of calf lung surfactant extracts for the prevention of hyaline membrane disease in extremely premature infants. Pediatrics 76: 585–592

Lafuma JE (1978) Cancers pulmonaires induits par differents emetteurs alpha inhales: evaluation de l'influence de divers parametres et comparison avec les donnees obtenues chez les mineurs d'uranium. In: Late biological effects of ionizing radiation (IAEA-SM-224/109), vol II. IAEA Vienna, 531–540

Lagrange JL, Brassard N, Costa A, Aubanel D, Hery M, Bruneton JN, Lalanne CM (1987) CT measurement of lung density: the role of patient position and value for total body irradiation. Int J Radiat Oncol Biol Phys 13: 941–944

Lambert BE, Phipps ML, Lindop PJ, Black A, Moores SR (1982) Induction of lung tumours in mice following the inhalation of 239 PuO2. In: Proc. Third International Symposium of the SRP, Inverness. Scotland I SRP Publ, Reading England, pp 370–375

Laurent GJ (1982) In vivo rates of collagen synthesis in lung, skin and muscle obtained by a simplified method using ^{3}H-proline. Biochem J 206: 535–544

Laurent GJ (1986) Lung collagen: more than scaffolding. Thorax 41: 418–428

Laurent GJ, McAnulty RJ (1983) Protein metabolism during bleomycin-induced pulmonary fibrosis in rabbits. Am Rev Respir Dis 128: 82–88

Laurent GJ, Sparrow MP, Bates PC, Millward DJ (1978) Muscle protein turnover in the fowl. Rates of protein synthesis in fast and slow skeletal, cardiac, and smooth muscle of the adult fowl (Gallus domesticus). Biochem J 176: 393–405

Laurent GJ, Cockerill P, McAnulty RJ, Hastings JRB (1981a) A simplified method for quantitation of the relative amounts of type I and type III collagen in small tissue samples. Anal Biochem 113: 301–312

Laurent GJ, McAnulty RJ, Corrin B, Cockerill P (1981b) Biochemical and histological changes in pulmonary fibrosis induced in rabbits with intratracheal bleomycin. Eur J Clin Invest 11: 441–448

Law MP (1981) Radiation induced vascular injury and its relation to late effects in normal tissues. Adv Radiat Biol 9: 37–73

Law MP (1985) Vascular permeability and late radiation fibrosis in mouse lung. Radiat Res 103: 60–76

Law MP, Hornsey S, Field SB (1976) Collagen content of lungs of mice after x-ray irradiation. Radiat Res 65: 60–70

Law MP, Ahier RG, Coultas PG (1986) The role of vascular injury in the radiation response of mouse lung. Br J Cancer [Suppl VII] 53: 327–329

Lehnert S (1985) Response of the lung to intermittent irradiation: the importance of average versus instantaneous dose rate. Int J Radiat Oncol Biol Phys 11: 2183–2184

Leonhardt H (1981) Histologie, Zytologie und Mikroanatomie des Menschen. Thieme, Stuttgart

Leroy EP, Leibner EJ, Jensik RJ (1966) The ultrastructure of canine alveoli after supervoltage irradiation of the thorax. Lab Invest 15: 1544–1558

Levitt SH, Perez CA (1987) Breast cancer. In: Perez CA, Brady CW (eds) Principles and practice of radiation oncology. Lippincott, Philadelphia, pp 731–792

Libshitz HI, Shuman LS (1984) Radiation-induced pulmonary change: CT findings. J Comput Assist Tomogr 8: 15–19

Libshitz HI, Southard ME (1974) Complications of radiation therapy: the thorax. Semin Roentgenol 9: 41–49

Libshitz HI, Brosof AB, Southard ME (1973) Radiographic appearance of the following extended field radiation therapy for Hodgkin's disease. Cancer 32: 206–215

Lin HS, Kuhn C, Chen DM (1982a) Effects of hydrocortisone acetate on pulmonary alveolar macrophage colony forming cells. Am J Respir Dis 125: 712–715

Lin HS, Kuhn C, Chen DM (1982b) Radiosensitivity of pulmonary alveolar macrophage colony forming cells. Radiat Res 89: 283–290

Lindahl U, Hook M (1978) Glycosaminoglycans and their binding to biological macromolecules. Annu Rev Biochem 47: 385–417

Lindop PJ, Rotblat J (1961) Long-term effects of a single whole-body exposure of mice to ionizing radiations. II. Cause of death. Proc R Soc Lond [Biol] 154: 350–368

Little JB, O'Toole WF (1974) Respiratory tract tumours in hamsters induced by benz (α) pyrene and polonium alpha radiation. Cancer Res 34: 3026–3029

Lopez Cardozo B, Hagenbeek K (1985) Interstitial pneumonitis following bone marrow transplantation: pathogenesis and therapeutic considerations. Eur J Cancer Clin Oncol 21: 43–51

Lopez Cardozo B, Zoetelief D, van Bekkum DW, Zurcher C, Hagenbeek A (1985) Lung damage following bone marrow transplantation: I. The contribution of irradiation. Int J Radiat Oncol Biol Phys 11: 907–914

Ludewig P, Lorenson E (1924) Untersuchungen der Grubenluft in den Schneebergen, Gruben auf den Gehalt und Radiumemanation. Strahlentherapie 17: 428–435

Lundgren DG, Halin SS (1979) Suppression of pulmonary clearance of staphylococcus aureus in mice that had inhaled either $^{144}CeO_2$ or $^{239}PuO_2$. Radiat Res 77: 361–376

Lundgren DL. McLennan RO, Thomas RL, Hahn FF, Sanchez A (1974) Toxicity of inhaled $^{144}CeO_2$ in mice. Radiat Res 58: 448–461

Lundin FE Jr, Lloyd JW, Smith EW, Archer VE, Holaday DA (1969) Mortality in uranium miners in relation to radiation exposure, hard-rock mining and cigarette smoking – 1950 through September 1967. Health Phys 16: 571–578

Mackie TR, El-Khatib E, Battista J, van Dyk J Cunningham JR (1985) Lung dose corrections for 6- and 15-MV x-rays. Med Phys 12: 327–332

Madrazo A,Suzuki Y, Churg J (1973) Radiation pneumonitis. Arch Pathol 96: 262–268

Mah K, van Dyk J (1988) Quantitative measurement of changes in human lung density following irradiation. Radiother Oncol 11: 169–179

Mah, K, van Dyk J, Keane T, Poon PY (1987) Acute induced pulmonary damage: a clinical study on the response to fractionated radiation therapy. Int J Radiat Oncol Biol Phys 13: 179–188

Maisin JR (1970) The ultrastructure of the lung of mice exposed to a supra-lethal dose of ionizing radiation on the thorax. Radiat Res 44: 545–564

Maisin JR (1973) Radiosensitivity of the lung. Strahlenschutz Forsch Prax 13: 49–64

Maisin JR (1974) Ultrastructure of the vessel wall. Curr Top Radiat Res Quart 10: 29–57

Mancini AM, Corinaldesi A, Tison V, Rimondi C, Ferracini R (1965) Immunological aspects of experimental pulmonary sclerosis due to ionizing radiations. Lancet 1397–1398

Margolis LW, Phillips TL (1969) Whole-lung irradiation for metastatic tumor. Radiology 93: 1173–1179

Marks JE, Haus AG, Sutton HC, Griesen ML (1974) Localisation error in the radiotherapy of Hodgkin's disease and malignant lymphoma with extended mantle fields. Cancer 34: 83–90

Martin M, Remy J, Daburon F (1986) In vitro growth potential of fibroblasts isolated from pigs with radiation-induced fibrosis. Int J Radiat Biol 49: 821–828

Martinet Y, Rom WN, Grotendorst GR, Martin GR, Crystal RG (1987) Exaggerated spontaneous release of platelet-derived growth factor by alveolar macrophages from patients with idiopathic pulmonary fibrosis. N Engl J Med 317: 202–209

Mathews MB (1965) The interaction of collagen and acid mucopolysaccharide. A model for connective tissue. Biochem J 96: 710–6

Mathews MB (1975) Connective tissue. Macromolecular structure and evolution. In: Kleinzeller A, Springer GF, Wittmann HG (eds) Molecular biology, biochemistry and biophysics. Springer, New York Berlin Heidelberg, 19: 212–217

McClellan RO, Benjamin SE, Boecker BB, Hahn FF, Hobbs CH, Johns RK, Lundgren DL (1976) Influence of variations in dose and dose rates on biological effects of inhaled beta-emitting radionuclides. In: Biological and environmental effects of low-level radiation. IAEA, Vienna, II, pp 3–19

McCullough EC (1978) Potentials of computed tomography in radiation therapy treatment planning. Radiology 129: 765–768

Metivier H, Nolibe D, Masse R, Lafuma J (1972) Cancers provoques chez le singe Babouin par inhalation de plutonium dioxide (translated by AA Howarth, LF-tr-80). CR Acad Sci (Paris) 275: Series D, 3069

Metivier H, Nolibe D, Masse R, Lafuma J (1974) Excretion and acute toxicity of plutonium-239 dioxide in baboons. Health Phys 27: 512–514

Metivier H, Junqua S, Masse R, Legendre N, Lafuma J (1980) Pulmonary connective tissue modifications induced in the rat by inhalation of $^{239}PuO_2$ aerosol. In: Sanders CL, Cross FT, Dagle GE, Mahaffey JA (eds) Pulmonary toxicology of respirable particles. US ERDA Symposium Series 53: 392–402

Mewhinney JA, Hobbs CH, Mo T (1976) Toxicity of inhaled polydisperse or monodisperse aerosols of $^{241}AmO_2$ in Syrian hamsters III. In: Boecker BB, Jones RK, Barnett NJ (eds) Annual Report of the Inhalation Toxicology Research Institute, Albuquerque for 1975–76. Albuquerque, NM, LF 56 251–258

Meyer KR, Ullrich RL (1981) Effects of x-rays and fission neutrons on an induced proliferative response in lung type II epithelial cells. Radiat Res 85: 380–389

Meyer KR, Witschi H, Ullrich RL (1980) Proliferative response of type 2 lung epithelial cells after x-rays and fission neutrons. Radiat Res 82: 559–569

Meyer OT, Dannenberg AM (1970) Radiation, infection and macrophage function. II. Effect of whole body irradiation on the number of pulmonary alveolar macrophages and their levels of hydrolytic enzymes. J Reticuloendothel Soc 7: 79–90

Meyers JD, Flournoy N, Wade JC, Hackman RC, McDougall JK, Neiman PE, Thomas ED (1983) Biology of interstitial pneumonia after marrow transplantation. In: Gale RP (ed) Recent advances in bone marrow transplantation. Alan R. Liss, New York, pp 405–423

Michalowski A (1981) Effects of radiation on normal tissues: hypothetical mechanisms and limitations of in situ assays of clonogenicity. Radiat Environ Biophys 19: 157–172

Miller G, Siemann DW, Scott P, Dawson D, Muldrew K, Trepanier P, McGann L (1986b) A semiquantitative probe for radiation-induced normal tissue damage at the molecular level. Radiat Res 105: 76–83

Molls M, van Beuningen D (1985) Strahlenbiologische Veränderungen der Lunge. In: Heuck F, Scherer E (eds) Strahlengefährdung und Strahlenschutz. Springer, Berlin Heidelberg New York (Handbuch der Medizinischen Radiologie, Vol XX, pp 379–402)

Molls M, Budach V, Bamberg M (1986) Total body irradiation: the lung as critical organ. Strahlenther Onkol 162: 226–232

Molls M, Bamberg M, Beelen DW, Mahmoud HK, Quast U, Schaefer UW (1987) Different TBI procedures in Essen: results and clinical considerations on the risk of leukemic relapse and interstitial pneumonitis. Strahlenther Onkol 163: 237–240

Molls M, Quast U, Schaefer UW et al. (1990) Clinical results and the Essen concept of TBI. Radiother Oncol 18, Suppl. 1: 121–124

Moore TN, Livingston R, Heilbrun L et al. (1978) An acceptable rate of complications in combined doxorubicin-irradiation for small cell carcinoma of the lung: a Southwest Oncology Group study. Int J Radiat Oncol Biol Phys 4: 675–680

Moores SR, Evans NH, Talbot RJ, Sykes SE, Black A, Coggle JE, Lambert BE (1983) The responses of pulmonary alveolar macrophages to inhaled plutonium dioxide particles. UKAEA Unclassified Report Harwell AERE-R 10635

Moores SR, Talbot RJ, Evans N, Lambert BC (1986) Macrophage depletion of mouse lung following inhalation of $^{239}PuO_2$. Radiat Res 105: 387–404

Moosavi H, McDonald S, Rubin P, Cooper R, Stuard D, Penney D (1977) Early radiation dose-response in lung: an ultrastructural study. Rad Oncol Biol Phys 2: 921–931

Morgan A, Black A, Belcher DR, Moores SR, Lambert BE, Hall WS, Scott DA (1983) Retention of ^{239}Pu in the mouse lung following inhalation of sized ^{239}Pu O_2. UKAEA Unclassified Report, Harwell AERE-R 10718

Morin M, Nenot JC, Masse R, Nolibe D, Metivier H, Lafuma JE (1976) Induction of cancers in the rat after inhalation of alpha emitting radionuclides. In: Biological and environmental effects of low level radiation (IAEA-SM-202/404), vol II. IAEA, Vienna, pp 109–119

Morin M, Masse R, Nenot JC, Metivier H, Nolibe D, Poncy JL, Lafuma J (1977) Etude experimentale des differents effets observes après inhalation de radionucleides emetteurs alpha. Relation dose effet. In: Recueil des Communications. IRPA Proceedings, vol 4, Paris, pp 1321–1328

Moss WT, Haddy FJ (1960) The relationship between oxygen tension of inhaled gas and the severity of acute radiation pneumonitis. Radiology 75: 55–58

Moyer RF, Riley RF (1969) Effects of whole body and partial body x-irradiation on the extractable cellular components of the lung with special consideration of the alveolar macrophage. Radiat Res 39: 716–730

Murray JC, Parkins CS (1987) Collagen metabolism in mouse lung after x-irradiation. Radiat Res 111: 498–510

Myers CE, Kinsella TJ (1985) Cardiac and pulmonary toxicity. In: DeVita VT, Hellman S, Rosenberg SA (eds) Cancer, principles and practice of oncology, 2nd edn. J.B. Lippincott, Philadelphia, pp 2022–2032

Naimark A, Newman D, Bowden DH (1970) Effect of radiation on lecithin metabolism, surface activity, and compliance of rat lung. Can J Physiol Pharmacol 48: 685–694

Newton KA, Spittle MF (1969) An analysis of 40 cases treated by total thoracic irradiation. Clin Radiol ZO: 19–22

Nicholas D, Down JD (1985) The assessment of early and late radiation injury to the mouse lung using x-rays computerised tomography. Radiother Oncol 4: 253–263

Nowell RC, Cole LJ (1959) Late effects of fast neutrons versus x-rays in mice. Radiat Res 11: 545–556

Obrink B (1973) The influence of glycosaminoglycans on the formation of fibers from monomeric tropocollagen in vitro. Eur J Biochem 34: 129–37

O'Donoghue JA (1986) Fractionated versus low dose-rate total body irradiation. Radiobiological considerations in the selection of regimes. Radiother Oncol 7: 241–247

Ogston AG (1970) The biological functions of the glycosaminoglycans. In: Balazs ES (ed) Chemistry and molecular biology of the intercellular matrix. Academic, New York, 3: 1231–1240

Okazaki I, Miura K, Kobayashi Y, Maruyama K, Yoshimatsu H, Tanaka T (1986) Serum type III procollagen peptide: indicator for pulmonary fibrosis. I. A tool for early detection of pulmonary fibrosis as a complication in cancer therapy. Keio J Med 35: 107–115

Oledzka-Slotvinska H, Maisin JR (1970) Electron microscopy and histochemical observation on the pulmonary alveolar surfactant in normal and irradiates mice. Lab Invest 22: 131–136

Otsuka K, Murota S-I, Mori Y (1977) Inhibitory effect of D-penicillamine on the fibrosis caused by bleomycin treatment in rat carrageenan granuloma. Chem Pharm Bull (Tokyo) 25: 1220–1224

Pagani JJ, Libshitz HI (1982) CT manifestations of radiation induced change in chest tissue. J Comput Assist Tomogr 6: 243–248

Palmer RF (1975) Inhalation hazards to uranium miners. In: Thompson RC (ed) Battelle Northwest Laboratory Annual Report for 1974 Part I. Richland, WA, 1975, BNWL-1950 115–123

Park JF, Bair WJ, Busch RH (1972) Progress in beagle dog studies with transuranium elements at Battelle-Northwest. Health Phys 22: 803–810

Parkins CS, Fowler JF (1985) Repair in mouse lung of multifraction x-rays and neutrons: extension to 40 fractions. Br J Radiol 58: 1097–1103

Parkins CS, Fowler JF, Maughan RL, Roper MJ (1985) Repair in mouse lung for up to 20 fractions of x-rays or neutrons. Br J Radiol 58: 225–241

Parkins CS, Whitsed CA, Fowler JF (1988) Repair kinetics in mouse lung after multiple x-ray fractions per day. Int J Radiat Biol 54: 429–443

Parris TM, Knight JG, Hess CE, Constable W (1979) Severe radiation pneumonitis precipitated by withdrawal of corticosteroids: a diagnostic and therapeutic dilemma. AJR 132: 284–286

Pattle RE (1963) The lining layer of the lung alveoli. Br Med Bull 19: 41–44

Peel DM (1979) Tumor induction and post-irradiation cell kinetics in the murine lung. Ph.D. Thesis, University of London

Peel DM, Coggle JE (1980) The effect of x-irradiation on alveolar macrophages in mice. Radiat Res 81: 10–19

Penney DP, Rubin P (1977) Specific early fine structural changes in the lung following irradiation. Int J Radiat Oncol Biol Phys 2: 1123–1132

Penney DP, Rosenkrans WA (1984) Cell-cell matrix interactions in induced lung injury. I. The effects of x-irradiation on basal laminar proteoglycans. Radiat Res 99: 410–419

Penney DP, Shapiro DL, Rubin P, Finkelstein J, Siemann DW (1981) Effects of radiation on the mouse lung and potential induction of radiation pneumonitis. Virchows Arch [B] 37: 327–336

Penney D, Siemann D, Rubin P, Shapiro DL, Finkelstein JN (1982a) Responses of the mouse lung to irradiation. Anat Rec 202: 147A

Penney D, Siemann D, Rubin P Shapiro D, Finkelstein J, Cooper R (1982b) Morphologic changes reflecting early and late effects of irradiation of the distal lung of the mouse: a review. Scan Electron Microsc Part I: 413–425

Penney DP, van Houtte P, Siemann DW, Rosenkrans Jr WA, Rubin P, Cooper Jr RA (1986) Long-term effects of radiation and combined modalities on mouse lung. Scan Electron Microsc Part I: 221–228

Peterkovsky B, Prockop DJ (1962) A method for the simultaneous measurement of the radioactivity of proline-14C and hydroxyproline-14C in biological material. Anal Biochem 4: 400–406

Peters LJ, Withers HR, Cundiff JH, Dicke KA (1979) Radiobiological considerations in the use of total-body irradiation for bone-marrow transplantation. Radiology 131: 243–247

Phan SH, Thrall RS, Ward PA (1980) Bleomycin-induced pulmonary fibrosis in rats: biochemical demonstration of increased rate of collagen synthesis. Am Rev Respir Dis 121: 501–506

Phillips TL (1966) An ultrastructural study of the development of radiation injury in the lung. Radiology 87: 49–54

Phillips TL, Margolis L (1972) Radiation pathology and the clinical response of lung and oesophagus. Front Radiat Ther Oncol 6: 254

Phillips TL, Margolis L (1974) Radiation pathology and the clinical response of lung and oesophagus. Front Radiat Ther Oncol 6: 254–273

Phillips TL, Wyatt JR (1980) Radiation fibrosis. In: Fishman AP (ed) Pulmonary diseases and disorders, vol I. McGraw-Hill, New York, pp 658–675

Phillips TL, Benak S, Ross G (1962) Ultrastructural and cellular effects of ionizing radiation. Front Radiat Ther Oncol 6: 21–43

Phillips TL, Wharam MD, Margolis L (1975) Modification of radiation injury to normal tissues by chemotherapeutic agents. Cancer 35: 1678–1684

Pickrell JA (1981) Sequence of events in pulmonary injury. In: Pickrell JA (ed) Lung connective tissue: location, metabolism and response to injury. CRC, Boca Raton, FL, pp 123–130

Pickrell JA, Mauderly JL (1981) Pulmonary fibrosis. In: Pickrell JA (ed) Lung connective tissue: location, metabolism and response to injury. CRC, Boca Raton, FL, pp 131–156

Pickrell JA, Harris DV, Hahn FF, Belasich JJ, Jones RK (1975a) Biological alterations resulting from chronic lung irradiation. III. Effect of partial ^{60}Co thoracic irradiation upon pulmonary collagen metabolism and fractionation in Syrian hamsters. Radiat Res 62: 133–144

Pickrell JA, Harris DV, Pfleger RC, Benjamin SA, Belasich JJ, Jones RK, McClellan RO (1975b) Biological alterations resulting from chronic lung irradiation. II. Connective tissue alterations following inhalation of ^{144}Ce fused clay aerosol in beagle dogs. Radiat Res 63: 299–309

Pickrell JA, Harris DV, Mauderly JL, Hahn FF (1976a) Altered collagen metabolism in radiation-induced interstitial pulmonary fibrosis. Chest 69: 311–316

Pickrell JA, Harris DV, Benjamin SA, Cuddihy RG, Pfleger RC, Mauderly JL (1976b) Pulmonary collagen metabolism after lung injury from inhaled ^{90}Y in fused clay particles. Exp Mol Pathol 25: 70–81

Pickrell JA, Schnizlein CT, Hahn FF, Snipes MB, Jones RK (1978) Radiation-induced pulmonary fibrosis: study of changes in collagen constituents in different lung regions of beagle dogs after inhalation of beta-emitting radionuclids. Radiat Res 74: 363–377

Pino Y, Torres JL, Bross DS, Lam WC, Wharam MD, Santos GW, Order SE (1982) Risk factors in interstitial pneumonitis following allogeneic bone marrow transplantation. Int J Radiat Oncol Phys 8: 1301–1307

Preston BN, Snowden JM (1973) Diffusion properties of model extracellular systems. In: Kulonen, Pikkarainen J (eds) Biology of the fibroblast. Academic, New York, pp 215–230

Puck TT, Marcus PI (1956) Action of x-rays on mammalian cells. J Exp Med 103: 653

Quast U (1986a) Physical problems of total body irradiation. Strahlenther Onkol 162: 233–236

Quast U (1986b) Problems of dose modification in total body irradiation. Strahlenther Onkol 162: 271–275

Quast U (1987) Total body irradiation – review of treatment techniques in Europe. Radiother Oncol 9: 1–16

Quast U, Glaeser L, Szy D (1986) Total body irradiation in Essen – dosimetry and physical treatment planning. Strahlenther Onkol 162: 240–242

Rall JE, Alpers JB, Lewallen CG, Sonnenberg M, Berman M, Rawson RW (1957) Radiation pneumonitis and fibrosis: a complication of radioiodine treatment of pulmonary metastases from cancer of the thyroid. J Clin Endocrinol 17: 1263–1276

Rappaport DS, Niewoehner DE, Kim TH, Song CW, Levitt SH (1983) Uptake of carbon monoxide by C3H mice following x-irradiation of lung only or total-body irradiation with ^{60}Co. Radiat Res 93: 254–261

Redpath JL, David RM, Colman M (1978) The effect of Adriamycin on radiation damage to mouse lung and skin. Int J Radiat Oncol Biol Phys 4: 229–232

Redpath JL, Zabilansky E, Colman M (1981) The effect of Adriamycin on repair of sublethal damage and slow repair in irradiated mouse lung. Int J Radiat Biol: 39, 157–161

Reiser KM, Last JA (1981) Pulmonary fibrosis in experimental acute respiratory disease. Am Rev Respir Dis 123: 58–63

Rennard SI, Hunninghake GW, Bitterman PB, Crystal RG (1981) Production of fibronectin by human alveolar macrophage: mechanism for the recruitment of fibroblasts to sites of tissue injury in interstitial lung disease. Proc Natl Acad Sci USA 78: 7147–7151

Rennard SL, Ferrans VJ, Bradley KH, Crystal RG (1982) Lung connective tissue. In: Witschi H, Nettelsheim P (eds) Mechanisms in respiratory toxicology, vol II. CRC, Boca Raton, FL, pp 115–153

Rider WD, Messner HA (1983) Magna-field irradiation: work in progress in bone marrow transplantation at the Princess Margaret Hospital, Toronto. Int J Radiat Oncol Biol Phys 9: 1967

Rohloff R, Naujokat B, Bender C, Haas R, Kolb K-J (1987) Results and side effects after total body irradiation for bone marrow transplantation in the Munich group. Strahlenther Onkol 163: 222–223

Rohloff R, Kolb K-J, Bender C, Haas R, Kantlehner R, Balk OA (1988) Methodik und Ergebnisse der Ganzkörperbestrahlung im Rahmen der Knochenmarktransplantation. Radiobiol Radiother 29: 289–290

Rosenblum LJ, Mauceri RA, Wellenstein DE, Bassano DA, Cohen WN, Heitzmann ER (1978) computed tomography of the lung. Radiology 129: 521–524

Rosenblum LJ, Mauceri RA , Wellenstein DE et al. (1980) Density patterns in the normal lung as determined by computed tomography. Radiology 137: 409–416

Rosenkrans WA, Penney DP (1985) Cell-cell matrix interactions in induced lung injury. II. x-irradiation mediated changes in specific basal laminar glycosaminoglycans. Int J Radiat Oncol Biol Phys 11: 1629–1637

Rosenkrans WA, Penney DP (1986) Cell-cell matrix interactions in induced lung injury. III. Long-term effects of x-irradiation on basal laminar proteoglycans. Anat Rec 215: 127–133

Rosenkrans WA, Penney D (1987) Cell-cell matrix interactions in induced lung injury. IV. Quantitative alterations in pulmonary fibronectin and laminin following x-irradiation. Radiat Res 109: 127–142

Rosenow EC (1972) The spectrum of drug-induced pulmonary disease. Ann Intern Med 77: 977–991

Ross R, Vogel A (1978) The platelet-derived growth factor. Cell 14: 203–210

Rubenstein JH, Richter MP, Moldofsky PJ, Solin LJ (1988) Prospective prediction of post-radiation therapy lung function using quantitative lung scans and pulmonary function testing Int. J Radiat Oncol Biol Phys 15: 83–87

Rubin P (1984) The Franz Buschke lecture: late effects of chemotherapy and radiation therapy: a new hypothesis. Int J Radiat Oncol Biol Phys 10: 5–34

Rubin P (1988) Prophets that don't predict. Int J Radiat Oncol Biol Phys 14: 212

Rubin P, Casarett GW (1968) Clinical radiation pathology. Saunders, Philadelphia

Rubin P, Shapiro DL, Finkelstein JN, Penney DP (1980) The early release of surfactant following lung irradiation of alveolar type II cells. Int J Radiat Oncol Biol Phys 6: 75–77

Rubin P, Siemann DW, Shapiro D, Finkelstein J, VanHoutte P, Penney D (1983) Surfactant release as an early measure of radiation pneumonitis. Int J Radiat Oncol Biol Phys 9: 1669–1673

Rubin P, Finkelstein JN, Siemann DW, Shapiro DL, Houtte van P, Penney DP (1986) Predictive biochemical assays for late radiation effects. Int Radiat Oncol Biol Phys 12: 469–476

Rüfer R, Merker HJ, Bublitz G (1973) Mechanik, Phospholipoidgehalt und Morphologie der Rattenlunge nach ^{60}Co-Bestrahlung. Strahlentherapie 145: 55–67

Said SI, Avery ME, Davis RK, Banerjee CM, El-Gohary M (1965) Pulmonary surface activity in induced pulmonary edema. J Clin Invest 44: 458–464

Salazar OM, Rubin P, Keller B, Sacrantino C (1978) Systemic (half body) radiation therapy: response and toxicity. Int J Radiat Oncol Biol Phys 4: 937–950

Sanders CL (1973) Carcinogenicity of inhaled plutonium-238 in the rat. Radiat Res 56: 540–553

Sanders CL, Dagle GE, Cannon WC, Powers GJ, Meier DM (1977) Inhalation carcinogenesis of high fired plutonium-238 dioxide in rats. Radiat Res 71: 528–546

Sanders CL, Dagle GE, Cannon WC, Craig DK, Powers GJ, Meier DM (1979) Inhalation carcinogenesis of high fired ^{239}PuO$_2$ in rats. Radiat Res 68: 349–360

Scheulen ME (1987) Reduction of pulmonary toxicity. Cancer Treat Rev 14: 231–243

Schmidtke JR, Dixon FJ (1971) The functional capacity of x-irradiated macrophages. J Immunol 108: 1624–1630

Schmidke JR, Dixon FJ (1973) The effect of in vivo irradiation on macrophage function. J Immunol 110: 848–854

Seyer JM, Kang AH, Rodnan G (1981) Investigation of type I and type II collagens of the lung in progressive systemic sclerosis. Arthritis Rheum 24: 625–631

Shank B, chu FCH, Dinsmore R et al. (1983) Hyperfractionated total body irradiation for bone marrow transplantation. Results in seventy leukemia patients with allogeneic transplants. Int J Radiat Oncol Biol Phys 9: 1607–1611

Shapiro DL, Finkelstein JN, Penney D, Siemann D, Rubin JP (1981) Sequential effects of irradiation on the pulmonary surfactant system. Int J Radiat Oncol Biol Phys 8: 879–882

Shapiro DL, Finkelstein JN, Rubin P, Penney DP, Siemann DW (1984) Radiation induced secretion of surfactant from cell cultures of type II pneumocytes: an in vitro model of radiation toxicity. Int J Radiat Oncol Biol Phys 10: 375–378

Sharplin J, Franko AJ (1982) Irradiation of mouse lungs causes a dose-dependent increase in lung weight. Int J Radiat Oncol Biol Phys 8: 1065–1069

Shorter RG, Titus JL, Divertie MB (1964) Cell turnover in the respiratory tract. Dis Chest 46: 138–142

Shorter RG, Titus JL, Divertie MD (1966) Cytodynamics in the respiratory tract of the rat. Thorax 21: 32–37

Shrivastava PH, Hans L, Concannon JP (1974) Changes in the pulmonary compliance and production of fibrosis in x-irradiated lungs of rats. Radiology 112: 439–440

Siemann DW, Hill RP, Bush RS (1980) Analysis of blood gas values in mice following pulmonary irradiation. Radiat Res 81: 303–310

Siemann DW, Hill RP, Penney DP (1982) Early and late pulmonary toxicity in mice evaluated 180 and 420 days following localized lung irradiation. Radiat Res 89: 396–407

Sikl H (1930) Lungenkrebs der Bergleute in Joachimstal (Tschechoslowakei). Z Krebsforsch 32: 609–613

Simnett JD, Heppleston AG (1966) Cell renewal in the mouse lung. The influence of sex, strain, and age. Lab Invest 15: 1793–1801

Skupinski W, Masse R, Lafuma J (1976) Etude experimentale de l'action de deux emetteurs beta inhales: le cerium-144 et le cerium-141. In: Biological and environmental effects of low level radiation, vol II. IAEA-SM-202/401, Vienna 35–44

Slanina J (1977) Untersuchungen über somatische Spätschäden nach ausgedehnter Strahlentherapie. Ergebnisse von 135 Patienten mit Hodgkin'scher Erkrankung in Langzeitremission (Freiburger Kollektiv, Behandlungsjahre 1948–1974). Habilitationsschrift

Slanina J, Musshoff K, Rahner T, Stiasny R (1977) Long-term side effects in irradiated patients with Hodgkin's disease. Int J Radiat Oncol Biol Phys 2: 1–19

Slanina J, Wannenmacher M, Bruggmoser G, Krüger H-U (1982) Die pulmonale Strahlenreaktion im Röntgenbild: Intensität und Häufigkeit röntgenmorphologischer Veränderungen der Lunge und des Mediastinums nach Mantelfeldbestrahlung mit 4-MeV Photonen und Satelitentechnik. Radiologe 22: 74–82

Sloane JP, Depledge MH, Powles RL, Morgenstern GR, Trickey BS, Dady PJ (1983) Histopathology of the lung after bone marrow transplantation. J Clin Pathol 36: 546–554

Smith CW, Lehan PH, Monks JJ (1963) Cardiopulmonary manifestation with high O$_2$ tensions at atmospheric pressure. J Appl Physiol 18: 849–853

Smith JC (1963) Radiation pneumonitis. A review. Am Rev Respir Dis 87: 647–655

Snihs JO (1974) The approach to radon problems in non-uranium mines in Sweden. In: Proceedings of the Third International Congress of the International Radiation Protection Association, USAEC, Washington, DC, pp 900–912

Soderland SC, Naum Y (1973) Growth of pulmonary macrophages in vitro. Nature 245: 150

Song CW, Kim TH, Kahn FM, Kersey YH, Levitt SH (1981) Radiobiological basis of total body irradiation with different dose rate and fractionation: repair capacity of hemopoietic cells. Int J Radiat Oncol Biol Phys 7: 1695

Sontag MR, Battista JJ, Bronskill MJ, Cunningham JR (1977) Implication of computed tomography for inhomogeneity correction in photon beam dose calculations. Radiology 124: 143–149

Speer CP, Harms K, Müller U, Schröter W, Curstedt T, Robertson B (1988) Behandlung des schweren Atemnotsyndroms Frühgeborener mit natürlichem Surfactant Monatsschr Kinderheilkd 136: 65–70

Spencer H, Shorter RG (1962) Cell turnover in pulmonary tissues. Nature 194: 880

Steel GG (1988) The search for therapeutic gain in the combination of radiotherapy and chemotherapy. Radiother Oncol 11: 31–53

Steel GG, Adams K, Peckham MJ (1979) Lung damage in C57Bl mice following thoracic irradiation: enhancement by chemotherapy. Br J Radiol 52: 741–747

Sterling KM jr, DiPetrillo T, Cutroneo KR, Prestayko A (1982) Inhibition of collagen accumulation by glucocorticoids in rat lung after intratracheal bleomycin instillation. Cancer Res 42: 405–408

Stevens RL, Colombo M, Gonzales JJ, Hollander W, Schmid K (1976) The glycosaminoglycans of the human artery and their changes in atherosclerosis. J Clin Invest 58: 470–81

Stone DJ, Schwartz MJ, Green RA (1956) Fatal pulmonary insufficiency due to radiation effect upon the lung. Am J Med 21: 211–226

Storb R (1983) Human bone marrow transplantation Transplant Proc 15: 1379–1383

Strandquist M (1944) Studien über die kumulative Wirkung der Röntgenstrahlen bei Fraktionierung. Acta Radiol [Suppl] 55.

Stratton CJ (1975) Multilamellar body formation in mammalian lung: an ultrastructural study utilizing three lipid-retention procedures. J Ultrastruct Res 52: 309–320

Stuart BE (1977) Inhalation hazards to uranium miners. In: Thompson RC (ed) Battelle Northwest Laboratory Annual Report for 1976, Part I. BNWL-2100 47–63

Stuart BO, Palmer RF, Filipy RE, Dagle GE (1978) Inhaled radon daughters and uranium ore dust in rodents. In: Wiley WR (ed) Pacific Northwest Laboratory Annual Report for 1977, Part I. Richland, WA, PNL-2500 3.65–3.72

Sweany SK, Moss WT, Haddy FJ (1959) The effects of chest irradiation on pulmonary function. J Clin Invest 38: 587–593

Talbot RJ, Moores SR (1985) The development and interlobar distribution of plutonium-induced pulmonary fibrosis in mice. Radiat Res 103: 135–148

Talbot RJ, Moores SR, Shewell J (1983) The time-course and interlobar distribution of pulmonary fibrosis in mice, induced by inhaled ^{239}Puo$_2$. UKAEA Unclassified Report Harwell AERE-R 10909

Tannock IF, Hayashi DS (1972) The proliferation of capillary endothelial cells. Cancer Res 32: 77–82

Tarbell NJ, Rosenblatt M, Amato DA, Hellman S (1986) The effects of N-acetylcysteine inhalation on the tolerance to thoracic radiation in mice. Radiother Oncol 7: 77–80

Tarbell NJ, M, Amato DA, Down JD, Mauch P, Hellman S (1987) Fractionation and dose rate effects in mice: a model for bone marrow transplantation in man. Int J Radiat Oncol Biol Phys 13: 1065–1069

Tarling JD, Coggle JD (1982a) Evidence for pulmonary origin of alveolar macrophages. J Reticuloendothelial Soc 31: 221–224

Tarling JD, Coggle JE (1982b) Evidence for the pulmonary origin of alveolar macrophages. Cell Tissue Kinet 15: 577–584

Tarling JD, Coggle JE (1982c) The absence of effect on pulmonary alveolar macrophage numbers during pro-

longed periods of monocytopenia. J Reticuloendothelial Soc 31: 221–224

Teates CD (1965) Effects of unilateral thoracic irradiation on lung function. J Appl Physiol 20: 628–636

Teates CD (1968) The effects of unilateral thoracic irradiation on pulmonary blood flow. AJR 102: 875–882

Temple LA, Marks S, Bair WJ (1960) Tumours in mice after pulmonary deposition of radioactive particles. Int J Radiat Biol 2: 143–156

Thames HD, Hendry JH (1987) Fractionation in radiotherapy. Taylor and Francis, London, p 72

Thames HD, Hendry JH, Moore JV, Ang KK, Travis EL (1989) The high steepness of dose-response curves for late-responding normal tissues. Radioth Oncol 15: 49–53

Thews G (1980) Lungenatmung. In: Schmidt RF, Thews G (eds) Physiologie des Menschen, 20th edn. Springer, Berlin Heidelberg New York, p 500

Thomas ED (1982) The use and potential of bone marrow allograft and whole-body irradiation in the treatment of leukemias. Cancer 50: 1449–1454

Thomas ED, Fefer A (1985) Bone marrow transplantation. In: DeVita VT, Hellman S, Rosenberg SA (eds) Cancer, principles and practice of oncology, 2nd ed. JB Lippincott, Philadelphia, pp 2320–2325

Thomas ED, Storb R, Brückner CD (1978) Total body irradiation in preparation for marrow engraftment. Transplant Proc 8: 591–593

Thomas ED, Clift RA Hersman J et al. (1982) Marrow transplantation for acute nonlymphoblastic leukemia in first remission using fractionated or single dose irradiation. Int J Radiat Oncol Biol Phys 8: 817–821

Thomas RL, Scott JK, Chiffelle TZ (1972) Metabolism and toxicity of inhaled ^{144}Ce in rats. Radiat Res 49: 589–610

Thrall RS, McCormick JR, Jack RM, McReynolds RA, Ward PA (1979) Bleomycin-induced pulmonary fibrosis in the rat. Inhibition by indomethacin. Am J Pathol 95: 117–130

Tichelli A, Gratwohl A, Speck B et al. (1986) Nebenwirkungen der Ganzkörperbestrahlung im Rahmen der Knochenmarktransplantation: Prophylaxe und Therapie. Schweiz Med Wochenschr 116: 1560–1566

Tombropoulos EG, Thomas JM (1970) Effect of 800 R thoracic x-irradiation on lung tissue biochemistry. Radiat Res 44: 76–86

Trask CWL, Joannides T, Harper PG et al. (1985) Radiation-induced lung fibrosis after treatment of small cell carcinoma of the lung with very high-dose-cyclophosphamide. Cancer 55: 57–60

Travis EL (1980a) The sequence of histological changes in mouse lungs after single doses of x-rays. Int J Radiat Oncol Biol Phys 6: 345–347

Travis EL (1980b) Early indicators of radiation injury in the lung: are they useful predicators for late changes? Int J Radiat Oncol Biol Phys 6: 1267–1269

Travis EL (1987) Relative radiosensitivity of the human lung. Advances in Radiation Biology 12: 205–238

Travis EL, De Luca AM (1985) Protection of mouse lung by WR-2721 after fractionated doses of irradiation. Int J Radiat Oncol Biol Phys 11: 521–526

Travis EL, Down JD (1981) Repair in mouse lung after split doses of x-rays. Radiat Res 89: 166–174

Travis EL, Fowler JF (1982) Protection against late and early damage in irradiated mouse lung by WR2721. Int J Radiat Oncol Biol Phys 8: 812

Travis EL, Hargove H, Klobukowski CJ, Feen JO, Frey

GD (1976) Alterations in vascular permeability following irradiation. Radiat Res 67: 539

Travis EL, Hartley RA, Fenn JO, Klobukowski CJ, Hargrove HB (1977) Pathological changes in the lung following single and multi-fraction irradiation. Int J Radiat Oncol Biol Phys 2: 475–490

Travis EL, Vojnovic B, Davies EE, Hirst DG (1979) A plethysmographic method for measuring function in locally irradiated mouse lung. Br J Radiol 52: 67–74

Travis EL, Down JD, Holmes SJ, Hobson B (1980) Radiation pneumonitis and fibrosis in mouse lung assayed by respiratory frequency and histology. Radiat Res 84: 133–143

Travis EL, Parkins CS, Down JD, Fowler JF, Maughan RL (1983a) Is there a loss of repair capacity in mouse lungs with increasing numbers of dose fractions? Int J Radiat Oncol Biol Phys 9: 691–699

Travis EL, Parkins CS, Down JD, Fowler JF, Thames HD (1983b) Repair in mouse lung between multiple small doses of x-rays. Radiat Res 94: 326–339

Travis EL, Meistrich ML, Finch-Neimeyer MV, Watkins TL, Kiss I (1985) Late functional and biochemical changes in mouse lung after irradiation: differential effects of WR-2721. Radiat Res 103: 219–231

Travis EL, Thames DL, Watkins TL, Kiss I (1987a) The kinetics of repair in mouse lung after fractionated irradiation. Int J Radiat Biol 52: 903–919

Travis EL, Curtis SB, Howard J (1987b) Repair not potentiation observed in mouse lung irradiated with neon ions. Radiat Res 112: 500–507

Travis EL, Newman RA, Helbing SJ (1987c) WR 2721 modification of type II cell and endothelial cell function in mouse lung after single doses of irradiation. Int J Radiat Oncol Biol Phys 13: 1355–1359

Trott KR (1987) Radiobiological aspects of total body irradiation following by bone marrow transplantation. Strahlentherapie und Onkologie 163: 212–213

Trott KR, Holler E, Kolb HJ (1981) Strahlenbiologische Überlegungen zur Weiterentwicklung der Ganzkörperbestrahlung bei der Behandlung akuter Leukämien mit anschließender. Knochenmarktransplantation. Strahlentherapie 157: 537–541

Tucker SL and Travis EL (1990) Comments on a time-dependent version of the linear-quadratic model. Radiother Oncol 18: 155–163

Ullrich RL (1980) Effects of split doses of x-rays or neutrons on lung tumor formation in RFM mice. Radiat Res 83: 138–145

Ullrich RL, Storer JB (1979) Influence of gamma irradiation on the development of neoplastic disease in mice. III. Dose rate effects. Radiat Res 80: 325–342

Ullrich RL, Jernigan MC, Cosgrove GE, Satterfield LC, Bowles ND, Storer JB (1976) The influence of dose and dose rate on the incidence of neoplastic disease in RFM mice after neutron irradiation. Radiat Res 68: 115–131

Ullrich RL, Jernigan MC, Adams LM (1979) Induction of lung tumors in RFM mice after localised exposures to x-rays or neutrons. Radiat Res 80: 464–473

UNSCEAR (1982) Report. Ionizing radiation: sources and biological effects, United Nations Publication Sales, no E.82.IX.8 06300, p 584

Upton AC, Furth J, Christenberry KW (1954) The late effects of thermal neutron irradiation in mice. Cancer Res 14: 682–690

Upton AC, Kimball AW, Furth J, Christenberry KW, Bennett WH (1960) Some delayed effects of atom-bomb radiations in mice. Cancer Res 20 (8, Pt 2): 1–62

Upton AC, Kastenbaum MA, Conklin JW (1963) Age specific death rates in mice exposed to ionizing radiation and radiomimetic agents. In: Harris RJC (ed) Cellular basis and etiology of late somatic effects of ionizing radiation. Academic, New York, pp 285–297

Upton AC, Randolph ML, Conklin JW (1970) Late effects of fast neutrons and gamma rays in mice as influenced by the dose rate of irradiation. Induction of neoplasia. Radiat Res 41: 467–491

van Bekkum DW, Bentvelsen P (1982) The concept of gene transfer – misrepair mechanism of radiation carcinogenesis may challenge the linear extrapolation model of risk estimation for low radiation doses. Health Phys 43: 231–237

van Beuningen D (1986) Some radiobiological aspects of total body irradiation (TBI). Strahlenther Onkol 162: 223–225

van den Brenk HAS (1971) Radiation effects on the pulmonary system. In: Berdjis CC (ed) Pathology of irradiation. Baltimore, Williams and Wilkins, pp 569–591

van der Maase H, Overgaard J, Valth M (1986) Effect of cancer chemotherapeutic drugs on radiation-induced lung damage in mice. Radiother Oncol 5: 245–259

van Dyk J (1983) Whole and partial body radiotherapy: physical considerations. In: Wright A, Boyer AL (eds) Advances in radiation therapy treatment planning. Med Phys Monogr 9: 403–426

van Dyk J (1985) Total and half body photon irradiation: review of AAPM task group 29, activities and recommendations. Med Biol Eng Comput 23: 589–590

van Dyk J (1987) Dosimetry for total body irradiation. Radiother Oncol 9: 107–118

van Dyk J, Hill RP (1983) Post-irradiation lung density changes measured by computerized tomography. Int J Radiat Oncol Biol Phys 9: 847–852

van Dyk J, Keane TJ, Kan S, Rider WD, Fryer CJ (1981) Radiation pneumonitis following large single dose irradiation: a reevaluation based on absolute dose to the lung. Int J Radiat Oncol Biol Phys 7: 461–467

van Dyk J, Mah K, Keane TJ (1989) Radiation-induced lung damage: dose-time – fractionation considerations Radioth Oncol 14: 55–69

van Dyk J, Mah K, Keane TJ (1990) Further comments on dose-time – fractionation considerations for lung damage; Letters to the Editor. Radioth Oncol 18: 183–184

van Rongen E, Madhuizen HT, Tan C HT, Durham SK, Gijbels MJJ (1990) Early and late effects of fractionated irradiation and the Kinetics of repair in rat lung. Radiother Oncol 17: 323–337

Varekamp AE, De Vries AJ, Zurcher C, Hagenbeek A (1987) Lung damage following bone marrow transplantation: II. The contribution of cyclophosphamide. Int J Radiat Oncol Biol Phys 13: 1515–1521

Vegesna SL, Withers HR, Thames HD, Mason KA (1985) Multifraction radiation response of mouse lung. Int J Radiat Biol 47: 413–422

Vegesna V, Withers HR, Taylor JMG (1989) Repair kinetics of mouse lung. Radioth Oncol 15: 115–123

Vitale V, Bacigalupo A, van Lint MT et al. (1983) Fractionated total body irradiation in marrow transplantation for leukemia. Br J Haematol 55: 547–554

Wahl SM (1985) Host immune factors regulating fibrosis. In: Fibrosis. Symposium No. 114, Ciba Foundation. London, pp 175–195

Walklin CM, Law MP (1986) Biosynthesis of collagen in the lung of the mouse after x-irradiation. Br J Cancer [Suppl VII] 53: 368–370

Walkin CM, Freedman RB, Law MP (1987) Biosynthesis and degradation of collagen in x-irradiated mouse lung. Radiat Res 112: 341–350

Wara WM, Phillips TL, Margolis LW, Smith V (1973) Radiation pneumonitis: a new approach to the deviation of time-dose factors. Cancer 32: 547–552

Ward WF, Shih-Hoellworth A, Tuttle RD (1983) Collagen accumulation in irradiated rat lung: modification by D-penicillamine. Radiology 146: 533–537

Ward WF, Molteni A, Ts'ao C-H (1984) Radiation injury in rat lung. IV. Modification by D-penicillamine. 98: 397–406

Ward WF, Molteni MD, Solliday NH, Jones GE (1985) The relationship between endothelial dysfunction and collagen accumulation in irradiated rat lung. Int Radiat Oncol Biol Phys 11: 1985–1990

Ward WF, Molteni A, Ts'ao C-H (1987) Functional responses of the pulmonary endothelium to thoracic irradiation in rats: differential modification by D-penicillamine. Int J Radiat Oncol Biol Phys 13: 1505–1513

Ward WF, Kim YT, Molteni A, Solliday NH (1988) Radiation-induced pulmonary endothelial dysfunction in rats: modification by an inhibitor of angiotensin converting enzyme. Int J Radiat Oncol Biol Phys 15: 135–140

Ward WF, Molteni A, Ts'ao C-H (1989) Radiation-induced endothelial dysfunction and fibrosis in rat lung: modification by the angiotensin converting enzyme inhibitor CL242817. Radiat Res 117: 342–350

Warren S, Spencer J (1940) Radiation reaction in the lung. AJR 43: 682–701

Wassermann TH, Kligerman M (1987) Chemical modifiers of radiation effects. In: Perez CA, Brady LW (eds) Principles and practice of radiation oncology. JB Lippincott, Philadelphia, pp 360–376

Watanabe S, Watanabe K, Ohishi T, Aiba M, Kageyama K (1974) Most cells in the rat alveolar septa undergo fibrosis after ionizing irradiation. Lab Invest 31: 555–567

Webster I (1970) Bronchogenic cancer in South African gold miners. In: Shapiro H (ed) Pneumonoconiosis: proceedings of the international conference, Johannesburg 1969. Oxford University Press, Oxford, pp 572–574

Weiner RS, Bortin MM, Gale RP et al. (1986) Interstitial pneumonitis after bone marrow transplantation. Ann Intern Med 104: 168–175

Weiss RB, Muggia FM (1980) Cytotoxic drug-induced pulmonary disease. Am J Med 68: 259–266

Wintz H (1923) Injuries from roentgen rays in deep therapy AJR 10: 140–147

Withers HR (1986) Predicting late normal tissue responses. Int J Radiat Oncol Biol Phys 12: 693–698

Withers HR (1987) Biological basis of radiation therapy. In: Perez CA, Brady CW (eds) principles and practice of radiation oncology. JB Lippincott, Philadelphia, pp 67–98

Withers HR, Peters LJ, Thames HD, Fletcher GH (1982) Hyperfractionation. Int J Radiat Oncol Biol Phys 8: 1807–1809

Wright ES, Couves CM (1977) The radiation-induced carcinoma of the lung. The St. Lawrence tragedy. J Thorac Cardiovasc Surg 74: 495–498

Wynne KM, Spector WG, Willoughby DA (1975) Macrophage proliferation in vitro induced by exsudates. Nature 253: 636

Yuhas JM, Storer JB (1969) Differential chemoprotection of normal and malignant tissues. J Natl Cancer Inst 42: 331

Yuhas JM, Walker AE (1973) Exposure-response curve for radiation-induced lung tumours in mouse. Radiat Res 54: 261–273

Yuile CL, Berke HL, Hull T (1967) Lung cancer following polonium-210 inhalation in rats. Radiat Res 31: 760–774

Zamboglou N, Fürst G, Pape H, Bannach B, Molls M, Schmitt G (1988) Ergebnisse der Ganzlungenbestrahlung und Chemotherapie im Vergleich zur Teillungenbestrahlung bei metastasierenden, undifferenzierten Weichteilsarkomen. Strahlenther Onkol 164: 386–392

Zuckerman JE, Hollinger MA, Giri SN (1980) Evaluation of antifibrotic drugs in bleomycin-induced pulmonary fibrosis in hamsters. J Pharmacol Exp Ther 213: 425–431

14 The Urinary Tract

F.A. Stewart and M.V. Williams

CONTENTS

14.1 The Kidney

14.1.1 Clinical Recognition of Radiation Nephropathy

The expression of renal radiation injury is usually delayed for months or years, with the result that some early reports erroneously suggested that the kidney is not a radiosensitive organ.

Radiation-related effects on the human kidney were first described in detail by WARTHIN (1907), who reported three cases of fatal nephritis following irradiation of lymph nodes and the spleen for leukemia. One patient died after a 6-month latent period during which he was well; tubular necrosis

F.A. STEWART, Ph.D. Division of Experimental Therapy, The Netherlands Cancer Institute, Antoni van Leeuwenhoek Huis, H6, Plesmanlaan 121, 1066 CX Amsterdam, The Netherlands

M.V. WILLIAMS, M.D., Radiotherapeutic Centre, Addenbrooke's Hospital, Hills Road, Cambridge CB2 2QQ, United Kingdom

was observed in necropsy material. By contrast the other two patients died within weeks of treatment, which in one case did not include the kidneys in the irradiated volume. The syndrome described was probably uric acid nephropathy and WARTHIN was therefore correct in ascribing it to the rapid destruction of white blood cells. This confusion possibly helped to delay the widespread recognition of nephritis as a *late* effect of irradiation, particularly as animal work on kidneys at the time concentrated on high dose acute effects such as proteinuria and minimal histological changes (see review by MOSTOFI 1966). Confusion continued into the 1920s, with several reports stating that the kidney is a radioresistant organ, based on inappropriate assays of early damage (STEPHAN 1920).

In 1926 O'HARE et al. reported that single doses of x-rays delivered to the exteriorized kidney of rabbits resulted in chronic nephritis, which developed over the ensuing months. Concurrent work by HARTMAN et al. (1926) demonstrated that a similar lesion could be produced in dogs by single exposures through the abdominal wall. Polyuria, diminished dye excretion, and nitrogen retention were all observed over follow-up periods of up to 13 months. These observations were confirmed in a later report in which the similarity to chronic interstitial nephritis in man was emphasized (HARTMAN et al. 1927). In a subsequent publication the same authors concluded that this experimental nephritis might be directly relevant to irradiation of the renal area in man (DOUB et al. 1927). Two cases of nephritis and hypertension were reported following such treatment, and a survey questionnaire yielded another 16 cases, of which 14 were reported by pathologists and only two by radiologists, indicating a continued ignorance of this late injury.

In 1944 DEAN and ABELS reported a case of hypertension occurring 8 years after irradiation of the left kidney. Unilateral impairment of renal function was demonstrated and the patient's hypertension was cured by nephrectomy; histological study showed marked tubular atrophy and sclerosis and extreme obliterative arteritis which was considered to be radiation induced. Nevertheless, so well established was the view that the kidneys were radioresistant organs, that Zuelzer et al. (1950) were most circumspect in suggesting that radiation damage was the cause of fatal nephritis in three children who had died of renal failure and hypertension 5–7 months after renal irradiation, despite previously normal renal function. In two cases normal histological appearances had been demonstrated in contralateral kidney excised with the primary tumor prior to irradiation.

The low limit of renal tolerance and the late time of appearance of injury were not generally accepted until the publication of the Christie Hospital experience. This was first reported by Paterson (1952), who described how attempts to increase the dose administered to abdominal metastases in patients with testicular tumors resulted in a progressive increase in the dose to the kidney. This led to a variety of clinical syndromes which were classified by Luxton (1953, 1961) into five groups:

1. *Acute radiation nephritis*: latent period 6–13 months; associated with proteinuria and hypertension
2. *Chronic radiation nephritis*: latent period 1.5–4 years; associated with protein and casts in the urine, nocturia, and failure of concentrating ability
3. *Benign hypertension*: latent period 1.5–5 years; associated with proteinuria
4. *Proteinuria*: sole evidence of renal damage in patients followed up for periods of 5–19 years. In one case subclinical renal impairment was manifested as a transient rise in blood urea following surgery
5. *Late malignant hypertension*: occurred at intervals of 1.5–11 years after treatment

Detailed analysis of the radiation distribution and dose to the kidneys established that if the whole of both organs was treated to a dose of 23 Gy in 30 fractions over 5 weeks then there was a significant risk of renal damage (Kunkler et al. 1952).

Partial or unilateral renal irradiation has been considered less dangerous because the loss of renal function can be compensated by contralateral hypertrophy. Le Bourgeois et al. (1979) studied the effects of irradiation of the left kidney in 74 lymphoma patients. Local renal damage was identified by isotope scans within 3–5 months of treatment and after doses as low as 15 Gy in 19 days. Transient proteinuria developed in three patients but there were no other clinically evident sequelae, no cases of hypertension, and no change in overall renal function during follow-up for 3–5 years. Clayman et al. (1968) reviewed 30 years' experience of using gastric irradiation in the treatment of peptic ulcer: a midline dose of 16 Gy in ten daily fractions was delivered through anterior and posterior fields which must have included a large part of the left kidney. No cases of renal disease or hypertension were observed in a series of almost 3000 cases. This would be a remarkable finding even in the normal population and is probably an indication of inadequate follow-up.

Luxton (1961) had indicated that the latent period for renal hypertension may be very long and this was confirmed by Thompson et al. (1971), who found that 31 of 84 patients who had received left renal irradiation during treatment of the stomach for peptic ulcer had evidence of nephritis or hypertension; the mean latent period was 9 years in their series. It does indeed seem that "the ultimate prognosis may thus be assessed only in terms of decades" (Luxton 1961); this is an important consideration in the treatment of young patients with early stage lymphoma (cf. Le Bourgeois et al. 1979) or seminoma.

The kidneys are now accepted as being radiosensitive organs which manifest radiation damage in a variety of ways, often with an extremely long latency. Their low tolerance limits the dose which can be administered to the whole abdomen in the radiation treatment of lymphoma, seminoma, and carcinoma of the ovary.

Combined modality therapy of cancer is becoming more common, which means that the kidneys may be exposed to the combined nephrotoxic insults of drugs and radiation. In the management of carcinoma of the ovary initial treatment is often with cisplatin-containing combination chemotherapy, and some patients may then be treated with whole abdominal irradiation including the kidneys. Read (1982) has reported two cases in which irradiation given in full doses following cisplatin resulted in irreversible renal failure. Animal experiments have also shown that the tolerance dose is reduced in these circumstances (see Sect. 14.1.6.5).

14.1.2 Clinical Management of Radiation Nephropathy

Good radiotherapy practice should minimize the risk of radiation nephropathy. The position of the kidneys should be considered in any pelvic, abdominal, or spinal treatment. Anomalies such as horseshoe or pelvic kidneys may place the kidneys at risk from what are normally safe treatments. In radical small volume treatment of the abdomen, care should be taken to exclude most of one kidney from the irradiated volume, particularly if there has been a contralateral nephrectomy, for example for renal carcinoma. Irradiation of the whole of one kidney or parts of both kidneys carries a risk of late nephritis and hypertension which is probably related to the volume of renal tissue irradiated. In many cases there will be no obvious clinical sequelae, despite renal atrophy (Fig. 14.1) or abnormal isotope scan appearances, and irradiation of a large part of the left kidney in the treatment of splenic Hodgkin's disease has become accepted practice in some centers (Le Bourgeois et al. 1979). Nevertheless, the long natural history of radiation nephritis means that these patients should be followed up closely and their blood pressure checked for life (Thompson et al. 1971; Kim et al. 1984; Willet et al. 1986).

Hypertension is an important consequence of renal irradiation because it is treatable. It is now established that hypertension results from renin

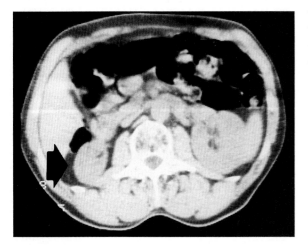

Fig. 14.1. CT scan of the abdomen showing gross reduction in the size of the right kidney (*arrow*) at 8 years after a dose of 32 Gy given in 16 fractions over 29 days for recurrent lymphoma. The patient remains asymptomatic, his blood pressure is normal, and there is no proteinuria

secretion from the juxtaglomerular apparatus (Shapiro et al. 1977). In man most of the vascular injury seen in irradiated kidneys is probably a secondary effect of hypertension (Wacholz and Casarett 1970). Irradiated vessels are particularly sensitive to such injury and early detection and control of hypertension are important. In the past the usual treatment of hypertension has been nephrectomy of the injured kidney (Dean and Abels 1944; Shapiro et al. 1977). However, with modern drugs it is usually possible to control the blood pressure medically (Kim et al. 1984; Willet et al. 1986). There has been a single case report of radiation-induced renal artery stenosis, which was relieved by transluminal angioplasty (Minton et al. 1986). This emphasizes the need for adequate investigation in all cases.

Established renal failure occurring after irradiation is managed in the usual way. The suitability of the patient for dialysis or transplantation will depend on whether the malignancy for which treatment was originally given has been eradicated.

14.1.3 Histological Changes and Pathogenesis of Radiation Nephropathy

The pathogenesis of radiation nephropathy has long been in dispute, with some authors favoring damage to the endothelial cells of the glomeruli or larger vessels as the critical lesion, while others are persuaded that tubular cell injury is more important. This difference of opinion is a reflection of the division between those who believe that vascular injury provides a general explanation of the late effects of radiotherapy (Rubin and Casarett 1968) and those who believe that parenchymal cell damage is more important (Withers et al. 1980; Michalowski 1981).

The first histological study of radiation-induced changes in the kidney was by Schulz and Hoffman in 1905. These authors reported atrophy of tubules and glomeruli with an associated increase in interstitial tissue after exposure of rabbit kidneys to irradiation. One of the most detailed early studies was carried out by Bolliger and Laidley (1930), who followed the progression of renal damage in dogs from hours to months after irradiation. These authors described five distinct phases of injury and correlated animal lethality with histological changes. Initially (0–48 h) there was a period of acute, transient congestion and edema. This was followed (1–8 days) by a latent

408 F.A. Stewart and M.V. Williams

period during which the kidneys appeared normal. From 5 to 32 days progressive tubular damage was noted, with degeneration of convoluted tubules, cast formation, and the beginnings of fibrous tissue invasion. In the fourth period (21–60 days), there was further degeneration of the parenchyma and progressive replacement with fibrous tissue; occasional islands of regenerating tubules were seen. The glomeruli were reported as mostly normal during this period. The final phase of damage (60–230 days) consisted of tubular depletion with distinct islands of regeneration, glomerular sclerosis or hyaline degeneration, and vascular tortuosity. Bolliger and Laidley (1930) described renal tubules as the initial site of damage, with glomeruli undergoing secondary degeneration in the later stages of disease. This observation is supported by more recent work of several authors (Phillips and Ross 1973; Jordan et al. 1978; Mason and Withers 1985; Michalowski 1986) but it is by no means a universal finding.

Phillips and Ross (1973) reported that the major histological change in mouse kidney (after unilateral irradiation with prior nephrectomy) was a loss of proximal and distal convoluted tubules which began at about 4 months. Glomerular changes were found to be minor and to occur later.

Madrazo and Churg (1976) reported progressive injury involving both tubules and glomeruli after unilateral irradiation of rat kidneys. The development of damage was considered to be essentially a degenerative process, with atrophy and fibrosis of the renal parenchyma leading to subsequent vascular damage and inflammation. In the glomeruli, mesangial thickening and wrinkling and thickening of the basement membrane occurred. Detachment of endothelial cells and a collapse of glomerular loops were also noted. Tubular changes included a characteristic thickening and layering of basement membranes, with cellular atrophy and necrosis at later times. Tubular degeneration was largely restricted to the cortex, with sparing of the medulla, which has also been observed by many other authors.

Jordan et al. (1978) developed a quantitative scoring system for the histological assessment of radiation-induced renal damage in mice which was entirely based on tubular changes (see Table 14.1). These tubular changes included nuclear enlargement of epithelial cells, thickening of the basement membrane, cellular atrophy, and cyst formation. Nuclear enlargement of the proximal tubular cells has subsequently been used by these

Table 14.1. Histopathological grading of tubular changes after renal irradiation (Jordan et al. 1978)

0 No significant tubular abnormality
1 Enlarged tubular epithelial nuclei
2 Tubular epithelial atrophy and cystic dilatation
3 Single tubular collapse or marked epithelial thinning with enlarged tubular epithelial nuclei
4 Focal tubular collapse
5 Extensive tubular collapse

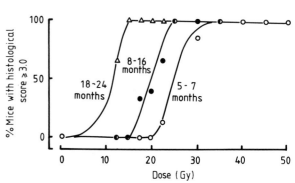

Fig. 14.2. The percentages of mice showing tubular collapse (histological grades >3.0) are compared at various doses and times following radiation. There is an inverse relation between time since irradiation and dose for a given level of damage. (Redrawn from Jordan et al. 1978)

authors and by others as a quantitative early predictor of the extent of renal damage (Jordan et al. 1984; Otsuka et al. 1988). Jordan et al. (1978) found that tubular changes were the most significant, and that glomerular damage was variable and less marked. Vascular injury was thought to be a secondary consequence of parenchymal cell loss. The scoring system developed by these authors gave good radiation dose–response relationships (Fig. 14.2) and correlated well with mortality and renal function tests.

Michalowski has recently undertaken a detailed study of sequential changes occurring in mouse kidneys after unilateral irradiation (Michalowski et al. 1986; Michalowski, personal communication, 1987). He found that the earliest changes (occurring as early as 2–4 weeks after irradiation) were in the proximal tubular cells of the juxtamedullary region of the cortex. Early damage was seen as a flattening of the epithelial cells with a wrinkling of the basement membrane. This progressed to tubular cell loss which was initially restricted to small foci clustered around the arcuate arteries and veins (Figs. 14.3, 14.4) but later affected the midcortical and superficial nephrons. During this period of tubular degeneration (1–3 months) the glomeruli, arterioles, and arteries were normal. Interstitial fibrosis and a chronic inflammatory response were sometimes observed but they were mild.

In contrast with the above-mentioned studies, several workers have concluded that the glomeruli or the fine vasculature are the principal targets for renal radiation damage. CASARETT (1964) described the pathogenesis of renal radiation injury in the rat as an arteriolonephrosclerotic process, with secondary progressive degeneration of glomeruli and tubules. Increased interstitial con-

nective tissue deposits and hyalinization were reported as the result of parenchymal degeneration but no tubular regeneration was seen. The fine vasculature was considered to be the primary target for damage, with endothelial degeneration followed by a period of regeneration, leading to vascular occlusion and sclerosis within 6–8 months. An early hyperemic response was also noted. Similar findings were subsequently reported by several other authors. RUBIN and CASARETT (1968) proposed that the fundamental mechanism for late radiation injury in tissues, including the kidney, is arteriolosclerotic vascular damage.

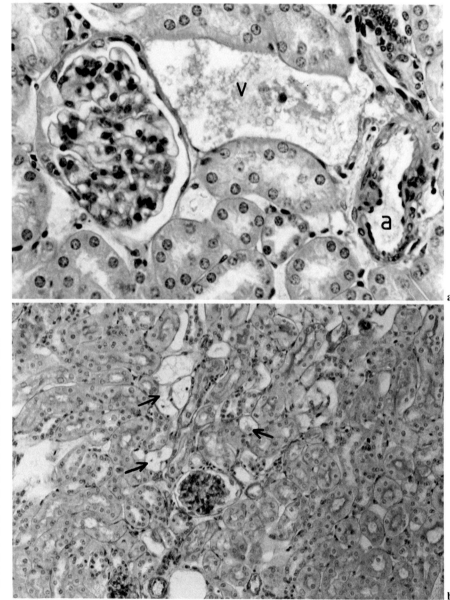

Fig. 14.3. a Cortex of a kidney from an untreated mouse showing a glomerulus surrounded by proximal and distal tubules. The artery (*a*) and vein (*v*) are also visible. **b** Twenty weeks after 14 Gy bilateral renal irradiation there are focal areas of tubular degeneration (*arrow*) whereas the glomeruli are essentially normal. **c, d** Forty weeks after 40 Gy there is extensive tubular loss with fibrinous replacement. At this time there is also extensive glomerular damage with contracted glomerular tufts and empty cystic spaces

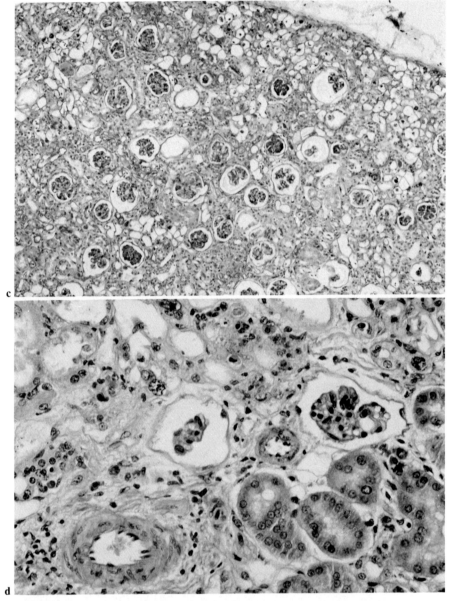

There are also several proponents of the theory that the glomerulus is the primary site for radiation injury in the kidney (LJUNG-QVIST et al. 1971; FAJARDO et al. 1976; GLATSTEIN et al. 1977). GLATSTEIN and co-workers followed the course of histopathological damage in mice after bilateral renal irradiation and concluded that the most striking changes occurred in the glomeruli. Atrophy and flattening of the cells lining Bowman's capsule, irregular distribution of nuclei within the glomerular tuft, increased glomerular density, and mesangial thickening were reported, beginning at 3 months after irradiation. There was subsequent progressive replacement of capillary walls and lumina by acidophilic, periodic acid-Schiff (PAS) positive material. These lesions increased in severity with time. Tubular damage occurred late and was considered to be less severe than glomerular damage (GLATSTEIN et al. 1977).

In summary, there is no real agreement between different authors about whether the primary target for renal radiation injury is tubular, vascular, or glomerular. Only tubular damage has yielded dose–response information, however, and similar results have been obtained by scoring slight or marked degrees of tubule enlargement or by identifying regenerating tubules. Radiation-induced glomerular injury has not been shown to

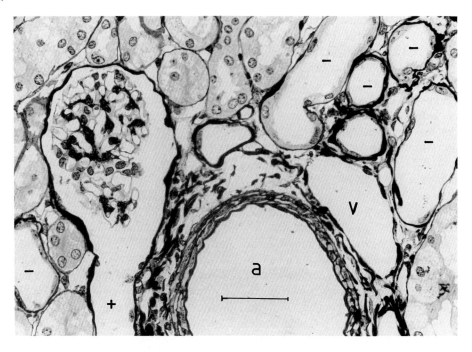

Fig. 14.4. The mouse left kidney 8 weeks after its exposure to a single dose of 15 Gy of x-rays. Denuded proximal tubule (+) communicating with the Bowman's space of an intact juxtamedullary glomerulus; *a* and *v* are cross-sections of the arcuate artery and vein, respectively. Other damaged tubules either lined with flattened epithelial cells or partially denuded are marked (-). The *bar* represents 50 μm. Perfusion fixation with formal saline; resin embedding; periodic acid methenamine silver staining after Jones (kindly provided by A. MICHALOWSKI)

be dose responsive, despite the use of scoring systems which can demonstrate temporal progression. Indeed, glomerular damage can be very variable, even within the same section.

It is clear that the interpretation of subtle histological changes is subjective and it is unlikely that this approach will permit identification of the critical target cell for radiation nephropathy. Nevertheless, there is agreement that early changes can be detected within a few weeks, that radiation nephropathy is slowly progressive, and that there is no true functional recovery at later times, despite epithelial proliferation and tubular regeneration.

14.1.4 Time of Expression of Damage and Recovery

Although some histological and functional changes can be observed within a few weeks of renal irradiation, the kidney is basically a late-responding tissue with functional impairment developing in a slowly progressive manner over months to years. This is partly because in clinical practice doses at the margin of tolerance are administered and the time of expression of renal damage is dose dependent, occurring late after low doses.

The tubular epithelium has been classed as an "F" type or flexible tissue (MICHALOWSKI 1981, 1986). In such tissues the functional cells also retain the capacity for cell proliferation although, in steady state conditions, they divide only rarely. In response to cell loss as a result of injury, however, all cells are capable of accelerated compensatory proliferation. The time of expression of radiation injury in F type tissues is inversely dose related, and progression of damage accelerates as more and more irradiated cells are triggered into a lethal mitosis; this has been termed the avalanche effect (MICHALOWSKI 1981). After low doses the apparent latency period before the expression of measurable functional impairment may be many months or years.

In mice the development of renal functional damage has been shown to be relentlessly progressive, even after low doses, with no indication of functional recovery at late times (GLATSTEIN 1973; PHILLIPS and ROSS 1973; STEWART et al. 1984b, 1986a; 1988a; MICHALOWSKI 1986). This is despite the fact that dose-dependent increases in the proliferation rate of renal tubular cells have been demonstrated at 3–4 months (SORANSON and DENEKAMP 1986; OTSUKA and MEISTRICH 1986) and regeneration of whole tubules has been observed at 15 months (WITHERS et al. 1986). This would suggest that either the extent of stimulated proliferation in the kidney is insufficient to match the progressive cell loss which occurs after irradiation, or that proliferation occurs without organization into functionally intact nephron units.

Acutely responding normal tissues such as skin and mucosa can proliferate in response to injury expressed during a course of irradiation. Prolonging overall treatment can then allow more time for proliferation and thus spare radiation injury. Since the kidney is a late-responding tissue, such factors would not be expected to influence its response. However, there are several reports in the literature of small to moderate increases in renal tolerance (for both mice and pigs) when the total irradiation time was protracted over several weeks (PHILLIPS and FU 1974; GLATSTEIN et al. 1975; HOPEWELL and WIERNIK 1977; WILLIAMS and DENEKAMP 1984a; WILLIAMS et al. 1985). These increases were generally attributed to a slow repair process or a transient hypoxia occurring as the result of radiation-induced edema, rather than cellular proliferation during treatment. However, there is a fundamental problem associated with the comparison of dose–effect curves from renal functional studies for treatments given in widely different overall times. Renal radiation damage develops progressively and the amount of damage is dependent both on radiation dose and on time since treatment. It is difficult to define time zero when the overall treatment is protracted, which means that direct comparison of the effects of treatments given in long and short overall times is complex. This problem has been discussed in detail by several authors (WILLIAMS et al. 1985; STEWART et al. 1988a; LEBESQUE et al. 1988). If the final rate of expression of injury is analyzed, it is possible to compare treatments satisfactorily, but dose precision is low and few experiments have collected the large amount of sequential data required for this type of analysis. It seems probable that much of the reported increase in renal tolerance with protracted irradiation schedules reflects a delay in the time of expression of damage rather than a reduction in the amount of tissue damage after the longer treatment times. Increases in overall treatment time are unlikely to lead to significant sparing of damage to the

kidneys either by proliferation or by any other mechanism.

The lack of renal functional recovery with increasing time would suggest that the kidneys may be very sensitive to reirradiation, even after periods of many months to years. Recent data from STEWART et al. (1988a) and MOULDER (1983) confirm that the tolerance of rodent kidneys to reirradiation after a 6-month interval is very poor. The studies of MOULDER demonstrated that the retreatment tolerance of previously irradiated rat kidneys was reduced to 25% of a full dose. STEWART et al. (1988a) found that there was no recovery of mouse kidneys within a 6-month period. Even low x-ray doses, which were insufficient to produce renal damage without retreatment, compromised tolerance to a second dose of irradiation after 6 months. These data strongly suggest that previously irradiated kidneys should not be reirradiated, even if the measured renal function appears to be normal.

One special circumstance in which apparent functional recovery can occur is when a single kidney is irradiated and the contralateral kidney removed after the onset of renal dysfunction. In the pig studies of ROBBINS et al. (1986), irradiated kidneys were judged to have no significant function by 24 weeks after unilateral irradiation with 8.8 Gy if the contralateral kidney was left in situ. After removal of the unirradiated kidney, the vascular supply and functional response (assessed by renography) of the irradiated kidney significantly improved (Fig. 14.5). It was concluded that the presence of an unirradiated kidney prevented recovery in the irradiated kidney, and that nephrectomy allowed a "revascularization" of the damaged kidney. It was suggested that tubular atrophy may be partly reversed by revascularization and that vasoactive agents could assist recovery (ROBBINS et al. 1986). The concept of a circulating renotrophic growth factor was also invoked to explain the increase in weight of the irradiated kidney after contralateral nephrectomy.

Alternatively, these results could perhaps be explained simply by the normal homeostatic control mechanisms which attempt to maintain total renal function. After unilateral irradiation there is no requirement for a damaged kidney to increase the workload per remaining nephron, since normal renal function can be performed by the unirradiated organ, which undergoes hypertrophy and hyperplasia to maintain a constant total renal mass (MICHALOWSKI 1986). However, after contra-

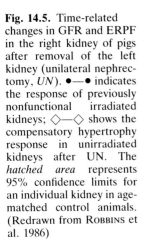

Fig. 14.5. Time-related changes in GFR and ERPF in the right kidney of pigs after removal of the left kidney (unilateral nephrectomy, *UN*). ●—● indicates the response of previously nonfunctional irradiated kidneys; ◇—◇ shows the compensatory hypertrophy response in unirradiated kidneys after UN. The *hatched area* represents 95% confidence limits for an individual kidney in age-matched control animals. (Redrawn from ROBBINS et al. 1986)

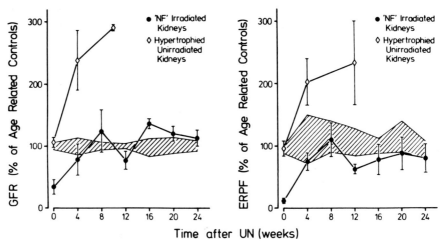

lateral nephrectomy the damaged kidney must respond by increasing the workload per nephron and this has been shown to occur within certain limits (ROBBINS et al. 1986; MICHALOWSKI 1986), although the total renal function of the animal decreases as a result of the nephrectomy. Thus the observed functional increase in an irradiated kidney after contralateral nephrectomy could simply represent the normal operation of homeostatic mechanisms, which demand that total renal function be maintained, rather than a true revascularization and recovery process.

14.1.5 Animal Models

14.1.5.1 Measurement of Functional Renal Damage

The mammalian kidney is an extremely complex organ with a multitude of regulatory and excretory functions, including control of blood volume and osmotic regulation of the plasma, excretion of metabolic waste products, and production of the active derivative of vitamin D, the enzyme renin, and the hormone erythropoietin. There are therefore many possibilities for the measurement of renal functional changes after irradiation. Several authors have measured a single physiological parameter and attempted to correlate this with damage to a specific cell type [e.g., polyuria has been attributed to tubular damage and decreased glomerular filtration rate (GFR) to glomerular damage]. It should be remembered, however, that homeostatic mechanisms ensure a very accurate balance between glomerular filtration and tubular

resorption in the kidney (control is mediated via the juxta-glomerular apparatus). This balance is maintained even in the face of disease or injury, and if there is severe damage to any part of a nephron then that whole unit will shut down (BRICKER et al. 1960; BRICKER and FINE 1981). As a consequence of a reduction in nephron number, the remaining nephrons must operate at an increased rate to maintain normal function. When renal damage becomes so severe that the remaining nephrons can no longer cope with the increased load, then this is reflected in decreased values for all parameters of renal function (regardless of the initial origin of the lesion). In the initial stages of damage the kidney may function normally under stable, nonstressed conditions but some reserve capacity will have been lost and the damaged kidney will be unable to respond to the requirements of the body in extreme situations (e.g., water deprivation or excessive salt intake). The concept of the "intact nephron" (BRICKER et al. 1960) should be borne in mind in interpreting results from functional studies, since these do not necessarily indicate the target cell population responsible for injury (WILLIAMS 1986).

Renal irradiation causes an initial hyperemic response within a few days. At later times there is a progressive, dose-dependent decrease in GFR and estimated renal plasma flow (ERPF) (see ROBBINS and HOPEWELL 1987, for review) with the deveolopment of polyuria, increased blood urea nitrogen (BUN) and creatinine levels, anemia, and hypertension (RUBIN and CASARETT 1968). The time of onset of functional damage is dose dependent, occurring earlier after high doses. Many authors report a delay of 4–6 months before the appearance of measurable renal dysfunction but this is probably partly due to the assay techniques used. Early (within 2 months) decreases in renal function have been measured in several studies, and a progressive decrease in renal wet weight has been demonstrated to begin within days of irradiation (Michalowski 1986).

Changes in ERPF and GFR can be measured either from the rate of clearance of tracer isotopes from the blood or by renography. This latter method has been extensively used for measurement of radiation-induced renal damage in the pig. Renography has also been used in rabbits, dogs, and rats.

Experiments with pigs using ^{99m}Tc-DTPA and ^{131}I-Hippuran renography to estimate GFR and ERPF respectively demonstrated dose-related decreases in function from 1 month after unilateral irradiation with 8.8 Gy. Maximum levels of damage were achieved within 6–12 weeks (Robbins et al. 1985). In dogs, changes in ERPF were observed from 4 to 6 weeks after unilateral irradiation with doses greater than 5 Gy (Gupp et al. 1967). In rats the onset of damage was slightly later, with normal renograms (^{131}I-Hippuran) until 16 weeks after 20 Gy and then a subsequent decline in function (Chauser et al. 1976). Renal function in rats was more recently investigated using ^{99m}Tc-DMSA (Landuyt et al. 1988), which is captured in the kidney proportionally to the number of patent nephrons. These studies demonstrated decreased renal function from 6 weeks after unilateral irradiation with a dose of 8 Gy. Radiation-induced decreases in renal blood flow have also been measured from 2 months after bilateral renal irradiation in mice, using the ^{86}Rb extraction technique (Glatstein 1973).

Clearance of ^{51}Cr-EDTA has been extensively used to measure changes in GFR after renal irradiation in rodents. The single sample method (Chantler et al. 1969), which dispenses with the need for prolonged isotope perfusion and urine collection, has been established as a simple and reliable method for assessment of renal function, although a precise measure of GFR is not obtained. Using ^{51}Cr-EDTA clearance several authors have demonstrated progressive renal dysfunction after single and fractionated irradiation. In most cases a minimum latent period of about 4 months was observed using this assay (Williams and Denekamp 1983; Stewart et al. 1984b).

Another functional change which occurs in the irradiated kidney is polyuria. In dogs polyuria and the loss of concentrating ability were observed within 10–15 days of renal irradiation after prior unilateral nephrectomy (Coburn et al. 1966). An increased output of dilute urine was also reported from 17 weeks after bilateral renal irradiation in mice (Williams and Denekamp 1983). These authors quantified the increased urinary output and constructed radiation dose–response curves. Cullen et al. (1986) found that polyuria developed even after unilateral irradiation, although a further increase in urinary output was observed after removal of the unirradiated kidney. Interestingly, these polyuric mice were still able to concentrate their urine if access to water was temporarily withheld.

Assays such as BUN and serum creatinine are also indicative of renal failure and have been used to measure radiation damage. They are, however, relatively insensitive and liable to be influenced by factors such as protein intake and liver function.

Hypertension is commonly associated with renal irradiation but there are clear species and strain differences. In man hypertension can follow unilateral or bilateral irradiation, whereas in the rat the presence of an untreated kidney exerts a protective effect against the development of hypertension (Redd 1960). It is now established that the hypertension of radiation nephritis results from increased renin secretion from the juxtaglomerular apparatus. Goldblatt et al. (1934) demonstrated that renal ischemia could stimulate renin secretion and this has subsequently been proposed as a mechanism for radiation-induced hypertension (Wacholz and Casarett 1970; Robbins and Hopewell 1987). Elevated blood pressure may develop in the absence of renal fibrosis and this can further exacerbate vascular injury already present in the kidney.

Another consequence of renal irradiation, which has been demonstrated both experimentally and clinically, is anemia (Kunkler et al. 1952; Stewart 1967; Alpen and Stewart 1984). The anemia of renal insufficiency is hypochromic to normochromic and is the result of both deficiencies in red blood cell production (due to insufficient production of erythropoietin) and a hemolytic defect. It has been suggested that renal anemia is partly due to damage to the juxtaglomerular apparatus, with an associated reduction in production of erythropoietin (Osnes 1959; Alpen and Stewart 1984), but fluorescent antibody labeling techniques appear to demonstrate that the site for erythropoietin production is located in the glomerular tuft rather than the juxtaglomerular apparatus (KURTZ et al. 1983).

14.1.5.2 Nonfunctional Assays of Renal Damage

Lethality assays have been used to measure renal radiation injury in animals but death is a very nonspecific endpoint and the interpretation of results is likely to be complicated by radiation-induced intestinal damage (WILLIAMS and DENEKAMP 1983), Kidney weight (either wet or dry weight) can, however, be used as a sensitive measure of renal damage and the results correlate well with functional and histological studies (MICHALOWSKI et al. 1986).

Radiation sensitivity of mouse kidney cells has been assessed using an in vitro colony assay (DESCHAVANNE et al. 1980; MALAISE et al. 1985). Kidney cells were either irradiated in vivo and subsequently removed for culture, or they were irradiated in vitro after disaggregation and plating. Both fibroblast and epithelial cell colonies could be identified (in the ratio 1:4) and colony counts were performed using both morphologies. D_0 values of 2 Gy after in vivo irradiation or 1.3 Gy after in vitro irradiation were found (Fig. 14.6).

An in vivo colony assay has also recently been described for renal tubular cells (MASON and

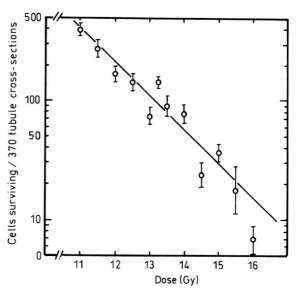

Fig. 14.7. Dose–survival curve for tubule-regenerating cells at 16 months after unilateral renal irradiation in the mouse. *Error bars* are SEM and the curve is a weighted linear regression, D_0 = 1.53 Gy (1.25–1.98 Gy, 95% confidehce limits). (Redrawn from WITHERS et al. 1986)

WITHERS 1985; WITHERS et al. 1986). Complete cross-sections of irradiated mouse kidneys were made at 30–70 weeks after unilateral irradiation and regenerating tubules were clearly visible among a background of parenchymal destruction. The number of healthy tubules in contact with the capsule was scored and this gave a dose-dependent relationship. It was argued by these authors that the intact tubules arose by regeneration from small (randomly distributed) numbers of surviving cells. This assay gave D_0 values for renal tubular cells of 1.5 Gy for single doses after in vivo irradiation (Fig. 14.7).

14.1.6 Modification of Radiation Response

14.1.6.1 Fractionation

The kidney has a large capacity for repair of sublethal radiation damage during fractionated treatments and the size of the dose per fraction markedly influences radiation tolerance. There are now several experimental studies which demonstrate the increase in total tolerance dose as the number of x-ray fractions is increased, and hence the size of each dose per fraction is decreased (e.g., Fig. 14.8).

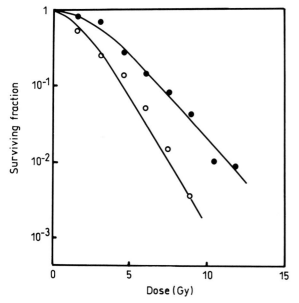

Fig. 14.6. Survival curves for murine kidney cells irradiated in vivo (●) in air-breathing mice and plated immediately afterwards, or plated and then irradiated in vitro 18 h later (○) (MALAISE et al. 1985)

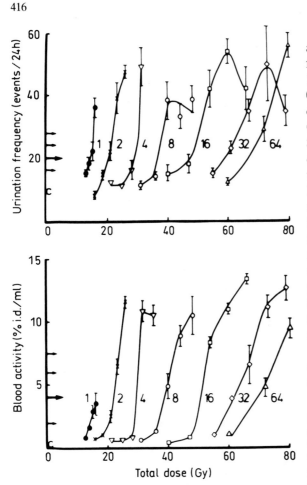

Fig. 14.8. Dose–response curves for urine output and ^{51}Cr-EDTA clearance at 26–27 weeks after fractionated bilateral renal irradiation in the mouse. The number of fractions is indicated against each curve and each point is the mean ±1 SEM of a group of four to six mice. There is clearly dose sparing with increasing fractionation. (STEWART et al. 1984b)

The early fractionation studies were analyzed according to an NSD (nominal standard dose) formulation – Total Dose = NSD $N^x \cdot T^y$ (ELLIS 1969) – and exponents for fraction number (N) of 0.4–0.5 were obtained for overall treatment times of 3–6 weeks (HOPEWELL and WIERNIK 1977; CALDWELL 1975; WILLIAMS and DENEKAMP 1984b; STEWART et al. 1984b, 1987b), with lower N exponents sometimes being obtained for the shorter overall treatment times (GLATSTEIN et al. 1975; HOPEWELL and BERRY 1975; WILLIAMS and DENEKAMP 1984b). Published data for changes in total isoeffective dose with fractionation are summarized in Fig. 14.9 and Table 14.2. It should be noted that most of the estimates of N for short overall treatment times were made from a comparison of only two or three different fractionation schedules over a limited range of doses per fraction; the reliability of some of these values may therefore be suspect.

It has recently become clear that a single N exponent cannot be fitted to fractionated kidney data over a wide range of doses per fraction, and

Fig. 14.9. Isoeffective doses as a function of fraction number from published studies on irradiation of kidneys of mice and pigs. Data sets where the N exponent is 0.4–0.5 are indicated with *solid lines*; those giving lower N exponents are shown with *dashed lines* (see Table 14.2). Data source: □, STEWART et al. 1984b; ■, STEWART et al. 1987b; ▲, WILLIAMS and DENEKAMP 1984b, overall treatment time 35 days; △, WILLIAMS and DENEKAMP 1984b, overall treatment time 4 days; X, JORDAN et al. 1981, 1985; ▼, GLATSTEIN et al. 1975, overall treatment time 18 days; ▽, GLATSTEIN et al. 1975, overall treatment time 4 days; ◊, PHILLIPS and FU 1974; ●, HOPEWELL and WIERNIK 1977; ○, HOPEWELL and BERRY 1975

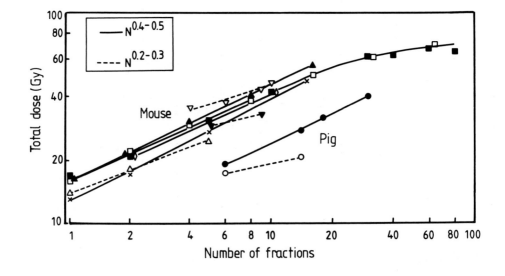

Table 14.2. Published studies of the fractionation response of irradiated kidney

Reference	Animal	Number of fractions	Overall time (days)	N exponent	α/β value (Gy)[b]
PHILLIPS and FU 1974	Mouse	2,10	1,11[a]	0.47	–
GLATSTEIN et al. 1975	Mouse	4,6,9,10	18	0.27	10.4
GLATSTEIN et al. 1975	Mouse	5,9	4	0.21	–
WILLIAMS and DENEKAMP 1984b	Mouse	1,2,4,8,16	35	0.42	2.8
WILLIAMS and DENEKAMP 1984b	Mouse	1,2,5	4	0.33	–
JORDAN et al. 1985	Mouse	1,2,5,15	1,4,14[a]	0.49	0.2
STEWART et al. 1984b	Mouse	1,2,4,8,16	21	0.42	2.7–3.2
STEWART et al. 1984b	Mouse	16,32,64	21	0.24	2.7–3.2
STEWART et al. 1987b	Mouse	1,2,5,10,30 (30,60,80)	28	0.42	1.9–2.3 (6.1)[c]
HOPEWELL and WIERNIK 1977	Pig	6,14,18,30	39	0.49	0.04
HOPEWELL and BERRY 1975	Pig	6,14	18	0.24	–
CALDWELL 1975	Rabbit	1,6,12,18,24	11–53[a]	0.54	−0.5

[a] Overall treatment time increased with fraction number.
[b] α/β values only calculated from experiments where there were at least three different fractionation schedules. All data obtained at doses per fraction >10 Gy are excluded from these calculations.
[c] Data in parentheses were analyzed separately. No single fit of all data to an LQ model was obtained. The α/β calculated for doses per fraction below 2 Gy was significantly increased (see text).

that the exponent of N tends to decrease as fraction number increases (see data from STEWART et al. 1987b in Fig. 14.9). Such a deviation from the Ellis fractionation formula would be expected if the dose response for damage is fitted by a linear–quadratic (LQ) expression. There is now substantial evidence to demonstrate that in the kidney, as with most other normal tissues, the dose fractionation response can be well described by an LQ formulation of the general format $E = \alpha d + \beta d^2$, where E is a defined level of damage and d is dose per fraction (DOUGLAS and FOWLER 1976; FOWLER 1984). The ratio α/β, which is obtained from an LQ analysis, gives a direct measure of the degree of curvature on the tissue radiation dose–response curve. Tissues with low α/β ratios have curvier dose–response curve shapes and are more sensitive to small changes in the size of the dose per fraction than tissues with high α/β ratios (WITHERS et al. 1982).

Recent multifraction data for mouse kidneys (WILLIAMS and DENEKAMP 1984b; STEWART et al. 1984b, 1987b; JORDAN et al. 1985; JOINER and JOHNS 1988) demonstrate that the LQ model

adequately describes the renal response to fractionation, at least for doses per fraction in the range 2–10 Gy. The α/β ratios obtained from these studies were invariably lower than 5 Gy (see Table 14.2), which indicates a strong dependence of renal tolerance on size of dose per fraction; this is consistent with the α/β values obtained in most other late-responding normal tissues (FOWLER 1984).

Experiments using very small doses per fraction with large fraction numbers (STEWART et al. 1987b) or a top-up design (JOINER and JOHNS 1988) have recently demonstrated that at doses below 1–2 Gy there is a major deviation of observed isoeffective doses from those predicted by the LQ model. At very low doses per fraction much less dose sparing with increased fractionation was observed than predicted. A part of this deviation could be explained by incomplete repair of sublethal damage between successive fractions if the $T_{1/2}$ for repair in the kidney was greater than 90 min (STEWART et al. 1987b). However, JOINER and JOHNS (1988) concluded that at doses per fraction below 1 Gy the LQ model did not fit renal fractionation data and that there was a substantial increase in the x-ray effectiveness at very low doses.

In summary, the kidney is extremely sensitive to changes in fraction number and the size of the dose per fraction. Large increases in total tolerance dose are obtained with increasing fractionation down to doses per fraction of about 1 Gy. This appears to be the limit for dose sparing with fractionation for kidney. No increased tolerance should be expected for protracted treatment times.

14.1.6.2 Radioprotection

Sulfydryl compounds have been shown to act as radioprotectors in a wide range of normal tissues, giving protection factors (PF) of up to 3 in some tissues such as bone marrow (YUHAS and STORER 1969). Radioprotection of the kidney by cysteamine (ASSCHER 1965) and its phosphorylated derivative WR-2721 [S-2-(3-aminopropylamino)-ethylphosphorothioic acid] has also been demonstrated, but relatively modest PFs of 1.1–1.5 were measured in the kidney using maximum tolerated drug doses (PHILLIPS et al. 1973; WILLIAMS and DENEKAMP 1984c; ROJAS et al. 1986). Fractionated studies by ROJAS et al. (1986) showed that there was no change in the extent of renal protection afforded by WR-2721 with fractionation.

14.1.6.3 Radiosensitization

The kidney is a well vascularized and well oxygenated organ receiving 25% of the cardiac output at rest. Nevertheless, a slight increase in the radiosensitivity of dog kidneys was observed in experiments where the kidneys of anesthetized aniamls were irradiated in hyperbaric oxygen (CONCANNON et al. 1964). Studies in mice using the hypoxic cell sensitizer misonidazole, however, showed no sensitization of the response of the kidneys to single or fractionated x-rays (WILLIAMS and DENEKAMP 1984c). This could reflect the lower efficiency of misonidazole than oxygen as a sensitizer.

14.1.6.4 High LET Irradiation

Relative biological effectiveness (RBE) values for renal damage after irradiation with high energy neutrons or pi–mesons (containing only a small component of high LET radiation) have been measured in rodent and large animal studies. After large single radiation doses (>10 Gy x-rays) RBE values of 1.7–2.3 were obtained for neutrons relative to 250 kV x-rays (GERACI et al. 1978; STEWART et al. 1984c; HOPEWELL et al. 1982), with a lower value of 1.1 after single doses of pi-mesons compared with 250 kV x-rays (JORDAN et al. 1981). The RBE for renal damage (as with other normal tissues) increases markedly with decreasing dose per fraction, and neutron RBEs [d(4)-Be neutrons] of up to 7.3 have been measured at x-rays doses per fraction of 1.5 Gy (JOINER and JOHNS 1987).

14.1.6.5 Combined Modalities

Abdominal irradiation (including the kidneys) in combination with chemotherapy is used in the treatment of several cancers, particularly testicular and ovarian. For these tumours one of the most effective drugs available is cis-diamminedichloroplatinum (II) (c-DDP), which is known to be nephrotoxic. In man renal toxicity from drug alone is dose limiting, despite the use of forced hydration and mannitol to promote diuresis. In rodents, renal damage develops rapidly, with tubular degeneration and epithelial necrosis evident within a few days and decreased renal function within 1–2 weeks (KOCIBA and SLEIGHT 1971; LEONARD et al. 1971; STEWART et al. 1986a). Experimental studies have also demonstrated a modest increase in late renal damage after combined treatment with radiation and c-DDP (STEWART et al. 1986a, 1988b; VAN RONGEN et al. 1988; MOULDER and FISH 1988). Dose enhancement factors of 1.1–1.3 were measured for both single and fractionated treatments (STEWART et al. 1988b), but most of this effect could be explained by independent, additive toxicities (see BEGG et al. 1989 for review).

Retreatment studies in which c-DDP was given at 3–12 months after renal irradiation have, however, shown a marked reduction in drug tolerance after previous irradiation, with a rapid onset of fatal nephropathy after drug doses which are normally well tolerated (Fig. 14.10 and STEWART et al. 1987a; MOULDER and FISH 1988; LANDUYT et al. 1988). The renal toxicity which results from c-DDP given several months after irradiation is much more severe than that seen when

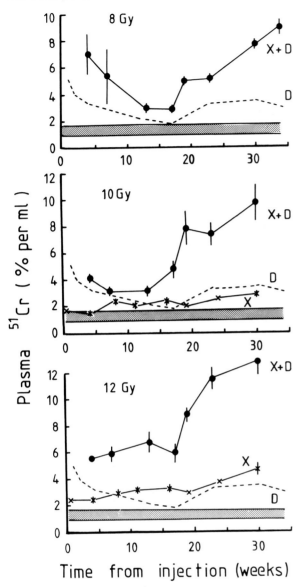

Fig. 14.10. Kidney damage in mice (measured from clearance of ^{51}Cr-EDTA) given c-DDP (6 mg/kg) at 6 months after bilateral renal irradiation with 8, 10, or 12 Gy. The response to drug alone (*D*) and development of damage after 10 and 12 Gy x-rays alone (*X*) are shown for equivalent testing periods, i.e., from 6 months after irradiation for a period of 30 weeks. Damage in previously irradiated mice was always much more severe than when drug was given to age-matched controls. This was true even for a low preirradiation dose of 8 Gy which alone did not cause measurable renal impairment. (STEWART et al. 1987a)

months after renal irradiation caused greater than additive cell killing (STEWART et al. 1987a; MOULDER and FISH 1988), which may be related to a reduced drug clearance rate in the previously irradiated animals (MOULDER et al. 1986). These data strongly suggest that c-DDP (or other nephrotoxic agents) should be avoided in retreatment schedules after previous renal irradiation.

Several other chemotherapeutic agents are also known to be nephrotoxic (e.g., mitomycin C, high dose methotrexate, and nitrosoureas), and both actinomycin D and Adriamycin appear to enhance renal radiation damage in man even in the absence of significant drug toxicity (RUBIN 1984; PHILLIPS and FU 1978).

14.2 The Bladder and Ureter

14.2.1 Clinical Picture of Radiation Damage

The bladder is routinely irradiated to tolerance in the clinical treatment of cancer of the bladder or prostate. In addition, its close proximity to the uterus means that high bladder doses are delivered in the radical treatment of cancer of the cervix. Similarly, the lower ureter is exposed to high irradiation doses as it enters the bladder.

In the treatment of carcinoma of the bladder the patient often has preexisting urinary symptoms such as frequency, dysuria, hematuria, or nocturia. These should improve as treatment proceeds and this may mask symptoms from radiation injury itself. Urinary frequency, dysuria, and referred penile pain are not uncommon side-effects of bladder irradiation. It is important to exclude urinary infection as a cause of these symptoms, and many radiotherapists request routine weekly cultures of the urine so that they can detect and treat subclinical infection.

Early clinical studies identified three separate phases of acute, subacute, and late bladder injury following irradiation (DEAN 1933; WATSON et al. 1947; GOWING 1960). It must be remembered that the early data were obtained before antibiotics were generally available and therfore include the complicating effects of infection. In the acute phase (4–6 weeks from the start of treatment) cystoscopy revealed a diffuse hyperemia with congestion and edema of the mucosa, sometimes accompanied by partial desquamation and ulceration. The early changes were usually reported as mild and transient, severe damage only occurring

the drug is given before irradiation (MOULDER and FISH 1988). This could be partly explained by drug cell killing adding to the slowly progressive radiation damage, resulting in the expression of previously subthreshold injury. It was generally concluded, however, that c-DDP given several

in association with a secondary bacterial infection. Also sometimes noted during this early phase were small calcareous deposits which form in the bladder in the presence of urea-splitting bacteria found in conditions of extensive necrosis (Dean 1933; Watson et al. 1947).

The subacute clinical phase (6 months to 2 years) has been principally described as one of vascular ischemia, leading to secondary epithelial denudation, the formation of ulcers, necrosis, and sometimes fistulation (Dean 1933; Gowing 1960). A chronic inflamatory infiltrate and extensive edema of the submucosa, plus the formation of calcareous deposits and calculi, may be noted during this phase. The late phase of clinical damage (1–10 years) consists of a reduced bladder capacity due to a combination of fibrosis (in the submucosa and muscle layers) and infection. Telangectasia (often at the site of the initial lesion) also occurs in the late phase (Gowing 1960; Morrison and Deeley 1965).

Long-term severe late effects have been documented in several studies and the incidence of late damage appears to correlate with the irradiated bladder volume and the dose delivered, particularly to the anterior wall (Dewit et al. 1983). Morrison (1975) performed a randomized study in which T_1 and T_2 bladder tumors were treated with 55 or 62.5 Gy to the bladder only in 20 daily fractions over 4 weeks. Major complications occurred in 35% of patients, but this figure includes bowel injury and fistula formation as well as bladder contraction and hemorrhage. Quilty et al. (1985) also undertook a dose-seeking study using the same fractionation schedule and giving 50 Gy through 10-cm fields or 57.5 Gy through 8-cm fields. Morbidity was assessed using the RTOG/EORTC criteria and the acute effects on bladder and bowel were comparable. However, severe late bladder injury occurred in 6% of those in the low dose group and 28% of the high dose group. They concluded that this was unacceptable and in further studies used a dose of 54 Gy in 20 fractions over 4 weeks, as previously recommended by Hope-Stone et al. (1981). It is clear that radical radiotherapy for bladder cancer can cause severe morbidity. This can be minimized either by limiting the dose or by restricting field sizes as much as possible. If tumor cure is to be achieved, the whole of the extravesical component of the tumor must be included and this can be facilitated using CT-directed planning.

Intracavitary therapy for carcinoma of the cervix gives a high local dose and this is an important factor in achieving high cure rates. However, beyond the immediate treatment volume the dose delivered is very variable and small areas of high dose may occur in the bladder, ureter, and rectum. Unal et al. (1981) showed that severe late effects could be related to a high x-ray dose and asymmetry of the insertion. Previous pelvic inflammation and surgery were also risk factors. There is now interest in using CT scanning (Hunter et al. 1986; Coltart et al. 1987) or ultrasound scanning (Mak et al. 1987) to localize pelvic organs accurately in relation to the radioactive sources. It is hoped that this will allow further individualization of treatment to reduce late injury.

The ureter descends retroperitoneally from the renal hilum to the bladder. Along its length it is in close relation to small bowel, which limits the dose prescribed in external beam treatments. In addition, tumors of the ureter itself are usually treated surgically, and it is therefore rare to see clinical problems arising from radiation damage to the ureter following external beam therapy alone. However, the ureter lies just 1.5 cm lateral to the vaginal fornix and a short portion receives a very high dose of radiation in the intracavitary treatment of carcinoma of the cervix. Nevertheless, the incidence of ureteric obstruction as a result of radiation damage is very low: Kottmeier (1964) reported 20 cases out of 3484 patients irradiated, and Slater and Fletcher (1971) reported 5 cases out of 1555 treated. These reports rightly exclude those patients in whom the cause of obstruction is recurrent tumor, and the ureters are therefore considered to be more radioresistant than the bladder (Bubin and Casarett 1968).

14.2.2 Clinical Management of Radiation Damage

Acute symptoms occurring during irradiation of the bladder are managed symptomatically. After infection has been excluded, alkalinization of the urine and a high fluid intake may help to relieve dysuria. Emepronium bromide (Cetiprin) 200 mg three times a day may relieve frequency and urgency of micturition, but these symptoms usually subside after the completion of treatment.

Late damage to the bladder is difficult to palliate. Long-term bladder symptoms after radical treatment for carcinoma of the cervix are surprisingly common. In a recent postal survey 56% of patients who replied had symptoms and these were severe in 26% (PARKIN et al. 1987). If symptoms are intolerable and the cancer has been controlled then surgery may be required. In all these operations wide margins and the use of unirradiated tissue in reconstruction are essential (KOTTMEIER 1964). If a contracted bladder develops then cystectomy and urinary diversion may be required.

Late effects on the ureter with stenosis and renal obstruction are rarely seen. If recurrent carcinoma can be excluded, urinary diversion can be considered as long as the irradiated lower third of the ureter is sacrificed (GOODMAN and DALTON 1982); in some cases it may be possible to dilate the ureter (SHINGLETON et al. 1969).

14.2.3 Morphological and Histological Changes After Irradiation

The bladder consists of a mucosa with three to five layers of transitional epithelium, beneath which is a collagenous lamina propria and additional loose connective tissue containing nerves and blood vessels (submucosa). The whole is surrounded by three smooth muscle layers containing the bladder sphincters. The epithelium is arranged in a pattern of increasing differentiation from small, diploid basal cells to large, poylploid surface cells. The surface cells have a unique plasma membrane at their luminal surface which enables contraction and expansion of the bladder and which maintains an effective osmotic barrier between the urine and blood.

Experimental animal studies have differed considerably in the time at which histological evidence of radiation-induced bladder damage (particularly epithelial denudation) was seen. In the studies of HUEPER et al. (1942) very early reactions were seen in dog bladders after irradiation with only low doses of 3×4 Gy. Acute edema and hyperemia of the mucosa occurred, followed by the development of large vacuoles and pyknotic nuclei in epithelial cells, lymphocytic infiltration of the submucosa, and the beginnings of epithelial degeneration and ulceration within 5 weeks. A generalized desquamation followed, leaving an edematous submucosa, covered only by a single layer of small, pyknotic, epithelial cells. Similar changes have been observed in mouse bladders (STEWART 1986 and unpublished data), but at much later times of 6–12 months after irradiation. In dog bladders, epithelial denudation was fol-

lowed by a period of rapid cell division and hyperplasia. By 10 months the mucosa was sometimes restored to near normal but in other specimens there remained large mucosal ulcers, and atrophic epithelium and a fibrotic submucosa (HUEPER et al. 1942).

The time scale for radiation damage in rodent bladders is much less rapid. The epithelium was found to remain essentially intact for the first 3 months after large single doses of 20–25 Gy (STEWART et al. 1978; STEWART 1986; ANTONAKOPOULOS et al. 1984), although the beginnings of pyknosis and some binucleate basal cells were seen during this period. Electron microscopy also revealed early subcellular changes such as edematous cytoplasm, an increased number of enlarged lysosomes, and minor changes in the blood vessels of the submucosa (ANTONAKOPOULOS et al. 1984). Epithelial damage occurred first in the basal cell layer, later spreading to other layers. From about 6 months after irradiation multifocal atypical hyperplasia, with extensive vacuolation of the epithelium, was seen in both rat (ANTONAKOPOULOS et al. 1984) and mouse studies (Fig. 14.11) (STEWART 1986). The superficial cells were small and immature and, by 12 months, most had lost their characteristic luminal membranes. Hyperplasia of endothelial cells was also noted, as well as perivascular fibrosis and degeneration of the muscle layers with collagen replacement. Bladder calculi were fairly common (up to 22%) in the irradiated mouse bladders at 1 year (STEWART et al. 1986b). In the rat study, but not in the mouse study, a large number of radiation-induced urothelial tumors were seen at 20 months (ANTONAKOPOULOS et al. 1984).

In an earlier study of the response of rat bladders to irradiation (ZHURAVLIEV 1963) a much more rapid degeneration of the urothelium was seen, with pyknotic or enlarged and deformed nuclei and the presence of binucleate basal cells within 8 days of irradiation. The rats used in this study were, however, infected with the parasitic roundworm *Trichosomoides crassicauda*, which causes the urothelium to be in a permanent state of irritation. Such an infection could explain the rapid onset of epithelial damage in this study. In general it appears that epithelial denudation, hyperplasia, and the formation of ulcers do not occur within the first 3 months after irradiation of rodent bladders, but such early changes can occur in dogs and in man.

The progression of damage in the irradiated

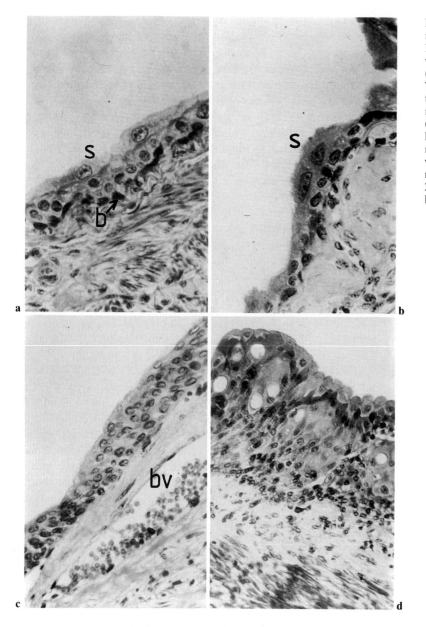

Fig. 14.11a-d. Epithelium and submucosa of mouse bladder. **a** Control. Note the well-defined basal layer with darkly staining basophilic cells (*b*) and two large surface cells (*s*). **b** Three months after 25 Gy. The epithelium is essentially intact. A normal, binucleate surface cell is visible (*s*). **c** Nine months after 25 Gy. Mild hyperplasia in the epithelium with no normal surface cells. Enlarged blood vessels (*bv*) can be seen in the submucosa. **d** Twelve months after 25 Gy. Marked hyperplasia with cellular vacuolation. (STEWART 1986)

ureter follows a similar pattern to that seen in the bladder and has been described by COSBIE (1941) and ALFERT and GILLENWATER (1972). An acute hyperemic phase is followed by epithelial degeneration and damage to the fine vasculature. The subacute phase is described as one of progressive vascular change with infiltration of inflammatory cells and epithelial degeneration. In the chronic phase (from 6 months after treatment) epithelial and muscular atrophy occur, possibly as the result of vascular deterioration.

14.2.4 Kinetic Changes After Bladder Irradiation

Under normal, unstressed conditions the bladder epithelium has a very slow cell turnover rate (LEVI et al. 1969; FARSUND 1975; STEWART et al. 1980) but these cells are capable of rapid turnover in response to injury. After chemical or mechanical damage a very early wave of proliferative activity can be measured in the epithelium within a few days (see STEWART 1986 for review). Stimulated proliferation of both epithelial and endothelial cells also occurs after irradiation but the response is delayed for many months.

The Urinary Tract   423

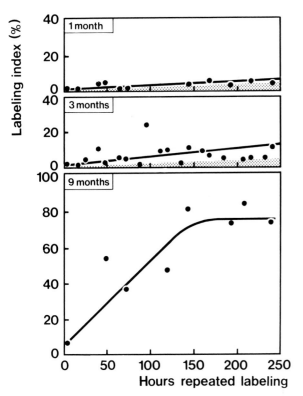

Fig. 14.12. Continuous labeling of mouse bladder epithelium at 1–9 months after irradiation with 25 Gy electrons. The labeling index is plotted as a function of time of exposure to ^{3}H-TdR. *Hatched areas* indicate a low rate of uptake of ^{3}H-TdR in controls. (Data from STEWART et al. 1980 and STEWART 1985)

In continuous labeling studies of the mouse bladder (STEWART et al. 1980; STEWART 1985) there was little or no increased proliferative activity until 3–6 months after irradiation. At 9 months, however, the epithelial cell turnover rate was reduced from a control value of about 1 year to only 9 days (Fig. 14.12). This coincides with the histological appearance of hyperplasia, which begins at around 6 months in mice and rats. Interestingly, in the experiments of STEWART and co-workers the proliferative activity (of both epithelium and endothelium) remained high for at least 19 months after irradiation, leaving the bladder in a permanent state of stimulated, rapid proliferation.

A much earlier onset of rapid proliferation was reported by SCHREIBER et al. (1969) after irradiation of rat bladders. In these experiments the labeling index of epithelial cells was increased within 3 days, and at 8 days after a dose of 20 Gy the labeling index was more than 100 times that of control bladders. There does not appear to be any obvious reason for this early proliferative activity,

since the labeling index in unirradiated bladders was only 0.1% (as reported in many other studies) and the rat bladders were reported to be free of parasites. In tissues with such a low labeling index, a much longer delay would be expected before onset of accelerated proliferation in response to radiation injury since radiation damage is only expressed as cells enter mitosis and attempt to divide. Subsequent studies on the kinetics of irradiated mouse bladder at early times after irradiation failed to support the findings of SCHREIBER et al. (REITAN and TVERA 1985).

14.2.5 Animal Models

The following assays have been developed to quantify the extent of radiation injury in the bladder: (a) bladder permeability to water and small ions, (b) urination frequency, and (c) bladder volume capacity under applied pressure. The incidence of hematuria has also been used to quantify the extent of bladder damage in mice after irradiation.

14.2.5.1 Permeability

The rate of transfer of ions across the bladder is normally very low (HLAD et al. 1956; LEVINSKY and BERLINER 1959). It has been suggested that the whole bladder acts as a passive barrier to the passage of water and small ions and that this barrier is dependent on an intact luminal membrane, as well as the presence of tight junctions between cells (HICKS 1966, 1975). Increases in bladder permeability have been observed when the luminal membrane is damaged, for example by treatment with chemical carcinogens (HICKS et al. 1974). Alterations in permeability of the human bladder have also been measured in patients with a history of bladder cancer or urinary infection (FELLOWS and MARSHALL 1972). Results showed an increased permeability of the bladder to water and sodium in the presence of undifferentiated tumor or urinary infection, but not at 6–50 months after radiotherapy in the absence of tumor.

Studies carried out in experimental animals demonstrated a marked increase in bladder permeability to sodium and lithium ions after mechanical or chemical trauma (TURNBULL 1973; TURNBULL and FELLOWS 1972; HICKS et al. 1974) but there have been no such studies to investigate permeability changes after irradiation. Water permeability was affected to much lesser extent.

14.2.5.2 Urination Frequency

Increased urination frequency and nocturia are common clinical symptoms of radiation-induced bladder damage. At late times after irradiation frequency is probably largely due to fibrosis and a reduction in bladder capacity. It is also possible that nerve damage may contribute, and indeed histological examination of irradiated human biopsy specimens has demonstrated the presence of nerve bundles "trapped" in a thickened collagenous submucosa (GOWING 1960). During the first few months after irradiation, before the onset of fibrosis, other factors such as epithelial desquamation, inflammation, and infection are likely to contribute to the increased frequency of urination.

Frequency has been used as a quantitative assay for measuring bladder damage in mice after irradiation (STEWART et al. 1978, 1981, 1984a) and after cyclophosphamide (STEWART 1985; EDREES et al. 1988). Urination frequency is calculated from the number of discrete urination events per test period and results can be expressed either as number of urinations per 24 h or as number of urinations per ml urine produced. This latter method is preferable since it corrects for any variation in urine production between mice.

Normal, healthy mice usually produce a total of 1.5–3.5 ml urine in a 24-h test period, voided in approximately 8–12 urination events. After bladder damage by radiation or cyclophosphamide the volume of urine produced remains unchanged except after very high doses of either agent, when the mice become generally sick or when secondary renal failure occurs as a result of ureteral obstruction (STEWART et al. 1981; EDREES et al. 1988). The *frequency* of urination, however, increases in proportion to the amount of damage incurred.

Increased urination frequency is not normally seen in mice earlier than 6 months after irradiation (Fig. 14.13). During the first 6 months there is no evidence of functional damage, no fibrosis or ulceration, and the epithelium remains essentially intact (STEWART et al. 1980; STEWART 1985, 1986). This differs from the clinical situation, where mild, transient frequency and referred pain are often seen towards the end of a 6-week course of radiotherapy. From about 6–9 months onwards a dose-related increase in urination frequency de-

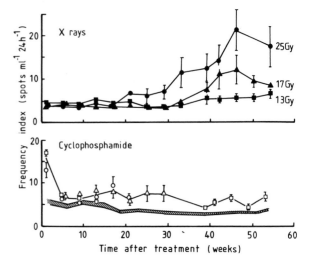

Fig. 14.13. Changes in urination frequency index (number of urination events in a 24-h test period, per ml urine produced) after x-rays or 100 mg/kg cyclophosphamide. Data points show the mean ± 1 SEM for groups of five to ten mice. After x-rays the onset of increased frequency is delayed until 30 weeks. After cyclophosphamide there is rapid development of increased frequency wihtin 1 week, and subsequent partial recovery. (EDREES et al. 1988)

velops in mice, with an earlier onset of damage after the highest radiation doses (Fig. 14.13). At 12 months after irradiation there is a correlation between increased frequency and reduced bladder capacity (STEWART et al. 1981), suggesting that fibrosis at least contributes to the late urination frequency response in mice. It is, however, possible to demonstrate marked increases in urination frequency in the absence of bladder fibrosis, e.g., within the first week of a dose of cyclophosphamide (Fig. 14.13). In these studies, early increased frequency coincided with a histological picture of extensive epithelial denudation and regeneration. It is possible that loss of the superficial epithelial cells in the bladder exposes the deeper, nonspecialized layers to the toxic effects of urine, causing bladder irritability and frequency (STEWART et al. 1980).

14.2.5.3 Bladder Capacity

At late times after irradiation an irreversible reduction in bladder volume capacity has been observed both clinically (DEAN 1933; GOWING 1960; MORRISON and DEELEY 1965) and experimentally (STEWART et al. 1981; LUNDBECK et al. 1987). This is at least in part due to the development of fibrosis. Early transient reductions in capacity have also been observed (LUNDBECK et al. 1987) which may be the result of edema or inflammation.

Bladder capacity has been used as an experimental model to quantify the extent of radiation-induced bladder damage in mice. In the experiments of STEWART and co-workers (1981) the bladders of newly killed mice were inflated via a transurethral catheter and the volume of the exposed bladder was serially measured at increasing applied pressure (5–40 mmHg). This technique produced a series of pressure volume curves with reduced bladder volumes after irradiation (Fig. 14.14). Bladder size at a given applied pressure can be used as quantitative measure of the extent of radiation injury. More recently LUNDBECK et al. (1987) have developed a technique to measure bladder capacity serially in live mice. For these studies catheters were inserted under anesthesia and saline was slowly introduced into the bladder (at a constant rate) while monitoring the intravesical pressure changes. The endpoint was a 50% reduction in bladder volume at a given pressure. Using this method an early, transient phase of damage was identified at 9–12 days after irradiation, as well as a second, irreversible, phase of reduced capacity from about 3 months.

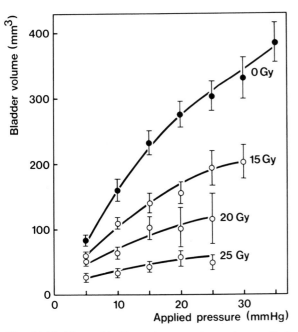

Fig. 14.14. Mouse bladder volumes at increasing applied pressure. Measured at 15 months after irradiation with 0–25 Gy electrons. (Data from STEWART et al. 1981)

14.2.5.4 Ureteral Stricture

Ureteral obstruction with consequent hydronephrosis is not a common radiation sequela but it does sometimes occur after combined surgery and radiation treatment for carcinoma of cervix (e.g., SHINGLETON et al. 1969). Recurrent tumor is often the cause of a ureteral blockage but radiation-induced stenosis in the absence of tumor has also been reported (ALFERT and GILLENWATER 1972; ALERT et al. 1980; GOODMAN and DALTON 1982).

An experimental system has recently been developed which allows precise, localized irradiation of the rat ureter without surgical intervention (KNOWLES 1985). Ureteral obstruction leading to hydronephrosis (detected by intravenous urography) developed progressively after a latency period which was inversely related to dose. The size of the irradiation field was found to have a marked influence on the incidence of stenosis (KNOWLES and TROTT 1987). The ED_{50} for hydronephrosis after irradiation of a 1.5 cm length of ureter was only 11.8 Gy but this increased to 29.6 Gy for a field size of 0.5 cm. For the small field size hydronephrosis after a dose of 30 Gy developed over the period 75–500 days but the onset was earlier (about 50 days) for a field size of 1.5 cm. The tissue sparing with the small field sizes was attributed to cellular migration and repopulation from the unirradiated margins (KNOWLES and TROTT 1987).

14.2.6 Modification of Radiation Response

14.2.6.1 Fractionation

The only experimental animal studies in which the response of the bladder to fractionated irradiation has been investigated are those of Stewart and co-workers (STEWART et al. 1981, 1984a). These studies used urination frequency and bladder capacity to measure functional damage after 1–20 fractions of irradiation, given in a total time of 1–2 weeks. A comparison of isoeffective doses from the different fractionation schedules demonstrated a large capacity for repair of sublethal damage, with total doses of 70 Gy in 20 fractions being equivalent to a single dose of 25 Gy (Fig. 14.15). An LQ analysis of the fractionated data gave an α/β value of 5–10 Gy for the bladder. This is

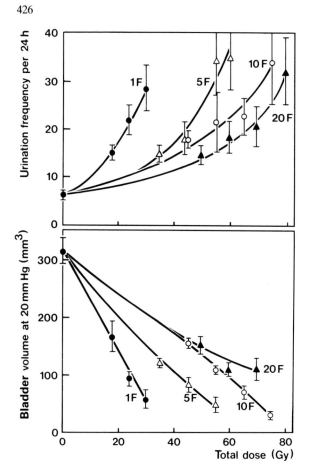

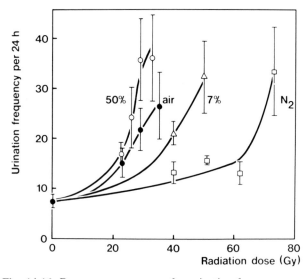

Fig. 14.16. Dose–response curves for urination frequency in mice at 9 months after electron irradiation in 50% O_2, air, 7% O_2, or N_2 (STEWART 1986)

Fig. 14.15. Radiation dose–response curves for urination frequency and bladder volume at an inflation pressure of 20 mmHg. The mean responses for groups of mice tested at 11–14 months after 1–20 fractions of electrons is shown. There is clear dose sparing with increasing fractionation. (Data from STEWART et al. 1984a)

rather higher than the α/β ratios obtained for most other late-responding tissues.

14.2.6.2 Radiosensitization and Radioprotection

The radiosensitivity of the mouse bladder can be modified by changing the irradiation conditions. Using an experimental system with fast electron irradiation, bladders have been irradiated while the mice were breathing nitrogen, air, or 95%, 50%, or 7% oxygen (STEWART 1986). The irradiations took a maximum of 40 s and the animals were rescued with an oxygen flush immediately after irradiation in nitrogen or 7% oxygen. These experiments demonstrated that the radiosensitivity of the bladder (assessed using the urination frequency assay) could be increased by raising the

oxygen content of the inspired gas (maximum enhancement ratio 1.2), or decreased by reducing the oxygen content (Fig. 14.16). An oxygen enhancement ratio of 2.5–2.7 was obtained by comparing the response of the mouse bladders irradiated in 95% oxygen and in nitrogen.

Radiation sensitivity of the mouse bladder can also be increased by misonidazole or decreased by the protector WR-2721 (STEWART 1986). The extent of misonidazole sensitization for irradiations in air was the same as that achieved by 95% oxygen (SER Sensitizer Enhancement Ratio = 1.2). Irradiation in air with WR-2721 gave PFs of 1.3–1.4 but in 50%–95% oxygen WR-2721 gave much greater protection (PF 1.9–2.0, Stewart, unpublished data). These studies would suggest that the mouse bladder is not normally fully oxygenated. This result is in line with clinical results of the MRC trial of irradiation in hyperbaric oxygen for carcinoma of the cervix, in which there was a slight increase in severe late bladder damage for patients irradiated in hyperbaric oxygen (WATSON et al. 1978).

14.2.6.3 High LET Irradiation

Several clinical trials have been carried out using neutron irradiation for the treatment of bladder cancer (BATTERMAN et al. 1981; LARAMORE et al. 1984; POINTON et al. 1985). Neutron therapy was found to be effective for the control of this disease

Fig. 14.17. Dose–response curves for urination frequency in mice after irradiation with electrons (●, ▲) or neutrons (○). The mean responses for groups of mice tested at 11–14 months after irradiation are shown and the RBEs for each fractionation schedule are written beside the curves. RBE increased with fractionation as the size of the dose per fraction was reduced

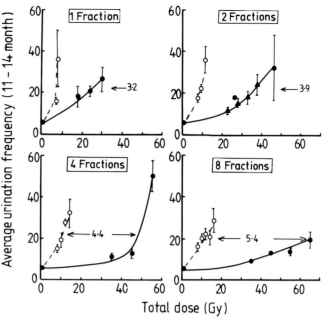

but severe late normal tissue damage occurred in some cases as the result of underestimating RBEs (BATTERMAN et al. 1981). Experimental studies in mice have demonstrated an RBE for bladder irradiations with d(4) + Be neutrons relative to 4 MeV electrons of 3.2 – for large single doses, increasing to 5.4 for fractionated doses of 5 Gy per fraction (Fig. 14.17, and STEWART et al. 1986b). RBEs using lower irradiation doses per fraction have not been experimentally measured but predictions based on an LQ analysis would suggest a maximum RBE of about 8 at low, clinically relevant doses (STEWART et al. 1986b), i.e., an RBE very similar to those measure in kidney at low doses per fraction (see Sect. 14.1.6.4).

14.2.6.4 Combined Modalities

Cyclophosphamide plus c-DDP is now being used in combination with pelvic irradiation for the treatment of ovarian cancer (RIZEL et al. 1985). Cyclophosphamide is also sometimes given with pelvic irradiation for treatment of rhabdomyosarcomas of the urogenital tract in children. Since cyclophosphamide is specifically toxic to the bladder such combined treatments carry the risk of increased bladder damage (frequency, dysuria, and hemorrhagic cystitis), as has been demonstrated both clinically (HUSTU et al. 1972; JAYALAKSHMAMMA and PINKEL 1976) and experimentally (STEWART 1985; EDREES et al. 1988).

Cyclophosphamide toxicity in the bladder is caused by the direct contact of its metabolites with the bladder epithelium as they are excreted in the urine. Ulceration, epithelial denudation, and hemorrhage appear within a few days, followed by a period of rapid compensatory proliferation in the surviving epithelial cells (see STEWART 1985, 1986 for reviews). Experimental studies in which cyclophosphamide was given at various intervals before or after bladder irradiation have demonstrated an increased early damage (1–3 months after treatment) after the combined treatments (EDREES et al. 1988). A part of this effect may be due to the precipitation of latent radiation injury by cyclophosphamide. Increased late bladder damage (9–12 months) was also seen with dose enhancement factors of 1.2–1.4. This appeared to be largely the result of additive toxicities from late radiation injury and persistent drug damage (EDREES et al. 1988).

There is no evidence from either clinical or experimental studies that cyclophosphamide sensitizes the bladder to irradiation. Enhanced damage after the combined treatments is probably the result of independent toxicities (possibly with different target cell populations) plus some precipitation of radiation damage due to rapid drug-induced proliferation.

Acknowledgments. We would like to express our thanks to Dr. Adam Michalowski for advice in the preparation of this manuscript and for allowing us to reproduce Figure 14.4. Drs. S. Jordan, M. Robbins, E. Malaise, and H. Withers have kindly given us permission to reproduce some of their published data. We would also like to thank Drs. H. Bartelink and A. Begg and Miss Thea Eggenhuizen for their help in the preparation of this manuscript.

References

Alert J, Jiminez J, Beldarrain L, Montalvo J, Roca C (1980) Complications from irradiation of carcinoma of the uterine cervix. Acta Radiol [Oncol] 19: 13–16

Alfert HK, Gillenwater JY (1972) The consequences of ureteral irradiation with special reference to subsequent ureteral injury. J Urol 107: 369–371

Alpen EL, Stewart FA (1984) Radiation nephritis and anaemia: a functional assay for renal damage after irradiation. Br J Radiol 57: 185–186

Antonakopoulos GN, Hicks RM, Hamilton E, Berry RJ (1984) Early and late morphological changes (including carcinoma of the urothelium) induced by irradiation of the rat urinary. Br J Cancer 46: 403–416

Asscher AW (1965) Prevention of renal damage by x-rays. Br J Radiol 38: 533–535

Batterman JJ, Hart GAM, Breur K (1981) Dose-effect relations for tumour control and complication rate after fast neutron therapy for pelvic tumours. Br J Radiol 54: 899–904

Begg AC, Stewart FA, Dewit D, Bartelink H (1990) Interaction between cisplatin and radiation in experimental rodent tumours and normal tissues. In: Hill B, Bellamy AS (eds), Antitumor drug-radiation interactions, CRC Press, Florida, pp 153–170

Bolliger A, Laidley JWS (1930) Experimental renal disease produced by x-rays. Histological changes in the kidney exposed to a measured amount of unfiltered rays of medium wavelength. Med J Aust 1: 136–147

Bricker NS, Fine LG (1981) The renal response to progressive nephron loss. In: Brenner BM, Rector FC (eds) The kidney. W.B. Saunders, London, p 1056

Bricker NS, Morrin PAF, Kime SW (1960) The pathologic physiology of chronic Bright's desease. Am J Med 28:77–98

Caldwell WL (1975) Time-dose factors in fatal post-irradiation nephritis. In: Alper T (ed) Cell survival after low doses of radiation. Theoretical and clinical implications. John Wiley, New York, pp 328–334

Casarett GW (1964) Pathology of single intravenous dose of polonium. In: Stannard J, Casarett GW (eds) Metabolism and biological effects on alpha emitter polonium 210. Radiat Res [Suppl] 5: 246–321

Chantler C, Garnett ES, Parsons V, Veall N (1969) Glomerular filtration rate measurement in man by the single injection method using ^{51}Cr-EDTA. Clin Sci 37: 169–180

Chauser BM, Hudson FR, Law MP (1976) Renal function in the rat following irradiation. Radiat Res 67: 86–97

Clayman CB, Palmer WL, Kirsner JB (1968) Gastric irradiation in the treatment of peptic ulcer. Gastroenterology 55: 403–407

Coburn JW, Rubini ME, Kleeman CR (1966) Renal concentrating defect in canine radiation nephritis. J Lab Clin 67: 209–223

Coltart RS, Nethersell ABW, Thomas S, Dixon AK (1987) A CT based dosimetry system for intracavitary therapy in carcinoma of the cervix. Radiother Oncol 10: 295–305

Concannon JP, Summers RE, Brewer R, Weil C, Hayeslip C (1964) High oxygen tension and radiation effect on the kidney. Radiology 82: 508–519

Cosbie WG (1941) The complications of irradiation treatment of carcinoma of the cervix. Am J Obst Gyn 42: 1003

Cullen BH, Burgin J, Reeves B, Michalowski A (1986) Functional assessments of radiation nephropathy. Br J Cancer 53 [Suppl VII]: 292–295

Dean AL (1933) Injury of the urinary bladder following irradiation of the uterus. J Urol 29: 559–575

Dean AL, Abels JC (1944) Study by the newer renal function tests of an unusual case of hypertension following irradiation of the kidney and the relief of the patient by nephrectomy. J Urol 52: 497–501

Deschavanne PJ, Guichard M, Malaise EP (1980) Radiosensitivity of mouse kidney cells determined with an in vitro colony method. Int J Radiat Oncol Biol Phys 6: 1551–1557

Dewit L, Ang KK, van der Schueren E (1983) Acute side effects and late complications after radiotherapy of localized carcinoma of the prostate. Cancer Treat Rev 10: 79–89

Doub HP, Bolliger A, Hartman FW (1972) The relative sensitivity of the kidney to irradiation. Radiology 8: 142

Douglas BG, Fowler JF (1976) The effects of multiple small doses of x-rays on skin reactions in the mouse and a basic interpretation. Radiat Res 66: 401–426

Edrees G, Luts A, Stewart F (1988) Bladder damage in mice after combined treatment with cyclophosphamide and x-rays. The influence of timing and sequence. Radiother Oncol 11: 349–360

Ellis F (1969) Dose, time and fractionation: a clinical hypothesis. Clin Radiol 20: 1–7

Fajardo LF, Brown JM, Glatstein E (1976) Glomerular and juxtaglomerular lesions in rediation nephropathy. Radiat Res 68: 177–183

Farsund T (1975) Cell Kinetics of mouse urinary bladder epithelium I. Virchows Arch [B] 18: 35–49

Fellows GJ, Marshall DM (1972) The permeability of human bladder epithelium to water and sodium. Invest Urol 9: 339–344

Fowler JF (1984) What next in fractionated radiotherapy. Br J Cancer 49 [Suppl VI]: 285–300

Geraci JP, Thrower PD, Mariano M (1978) Cyclotron fast neutron RBE for late kidney damage. Radiology 126: 519–520

Glatstein E (1973) Alterations in rubidium-86 extraction in normal mouse tissue after irradiation. Radiat Res 53: 88–101

Glatstein E, Brown RC, Zanelli GO, Fowler JF (1975) The uptake of rubidium-86 in mouse kidneys irradiated with fractionated doses of x-rays. Radiat Res 61: 417–426

Glatstein E, Fajardo LF, Brown JM (1977) Radiation injury in the mouse kidney – I. Sequential light microscopic study. Int J Radiat Oncol Biol Phys 2: 933–943

Goldblatt H, Lynch J, Hanzal RF, Summerville WW (1934) Studies on experimental hypertension. 1. The production of persistent elevation of systolic blood pressure by means of renal ischaemia. J Exp Med 59: 347

Goodman M, Dalton JR (1982) Ureteral strictures following radiotherapy: incidence, etiology and treatment guidlines. J Urol 128: 21–24

Gowing NFC (1960) Pathological changes in the bladder following irradiation. Br J Radiol 33: 484–487

Gupp AK, Schlegel JV, Caldwell T, Schosser J (1967) Effect of irradiation on renal function. J Urol 97: 36–39

Hartman FW, Bolliger A, Doub HP (1926) Experimental nephritis produced by irradiation. Am J Med Sci 172: 39–39

Hartman FW, Bolliger A, Doub P (1927) Functional studies throughout the course of roentgen-ray nephritis in dogs. JAM A 88: 139–145

Hicks RM (1966) The permeability of rat transitional epithelium. J Cell Biol 28: 21–31

Hicks RM (1975) The mammalian urinary bladder: an accommodating organ Biol Rev 50: 215–246

Hicks RM, Ketterer B, warren RC (1974) The ultrastructure and chemistry of the luminal plasma membrane of the mammalian urinary bladder: a structure with low permeability to water and ions. Philos Trans R Soc Lond [Biol] 268: 23–38

Hlad CJ, Nelson R, Holmes JH (1956) Transfer of electrolytes across the urinary bladder in the dog. Am J Physiol 184: 406–411

Hope-Stone HF, Blandy JP, Oliver RTD, England HS (1981) Radical radiotherapy and salvage cystectomy in the management of invasive carcinoma of the bladder. In: Oliver RTD, Herdns WF, Bloom HJG (eds) Bladder cancer: Principles of combination therapy. Butterworths, London, pp 127–138

Hopewell JW, Berry RJ (1975) Radiation tolerance of the pig kidney: a model for determining overall time and fraction factors for preserving renal function. Int J Radiat Oncol Biol Phys 1: 61–68

Hopewell JW, Wiernik G (1977) Tolerance of the pig kidney to fractionated x-irradiation. In: Radiobiological research and radiotherapy. IAEA, Vienna, pp 65–73

Hopewell JW, Barnes DWH, Goodhead DT, Knowles JF, Wiernik G, Young CMA (1982) The relative biological effectiveness of fast neutrons 42 Me Vd-Be for early and late normal tissue injury in the pig. Int J Radiat Oncol Biol Phys 8: 2077–2081

Hueper WC, Fisher CV, De Carvajal-Forero J, Thompson MR (1942) The pathology of experimental roentgen cystitis in dogs. J Urol 47: 156–167

Hunter RD, Wong F, Moore C, Notley HM, Wilkinson J (1986) Bladder base dosage in patients undergoing intracavitary therapy. Radiother Oncol 7: 189–197

Hustu H, Pinkel D, Pratt CB (1972) Treatment of clinically localized Ewing's sarcoma with radiotherapy and combination chemotherapy. Cancer 30: 1522–1527

Jayalakshmamma B, Pinkel D (1976) Urinary bladder toxicity following pelvic irradiation and simultaneous cyclophosphamide therapy. Cancer 38: 701–707

Joiner MC, Johns H (1987) Renal damage in the mouse: the effect of d(4)-Be neutrons. Radiat Res 109: 456–468

Joiner MC, Johns H (1988) Renal damage in the mouse: the response to very small doses per fraction. Radiat Res 114: 385–398

Jordan SW, Key CR, Gomez LS, Agnew J, Barton SL (1978) Late effects of radiation on the mouse kidney. Exp Mol Path 29: 115–129

Jordan SW, Yuhas JM, Butler JLB, Kligerman MM (1981) Dependence on fraction size for negative pimeson induced renal injury. Int J Radiat Oncol Biol Phys 7: 223–227

Jordan SW, Brayer JM, Bartels PH, Olson GB, Anderson RE (1984) Computer-assisted morphometric analysis of the late renal radiation injury. Monogr Clin Cytol 9: 117–147

Jordan SW, Anderson RE, Lane RG, Brayer JM (1985) Fraction size, dose and time dependence of x-ray induced late renal injury. Int J Radiat Oncol Biol Phys 11: 1095–1101

Kim TH, Somerville PJ, Freeman CR (1984) Unilateral nephropathy – the long term significance. Int J Radiat Biol Oncol Phys 10: 2053–2059

Knowles JF (1985) Radiation-induced hydronephrosis in the rat: a new experimental model. Int J Radiat Biol 48: 737–744

Knowles JF, Trott KR (1987) Experimental irradiation of the rat ureter: the effects of field size and the presence of contrast medium on incidence and latency of hydronephrosis. Radiother Oncol 10: 59–66

Kociba RJ, Sleight SD (1971) Acute toxicological and pathological effects of cis-diammine dichloroplatinum (NSC-119875) in the male rat. Cancer Chemother Rep 55: 1–8

Kottmeier HL (1964) Complications following radiation therapy in carcinoma of the cervix. Am J Obstet Gynecol 88: 854–866

Kunkler PB, Farr RF, Luxton RW (1952) The limit of renal tolerance to x-rays. Br J Radiol 25: 190–201

Kurtz A, Jelkmann W, Bauer C (1983) Insulin stimulates erythroid colony formation independently of erythropoietin. Br J Haematol 53: 311–316

Landuyt W, van der Kogel AJ, De Roo H, Hoogmartens H, Ang KK, van der Schueren E (1988). Unilateral kidney irradiation and late retreatments with cis-dichlorodiammineplatinum. (II) Functional measurements with 99m technetium-dimercaptosuccinic acid. Int J Radiat Oncol Biol Phys 14: 95–101

Laramore GE, Davis RB, Hussay DH et al. (1984) Radiation therapy oncology group phase I-II study on fast neutron teletherapy for carcinoma of the bladder. Cancer 54: 432–439

Lebesque JV, Hart AM, Stewart FA (1988) Reirradiation at long time intervals in mouse kidney: a comparison between experimental results and predictions of the F type tissue model. Int J Radiat Biol 53: 417–428

Le Bourgeios HP, Meigvan M, Parmentier C, Tubiana M (1979) Renal consequences of irradiation of the spleen in lymphoma patients. Br J Radiol 52: 56–60

Leonard BJ, Eccleston E, Jones D, Todd P, Walpole A (1971) Antileukaemic and nephrotoxic properties of platinum compounds. Nature 234: 43–45

Levi PE, Cowan DM, Cooper EM (1969) Induction of cell proliferation in the mouse bladder by 4-ethylsulphonylnaphthalene-1-sulphonamide. Cell Tissue Kinet 2: 249–262

Levinski NG, Berliner RW (1959) Changes in composition of the urine in ureter and bladder at low urine flow. Am J Physiol 196: 549–553

Ljung-Qvist A, Unge G, Lagergren C, Notter G (1971) The intrarenal vascular alterations in radiation nephritis and their relationships to the development of hypertension. Acta Pathol Microbiol Scand [A] 79: 629–638

Lundbeck F, Ulso N, Overgaard J, Djurhuus JC (1987) Cytometry in mice: an in vivo model for evaluating early and late radiation damage to the urinary bladder. In: Fielden EM, Fowler JF, Hendry JH, Scott D (eds) Proceedings of the 8th International Congress of Radiation

Luxton RW (1953) Radiation nephritis. Q J Med 22: 215–242

Luxton RW (1961) Radiation nephritis: a long term study of 54 patients. Lancet II: 1221–1224

Madrazo A, Churg J (1976) Radiation nephritis: chronic changes following moderate doses of radiation. Lab Invest 34: 283–290

Mak ACA, Van 't Riet A, Ypma AFGVM, Veen RE, Slooten FHS (1987) Dose determination in bladder and rectum during intracavitary irradiation of cervix carcinoma. Radiother Oncol 10: 97–100

Malaise EP, Guichard M, Deschavanne PJ (1985) Primary cultures from lung and kidney. In: Potten W, Hendry JH (eds) Cell clones. Churchill Livingstone, Edinburgh, p 175

Mason KA, Withers HR (1985) Kidney tubules. In: Potten W, Hendry JH (eds) Cell clones. Churchill Livingstone, Edinburgh, p 152

Michalowski AS (1981) Effects of radiation on normal tissues: hypothetical mechanisms and limitations of in situ assays of clonogenicity. Radiat Environ Biophys 19: 157–172

Michalowski A (1986) The pathogenesis of the late side-effects of radiotherapy. Clin Radiol 37: 203–207

Michalowski A, Cullen BM, Burgin J, Rogers MA (1986) Development of structural renal damage and its quantitation. Br J Cancer 53 [Suppl VII]: 295–298

Minton MJ, McIvor J, Capuccio FP, MacGregor GA, Newlands ES (1986) Renovascular hypertension following radiotherapy and chemotherapy treated by transluminal angioplasty. Clin Radiol 37: 399–401

Morrison R (1975) The results of treatment of cancer of bladder. A clinical contribution to radiobiology. Clin Radiol 26: 67–75

Morrison R, Deeley TJ (1965) The treatment of carcinoma of the bladder by supervoltage x-rays. Br J Radiol 38: 449–458

Mostofi FK (1966) Radiation effects on the kidney. In: Mostofi FK (ed) The kidney. International Academy of Pathology, Monograph 6, Williams & Wilkins, Baltimore, pp 338–386

Moulder JE (1983) Kidney tolerance in split-course radiation schedules (abstr). Int Radiat Oncol Biol Phys 9: 107

Moulder JE, Fish BL (1988) Effects of sequencing on combined toxicity of renal irradiation and cisplatin. NCI Monogr 6: 35–41

Moulder JE, Holcenberg JS, Kamen BA et al. (1986) Renal irradiation and the pharmacology and toxicity of methotrexate and cisplatinum. Int J Radiat Oncol Biol Phys 12: 1415–1418

O'Hare JP, Althow H, Christian TD Jr, Calhoun AW, Sosman MC (1926) Chronic nephritis produced by x-ray. Boston Med Surg J 194: 43–45

Osnes S (1959) Experimental study of an erythropoietic principle produced in the kidney. Br Med J 10: 650–658

Otsuka M, Meistrich ML (1986) Late irradiation effects on renal tubular cells. Abstracts of papers for 34th Annual Meeting, Radiation Research

Otsuka M, Meistrich ML, Brock WA (1988) Characterization of abnormal nuclei in renal proximal tubules after irradiation. Radiat Res 115: 161–175

Parkin DE, Davis JA, Symonds RP (1987) Long-term bladder symptomatology following radiotherapy for cervial carcinoma. Radiother Oncol 9: 195–199

Paterson R (1952) Renal damage from radiation during treatment of seminoma testis. J Fac Radiol (London) 3: 370–374

Phillips T, Fu K (1974) Derivation of time-dose factors for normal tissues using experimental endpoints in the mouse. In: Caldwell WL, Tolbert DD (eds) Proceedings of the Conference on Time-Dose Relationships in Clinical Radiotherapy University of Wisconsiw pp 42–47

Phillips T, Fu K (1978) The interaction of drug and radiation effects on normal tissues. Int J Radiat Oncol Biol Phys 4: 59–64

Phillips TL, Ross G (1973) A quantitative technique for measuring renal damage after irradiation. Radiology 109: 457–462

Phillips TL, Kane L, Utley JF (1973) Radioprotection of tumour and normal tissues by thiophosphate compounds. Cancer 32: 528–535

Pointon RS, Read G, Greene D (1985) A randomised comparison of photons and 15 MeV neutrons for the treatment of carcinoma of the bladder. Br J Radiol 58: 219–224

Quilty PM, Duncan W, Kerr GR (1985) Results of a randomized study to evaluate influence of dose on morbidity in radiotherapy for bladder cancer. Clin Radiol 36: 615–618

Read G (1982) Reduction in renal radiation tolerance by combination chemotherapy including cis-platinum (abstr). Br J Cancer 45: 635

Redd BL (1960) Radiation nephritis; review, case report and animal study. AJR 83: 88–106

Reitan JB, Tvera K (1985) Some short-term cell kinetic effects of ionizing radiation on the mouse bladder urothelium. Cell Tissue Kinet 18: 631–639

Rizel S, Biran S, Anteby S et al. (1985) Combined modality treatment for stage III ovarian carcinoma. Radiother Oncol 3: 237–244

Robbins MEC, Hopewell JW (1978) Radiation-related renal damage. In: Bach PH, Lock EA (eds) Nephrotoxicity in the experimental and clinical situation. Martinus Nijhoff, Dordrecht, p 817

Robbins MEC, Hopewell JW, Gunn Y (1985) Effects of single doses of x-rays on renal function in unilaterally irradiated pigs. Radiother Oncol 4: 143–151

Robbins MEC, Hopewell JW. Golding SJ (1986) Functional recovery in irradiated kidneys following removal of the unirradiated contralateral kidney. Radiother Oncol 6: 309–316

Rojas A, Stewart FA, Sorenson JA, Smith KA, Denekamp J (1986) Fractionation studies with WR-2721: normal tissue and tumour. Radiother Oncol 6: 51–60

Rubin P (1984) Late effects of chemotherapy and radiation therapy: a new hypothesis. Int J Radiat Oncol Biol Phys 10: 5–34

Rubin P, Casarett G (1968) Clinical radiation pathology as applied to curative radiotherapy. Cancer 22: 767–778

Schreiber H, Oehlert W, Kugler K (1969) Regeneration and Proliferationskinetik des normalen und strahlengeschädigten Urothels der Ratte. Virchows Arch [B] 4: 30–44

Schulz A, Hoffman B (1905) Zur Wirkungsweise der Roentgenstrahlen. Dtsch Z Chir 79: 350–362

Shapiro AP, Cavallo T, Cooper W, Lapenas D, Bron K, Berg G (1977) Hypertension in radiation nephritis. Arch Intern Med 137: 848–851

Shingleton HM, Fowler WC, Pepper FD, Palumbo L (1969) Ureteral structure following therapy for carcinoma of the cervix. Cancer 24: 77–83

Slater JM, Fletcher GH (1974) Ureteral strictures after radiation therapy for carcinoma of the uterine cervix. AJR 111: 269–272

Soranson J, Denekamp J (1986) Precipitation of latent renal radiation injury by unilateral nephrectomy. Br J Cancer 53: 268–272

Stephan O (1920) Ueber die Steigerung der Zellfunktion durch roentgenenergie. Strahlentherapie 11: 517–562

Stewart FA (1985) The proliferative and functional response of mouse bladder to treatment with radiation and cyclophosphamide. Radiother Oncol 4: 353–362

Stewart FA (1986) Mechanism of bladder damage and repair after treatment with radiation and cytostatic drugs. Br J Cancer 53 [Suppl VII]: 280–291

Stewart FA, Michael BD, Denekamp J (1978) Late radiation damage in the mouse bladder as measured by increased urination frequency. Radiat Res 75: 649–659

Stewart FA, Denekamp J, Hirst DG (1980) Proliferation kinetics of the mouse bladder after irradiation. Cell Tissue Kinet 13: 75–89

Stewart FA, Randhaẁa VS, Denekamp J (1981) Repair during fractionated irradiation of the mouse bladder. Br J Radiol 54: 799–804

Stewart FA, Randhawa VS, Michael BD (1984a) Multifraction irradiation of mouse bladders. Radiother Oncol 2: 131–140

Stewart FA, Soranson JA, Alpen EL, Williams MV, Denekamp J (1984b) Radiation-induced renal damage. The effects of hyperfractionation. Radiat Res 98: 407–420

Stewart FA, Soranson JA, Maughan R, Alpen EL, Denekamp J (1984c) The RBE for renal damage after irradiation with 3 MeV neutrons. Br J Radiol 57: 1009–1021

Stewart FA, Bohlken S, Begg A, Bartelink H (1986a) Renal damage in mice after treatment with cisplatinum alone or in combination with x-irradiation. Int J Radiat Oncol Biol Phys 12: 927–933

Stewart FA, Randhawa VS, Maughan R (1986b) The RBE for mouse bladders after irradiation with 1 to 8 fractions of 3 MeV neutrons. Br J Radiol 59: 61–68

Stewart FA, Luts A, Begg AC (1987a) Tolerance of previously irradiated mouse kidneys to cisplatinum. Cancer Res 47: 1016–1021

Stewart FA, Oussoren Y, Luts A, Begg AC, Dewit L, Lebesque J, Bartelink H (1987b) Repair of sublethal radiation injury after multiple samll doses in mouse kidney: an estimate of flexure dose. Int J Radiat Oncol Biol Phys 13: 765–772

Stewart FA, Lebesque JV, Hart AAM (1988a) Progressive development of radiation damage in mouse kidneys and the consequences for reirradiation tolerance. Int J Radiat Biol 53: 405–415

Stewart FA, Luts A, Oussoren Y, Begg AC, Dewit L, Bartelink H (1988b) Renal damage in mice after treatment with cisplatin and x-rays: comparison of fractionated and single dose studies. NCI Monogr 6: 23–27

Stewart JH (1967) Haemolytic anaemia in acute and chronic renal failure. Q J Med 141: 85–105

Thompson PL, Mackay IR, Robson GSM, Wall AJ (1971) Late radiation nephritis after gastric x-irradiation for peptic ulcer. Q J Med 40: 145–157

Turnbull GJ (1973) Ultrastructural basis of the permeability barrier in urothelium. Invest Urol 11: 198–204

Turnbull GJ, Fellows GJ (1972) Permeability of the urinary

bladder of the rabbit. Rev Eur Etud Clin Biol 17: 745–749

Unal A, Hamberger AD, Seski JC, Fletcher GH (1981) An analysis of the severe complications of irradiation of carcinoma of the uterine cervix: treatment with intracavitary radium and parametrial irradiation. Radiat Oncol Biol Phys 7: 999–1004

Van Rongen E, Kuijpers C, Van der Kogel AJ (1988) Interaction of cisplatin and x-rays in rat kidney. NCI Monog 6: 19–23

Wacholz BW, Casarett GW (1970) Radiation hypertension and nephrosclerosis. Radiat Res 41: 39–56

Warthin AS (1907) The changes produced in the kidneys by roentgen irradiation. Am J Med Sci 133: 736–746

Watson ER, Herger CC, Sauer HR (1947) Irradiation reactions in the bladder. Their occurrence and clinical course following the use of x-rays and radium in the treatment of female pelvic disease. J Urol 57: 1038–1053

Watson ER, Halnan KE, Dische S et al. (1978) Hyperbaric oxygen and radiotherapy: a medical research council trial in carcinoma of the cervix. Br J Radiol 51: 879–887

Willet CG, Tepper JE, Orlow EL, Shipley WU (1986) Renal complications secondary to radiation treatment of upper abdominal malignancies. Int J Radiat Biol Phys 12: 1601–1604

Williams MV (1986) The cellular basis of renal injury by radiation. Br J Cancer 53 [Suppl VII]: 257–264

Williams MV, Denekamp J (1983) Sequential functional testing of radiation induced renal damage in the mouse. Radiat Res 94: 305–317

Williams MV, Denekamp J (1984a) Radiation induced renal damage in mice: influence of overall treatment time. Radiother Oncol 1: 355–367

Williams MV, Denekamp J (1984b) Radiation induced renal damage in mice: influence of fraction size. Int J Radiat Oncol Biol Phys 10: 885–893

Williams MV, Denekamp J (1984c) Modification of the radiation response of the mouse kidney by misonidazole and WR-2721. Int J Radiat Biol Oncol Phys 9: 173–176

Williams MV, Stewart FA, Soranson JA, Denekamp J (1985) The influence of overall treatment time on renal injury after multifraction irradiation. Radiother Oncol 4: 87–96

Withers HR, Peters LJ, Kogelnik HD (1980) The pathobiology of late effects of irradiation. In: Meyn RE, Withers HR (eds) Radiation biology in cancer research. Raven, New York, p 439

Withers HR, Thames HD, Peters LJ (1982) Differences in the fractionation response of acutely and late-responding tissues. In: Kaercher KH (ed) Progress in radio-oncology II. Raven, New York, p 287

Withers HR, Mason KA, Thames HD (1986) Late radiation response of kidney assayed by tubule-cell survival. Br J Radiol 59: 587–597

Yuhas JH, Storer JG (1969) Chemoprotection against three modes of radiation death in the mouse. Int J Radiat Biol 15: 233–237

Zhuravliev AV (1963) Changes in transitional epithelium subject to ionizing radiation. Arkh Anat Gistol Embriol 45: 59–66

Zuelzer NW, Palmer HD, Newton WA (1950) Unusual glomerulonephritis in young children, probably radiation nephritis; reports of three cases. Am J Pathol 26: 1019–139

15 Reproductive Organs

H.-A. LADNER

CONTENTS

15.1 Introduction

The aim of this article is to update earlier reviews and monographs on this subject to take account of the enormous increase in our knowledge that has occurred during the last 20 years. The following summarizing publications will be referred to frequently[1]:

H.A. LADNER, M.D., Professor der Radiologie, Klinikum der Albert-Ludwigs-Universität, Abteilung Gynäkologische Radiologie, Hugstetterstraße 55, 7800 Freiburg i.Br., FRG

Ovaries:	BAKER and NEAL 1977	$= R_1$
Testes:	OAKBERG 1975	$= R_2$
Ovaries and Testes:	CARLSON and GASSNER 1964	$= R_3$
	MANDL 1964	$= R_4$
	OAKBERG and LORENZ 1972	$= R_5$

These five reviews are indispensable when conducting a literature search in this field. For the sake of better comparison I shall retain the structure used in the reviews, distinguishing between morphological and functional changes after exposure of the ovaries and testes to radiation, even though the borders between morphology and function are no longer so clear-cut. Observations in humans will be summarized separately; it will thereby be shown that results from animal studies have only limited relevance for humans. In the discussion on species-specific radiation effects on reproductive organs, the increased sensitivity of germ cells during certain stages in their development will be pointed out. Central topics in the survey will be the discovery of radioresistant stem cells as a result of more refined morphological methods and the endocrinological problems that arise after radiation exposure. Finally, those factors which can modify the radiation effects on reproductive organs [fractionation, dose rate, relative biological effectiveness (RBE), chemical agents, and radionuclides] will be discussed.

Since the five reviews mainly cover the Anglo-American literature, some older studies from German journals are also referred to. However, results in the fields of radiation genetics (SANKARA-NARAYANAN 1982), teratology (BRENT 1977), and mutation research could not be included. The influence of recovery processes on the radiation reactions of ovaries and testes is not discussed in

---

[1] When a reference citation is followed by R_1-R_5, full details of the publication concerned can be found in these original reviews.

detail. Examination of literature of the past 20 years in this field reveals that publications dealing with radiation effects on the testes predominate. However, due to the importance of radiation effects on the ovaries described in recent papers, I shall quote about the same number of publications on each topic.

15.2 History

Soon after the discovery of x-rays by C.F. Roentgen in 1896, macroscopic and microscopic changes in the ovaries and testes after radiation were described. Early research focused on the discovery of azoospermia and the development of sterility (in male rabbits: ALBERS-SCHOENBERG 1903, R_3) and thus on functional disturbances after radiation exposure. Other problems which are still relevant in radiation research today were already becoming evident at that time. REGAUD's observations on the relative radiation reactions of the testes and scrotal skin were based on the phenomenon of fractionation. The so-called law of Bergonnie and Tribondeau is the result of studies with irradiated testes. As early as 1904 PHILIPP reported on the regenerative capacity of the testes after radiation. The death of oocytes, as well as differences in radiosensitivity of primordial oocytes in different species, was described by REIFFERSCHEID in 1914. The marked germ cell damage that occurs within a short period of exposure led to consideration of the gonadal effects of diagnostic and therapeutic radiation, and JACOX reported in 1939 that 5 Gy to the ovaries produced permanent castration in most patients. Further research initiatives were stimulated by MUELLER's discovery in 1927 that x-rays can elicit mutations, and even more so by the recognition of the sequelae of the two nuclear explosions in Japan in 1945.

15.3 Indirect Influences on the Effect of Irradiation

Some findings suggest the existence of other, as yet unexplained, mechanisms for the development of sex-specific differences in radiosensitivity, especially after total body irradiation (TBI) or irradiation of the head. After TBI of male mice the hormonal performance of the gonads was virtually unaffected; in female mice, on the other hand, late effects were seen in nearly all endocrine organs, including the ovaries (COTTIER 1961). Additional hormone applications in male mammals appeared to alter the radiation response, e.g., spermatogenesis (KONDRATENKO et al. 1978), while in females such alteration was not observed (BAGER 1982). Irradiation of the head in adult male guinea pigs had no effect on semen production (FREUND and BORELLI 1965). In contrast, irradiation of the head with 300–600 R in 2-day-old male rats influenced fertility and spermatogonia counts in a dose-dependent manner (only 30% of male rats were fertile after 600 R). These lasting effects are attributed to disturbances of the endocrine system (SAVKOVIC et al. 1966), such as have been described after irradiation of the head (WIGG et al. 1982).

Another finding worthy of mention is the decrease in luteinizing hormone (LH) and testosterone plasma levels, as seen only in male rats 3–4 days after TBI, head, and abdominal irradiation (McTAGGART and WILLS 1977), which can be blocked by prior injection of testosterone. This phenomenon can be a result of a radiation-induced disturbance of testosterone synthesis at cleavage of the side chain of hydroxyprogesterone in the liver (BERLINER et al. 1964). This impairment of liver enzymes can elicit irradiation-induced interactions between the testes, anterior pituitary, liver, and hypothalamus.

15.4 Findings in Humans

Reviews of findings in humans have been made by ZUCKERMAN (1965, R_1), SANDEMAN (1966), BAKER (1971a, R_1), LUSHBAUGH and RICKS (1972), LUSHBAUGH and CASARETT (1976), ASH (1980), GREINER (1982), and CLIFTON and BRENNER (1983). Our knowledge is based mainly on past radiation accidents and on radiotherapy data, where the reconstruction of the actual dose is sometimes difficult. It should be mentioned that progress in medical radiation protection has improved our ability to determine the gonadal dose in men and women [for example, in respect of radiation therapy in men see FUCHS and HOFBAUER (1969), GREEN and BUSHONG (1971), and FRAASS et al. (1985), and in women, SCHERHOLZ et al. (1978) and Sobels (1969: radioiodine therapy)]. Thus the gonadal dose can be reduced more than in earlier years.

15.4.1 Changes in Female Gonads After Irradiation

Data exist on the morphological changes caused by irradiation and combined chemotherapy in children aged between 5 months and 7 years (HIMELSTEIN-BRAW et al. 1977) and in sexually mature individuals (CIANCI et al. 1968). However, it is not clear to what extent these morphological changes are correlated with reduced fertility. STILLMAN et al. (1981) found that in 12% of 182 long-term survivors of childhood malignancy there was ovarian failure as a sequela of abdominal irradiation or chemotherapy. SEIGEL (1966), BLOT and SAWADA (1972), and BLOT et al. (1975) found no significant differences in fertility between normal controls and female survivors of the atomic bombs of Hiroshima and Nagasaki. Today ovarian irradiation is no longer used in the treatment of hemorrhagic metrorrhagia or sterility: According to DOLL and SMITH (1968), amenorrhea was found in only 97% of patients after the application of 3.6–7.2 Gy x-rays to the ovary (it is estimated that after 6 Gy about 50% of primary follicles in premenopausal women are destroyed). In 1958 KAPLAN reported that after 150–225 R (3x 75 R) to the ovary, 75% of amenorrheic women started to menstruate regularly; 52% of these women became pregnant and 84% of them gave birth to healthy children.

There is no clear indication as to which minimum dose elicits permanent infertility. It is known, however, that this radiation effect depends on the age of the woman (PECK et al. 1940). In young women 200 R to the ovaries led to temporary amenorrhea. After 500 R permanent amenorrhea was observed in only 30% of women aged between 30 and 35 years, but in 80% of women in the 35–40 year age group. Generally speaking it was found that for women aged between 35 and 40, the ovarian dose which led to temporary amenorrhea was nearly equivalent to the dose which caused permanent infertility (ICRP 1969).

The situation is different after continuous irradiation over a period of several hours at a low dose rate (radium) or after fractionated x-ray or megavoltage irradiation. Normal pregnancies have been reported several years after treatment of carcinoma of the cervix (WHELTON and McSWEENY 1964; PRICE and ROMINGER 1965; FRANCIS and STEVENS 1965; VUKSINOVIC 1966, R₁, R₃) or of dysgerminoma (GANS et al. 1963, R₁, R₂; AYERST and

Table 15.1. Data regarding the sensitivity of human gonads to irradiation (modified from LUSHBAUGH and RICKS 1972; see reference list in that article)

	Temporary sterility	Permanent sterility	Authors
Female	170R	320 R	GLUCKSMANN (1947)
	400 R	400 R (>40 years)	PATERSON (1963)
		1200 R	
		625 R	PECK et al. (1949)
	640 R	2000 R	JACOX (1939)
		800–1000 R	LACASSAGNE et al. (1962)
Male	78 R		ROWLEY et al. (1974)
	15–300 rad (20 rad/min)	600 R	HELLER (1967)
		600 R	HELLER and ROWLEY (1970)
	250 R	500–600 R	GLUCKSMANN (1947)
	416 R		OAKES and LUSHBAUGH (1952)
		950 R	CALLAWAY et al. (1947)

JOHNSON 1959; McCARTHY and MILTON 1975). This suggests that irradiation of the ovary is better tolerated when the total dose is administered (fractionated) over a period of 4–6 weeks. The dose required to induce menopause in women is reported to range between 10 and 20 Gy, depending on the age (BARBER 1981). Doses of 12 Gy over 4 days or 20 Gy over 2 weeks are recommended for the induction of menopause in breast cancer patients (DELCLOS and MONTAGUE 1973). According to the data in Table 15.1, the radiation doses required to reduce fertility are higher in women than in men. This is supported by the results of studies on ovarian function in patients with Hodgkin's disease or carcinoma of the cervix in whom the ovaries were relocated by oophoropexy or lateral ovarian transposition before radiotherapy (TRUEBLOOD et al. 1970; HODEL et al. 1982; HUSSEINZADEH et al. 1984; GAETINI et al. 1987; LEPORRIER et al. 1987); several such patients subsequently gave birth to apparently healthy children despite gonadal doses and FSH elevation (BIELER et al. 1976b; THOMAS et al. 1976; GUGLIELMI et al. 1980; HODEL et al. 1982; BARBER 1981; SLANINA et al. 1985). Following inverted Y radiotherapy for Hodgkin's disease in Freiburg, 39 of 122 women (32%) became pregnant at least once [cf. HORNING et al. (1981): 19% (20/103); THOMAS et al. (1976): 23% (5/22)] – data obtained from a questionnaire inquiry.

15.4.2 Changes in Male Gonads After Irradiation

Only a few data are available on the situation after a single small or medium radiation dose (Heller et al. 1968; Rowley et al. 1974: single local dose of 15–400 R in healthy males). These data, as well as those obtained after irradiation accidents, show to what extent the cell renewal system of the male can compensate radiation damage to the testes (Hempelman et al. 1952, R_2, R_5; Dames and Lushbaugh 1952, R_2, R_3; Beninson et al. 1969). After local irradiation with 15–400 R the number of sperm decreased; 15 R caused oligospermia, but aspermia was not observed during the 6-month observation period. A dose of 50 R mainly affected the spermatogonia; 400 R, on the other hand, showed a greater effect on the later stages in spermatogenesis, e.g., spermatocytes (Table 15.1). The recovery period was 30 months after a single local dose of 200 R; after 400–600 R it was 60 months upwards. After 10–12 Gy (Deschner et al. 1969) partial recovery of spermatogenesis is possible. After an accident at a nuclear reactor plant (390 R TBI) sterility lasted 7 months. Only 50 months later did the spermiograms return to normal and a healthy child was procreated.

Up to 10 months after application of neutron radiation in a 26-year-old man no sperm were found in the ejaculate and a biopsy of the testes showed only a few spermatogonia; then, however, there was a rapid recovery in the sperm count (Robinson and Eagle 1949). Similar recovery rates were described by Kumatori et al. (1980) in their long-term study on Japanese fisherman exposed to radioactive fall-out in 1954, although acute disturbances of spermatogenesis were described as severe (Shimizu et al. 1956). The following reviews report on the dose-related occurrence of reversible and irreversible azoospermia after radiation therapy of the pelvic lymph nodes subsequent to surgery of testicular tumors: Amelar et al. (1971), Orecklin et al. (1973), Weissbach et al. (1974a, b), Hahn et al. (1976), Greiner and Meyer (1977), Greiner (1982), Nader et al. (1983), and Berthelsen (1984). By performing a sperm analysis before radiotherapy one can establish whether the tumor itself has led to infertility (Haubrich and Harms 1973) and whether ejaculation disorders exist as a result of retroperitoneal lymph node dissection (Nijiman et al. 1982; Thüroff 1982). Other disturbances in gonadal function in patients with testicular cancer also have to be taken into consideration (Fossa et al. 1982; Berthelsen and Skakkebaeck 1983; Willemse et al. 1983; Freund et al. 1987). Of 273 patients with testicular cancer who received pelvic lymph node radiotherapy, 18 subsequently fathered apparently healthy children (n = 22) (Sandeman 1966; Fossa et al. 1986). In this context it is not without importance whether the radiotherapy is prepubertal (8–14 years) or postpubertal (17–36 years), as indicated by certain endocrinological parameters and the occurrence of azoospermia (Shalet et al. 1978; Brauner et al. 1983, 1988). Sperm analyses from patients with Hodgkin's disease receiving pelvic radiotherapy demonstrated that fractionated irradiation has a stronger impact on spermiogenesis than the same single dose (Speiser et al. 1973; Slanina et al. 1977; Pedrick and Hoppe 1986). The critical dose to the testes with usual fractionation appears to be 1.5 Gy (Greiner 1982, 1985). For a long time it was unclear whether azoospermia must be considered irreversible after both single and fractionated irradiation. Up to 7.5 months after local irradiation with 600 R repair processes were observed histologically, and up to 24 months living spermatozoa were found in the ejaculate (Rowley et al. 1974). After fractionated irradiation during radiotherapy, initial signs of recovery could be observed in the spermiogram within 24 months, even if spermatogenesis was only partially restored (Greiner 1982, 1985; Hahn et al. 1982). About 3 years after the termination of radiotherapy a definite conclusion can be drawn regarding the damage to spermatogenesis. Hormonal pretreatment with LH-RH analogues during fractionated irradiation had no protective effect on stem cell survival in rats (van Kroonenburgh et al. 1987).

15.5 Difficulties in the Transfer of Data from Animal Studies to Man

15.5.1 Reactions of Oocytes and Sterility After Irradiation

There are large variations in the radiosensitivity of the oocytes:

(a) during development,
(b) in different animal strains, and
(c) in different species.

a) Application of 20 R 1 day after birth (pachytene and diplotene stages) killed about 50% of mouse oocytes; administration 8 days later killed 86%, while administration on the 21st day killed 92%. Afterwards the oocytes became more resistant, so that 12% survived administration of 20 R in the 7th week (OAKBERG and CLARK 1964, R_3; FRITZ-NIGGLI 1972; OAKBERG 1975, R_2).

b) The time of maximal radiosensitivity also varies in different animal strains: In the Bagg strain (mouse) this phase is observed at the age of 2 weeks, whereas in the Street strain it occurs at 3 weeks (PETERS 1968, R_1). Similar variations exist between rat strains. In mice the absolute numbers of oocytes vary considerably from strain to strain, e.g., from 6000 at birth in the Street strain (PETERS 1966, R_1) to 3000 in the CBA strain (NILSSON and HENDRICSON 1969, R_1). In the Street strain numbers are reduced to one-third within the first 7 weeks of life, while in the CBA strain they are reduced to one-half (RÖNNBÄCK et al. 1971; RÖNNBÄCK 1979).

c) The small primary follicles are considerably more radiosensitive than the later graafian follicles, which are killed only after 800–2000 R in mice, and only after 4000–5000 R in rats and monkeys. During preovulatory maturation the radiosensitivity increases, becoming maximal between metaphase I and II (these phases vary in duration between mice and man, lasting 12 and 36 h respectively). IOANNOU (1963, R_1) reported that the radiation dose required to kill primordial oocytes in guinea pigs was ten times that required in mice and rats. Similar differences were found by BAKER (1969, R_1) after in vitro irradiation of tissue cultures: 4000–5000 R was required to kill oocytes of monkeys and humans, whereas 100–150 R was sufficient to reduce the numbers of oocytes of rats and mice considerably. In addition, the radiation doses required to destroy all germ cells in the fetal ovaries of humans were significantly higher than those necessary to achieve the same effect in the fetal ovaries of monkeys (BAKER and BEAUMONT 1967, R_1; for further data see DOBSON and FELTON 1983).

The major differences in the number of oocytes between animal species and the variation in radiation effects on multilayered and graafian follicles as well as on interstitial tissue make apparent the limitations in transferring results from studies with small animals to humans.

With regard to infertility, studies in different species indicate that as little as 50–100 R is sufficient to reduce the number of offspring in rats or mice and subsequently to produce lasting sterility. In guinea pigs and dogs, however, 300–400 R had no major influence on fertility. Besides the varying radiation reactions of certain oocyte stages, other factors may play a role in generating these differences, i.e., characteristics of the nucleus in "resting oocytes" and the normal rate of oocyte destruction (R_1). Further reasons for these species differences remain unknown.

15.5.2 Radiation Reactions of Spermatogonia

There is also considerable variation in radiosensitivity in males depending on (a) stage of development, (b) animal strain, and (c) species.

a) In immature rat testes three phases of high radiosensitivity can be distinguished: The first phase occurs in the 13.5- to 17.5-day-old embryo with its high mitotic activity of primordial germ cells. The second phase is entered at around the time of birth (day 19 of gestation up to the 2nd day postpartum), with the occurrence of type A spermatogonia. Subsequently a radiation-resistant phase is reached with the division of type A spermatogonia, giving way to a third radiosensitive stage at the 17th day postpartum (OAKBERG 1975). Comparable developmental phases in human fetal and prepubertal testes are well documented.

b) In C3H mice testicular stem cells showed better survival after intermittent irradiation for 24 h than after a single application of the total dose; however, this could not be observed in CBA mice (LU et al. 1980). Differences in radiosensitivity of spermatogonia and during stem cell proliferation are seen in several mouse and rat strains (VALENTIN 1978; BIANCHI et al. 1985; DELIC et al. 1987a).

c) The time required for the development of type A spermatogonia also varies according to the species investigated. These times are:

In *mice* $35 + 8.6 = 43$ days
In *rats* $52 + 13 = 65$ days
In *humans* $72 - 74$ days

These times are constant for each species, and only appear to be slightly less in younger individuals. In the mouse and Chinese hamster, differences in the number of spermatogonial stem cells were found in different animals, but these differences were never as large as those among rhesus monkeys (van Alphen et al. 1988a). There also seem to be large variations between man and mouse in respect of the relation between dose used and cell repopulation processes. In mice one finds dose-related reactions of type A spermatogonia during the first 10 days after x-ray irradiation with 200, 300, or 600 R. Whereas the disappearance of spermatogonia in the mouse is mainly the result of cell death, in humans it appears that differentiation into more mature cell types is of importance for the radiation effects. Repopulation of the testicular endothelium is slower in humans than in mice, the difference being greater than would be expected from the duration of spermatogenesis (72 days in humans, 36 days in mice).

According to the existing experimental data man seems to be more radiosensitive than mouse (by a factor of 2.7–7 according to Meistrich and Samuels 1985) with regard to the depression of spermatogonia (5–7 days in mice, 90–200 days in humans). When using the reduction of testicular weight as a parameter for radiation effects (which was more frequently the practice in earlier studies) one has to realize that the ratio between testicular weight and body weight is inversely proportional to body weight. This ratio is 0.0058 in mice, 0.0015 in dogs, and 0.00057 in humans. Such differences have to be taken into consideration when making comparisons, e.g., regarding the effects of ^{239}Pu accumulation in mouse and human testes: these effects should be more pronounced in humans than in mice (Russel and Lindenbaum 1979).

15.6 Morphological Changes

15.6.1 Morphological Changes in the Ovary

The histomorphological radiation sequelae originally described by Reifferscheid (1914) and Halberstaedter (1952, R_1) have been confirmed by numerous authors (reviews: Jostes 1963; Jostes and Scherer 1961). The cells in the ovary and their functional units were found to vary in their radiosensitivity. It remains uncertain whether a different radiosensitivity exists, since whether follicle cells during certain stages are more sensitive than oocytes depends on the species. To the surprise of several research groups, even after high dose irradiation of the ovaries, complete sterilization could not always be observed (e.g., following 3500 R in rabbits:

Lacassagne and Gicouroff 1941, quoted by Jostes 1963); some primitive eggs began to develop afterwards. In many laboratory animals, including monkeys, developing follicles were radiosensitive, mature follicles were more resistant, and primordial follicles were most resistant. Thus, considerable species differences exist, whereby the stage in development is also of significance. Primordial oocytes of mice and rats are very radiosensitive: doses that destroy the germ cells have little effect on granulosa cells (Mandl 1964; Peters 1969; Baker and Neal 1969, 1975, R_1). However, in monkeys and guinea pigs the primordial oocytes (in the diplotene phase) are very radioresistant. Granulosa cells in these species, which are of similar radiosensitivity to those in rats, are destroyed long before the oocytes (Baker 1966, R_1; Iannou 1969, R_4). On the other hand the radiosensitivity of multilayered and graafian follicles appears more uniform among species. Only the mouse was twice as sensitive as rat, guinea pig, and monkey (2000 R as against 4000–5000 R; Mandl 1964; Baker 1971, R_1).

Examining radiation-induced tumorigenesis in mice or in transplanted ovaries, Covelli et al. (1982) observed the radiosensitivity of various ovarian tissues to differ. Increasing doses of radiation (10–60 Gy) to the exteriorized rat ovary caused a reduction in ovarian follicles and an increase in luteinized tissues (Jarrell et al. 1986). Quantitatively there was a reduction in antral follicles, with no difference in preantral follicles. The point in time at which morphological changes occur after exposure to radiation mainly depends on the dose. After higher doses (1500 R) severe disturbances can be seen within 1 h; early damage to the nucleus of the germ cells was observed with subsequent condensation of the chromosomes and destruction of the nuclear membrane (Jostes and Scherer 1961; Beaumont 1965, R_1; Baker 1966, R_1). Changes in the cell nucleus were found within 1 h after single-dose TBI with 400 R, within 10 h after TBI with 100 R, and within 7 weeks after long-term irradiation with 1.2 R/day (radium, 59 R). Cytoplasmic edema of the follicle cells and changes in the endoplasmic reticulum and mitochondria, however, occurred earlier and were more pronounced. Besides aging processes involving the nucleus, cytoplasmic alterations appeared after 2–3 months and underwent only partial repair. These repair processes were more impressive during a long-term experiment with 1.2 R/day, even though the number of follicles was reduced

(JOSTES and SCHERER 1967). The membrane of the oocytes in mice is probably radiosensitive (DOBSON and FELTON 1983). Studies on immature oocytes in mice also show that these extremely sensitive cells (γ-ray LD_{50} ≤ 0.08 Gy in juvenile animals: DOBSON and KWAN 1977) are killed by a mechanism other than nuclear or DNA damage (DOBSON and FELTON 1983; STRAUME and DOBSON 1985; STRAUME et al. 1987); previous target studies (STRAUME et al. 1989) with low energy neutrons and with tritium implicate the oocyte plasma membrane. For further data see the reviews.

15.6.1.1 Electron Microscopic Studies

Ultrastructural alterations in oocytes have been described in the mouse and rat. *Mouse*: PEARSONS (1962, R_1: TBI with 7–200 R at the age of 4 days), BOJADJIEVA MIHAILOVA (1964, R_1: 600–1200 R), and JOSTES and SCHERER (1967: TBI with 100–300 R, 1.2 R/day); *rat*: PARKIN (1970, R_1). For further details see BAKER and NEAL (1975, R_1), BAKER and BEAUMONT (1967, R_1), and BAKER and FRANCHI (1972a,b, R_1). Differences in the arrangement of chromosomes have been found (R_1). Electron microscopic studies have also been performed after radiotherapy (GRÖNROOS et al. 1982). Electron microscopic autoradiography was used to localize ^{241}Pu within various cellular components of the testes of dogs, guinea pigs, and rats (MILLER 1982, 1989).

15.6.2 Morphological Changes in the Testis

The measurement of testicular weight after radiation exposure is still carried out today, although mainly in combination with other morphological and functional parameters. In this context it should be noted that the testicular weight loss described by KOHN and KALLMAN (1954, R_5) as an exponential function of the radiation dose correlates with histological changes.

While type A spermatogonia with their short cell cycle are considered very radiosensitive, all cells which survive irradiation with 3 Gy have a slower cell cycle (OAKBERG 1971, R_5; HUCKINS 1978a,b; OAKBERG and HUCKINS 1976; HUCKINS and OAKBERG 1978). On the basis of a number of contributions from other authors (R_1; R_2; R_5; OAKBERG and LORENZ 1972, R_5; RUITER-BOOTSMA 1977; ERICKSON 1976, 1981; ERICKSON and HALL

1983; see also GREINER 1982), a generally recognized model for the source of spermatogenesis has been developed. The data of ALPHEN et al. (1988a) suggest that after irradiation the dark type A spermatogonia gradually transform into pale type A spermatogonia and then start to proliferate. There are no fundamental differences between spermatogenesis in man and rodents. The only distinctions are the previously described varying duration of spermatozoal development and different behavior in the regeneration and repopulation of testicular tubuli. Several publications have attempted to elucidate the sensitivity of spermatogenesis, and especially that of spermatogonia. Depletion and repopulation of the spermatogonia from the seminiferous epithelium of the rhesus monkey occurred after local irradiation with 0.5–4 Gy x-rays (ALPHEN et al. 1988a,b). Besides the sequelae of continuous radiation and the question of borderline doses which only just result in an alteration in kinetics, the following topics are of special interest with respect to clinical application.

Continuous irradiation: Continuous irradiation with 0.00009 Gy/min (= ca. 0.13 Gy/day) appears to be the borderline dose rate (OAKBERG and CLARK 1964, R_3) for which a steady state (between cell destruction and cell renewal) is reached at 80% of the normal cell number. With 0.0004 Gy/min a threshold dose rate was found; at a higher dose rate it is the total dose which is decisive for radiation sequelae. It was also seen in studies on dogs (CASARETT 1970) that 0.00065 Gy daily to total doses of 0.6 Gy resulted in a lower spermatozoa concentration, while when given daily to a total dose of 1.5 Gy it caused oligospermia in ejaculates. If 0.02 Gy, when given over more than ten generations, is exceeded, a continuous loss of spermatozoa is observed, extending to infertility (DE BOER 1964, R_3).

Threshold doses: The differentiated spermatogonia, which are especially radiosensitive in spermatogenesis, are reported to have an LD_{50} of 0.2–0.24 Gy in mice (OAKBERG, R_3, R_5). According to investigations by OAKBERG (1971), 72 h after 1 Gy 22% of type A_1 and 5% of type A_{2-4} spermatogonia were still alive, whereas after 1.5 Gy only stem cells and preleptotene spermatocytes were found to be living. The results of studies in man using differing single doses indicate a similar situation in humans (HELLER et al. 1968; ROWLEY

1974). Recovery originating from the subpopulation in the pool of spermatogonial stem cells is likely to occur after the following single doses: 6 Gy (man), 8 Gy (bull), and more than 0.2 Gy in other test animals (dog: CASARETT 1980). WATTENWYL 1980).

Fractionation: The tolerance doses suggested by RUBIN and CASARETT (1972) have to be corrected – for spermatogonial stem cells an $LD_{5/5}$ of 1 Gy and an $LD_{50/5}$ of 2 Gy can now be assumed (LUSHBAUGH and CASARETT 1976). According to data concerning radiotherapy in 58 patients (GREINER 1982), the recovery of spermatogenesis was not jeopardized by daily doses of 0.03–0.05 Gy up to a total dose of 1 Gy; daily doses of 1.5 Gy, however, made recovery impossible. Thus, the survival of stem cells was used to assess the RBE (see Sect. 15.8.3) of different types of radiation: neutrons (e.g., CLOW and GILLETTE 1970; COGGLE et al. 1977; GERACI et al. 1975, 1977, 1980) or high LET-charged particles (ALPEN and POWERS-RISIUS 1981).

Time of repopulation or recovery: ROWLEY et al. (1974) and OAKBERG (1975) found first signs of recovery in the number of ADL spermatogonia 200 days after 1 Gy x-rays. CLIFTON and BRENNER (1983), referring to data from ROWLEY et al. (1974) and PAULSEN (1973), described an increase in the total number of Ad and Ap spermatogonia at approximately the same time after irradiation. In contrast, the repopulation of the seminiferous epithelium in nonprimates proceeds much faster: 80 days (DYM and CLERMONT 1970) after 3 Gy in the rat and 2.4 and 14 weeks after 1.5 and 10 Gy (x-rays), respectively, in the mouse (ITO and ITAGAKI 1963). In addition to the heterogeneity of the stem cells and the varying duration of spermatogenesis in mice, rats, and man (35, 42, and 72 days respectively), it was shown long ago (OAKBERG 1955, R_2, R_5) that irradiation does not influence the time required by the surviving cells to reach the ejaculate. Mitotic arrest was also not significantly prolonged after spermatogonial irradiation; for type B spermatogonia the mitotic delay is supposed to last about 2.5 h after 20–50 R and about 6 h after 200–300 R. The morphological sequelae of low dose preirradiation and subsequent high dose TBI were studied in rats by DIETHELM and LORENZ (1964). Differing radiation responses of peripheral and central tubuli after γ-irradiation of mouse testes were described by BHATIA et al. (1982).

Contradictory results exist regarding the direct influence of ionizing radiation on sperm motility (frequently investigated after direct irradiation of semen) in different animal species. Whereas RIKMENSPOEL and VAN HERPEN (1969, 1975: bulls), NIEDETZKY and LAUTAI (1969: frogs), BRUCE et al. (1974: mice), and MAKLER et al. (1980: man) described reduced sperm motility over a wide dose range, OVERSTREET and ADAMS (1971: rabbits) observed no significant effects. CASARETT (1964, R_2), WU and PRICE (1964, R_3), and LAWSON et al. (1967) reported on the radiation effects on the sperm composition. Changes in the vascularization of mouse testes days after local irradiation (10 Gy) were observed by KOCHAR and HARRISON (1971a; see also WANG et al. 1983). The significance of the other testicular components with respect to the radiation response has also been clarified. Besides the spermatogonia, the Sertoli cells under the influence of the endocrine system (FAKUNDING et al. 1976; DEDOV and NOREC 1982; WANG et al. 1983) and the Leydig cells (ABBOTT 1959, R_5; ERICKSON 1964; BRAUNER et al. 1983, 1988) are important for the recovery processes.

Finally it should be mentioned that morphological alterations after radiation have been studied in several other species, too. For example, PRASAD et al. (1977) reported on the opossum, HYODO-TAGUCHI and EGAMI (1977) on alterations in spermatogonia in fish after irradiation with tritiated water, and ASHRAF et al. (1974) on th bollworm.

15.7 Functional Changes

Knowledge of the functional changes caused by irradiation of the ovary has been improved over the last 20 years mainly through three lines of research:

1. While radiation-induced sterility in adult small animals was the main area of study until 1965, this parameter is now mainly assessed after irradiation of developing gonads, since the influence of radiation on the number of offspring, the duration of sterility, and the ability to reproduce as a whole is more pronounced and prolonged at this stage than in adult organisms. BAKER and NEAL (1972, R_1) described such functional changes on the basis

of a large number of observations. Thereby, it became clear that although a substantial loss of germ cells occurred, high dose acute irradiation could never totally suppress the ability to reproduce. However, exact assessment of the number of offspring during the entire reproductive phase is possible only for rodents, as a number of factors (life expectancy, individual differences, number of offspring) make it impossible to document the reproductive ability in large animals comprehensively. As yet, corresponding studies in humans are difficult to evaluate (MONDORF and FABER 1968).

2. Studies with large animals have partially confirmed the results obtained in mice and rats. In addition to the differences between species, it became apparent that higher doses of radiation (single exposure) are required in large animals to elicit effects similar to those observed in rodents. A summary of these results is found in BAKER and NEAL (1975, R_1).

3. Besides studies with large animals, clinical investigations employing endocrinological methods have contributed to a better understanding of the significance of functional changes after radiation exposure. However, it is known that in large animals and in humans stress factors can also lead to menstrual disturbances or to alterations in endocrinological parameters (RICHTER 1982), whereas such effects are negligible in rodents. Two observations have to be mentioned in this context: The extent of radiation effects after continuous irradiation with low and medium doses differs substantially from that seen after single-dose irradiation. Furthermore, the maturation of oocytes is obviously accelerated by irradiation, so that so-called superovulation occurs. Low doses of ^{90}Sr, which do not impair the function, led to an increase in the number of mature oocytes in mice (HENDRICSON and NILSSON 1970). A 10%–15% increase in fertility after prenatal exposure to low doses of x-rays (MEYER and TONASCIA 1973; MEYER et al. 1976), together with additional results from animal studies and the results of radiotherapy in gynecology and in female patients with Hodgkin's disease, also can be related to radiation-induced superovulation.

15.7.1 Sterility and Reproductive Capacity in the Male

As pointed out in the reviews R_2–R_5 and in Sect. 15.4.2, the assessment of sterile periods was in the past mainly carried out with specific questions in mind, i.e., regeneration and repopulation (MEISTRICH et al. 1978) and the effects of fractionated irradiation (CATTANACH 1974; SHERIDAN 1971), even if the relationship between the dose and the duration of sterile periods was also dealt with in these studies. Up to a total dose of 400 R, there was no difference in the duration of sterile periods after fractionated irradiation or single-dose irradiation. After a total dose of 600 R, however, the sterile period was shorter after fractionated irradiation, only to become longer again (compared with single-dose irradiation) after an even higher total dose.

Permanent infertility seems to appear in small laboratory animals after exposure to radiation at the LD90 level. CLOW and GILLETTE (1970) concluded from their investigations that permanent sterility in the rat can be observed when the survival of type A spermatogonia is reduced to 6%–8% of the control values. MEISTRICH et al. (1978) and PINON-LATAILLADE and MAAS (1985) are of the opinion that 10%–15% of the normal sperm production is sufficient to maintain fertility in the rat. It is thereby clear that the radiation dose required to achieve permanent sterility is larger in small laboratory animals than in dogs, monkeys, and humans. This work and the radiation effects on the endocrine system, as discussed in the following sections, demonstrate that today it is more useful to examine in combination the morphological and functional changes that occur after radiation.

15.7.2 Biochemical Changes in the Male and Female

Several factors make it difficult to describe and evaluate systematically the biochemical changes in metabolism in the ovary and testes that occur after irradiation.

a) The basic biochemical knowledge of metabolic processes in the intact ovary and testes has only been established during the last two decades.

b) The differences in radiosensitivity between germ and interstitial cells, as well as their dependence on the pituitary and diencephalon and the associated hormonal changes, have led to results which only now can be brought together systematically.

c) Progress in relating biochemical disturbances to morphological changes is slow due to the fact that radiation processes are influenced by several additional factors, e.g., time, recovery mechanisms, and medications.

Several methods were used in the past to measure changes in DNA and RNA content and synthesis in the testes (MEYHÖFER et al. 1971; GERACI et al. 1977; LU et al. 1980; HACKER et al. 1980, 1981, 1982; HILSCHER et al. 1982; GUPTA and BAWA 1975; GERACI et al. 1975; PINKEL et al. 1983; JOSHI et al. 1990).

The increase in the metabolic activity (oxygen consumption) of locally irradiated (6 Gy, mouse) testes occurs concurrently with testicular weight loss but is evident only after a quiescent period of 2 weeks following exposure; the use of adenosine triphosphate suggests that metabolic control in regenerating testes may be highly modified (Pogany 1983).

Several studies have described changes in enzyme activity in testicular tissue, mainly after local irradiation of rats. Radiation-induced alterations in enzyme activity in various metabolic pathways have been reported, sometimes in combination with histological changes (GUPTA and BAWA 1971–1979; HORI et al. 1970; ITO 1966; KOCHAR and HARRISON 1971b). As well as alterations in 5-nucleotidase and adenosine triphosphatase activity (GUPTA and BAWA 1975, 1978a), changes in the activity of the following enzymes have been demonstrated: malic dehydrogenase, lactate dehydrogenase, sorbitol dehydrogenase, glucose-6-phosphatase dehydrogenase, and isocitric dehydrogenase (GUPTA and BAWA 1971, 1978a, 1979; see also HORI et al. 1970). Furthermore, an increase in prostaglandin synthetase activity has been described 15 min after TBI with 9 Gy (NIKANDROVA et al. 1981). As the uptake of zinc by the testis or its neighboring organs is influenced by gonadotropins and testosterone, and as zinc is important for spermatogenesis, GUPTA and BAWA (1975) investigated the uptake of ^{65}Zn after lower abdominal irradiation of rats.

15.7.3 Endocrinological Changes

Several authors have examined endocrinological parameters as well as morphological and function-

al changes after exposure to radiation (i.e., BIELER et al. 1976a, b; HOPKINSON et al. 1978; KALISNIK et al. 1978; MURAMATSU et al. 1978; GRÖNROOS et al. 1982; WANG et al. 1983). In the process, questions concerning the endocrine control of ovarian and testicular function were more intensely studied than previously, even though they were considered to be secondary effects. The blockage of hormone effects seems to be of increasing importance.

15.7.3.1 Endocrinological Changes in the Female

Under the control of the hypothalamus (via releasing hormones or inhibiting factors) the anterior pituitary releases, in addition to four other hormones, follicle-stimulating hormone (FSH) and luteinizing hormone (LH or ICSH: interstitial cell stimulating hormone); together these two hormones are referred to as the gonadotropins. After removal or destruction of the pituitary, the ovaries (and testes in the case of the male) will degenerate. FSH is responsible for the initial growth of the ovarian follicle in the female. LH stimulates maturation of the follicles and hormone secretion by the ovaries, as well as ovulation, formation of the corpus luteum, and secretion of progesterone. The sex steriods which are released from the ovary regulate and modulate the function of the hypothalamus, and even more so that of the pituitary, via a negative and a positive feedback action.

After both surgical and radiological elimination of the ovaries (e.g., castration of a premenopausal patient with metastasizing breast cancer) the release of gonadotropins is increased. A significant elevation of LH and FSH levels in plasma and increased excretion of gonadotropins in the urine have been described (LORAINE 1957; JANSON et al. 1981). This corresponds to the typical picture of hypergonadotropic insufficiency of the ovary as observed after other diseases of the organ (BRECKWOLDT et al. 1981). The actual dysfunctions are situated in the ovary itself; the increase in gonadotropin levels in plasma after radiological castration occurs later and is less profound than after surgical removal of the organ (CZYGAN and MARUHN 1972). The time course of the changing estradiol, FSH, and LH levels in serum depends on the ovarian dose after radiological castration (NAUJOKAT et al. 1988). This well-known clinical observation was confirmed in experiments with calves and rhesus monkeys (ATKINSON et al. 1970, R_1; DRIANCOURT et al. 1983); however, gradual differences were noticed (HOBSON and BAKER 1979). HALAWA et al. (1981), BIELER et al. (1976a, b), and GRÖNROOS et al. (1981, 1982) have described the early changes in FSH, LH, and estradiol 7 days after pelvic irradiation or 40 days after radium application in patients with gynecological carcinomas.

SANDERS et al. (1983) and BARRETT et al. (1987) have reported on ovarian failure with low levels of β-estradiol and raised FSH and LH values in girls as late effects of TBI conditioning before bone marrow transplantation in childhoood acute leukemia.

In humans estrogen synthesis was unaffected by radiotherapy of the ovaries up to a total dose of 20 Gy. Estrogen excretion was reduced in young women (aged 24–38 years) undergoing radiotherapy (JANSON et al. 1981). but was found to be higher than after ovariectomy (DIEZ-FALUSY et al. 1959). Metabolism and conjugation of estradiol in the kidney and small gut were impeded. The conversion of testosterone into estrogen is reduced shortly after TBI of rats, but it normalizes quickly. Even after investigations by SHELTON (1961) it was not clear whether androgen secretion in the adult rat is impaired after x-irradiation of the ovary. Findings after LH stimulation in irradiated rats have been described by SPALDING et al. (1957) and CHRISTIANSEN et al. (1970).

In Sprague-Dawley rats in which the ovaries were exteriorized and subjected to increasing doses of radiation (10–60 Gy) there were increases in ovarian follicular atresia and in FSH levels, but no change in serum LH levels (JARRELL et al. 1986). Interesting aspects of hormone effects emerged following the discovery of hormone receptors, but with respect to irradiation only a few reports exist (BLANKENSTEIN et al. 1981; JANSSENS et al. 1981), according to which a significant reduction in the estrogen receptor concentration in the rat tumor occurs after 20 Gy.

15.7.3.2 Endocrinological Changes in the Male

In the male, too, the hypothalamus controls the secretion of the gonadotropins by the anterior pituitary. FSH and LH regulate the function of the gonads. Apart from FSH, testosterone also stimulates spermatogenesis. The secretion of testoster-

one, synthesized from cholesterol in the Leydig cells, is controlled by LH; testosterone and other androgens exert a negative feedback effect on LH secretion by the anterior pituitary. Androgen binding protein, as a specific product of the Sertoli cells, also influences spermatogenesis. In addition the Sertoli cells produce inhibin, which inhibits FSH secretion by the anterior pituitary. Simultaneous occurrence of oligo-and azoospermia and an increase in FSH and LH levels in plasma can be observed after irradiation accidents (WAKABAYASHI et al. 1974), after irradiation of the testes during radiotherapy (ASBJORNSEN et al. 1976; CLUBB and CARTER 1976; SHALET et al. 1978, 1985; FLECK et al. 1981; TOMIC et al. 1983), after ^{131}I therapy for thyroid carcinoma (HANDELSMAN and TURTLE 1983), and after local irradiation of healthy men (ROWLEY et al. 1974; HELLER et al. 1968). A local dose to the testis of 12 R (accidental irradiation) was sufficient to achieve an increase in FSH, whereas 75 R was required to cause an elevation in plasma LH levels in healthy men (FREUND et al. 1987). Plasma FSH levels in humans increased shortly after irradiation with 0.75–6 Gy while plasma LH levels increased after approximately 1 month (ROWLEY et al. 1974). The amount of testosterone excreted in the urine was reduced in correspondence with the irradiation dose, especially after 1500 R local irradiation (BIRKE et al. 1956); however, this reduction was more pronounced after orchiectomy. The elevation of FSH in serum appeared to be higher after postoperative irradiation of patients with renal tumors aged between 17 and 36 years than in comparable patients aged between 8 and 14 years (SHALET et al. 1978).

Leydig cell dysfunction following direct high dose testicular irradiation in childhood for acute leukemia is usually severe (BRAUNER et al. 1983, 1988; CARRASCOSA et al. 1984; GREINER 1985; SHALET et al. 1985) and androgen replacement is often required to make possible normal pubertal development. A possible disturbance in Leydig cell function was further demonstrated by increased LH values in eight of nine patients receiving radiotherapy because of seminomas found several years after irradiation (NADER et al. 1983). A few experimental studies performed in immature animals (RUSH and LIPNER 1979; SUZUKI et al. 1973; WALL 1961) have failed to provide information on dose–response relationships; the results of DELIC et al. (1986b) support the clinical view that the Leydig cells in the boy are more radioresponsive than those in the adult (Brauner et al. 1983, 1988; Shalet et al. 1985). Shamberger et al. (1981) have reported an age-related elevation in LH and FSH after combination of chemotherapy and radiation therapy; patients younger than 40 years showed a smaller increase. Testosterone levels remained stable during the adjuvant postoperative treatment. These changes in hormone levels appeared to be therapy induced. They normalized quickly if the remaining testis was functioning properly. There is increasing interest in the combined effects of radio- and chemotherapy, e.g., in cases of testicular germ cell cancer (Berthelsen 1984). Whether the elevation of LH and FSH plasma levels is more pronounced after higher doses, as assumed by Hahn et al. (1982), remains unclear. Popescu et al. (1975) demonstrated that in 27 of 57 workers with occupational exposure to irradiation the gonadotropin concentration in 24-h urine samples was higher than in the control group.

The time and mode of irradiation influence the alterations induced in hormone production and levels in small animals. The decrease in LH and testosterone concentrations in the plasma 3–4 days after TBI or head or abdominal irradiation with 8.5–15 Gy has so far only been observed in rats (McTaggart and Wills 1977; Thithapandha et al. 1979); a connection with the irradiation-induced alteration of liver enzyme activity has been discussed. A reduction in testosterone accompanied by a rise in FSH and LH levels in plasma was demonstrated by Ivanov and Maleeva (1980) after TBI of rats with doses between 50 and 60 γ-R. After a local testicular irradiation dose of 6 Gy (either as a single dose or as two 3-Gy doses) in the rat no alterations were observed in the serum concentrations of FSH, LH, and testosterone at different time intervals ranging from 8 to 72 h (van Kroonenburgh et al. 1987). After irradiation of the testes of rats, especially with high doses, a distinct rise in FSH in the blood was found, whereas LH concentrations showed only a very small or delayed increase 39–45 days postirradiation (150 R: Verjans and Eik-Nes 1976; 400 R: Bain and Keene 1975; 300 R: Hopkinson et al. 1978). The testosterone levels remained mostly unchanged. Androgen synthesis was altered by TBI as well as by irradiation of the lower half of the body in both rats (1000 R: Binhammer 1967; Schoen 1964) and mice (Berliner et al. 1964; Ellis and Berliner 1967); Suzuki et al. (1973) found prepubertal irradiation of the testes in rats

to have a similar effect. In dogs comparable effects on androgen synthesis were observed after the application of several radionuclides (Ellis and Berliner 1967). After local irradiation of rhesus monkey testes with 0.5–4 Gy x-rays, serum FSH levels increased during the first week, while serum LH levels increased between 18 and 25 days after irradiation; serum testosterone levels did not change at all (van Alphen et al. 1988a,b). The increase in FSH, which is a common feature when spermatogenesis is severely impaired, was probably due to a decrease in inhibin production by Sertoli cells (Cunningham and Huckins 1978). The reason for the increase in LH is unknown as yet.

Irradiation has an effect on enzymes important for androgen synthesis, and the conversion of progesterone or 5-pregnenolone into testosterone was impaired. The different times of irradiation (Dierickx and Verhoeven 1980: rat, 20th day of gestation; De Jong and Sharpe 1977: pre- and postnatal TBI with 150 R) were chosen to clarify the role of interstitial cells in the development of radiation-induced hormone changes. The increase in FSH and LH levels in plasma runs parallel to a relatively strong reduction in spermatid numbers but not to the slight decrease in the number of spermatogonia; this suggests a connection with the reduced inhibin secretion by Sertoli cells (Cunningham and Huckins 1978; Hopkinson et al. 1978). After irradiation in the fetal period, the testis is enriched with Sertoli cells. This situation is used as a test model for the evaluation of the role of Sertoli cells in the change in endocrinological parameters (Fakunding et al. 1976). The threshold dose for Sertoli cell dysfunction, as assessed by serum androgen-binding protein (ABP) concentrations in rats, was estimated to be 5 Gy (Delic et al. 1986a). After fetal irradiation (250 R TBI on the 20th day of gestation, Rich and de Kreter 1977), the increase in ABP in the testes provides indirect evidence of impairment in the secretory function of the Sertoli cells. After 30 and 60 days the ABP content of the testes was significantly reduced (Cunningham and Huckins 1978). In this context studies have to be mentioned which elucidate the role of Leying interstitial cells. These cells also participate in the regulation of the testicular endocrine function (Abbott 1959, R4; Wall 1961, R4). Results after irradiation of the pubertal rat testis indicate that the Leydig cells in this age group are more radioresponsive than those in the adult (Delic et al. 1986b). Other experimental studies were performed in immature animals (RUSH and LIPNER 1979; SUZUKI et al. 1973; WALL 1961, R₄; JANSZ and POMERANTZ 1984).

15.8 Factors That Can Modify Radiation Effects on Reproductive Organs

15.8.1 Fractionation

In respect of irradiation of testes with two fractions of 300, 400, or 500 R, SHERIDAN (1971) was able to show that intervals of 24, 48, and 72 h significantly prolong the duration of infertility in mice in comparison with single-dose irradiation or an interval of 144 h. This confirmed the results of RUSSELL (1962). LEIDL and ZANKL (1970) investigated the influence of the interval during split-dose local irradiation (x-rays) of the germinative epithelium of rabbits. Such results are better understood today, following OAKBERG's (1975, R₂) description of A_s spermatogonia as true stem cells and as especially radioresistant. After dose splitting, SHERIDAN (1971) and DE RUITER-BOOTSMA et al. (1977) found reduced survival of stem cells, whereas WITHERS et al. (1974) showed the opposite. Mice that received a daily dose of 1.8 R showed a transient adaptation in the kinetics of the cell cycle, a regulatory mechanism stabilizing the cell population; increasing the daily dose to 2 R led to a loss of this compensatory reaction (FABRIKANT 1972). According to HELLER and CLERMONT (1964, R₅) human stem cells retain their pattern of differentiation and proliferation for at least 14 days after irradiation. OAKBERG (1978) and CATTANACH (1974) observed no significant changes in stem cell survival due to dose splitting. Cellular repopulation of the tubuli within the testes of mice 11 weeks after single-dose or fractionated total body irradiation was investigated by KRAMER et al. (1974); they found it to be less impaired with 12- to 14-day intervals between radiation doses than with daily irradiation. In addition to the length of infertility and stem cell survival, LU et al. (1980) used three further parameters to study the impact of dose splitting: the colony test, the activity of the x-isoenzyme of lactate dehydrogenase, and the number of spermatozoa in testicular homogenates (see also MEISTRICH et al. 1978, 1984b). The survival of testicular stem cells of C₃H mice was

better after split-dose irradiation with a 24-h interval than after single-dose irradiation. This was not found to be the case in CBA mice, demonstrating that there will be differences even between strains, and making it even more difficult to transfer results from investigations in mice to man. Few experimental data on the effect of dose fractionation in females are available from animal studies. However, observations after clinical radiotherapy demonstrate pronounced differences between the effects of single-dose and fractionated irradiation with a marked reduction of effect by fractionation.

15.8.2 Low Dose Rate (Protracted Irradiation)

Studies in small and large animals have shown that in both female and male animals the effects of irradiation are dependent on the dose rate and the total dose (see R₂-R₅). Testicular weight remained unchanged after continuous irradiation with 1 R/day (ESCHENBRENNER et al. 1948, R₅). In dogs, however, testicular weight and spermatogenesis were reduced after only 0.17 R/day (FEDEROVA 1976; according to Erickson 1978).

Histopathological findings about the effect of dose rate have been presented frequently in *female* animals [MOAWAD et al. 1965, R₁; SAMUELS 1966; RAO and SRIVASTAVA 1967; JOSTED and SCHERER 1967; VORISEK and JIRASEK 1967; VORISEK and VONDRACEK 1968 (postnatal); JONES et al. 1980; SEARLE et al. 1980 (^{239}Pu)] and in *male* animals (ERICKSON et al. 1972; GERACI et al. 1975, 1977; HSU and FABRIKANT 1976; ERICKSON 1978; UNGER 1980; DELIC et al. 1987a). It seems from these studies that in the case of neutron radiation the dose rate is of minor importance (GERACI et al. 1975, 1977).

Other investigators examined simultaneously the influence of low dose rate irradiation on testicular weight and gametogenesis (LAMERTON 1966, 1967; FABRIKANT 1972; ERICKSON and MARTIN 1972; MURAMATSU et al. 1978; PINON-LATAILLADE and MAAS 1985). After continuous irradiation for a week far greater differences between strains were found than after single-dose irradiation (MOLE 1959, R₁; DOBSON and FELTON 1983). This seems also to be the case in respect of the elicitation of mutations in hybrid mice (RUSSELL et al. 1957, R₁). Here reference should again be made to the reaction after radium exposure (total dose applied within several hours or days), because the effects are far milder than after single-dose irradiation

15.8.3 Relative Biological Effectiveness (RBE)

To assess the RBE in mice, the degree of destruction of spermatogonia and testicular weight were measured.

For spermatogonial killing, ^{137}Cs γ-irradiation, x-rays, and 730 MeV neutrons appear similarly effective. For 2.5 and 14 MeV neutrons an RBE value of about 2 has been reported (Oakberg 1964, 1975, R_4; Gasinska et al. 1987), while values of between 2 and 3.6 have been published for 22–35 MeV neutrons, pions, and high LET-charged particles (Bianchi et al. 1969, 1974; Coggle et al. 1977; Geraci et al. 1977, 1980; Lu et al. 1980; Montour and Wilson 1979; Alpen and Powers-Risius 1981). If colony formation is used to monitor spermatogonial stem cell survival, RBE values of between 4 and 6 are measured (De Ruiter-Bootsma et al. 1974, 1976, 1977; Withers et al. 1974; van den Aardweg et al. 1982). These values are higher than those obtained for stem cells of the hematopoetic tissue (2.4) or the small intestine (3.3) as reported by Davids (1973). Measurement of testicular weight is a suitable method for determining RBE (Batchelor et al. 1964; Bianchi et al. 1972: electrons; Hornsey et al. 1977: 7.5 MeV neutrons; Geraci et al. 1977: 16–50 MeV deuterons; Montour and Wilson 1979: 35 MeV neutrons, di Paola et al. 1980: 1–600 MeV neutrons). Hwang et al. (1984) studied the effects of low dose rate ^{252}Cf and its mixed neutron plus γ-radiation and compared it with acute ^{60}Co radiation and low dose rate ^{137}Cs to determine RBE: ^{252}Cf neutron RBE (n + γ) was 3.7 for testicular weight loss, while RBE for the neutrons only was 5.1.

As first described by Kohn and Kallman 1954, R_2, the dose–response curve of testis weight loss is biphasic. The initial steep part is considered independent of dose rate and very radiosensitive (Oakberg 1975, R^2). However, the mode of irradiation used by the investigators differed markedly: TBI was used by Bateman et al. (1968, R_2: 0.62–12 MeV neutrons), Kramer et al. (1974: 1 MeV neutrons), de Ruiter-Bootsma et al. (1976: 1 MeV fusion neutrons), and Geraci et al. (1977: 16–50 MeV deuterons). Local irradiation of the testes was used by Abbott (1959, R_5), Börner et al. (1956: rat, 6 MeV electrons), and

Verjans and Eik-Nes (1976), while irradiation of the lower abdomen was used by Hornsey et al. (1977) and Alpen and Powers-Risius (1981). For ^{252}Cf fission neutrons (2.15 MeV) the values are intermediated between those for 0.43 and 15 MeV neutrons (Straume et al. 1987). Mouse age at exposure does affect neutron RBE values for oocyte killing.

15.8.4 Radionuclides

Radionuclides can elicit effects on the ovaries and testes. Baker and Neal (1977) and ICRP (1979, 1988) give lists of publications over the last 20 years covering this topic.

1. Tritium; ^3H: In mouse testes the RBE of tritiated water, in comparison to ^{60}Co γ-irradiation, is 1.43; for tritiated thymidine a value of 2.07 has been found (Carr and Nolan 1979). The effects of tritiated water on fish spermatogonia or medaka embryos were reported in studies by Hyodo-Taguchi and Egami (1977) and Etoh and Hyodo-Taguchi (1983).

The RBE value of ^{3}H in relation to ^{60}Co γ-rays was suggested to be close to 2 or more (Kapoor and Srivastava 1980; Feinendegen et al. 1980; Dobson and Kwan 1976; Kellerer and Rossi 1978). Following the administration of doses of tritiated water 16–1000 times higher than allowed for humans, Jones et al. (1980) demonstrated a high sensitivity of monkey oocytes. Other authors reported findings in mice (Dobson and Cooper 1974; Dobson and Kwan 1974; Dobson and Felton 1983; Kapoor et al. 1985; Satow et al. 1989), in which radiosensitivity was found to vary with age. In a study comparing the responses of oocytes and spermatogonia after injection of tritiated water at different times during gestation, a 50%–100% impairment of fertility in the following generation was observed (Török et al. 1979). The sensitivity of prenatal germ cells to irradiation was greater in the male than in the female mouse: the spermatogonia kept their ability to divide longer than did the oocytes. Further data about the effect of tritiated water on fertility, testes, and fetal development are to be found in Cahill and Yuile (1970), Laskey et al. (1973), Cahill et al. (1975), and Török et al. (1979), and on oocytes in Haas et al. (1973) and Pietrzak-Fils (1982).

Bhatia and Srivastava (1982) investigated the tritium toxicity in mouse testes during pre- and postnatal development (see also DOBSON and FELTON 1983).

2. Phosphorus, ^{32}P: In a study comparing the sensitivity of spermatogonia and oocytes to the administration of 1 μCi ^{32}P, 30% of the spermatogonia were killed (REDDI et al. 1980). ^{32}P, like ^{131}I, is enriched in granulosa cells of the growing follicles; following intravenous injection of up to 0.8 μCi/g in rats no morphological changes could be found after 30 days. However, 3 days after administration of 1.2 μCi/g, degenerative changes were seen, especially in granulosa cells; immature graafian follicles showed extensive alterations after 30 days (see also REITHER and LANG 1955, R_5). According to REDDI et al. (1968, R_1) and OAKBERG (1968, R_2, R_5), cuboid granulosa cells in the proximity of the oocyte during stage II of follicle growth are supposed to be more sensitive towards ^{32}P than are flat granulosa cells during stage I.

3. Selenium methionine 75: Relatively small activities (1.22×10^4 Bq/g body weight) of selenium methionine 75 led to dramatic changes in the ultrastructure of Sertoli and Leydig cells in rats. Furthermore a significant reduction in plasma levels of testosterone was observed, together with impaired fertility. However, no visible changes in the spermatogonial epithelium could be demonstrated (DEDOV and NOREC 1982). This radionuclide was also found to be enriched in the germ cells of rats (CHAIT and NOREC 1979, quoted by DEDOV and NOREC 1982).

4. Strontium, ^{90}Sr: A Scandinavian group looked into the effects of intravenous ^{90}Sr injections between the 11th and 17th days of gestation on mouse oocytes (NILSSON and HENDRIKSON 1969, R_1; RÖNNBÄCK et al. 1971; RÖNNBÄCK 1979). The effects of irradiation from ^{90}Sr on spermatogenesis in the teleost were described by YOSHIMURA et al. (1969).

5. Technetium, ^{99m}Tc: MIAN et al. (1977) reported on the damage to mouse testis cells after administration of ^{99m}Tc-pertechnetate.

6. Iodine, ^{131}I: Iodine is found to be accumulated in the ovaries as well as in the thyroid. REDDI (1971, 1973, R_1) found an enrichment of ^{131}I in the walls of multilayered follicles in mice and cows, as had BENGTSSON et al. (1963, R_1) in rats, rabbits, and cats. However, not only these follicles were damaged; also the oocytes and granulosa cells of the neighboring smaller follicles were affected (SARKAR et al. 1976; HANDELSMAN 1980; HANDELSMAN and TURTLE 1983). Rösler and Moser (1984) reported on testicular damage, alterations in the endocrine system, and pregnancies after ^{131}I therapy for thyroid cancer.

7. Thorotrast: Only a few morphological ovarian changes were registered 23 years after exposure in a Thorotrast patient who developed menstruation anomalies and early menopause at 41 years of age (MATTHES and KRIEGEL 1958). Similar results were obtained in nine rabbits 18 months after intravenous Thorotrast injections. HEITE (1951) reported on the fertility of thorium X patients.

8. Plutonium, ^{239}Pu: The distribution of ^{239}Pu in the mouse ovary over a period of 6 months after intravenous injection was investigated by GREEN et al. (1975, 1977) and TAYLOR (1977). In testes, RUSSEL and LINDENBAUM (1979) found about 50% of the ^{239}Pu activity in the interstitial cells, even though these cells represent only 5% of the testicular volume. As a consequence a pronounced reduction in androgen synthesis is to be expected. In relation to fertility, the RBE of the α-radiation from ^{239}Pu was found to be 2.5 in comparison to ^{60}Co; in relation to testicular weight loss even higher values were observed (SEARLE et al. 1980, 1982). Comparative studies in several animal species looking into the differences in the distribution of ^{239}Pu have been published by BROOKS et al. (1979), MILLER (1982), MILLER et al. (1985; rat and 1989: beagle; testis), RICHMOND and THOMAS (1975: ovary and testis), and THOMAS et al. (1985: ovary and testis).

15.8.5 Radioprotective Substances

Various substances have been tested for their ability to alleviate radiation effects in the ovary and testis. Numerous investigations have been carried out with sulfhydryl-containing compounds: MAISIN et al. (1956, R_4), RUGH (1958, R_4), STARKIE (cysteamine, 1961, R_4), SAHARAN and DEVI (1977), GOYAL and DEV (testis, 1982), and KUMAR and DEVI (ovary, 1982, 1983). Others have used sedatives, like chlorpromazine (RUPKEY et al. 1963, R_4), or biological amines, like serotonin (ABE and LANGENDORFF 1964), sometimes with marked effects. Although histamine and serotonin have specific effects on ovarian vessel permeability and steroidogenesis, the specific cell types which bind histamine and serotonin remain largely unknown (receptor type?). MILAS et al. (1982), MEISTRICH et al. (1984), BHARTIYA and PAREEK (1984), and BHARTIYA (1986) reported on the radioprotective substance WR-2712. DOBSON and FELTON (1983) reported on the destruction of primordial oocytes in juveniles by radiation and several chemical compounds. The application of radiation protectors and their influence on the sequelae of radiation of reproductive organs also has to be mentioned (BRADY et al. 1981). In dogs GnRH analogues exhibit a protective effect for the germinal epithelium (NSEYO et al. 1985). Hormonal pretreatment with an LH-RH analogue depot preparation during split-dose irradiation had no protective effect on stem cell survival after local testicular irradiation in rats (VAN KROONENBURGH et al. 1987).

15.8.6 Chemotherapy and the Combination with Radiotherapy

In recent years many studies have investigated the effects of cytotoxic drugs on testis and ovary. Late effects of combined chemo- and radiotherapy in long-term survivors, particularly children, can be divided into two categories (BARRETT et al. 1987): those affecting hormonal status and those affecting specific organ function (*females*: low levels of estradiol and raised FSH and LH values; *males*: raised FSH and LH values and normal testosterone levels, with azoospermia in most patients; *children*: delayed puberty, can be overcome by hormone replacement). Most reports on males have described effects on spermatogenesis rather than on Leydig cell function and the production of androgens. However, some reports have been published recently on the dysfunction of the Leydig cells after chemo- and radiotherapy (SHAMBERGER et al. 1984; NADER et al. 1983; TOMIC et al. 1983; CARRACOSA et al. 1984). There are a number of publications dealing with the effect of combined ionizing irradiation and chemotherapy on the ovary (CIANCI et al. 1968; CHRISTOV and RAICHEV 1973; HIMELSTEIN-BRAW et al. 1977; SHAMBERGER et al. 1981; STILLMAN et al. 1981; BARBER1981; DOBSON and FELTON 1983; GREINER 1983; DAMEWOOD and GROCHOW 1986; GRITZ et al. 1989) or the testis (BARBER 1981; GREINER 1983; BERTHELSEN 1984; CARRASCOSA et al. 1984; DELIC

et al. 1986a; PEARSON and STEEL 1984: mouse; GRITZ et al. 1989; SKLAR et al. 1990).

Banking of gametes, such as sperm banking, ovulation induction, oocyte retrieval, and cryopreservation offer some prospect of maintaining fertility in patients who may develop permanent gonadal failure after chemo- and/or radiotherapy for neoplastic disease. Treatment of the gonadal damage may alleviate some of the emotional consequences of cancer therapy for those patients afflicted not only with a malignant disease but also with possible impairment of their reproductive potential (CHAPMAN 1982; DAMEWOOD and GROCHOW 1986).

15.9 Conclusions

Discussion within this chapter has of necessity been restricted to the description of new trends in research on a few central topics. Essentially new findings and results in eight fields of research improved our understanding of radiation reactions and sequelae in the gonads:

1. Specific differences of female and male gametogenesis in radiosensitivity
2. Species-specific differences between small and large animals, which have been elucidated through the preference for the use of larger animals in experimental studies
3. Supplementation of medical data by evaluation of radiation accidents and radiotherapeutic effects
4. The differing radiosensitivity of gonads at the various stages of development
5. Morphology and turnover of stem cells and Sertoli or Leydig cells
6. Correlations between morphology and function of the gonads
7. Endocrine regulation of ovarian and testicular function
8. Changes in radiosensitivity due to various factors (e.g., fractionation, dose rate, radioisotopes, chemical agents)

During the last 25 years a vast amount of knowledge has accumulated on radiation-induced somatic reactions and sequelae in gonads. Today this knowledge is far more extensive than the understanding of the influence of other noxious agents, drugs, and chemicals. In this review only an outline of the new findings could be given. Further progress, evolving from scientific and practical initiatives as well as from technical and methodological innovations, will complete this knowledge for the benefit of our patients.

References

Abe M, Langendorff H (1964) Untersuchungen über einen biologischen Strahlenschutz. 60. Mitt. Das Verhalten des Hodengewebes von Mäusen bei einmaliger oder wiederholter lokaler Bestrahlung unter Serotonin-Schutz. Strahlentherapie 125: 358–370

Adler ED (1977) Stage-sensitivity and dose-response study after gamma-irradiation of mouse primary spermatocytes. Int J Radiat Biol 31: 79–85

Alpen EL, Powers-Risius P (1981) The relative biological effect of high-Z, high-LET charged particles for spermatogonial killing. Radiat Res 88: 132–143

Amelar RD, Dubin L, Hotchkiss RS (1971) Restoration of fertility following unilateral orchiectomy and radiation therapy for testicular tumors. J Urol 106: 714–718

Andersen AC, Nelson VG, Simpson ME (1972) Fractionated x-radiation damage to developing monkey ovaries. J Med Primatol I: 318–325

Andersen AC, Hendrickx AG, Momeni MH (1977) Fractionated x-radiation damage to developing ovaries in the bonnet monkey (Macaca radiata). Radiat Res 71: 398–405

Asbjornsen G, Moline K, Klepp O, Aakvaaz A (1976) Testicular function after radiotherapy to inverted "Y" field for malignant lymphoma. Scand J Haematol 17: 96

Ash P (1980) The influence of radiation on fertility in man. Br J Radiol 53: 271–278

Ashraf M, Anwar M, Siddiqui QH (1974) Histopathological effects of gamma radiation on testes of the spotted bollworm of cotton, Eariax insulana (Lepidoptera: Arctüdae). Radiat Res 37: 80–87

Ayerst RI, Johnsen CG (1959) Dysgerminoma. Report of a case treated by surgery and x-ray therapy and followed by term pregnancy. Obstet Gynecol 14: 685–687

Bager S (1982) Radiation sensitivity of small oocytes in immature mice. Effect of gonadotropin treatment. Correspondence. Radiat Res 89: 420–423

Bain J, Keene J (1975) Further evidence for inhibin: change in serum luteinizing hormone and follicle stimulating hormone levels after irradiation of rat testes. J Endocrinol 66: 279–280

Baker TG, Neal P (1977) Action of ionizing radiations of the mammalian ovary. In: Zuckerman L, Weir BJ (eds) The ovary, vol III. Academic, New York, pp 1–58

Barber HRK (1981) The effect of cancer and its therapy upon fertility. Int J Fertil 26: 250–259

Barrett A, Nicholls J, Gibson B (1987) Late effects of total body irradiation. Radiother Oncol 9: 131–135

Batchelor AL, Mole RH, Williamson FS (1964) The effect on the testis of the mouse of neutrons of different energies. In: Biological effects of neutrons and proton irradiations, vol II, IAEA, Vienna, pp 303–310 (STI/PUB 807)

Beaumont HM (1969) Effect of hormonal environment on the radiosensitivity of oocytes. In: Sikov MR, Mahlum DD (eds) Radiation biology of the fetal and juvenile mammal. USAEC Division of Technical Information Service, Oak Ridge

Beninson D, Placer A, van der Elst E (1969) Estudio de un caso de irradiation humana accidental. In: Handling of radiation accidents. Pro Symp Vienna Int Atomic Energy Agency, pp 415–429

Berliner DL, Ellis LC (1965) The effects of ionizing radiations on endocrine cells. IV. Increase production of 17α-, 20α-dihydroxyprogesterone in rat testes after irradiation. Radiat Res 24: 368–373

Berliner DL, Ellis LC, Taylor GN (1964) The effects of ionizing radiations on endocrine cells. II. Restoration of androgen production with a reduced nicotinamide adenine dinucleotide phosphate-generating system after irradiation of rat testes. Radiat Res 22: 345–356

Berthelsen JG (1984) Sperm counts and serum follicle-stimulating hormone levels before and after radiotherapy and chemotherapy in man with testicular germ cell cancer. Fertil Steril 41: 281–286

Berthelsen JG, Skakkebaek NE (1983) Gonadal function in men with testis cancer. Fertil Steril 39: 68–75

Bhartiya HC (1986) Inhibition of reduction in the testicular weight by WR-2721 in relation to the body weight after whole-body gamma irradiation. Strahlentherapie 162: 68–70

Bhartiya HC, Pareek BP (1984) Effects of S-2 (3-aminopropylamino) ethyl-phosphorothioic acid (WR 2721) on the sensitivity of mouse spermatogonia A to radiation. Acta Radiol Ther 23: 65–68

Bhatia AL, Srivastava PN (1982a) Tritium toxicity in mouse testis: effect of continuous exposure during pre- and postnatal development. Strahlentherapie 158: 752–755

Bhatia AL, Saharan BR, Mathur KM (1982b) Radioresponse of spermatogenic cell population and tubular diameter in mice testes to external 60 Co gamma rays. Radiobiol Radiother 23: 699–704

Bianchi M, Quintiliani M, Baarli J, Sullivan AH (1969) Survival of mouse type-B spermatogonia for the study of the biological effectiveness of very high-energy neutrons. Int J Radiat Biol 15: 185–189

Bianchi M, Ebert M, Keene JP, Quintiliani M (1972) Survival of type A and B spermatogonia in the mouse testis after exposure to high dose rates of electrons. Int J Radiat Biol 22: 191–195

Bianchi M, Baarli J, Sullivan AH, Di Paola M, Quintiliani M (1974) RBE values of 400 MeV and 14 MeV neutrons using various biological effects. In: Biological effects of neutrons irradiation. IAEA 179/6, Vienna, pp 349–357

Bianchi M, Delic JI, Hurtado-de-Catalfo G, Hendry JH (1985) Strain differences in the radiosensitivity of mouse spermatogonia. Int J Radiat Biol 48: 579–588

Bieler EU, Schnabel T, Knobel J (1976a) The influence of pelvic irradiation on the formation and function of the human corpus luteum. Int J Radiat Biol 30: 283–285

Bieler EU, Schnabel T, Knobel J (1976b) Persisting cyclic ovarian activity in cervical cancer after surgical transposition of the ovaries and pelvic irradiation. Br J Radiol 49: 875

Binhammer RT (1967) Effect of increased endogenous gonadotrophin on testes or irradiated immature and mature rats. Radiat Res 30: 676

Birke G, Franksson C, Hultborn KA, Plantin LO (1956) The effect of roentgen irradiation on the steroid production of the testicles. Acta Chir Scand 110: 469–476

Blankenstein MA, Mulder E, Broerse JJ, van der Molen

HJ (1981) Oestrogen receptors in rat mammary tissue and plasma concentrations of prolactin during mammary carcinogenesis induced by oestrogen and ionizing radiation. J Endocrinol 88: 233–241

Blot WJ, Sawada H (1972) Fertility among female survivors of the atomic bombs of Hiroshima and Nagasaki. Am J Hum Genet 24: 613–622

Blot WJ, Shimizu Y, Kato H, Miller RW (1975) Frequency of marriage and life birth among survivors prenatally exposed to the atomic bomb. Am J Epidemiol 102: 128

Börner W, Neff V, Ricmann H, Wachsmann F (1956) Die Wirkung von 180 kV-Röntgenstrahlen und 6-MeV-Elektronen auf das Hodengewebe der Ratte. Strahlentherapie 101: 101–109

Brady LW, Philips TL, Wasserman TH (1981) The potential for radiation sensitizers and radiation protectors combined with radiation therapy in gynecologic cancer. Cancer 48: 650–657

Brauner R, Czernichow P, Cramer P, Schaison G, Rappaport R (1983) Leydig-cell function in children after direct testicular irradiation for acute lymphoblastic leukemia. N Engl J Med 309: 25–28

Brauner R, Caltabiano P, Rappaport R, Leverger G, Sehaison G (1988) Leydig cell insufficiency after testicular irradiation for acute lymphoblastic leukemia. Horm Res 30: 111–114

Breckwoldt M, Siebers JW, Müller U (1981) Die primäre Ovarialinsuffizienz. Gynäkologe 14: 131–144

Brent RL (1977) Radiations and other physical agents. In: Wilson JG, Fraser C (eds) Handbook of teratology, vol I. Plenum, New York, pp 153–223

Brooks AL, Diel JH, McClellan RO (1979) The influence of testicular microanatomy on the potential genetic dose internally deposited ^{239}Pu citrate in Chinese hamster, mouse and man. Radiat Res 77: 292–302

Bruce WR, Furrer R, Wyrobek AJ (1974) Abnormalities in the shape of murine sperm after acute testicular x-irradiation. Mutat Res 23: 381–386

Cahill DF, Yuile C (1970) Tritium: some effects of continuous exposure in "utero" on mammalian development. Radiat Res 44: 727

Cahill DF, Wright JF, Godbold FH (1975) Neoplastic and lifespan effects of chronic exposure to tritium II. Rats exposed in utero. J Natl Cancer Inst 55: 1165–1169

Carlsson WD, Gassner FX (eds) (1964) Effects of radiation on the reproductive system. Pergamon, Oxford

Carr TEF, Nolan J (1979) Testis mass loss in the mouse induced by tritiated thymidine, tritiated water, and ^{60}Co gamma irradiation. Health Phys 36: 135–145

Carrascosa A, Audi L, Ortega JJ, Javier C, Toran N (1984) Hypothalamo-hypophyseal-testicular function in prepubertal boys with acute lymphoblastic leukaemia following chemotherapy and testicular radiotherapy. Acta Paediatr Scand 73: 364–371

Casarett GW (1970) Pathological changes after protracted exposure to low dose radiation. In: Fry RJM, Grahn D. Griem ML, Rust JH (eds) Late effects of radiation. Taylor & Francis. London, pp 85–100

Casarett GW (1980) Radiation histopathology, vol II. CRC, Boca Raton, pp 75–94

Cattanach BM (1974) Spermatogonial single and fractionated x-ray dosis, as assessed by length of sterile period. Mutat Res 25: 53–62

Cattanach BM, Moseley H (1974) Sterile period, translocation and specific locus mutation in the mouse following fractionated x-ray treatments with different fractionation intervals. Mutat Res 25: 63–72

Chapman RM (1982) Effects of cytotoxic agents on sexuality and gonadal function. Semin Oncol 9: 84

Christiansen JM, Keyes PL, Armstrong DT (1970) x-irradiation of the rat ovary luteinized by exogenous gonadotropins: influence on steroidogenesis. Biol Reprod 3: 135–139

Christov K, Raichev R (1973) Proliferative and neoplastic changes in the ovaries of hamsters treated with 131-iodine and methylthiouracil. Neoplasma 20: 511–516

Cianci S, Marotta N, Nigro SC (1968) Effecti delle radiazioni ionizzanti sull'ovaio umano. Clin Ginecol 10: 1082–1098

Clayton PE, Shalet SM, Price DA (1988) Gonadal function after chemotherapy and irradiation for childhood malignancies. Hormone Res 30: 104–110

Clifton DK, Brenner WJ (1983) The effect of testicular x-irradiation on spermatogenesis in man: a comparison with the mouse. J Androl 4: 387–392

Clow DJ, Gillette EL (1970) Survival of type A-spermatogonia following x-irradiation. Radiat Res 42: 397–404

Clubb B, Carter J (1976) Effects of testicular radiation. Aust Radiol 20: 64–67

Coggle JE, Lambert BE, Peel DM, Davies RW (1977) Negative pion irradiation of the mouse testis. Int J Radiat Biol 32: 397–400

Coniglio JG, Culp FB, Davis J, Ford W, Windler F (1963) The effect of total body x-irradiation on fatty acids of testes of rats. Radiat Res 20: 372–382

Cottier H (1961) Strahlenbedingte Lebensverkürzung. Pathologische Anatomie somatischer Spätwirkungen der ionisierenden Ganzkörperbestrahlung auf den erwachsenen Säugetierorganismus. Springer, Berlin Göttingen Heidelberg

Covelli V, di Majo V, Bassani B, Metalli P, Silini G (1982) Radiation induced tumors in transplanted ovaries. Radiat Res 90: 173–186

Crone M (1970) Radiation stimulated incorporation of ^{3}H-thymidine into diplotene oocytes of the guinea-pig. Nature 228: 460

Cunningham GR, Huckins C (1978) Serum FSH, LH and testosterone in ^{60}Co gamma-irradiated male rats. Radiat Res 76: 331–338

Czygan PJ, Maruhn G (1972) Einfluß ablativer gynäkologischer Maßnahmen auf den Serum-Gonadotropingehalt. Arch Gynaekol 212: 176–188

Damewood MD, Grochow LB (1986) Prospects for fertility after chemotherapy or radiation for neoplastic disease. Fertil Steril 45: 443–459

Davids JAG (1973) Acute effects of 1 MeV fast neutrons on the haematopoetic tissues, intestinal epithelium and gastric epithelium in mice. In: Duplan JF, Shapiro A (eds) Advances in radiation research. Biology and medicine, vol II. Gordon & Breach, New York, pp 565–576

Dedov VI, Norec TA (1982) Die reproduktive und hormonale Hodenfunktion bei Ratten unter den Bedingungen einer inneren Dauerbestrahlung. Radiobiol Radiother 23: 159–166

de Jong FH, Sharpe RM (1977) Gonadotropins, testosterone and spermatogenesis in neonatally irradiated rats: evidence for a role of the Sertoli cell in follicle-stimulating hormone feedback. J Endocrinol 75: 209–219

Delclos L, Montague ED (1973) Metastasis from breast cancer. In: Fletcher GH (ed) Textbook of radiotherapy. Lea & Febiger, Philadelphia, pp 493–496

Delic JI, Bush C, Steel GG (1986a) Influence of timing

of cytotoxic drug treatment on the response of murine clonogenic spermatogonia to x-irradiation. Radiother Oncol 7: 341–348

Delic JI, Hendry JH, Morris ID, Shalet SM (1986b) Leydig cell function in the pubertal rat following local testicular irradiation. Radiother Oncol 5: 29–37

Delic JI, Schlappack OK, Harwood JR, Stanley JA (1987a) Comparative effects of x-irradiation on the testes of adult Sprague-Dawley and Wistar rats. Radiat Res 112: 99–104

Delic JI, Schlappack OK, Steel GG (1987b) Effects of dose-rate on the survival of murine spermatogonia following ^{60}Co irradiation. Radiother Oncol 8: 345–352

de Ruiter-Bootsma AL, Davids JA (1981) Survival of spermatogonial stem-cells in the CBA mouse after combined exposure to 1-MeV fission neutrons and hydroxyurea. Radiat Res 85: 38–46

de Ruiter-Bootsma AL, Kramer MF, Rooij DG, Davids IAG (1974) Survival of spermatogonial stem cell in the mouse after exposure to 1 MeV fast neutrons. In: Biological effects of neutron irradiation. IAEA, Vienna, pp 325–334

de Ruiter-Bootsma AL, Kramer MF, Rooij DG (1976) Response of stem cells in the mouse testis to fission neutrons of 1 MeV energy and 300 kV x-rays. Methodology, dose-response studies, relative biological effectiveness. Radiat Res 67: 56–68

de Ruiter-Bootsma AL, Kramer MF, Rooij DG (1977) Survival of spermatogonial stem cells in the mouse after split-dose irradiation with fission neutrons of 1 MeV mean energy or 300 kV x-rays. Radiat Res 71: 579–592

Deschner EE, Rugh R, Grupp E (1969) A cytological and cytochemical study of x-irradiated human testes. Milit Med 125: 447–462

Dierickx P, Verhoeven G (1980) Effect of different methods of germinal cell destruction on rat testis. J Reprod Fertil 59: 5–9

Diethelm L, Lorenz W (1964) Über Unterschiede des strahlengeschädigten Rattenhodens. Eine histologische und zytologische Studie am 2. und 8. Tag nach 600 R-Röntgen-Ganzkörperbestrahlung und zehntägiger Tumorbestrahlung mit täglich 3 R. Strahlentherapie 123: 207–225

Diez-Falusy E, Notter G, Edsmyr F, Westmann A (1959) Estrogen excretions in breast cancer patients before and after ovarian irradiation and oophorectomy. J Clin Endocrinol Metab 19: 1230

di Paola M, Caffarelli V, Coppola M, Porro F, Quintiliani M (1980) Biological responses to various neutron energies from 1 to 600 MeV. I. Testes weight loss in mice. Radiat Res 84: 444–452

Dobson RL, Cooper MF (1974) Tritium toxicity: effects of low-level ^{3}HOH exposure on developing female germ cells in the mouse. Radiat Res 58: 91–100

Dobson RL, Felton JS (1983) Female germ cell loss from radiation and chemical exposures. Am J Ind Medic 4: 175–190

Dobson RL, Kwan TC (1974) Low-level exposure to tritium and gamma-irradiation compared in mouse oocytes. Radiat Res 59: 62

Dobson RL, Kwan TC (1976) The RBE of tritium radiation measures in mouse oocytes: increase at low exposure levels. Radiat Res 66: 615–625

Dobson RL, Kwan TC (1977) The tritium RBE at low-level exposure – variation with dose, dose rate, and exposure duration. Curr Top Radiat Res Q 12: 44–62

Doll R, Smith PG (1968) The long-term effects of x-irradiation in patients treated for metropathia haemorrhagica. Br J Radiat 41: 362–368

Driancourt MA, Blanc MR, Mariana JC (1983) Hormonal levels after ovarian x-irradiation of ewes. Reprod Nutr Dev 23: 775–781

Dym M, Clermont Y (1979) Role of spermatogonia in the repair of the seminiferous epithelium following x-irradiation of the rat testis. Am J Anat 127: 265–282

Ellis LD, Berliner DL (1967) The effects of ionizing radiations on endocrine cells. VI. Afterloadings in androgen biosynthesis by canine testicular tissue after the internal deposition of some radionuclides. Radiat Res 32: 520–537

Erickson BH (1976) Effect of ^{60}Co gamma-radiation on the stem and differentiating spermatogonia of the postpubertal rat. Radiat Res 68: 433–448

Erickson BH (1978) Effect of continuous gamma-radiation of the stem and differentiating spermatogonia of the adult rat. Mutat Res 52: 117–128

Erickson BH (1981) Survival and renewal of murine stem spermatogonia following ^{60}Co gamma-radiation. Radiat Res 86: 34–51

Erickson BH, Blend MJ (1976) Response of the Sertoli cell and stem cell to Co^{60} radiation (dose and dose rate) in testes of immnature rats. Biol Reprod 14: 641–650

Erickson BH, Hall GG (1983) Comparison of stem-spermatogonial renewal and mitotic activity in the irradiated mouse and rat. Mutat Res 108: 317–335

Erickson BH, Martin PG (1972) Effect of dose-rate (gamma-radiation) on the mitotically-active and differentiating germ cell of the prenatal male rat. Int J Radiat Biol 22: 517–524

Erickson BH, Martin PG (1973) Influence of age on the response of rat stem spermatogonia to gamma-radiation. Biol Reprod 8: 607–612

Erickson BH, Martin PG (1976) Effects of continuous prenatal radiation on the pig and rat. In: Biological and environmental effects of low-levels radiation, vol. I. Proc Symp Chicago, 3–7 Nov 1975, Vienna 1, pp 111–117

Erickson BH, Reynolds RA (1978) Oogenesis, follicular development and reproductive performance in the prenatally irradiated bovine. In: Late biological effects of ionizing radiation, vol II. IAEA, Vienna, Symposium 13–17 March

Erickson BH, Reynolds RA, Brooks FT (1972) Differentiation and radioresponse (dose and dose rate) of the primitive germ cell of the bovine testis. Radiat Res 50: 388–400

Erickson BH, Reynolds RA, Murphree RL (1976) Late effects of ^{60}Co gamma-radiation of the bovine oocyte as reflected by oocyte survival, follicular development, and reproductive performance. Radiat Res 68: 132–137

Etoh H, Hyodo-Taguchi Y (1983) Effects of tritiated water on germ cells in medaka embryos. Radiat Res 93: 332–339

Fabrikant JI (1972) Cell population kinetics in the seminiferous epithelium under low dose irradiation. AJR 114: 792–802

Faizi-Gorn R (1990) Critical sensitivity periods in embryofetal germ cells. Radiat Environ Biophys (in press)

Fakunding JL, Tindall DJ, Dedman JR, Mesa CR, Means AR (1976) Biochemical actions of follicle stimulating hormone in the Sertoli cell of the rat testis. Endocrinology 98: 392–402

Feinendegen LE, Cronkite EP, Bond VP (1980) Radiation problems in fusion energy production. Radiat Environ Biophys 18: 157

Feingold SM, Hahn W (1972) Postconception development of rat ova following x-ray induced superovulation. Radiat Res 51: 110–120

Fleck H, Stahl F, Mau S (1981) Studies on the interruption of testicular testosterone production through testicular irradiation in prostate cancer patients. Z Urol Nephrol 74: 443–446

Fossa SD, Klepp O, Moine K, Aakvaag A (1982) Testicular function after unilateral orchiectomy for cancer and before further treatment. Int J Androl 5: 179–184

Fossà SD, Almaas B, Jetne V, Bjerkedal T (1986) Paternity after irradiation for testicular cancer. Acta Radiol Oncol 25: 33–36

Fraass, BA, Kinsella TJ, Harrington FS, Glatstein E (1985) Peripheral dose to the testes: the design and clinical use of a practical and effective gonadal shield. Int J Radiat Oncol Biol Phys 11: 609–616

Francis O, Stevens RD (1965) Pregnancy after primary irradiation for carcinoma of cervix. Br Med J 2: 342–343

Freund I, Zenzes MT, Müller RP, Pötter R, Knuth UA, Nieschlag E (1987) Testicular function in eight patients with seminoma after unilateral orchidectomy and radiotherapy. Int J Androl 10: 447–456

Freund M, Borelli FJ (1965) The effects of x-irradiation on male fertility in the guinea pig: semen production after x-irradiation of the testis, of the body or of the head. Radiat Res 24: 67–80

Fritz-Niggli H (1972) Strahlenbedingte Entwicklungsstörungen. In: Hug O, Zuppinger A (ed) Strahlenbiologie. Handbuch der medizinischen Radiologie, Vol II/3, pp 235–297. Springer, Berlin Heidelberg New York

Fritz-Niggli H (1973) Strahlenempfindlichkeit der Gonaden. In: Braun H, Heuck F, Ladner HA, Messerschmidt O, Musshoff K, Streffer C (eds) Strahlenempfindlichkeit von Organen und Organsystemen der Säugetiere und des Menschen. Thieme, Stuttgart, pp 107–122

Fritz K, Weissbach L (1985) Sperm parameters and ejaculation before and after operative treatment of patients with germ-cell testicular cancer. Fertil Steril 43: 451–454

Fuchs G, Hofbauer J (1969) Gonadendosen und genetische Strahlenbelastung in der Telekobalttherapie. Strahlentherapie 138: 178–180

Gaetini A, Resegotti A, Urgesi A, Rossi G, Levis A, de Simone M, Monetti U (1987) Lateral high abdominal ovariopexy. An effective surgical method for gonadal protection in young women during radiation therapy for Hodgkin's disease. Haematologia (Budap) 72: 186

Gagnon C, Axelrod J, Musto N, Dym M, Bardin CW (1979) Protein carboxyl-methylation in rat testes: a study of inherited and x-ray-induced seminiferous tubule failure. Endocrinology 105: 1440-1445

Gasinska A (1985) Mouse testis weight loss and survival of differentiated spermatogonia following irradiation with 250 kV x-rays and 5.5 MeV fast neutrons. Neoplasma 32: 443–450

Gasinska A, de Ruiter-Bootsma A, Davids J AG, Folkard M, Fowler JF (1987) Survival of mouse type B spermatogonia for the study of the biological effectiveness of 1 MeV, 2,3 MeV and 5,6 MeV fast neutrons. Int J Radiat Biol 52: 237–244

Geller FC (1925) Über die Wirkung schwacher Eierstockbestrahlung auf Grund tierexperimenteller Untersuchungen. Strahlentherapie 19: 22–61

Geraci JP, Jackson KL, Thrower PD, Fox MS (1975) An estimate of the patient risk in cyclotron neutron radio-

therapy using mouse testes as a biological test system. Health Phys 29: 729–737

Geraci JP, Jackson KL, Christensen GM, Thrower PD, Weyer BJ (1977) Mouse testes as a biological test system for intercomparison of fast neutron therapy beams. Radiat Res 71: 377–386

Geraci JP, Decello JF, Eanmaa J, Jackson KL, Thrower PD, Mariano MS (1980) Comparative effects of negative pions, neutrons and photons on testes weight loss and spermatogenic stem cell survival in mice. Radiat Res 82: 579–587

Gibbons AFE, Chang MC (1973a) Indirect effects of x-irradiation on embryonic development: irradiation of the exteriorized rat uterus. Biol Reprod 9: 133–141

Gibbons AFE, Chang MC (1973b) The effects of x-irradiation of the rat ovary on implantation and embryonic development. Biol Reprod 9: 343–349

Glucksmann A (1947) The effects of radiation on reproductive organs. Br J Radiol 1: 101–109

Goyal PK, Dev PK (1982) Weight loss of mouse testes after gamma irradiation in utero and its modification by MPG (2-mercaptopropionglycine). Radiobiol Radiother 23: 283–286

Gragg RL, Humphrey RM, Meyn RE (1976) The response of Chinese hamster ovary cells to fast neutron radiotherapy beams. I. Relative biological effectiveness and oxygen enhancement ratio. Radiat Res 65: 313–334

Green AD, Bushong SC (1971) Gonadal dose in male radiotherapy patients. Radiology 98: 661–663

Green AD, Howells GR, Humphreys ER, Vennart J (1975) Localisations of plutonium in mouse testes. Nature 255: 77

Green D, Howells G, Vennart J, Watts R (1977) The distribution of plutonium in the mouse ovary. Int J Radiat Isotop 28: 487–501

Greiner R (1982) Die Erholung der Spermatogenese nach fraktionierter, niedrig dosierter Bestrahlung per männlichen Gonaden. Strahlentherapie 158: 342–355

Greiner R (1983) Tumortherapien, Fertilität und Sexualität. Schweiz Rundsch Med Prax 72: 1293–1298

Greiner R (1985) Die Hodenfunktion nach Einwirkung ionisierender Strahlen. In: Ladner H-A, Reiners C, Börner W, Schütz J (eds) 25 Jahre medizinischer Strahlenschutz. Thieme, Stuttgart, pp 114–121

Greiner R, Meyer A (1977) Reversible und irreversible Azoospermie nach Bestrahlung des malignen Hodentumors. Strahlentherapie 153: 257–262

Griffiths TD (1970) x-ray response of Chinese hamster ovary cells during the latter part of G_2. Biophys J 28: 497–501

Gritz ER, Wellisch DK, Wang H-J, Siau J, Landsverk JA, Cosgrove MD (1989) Long-term effects of testicular cancer on sexual functioning in married couples. Cancer 64: 1560–1567

Grönroos M, Kauppila O, Pulkikinen M, Turunen S, Salmi T, Raekallio J (1981) Pituitary-ovarian hormones after low dose endometrial afterloading irradiation. Int J Gynecol Obstet 19: 375–380

Grönroos M, Klemi P, Piiroinen O, Erkkola R, Nikkanen V, Routsalainen P (1982) Ovarian function during and after curative intracavitary high-dose-rate irradiation: steroidal output and morphology. Eur J Obstet Gynecol Reprod Biol 14: 13–21

Guglielmi R, Calzavara F, Pizzi BG (1980) Ovarian function after pelvic lymph node irradiation in patients with Hodgkin's disease submitted to oophoropexy during laparotomy. Eur J Gynecol Oncol 41: 99–107

Gupta GS, Bawa SR (1971) Phosphatases in testes and epididymides of albino rats after partial body irradiation. J Reprod Fertil 27: 451–454

Gupta GS, Bawa SR (1975) Radiation effects on testes VI. 5-Nucleotidase and adenosine triphosphatase following partial body gamma irradiation. Radiobiol Radiother 2: 221–234

Gupta GS, Bawa SR (1978a) Radiation effects on testes XIII. Studies on isocitrate dehydrogenases following partial-body gamma irradiation. Radiat Res 73: 476–489

Gupta GS, Bawa SR (1978b) Radiation effects on testes. XIV. Studies on glucose 6-phosphatase dehydrogenase following partial-body gamma irradiation. Radiat Res 73: 490–501

Gupta GS, Bawa SR (1979) Radiation effects on testes. Strahlentherapie 155: 287–292

Haas RJ, Schreml W, Fliedner TM, Calvo W (1973) The effect of tritiated water on the development of the rat oocyte after maternal infusion during the pregnancy. Int J Radiat Biol 23: 603

Hacker U, Schumann J, Göhde W (1980) Effects of acute gamma-irradiation on spermatogenesis as revealed by flow cytometry. Acta Radiol Oncol 19: 361

Hacker U, Schumann J, Göhde W, Müller K (1981) Mammalian spermatogenesis as biologic dosimeter for radiation. Acta Radiol Oncol 20: 279–282

Hacker U, Schumann J, Göhde W (1982) Mammalian spermatogenesis as a new system for biologic dosimeter of ionizing irradiation. Acta Radiol Oncol 21: 349

Hahn EW, Feingold SM (1973) Unilateral reduction of ovulations following selective ovarian x-irradiation. Endocrinology 92: 1447–1450

Hahn EW, Ward WF (1971) Changes in ovarian intravascular compartment prior to superovulation in x-irradiated rats. Radiat Res 46: 192–198

Hahn EW, Feingold SM, Nisce L (1976) Aspermia and recovery of spermatogenesis in cancer patients following incidental gonadal irradiation during treatment: a progress report. Radiology 119: 223–225

Hahn EW, Feingold SM, Simpson L, Batata M (1982) Recovery from aspermia induced by low-dose radiation in seminoma patients. Cancer 50: 337–340

Halawa B, Wawrzkiewicz M, Mazurek W, Kasprzak J, Kornafel J (1981) The behaviour of pituitary gonatropins and estrogens in blood serum of gamma-Ra 226 irradiated patients. Radiobiol Radiother 22: 214–218

Hamaguchi S, Egami N (1975) Post-irradiation changes in oocyte populations in the fry of the fish Oryzias latipes. Int J Radiat Biol 28: 279–284

Handelsman DJ (1980) Azoospermia after iodine – 131 treatment for thyroid carcinoma. Br Med J 281: 1527

Handelsman DJ, Turtle JR (1983) Testicular damage after radioactive iodine (I-131) therapy for thyroid cancer. Clin Endocrinol 18: 465–472

Hassenstein E, Nüsslin F (1976) Die Gonadenbelastung bei der ^{60}Co-Bestrahlung peripherer, mediastinaler und retroperitonealer Lymphknotenstationen. Strahlentherapie 152: 427–432

Haubrich R, Harms I (1973) Unfruchtbarkeit beim einseitigen Hodenkrebs. Strahlentherapie 146: 94–103

Heite HJ (1951) Fertilitätsuntersuchungen bei behandelten Patienten mit Thorium. Med Klin 1297

Heller CG, Heller GV, Warner GA, Rowley MJ (1968) Effect of graded doses of ionizing radiation on testicular cytology and sperm count in man. Radiat Res 35: 493–494

Henricson B, Nilsson A (1970) Roentgen ray effects on the ovaries of foetal mice. Acta radiol (Ther.) 9: 443–448

Hilscher WM, Trott KR, Hilscher W (1982) Cell progression and radiosensitivity of T_1-prospermatogonia in Wistar rats. Int J Radiat Biol 41: 517–524

Himelstein-Braw R, Peters H, Faber M (1977) Influence of irradiation and chemotherapy on the ovaries of children with abdominal tumours. Br J Cancer 36: 269–275

Hobson BM, Baker TG (1979) Reproductive capacity of rhesus monkeys following bilateral ovarian x-irradiation. J Reprod Fertil 55: 471–480

Hodel K, Rich WM, Austin P, Di Saia PJ (1982) The role of ovarian transposition in conservation of ovarian function in radical hysterectomy followed by pelvic radiation. Gynecol Oncol 13: 195–202

Hopkinson CRN, Dulisch B, Gaus G, Hilscher W, Hirschhäuser C (1978) The effects of local testicular irradiation on testicular histology and plasma hormone levels in the male rat. Acta Endocrinol (Copenh) 87: 413–423

Hori Y, Takamori Y, Nisshio K (1970) The effect of x-irradiation on lactic hydrogenase isoenzymes in plasma and in various organs of mice. Radiat Res 43: 143–151

Horning SJ, Hoppe RT, Kaplan HS, Rosenberg SA (1981) Female reproductive potential after treatment for hodgkin's disease. N Engl J Med 304: 1377–1382

Hornsey S, Myers R, Warren P (1977) RBE for the two components of weight loss in the mouse testis for fast neutrons relative to x-rays. Int J Radiat Biol 32: 297–301

Hovatta O, Kormano M (1974) Development of the seminiferous tubules following prepuberal whole body x-irradiation. Andrologia 6: 277–285

Hsu AC, Folami AO, Bain J, Rance CP (1979) Gonadal function in males treated with cyclophosphamide for nephrotic syndrome. Fertil Steril 31: 173–177

Hsu THS, Fabrikant JL (1976) Spermatogonial cell renewal under continuous irradiation of 1, 8 and 45 rads per day. In: Biological and environmental effects of low-level radiation, vol I. IAEA, Vienna, p 157

Huckins C (1978a) Spermatogonial intercellular bridges in whole-mounted seminiferous tubules from normal and irradiated rodent testes. Am J Anat 153: 97–122

Huckins C (1978b) Behavior of stem cell spermatogonia in the adult rat irradiated testis. Biol Reprod 19: 742–760

Huckins C, Oakberg EF (1978) Morphological and quantitative analysis of spermatogonia in mouse testes using whole mounted seminiferous tubules. Anat Res 192: 529–542

Hugue H, Ashraf J (1973) Effect of gamma radiation on the ovaries of desert locust Schistocerca gregaria. Zentralbl Radiol 109: 491

Husseinzadeh N, Nahhas WA, Velkley DE, Whitney CW, Mortel R (1984) The preservation of ovarian function in young women undergoing pelvic radiation therapy. Gynecol Oncol 18: 373–379

Hwang HN, Feola JM, Beach JL, Maruyma Y (1984) RBE of CF-252 neutrons by mouse testes weight loss. J Radiat Oncol Biol Phys 10: 901–905

Hyodo-Taguchi Y, Egami N (1976) Effect of irradiation on spermatogonia of the fish, Oryzias latipes. Radiat Res 67: 324–331

Hyodo-Taguchi Y, Egami N (1977) Damage to spermatogenic cells in fish kept in tritiated water. Radiat Res 71: 641–652

Hyodo-Taguchi Y, Etoh H (1986) Effects of tritiated water on germ cells in medaka. Radiat Res 106: 321–330

ICRP (1969) Radiosensitivity and special distribution of dose. ICRP Publication 14. Pergamon, Oxford

ICRP (1979) Limits for intakes of radionuclides by workers. ICRP Publication 30, part I, Pergamon, Oxford

ICRP (1980) Biological effects of inhaled radionuclides. ICRP publication 31. Pergamon, Oxford

Israel SL (1958) The repudiation of low-dosage irradiation of the ovaries. Am J Obstet Gynecol 76: 443–446

Ito M (1966) Histochemical observations of oxidative enzyme in irradiated testis and epididymis. Radiat Res 28: 266

Ito T, Itagaki G (1963) The effects of 1000R of x-rays on spermatogensis in the mouse. Bull Faculty Agric Hirosaki Univ 59–65

Ivanov B, Maleeva A (1980) Effect of different doses of gamma-radiation on the concentration of testosterone, follicle-stimulating and luteinizing hormones in the blood plasma of rats. Radiobiology 20: 285–288

Ivey JR (1963) Preconception radiation for carcinoma of the cervix. J Obstet Gynecol Br Emp 70: 128–129

Jablon S, Kato H (1971) Sex ratio in offspring of survivors prenatally to the atomic bombs in Hiroshima and Nagasaki. J Epidemiol 93: 253–258

Jacox HW (1939) Recovery following human ovarian irradiation. Radiology 32: 538–545

Janson PO, Jansson I, Skryten A, Damber JE, Lindstedt G (1981) Ovarian endocrine function in young women undergoing radiotherayp for carcinoma of the cervix. Gynecol Oncol 11: 218–223

Janssens PJ, Wittevrongel C, van Dam J, Goddeeris P, Lauwerijns KM, De Loecker W (1981) Effects of ionizing irradiation on the estradiol and progesterone receptors in rat mammary tumors. Cancer Res 41: 703–707

Jansz GF, Pomerantz DK (1984) Fetal irradiation increases androgen production by dispersed Leydig cells in the rat. J Androl 5: 344–350

Jarrell J, YoungLai V, Barr R, O'Connoll G, Belbeck L, McMahon A (1986) An analysis of the effects of increasing doses of ionizing radiation to the exteriorized rat ovary on follicular development, atresia, and serum gonadotropin level. Am J Obstet Gynecol 154: 306–309

Johnson MI, Newman L (1976) Radiation-induced fetal testicular damage in the monkey (*Macaca radiata*). J Med Primatol 5: 195–199

Jones DCL, Krebs JS, Sasmore DP, Mitoma C (1980) Evaluation of neonatal squirrel monkeys receiving tritiated water throughout gestation. Radiat Res 83: 592–606

Joshi DS, Yick J, Murray D, Meistrich ML (1990) Stage-dependent variation in the radiosensitivity of DNA in developing male germ cells. Radiat Res 121: 274–281

Jostes E (1963) Ovar. In: Stender H, Scherer E (eds) Strahlentherapie der Zelle. Thieme, Stuttgart, pp 209–219

Jostes E, Scherer E (1961) Beitrag zur Morphologie röntgen- und radiumbestrahlter Mäuseovarien. Strahlentherapie 115: 337–365

Jostes E, Scherer E (1967) Beitrag zur Morphologie röntgen- und radiumbestrahlter Mäuseovarien. II. Mitt. Beobachtungen an Follikel-, Theka- und Luteinzellen. Strahlentherapie 132: 59–78

Kalisnik M, Vraspir O, Skrk J et al. (1978) Histological and stereological analysis of some endocrine and lymphatic organs in mice after whole-body-radiation. In: Late biological effects of ionizing radiation, vol II. IAEA, Vienna, pp 137–146

Kaplan I (1958) The treatment of female sterility with x-ray therapy directed to the pituitary and ovaries. Am J Obstet Gynecol 76: 447–453

Kapoor G, Srivastava PN (1980) J Radiat Res 21: 163

Kapoor G, Sharan RN, Srivastava PN (1985) Histopathological changes in the ovary following acute and chronic low-level tritium exposure to mice in vivo. Int J Radiat Biol 47: 197–204

Kashiwabara T, Tanaka R, Stern C (1971) The effects of radiation (x-, gamma-, neutron rays) on male fertility in the mouse, domestic fowl and drosophila. In: Excerp Med Amsterdam 1973, Proceedings of the VIIth. World Congress 1971 Tokyo and Kyoto, Japan. Elsevier, New York

Kellerer AM, Rossi HH (1978) A generalized formulation of dual radiation action. Radiat Res 75: 471

Kimler BF, Leeper DB, Schneiderman MH (1981) Radiation-induced division delay in Chinese hamster ovary fibroblasts and carcinoma cells: dose effect and ploidy. Radiat Res 85: 270–280

Kochar NK, Harrison RG (1971a) The effect of x-rays on the vascularization of the mouse testis. Fertil Steril 22: 53–57

Kochar NK, Harrison RG (1971b) The effects of x-rays on lipids, phospholipids and cholesterol of the mouse testis. J Reprod Fertil 27: 159–165

Kondratenko VG, Ganzenko LF, Stakanov VA (1978) Cytological and cytochemical analyses of the influence of hormones on the postirradiation changes in testicular sex and incretory cell. Radiobiologiia 18: 347–352

Kormano U, Hovatta O (1972) In vitro contractility of seminiferous tubules following 400 R whole-body irradiation. Strahlentherapie 144: 713–718

Kramer MF, Davids JAG, von der Ven TPA (1974) Effect of 1 MeV fast-neutron irradiation on spermatogonial proliferation in mice; influence of dose fraction with different intervals. Int J Radiat Biol 25: 253–260

Krebs JS (1968) Analysis of the radiation induced loss of testes and weights in terms of stem cell survival. USNRDL Tech Rep 18: 68–104

Krehbiel RH, Plagge JC (1963) Number of rat ova implanting after substerilizing x-irradiation of one or both ovaries. Anat Res 146: 257–261

Kriegel H, Schmahl W, Kistner G, Stieve FE (eds) (1982) Development effects of prenatal irradiation. Fischer, Stuttgart

Kumar A, Devi U (1982) Chemoprotection of ovarian follicles of mice against gamma irradiation by MPG (2-mercaptopropinylglycine). J Radiat Res 23: 306–312

Kumar A, Devi u (1983) Chemical radiation protection of ovarian follicles of mice by MPG (2-mercaptopropionylglycine). J Nucl Med 27: 9–12

Kumatori T, Ishihara T, Hirashima K, Sugiyma H, Ishii S, Miyoshi K (1980) Follow-up studies over a 25-year period on the Japanese fishermen exposed to radioactive fallout in 1954. In: Hübner KF, Fry SA (eds) The medical basis for radiation accident preparedness. Elsevier, North Holland, pp 33–54

Lacassagne A (1936) Untersuchungen über die Radiosensibilität des Corpus luteum und der Uterusschleimhaut mit Hilfe eines künstlich erzeugten Deziduums beim Kaninchen. Strahlentherapie 56: 621–625

Lacassagne A, Duplan JF, Marcovich H, Raynaud A (1962) The action of ionizing radiations on the mammalian ovary. In: Zuckerman S (ed) The ovary, vol II. Academic, New York, p 463

Ladner HA (1985) Somatische Strahlenreaktionen an

Generationsorganen. In: Heuck F, Scherer E (eds) Strahlengefährdung und Strahlenschutz. Springer, Berlin Heidelberg New York Handbuch der medizinischen Radiologie, Vol XX, pp 123–170

Lamerton LF (1966) Cell proliferation under continuous irradiation. Radiat Res 27: 119–138

Lamerton LF (1967) Response of mammalian cell populations to continuous irradiation. In: Silini H (ed) Radiation research. North Holland, Amsterdam, pp 658–664

Langendorff M, Stevenson AEF (1981) Murine spermatogonial regeneration after exposure to either x-rays or 15 MeV-neutrons. Radiat Environ Biophys 19: 41–49

Langendorff M, Langendorff H, Neumann GK (1972) Die Wirkung einer fraktionierten Röntgenbestrahlung auf die Fertilität von in utero bestrahlten Mäusen. Strahlentherapie 144: 324–337

Laskey JW, Parrish JL, Cahill DF (1973) Some effects of lifetime parenteral exposure to low levels of tritium on the F_2-generation. Radiat Res 56: 171–179

Laughlin TJ, Taylor JH (1980) The effects of x-ray on DNA synthesis in synchronized Chinese hamster ovary cells. Radiat Res 83: 205–209

Lawson RL, Krise GM, Brown SO, Sorensen AM Jr (1967) Effects of single, continuous, and fractionated gamma irradiation on semen quality in albino rats. Radiat Res 31: 273–280

LeFloch A, Donaldson SS, Kaplan HS (1976) Pregnancy following oophoropexy and total nodal irradiation in women with Hodgkin's disease. Cancer 38: 2263–2268

Leichner PK, Roenshein NB, Leibel SA, Order SE (1980) Distribution and tissue dose of intraperitoneally administered radioactive chromic phosphate in New Zealand white rabbits. Radiology 134: 729–734

Leidl W, Zankl H (1970) Untersuchungen über den Einfluß der Pausendauer bei fraktionierter Röntgenbestrahlung am Modell des Kaninchenhodens. Strahlentherapie 139: 548–552

Leporrier M, v Theobald P, Roffe JL, Muller G (1987) A new technique to protect ovarian function before pelvic irradiation Cancer 60: 2201–2204

Lindop PJ (1969) The effects of radiation on rodent and human ovaries. Proc Soc Med 62: 144–148

Loraine JA (1957) Recent work on the quantitative determination of pituitary gonadotrophins in urine. Acta Endocrinol 31: 75–84

Lu CC, Meistrich ML, Thames AD (1980) Survival of mouse testicular stem cells after gamma- or neutron irradiation. Radiat Res 81: 402–425

Lushbaugh CC, Casarett GW (1976) The effects of gonadal irradiation in clinical radiation therapy: a review. Cancer 37: 1111–1120

Lushbaugh CC, Ricks RC (1972) Some cytokinetic and histopathologic considerations of irradiated male and female gonadal tissues. Front Radiat Ther Oncol 6: 228–248

Makler A, Tatcher M, Velinsky A, Brandes JM (1980) Factors affecting sperm motility. III. Influence of visible light and other electromagnetic radiation on human sperm velocity and survival. Fertil Steril 33: 439–444

Mandl AM (1964) The radiosensitivity of germ cells. Biol Rev 39: 288–371

Martius H (1961) Strahlentoleranzdosis der Eierstöcke. Dtsch Med Wochenschr 86: 888–890

Matthes T, Kriegel H (1958) Über die Speicherung von Thoriumdioxyd in den Keimdrüsen von Kaninchen und beim Menschen. Strahlentherapie 105: 441–449

McCarthy TG, Milton PJD (1975) Successful pregnancy after conservative surgery and radiotherapy for dysgerminoma of the ovary. Br J Obstet Gynecol 82: 64–67

McTaggart J, Wills ED (1977) The effects of whole and partial body irradiation on circulating anterior pituitary hormones and testosterone and the relationship of these hormones to drug-metabolizing enzymes in the liver. Radiat Res 72: 122–133

Meistrich ML, Hunter NR, Suzuki N, Trostle PK, Withers HR (1978) Gradual regeneration of mouse testicular stem cells after exposure of ionizing radiation. Radiat Res 74: 349–362

Meistrich ML, Finch MV, Hunter N, Milas L (1984a) Protection of spermatogonial survival and testicular function by WR-2721 against high and low dose radiation. Int J Radiat Oncol Biol Phys 10: 2099–2107

Meistrich ML, Finch M, Lu CC, de Ruiter-Bootsma AL, de Rooij DG, Davids JAG (1984b) Strain differences in the response of mouse testicular stem cells to fractionated radiation. Radiat Res 97: 478–487

Meistrich ML, Samuels RC (1985) Reduction in sperm levels after testicular irradiation of the mouse: a comparison with man. Radiat Res 102: 138–147

Meyer MB, Tonascia JA (1973) Possible effects of x-ray exposure during fetal life on the subsequent reproductive performance of human females. Am J Epidemiol 114: 304–316

Meyer MB, Merz T, Diamond EL (1969) Investigation of the effects of prenatal x-ray exposure of human oogonia oocytes as measured by later reproductive performance. Am J Epidemiol 89: 619–635

Meyer MB, Tonascia JA, Merz T (1976) Long term effects of prenatal x-rays on development and fertility of human females. In: Biological and environmental effects of low-level radiation, vol II. Proceedings of symposium, Chicago, 3–7 Nov 1975. International Atomic Energy Agency, Vienna

Meyhöfer W, Hülsmann B, Morchek H (1971) Der Einfluß von Röntgenstrahlen auf die Spermiogenese der Maus (DNS- und Histonproteine in Spermatozoien). Fortschr Fertil Forsch 2: 58–62

Mian TA, Suzuki N, Glenn HJ, Hayne TP, Meistrich M (1977) Radiation damage to mouse testis cells from (^{99m}Tc) pertechnetate. J Nucl Med 18: 1116–1122

Milas L, Hunter N, Reid BO (1982) Protective effects of WR-2721 against radiation-induced injury of murine gut, testis, lung, and lung tumor nodules. Int J Radiat Oncol Biol Phys 8: 535–538

Miller SC (1982) Localization of plutonium-241 in the testis. An interspecies comparison using light and electron microscope autoradiography. Int J Radiat Biol 41: 633–643

Miller SC, Rowland HG, Bowman BM (1985) Distributions of cell populations within α-particle range of plutonium deposits in the rat and beagle testis. Radiat Res 101: 102–110

Miller SC, Bruenger FW, Williams FW (1989) Influence of age at exposure on concentrations of Pu-239 in beagle gonads. Health Phys 56: 485–492

Mondorf L, Faber M (1968) The influence of radiation on human fertility. J Reprod Fertil 15: 165–169

Montour JL, Wilson JD (1979) Mouse testis weight loss following high energy neutron or gamma irradiation. Int J Radiat Biol 36: 185–189

Mroueh AM (1971) The excretion of radioiodine in human semen. Fertil Steril 22: 61–63

Müller C, Kubat K, Marsalek J (1962) Der Einfluß des Arbeitsrisikos auf die Generationsfunktionen der beim Fördern und Aufbereiten von radioaktiven Rohstoffen beschäftigten Frauen. Zentralbl Gynaekol 15: 561–568

Müller J, Hertz H, Skakkebaeck NE (1988) Development of the seminiferous epithelium during and after treatment for acute lymphoblastic leukemia in childhood. Horm Res 30: 115–120

Müller W (1915) Beitrag zur Frage der Strahlenwirkung auf tierische Zellen, besonders die der Ovarien. Strahlentherapie 5: 155–147

Muramatsu S, Tsuchiya T, Hanada H (1978) Effects of continuous gamma radiation on the reproductivity of mice. In: Late biological effects of ionizing radiation, vol II. IAEA, Vienna, pp 191–198

Nader S, Schultz PN, Cundiff JH, Hussey PH, Samaan NA (1983) Endocrine profiles of patients with testicular tumours treated with radiotherapy. Int J Radiat Oncol Biol Phys 9: 1723–1726

Naujokat B, Rohloff R, Willich N, Eiermann W (1988) Veränderungen der Serumspiegel weiblicher Geschlechtshormone nach Strahlenkastration mit unterschiedlicher Gesamtdosis. Strahlenther Onkol 164: 208–213

Nebel BR, Murphy CJ (1960) Damage and recovery of mouse testis after 1000 r acute localized x-irradiation, with reference to restitution cells, Sertoli cell increase and type A spermatogonial recovery. Radiat Res 12: 626–641

Niedetzky A, Lautai CS (1969) Effect of radioactive radiations on the lifetime of sperms. Acta Biochem Biohys 211–216

Nijiman JM, Jager S, Boer PW, Kremer J, Oldhoff J, Koops HS (1982) The treatment of ejaculation disorders after retroperitoneal lymph node dissection. Cancer 50: 2967–2971

Nikandrova TI, Zhulanova ZI, Romatsev EF (1981) Prostaglandin synthase activity in the liver, brain and testicles of (CBA C57 B1) mice under irradiation. Radiobiology 21: 265–269

Nseyo UO, Huben RT, Klioze SS, Pontes JE (1985) Protection of germinal epithelium with luteinizing hormone-releasing hormone analogue. J Urol 34: 187–190

Oakberg EF (1968) Mammalian gametogenesis and species comparisons in radiation response of the gonads. In: Effects of radiation on meiotic systems. IAEA, Vienna, pp 3–15

Oakberg EF (1975) Effects of radiation on the testis. In: Hamilton DW, Greep RO (eds) Male reproductive system. William & Wilkins, Baltimore (Handbook of Physiology, Sect 7, vol V, pp 233–243)

Oakberg EF (1978) Differential spermatogonial stem-cell survival and mutation frequency. Mutat Res 50: 327–340

Oakberg EF (1979) Timing of oocyte maturation in the mouse and its relevance to radiation-induced cell killing and mutational sensitivity. Mutat Res 59: 39–48

Oakberg EF, Huckins C (1976) Spermatogonial stem cell renewal in the mouse as revealed by ^{3}H-thymidine labeling and irradiation. In: Cairne AB, Lala PK, Osmond DG (eds) Stem cells of renewing cell population. Academic, New York, pp 287–302

Oakberg EF, Lorenz EC (1972) Irradiation of generative organs. In: Hug O, Zuppinger A (eds) Strahlenbiologie 3. Springer, Berlin Heidelberg New York (Handbuch der medizinischen Radiologie, Vol II/3, pp 217–233)

O'Brien CA, Hupp EW, Sorensen AM, Brown SO (1966) Effects of prenatal gamma radiation on the reproductive physiology of the Spanish goat. Am J Vet Res 27: 711

Orecklin JR, Kaufmann JJ, Thompson RW (1973) Fertility in patients treated for malignant testicular tumors. J Urol 109: 293–295

Overstreet JW, Adams CE (1971) Mechanisms of selective fertilization in the rabbit: sperm transport and viability. J Reprod Fertil 26: 219

Paulsen CA (1973) The study of radiation effects on the human testis: including histology, chromosomal and hormonal aspects. Final progress report of AEC contract AT (45–1)–2225, task agreement 6, RLO-2225–2

Pearson AE, Steel GG (1984) Chemotherapy in combination with pelvic irradiation: a time-dependence study in mice. Radiother Oncol 2: 49–55

Pearson AK, Licht P, Nagy KA, Medica PA (1978) Endocrine function and reproductive impairment in an irradiated population of the lizard Ute stansburiana. Radiat Res 76: 610–623

Peceski J, Malcic K (1969) The effect of local irradiation of the gonads of infantile and adult male rats on the survival and regeneration of reproductive organs. Strahlentherapie 137: 394–498

Peck WS, McGreer JT, Kretzschmar NR, Brown WE (1940) Castration of the female by irradiation. Radiology 34: 176–186

Pedrick J, Hoppe RT (1986) Recovery of spermatogenesis following pelvic irradiation for Hodgkin's disease. Int J Radiat Oncol Biol Phys 12: 117–121

Peters H (1969) The effect of radiation in early life on the morphology and reproductive function of the mouse ovary. In: McLaren A (ed.) Advances in reproductive physiology, 4149. Logos-Academic, London

Philipp F (1904) Die Röntgenbestrahlung der Hoden des Mannes. Fortschr Roentgenstr 8: 114–119

Philipp F (1932) Erhaltung der Genitalfunktion nach Bestrahlung wegen Uteruskarzinom. Zentralbl Gynaekol 56: 1409–1412

Pietrzak-Fils Z (1982) Effects of chronically ingest tritium on the oocytes of two generations of rats. In: Kriegel H (eds) Developmental effects of prenatal irradiation. Fischer, Stuttgart, pp 111–115

Pinkel D, Gledhill BL, van Dilla MA, Lake S, Wyrobek AJ (1983) Radiation-induced DNA content variability in mouse sperm. Radiat Res 95: 550–565

Pinon-Lataillade G, Maas J (1985) Continuous gamma-irradiation of rats: dose-rate effect on loss and recovery of spermatogenesis. Strahlentherapie 161: 421–426

Pogany GC (1983) Oxygen consumption in gamma irradiated mouse testes. J Radiat Res 24: 173–183

Popescu HI, Klepsch I, Lancranja J (1969) Utility of urinary total gonadotrophin excretion determination after acute irradiations by penetrating rays. Radiat Res 40: 544–551

Popescu HI, Klepsch I, Lancrangan J (1975) Elimination of pituitary gonadotropic hormones in men with protracted irradiation during occupational exposure. Health Phys 29: 385–389

Prasad N, Prasad R, Bushong SC, North LB (1977) Effect of irradiation on testicular cells of opossum. Strahlentherapie 153: 470–473

Price JJ, Rominger J (1965) Carcinoma of the cervix treated during pregnancy and followed by successful pregnancy. Obstet Gynecol 26: 272–274

Rao RA, Srivastava PN (1967) Ovarian changes induced by chronic gamma radiation emitted by sealed cobalt-60 source placed inside the abdomen in the Indian desert gerbil. Strahlentherapie 133: 594–601

Rao LRA, Srivastava PN (1982) Oocyte depopulation pattern in adult Indian desert gerbil exposed to internally deposited ^{32}P, ^{60}Co and ^{45}Ca. J Radiol Res 23: 176–186

Rassow J, Strüter HD (1970) Systematische Untersuchungen mit LiF-Thermolumineszenzdetektoren TLD 100 am Alderson-Phantom zur Gonadenbelastung bei der Therapie mit konventionellen Röntgenstrahlen (60–300 kV), Telegammastrahlen (^{137}Cs und ^{60}Co) sowie Betatronbems- und Elektronenstrahlen von 20 und 43 MeV-grenzenergie. Strahlentherapie 139: 446–458

Rathenberg, R, Schwegler H, Miska W (1976) Comparative investigations on cytogenetic effects of x-irradiation on the germinal epithelium of male mice Chinese hamsters. Hum Genet 34: 171–183

Regaud C (1977a) The influence of the duration of irradiation on the changes produced in the testicle by radium. Übers C R Soc Biol (Paris) (1922) 86: 787–789 Int J Radiat Oncol Biol Phys 2: 565–567

Regaud C (1977b) The alternating rhythm of cellular mitoses and the radiosensitivity of the testis. Übers C R Soc Biol (Paris) (1922) 86: 822–824. Int J Radiol Oncol Biol Phys 2: 569–570

Reifferscheid K (1914) Die Einwirkung der Röntgenstrahlen auf tierische und menschliche Eierstöcke. Strahlentherapie 5: 407–425

Rich KA, de Kreter DM (1977) Effect of differing degrees of destruction of the rat seminiferous epithelium on levels of serum follicle stimulating hormone and androgen binding protein. Endocrinology 101: 959–968

Richmond CR, Thomas RL (1975) Plutonium and other actinide elements in gonadal tissue of man and animals. Health Phys 29: 241–250

Richter D (1982) Psychosomatisch und endokrinologisch orientierte Diagnostik und Therapie des sekundären Amenorrhoe-Syndroms. Gynaekologe 15: 173–189

Rikmenspoel R (1975) III. Further x-ray studies. Biophys J 15: 831–841

Rikmenspoel R, van Herpen G (1969) Radiation damage to bull sperm motility. II. Proton irradiation and respiration measurements. Biophys J 9: 833

Robinson JN, Engle ET (1949) Effect of neutron radiation on the human testes: a case report. J Urol 61: 781–784

Rönnbäck C (1979) Effect of ^{90}Sr on ovaries of foetal mice depending on time for administration during pregnancy. Acta Radiol (Oncol) 18: 225–234

Rönnbäck C (1981) Influence of ^{90}Sr-contaminated milk on the ovaries of foetal and young mice. Acta Radiol (Oncol) 20: 131–135

Rönnbäck C, Henricson B, Nilsson A (1971) Effect of different doses of 90-Sr on the ovaries of the foetal mouse. Acta Radiol 310: 200–209

Rooij DG (1978) The effect of x-irradiation on spermatogenesis in the rhesus monkey. Int J Radiat Biol 34: 565–566

Rösler H, Moser M (1984) Schwangerschaft nach hochdosierter Radiojod-Therapie. In: Schmidt HAE, Adam WE (eds) Nuklearmedizin. 21.Jahrestagung Gesellschaft Europa 13–16.9.1983, Ulm. Schattauer, Stuttgart, pp 920–923

Rowley MJ, Leach DR, Warner GA, Heller CG (1974) Effect of graded doses of ionizing radiation on the human testis. Radiat Res 59: 665–678

Rubin P, Casarett G (1972) A direction for clinical radiation pathology. The tolerance dose. Front Radiat Ther Oncol 6: 1–16

Rugh R, Budd RA (1975) Does x-radiation of the preconceptional mammalian ovum lead to sterility and/or congenital anomalies? Fertil Steril 26: 560–572

Rugh R, Clugston H (1955) Radiosensitivity with respect to the estrous cycle in the mouse. Radiat Res 2: 227–236

Rugh R, Skaredorf L (1971) The immediate and delayed effects of 1000 R x-rays on the rodent testis. Fertil Steril 22: 73–82

Rush ME, Lipner H (1979) Effect of bovine testicular extracts on plasma gonadotrophins of x-irradiated rats. Proc Soc Biol Med 162: 85–89

Russel JJ, Lindenbaum A (1979) One-year study of nonuniformly distributed plutonium in mouse testis as related to spermatogonial irradiation. Health Phys 36: 153–157

Russell WL (1962) An augmenting effect of dose fractionation on radiation-induced mutation rate in mice. Proc Natl Acad Sci (us) 48: 1724–1727

Saharan BR, Devi PU (1977) Radiation protection of mouse testes with 2-mercaptopropionylglycine. J Radiat Res (Tokyo) 18: 308

Sandeman TF (1966) The effects of x-irradiation on male human fertility. Br J Radiol 39: 901–907

Sanders JE, Buckner CD, Leonard JM (1983) Late effects on gonadal function of cyclophosphamide, total body irradiation and marrow transplantation. Transplantation 36: 252–255

Sankaranarayanan K (1982) Genetic effects of ionizing radiation in multicellular eukaryotes and the assessment of genetic radiation hazards in man. Elsevier Biomedical, Amsterdam

Sarkar SD, Beierwaltes WH, Gill SP, Cowley BJ (1976) Subsequent fertility and birth histories of children and adolescent treated with I-131 for thyroid cancer. J Nucl Med 17: 460

Satow Y, Hori H, Lee YL, Ohtaki M et al. (1989) Effect of tritiated water on gemale germ cells: mouse oocyte killing and RBE. Int J Radiat Biol 56: 293–300

Savkovic N, Kacaki J, Andjus R, Malkic K (1966) The effect of local irradiation of the head of rats in the infantile period on spermatogenesis. Strahlentherapie 130: 432–436

Scherholz KP, Frommhold H, Barwig P (1978) Strahlenbelastung der Ovarien bei Bestrahlung der paraaortalen, iliakalen und inguinalen Lymphknoten mit Telekobalt sowie mit Photonen der Energie 42 MeV. Strahlentherapie 154: 844–851

Schoen EJ (1964) Effect of local irradiation on testicular androgen biosynthesis. Endocrinology 75: 56–65

Schreiber H, Plishuk Z (1956) The effect of x-rays on the ovaries in childhood and adolescence. Br J Radiol 29: 687

Searle AG, Beechey CV, Green D, Howells GR (1980) Comparative effects of protracted exposures to ^{60}Co x-radiation and ^{239}Pu x-radiation on breeding performance in female mice. Int J Radiat Biol 37: 189–200

Searle AG, Beechy CV, Green D, Howells GR (1982) Dominant lethal and ovarian effects of plutonium-239 in female mice. Int J Radiat Biol 42: 235–244

Seigel DG (1966) Frequency of live births among survivors of Hiroshima and Nagasaki atomic bombings. Radiat Res 28: 278

Shalet SM, Beardwell CG, Morris PH, Pearson D, Orrell DH (1976) Ovarian failure following abdominal irradiation in childhood. Br J Cancer 33: 655–658

Shalet SM, Beardwell CG, Jacobs HS, Pearson D (1978) Testicular function following irradiation of the human prepubertal testis. Clin Endocrinol 9: 483–490

Shalet SM, Horner A, Ahmed SR, Morris-Jones PH (1985) Leydig cell damage after testicular irradiation for acute lymphoblastic leukaemia. Med Pediatr Oncol 13: 65–68

Shamberger RC, Sherins RJ, Rosenberg SA (1981) Effects of postoperative adjuvant chemotherapy and radiotherapy on testicular function in man undergoing treatment for soft tissue sarcoma. Cancer 47: 2368–2374

Shehata N (1983) The effect of gamma rays on the gonads of the olive fruit fly, Dacus oleae (Gmelin). Int J Radiat Biol 43: 169–173

Shelton M (1961) The secretion of androgen by the x-irradiated ovary of the adult rat. Acta Endocrinol 37: 529–540

Sheridan W (1971) The effects of the time interval in fractionated x-ray treatment of mouse spermatogonia. Mutat Res 13: 163–169

Shimizu K, Ishikava K, Nakamurak K, Sato I (1955) Study on the spermatogenesis of the Bikini victims. J Jpn Surg Ass 55: 1221–1230

Shimizu K, Ishikawa K, Saito Y et al. (1956) Some observations on the victims of the Bikini-H-bomb-test explosions. In: Research in the effects and influences of the nuclear bomb test, vol II. Japan Society for the Promotion of Science. Tokyo, 1333–1351

Sklar, CA, Robinson LL, Nesbit ME, Sather HN, Meadows AT, Ortega JA, Kim TH, Hammond GD (1980) Effects of radiation on testicular function in long-term survivors of childhood acute lymphoblastic leukemia. A report from the children's cancer study group. J Clin Oncol 8: 1981–1987

Slanina J, Musshoff K, Rahner T, Stiasny R (1977) Long-term side effects in irradiated patients with Hodgkin's disease. Int J Radiat Oncol Biol Phys 2: 1–19

Slanina J, Wannenmacher M, Spratler J (1985) Schwangerschaft und Kindesentwicklung nach Therapie des Morbus Hodgkin. Strahlentherapie 161: 558–564

Smith P, Doll R (1976) Late effects of x-irradiation treated for metropathia haemorrhagica. Br J Radiol 49: 244

Smithers DW, Wallace DN, Austin DE (1973) Fertility after unilateral orchidectomy and radiotherapy for patients with malignant tumors of the testis. Br J Med 4: 77–79

Sobels FH (1969) Estimation of the genetic risk resulting from the treatment of women with [131]iodine. Strahlentherapie 138: 172–177

Sommers SC (1953) Endocrine changes after hemiadrenalectomy and total body irradiation in parabiotic rats. J Lab Clin Med 42: 396–407

Spalding JF, Wellnitz JM, Schweitzer WH (1957) The effects of high-dosage x-rays on the maturation of the rat ovum, and their modification by gonadotropins. Fertil Steril 8: 80–88

Speiser B, Rubin P, Casarett G (1973) Aspermia following lower truncal irradiation in Hodgkin's disease. Cancer 32: 692–698

Spiro G, Wachsmann F (1962) Über die Wirkung einzeitig und fraktioniert verabreichter Röntgenstrahlen auf Rattenhoden. Strahlentherapie 118: 153–158

Srivastava PN, Rao AR (1967) Co^{60}-induced radiation changes in the ovary of unilaterally ovariectomized Indian desert gerbil, Meriones hurrianae Jerdon. Strahlentherapie 134: 452–456

Stillman RJ, Schinfeld JS, Schiff I et al. (1981) Ovarian failure in long-term survivors of childhood malignancy. Am J Obstet Gynecol 139: 62–66

Straume T, Dobson RL (1985) Mouse oocyte killing by neutrons: target considerations. Radiat Prot Dosim 13: 215–227

Straume T, Dobson L, Kwan TC (1987) Neutron RBE's and the radiosensitive target for mouse immature oocyte killing. Radiat Res 111: 47–57

Straume T, Dobson RL, Kwan TC (1989) Size of lethality target in mouse immature oocytes determined with accelerated heavy ions. Radiat Environ Biophys 28: 131–139

Suzuki K, Inano H, Tamaoki B (1973) Testicular function at puberty following prepubertal local x-irradiation in the rat. Biol Reprod 9: 1–8

Tabuchi A, Nakagawa S, Hirai T et al. (1967) Fetal hazards due to x-ray diagnosis during pregnancy. Hiroshima J Med Sci 16: 49–66

Taylor DM (1977) The uptake, retention and distribution of plutonium-239 in rat gonads. Health Phys 32: 29–31

Thithapandha A, Chanachai W, Suriyachon D (1979) Effects of γ-irradiation on plasma testosterone levels and hepatic drug metabolism. Radiat Res 79: 203–207

Thomas PRM, Winstanly D, Peckham MJ, Austin DE, Murray MAF, Jacobs HS (1976) Reproductive and endocrine function in patients with Hodgkin's disease: effects of oophoropexy and irradiation. Br J Cancer 33: 226

Thomas RG, Healy JW, McInroy JF (1985) Plutonium in gonads: a summary of the current status. Health Phys 48: 7–18

Thorslund TM, Paulsen CA (1972) Effects of x-ray irradiation on human spermatogenesis. In: Warman EA (ed) Nat symp natural manmade radiat Sp. NASA TMX 2440, pp 229–232

Thüroff JW (1982) Fertilitätsstörungen nach retroperitonealer Lymphadenektomie. Dtsch Med Wochenschr 107: 834

Tindall DJ, Vitale R, Means AR (1975) Androgen binding protein as a biochemical marker of formation of the blood-testis barrier. Endocrinology 97: 636–648

Tomic R, Bergman B, Damber JE, Littbrand B, Lofroth PO (1983) Effects of external radiation therapy for cancer of the prostate on the serum concentrations of testosterone, follicle-stimulating hormone, luteinizing hormone and prolactin. J Urol 130: 287–289

Török P, Schmahl W (1982) Einfluß von 5-Azazytidin und akuter Röntgenbestrahlung auf Mäusetestes während der sexualen Differenzierung in utero. In: Kriegel H, Schmahl W, Kistner G, Stieve FE (eds) Entwicklungsstörungen nach pränataler Bestrahlung. Fischer, Stuttgart, pp 305–308

Török P, Schmahl W, Meyer I, Kistner G (1979) Effects of a single injection of tritiated water during organogeny on the prenatal and postnatal development of mice. In: Biological implications of radionuclides released for nuclear industries. Int Atomic Energy Agency 1, Vienna

Trautmann J (1963) Hoden. In: Scherer E, Stender HS (eds) Strahlentherapie der Zelle. Thieme, Stuttgart, pp 195–208

Trautmann J, Millin G (1962/63) Wirkungen subletaler Strahlendosen auf den Zyklus und Oestrus der weißen Laboratoriumsmaus. I. und II. Mitteilung. Strahlentherapie 118: 67–76; 122: 558–564

Trueblood HW, Enright LP, Ray GR, Kaplan HS, Nelsen TS (1970) Preservation of ovarian function in pelvic radiation for Hodgkin's disease. Arch Surg 100: 236–237

Unger E (1976) Histologische Untersuchungen nach experimenteller Rasterstrahlung. Befunde von Kaninchenhoden. Strahlentherapie 132: 255–267

Unger E (1980) Histological effects of low-dose-rate gamma-irradiation. Strahlentherapie 156: 46–50

Vahlensieck W, Weissbach L (1974) Vergleich andrologischer Befunde bei jüngeren und älteren Männern mit Hodentumoren. Ref Congr Urol et Nephrol, Budapest, 17–19.10.1974

Valenta M, Kolousek J, Fulka J (1963) The influence of ionizing radiation on nucleic acids, vitality and fecundating ability of male sexual cells. Int J Radiat Biol 6: 81–91

Valentin K (1978) Normal stem cell proliferation and cell depletion after x-irradiation of spermatogonia of inbred and hybrid mice. Hereditas 88: 117–126

van Alphen MMA, van de Kant HJG, de Rooij DG (1988a) Depletion of the spermatogonia from the seminiferous epithelium of the rhesus monkey after x-irradiation. Radiat Res 113: 473–486

van Alphen MMA, van de kant HJG, de Rooij DG (1988b) Repopulation of the seminiferous epithelium of the rhesus monkey after x-irradiation. Radiat Res 113: 487–500

van Beek MEAB, Davids JAG, van de kant HJG, de Rooij DG (1984) Response to fission neutron irradiation of spermatogonial stem cells in different stages of the cycle of the seminiferous epithelium. Radiat Res 97: 556–569

van Beek MEAB, Davids JAG, de Rooij DG (1986) Nonrandom distribution of mouse spermatogonial stem cells surviving fission neutron irradiation. Radiat Res 107: 11–23

van den Aardweg GJMJ, de Ruiter-Bootsma AL, Kramer MF (1982) Growth of spermatogenetic colonies in the mouse testis after irradiation with fission neutrons. Radiat Res 89: 150–165

van den Aardweg GJMJ, de Ruiter-Bootsma AL, Kramer MF, Davids JAG (1983) Growth and differentiation of spermatogenic colonies in the mouse testis after irradiation with fission neutrons. Radiat Res 94: 447–463

van Kroonenburgh MJPG, Vandaal WAJ, Beck JL, Vemer HM, Rolland R, Herman CJ (1987) Survival of spermatogonial stem cells in the rat after split dose irradiation during LH-RH-analogue treatment. Radiother Oncol 9: 67–71

van Wagenen G, Gardner WU (1960) x-irradiation of the ovary in the monkey. Fertil Steril 11: 291–302

van Vermande-Eck GJ (1959) Effect of low-dosage x-irradiation upon pituitary gland and ovaries of the rhesus monkey. Fertil Steril 10: 190–202

Verjans HJ, Eik-Nes KB (1976) Hypothalamic-pituitary-testicular system following testicular x-irradiation. Acta Endocrinol 83: 190–200

Vorisek P, Jirasek JE (1967) Morphologische Veränderungen an intrauterin mit kontinuierlichen kleinen Dosen bestrahlten Ovarien. Strahlentherapie 132: 79–89

Vorisek P, Vondracek J (1968) Der Mechanismus der postnatalen Veränderungen des Follikelapparates bei intrauterin mit kleinen Dosen bestrahlten Ovarien. Strahlentherapie 135: 602–609

Wakabayashi K, Isurugi K, Tamaoke B, Akaboshi S (1974) Serum levels of luteinizing hormone (LH) and follicle stimulating hormone (FSH) in subjects accidentally exposed to 192-Ir gamma rays. J Radiat Res 14: 297

Wall PG (1961) Effects of x-irradiation on differentiating Leydig cells of the immature rat. J Endocrinol 23: 291–301

Walther G, Schmidt KJ, Ladner HA (1968) Das histochemische Verhalten der Isocitrat-. Succinat- und Malathydrogenase sowie der Cytochromoxydase in Rattenorganen nach Ganzkörperbestrahlung. Strahlentherapie 136: 500–507

Wang J, Galil KAA, Setchell BP (1983) Changes in testicular blood flow and testosterone production during aspermatogenesis after irradiation. J Endocrinol 98: 35–46

Weissbach L, Lange CE, Meyhofer W (1974a) Hodenhistologie, Ejakulat und Nukleoproteingehalt der Spermatozoen behandelter Hodentumorpatienten. Andrologia 5: 135–146

Weissbach L, Lange CE, Rodermund OE, Zwicker H, Gropp A, Pothmann W (1974b) Fertilitätsstörungen bei behandelten Hodentumorpatienten. Urologie 13: 80–85

Whelton JA, McSweeney DJ (1964) Successful pregnancy after radiation for carcinoma of cervix. Am J Obstet Gynecol 88: 443–446

Wigg DR, Murray ML, Koschel K (1982) Tolerance of the central nervous system to photon irradiation. Endocrine complications. Acta Radiol (Onkol) 21: 49–60

Wigoder SB (1929) The effect of x-rays on the testis. Br J Radiol 2: 213–221

Willemse PHB, Sleijfer DT, Sluiter WJ, Koops HS, Doorenbos H (1983) Altered Leydig cell function in patients with testicular cancer: evidence for a bilateral testicular defect. Acta Endocrinol (Copenh) 102: 616–624

Withers HR, Hunter N, Barkley HT Jr, Reid BO (1974) Radiation survival and regeneration characteristics of spermatogenic stem cell of mouse testis. Radiat Res 54: 88–103

Yoshimura N, Etoh H, Egami N, Asami K, Yamada T (1969) Note on the effects of β-rays from ^{89}Sr-^{90}Y on spermatogenesis in the teleost, Oryzias latipes. Anat Zool Jpn 42: 75–79

Zollinger HU (1960) Radio-Histologie und Radio-Histopathologie. In: Roulet F (ed) Strahlung und Wetter. (Handbuch der allgemeinen Pathologie, Vol X/1, pp 209–215) Springer, Berlin Göttingen Heidelberg

Zuckerman S (1965) The sensitivity of the gonads to radiation. Clin Radiol 16: 1–15

16 Radiotherapy in Childhood: Normal Tissue Injuries and Carcinogenesis

M. MOLLS and M. STUSCHKE

CONTENTS

16.1 Introduction

Radiotherapeutic treatment contributes to long-term survival after cancer in childhood, especially in cases of Hodgkin's disease, acute lymphocytic leukemia (ALL), Wilms' tumor, and soft tissue and Ewing's sarcoma (PEREZ and BRADY 1987; HAVERS 1987). Like other treatment modalities, irradiation induces early and late side-effects. In general, the early effects are reversible and the related symptoms can be treated effectively. Moreover, children often tolerate the acute local side-effects of radiotherapy better than do adults (PIZZO et al. 1985). The persistent late effects are more critical; their clinical significance is variable.

M. MOLLS, Priv.-Doz., Dr. med., Oberarzt, Radiologisches Zentrum, Universitätsklinikum Essen, Hufelandstraße 55, 4300 Essen 1, FRG

M. STUSCHKE, Dr. med., Radiologisches Zentrum, Universitätsklinikum Essen, Hufelandstraße 55, 4300 Essen 1, FRG

In general, the frequency and the degree of radiation-induced sequelae depend on the total radiation dose, dose fractionation, and the irradiated volume. Furthermore, reduction of the dose rate in the case of total body irradiation decreases the risk of early and late effects. In principle, a shrinking field technique reduces the volume of critical tissues affected and may be beneficial. Until now the influence of the age of the child on radiation sensitivity has not been very precisely defined.

Some major problems arise in the analysis of normal tissue effects after irradiation of children. The therapeutic concepts in pediatric oncology are relatively new and are still under going development. Thus, it is rather difficult to find larger and homogeneously treated patient populations with a substantial follow-up period. Besides irradiation, chemotherapy and other factors may contribute to the long-term alterations (RUBIN 1984; MOLLS et al. 1986). In this article we have tried to take into consideration as far as possible observations after irradiation alone.

16.2 Mechanisms

On the basis of general radiobiological considerations it appears reasonable to assume that the radiosensitivity of children is relatively high during periods of organ growth. This assumption is of some practical value in clinical situations, in which the risk of side-effects has to be considered in an individual child. The most rapid organ growth is observed during the postnatal period and puberty. However, organ growth is not due to cell proliferation alone. In the brain the neuroblasts lose their capacity to divide at the time of birth or during the first 2 postnatal years (SINCLAIR 1969). During the postnatal growth of the CNS, processes of maturation such as the increase in the diameter and length of nerve fibers and myelinization are the fundamental events (BRASEL et al. 1978). Experimentally in the rat three phases of organ growth have been identified. After birth organs grow primarily by cell multiplication. The amount of DNA increases rapidly. Thereafter, a phase follows in which cell proliferation is slower than protein synthesis. Finally cell proliferation stops or is slow (ENESCO and LEBLOND 1962; WINIEK and NOBLE 1965). These facts may be of some relevance to changes in the radiosensitivity of any organ during childhood (RUBIN et al. 1982). However, the radiosensitivity of an organ is not closely related to its parenchymal cells. Especially with regard to late organ injuries, radiation-induced alterations of the vascular-connective tissue play an important role. The occlusion of capillaries and the reduction in microcirculation lead to damage of connective and parenchymal tissue. Fibroblasts are activated and the fibrillar density increases (CASARETT 1980).

Repair of radiation damage is another fundamental biological phenomenon found at the molecular, cellular, and tissue level. A set of enzymes repair radiation-induced DNA lesions such as strand breaks within a few hours. Within days after irradiation repopulation occurs at the cellular level. An increased, compensatory cell proliferation counteracts cell loss (STREFFER and VAN BEUNINGEN, this volume; MOLLS et al. 1982). DNA repair and repopulation constitute the process of *restitutio ad integrum*. By contrast, a *functio laesa* can be observed when fibrosis and cicatrization, which represent secondary repair at the tissue level, take place.

From a biological and also a clinical point of view it is interesting to ask whether the repair capacity in children differs from that in adults. In cell culture experiments, the decrease in mitotic activity in late-passage human fibroblasts was the criterion of aging. In these cells, DNA repair was comparatively less efficient (HART and SETLOW 1976). Further evidence of a more efficient DNA repair in children might be the fact that in babies the frequency of spontaneous chromosomal aberrations is lower than in adults (TONOMURA et al. 1983). Repopulation in organs of children and adults after application of isodoses has not been studied to date. However, there is some evidence that in children repair of radiation damage might be better than in adults. This question needs to be further clarified in experimental investigations.

16.3 Normal Tissue Injury

In this section we describe radiation effects on the structure and function of normal tissues. We have tried to concentrate on the critical radiation doses or dose ranges for the different organs. As pointed out in the introduction, it must be kept in mind that in situations in which irradiation has been combined with chemotherapy it is difficult to estimate exactly the quantitative contribution of each agent to the injury of organs.

16.3.1 Brain

At the age of 3 years, the weight of a child's brain is about 75% that of an adult's brain. The DNA content of the brain increases into the 2nd year of life due to cell division of glial cells (DOBBING and SANDS 1973). Neuronal cell division predominantly occurs prenatally.

The most frequent indications for irradiation of the brain in childhood are primary brain tumors and prophylactic whole brain irradiation in diseases such as ALL and malignant lymphomas. These account for more than 50% of all childhood malignancies (KAATSCH and MICHAELIS 1985). Only late structural and functional radiation-induced changes will be reported here.

16.3.1.1 Brain Necrosis

There is evidence that the age of the child influences the radiosensitivity of the brain. On the bases of (a) what is known about human brain development and the radiosensitivity of the central nervous system in young experimental animals and (b) clinical experience, BLOOM et al. (1969) arbitrarily restricted the total dose for local brain irradiation in children under the age of 3 years to 40–45 Gy in 6–7 weeks. In irradiation of optic gliomas, BLOOM (1982) recommended maximum total doses of 50–55 Gy in 7–8 weeks (1.4 Gy daily doses 5 times a week) for older children in order to avoid damage to normal CNS tissue, especially optic nerve fibers. For children aged between 2 and 5 years the recommended total dose was lower, 45–50 Gy in 6.5–7 weeks, and for those less than 2 years it was 40–45 Gy in 6–6.5 weeks (BLOOM 1982).

In 43 children under 15 years of age and 31

children of the same age group, doses of 50–60 Gy and 60–79 Gy respectively were tolerated without any signs of necrosis when given in fractions over 6–10 weeks (Onoyama et al. 1975). On the other hand, Cumberlin et al. (1979) described the case of an 8.5-year-old boy with a medulloblastoma who received 57.4 Gy in 34 fractions within 70 days to the posterior fossa and 40.2 Gy to the remaining CNS over 5.5 weeks. Before irradiation the child suffered from postoperative meningitis which was cured with antibiotics. The patient died 1 year after radiotherapy, and massive necrosis of the pons, the medulla oblongata, and the upper cervical medulla was seen at autopsy.

A total dose of 52 Gy with conventional fractionation (2 Gy per fraction, five daily fractions per week) is considered to be tolerable in adults (Sheline et al. 1980). The rate of brain necrosis at that dose level was estimated to be 0.04%–0.4% (Sheline 1980). A strong influence of the size of dose per fraction became apparent in her isoeffect analysis of brain necrosis after radiotherapy of extracranial tumors (predominantly of the paranasal sinuses and skin) and brain tumors. The lower the dose per fraction, the better the fractionation schedule was tolerated. The onset of symptoms of brain necrosis can be as early as 6 months after treatment. The peak time of presentation is between 1 and 2 years after therapy. The age-dependent maximum tolerable dose has not been determined up to now. Bloom et al. (1969) assumed that the total dose tolerated by the CNS in children less than 3 years old is 10%–20% lower than in adults. According to a more recent publication by Bloom (1982), the radiation dose for children 3–5 years old has to be reduced by 20%, and that for children up to 3 years old, by 33%

A late side-effect occurring after combined treatment with radiotherapy and methotrexate is leukoencephalopathy. Clinically, symptoms such as seizures, spasticity, paresis, ataxia, and lethargy are dominant. Leukoencephalopathy is morphologically characterized by diffuse reactive astrocytosis of telencephalic white matter and by multiple noninflammatory foci containing varying amounts of mineralized cellular debris. In a literature survey Bleyer and Griffin (1980) stated that there are no reports of leukoencephalopathy after irradiation of the neurocranium alone, with fractionated total doses of 18–24 Gy. The interaction between radio- and chemotherapy is considered to be responsible for the development of leukoencephalopathy after treatment of ALL (Price and Jamieson 1975). This latter study suggested as a possible mechanism the ability of chemotherapeutic agents to diffuse better through the blood–brain barrier following CNS irradiation with 20 Gy or more.

White matter changes after radiation therapy of the brain can be detected most sensitively by magnetic resonance imaging (Constine et al. 1988). It was found that children had less severe abnormalities after treatment of primary brain tumors than did adults. This might be due to the lower total radiation doses used for children (mean: 54.4 Gy) than for adults (mean: 63.7 Gy).

16.3.1.2 Endocrinological Changes

Growth Hormone

Undisturbed growth hormone (GH) secretion in children is necessary of normal growth. GH affects the formation of somatomedin in the liver and kidneys, which in turn stimulates DNA synthesis and division of the cells of the columnar cartilage, resulting in elongation and thickening of long bones (Fisher and Rhomes 1982). Irradiation of the neurocranium can exert both acute and chronic effects on GH release.

The most sensitive endocrinological target are the cells producing the growth hormone releasing hormone (GHRH) in the hypothalamus. Lannering and Albertsson-Wikland (1987) were able to show that of 19 children who had received a radiation dose of 37–60 Gy (4 × 2 Gy/week) to the hypothalamic–hypophysial region at the age of 1.7–16.9 years, all 19 showed severely impaired spontaneous secretion of GH over a 24-h period. After intravenous application of GHRH, 13 children showed an immediate increase in GH serum levels, indicative of a primary disturbance of hypothalamic function.

Growth hormone deficiency is dose dependent. Shalet et al. (1976c) found a highly significant inverse correlation between the radiation dose and the peak plasma level of GH following insulin-induced hypoglycemia in a total of 56 children with brain tumors or acute leukemia who had received radiotherapy. Of 41 children irradiated with total doses of more than 29 Gy, 36 showed an inadequate GH response 24 months or later after therapy, as compared with only 1 of 15 with total doses less than 29 Gy. Onoyama et al. (1975) obtained similar results. They observed a shortened elongatory growth in 47% of children with brain tumors (craniopharyngiomas and hypophysial tumors) who had been irradiated with total doses of more than 30 Gy to the hypothalamic–hypophysial region but in only 7% of children who had received doses below 30 Gy. Measurements of GH release were not carried out in this latter study.

The significance of the total dose for impairment of GH release can also be demonstrated by comparing the data after irradiation for medulloblastoma (total dose $\geq$30 Gy) and ALL (total dose 18 or 24 Gy). Children with medulloblastomas or other primary brain tumors receive total doses of 30 Gy or more to the hypothalamic–hypophysial region within 5 weeks. GH deficiency has been found in 60%–100% of cases in several studies (ABAYOMI and SADEGHI-NEJAD 1986; DUFFNER et al. 1985; RAPPAPORT et al. 1982). The deficiency progressed with time but was sometimes already apparent at the first follow-up examination 3 months after the end of therapy (DUFFNER et al. (1983). Spontaneous recovery of GH deficiency was not seen in any of 20 patients 1–8 years after therapy.

There is conflicting information concerning the impairment of GH release in children with ALL after chemotherapy and cranial irradiation. Whereas SHALET et al. (1976b) and DICKINSON et al. (1978) reported reduced stimulation of GH release by hypoglycemia 8 months or later after the commencement of therapy, other investigators did not observe such changes (FISHER and RHOMES 1982; SWIFT et al. 1978; WELLS et al. 1983). In the study by SHALET et al. (1976), 11 of 15 patients with total brain doses of 25 Gy given in ten fractions over 2.5 weeks had lowered GH peak plasma levels, compared with none of seven children given 24 Gy in 20 fractions over 4 weeks in the insulin tolerance test. The children given the higher single and total doses, however, had a longer follow-up period. This would be of significance if GH deficiency were to progress with time. Moreover in a later publication the same authors reported on two patients who did show decreased secretion of GH after prophylactic cranial irradiation totalling 24 Gy (AHMED et al. 1986).

In a prospective study DACOU-VOUTETAKIS et al. (1975) determined the daily GH profiles before and after prophylactic cranial irradiation of children with ALL (total dose: 24 Gy). After irradiation, the initially normal plasma values were markedly decreased but they recovered 6–12 months later. This underlines that the clinical significance of GH deficiency after cranial irradiation in cases of ALL remains to be determined. Fractionated total doses of 24 Gy in 3 weeks or lower doses only exceptionally led to substantial changes in growth (CHESSELLS 1985). Height and growth were studied in 21 children with ALL after randomization into treatment arms with and without whole brain irradiation (WELLS et al. 1983). The irradiated patients showed decreased elongatory growth over a period of 36 months after the commencement of therapy. After that, this difference no longer existed. However, no significant decrease in absolute height in comparison with the normal population resulted from the temporarily reduced elongatory growth. The initial changes were attributed to acutely lowered secretion levels of GH, although these were not studied systematically. Despite clear biochemical alterations of the GH response in the insulin tolerance test, SHALET et al. (1979) rarely found a clinical growth deficiency in children with ALL after prophylactic cranial irradiation either with 25 Gy in ten fractions over 2.5 weeks or 24 Gy in 20 fractions over 4 weeks.

With total doses of 18 Gy in ten fractions and 24 Gy in 12 fractions, CIOGNANI et al. (1988) found different effects of cranial irradiation on growth rate and GH release in children with prolonged survival after ALL. Two years after irradiation only children who had received 24 Gy cranial irradiation showed standard deviation scores for height that were significantly lower than at diagnosis and an impaired GH response to the arginine and levodopa tests. Children who had received 18 Gy had complete growth recovery and normal GH responses to the pharmacological tests. This indicates that the threshold dose for the impairment of GH secretion is between 18 and 24 Gy in fractions of 1.8 and 2 Gy. Near the threshold total dose, BRÄMSWIG et al. (1989) found a significant fractionation effect for cranial irradiation. Whereas children with ALL who received 24 Gy cranial irradiation in 16–26 fractions (DAL-70 and BMF-70 protocols) showed normal growth, children given the same total dose in 11–14 fractions (BFM-70 protocol) had a significantly reduced standard deviation score for height. Growth hormone release was not tested in this study.

A possible age dependence of the radiation effect on GH secretion is suggested by the retrospective analysis by SHALET et al. (1976c). Among GH-deficient patients the number of individuals older than 13 years was disproportionately high. This was seen in the insulin tolerance test at total doses of more than 29 Gy. According to the authors it remains to be discussed whether the result can be attributed in part to a relatively better stimulatory capacity of GH release under hypoglycemic conditions in children under 13.

In summary, the findings indicate that there is a dose-dependent and probably also an age-dependent effect of radiation on GH secretion. The critical threshold dose for the at least temporary impairment of GH secretion ranges from about 18 to 24 Gy with conventional fractionation as applied in prophylactic brain irradiation for ALL. Most data have been derived from retrospective studies. It must be emphasized that the reduced GH secretion after irradiation can also be due, in part, to other factors such as steroid application, emotional disturbances, increased brain pressure, and chemotherapy.

Further Endocrinological Deficiencies Related to the Hypophysis or Hypothalamus

In contrast to GH, disturbances of the secretion of glandotropic hormones of the hypophysis and of antidiuretic hormone (ADH) only occur at higher doses. DUFFNER et al. (1985) found no pathological changes in either the serum or the plasma thyroid-stimulating hormone (TSH) and prolactin levels or in follicle-stimulating hormone (FSH) and luteinizing hormone (LH) excretion in the urine up to 1 year after irradiation of ten children with brain tumors with total doses of 39 Gy to the hypothalamic–hypophysial region. HIRSCH et al. (1979) found no alterations in adrenocorticotropic hormone (ACTH) secretion or in antidiuretic function after irradiating 17 children with medulloblastomas. Secondary or tertiary hypothyroidism was similarly not observed. The Manchester Group (AHMED et al. 1983) found no changes in gonadotropin levels in irradiated medulloblastoma patients without long-term chemotherapy (30 Gy in 20 fractions to the neurocranial axis; 15 Gy boost to the posterior fossa in ten fractions). In addition three groups have reported normal hypothalamic–hypophysial function after prophylactic cranial irradiation in ALL (FISHER and RHOMES 1982; VON MÜHLENDAHL et al. 1976; SWIFT et al. 1978). Only one of 25 children showed abnormal TSH and ACTH secretion after treatment for acute leukemia including prophylactic cranial irradiation (SHALET et al. 1977a).

Disturbances have been found after higher radiation doses. RICHARDS et al. (1976) reported on four children with brain tumors who received total doses higher than 40 Gy to the hypothalamic–hypophysial axis. In addition to GH deficiency, was deficient in TSH, ACTH, and gonadotropin. In the study by RAPPOPORT et al. (1982), 5 of 45 children with brain tumors developed gonadotropin deficiency. Two of them with frontal and temporal astrocytomas were given total doses of 55 Gy to the critical region. The remaining three children were medulloblastoma patients. They received lower radiation doses (35 or 45 Gy) and additional chemotherapy. All these five patients were GH deficient.

16.3.1.3 Effects on Neuropsychological Functions

The considerable emotional and social problems of the frequently very young children with cancer who undergo radiotherapy of the cranium as well as the lengthy follow-up period might affect intellectual development. Many of the published studies concerning neuropsychological changes are retrospective and are based on a small number of patients. In more recent studies, psychological tests have also been used to assess quantitatively slight alterations in the neuropsychological functions of children after brain irradiation.

Up to now, no clear dose–response relationship has been established for impairment of intellectual functions. RON et al. (1982) investigated the effects of small doses, on average 1.3 Gy, on mental function in a large group of 10 842 children suffering from tinea capitis. They had been irradiated at the age of 1–15 years. In comparison to a control group of ethnic-, sex-, and age-matched individuals from the general population as well as a control group of siblings, the children who had received epilation irradiation (Adamson Kienbock technique) achieved lower scores on a high school aptitude test, completed fewer school grades, had lower scores on intelligence and psychological tests, and had a slight excess of mental hospital admissions. Not all comparisons were statistically significant, but there was a consistent trend for the irradiated subjects to exhibit signs of impairment more often than their comparison groups. The dose given to the above-mentioned patients is the lowest that has been reported to lead to functional neuropsychological disturbances after irradiation in childhood. At present, it is difficult to identify mechanisms which could explain these functional changes after very low radiation doses.

A considerable body of observations exists after application of higher total doses (18–24 Gy with daily fractions of 1.5–2.0 Gy) for prophylactic cranial irradiation in ALL. However, apart from radiation, children with ALL receive a lengthy course of chemotherapy and, therefore, the effect of prophylactic cranial irradiation on cognitive development is difficult to analyze. Possible interactions of the side-effects of both therapeutic modalities cannot be excluded.

In a prospective study, SONI et al. (1975) did not observe any great differences in neurological and psychological functions between children with ALL whose treatment included cranial irradiation and a control group with tumors outside the CNS who had not received cranial irradiation. Children of both groups achieved similar scores in various intelligence tests as well as in reading, spelling, and arithmetic tests of the wide range achievement test. VEROZOSA et al. (1976) found no neuropsychological abnormalities in cranially irradiated children with leukemia 5 years after therapy. No psychometric tests were used in this study.

However, the number of reports with unfavorable results after prophylactic cranial irradiation in the treatment of ALL has increased in recent years (BRECHER et al. 1983; EISER 1978, 1980; EISER and LANSDOWN 1977; JANNOUN 1983; LADAVAS et al. 1985; MCINTOSH et al. 1976; MEADOWS et al. 1981; Moss et al. 1981; TWADDLE et al. 1983). LADAVAS et al. (1985) found subtle decreases in intellectual function, particularly in the verbal intelligence relating to information, experience, distractability, and late memory, in children with ALL after irradiation and systemic chemotherapy compared with children with solid tumors who had been treated with chemotherapy and only extracranial irradiation. Moss et al. (1981) compared the performance scores of children with ALL after therapy with and without prophylactic cranial irradiation with those of their siblings. After irradiation, the performance as well as the verbal intelligence quotient was significantly lower than in the healthy counterparts, although the performance of treated children was within the normal limits of these tests. No such differences were seen in the group subjected to chemotherapy alone compared with the controls. The mean interval between the commencement of CNS prophylaxis and initial psychological testing was 3 years 11 months in this study. An interesting result concerning the temporal sequencing of therapy was obtained by EISER (1980). She found worse intellectual abilities using psychometric tests in children with ALL who had received prophylactic cranial irradiation within 2 months after diagnosis than in those with delayed cranial irradiation given 6 months after diagnosis or those without irradiation. The disturbances, however, were slight. Thus, this group of very young irradiated children also showed performances corresponding to the lower normal range. The study indicates that the development of functional disturbances may result from interactions of radio- and chemotherapy.

The effect of age on the extent of the disturbances of intellectual functions in cases of ALL has been studied by several groups. There is some evidence that chemotherapy combined with irradiation tends to impair such functions to a greater extent in younger children (<5 years) than in older ones (EISER et al. 1977, 1978, 1980; JANNOUN 1983; Moss et al. 1981). Differing from these results, LADAVAS et al. (1985) observed worse performance in children over 5 years old than in the younger age group. However, the group of patients was relatively small.

The investigations that have emphasized prophylactic irradiation as the etiological factor responsible for the diminution of intellectual functions need to be further substantiated by means of prospective studies. Such studies are imperative especially since changes such as ventricular dilatation and cortical atrophy, diffuse white matter hypodensity, and intracerebral calcifications have been observed with computer tomography at the same frequency in patients with ALL who received radiotherapy as part of their CNS prophylaxis and those receiving only methotrexate (ESSELTINE et al. 1981; OCHS et al. 1983).

Children with primary brain tumors receive the highest total doses to the neurocranium, i.e., up to 60 Gy. Clinically, the neuropsychological function of the majority of them appears fairly satisfactory (BLOOM et al. 1969). Eighty-two percent of long-term survivors among children with medulloblastomas and 75% of children with gliomas, who had received total doses of between 50 and 60 Gy in conventional fractions to parts of the brain, were found to "lead active lives" (BLOOM et al. 1969; BOUCHARD and PEIRCE 1960). It was the impression of BOUCHARD and PEIRCE (1960) that following radiotherapy of brain tumors the quality of life was slightly better in long-term surviving children than in adults. Using more elaborate testing methods, several more recent and more quantitative investigations found slight mental defects and emotional disturbances. However, these were often compatible with a relatively intact overall function (BAMFORD et al. 1976; HIRSCH et al. 1979; SPUNBERG et al. 1981; KUN et al. 1983; LI et al. 1984). Of 102 patients irradiated for primary brain tumors in childhood, 78 had mild or no gross deficits (LI et al. 1984). Forty-six of the children were attending school at the time of the survey, and 71 had completed school and attained educational levels. Follow-up in this study ranged from 5 to 47 years (median, 18 years).

In most retrospective studies on children with primary brain tumors, the effect of radiotherapy on neuropsychological functions cannot be differentiated from the effects of the tumor itself, of surgery, of educational deficiencies, and of the emotional stress caused by the frequently long-lasting treatment. Indications of the importance of radiotherapy for the alterations in intellectual function of children have come from comparative studies involving medulloblastoma patients treated with surgery, radiation, and in some cases chemotherapy and, on the other hand, patients with tumors of similar location (cerebellar astrocytomas) treated with surgery alone (HIRSCH et al. 1979; RAIMONDI and TOMITA 1979). The medulloblastoma patients had significantly lower intelligence quotients than the children in the control group; 58% of the children had IQs between 70 and 90 and 31% had values lower than 70. Behavioral disturbances were seen in 82% of patients as against 59% of controls (HIRSCH et al. 1979). The doses given to the overall cerebrospinal axis of medulloblastoma patients totalled 35 Gy. A boost of 15 Gy was given to the posterior fossa (total dose: 50 Gy). Total treatment time was 6 weeks.

There are hints that younger children more frequently show mental defects than older ones after irradiation of primary brain tumors (BAMFORD et al. 1976; Danoff et al. 1982; SILVERMAN et al. 1984; SPUNBERG et al. 1981). However, from the reported data, age dependence of the radiosensitivity of the brain cannot be derived in a more quantitative manner.

Summarizing, the cited retrospective studies do not permit a quantitative assessment of the dependence of neuropsychological disturbances on radiation dose. On the one hand, this is largely due to the heterogeneity of the patient populations and the irradiation techniques. On the oter hand, data obtained after standardized radiotherapy as applied in medulloblastoma are insufficient to establish a dose–response relationship because of the small range of total doses used. Apart from these considerations it must be stressed that in treatments with curative intent the radiation dose should not be compromised. The disabilities arising after combined therapy, usually consisting of surgery and irradiation, must be seen against the background of improved prognosis for children with brain tumors. Only by means of high dose radiotherapy has it been possible to improve the prognosis for medulloblastoma from a 5-year survival rate of 0% after surgery alone (CUSHING 1930) to about 50% (BAMBERG 1987; STUSCHKE et al. 1988). Finally, the clinical experience also shows that during follow-up the intellectual performance improves in a considerable proportion of children (KUN et al. 1983). This indicates possible benefits of remedial treatments after tumor therapy (DUFFNER et al. 1985).

16.3.2 Skeletal System

The skeleton shows a growth spurt during the postnatal period and again during puberty (WATZKA 1964). Only the jaw, the clavicle, and the cranial and facial bones develop by direct ossification of the mesenchyma (LEONHARDT 1977). The other bones, including the tubular bones, show enchondral ossification. Growth is characterized by processes of composition and decomposition in which cells of the mesenchyma, chondroblasts, osteoblasts, and osteoclasts participate (RIEDE et al. 1981). In addiation, proliferation of capillary endothelium takes place. Due to the complexity of bone growth late effects may result from damage to different cell types and radiation effects on the vascular-connective tissue.

Radiation effects on the skeleton of children have been investigated extensively in the vertebral column. NEUHAUSER et al. (1952) studied 45 children who had been given fractionated x-irradiation (200 kV) at ages ranging from 0.1 to 9.8 years. Total doses of less than 10 Gy resulted in either no or only slight changes to the vertebral bodies. This finding also applies to very young children less than 1 year of age. Total doses of more than 20 Gy produced severe deformation of the vertebral body contours, with marked height reduction in most cases. Doses between 10 and 20 Gy led to slight deformations which could be subdivided into two degrees of severity. The more subtle changes were irregular ossifications of the ring apophyses, associated with height reduction. The more severely damaged vertebral bodies additionally showed gross irregularities or scalloping of the vertebral epiphyseal plates with marked height reduction. Despite the limitation that most of the children in this study were less than 6 years old at the time of therapy and that those under the age of 2 had been given the higher doses, the authors concluded that the radiogenic growth disturbances of the spinal column were directly related to dosage and inversely related to age.

Regarding the dose deposition in bone, one has to be aware that it is dependent on the energy spectrum of the photon beam. At beam energies of 200 Kilovolt (kV) and higher the absorption coefficient of bone does not vary, whereas it increases at lower energies. At 200 kV and higher the roentgen to rad conversion factor for bone is about 1 (Purdy et al. 1987).

Probert and co-workers examined the growth of spinal column after megavoltage irradiation in children with Hodgkin's disease, medulloblastoma, and ALL (Probert et al. 1973; Probert and Parker 1975). The sitting height was decreased by more than two standard deviations below the mean normal values only in those patients irradiated (a) under the age of 6 years or (b) during the adolescent growth spurt; this finding was obtained in both the high (>35 Gy) and the low (<25 Gy) dose group. It was concluded that maximal radiosensitivity occurs at the time when enchondral bone formation is greatest.

Riseborough et al. (1976) followed a group of 81 patients with Wilms' tumors after irradiation at ages ranging from 1 week to 13 years. The mean total dose was 30.7 Gy (range: 15.3–61.6 Gy). Although the entire vertebral body was irradiated, 38 children developed scoliosis and 19 showed kyphoscoliosis. These skeletal alterations (especially the scolioses) were the consequence of defects in the growth of the irradiated muscles on the side of the tumor. A rapid worsening of the scoliosis frequently developed during the adolescent growth spurt. The more severe vertebral deformities were seen in patients irradiated at a younger age and with higher total doses.

Shalet et al. (1987) studied the elongatory growth of children with brain tumors after neurocranial irradiation. The total doses given to the vertebral bodies ranged from 27 to 35 Gy in 17–20 fractions. The control group consisted of children with cranial irradiation alone. This allowed the effect of GH deficiency following irradiation of the hypothalamic–hypophysial region in the control group to be taken into account too. The disproportionate shortening of the spinal column after craniospinal irradiation decreased significantly with increasing age. The authors estimated growth reduction to be 9, 7, and 5.5 cm when the spinal column was irradiated at the ages of 1, 5, and 10 years, respectively. This study does not confirm the hypothesis of Probert and co-workers, that irradiation of the spine during puberty is particularly likely to impair spinal growth.

The age and dose dependence of capital femoral slippage was studied by Silverman et al. (1981). Children under the age of 4 years at the time of irradiation were at higher risk (7/15 patients, 47%) than the older ones (1/21, 4.7%). No slippage occurred at total radiation doses lower than 25 Gy. Above this threshold, the incidence of capital femoral slippage varied only slightly with dose. Most abnormalities occurred at ages between 8 and 10 years. The latency time from radiation therapy to epiphyseal slippage ranged from 1 to 10 years. Of the children in this study, 80% received chemotherapy, in most cases dactinomycin. Libshitz and Edeiken (1981) described eight additional cases of radiation-induced abnormalities of femoral heads and epiphyses (six aseptic necroses, four of them bilateral; three slipped epiphyses) after radiotherapy in childhood. Four children were treated for Hodgkin's disease, two for rhabdomyosarcoma, one for neuroblastoma, and one for Ewing's sarcoma. The total dose to the hip was 30 Gy in four children. The remaining children received higher doses, 34–55 Gy, with conventional fractionation. Latency times to aseptic necrosis ranged from 1.4 to 13.2 years and for epiphyseal slippage from 4.5 to 10 years.

Gonzales and Breur (1983) studied the growth of irradiated long bones in children. They found that the absolute shortening of long bones after irradiation compared with the unirradiated bones depended on the total radiation dose and the age at the time of irradiation. Long bones of children irradiated under 1 year of age showed the greatest shortening at each dose level, followed by the age group from 1 to 5 years and that older than 11 years. However, when the remaining growth was considered the age at irradiation was not of significance, the irradiation dose being the most important factor.

In conclusion the growing bone is quite radiosensitive. A total dose as low as 10 Gy given in daily fractions of 2 Gy can lead to growth disturbances of the vertebral bodies. Total doses lower than 4 Gy probably do not induce abnormalities in the growing spine, even in children under 1 year old (NEUHAUSER et al. 1952; TEFFT 1972). The age dependence of the effect of irradiation on growing bone has not yet been definitely established.

In addition, there are case reports of growth disturbances to the facial bones and dental development (HARRIS et al. 1986), to the long bones (DAWSON et al. 1968), and to the ossicular chain (KVETON and SOTELO-AVILA 1986) after irradiation, as well as of slipped capital femoral epiphyses (SABIO et al. 1987; SILVERMAN et al. 1981).

16.3.3 Testes

The prepubertal testicular constituents are quiescent by morphological and biochemical criteria (KERR and DE KRETSER 1981). In the course of childhood, the male gonads show little growth change but rapid development occurs before and during puberty. In the testicles of the newborn the testicular canals are still present as solid epithelial strands. They contain only two types of cells. Small round cells give rise to the Sertoli cells. Single large cells correspond to the spermatogonial stem cells. Although these are able to proliferate prior to puberty, actual spermatogenesis only sets in at the start of puberty (LEONHARDT 1977).

Data are available on the radiosensitivity of male gonads in childhood particularly after irradiation of the testes in cases of ALL. Six months after testicular irradiation of prepubertal boys (4–10 years) with total doses of 24 Gy in 10–12 fractions over 14–16 days because of testicular relapses, LEIPER et al. (1983) found significantly lower basal and peak testosterone values after application of 1000 units of HCG than in a control group with cranial irradiation and chemotherapy given over 2–3 years. Furthermore, the peak FSH levels were significantly higher after administering luteinizing hormone releasing hormone (LHRH) to boys given testicular irradiation. The results suggest that the testosterone-producing Leydig cells suffered radiation damage. Of the 13 boys

examined, 7 showed a distinct delay or an arrest in pubertal development. Testicular irradiation with the above-mentioned doses can result in permanent and pronounced damage to the Leydig cells in ALL patients (BRAUNER et al. 1983; LEIPER et al. 1986), thus making testosterone replacement necessary. The risk appears to decrease with age between 4 and 12 years (LEIPER et al. 1986).

Following whole-body irradiation with single doses of 7.5 Gy in preparation for bone marrow transplantation in a small group of five boys aged 12.8–17.3 years, SKLAR et al. (1984) found a decreased plasma testosterone level in one case and in two cases raised LH levels with normal amounts of plasma testosterone. This indicates slight damage to the Leydig cells.

Chemotherapy, given simultaneously with testicular radiation, may have an additional negative effect. However, two studies have shown that the function of the Leydig cells in children given chemotherapy for ALL including the agents (6-mercaptopurine, methotrexate, vincristine, or BCNU) is hardly affected by chemotherapy (BLATT et al. 1981; SHALET et al. 1981).

Spermatogonia are clearly much more radiosensitive than the Leydig cells (SHALET et al. 1978; ROWLEY et al. 1974; GREINER 1982). However, broader clinical experience regarding the details of the radiosensitivity of spermatogonia in childhood is lacking.

16.3.4 Ovaries

In the ovaries of newborn girls, several hundred thousand oocytes exist as primary follicles. Most of these will have perished by the time of puberty. Starting at puberty and later, a portion of the remaining 40000 primary follicles develop into secondary follicles. Differentiation of the follicle-surrounding connective tissue occurs at the time of development into secondary and subsequently tertiary follicles (LEONHARDT 1977). In contrast to the male gonads, replication of stem cells in the ovaries no longer takes place after birth.

Ovarian failure, defined as amenorrhea accompanied by a persistent increase in the gonadotropins FSH and LH, is observed after irradiation of the ovaries during childhood. STILLMAN et al. (1981) found ovarian failure in 17 of 25 girls who had received a median gonadal total dose of 32 Gy (12–50 Gy) at the age of 6–17 years for abdominal tumors, mostly Wilms' tumors and lymphomas. In

addition, 23 of the 25 girls had received chemotherapy, in most cases involving combinations
of three or more agents (actinomycin D, chlorambucil, cyclophosphamide, methotrexate, vincristine, nitrogen mustard). In the same study no
cases of amenorrhea were observed in a group of
75 girls treated with chemotherapy only. Of 35
girls in the same study whose ovaries were located
at the periphery of the radiation field [dose to
ovary: median 2.9 Gy (0.9–10 Gy)], five developed ovarian failure. The only significant risk
factor in this study for the development of
amenorrhea was the radiation dose; the age of the
girls at therapy and the number of chemotherapeutic agents had no significant effect. However,
it appears possible that there was an interaction
between radio- and chemotherapy.

In a further study ovarian function was examined in 16 girls after irradiation of the abdomen
and pelvis at the age of 1–13 years, in most cases
for the treatment of Wilms' tumors (SHALET et al.
1976a). Total doses of 20–30 Gy were given in
25–44 days and six received additional chemotherapy (actinomycin D with or without vincristine or
cyclophosphamide and vincristine). All patients
older than 13 years at the time of last follow-up
had primary or secondary amenorrhea. FSH levels
were raised in all patients.

Further information on female reproductive
potential after ovarian irradiation in childhood or
adolescence has been derived from patients treated for Hodgkin's disease. HORNING et al. (1981)
found that 18 of 19 patients who had received total
nodal irradiation at the age of 13–28 years
(median: 22 years) later had menstruation. Of
these 18, nine had regular menstruation and seven
bore nine healthy children. Only one female
developed amenorrhea. All 19 patients had undergone midline ovariopexy at staging laparotomy. A
10-cm midline block was used to shield ovaries.
Under these conditions the minimal gonadal dose
was estimated to be 2.6–6.6 Gy in 4–6 weeks
(dosimetry: RAY et al. 1970). The median interval
between completion of therapy and start of examination was 64 months (range: 9–124 months).
In the 13–28 year age group, younger patients had
a significantly higher probability of achieving
regular menses and pregnancy than older ones.
This can be explained by the larger number of
stem cells in child ovaries (BAKER 1971).

HORNING et al. (1981) found evidence of increasing damage to the ovaries as a result of
combined radiation and chemotherapy [MOP(P),

nitrogen mustard, vincristine, and procarbazine
with or without prednisone, or procarbazing with
L-phenylalanine mustard and vinblastine] in the
treatment of Hodgkin's disease. Regular menses
were seen in 47% of women after total nodal
irradiation, in 56% after chemotherapy without
pelvic irradiation, and in only 20% after chemotherapy and pelvic irradiation.

Information about ovarian dysfunction after
bone marrow transplantation is available. SKLAR et
al. (1983) found secondary amenorrhea and increased gonadotropin levels 1.5 years after whole-
body irradiation with a single fraction of 7.5 Gy
and high dose cyclophosphamide chemotherapy in
four women aged between 15.9 and 22.5 years.
These data show that there is marked ovarian
sensitivity towards combined single dose irradiation and short-term high-dose chemotherapy in
younger women.

In larger studies it was found that rates of fetal
wastage and malformations were not increased
after total lymphoid irradiation and ovariopexy
(HORNING et al. 1981; THOMAS et al. 1976; HOLMES
and HOLMES 1978). However, there may be an
increased genetic risk after combined radio- and
chemotherapy. HOLMES and HOLMES (1978) and
McKEEN et al. (1979) observed an increased rate
of inherited defects in 13 and 44 pregnancies
respectively; in both studies, five malformations
were found.

16.3.5 Mammary Glands

The mammary glands begin to develop prior to
achievement of sexual maturity. Proliferation of
the glandular system and the interstitial connective
tissue occurs 3–5 years before menarche. The few
branched glandular ducts found in newborn girls
can be considered to be a stem cell epithelium.
This is stimulated to proliferate through the effects
of hormones before puberty (THURLBECK 1975).

KOLAR et al. (1957) observed severe right-sided
breast hypoplasia after irradiation of a 9-year-old
girl with a hemangioma in the pectoral region.
Irradiation was performed three times within 3
years with a total dose of about 24 Gy. According
to RUBIN and CASARETT (1968), doses above 10 Gy
with conventional fractionation can lead to disturbances in the normal development of the
mammary glands. A further study by KOLAR et al.
(1967) described in more detail the high sensitivity
of the infant breast. A dose of 3 Gy during the 1st

year of life interfered with a normal development. However, no changes were observed in three girls who received doses of 1 Gy or less.

16.3.6 Thyroid

The growth of the thyroid roughly parallels body growth. The average weight of the gland increases from about 1.5 g at birth to 2.5, 6.1, 8.7, and 15.8 g at 1, 5, 10, and 15 years of age, respectively. In the adult a median value of 20 g is measured. Thyroid iodine clearance (per gram tissue) decreases progressively with age. This suggests a decreasing activity of the gland which would be in accordance with the decrease in thyroxine turnover with increasing age (FISHER 1982).

Most experience regarding radiation-related functional changes in thyroids of children has been gained from the treatment of Hodgkin's disease. SHALET et al. (1977b) found a decreased serum level of thyroid hormones in 16% of patients. Minor alterations were found more often. Fifty-three percent of patients showed normal T_3 and T_4 values with raised basal levels of TSH, and a further 22% were euthyroid with a normal basal TSH level but an augmented TSH response to TRH. All patients were asymptomatic. Irradiation of the thyroid region was performed at the age of 4–15 years with total doses of 25–34 Gy in 19–25 days.

In a further study of children and adult patients with Hodgkin's disease, SCHIMPFF et al. (1980) found elevated TSH serum levels in 66% of cases and in 26% an additional lowering of the T_4 level after mantle field irradiation with total doses of 40 Gy to the thyroid region. Some patients also received chemotherapy. The high rate of thyroid hypofunction developed slowly and reached a plateau 6 years after therapy.

Lymphography is an additional risk factor in the development of hypothyroidism after radiotherapy, as has also been observed in children (FUKS et al. 1975; GLATSTEIN et al. 1970; SCHIMPFF et al. 1980; SHALET et al. 1977b; SMITH et al. 1981). The mechanism by which the prolonged release of fat-soluble organic iodide can increase the sensitivity of the thyroid to radiation remains unknown (FUKS et al. 1975).

Additional information on the frequency of thyroid dysfunctions after radiotherapy has derived from medulloblastoma patients. The radiation technique used in the treatment of this tumor

entity varies only slightly. BROWN et al. (1983) studied 13 children who, at the age of 4.7–13.3 years, had received a total dose of 20–40 Gy to the thyroid region during irradiation of the neuroaxis. Three patients received additional polychemotherapy. An increase in basal TSH levels and an enhanced TSH response to TRH, and thus compensated hypothyroidism, were seen in 54% of children. However, it is important to note that no child showed clinical evidence of hypothyroidism. HIRSCH et al. (1979) observed high basal TSH levels and an increased TSH response to TRH in 59% of children followed up after irradiation of neuroaxis. In addition, one patient had lowered T_3 and T_4 plasma levels. Increased TSH plasma levels were observed in 20% of cases treated for medulloblastoma in a study by AHMED et al. (1983). All patients received concomitant polychemotherapy.

The effect of age on the development of a dysfunction of the thyroid after irradiation is a matter of controversy. Whereas GLATSTEIN et al. (1970) and GREEN et al. (1980) observed enhanced radiosensitivity of the thyroid in younger patients, others found no significant age effect (DEVNEY et al. 1984; NELSON et al. 1978; SCHIMPFF et al. 1980; SMITH et al. 1981). GLATSTEIN et al. (1970) found the level of TSH to be raised in 48% of irradiated patients under 20, but in only 33% of older patients. However, no multivariance analysis of the different factors was carried out. The possibility that the thyroid is more radiosensitive in childhood is also supported by the high rates of increase in TSH levels – 53% and 80% respectively – found in the studies by SHALET et al. (1977b) and DEVNEY et al. (1984). In the children aged 4–16 years studied by SHALET et al. (1977b) comparatively low total doses of 25–30 Gy over 3 weeks were applied.

The various studies show that hypothyroidism is dose dependent (GLATSTEIN et al. 1970; NELSON et al. 1978). The study by GLATSTEIN et al. (1970) was on children with malignant lymphoma. No patient had an elevated level of TSH after total doses of 15 Gy. In contrast, elevated levels were seen in 44% of cases after doses of 40–45 Gy to the whole neck.

CONSTINE et al. (1984) found thyroid abnormalities in 17% of children who received 26 Gy or less and in 78% who received greater radiation doses to the thyroid during treatment for Hodgkin's disease. In all but three of the 119 children studied the abnormality included the development of elevated TSH levels. Age, sex, and administration of chemotherapy were not significant factors in development of thyroid dysfunction in this study.

It should be emphasized that the endocrinological changes are often not associated with any clinical signs. After polychemotherapy alone for Hodgkin's disease, dysfunctions of the thyroid were rarely observed (Devney et al. 1984; Schimpff et al. 1980).

16.3.7 Lung

The most rapid phase of alveolar multiplication and cellular proliferation occurs during the first 3 years of life, and especially in the first postnatal months. A period of comparatively slower growth follows. The number of alveoli increases from 20 millions at birth to above 300 millions at the age of 8 years. Later, the growth of the gas exchanging surface is characterized by an increase in volume but not in the number of alveoli. The vascular system grows in parallel with proliferation of the alveoli (Brasel and Gruen 1978; Hodson 1977; Simon et al. 1972; Thurlbeck 1975).

A specific radiation effect in children can be the disturbance or impairment of the formation of new alveoli (Rubin et al. 1982). Furthermore, radiogenic muscular atrophy or radiation effects on the growing cartilage and bones may lead to failures in the development of the thoracic skeleton and thus to a reduced size of the lung (Benoist et al. 1982; Rubin et al. 1982). Generally from a clinical point of view the lung is more sensitive than other tissues of the thorax, particularly the spinal cord, esophagus, and heart (Travis 1987).

Data in children are comparable with observations in adults (Molls and van Beuningen, this volume). Forty-four patients, most of them young (nine patients younger than 10 years, 21 between 10 and 15 years, nine between 15 and 20 years, and five patients older than 20 years), received irradiation of the lungs as adjuvant therapy in the treatment of osteosarcoma. The total dose delivered to the lungs was 20 Gy within 12 days, five fractions per week. This procedure caused no clinical symptoms of impairment of lung function in any of the patients, of whom 60% were still alive 2 years after treatment (Breur et al. 1978).

In a recently published study whole lung irradiation with or without Adriamycin was given to treat pulmonary micrometastases in osteosarcoma patients (Zaharia et al. 1986). The mean age of the comparatively young individuals was 15.2 years. All patients received 20 Gy tissue dose with daily doses of 1.5 Gy, five times a week. The mean lung radiation dose was 20.7 Gy. No significant clinical side-effects occurred. After mantle field irradiation the incidence of pulmonary reactions among children was 4% ($n = 6$), which was no higher than among adults (Donaldson and Kaplan 1982). The aforementioned study involved 153 children with Hodgkin's disease who were treated at Stanford University and followed up over a period of 20 years.

Comparing the clinical and radiographic observations in irradiated children and adults one can conclude that the level of tolerance is similar for both groups. According to Philips and Margolis (1972) the dose required to cause clinical pneumonitis in 5% of patients is about 26.5 Gy delivered in 20 fractions. However, investigations on pulmonary functions reveal alterations which seem to occur especially when irradiation has been performed relatively early during infancy.

Forty-eight children (age: 1–13 years; mean: 4 years) were treated for Wilms' tumors and metastases in the study by Benoist et al. (1982). They received bilateral lung irradiation. The total dose was 20 Gy given in 3 weeks. In five patients Actinomycin D was given concomitantly with irradiation. Lung function tests were performed before irradiation and were repeated annually. The follow-up was 2–17 years. Static pressure volume curves, blood gases, and carbon monoxide transfer were normal but reductions in lung volume and dynamic compliance were observed. In some patients these changes occurred during the initial months following irradiation; in most cases the decreases progressed over longer periods. It was concluded that involvement of pulmonary fibrosis was unlikely. Another explanation was an injury to alveoli and peripheral airways. In particular they may have failed to develop at this age of alveolar multiplication. In addition disturbed growth and function of the chest wall was discussed as a reason for the progressive diminution of lung volume. Comparable functional alterations have been found in a previous, small series of children with Wilms' tumor and prophylactic lung irradiation (doses lower than 14 Gy) (Littman et al. 1976). The data suggested moderately reduced lung volumes. However, as in the study by Benoist et al. (1982), these changes were not generally severe.

With regard to the question of whether differences in sensitivity exist between children and adults, some new aspects have emerged recently. In a retrospective study WEINER et al. (1986) analyzed data from 920 patients with leukemia who had received bone marrow transplants after conditioning by means of chemotherapy and total body irradiation. Unfortunately, the report of this multi-institutional study did not give full details of the radiation modalities. The mean lung doses were in the range 5.6–12.8 Gy. Some patients received 12 Gy in five or six fractions, others 10 Gy in one fraction. The dose rates varied between 0.02 and 1.08 Gy/min (in 358 patients the dose rate was lower than 0.1 Gy/min). Five factors were associated with an increased risk of interstitial pneumonitis: use of methotrexate rather than cyclosporine to prevent graft-versus-host disease, a long interval from diagnosis to transplantation, Karnofsky indices before transplantation of less than 100%, high dose rate irradiation in patients given methotrexate after transplantation, and older age. With regard to the last-mentioned factor, the incidence of interstitial pneumonitis increased with age from about 20% (1–10 years) and 22% (11–20 years) to about 34% (21–30 years), 36% (31–40 years), and 43% (41–59 years).

One has to be very careful when interpreting these data. Besides irradiation many factors are involved in the development of interstitial pneumonitis (MOLLS et al. 1986; MOLLS and VAN BEUNINGEN, this volume). The significance of these factors may differ between children and adults. The facultative adverse effects of chemotherapy with regard to morbidity of the lung are known. They may add to the effect of irradiation (RUBIN et al. 1982). WEINER et al. (1986) discussed the possibility that the lower incidence of interstitial pneumonitis in younger patients could be related to differences in previous lung damage or to age-related differences in drug metabolism, toxicity, tissue resistance to radiation and chemotherapeutic agents, or ability to repair tissue injury. According to WEINER et al. (1986) the difference might also reflect the increased likelihood of older patients having had prior exposure to cytomegalovirus (with reactivation after transplantation). This assumption was supported by the observation that cytomegalovirus pneumonia occurred in only 6% of the 451 patients younger than 21 years of age whereas the incidence was 15% in the 478 older patients. Thus, the association of age with the risk of pneumonitis was strong among patients with cytomegalovirus-associated disease. However, it was pointed out that the age

of the patient was also an important risk factor for idiopathic interstitial pneumonitis, in which no infectious agent can be identified and which at least in part is related to irradiation and possibly to chemotherapy

Summarizing the observations after irradiation of children and with regard to radiation pneumonitis, there is a lot of evidence that the lung in children is no more sensitive than the lung in adults. Moreover, the data suggest that the lung in children in fact may be comparatively more resistant than the lung in adults. This could be due to a better repair capacity (RUBIN and CASARETT 1972). This hypothesis might be favored by the above-described observations after total body irradiation and bone marrow transplantation (WEINER et al. 1986). On the other hand, especially when irradiating very young children one has to take into account the fact that disturbances of cell proliferation in the growing lung and thoracic skeleton may lead to reduced lung volume and late functional injuries.

16.3.8 Other Organs Which May Limit Radiation Therapy in Childhood Cancer

16.3.8.1 Kidney

The development of nephrons is completed at the time of birth (DARMADY and MACIVER 1980). Postnatally, the growth of the kidney is characterized by hypertrophism.

There are no clinical data indicative of a particularly high radiosensitivity of the kidney during childhood. RUBIN (1984) indicated the tolerance doses for 5% acute nephritis and chronic nephrosclerosis within 5 years to be 15 and 20 Gy total dose, respectively, with conventional dose fractionation. Similarly, the recommendations of the national Wilms' tumor study number 1 were not to exceed 15 Gy total dose in daily fractions of 2 Gy to the remaining single kidney (TEFFT 1977a). MITUS et al. (1969) examined renal function in children with Wilms' tumors, neuroblastomas, and renal cell carcinomas following one-sided nephrectomy, radiotherapy, and chemotherapy with dactinomycin. No information about dose fractionation was given. Reduced creatinine clearance was seen in 18% of children who had received total doses of less than 12 Gy. At doses of 12–24 Gy and more than 24 Gy the corresponding values were 33% and 76%, respectively. No evidence for increased radiosensitivity of the child organ compared with that of the adult can be deduced from this large group of, in part, very young children (median 6.5 years; range 0.5–18 years). This is especially true considering that the children received radiation in combination with chemotherapy, which can enhance the side-effects in the kidney (Rubin 1984).

16.3.8.2 Liver

The liver grows slowly until puberty. At birth all the cells have a diploid nucleus. At the beginning of puberty the number of liver cells with two nuclei increases. In addition tetraploid and octaploid nuclei occur (Ahmed 1967).

Two larger studies on the radiosensitivity of the liver in childhood are available. In 1970, Tefft et al. published a review involving 115 children who had received liver irradiation (250 kV x-rays, 10 Gy per week in five or six equal fractions). The total doses were arranged in three classes (less than 25 Gy, from 25 to 35 Gy, and more than 35 Gy) given to either a partial volume or the whole organ. All children received additional chemotherapy – 108 Actinomycin D, six an alkylating agent, and one 5-fluorouracil – so that the effect of radiotherapy alone could not be distinguished. The authors observed a slight trend towards higher radiosensitivity in children under 1 year of age for the early phase of liver damage within 6 months after therapy. No influence of age was seen in the chronic phase more than 6 months after radiation, which is characterized by abnormalities in liver function tests, in serum enzymes (in particular alkaline phosphatase), or on liver scintigrams.

Radiogenic coinduced liver damage in 17 of 263 irradiated children was seen in the national Wilms' tumor study number 1 (Tefft 1977a). The administered drugs were Actinomycin D and vincristine. Of these 17 patients with liver damage, ten showed clinically evident signs with liver enlargement, ascites, or liver failure; the others developed temporary abnormalities in liver function tests without clinical symptoms. Liver damage was manifest in all patients within 2–4 months after the start of radio- and chemotherapy. Recovery occurred in 12 cases within a further 2–4 months. In general, the degree and frequency of liver damage were dependent on the dose and liver volume irradiated.

The following details of this study are interesting with regard to the dose and volume dependency of liver damage. Three patients who received total doses below 15 Gy to the whole liver had a boost to a portion of the liver to more than 30 Gy. Two of them showed liver toxicities. Liver toxicities developed in two of ten children who received a total dose to the entire liver of between 15 and 24 Gy, in one of 12 who received 24–30 Gy, and in two of three who received more than 30 Gy. A minority of these children received a boost to more than 30 Gy to parts of the liver. Dose fractions of 2 Gy were given five times per week. Since the total dose given was age dependent, no definite statements as to the age dependence of the radiosensitivity of the liver could be made. However, the impression arose that in very young children (below 1.5 years) this organ was comparatively more sensitive, even though they had received total doses smaller than 15 Gy.

16.3.8.3 Heart

The development of the heart is characterized by hypertrophic growth of the muscle cells (Riede et al. 1981). Morphologically, an increase in the diameter and the number of myofibrils is observed. From birth until the age of 7 years 90% of the cell nuclei are diploid. Then, the DNA content per cell doubles, and most of the cells of the adult heart show a tetraploid genome. The weight of the heart increases from 20 g at birth to about 300 g in the adult (Riede et al. 1981).

In the heart three different tissues have to be considered as radiation targets: the myocardium, the endocardium, and the epicardium. While the muscle cells, which are largely postmitotically fixed, are rather insensitive to direct action of irradiation, the fine vasculature is only moderately resistant. Damage to the fine vasculature leads to alterations of the connective tissue and indirectly of the heart muscle (Casarett 1980).

The following diseases may occur after irradiation of the heart: acute pericarditis (increased vascular permeability, plasmatic transudation, fine vascular obstruction, acute inflammation), chronic pericarditis (pericardial effusion and fibrosis, constrictive pericarditis associated with myocardial fibrosis and endocardial fibroelastosis, adhesions, constricting fibrosis), coronary artery disease with myocardial infarction, mitral valve insufficiency, and myocardial disease. Heart injury is related to radiation dose, dose rate, and volume treated.

Among 120 children with Hodgkin's disease who received high dose mantle field irradiation, 16 developed signs or symptoms of carditis (DONALDSON and KAPLAN 1982). After this experience the authors refined the radiotherapy technique, including cardiac and subcarinal blocks and modification of the total dose. Carditis related to radiation alone was no longer observed. According to DONALDSON and KAPLAN (1982), the low incidence of arterial vascular injury following high dose mantle field irradiation with subsequent development of premature coronary artery disease is of particular concern. In the Stanford University pediatric experience there have been two such cases, one of which was lethal. A 15-year-old boy died of myocardial infarction 16 months after receiving 40 Gy to the supradiaphragmatic lymph nodes for Hodgkin's disease. There was no known familial or metabolic predisposition to atherosclerosis. Autopsy revealed intimal proliferation and atheromatous deposits in the coronary arteries with a fresh myocardial infarction (STEWART et al. 1967).

However, as pointed out by FAJARDO (1977), coronary artery disease should not be an important consideration when planning a course of radiotherapy because the incidence of coronary disease appears to be very low. In the majority of cases radiation-induced heart injury will be mild and confined to the pericardium (FAJARDO 1977). Late complications in the heart are a particular concern when chemotherapy (especially anthracyclines) is administered in addition to radiotherapy (DONALDSON and KAPLAN 1982).

16.4 Carcinogenesis

A severe late complication following irradiation during childhood is the development of neoplasia. In the following, only those studies are taken into consideration that have analyzed data from larger groups of children irradiated for malignant diseases during childhood. Assessment of the risk is especially difficult because children are mostly treated with radio- and chemotherapy, and separation of the effects of the two modalities is necessary. Furthermore, data from large, well-characterized patient populations are scant at present. Data concerning children with retinoblastomas are not considered here because of such children's particular genetic disposition to

the induction of second tumors (TUCKER et al. 1987a).

16.4.1 Leukemia

MIKE et al. (1982) analyzed the incidence of second malignant neoplasms after therapy for pediatric cancer in a population of almost 15000 patients from ten centers of the late effect study group with 77460 person-years (PY, product of the number of patients and the mean follow-up period) at risk. A total of 13 leukemias were observed as second tumors. This corresponds to an incidence of $16.8/10^5$ PY. The highest incidences of leukemia of $84/10^5$ PY and $30.6/10^5$ PY were found after therapy for Hodgkin's disease and Wilms' tumor respectively. In the normal population the incidence in children is estimated to be $3/10^5$ PY. The person-year concept assumes a constant incidence of leukemia during the follow-up period. From other studies it is known that the peak incidence of radiation-induced leukemia occurs 7–8 years after exposure (FINCH 1984). Of the above 13 children, 70% received radiation during primary therapy. All leukemias in irradiated children were classified as radiation associated, since the bone marrow was exposed at least to scattered irradiation. In this review the risk factors for the development of leukemias as second tumors could not be established because of the multitude of therapeutic parameters involved in the treatment of the various primary tumors. Contributions of familial or genetic predisposing conditions as possible risk factors could not be determined. This study shows an association between the incidence of leukemia and therapy for childhood cancer, but not a causal dependence of leukemia induction on irradiation.

Further data concerning the incidence of leukemia, mainly acute myeloblastic leukemia (AML) after therapy for childhood cancer, derived from centers of the late effect study group and were reported by TUCKER et al. (1984). The risk of AML increased 89-, 13-, and 62-fold respectively after therapy for Hodgkin's disease, Wilms' tumor, and Ewing's sarcoma. The number of patients irradiated for the individual tumor entities were not given. The effects of the age of the child at therapy and the radiation dose were not analyzed.

An analysis of the influence of the dose of alkylating agents, doxorubicin, and radiation on leukemia risk in long-term surviving children from the late effect study group showed a strong dose–response relationship between leukemia risk and dose of alkylating agents (TUCKER et al. 1987b). The relative risk of leukemia reached a factor of 23 in the highest dose group. A lower risk was seen for doxorubicin. The radiation dose had no influence on the leukemia risk. An analysis of cases of leukemia after therapy for Hodgkin's disease at Stanford University also showed an enhanced leukemia risk which was associated with MOP (P) chemotherapy and which was largely independent of radiation dose (ROSENBERG and KAPLAN 1985).

Thus, the radiation dose does not appear to be a major risk factor for leukemia in the currently used combined therapy schedules for childhood tumors.

16.4.2 Bone and Soft Tissue Sarcoma

Bone and soft tissue sarcomas are the most frequent secondary tumors following cancer therapy in childhood (MIKE et al. 1982; TUCKER et al. 1984, 1987a). The risk of bone and soft tissue sarcomas is increased 133- and 41-fold respectively in children after tumor therapy as compared with the untreated normal population (TUCKER et al. 1984, 1987a). A steep dose–response relationship for the development of bone sarcomas in the radiation field was found for increasing radiation doses from 0 to 80 Gy. At doses higher than 80 Gy the risk decreased; probably those cells which underwent malignant transformation were also killed. Upon separating the carcinogenic effect of radiotherapy from that of alkylating agents the risk also increased with cumulative drug dose.

16.4.3 Thyroid Carcinoma

According to two reports of the late effect study group (MIKE et al. 1982; TUCKER et al. 1984), the frequency of thyroid carcinomas ranks second or third behind bone and soft tissue sarcomas after irradiation for childhood cancer. MIKE et al. (1982) found 17 thyroid carcinomas in a total of almost 15 000 child tumor patients who had been treated during the period 1950–1970. TUCKER et al. (1984) found a 53-fold risk (female: 45-fold, male: 75-fold) for the development of a thyroid carcinoma after tumor therapy in childhood. In both studies, the highest relative risks were seen in

patients with Hodgkin's disease, neuroblastoma, and Wilms' tumor. KAPLAN et al. (1983) found three thyroid carcinomas during a follow-up period of 5–34 years in a much smaller group of 95 patients. The frequency of benign and malignant palpable thyroid abnormalities increased with duration of follow-up but was dependent neither on the radiation dose (30–50 Gy) to the thyroid region nor on the level of TSH. It is important to recognize that thyroid carcinomas have a markedly better prognosis than the other radiation-induced cancers mentioned.

16.5 Final Remarks

This review has concentrated on chronic side-effects after irradiation of children. Whereas morphological and functional alterations of the normal tissues occur after exceeding organ-specific threshold doses (Table 16.1), radiation-induced malignant tumors can develop even after comparatively low doses. The observations reported here show that considerable knowledge has accumulated concerning the risk of irradiation during childhood. However, studies in children treated for cancer with combined modalities entail the difficulty of estimating the quantitative contribution of each treatment to adverse reactions. In most cases the adverse effects of radio- and chemotherapy will be more severe than would be expected for radiotherapy alone. Furthermore, there are situations in which a late effect is mainly related to chemotherapy and only to a minor degree to radiation. This is true for second malignancies after treatment for Hodgkin's disease.

The radiotherapist is well acquainted with the possibilities to minimize radiation-induced normal tissue damage. Concerning late effects, the appropriate spatial dose distribution (shrinking field technique; symmetrical irradiation of the skeleton) decreases failures in the growth of bones. Most important is the reduction in the dose per fraction as practiced for example in very young children receiving cranial irradiation for brain tumors. In total body irradiation prior to bone marrow transplantation, low dose rate irradiation ($<0.06–0.1$ Gy/min; MOLLS and VAN BEUNINGEN, this volume) is beneficial with regard to pulmonary morbidity. However, lowering the dose per fraction may also spare tumors, which can have large

Table 16.1. Critical doses of normal tissues in children and adults[a]

Organ	Effect	Children[b]	Adults
Brain	Necrosis	50–55 Gy* (>5 years) 45–50 Gy* (3–5 years) 40–45 Gy* (< 3 years)	50–55 Gy
	Growth hormone deficiency	18–24 Gy	
	Other hypophysial defiencies	>30 Gy	
	Neuropsychological changes	~20 Gy (ALL)	
Lens	Cataract	~8 Gy	8 Gy
Skeleton	Necrosis, fracture		60 Gy
	Minor growth disturbances	>10 Gy	
	Significant growth disturbances	>20 Gy	
Lung	Pneumonitis, fibrosis		40 Gy (lobe)
		20 Gy (whole organ)	20 Gy (whole organ)
Heart	Pericarditis	40 Gy (whole organ)	40 Gy (whole organ)
Kidney	Nephritis		20 Gy (whole organ)
	Lowered creatinine clearance	12–20 Gy	
Testes	Severe impairment of Leydig cell function	24 Gy	
	Azoospermia		1.5 Gy
Ovaries	Menstruation irregularities	3 Gy	2–3 Gy
Mammary glands	Hypoplasia	10–20 Gy	
Thyroid	Dysfunction	20–40 Gy	40 Gy

[a] The table gives critical total doses or dose ranges for which radiation-induced organ injuries have been reported. The radiation effects were observed in a small percentage of irradiated individuals. Doses per fraction were 1.8–2.0 Gy (conventional fractionation) or lower. In the latter case, the tissues under consideration (lens, ovary, testes) were either outside the target volume and did not receive the full dose or the dose per fraction was lowered due to the very young age of the children (brain). The critical total doses for children are deduced from the literature as reviewed in this article and from textbooks of pediatric oncology (RIEHM 1986; GUTJAHR 1987). Most of the values for adults were published by RUBIN and CASARETT (1968) or are in accordance with broad clinical experience in radiotherapy. The value for azoospermia was reported by GREINER (1982).
[b]* whole brain irradiation.

repair capacities (STUSCHKE et al. 1989). The therapeutic gain which can be expected from superfractionation (small dose per fraction; higher total dose than in conventional regimes, same level of side-effects; constant overall treatment time) still remains to be established for pediatric tumors.

Modern clinical and experimental radiotherapy is contributing to the improvement of cure rates in pediatric oncology and striving for a further reduction in side-effects, which means further optimization of the therapeutic ratio. However, if after treatment chronic alterations develop they have to be detected as early as possible for prompt alleviation of symptoms by either conservative or surgical means. The radiotherapist is familiar with these problems on a clinical and radiobiological basis. Therefore it is necessary that he cooperates in the follow-up programs with the pediatric oncologist.

References

Abayomi OK, Sadeghi-Nejad A (1986) The incidence of late endocrine dysfunction following irradiation for childhood medulloblastoma. Int J Radiat Oncol Biol Phys 12: 945–948

Ahmed MM (1967) Age and sex differences in the structure of the tunica media of the human aorta. Acta Anat (Basel) 66: 45–58

Ahmed SR, Shalet SM, Campbell RH, Deakin DP (1983) Primary gonadal damage following treatment of brain tumors in childhood. J Pediatr 103: 562–565

Ahmed SR, Shalet SM, Beardwell CG (1986) The effects of cranial irradiation on growth hormone secretion. Acta Paediatr Scand 75: 255–260

Baker TG (1971) Radiosensitivity of mammalian oocytes with reference to the human female. Am J Obstet Gynecol 110: 746–761

Bamberg M (1987) Nervensystem. In: Scherer E (ed) Strahlentherapie, Radiologische Onkologie. Springer, Berlin Heidelberg New York

Bamford FN, Jones PM, Pearson D et al. (1976) Residual

disabilities in children treated for intracranial space-occupying lesions. Cancer 37: 1149–1151

Benoist MR, Lemerle J, Jean R, Rufin P, Scheinmann P, Panpe J (1982) Effects on pulmonary function of whole lung irradiation for Wilm's tumour children. Thorax 37: 175–180

Blatt J, Poplack DG, Shering, RJ (1981) Testicular function in boys after chemotherapy for acute lymphoblastic leukaemia. N Engl J Med 304: 1121–1124

Bleyer WA, Griffin TW (1980) White matter necrosis, mineralizing microangiopathy, and intellectual abilities in survivors of childhood leukaemia; association with central nervous system irradiation and methotrexate therapy. In: Gilbert HA, Kagan AR (eds) Radiation damage to the nervous system. Raven, New York, pp 155–174

Bloom HJG (1982) Intracranial tumors: response and resistance to therapeutic endeavors, 1970–1980. Int J Radiat Biol Phys 8: 1083–1113

Bloom HJG, Wallace ENK, Henk JM (1969) The treatment and prognosis of medulloblastoma in children. AJR 105: 43–62

Bouchard J, Peirce CB (1960) Radiation therapy in the management of neoplasms of the central nervous system with special note in regard to children: Twenty years' experience, 1939–1958. AJR 84: 610–628

Brasel JA, Gruen RK (1978) Cellular growth: Brain, liver, muscle and lung. In: Falkner, Tanner (eds) Human growth, vol 2. Potential growth. Plenum, New York, pp 3–19

Brämswig JH, Wegele M, von Lengerke, HJ, Müller RP, Schellong G (1989) The effect of the number of fractions of cranial irradiation on growth in children with acute lymphoblastic leukaemia. Acta Paediatr Scand 78: 269–302

Brauner R, Czernichow P, Cramer P et al. (1983) Leydig cell function in children after direct testicular irradiation for acute lymphoblastic leukaemia. N Engl J Med 309: 25–28

Brecher ML, Freeman AI, Glicksman AS et al. (1983) Long-term toxicity of central nervous system prophylaxis in acute lymphoblastic leukaemia. In: Freeman AI, Pochely C (eds) Controversies in pediatric and adolescent haematology/oncology. Massen,

Breur K, Cohen P, Schweisguth O, Hart AMM (1978) Irradiation of the lungs as an adjuvant therapy in the treatment of osteosarcoma of the limbs. Eur J Cancer 14: 461–471

Brown H, Lee TJ, Eden OB, Bullimore JA, Savage DCL (1983) Growth and endocrine function after treatment for medulloblastoma. Arch. Dis. Child 58: 722–727

Casarett GW (1980) Radiation histopathology, vols I and II. CRC, Boca Raton, Fl.

Chessells M (1985) Cranial irradiation in childhood lymphoblastic leukaemia: time for reappraisal? Br Med J 291: 686–687

Cicognani A, Cacciari E, Vecci V, Cau M, Balsamo A, Pirazzoli P, Tosi MT, Rosito P, Paolucci G (1988) Differential effects of 18- and 24-Gy cranial irradiation on growth rate and growth hormone release in children with prolonged survival after acute lymphocytic leukemia. A.J. Dis. Child. 142: 1199–1202

Constine LS, Donaldson SS, McDougall R, Cox RS, Link MP, Kaplan HS (1984) Thyroid dysfunction after radiotherapy in children with Hodgkin's disease. Cancer 53: 878–883

Constine LS, Konski A, Ekholm S, McDonald S, Rubin P (1988) Adverse effects of brain irradiation correlated with MR and CT imaging. Int J Radiat Biol Phys 15: 319–330

Cumberlin RL, Luk KH, Wara WM, Sheline EG, Wilson CB (1979) Medulloblastoma: treatment results and effects on normal tissues. Cancer 43: 1014–1020

Cushing H (1930) Experience with cerebellar medulloblastoma: Critical review. Acta Pathol Microbiol Scand 7: 1–86

Dacou-Voutetakis C, Haidas S, Zannos-Mariolea L (1975) Radiation and pituitary function in children. Lancet II: 1206–1207

Danoff BF, Cowchock FS, Marquette C et al. (1982) Assessment of the long-term effects of primary radiation therapy for brain tumors in children. Cancer 49: 1580–1586

Darmady EM, MacIver AG (1980) Renal pathology. Butterworths, London, Boston, p 43

Dawson WB (1968) Growth impairment following radiotherapy in childhood. Clin Radiol 19: 241–256

Devney RB, Sklar CA, Nesbit ME, Kim TH, Williamson JF, Robison LL, Ramsay NK (1984) Serial thyroid function measurements in children with Hodgkin's disease. J Pediatr 105: 223–227

Dickinson WP, Berry DH, Dickinson L et al. (1978) Differential effects of cranial radiation on growth hormone response to arginine and insulin infusion. J Pediatr 92: 754–757

Dobbing J, Sands J (1973) The quantitative growth and development of the human brain. Arch Dis Child 48: 757–767

Donaldson SS, Kaplan SS (1982) Complications of treatment of Hodgkin's disease in children. Cancer Treat Rep 66: 977–989

Duffner PK, Cohen ME, Anderson SW et al. (1983) Long-term effects of treatment on endocrine function in children with brain tumors. Ann Neurol 14: 528–532

Duffner PK, Cohen ME, Voorhess ML (1985) Long-term effects of cranial irradiation on endocrine function in children with brain tumors. Cancer 56: 2189–2193

Eiser C (1978) Intellectual abilities among survivors of childhood leukaemia as a function of CNS irradiation. Arch Dis Child 53: 391–395

Eiser C (1980) Effect of chronic illness on intellectual development. Arch Dis Child 55: 766–770

Eiser C, Lansdown R (1977) Retrospective study of intellectual development in children treated for acute lymphoblastic leukaemia. Arch Dis Child 52: 525–529

Enesco M, Leblond CP (1962) Increase in cell number as a factor in the growth of the organs and tissues of the young male rat. J Embryol Exp Morphol 10: 530 ff.

Esseltine DW, Freeman CR, Chevalier R et al. (1981) Computed tomography brain scans in long-term survivors of childhood acute lymphoblastic leukaemia. Med Pediatr Oncol 9: 429–438

Fajardo LF (1977) Radiation induced coronary artery disease. Chest 71: 563–564

Finch SC (1984) Leukemia and lymphomas in atomic bomb survivors. In: Boice JD, Fraumeni JF (eds) Radiation carcinogenesis: epidemiology and biological significance. Raven, New York, pp 37–44

Fisher DA (1982) Thyroid physiology and function tests in infancy and childhood, In: The thyroid, a fundamental clinical text, Harper and Row, Hagerstown, pp 375–383

Fisher JN, Rhomes JA (1982) Endocrine assessment in

childhood acute lymphocytic leukemia. Cancer 49: 145–151

Fuks Z, Glatstein E, Marsa GW, Bagshaw MA, Kaplan HS (1975) Long-term effects of external radiation on the pituitary and thyroid glands. Cancer 37: 1152–1161

Glatstein E, McHardy-Young S, Brast N, Eltringham JR, Kriss JP (1970) Alterations in serum thyrotropin (TSH) and thyroid function following radiotherapy in patients with malignant lymphoma. J Clin Endocrinol 32: 833–841

Gonzales D, Breur K (1983) Clinical data from irradiated growing long bones in children. Int J Radiat Oncol Biol Phys 9: 841–846

Green EM, Grecher ML, Yakar D et al. (1980) Thyroid function in pediatric patients after neck irradiation for Hodgkin's disease. Med Pediatr Oncol 8: 127 ff.

Greiner R (1982) Die Erholung der Spermatogenese nach fraktionierter, niedrig dosierter Bestrahlung der männlichen Gonaden. Strahlentherapie 158: 342–355

Gutjahr P (1987) Krebs bei Kindern und Jugendlichen. Deutscher Ärzte-Verlag, Köln

Harris AMP, Nortje CJ, Luchhesi MV (1986) Some effects of radiation therapy during early childhood on facial growth and tooth development. J Dent Assoc South Africa 41: 681–686

Hart RW, Setlow RB (1976) DNA repair in late-passage human cells. Mech Ageing Dev 15: 67–77

Havers W (1987) Maligne Erkrankungen im Kindesalter. In: Scherer E (ed) Strahlentherapie, Radiologische Onkologie. Springer, Berlin Heidelberg New York, pp 1333–1354

Hirsch JF, Renier D, Czernichow P et al. (1979) Medulloblastoma in childhood. Survival and functional results. Acta Neurochir (Wien) 48: 1–15

Hodson W (1977) Development of the lung. Dekker, New York

Holmes GE, Holmes FF (1978) Pregnancy outcome of patients treated for Hodgkin's disease: a controlled study. Cancer 41: 1317–1322

Horning SJ, Hoppe RT, Kaplan HS, Rosenberg SA (1981) Female reproductive potential after treatment for Hodgkin's disease. N Engl J Med 304: 1377–1382

Jannoun L (1983) Are cognitive and eductional development affected by age at which prophylactic therapy is given in acute lymphoblastic leukaemia? Arch Dis Child 58: 953–958

Kaatsch P, Michaelis J (1985). Jahresbericht 1984 über die kooperative Dokumentation von Malignomen im Kindesalter. Institut für medizinische Statistik und Dokumentation, Universität Mainz

Kaplan MM, Garnick MB, Gelber R et al. (1983) Risk factors for thyroid abnormalities after neck irradiation for childhood cancer. Am J Med 74: 272–280

Kerr JB, De Kretser DM (1981) The cytology of human testis. In: Burger H, De Kretser DM (eds) The testis, vol 4. Raven, New York, pp 141–169

Kolar J, Vrabec R, Bek V (1957) Entwicklungsstörungen der weiblichen Brust nach Röntgenbestrahlung im Kindesalter. Strahlentherapie 104: 596–599

Kolar J, Bek V, Vrabec R (1967) Hypoplasia of the growing breast. Arch Dermatol 96: 427–432

Kun LE, Mulhern RK, Crisco JJ (1983) Quality of life in children treated for brain tumors. J Neurosurg 58: 1–6

Kveton JF, Sotelo-Avila C (1986) Osteoradionecrosis of the ossicular chain. Am J Otol 7: 446–448

Ladavas E, Missiroli G, Rosito P, Serra L, Vecchi V (1985)

Intellectual function in long-term survivors of childhood acute lymphoblastic leukaemia. Int J Neurol Sci 6: 451–455

Lannering B, Albertsson-Wikland K (1987) Growth hormone release in children after cranial irradiation. Horm Res 27: 13–22

Leiper AD, Grant DB, Chessels JM (1983) The effect of testicular irradiation on Leydig cell function in prepubertal boys with acute lymphoblastic leukaemia. Arch Dis Child 58: 906–910

Leiper AD, Grant DB, Chessels JM (1986) Gonadal function after testicular irradiation for acute lymphoblastic leukaemia. Arch Dis Child 61: 53–56

Leonhardt H (1977) Histologie, Zytologie und Mikroanatomie des Menschen. Thieme, Stuttgart

Li, F.P., Winston, K.R., Gimbrere, K. (1984) Follow up of children with brain tumors. Cancer 54, 135–138

Libshitz HI, Edeiken BS (1981) Radiotherapy changes of the pediatric hip. AJR 137: 585–588

Littman P, Meadows AT, Polgar G, Borns PF, Rubin E (1976) Pulmonary function in survivors of Wilm's tumor. Cancer 37: 2773–2776

McIntosh S, Klatskin EH, O'Brien RT (1976) Chronic neurologic disturbance in childhood leukaemia. Cancer 37: 853–857

McKeen EA, Mulvihill JJ, Rosner F, Zarrabi MH (1979) Pregnancy outcome in Hodgkin's disease. Lancet II: 590

Meadows AT, Massari DJ, Ferguson J et al. (1981) Declines in IQ scores and cognitive dysfunctions in children with acute lymphocytic leukaemia treated with cranial irradiation. Lancet II: 1015–1018

Mike V, Meadows AT, D'Angio GJ (1982) Incidence of second malignant neoplasms in children: results of an international study. Lancet II: 1326–1331

Mitus A, Tefft M, Fellers FX (1969) Long-term follow-up of renal functions of 108 children who underwent nephrectomy for malignant disease. Pediatrics 44: 912–921

Molls M, Streffer C, van Beuningen D, Zamboglou N (1982) x-irradiation in G_2 Phase of two-cell mouse embryos in vitro: cleavage, blastulation, cell kinetics and fetal development. Radiat Res 91: 219–234

Molls M, Budach V, Bamberg M (1986) Total body irradiation: the lung as critical organ. Strahlenther Onkol 162: 226–232

Moss HA, Nannis ED, Poplack DG (1981) The effects of prophylactic treatment of the central nervous system on the intellectual functioning of children with acute lymphoblastic leukaemia. Am J Med 71: 47–52

Nelson DF, Reddy KV, O'Mara RE, Rubin P (1978) Thyroid abnormalities following neck irradiation for Hodgkin's disease. Cancer 42: 2553–2562

Neuhauser EBD, Wittenborg MH, Berman CZ, Cohen J (1952) Irradiation effects of roentgen therapy on the growing spine. Radiology 59: 637–650

Ochs JJ, Parvey LS, Whitaker JN et al. (1983) Serial cranial computed tomography scans in children with leukaemia given two different forms of central nervous therapy. J Clin Oncol 1: 793–798

Onoyama Y, Abe M, Takahashi M et al. (1975) Radiation therapy of brain tumors in children. Radiology 115: 687–693

Perez CA, Brady CW (eds) (1987) Principles and practice of radiation oncology. JB Lippincott, Philadelphia

Philips TL, Margolis L (1972) Radiation pathology and the

clinical response of lung and esophagus. Front Radiat Ther Oncol 16: 254–273

Pizzo PA, Miser JS, Cassady JR, Filler RM (1985) Solid tumors of childhood. In: De Vita VT Jr, Hellman S, Rosenberg SA (eds) Cancer principles and practice of oncology. JB Lippincott, Philadelphia pp 1511–1589

Price RA, Jamieson PA (1975) The central nervous system in childhood leukaemia II. Subacute leukencephalopathy. Cancer 35: 306–318

Probert JC, Parker BR (1975) The effects of radiation therapy on bone growth. Radiology 114: 155–162

Probert JC, Parker BR, Kaplan HS (1973) Growth retardation in children after megavoltage irradiation of the spine. Cancer 32: 634–639

Purdy JA, Lightfoot DA, Glasgow GP (1987) Principles of radiologic physics, dosimetry and treatment planning. In: Perez CA, Brady LW (eds) Principles and practice of radiation oncology. JB Lippincott, Philadelphia, pp 129–158

Raimondi AJ, Tomita T (1979) Advantages of total resection of medulloblastoma and disadvantages of full head postoperative radiation therapy (abstr). Childs Brain 5: 550–551

Rappaport R, Brauner R, Czernichow P, Thiabud E, Renier D, Zucker JM, Lemerle J (1982) Effect of hypothalamic and pituitary irradiation on pubertal development in children with cranial tumors. J Clin Endocrinol Metab 54: 1164–1168

Ray GR, Trueblood HW, Enright LP, Kaplan HS, Nelson TS (1970) Oophoropexy: a means of preserving ovarian function following pelvic megavoltage radiotherapy for Hodgkin's disease. Radiology 96: 175–180

Richards GE, Wara WM, Grumbach MM et al. (1976) Delayed onset of hypopituitarism: sequelae of therapeutic irradiation of central nervous system, eye and middle eye tumors. J Pediatr 89: 553–559

Riede UN, Rohrbach R, Adler C-P, Sandritter W, Thomas C, Mittermayer C (1981) Störungen des Wachstums. In: von Sandritter W (ed) Allgemeine Pathologie. FK Schattauer, Stuttgart, p. 627

Riehm H (1986) Malignant neoplasms in children and adolescence. In: Falkner F, Kretchmer N, Rossi E (eds) Monographs in paediatrics. Karger, Basel

Riseborough EJ, Grabias SL, Burton RI, Jaffe N (1976) Skeletal alterations following irradiation for Wilms' tumor. J Bone Joint Surg 58A: 526–536

Ron E, Modan B, Floro S, Harkedar I, Gurewitz R (1982) Mental function following scalp irradiation during childhood. Am J Epidemiol 116: 149–160

Rosenberg SA, Kaplan HS (1985) The evolution and summary results of the Stanford randomized clinical trials of the management of Hodgkin's disease: 1962–1984. Int J Radiat Oncol Biol Phys 11: 5–22

Rowley ML, Leach DR, Warner GA (1974) Effect of graded doses of ionizing radiation on the human testis. Radiat Res 59: 665–678

Rubin P (1984) The Franz Buschke Lecture: late effects of chemotherapy and radiation therapy: a new hypothesis. Int J Radiat Oncol Biol Phys 10: 5–34

Rubin P, Casarett GW (1968) Clinical radiation pathology, vols I and II. WB Saunders, Philadelphia

Rubin P, Casarett GW (1972) Front Radiat Ther Oncol 6: 1–16

Rubin P, van Houtte P, Constine L (1982) Radiation sensitivity and organ tolerances in pediatric oncology: a new hypothesis. Front Radiat Ther Oncol 16: 62–82

Sabio H, Sussmann M, Levin M (1987) Postradiation slipped capital femoral epiphyses. J Surg Oncol 36: 45–47

Schimpff SC, Diggs CH, Wiswell JG, Salvatore PC, Wiernik PH (1980) Radiation-related thyroid dysfunction: implications for the treatment of Hodgkin's disease. Ann Intern Med 92: 91–98

Shalet SM, Beardwell CG, Morris-Jones PH, Pearson D, Orrell DH (1976a) Ovarian failure following abdominal irradiation in childhood. Br J Cancer 33: 655–658

Shalet SM, Beardwell CG, Morris-Jones PH, Pearson D (1976b) Growth hormone deficiency after treatment for acute leukaemia in children. Arch Dis Child 51: 489–493

Shalet SM, Beardwell CG, Pearson D, Morris-Jones HP (1976c) The effect of varying doses of cerebral irradiation on growth hormone production in Childhood. Clin Endocrinol 5: 287–290

Shalet SM, Beardwell CG, Twomey JA (1977a) Endocrine function following the treatment of acute leukemia in childhood. J Pediatr 6: 920–923

Shalet SM, Rosenstock JD, Beardwell CG, Pearson D, Morris-Jones PH (1977b) Thyroid dysfunction following external irradiation to the neck for Hodgkin's disease in childhood. Clin Radiol 28: 511–515

Shalet SM, Beardwell CG, Jacobs HS (1978) Testicular function following irradiation of the human prepubertal testis. Clin Endocrinol 9: 483–490

Shalet SM, Price DA, Beardwell CG, Morris-Jones PH, Pearson D (1979) Normal growth despite abnormalities of growth hormone secretion in children treated for acute leukemia. J Pediat 94: 719–722

Shalet SM, Hann IM, Lendon M et al. (1981) Testicular function after combination chemotherapy in childhood for acute lymphoblastic leukaemia. Arch Dis Child 56: 275–278

Shalet SM, Gibson B, Swindell R, Pearson D (1987) Effect of spinal irradiation on growth. Arch Dis Child 62: 461–464

Sheline GE (1980) Irradiation injury of the human brain, a review clinical experience. In: Gilbert HA, Kagan AR (eds) Radiation damage to the nervous system. Raven, New York,

Sheline GE, Wara WM, Smith V (1980) Therapeutic irradiation and brain injury. Int J Radiat Oncol Biol Phys 6: 1215–1218

Silverman CL, Thomas PRM, McAlister WH, Walker S, Whiteside LA (1981) Slipped femoral capital epiphyses in irradiated children: dose, volume and age relationships. Int J Radiat Oncol Biol Phys 7: 1357–1363

Silverman CL, Plakes H, Talent B (1984) Late effects of radiotherapy on patients with cerebellar medulloblastoma. Cancer 54: 825–829

Simon G, Reiol L, Tanner SM, Goldstein H, Benjamin B (1972) Growth of radiobiologically determined heart diameter, lung width and lung length from 5–19 years with standard for clinical use. Arch Dis Child 47: 373–382

Simpson CL, Hempelmann LH, Fuller LM (1955) Neoplasia in children treated with x-rays in infancy for thymic enlargement. Radiology 64: 840–845

Sinclair D (1969) Human growth after birth. Oxford University Press, London

Sklar CA, Kim TH, Williamson JF, Ramsay NK (1983) Ovarian function after successful bone marrow transplantation in postmenarcheal females. Med Pediatr Oncol 11: 361–364

Sklar CA, Kim TH, Ramsay NK (1984) Testicular function following bone marrow transplantation performed during or after puberty. Cancer 53: 1498–1501

Smith E, Adler RA, Clark P et al. (1981) Thyroid function after mantle irradiation in Hodgkin's disease. JAMA 245: 46–49

Soni SS, George MA, Marten W, Pitner SE, Duenas DA, Powasek M (1975) Effects of central-nervous-system irradiation on neuropsychologic functioning of children with acute lymphocytic leukemia. N Engl J Med 293: 113–118

Spunberg JJ, Chang CH, Goldman M et al. (1981) Quality of long-term survival following irradiation for intracranial tumors in children under the age of two. Int J Radiat Oncol Biol Phys 7: 727–736

Stewart JR, Cohn KE, Fajardo LF, Hancock EW, Kaplan HS (1967) Radiation-induced heart disease, a study of twenty-five patients. Radiology 89: 302–310

Stillman RJ, Schinfeld JS, Schiff I (1981) Ovarian failure in long-term survivors of childhood malignancy. Am J Obstet Gynecol 139: 62–66

Stuschke M, Sauerwein W, Bamberg M, Havers W, Nau E (1988) Multivariante Analyse von Einflußfaktoren auf die Prognose des Medulloblastoms. In: Bamberg M, Sack H (eds) Therapie primärer Hirntumoren, Zuckschwerdt, Munich, pp 406–410

Stuschke M, Budach V, Budach W, Erhard J, Sack H (1989) Multicellular spheroids from human soft tissue sarcomas: radiocurability and dose fractionation effect. Int J Radiat Biol 56: 549–552

Swift PGF, Kearney PJ, Dalton RG et al. (1978) Growth and hormonal status of children treated for actue lymphoblastic leukemia. Arch Dis Child 53: 890–894

Tefft M (1977) Radiation related toxicities in national Wilms' tumor study number 1. Int J Radiat Oncol Biol Phys 2: 455–463

Tefft M (1972) Radiation effect on growing bone and cartilage. Front Radiat Ther Oncol 6: 289–311

Tefft M, Mitus A, Das L, Vawter GF, Filler RM (1970) Irradiation of the liver in children: review of experience in the acute and chronic phases, and in the intact normal and partially resected. AJR 108: 365–385

Thomas PRM, Horning SJ, Le Floch O, Donaldson SS, Kaplan HS (1976) Pregnancy following oophoropexy and total nodal irradiation in women with Hodgkin's disease. Cancer 38: 2263–2268

Thurlbeck WM (1975) Postnatal growth and development of the lung. Am Rev Respir Dis 111: 803–843

Tonomura A, Kishi K, Saito F (1983) Types and frequencies of chromosome aberrations in peripheral lymphocytes of general population. In: Ishihara T, Sasaki MS (eds) Radiation-induced chromosome damage in man. Alan R. Liss, New York

Travis EL (1987) Relative radiosensitivity of the lung. Adv Radiat Biol 12: 205–239

Tucker MA, Meadows AT, Boice JD, Hoover RN, Fraumeni JF (1984) Cancer risk following treatment of childhood cancer. In: Radiation carcinogenesis: epidemiology and biological significance. Boice JD, Fraumeni JF (eds) Raven, New York, pp 211–224

Tucker MA, D'Angio GJ, Boice JD et al. (1987a) Bone sarcomas linked to radiotherapy an chemotherapy in children. N Engl J Med 317: 588–593

Tucker MA, Meadows AT, Boice JD et al. (1987b) Leukemia after therapy with alkylating agents for childhood cancer. J Natl Cancer Inst 78: 459–464

Twaddle V, Britton PG, Craft AC et al. (1983) Intellectual function after treatment for leukaemia or solid tumours. Arch Dis Child 58: 949–952

Verozosa MS, Rhomes JA, Aur JA, Simone JV, Hustu HO, Pinkel DP (1976) Five years after central nervous system irradiation of children with leukemia. Int J Radiat Oncol Phys 1: 209–215

von Mühlendahl KE, Gardner H, Riehm H, Helge H, Weber B, Müller-Hess R (1976) Endocrine function after antineoplastic therapy in 22 children with acute lymphoblastic leukemia. Helv Paediatr Acta 31: 463–471

Watzka M (1964) Kurzlehrbuch der Histologie und mikroskopischen Anatomie des Menschen. FK Schattauer, Stuttgart

Weiner RS, Bortin MM, Gale RP et al. (1986) Interstitial pneumonitis after bone marrow transplantation. Ann Intern Med 104: 168–175

Wells RJ, Foster MB, D'Ercole J, Campbell W, McMillian W (1983) The impact of cranial irradiation on the growth of children with acute lymphoblastic leukemia. Am J Dis Child 137: 37–39

Winiek M, Noble A (1965) Quantitative changes in DNA, RNA and protein during prenatal and postnatal growth in the rat. Dev Biol 12: 451ff

Zaharia M, Caceres E, Valdivia S, Moran M, Tejada F (1986) Postoperative whole lung irradiation with or without adriamycin in osteogenic sarcoma. Int J Radiat Oncol Biol Phys 12: 907–910

Subject Index

List of Contributors

Privatdozent Dr. W. ALBERTI
Klinik für Strahlentherapie und
Nuklearmedizin
Alfried Krupp Krankenhaus
Alfried-Krupp-Straße 21
W-4300 Essen 1
FRG

K.K. ANG, MD
The University of Texas
M.D. Anderson Cancer Center
1515 Holcombe Blvd.
Houston, TX 77030
USA

Professor Dr. W. CALVO
Abt. für Klin. Physiologie
Universität Ulm
Oberer Eselsberg
W-7900 Ulm
FRG

Professor Dr. W. GÖSSNER
Institut für Allgemeine Pathologie und
Pathologische Anatomie
der Technischen Universität
Ismaninger Straße 22
W-8000 München 80
FRG

Professor Dr.med. H. GROSSE-WILDE
Institute für Immungenetik
Universitätsklinikum Essen
Hufelandstraße 55
W-4300 Essen
FRG

Doz. Dr.sc.med. T. HERRMANN
Medizinische Akademie
"Carl Gustav Carus"
Klinik für Radiologie
Abt. f. Strahlentherapie
Fetscherstraße 74
O-8019 Dresden
FRG

Professor Dr. F. HEUCK
Hermann-Kurz-Straße 5
W-7000 Stuttgart 1
FRG

Dr. J.W. HOPEWELL
Research Institute
University of Oxford
Oxford
UK

Dr. L. KEILHOLZ
Strahlentherapeutische Klinik
und Poliklinik der Universität
Erlangen-Nürnberg
Universitätsstraße 27
W-8520 Erlangen
FRG

Dr. A. KEYEUX
Unité de Radiobiologie
U C L
Brussels
Belgium

Dr. J. KUMMERMEHR
Abt. für Strahlenbiologie der
Gesellschaft für Strahlen- und
Umweltforschung
W-8042 Neuherberg
FRG

Professor Dr. H.-A. LADNER
Klinikum der Universität
Universitäts-Frauenklinik
Strahlenabteilung
Hugstetter Straße 55
W-7800 Freiburg i. Brsg.
FRG

Privatdozent Dr. A. LUZ
Gesellschaft für Strahlen- und
Umweltforschung mbH
Institut für Biologie
Abteilung für Pathologie
Ingolstadter Landstraße 1
W-8042 Neuherberg
FRG

Privatdozent Dr. med. M. MOLLS
Oberarzt
Radiologisches Zentrum
Universitätsklinikum Essen
Hufelandstraße 55
W-4300 Essen 1
FRG

Professor Dr. W. NOTHDURFT
Universität Ulm, Klinikum
Institut für Arbeits- und Sozialmedizin
Oberer Eselsberg, M 24
W-7900 Ulm/Donau
FRG

Dr. H.S. REINHOLD
T N O Radiobiological Institute
Lange Kleiweg 151
P.O. Box 5815
2280 GJ Rijswijk
The Netherlands

Dr. H. REYNERS
Dept. de Radiobiologie
CEN/SCK
Mol
Belgium

Professor Dr. R. SAUER
Strahlentherapeutische Klinik
und Poliklinik der Universität
Erlangen-Nürnberg
Universitätsstraße 27
W-8520 Erlangen
FRG

Professor Dr.med. U. SCHAEFER
Innere Klinik und Poliklinik
(Tumorforschung)
Universitätsklinikum Essen
Hufelandstraße 55
W-4300 Essen 1
FRG

Professor (em.) Dr. E. SCHERER
Universitätsklinikum der
Gesamthochschule
Radiologisches Zentrum,
Strahlenklinik und Poliklinik
Hufelandstraße 55
W-4300 Essen 1
FRG

T.E. SCHULTHEISS, MD
The University of Texas
M.D. Anderson Cancer Center
1515 Holcombe Blvd.
Houston, TX 77030
USA

Dr. med. S. Schultz-Hector
Institut für Strahlenbiologie der
Gesellschaft für Strahlen- und
Umweltforschung mbH
Ingolstädter Landstraße 1
W-8042 Neuherberg
FRG

L.C. Stephens, DVM, PhD
Associate Professor and Chief
Veterinary Pathology
The University of Texas
M.D. Anderson Cancer Center
1515 Holcombe Blvd.
Houston, TX 77030
USA

Dr. F.A. Stewart
Division of Experimental Therapy
The Netherlands Cancer Institute
Antoni van Leeuwenhoek Huis
H6, Plesmanlaan 121
1066 CX Amsterdam
The Netherlands

Professor Dr.rer.nat. C. Streffer
Universitätsklinikum der
Gesamthochschule
Institut für Medizinische
Strahlenphysik und Strahlenbiologie
Hufelandstraße 55
W-4300 Essen 1
FRG

Dr. med. M. Stuschke
Radiologisches Zentrum
Universitätsklinikum Essen
Hufelandstraße 55
W-4300 Essen 1
FRG

Professor Dr. K.-R. Trott
Dept. of Radiation Biology
Medical College of St. Bartholomew's
Hospital
University of London
Charterhouse Square
London EC1M 6BQ
UK

Prof. Dr. D. van Beuningen
Oberfeldarzt
Akademie des Sanitäts-
und Gesundheitswesen
der Bundeswehr
Neuherbergstraße 11
W-8000 München 45
FRG

A.J. van der Kogel, PhD
Professor of Radiobiology
Institute of Radiotherapy
University of Nijmegen
Geert Grooteplein Zuid 32
6525 GA Nijmegen
The Netherlands

Dr. M.V. Williams
Radiotherapeutic Centre
Addenbrooke's Hospital
Hills Road
Cambridge CB2 2QQ
UK

MR Medical Radiology

Diagnostic Imaging and Radiation Oncology

Series Editors:
L. W. Brady, M. W. Donner, H.-P. Heilmann, F. Heuck

This series recognizes the demand for an international state-of-the-art account of the developments reflecting the progress in the radiological sciences. Each volume conveys an overall picture of a topical theme so that it can be used as a reference work without taking recourse to other volumes.

The contents of the volumes concentrate on new and accepted developments in a manner appropriate for review by physicians engaged in the practice of radiology.

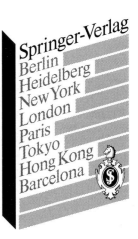

Springer-Verlag
Berlin
Heidelberg
New York
London
Paris
Tokyo
Hong Kong
Barcelona

C. W. Scarantino (Ed.)

Lung Cancer

Diagnostic Procedures and Therapeutic Management with Special Reference to Radiotherapy

1985. XI, 173 pp. 42 figs. Hardcover.
ISBN 3-540-13176-0

H. R. Withers, University of California, Los Angeles, CA; L. J. Peters, University of Texas, Houston, TX (Eds.)

Innovations in Radiation Oncology

1987. XVII, 329 pp. 111 figs. Hardcover.
ISBN 3-540-17818-X

G. E. Laramore, University of Washington, Seattle, WA (Ed.)

Radiation Therapy of Head and Neck Cancer

1989. XII, 237 pp. 123 figs. Hardcover.
ISBN 3-540-19360-X

J. H. Anderson, The Johns Hopkins University, Baltimore, MD (Ed.)

Innovations in Diagnostic Radiology

1989. XIII, 213 pp. 144 figs. some in color.
Hardcover. ISBN 3-540-19093-7

R. R. Dobelbower Jr., Toledo, OH (Ed.)

Gastrointestinal Cancer

Radiation Therapy

1990. XV, 301 pp. 76 figs. 90 tabs. Hardcover.
ISBN 3-540-50505-9

E. Scherer, C. Streffer, University of Essen;
K.-R. Trott, London (Eds.)

Radiation Exposure and Occupational Risks

1990. XI, 150 pp. 32 figs. 55 tabs. Hardcover.
ISBN 3-540-51174-1

S. E. Order, The Johns Hopkins University, Baltimore, MD; S. S. Donaldson, Stanford University, Stanford, CA

Radiation Therapy of Benign Diseases

A Clinical Guide

1990. VIII, 214 pp. 103 tabs. Hardcover.
ISBN 3-540-50901-1

R. Sauer, University of Erlangen-Nürnberg, Erlangen (Ed.)

Interventional Radiation Therapy Techniques – Brachytherapy

1991. XII, 388 pp. 193 figs. Hardcover.
ISBN 3-540-52465-7

M. Rotman, C. J. Rosenthal, State University of New York, NY (Eds.)

Concomitant Continuous Infusion Chemotherapy and Radiation

1991. Approx. 295 pp. 43 figs. Hardcover.
ISBN 3-540-52545-9